The
MEDICAL and HEALTH ENCYCLOPEDIA

The
MEDICAL and HEALTH
ENCYCLOPEDIA

EDITED BY
RICHARD J. WAGMAN, M.D., F.A.C.P.
Associate Clinical Professor of Medicine
Downstate Medical Center
New York, New York

J. G. FERGUSON PUBLISHING COMPANY • CHICAGO, ILLINOIS

Portions of *The New Complete Medical and Health Encyclopedia* have
been previously published under the title of *The Complete Illustrated
Book of Better Health,* and *The Illustrated Encyclopedia of Better
Health,* edited by Richard J. Wagman, M.D.

International Standard Book Number 0-89434-138-3
Library of Congress Catalog Card Number 77-81669
Printed in the United States of America
P-7

Editor

Richard J. Wagman, M.D.,
F.A.C.P.
Associate Clinical Professor of
Medicine
Downstate Medical Center
New York, New York

Consultant in Gynecology

Douglas S. Thompson, M.D.
Clinical Professor of Obstetrics and
Gynecology and Clinical Associate
Professor of Community Medicine
University of Pittsburgh School of
Medicine
Pittsburgh, Pennsylvania

Consultant in Pediatrics

Charles H. Bauer, M.D.
Clinical Associate Professor of
Pediatrics and Chief of Pediatric
Gastroenterology
The New York Hospital-Cornell
Medical Center
New York, New York

Consultants in Psychiatry

Julian J. Clark, M.D.
Assistant Professor of Psychiatry
and
Rita W. Clark, M.D.
Clinical Assistant Professor of
Psychiatry
Downstate Medical Center
New York, New York

Contents

INTRODUCTION

THE MEDICAL AND HEALTH ENCYCLOPEDIA provides for you answers to your health questions. This encyclopedia can serve as a guide for you in learning about and understanding the medical terms and conditions that you or your family may experience during your life. The books cover a wide range of topics, from skin care to how to choose a daycare center for your toddler.

We have compiled the most up-to-date information on health care, medicine, and treatment of diseases and illnesses. We give you thorough coverage on major diseases such as cancer and heart problems. We also cover the day-to-day changes that you experience from growing older. THE MEDICAL AND HEALTH ENCYCLOPEDIA takes you from health care for newborns through early childhood, to adolescence, adulthood, and the concerns of the middle and later years in life. Each stage provides fundamental information about what to expect, what happens, and how to find out if something is wrong.

To understand your health needs and problems, you need to have some knowledge of how your body works. We start the encyclopedia with a basic guide to your body and all its functioning parts. If you come across something in the chapters following, you can turn back to the first chapter to learn about that particular part of your body.

From there you can look up whatever concerns you about your health or your family's health. Simple problems like treating poison ivy rashes are explained. Problems that are serious or difficult to understand are also explained, like mastectomies and breast cancer. After you discuss a problem with your doctor, you can turn to THE MEDICAL AND HEALTH ENCYCLOPEDIA to see diagrams and illustrations of the body part affected and the types of surgery involved. This helps you to understand what is being discussed, and may also provide for you guidance for some questions you may have for the doctor.

The key to better health is preventing injuries and illness whenever possible. By following a healthy diet, combined with some exercise, you set yourself on a good start. THE MEDICAL AND HEALTH ENCYCLOPEDIA can give you some guidance about your diet and exercise needs. It also provides guidance for making you home a safe environment. The Medical Emergency section, edged in color for easy finding, includes how to provide first aid for injuries. It also guides you through making your home emergency-free. The chapter shows you how to eliminate some of the dangers you may have in your home without realizing it.

The best thing you can do for your family's and your own health is to learn about it. This set of books can give you the information you need about what to ask and what to expect of your doctor and your medical care. It can give you a good start on providing a safe, healthy, and happy life for you and those you love.

1

Your Body

The Skeleton

Say "skeleton" to children and you probably conjure up in their minds a rickety structure of rigid sticks, or, to the more fanciful child, a clickety-clacketing collection of rattling bones cavorting under a Halloween moon. A look at almost any anatomical drawing of the human skeletal system bears out the child's image: dry sticks of bones, stripped of skin and flesh, muscle and tendon—a grotesque caricature of a living human being.

Our living bones are something quite different. They are rigid, yes, but not entirely so: they also may bend a little and grow and repair themselves; and they are shaped and fitted so that—rather than the herky-jerky motions of a wooden puppet—they permit the smooth grace and coordination power displayed by an accomplished athlete or a prima ballerina.

Our bones do not do just one thing but many things. Some bones, like the collarbone or *clavicle,* mainly give support to other body structures. Others, like the skull and ribs, encase and protect vulnerable organs. Still others, like the *metacarpus* and *phalanges* that make up our hands and fingers, give us mechanical advantages—leverage and movement. There are even bones, the tiny *ossicles* in the middle ear, whose vibrations enable us to hear.

Finally, to think of bone simply as a structural member, like a solid steel girder in a skyscraper, ignores the fact that bone is living tissue. It is one of the busiest tissues in our bodies, a chemical factory that is continually receiving, processing and shipping a wide variety of mineral salts, blood components, and a host of other vital materials.

How the Bones of the Skeletal System Fit and Work Together

Medical textbooks name a total of 206 bones making up the skeletal system of the normal, adult human being. The words "normal" and "adult" are significant. A newborn baby normally has 33 vertebrae making up its backbone (also called *spinal column* or simply *spine*); but by the time a person reaches adulthood, the number of individual vertebrae has shrunk to 26. The explanation: during the growth process, the nine bottom vertebrae fuse naturally into just two. In like fashion, we "lose" some 60 bones as we grow up. Some otherwise perfectly normal adults have "extra" bones or "missing" bones. For example, although the normal number of ribs is 12 pairs, some adults may have 11; others may have 13 pairs.

Even a practicing physician might be hard-pressed to identify each of our 200-plus bones and describe its function. An easier way to gain a general understanding of the various functions, capabilities—and weaknesses, too—of our bones is to visualize the skeletal system as a standing coatrack, say, about six feet high.

Call the central pole the backbone. About ten inches down from its top (the top of your skull) is a horizontal crossbar (your shoulders—collarbones and shoulder blades), approximately a foot-and-a-half across. Sixteen or so inches below the bottom of the top crossbar is another, shorter crossbar, broader and thicker—the *pelvic girdle.* The coatrack with its two crossbars is now a crude model of the bones of the head and trunk, collectively called the *axial skeleton.* Its basic unit is the backbone, to which are attached the skull at the top, then the bones of the shoulder girdle, the ribs, and at the bottom, the bones of the pelvic girdle.

By hanging down (or appending) members from the two ends of the top crossbar, and doing the same at the lower crossbar, we would simulate what is called the *appendicular skeleton*—arms and hands, legs and feet.

Now, make the coatrack stand on its new legs, cut off the central pole just below the lower bar (if you wish, calling it man's lost tail), and you have the two main components of the skeletal system, joined together before you. Let us look at each more closely.

The Axial Skeleton

Within the framework of the axial skeleton lie all the most vital organs of the body. People have gone on living with the loss of a hand or a leg—indeed, with the loss of any or all of their limbs. But nobody can live without a brain, a heart, a liver, lungs, or kidneys—all of which are carried within the framework of the axial skeleton.

The Skull

The bones of the skull have as their most important function the protection of the brain and sense organs.

There are also, of course, the jawbones that support the teeth and gums and which enable us to bite and chew our food.

Most of the skull appears to consist of a single bone—a hard, unbroken dome. Actually, the brain cage or *cranium* consists of eight individual platelike bones which have fused together in the process of growth. At birth, these bones are separated, causing the soft spots or *fontanelles* we can readily feel on a baby's head. As the baby's brain enlarges, the bones grow along their edges to fill in the fontanelles, finally knitting together in what are called *suture lines,* somewhat resembling inexpertly mended clothes seams. Along the suture lines, the skull bones continue to grow until the individual's mature skull size is reached.

Teeth

The hardest substance in the human body is the *enamel* that covers the exposed surface of a tooth. Below the gum, the tooth's outside surface is composed of somewhat softer *cementum.* Beneath enamel and cementum is a bonelike substance, called *dentin,* which covers the soft interior of the tooth, called *pulp.* Pulp is serviced by blood vessels and nerves through the root or roots of the tooth. The passageway of nerves and blood vessels that lead up through the tooth from the gum sockets is called a *root canal.* Tooth and gum are stuck to each other by a tough, adhesive tissue called *periodontal* (or peridental—"surrounding the tooth") *membrane.* See Ch. 22, *The Teeth and Gums,* for further information on teeth.

The Backbone

At the base of the skull, the backbone begins. The skull is supported by the

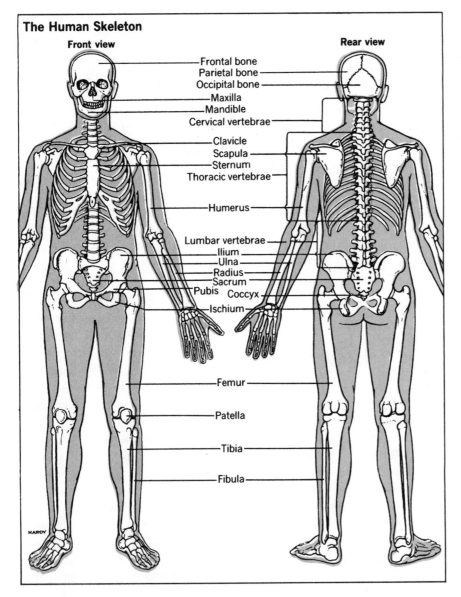

The Human Skeleton

Front view

Rear view

Frontal bone
Parietal bone
Occipital bone
Maxilla
Mandible
Cervical vertebrae
Clavicle
Scapula
Sternum
Thoracic vertebrae
Humerus
Lumbar vertebrae
Ilium
Ulna
Radius
Sacrum
Pubis   Coccyx
Ischium
Femur
Patella
Tibia
Fibula

topmost *cervical* (neck) vertebra. The curious thing about a backbone is that the word has come to suggest something solid, straight, and unbending. The backbone, however, just isn't like that: it consists of 26 knobby, hollowed-out bones—*vertebrae,* rather improbably held together by muscles, ligaments, and tendons. It is not straight when we stand, but has definite backward and forward curvatures; and even some of its most important structures (the disks between the vertebrae) aren't made of bone, but of cartilage.

All in all, however, the backbone is a fairly well designed structure in terms of the several different functions it serves—but with some built-in weaknesses. For a discussion of backache, see Ch. 23, *Aches, Pains, Nuisances, Worries.*

The Vertebrae

Although they will have features in common, no two of our 26 vertebrae are exactly alike in shape, size, or function. This is hardly surprising if we consider, for example, that the cervical vertebrae do not support ribs, while the *thoracic* vertebrae (upper trunk, or chest) do support them.

But for a sample vertebra, let us pick a rib-carrying vertebra, if for no other reason than that it lies about midway along the backbone. If viewed from above or below, a thoracic vertebra, like most of the others, would look like a roundish piece of bone with roughly scalloped edges on the side facing inward toward the chest and on the side facing outward toward the surface of the back, and would reveal several bony projections. These knobby portions of a vertebra—some of which you can feel as bumps along your backbone—are called *processes.* They serve as the vertebra's points of connection to muscles and tendons,

to ribs, and to the other vertebrae above and below.

A further conspicuous feature is a hole, more or less in the middle of the typical vertebra, through which passes the master nerve bundle of our bodies, the spinal cord, running from the base of the skull to the top of the pelvis. Thus, one of the important functions of the backbone is to provide flexible, protective tubing for the spinal cord.

Between the bones of one vertebra and the next is a piece of more resilient cartilage that acts as a cushion or shock absorber to prevent two vertebrae from scraping or bumping each other if the backbone gets a sudden jolt, or as the backbone twists and turns and bends. These pieces of cartilage are the intervertebral disks—infamous for pain and misery if they become ruptured or slipped disks.

Regions of the Backbone

The backbone can be divided into five regions, starting with the uppermost, or *cervical* region, which normally has seven vertebrae. Next down is the *thoracic* (chest) section, normally with 12 vertebrae. From each vertebra a rib extends to curl protectively around the chest area. Usually, the top ten ribs come all the way around the trunk and attach to the breastbone (or *sternum*); but the bottom two ribs do not reach the breastbone and are thus called floating ribs. The thoracic section also must support the shoulder girdle, consisting of the collarbones (*clavicles*) and shoulder blades (*scapulas*). At the end of each shoulder blade is a shoulder joint—actually three distinct joints working together—where the arm connects to the axial skeleton.

Below the thoracic vertebrae come the five vertebrae of the *lumbar* sec-

tion. This area gets a good deal of blame for back miseries: lower back pain often occurs around the area where the bottom thoracic vertebra joins the top lumbar vertebra. Furthermore, the lumbar region or small of the back is also a well-known site of back pain; indeed, from the word "lumbar" comes *lumbago,* medically an imprecise term, but popularly used to describe very real back pain.

Below the lumbar region are two vertebrae so completely different from the 24 above them—and even from each other—that it seems strange they are called vertebrae at all: the *sacrum* and the *coccyx.* These two vertebrae are both made up of several distinct vertebrae that are present at birth. The sacrum is a large bone that was once five vertebrae. The coccyx was originally four vertebrae—and, incidentally, is all that remains of man's tail in his evolution from the primates.

The Pelvic Girdle

The sacrum is the more important of these two strange-looking vertebrae. It is the backbone's connection to the *pelvic girdle,* or pelvis. On each side of the sacrum, connected by the sacroiliac joint, is a very large, curving bone called the *ilium,* tilting (when we stand) slightly forward and downward from the sacrum toward the front of the groin. We feel the top of the ilium as the top of the hip—a place mothers and fathers often find convenient for toting a toddler.

Fused at each side of the ilium and slanting toward the back is the *ischium,* the bone we sit on. The two *pubis* bones, also fused to the ilium, meet in front to complete the pelvic girdle. All the bones of the pelvis—ilium, ischium, and pubis—fuse together so as to form the hip joint (*acetabulum*), a deep socket into which the "ball" or upper end of the thigh-bone fits.

The Appendicular Skeleton

The bones of the appendages—arms, hands, and fingers; legs, feet, and toes—allow human beings to perform an astonishing array of complex movements, from pushing themselves through the physical rigors of the Olympic decathlon to creating an elaborate piece of needlework. The key points in the appendicular skeleton, as indeed, in the axial skeleton, are where the ends or edges of bones lie close together and must work with or against one another in order to achieve coordinated movement. These key points are the *joints*—not really bones at all but the non-bony spaces between bones.

The Joints

A typical joint consists of several different structures. First, there are the bones themselves—two, three, four, or more almost touching in the area of the joint—with their ends or edges shaped to fit in their respective niches. Between the bones of an appendage joint (as between the verte-

Joint

Skin
Bone
Synovial fluid
Cartilage
Tissue producing synovial fluid

All of the body's joints allow movement of the bones through this combination of ball and socket contours. Cartilage allows the bones to move without scraping or catching. Synovial fluid helps reduce friction in the movement.

brae of the back) is the smooth, resilient material called *cartilage* that allows the bones to move over one another without scraping or catching. At the joint, the bones, with their layer of cartilage between them, are held together by tough bonds of muscle. *Bursas,* tiny sacs containing a lubricating fluid, are also found at joints; they help to reduce the friction between a joint's moving parts.

The Hip and Knee

The hip joint must not only support the weight of the head and trunk, but must allow for movement of the leg and also play a part in the constant balancing required to maintain upright posture. Similar stresses and strains, often literally tending to tear the joint apart, are placed on every joint in the body.

The notoriety of athletes' bad knees attests to the forces battering at the knee joint, the largest in the human body. Sports involving leaping or sudden changes in direction, such as basketball, are especially hard on the knee. However, the fact that there are not more disabled sports heroes speaks well for the design of the knee joint. The same can be said of the ankle joint and the joints of the foot and toes.

The Shoulder, Elbow, and Wrist

The counterpart of the hip joint in the upper trunk is the shoulder joint. Free of weight-bearing responsibilities, the shoulder has a system of three interconnected joints that allow it and the arm far more versatile movements than the hip and leg.

The elbow connects the upper arm bone (*humerus*) with the two bones of the lower arm (*radius* and *ulna*). Like the knee, it is basically a hinge joint, which allows the lower arm to be

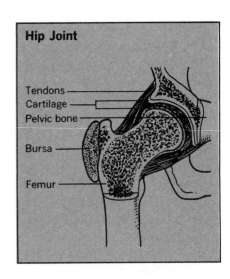

Hip Joint

Tendons
Cartilage
Pelvic bone
Bursa
Femur

raised and lowered. The elbow is also constructed to allow some rotation by the hand; likewise, the knee joint allows us to waggle the foot.

Of all our body parts, the wrist, hand, and fingers are perhaps the most elegantly and finely jointed—witness the performance of a concert pianist—and our ankles, feet, and toes probably the most subject to everyday misery.

Bone as Living Tissue

Our bones, like all our tissues, change as we grow up, mature, and finally grow old. There are changes in the chemical activity and composition of bone representative of each stage of life.

In young children, the ends and edges of bones are mainly cartilage, forming a growing surface on the bone that is gradually replaced by hard bone as full size is attained. The bones of a child are more pliable and less likely to break than those of a full-grown adult.

Similarly, as an adult ages, the bones turn from a resilient hardness to a more brittle hardness. This accounts for the much greater danger of broken bones in older people.

These changes with age are an indication of the great amount of chemical activity going on within bone. We sometimes forget that our bones are amply supplied and penetrated by blood vessels. There is a constant building up and breaking down, an interchange of materials between blood and bone.

The Composition of Bone

A living bone does not have a single uniform composition, but instead is composed of several different kinds of tissue. To begin with, there are actually two types of bone tissue in the same bone: compact and spongy. In addition, bone is sheathed in a tough membranous tissue called the *periosteum,* interlaced with blood vessels. Finally, within most of the larger and longer bones of the body, as well as in the interior of the skull bones and vertebrae, are two more kinds of tissue: red marrow and yellow marrow.

Marrow

Within the spongy bone areas, *red marrow* produces enormous numbers of red blood cells, at a rate of millions per minute. These are needed for growth as well as for replacement of red cells, which also die in enormous numbers. Children's bones contain greater proportions of red marrow than adults'. With age, *yellow marrow,* composed mainly of fat cells, begins to fill the interior bone cavities formerly occupied by red marrow.

Calcium

Bone also serves as a storage and distribution center for one of the most important elements in our body. Calcium, in the form of calcium phosphate, is the basic chemical of bone tissue, but this element also must always be present in the bloodstream at a certain level to ensure normal heartbeat, blood clotting, and muscle contraction. When the calcium level in the blood is deficient, the bones release some calcium into the bloodstream; when the blood has a surplus of calcium, the bones reabsorb it.

Fractures

Like most other tissues, broken bone can repair itself, and it is a remarkable process to observe. It is a process, however, that will proceed even if the ends are not aligned or set—an important reason why any suspected fracture should be checked by a physician.

A break in a bone causes a sticky material to be deposited by the blood around the broken ends. This material begins the formation of a kind of protective, lumpy sleeve, called a *callus,* around the broken ends. Mainly cartilage, the callus hardens into spongy bone, normally within a month or two. Then, the spongy bone begins to be reduced in size by bone-dissolving cells produced in the marrow, while at the same time the spongy bone in the area of the break is beginning to be replaced by hard bone.

Depending on the particular bone involved and the severity of the fracture, the broken bone can be completely healed within four to ten months.

Potential Trouble Spots

Essentially there are two kinds of things that can go wrong with the skeletal system and cause trouble.

Mechanical Difficulties

A healthy bone's main mechanical functions—support, movement, protection—can be impaired. This can happen as a result of a physical injury resulting in a fracture or dislocation.

The stack of vertebrae called the backbone is vulnerable to a number of painful conditions from top to bottom, especially in the region of the lower back. Unfortunately, man seems to have evolved relatively quickly from a four-footed creature, and his backbone is not ideally suited for standing and walking on two feet. Back troubles become increasingly common with age.

Areas where bones interact are also very susceptible to injury because of the stresses and strains they undergo even in people who are not

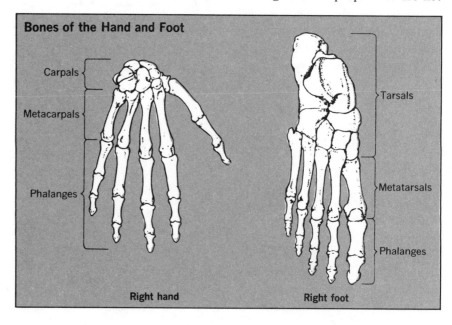

Bones of the Hand and Foot

Carpals
Metacarpals
Phalanges
Right hand

Tarsals
Metatarsals
Phalanges
Right foot

especially active. Normal wear and tear also takes its toll on our bones and joints; for example, the bones' structure or their alignment at a joint may be altered slightly with age, making one bone or another prone to slipping out of the joint causing a dislocation. In any case, it is not advisable to make the same demands on our skeletal system at 40 as we did at 20. Joints are also the site of arthritis.

Disease

Second, and generally more serious if untreated, the interior bone tissues themselves may become infected and diseased. This can lead as a secondary effect to impairment of the bones' mechanical functions. *Osteomyelitis,* for example, a bacterial infection of bony tissues, can destroy large portions of bone unless antibiotics are started at once.

Fortunately, disorders of the skeletal system generally reveal themselves early and clearly by pain. Any severe or lingering pain of the joints or bones should be reported to a physician. For example, some people may feel that aching feet are unavoidable—and a little undignified. But a foot is not meant to hurt, nor is any part of the skeletal system. Consulting a physician could prevent much present and future misery. See also Ch. 7, *Diseases of the Skeletal System.*

The Muscles

Some 600 muscles of all sizes and shapes are attached to the framework of the skeletal system. Altogether these muscles make up nearly half of a normal adult's weight. They hold the skeleton together and, on signals originating in the brain, empower its various parts to move. Everywhere throughout the skeletal system, muscles work together with bones to protect the body's vital organs and to support and move its parts.

Skeletal Muscle

Such muscles are called, collectively, *skeletal muscle.* They are also called *voluntary muscles* because, for the most part, we can choose when we want them to act and what we want them to do—drive a car, kick a football, turn a page, jump a brook, ride a bicycle. Skeletal muscle also goes by two other names, based on its appearance under a microscope—striped and striated.

Skeletal, voluntary, striped, striated—all refer to the same general type of muscle. To avoid confusion, the term used throughout this section is skeletal muscle.

Smooth Muscle

There are two other general types of muscle. One is called *smooth muscle* because, under the microscope, it lacks the clearly defined stripes of skeletal muscle. Smooth muscle has another name, *involuntary muscle,* so called because the brain does not voluntarily control its actions. Smooth muscle is responsible for movements such as the muscular action that moves food and waste along the

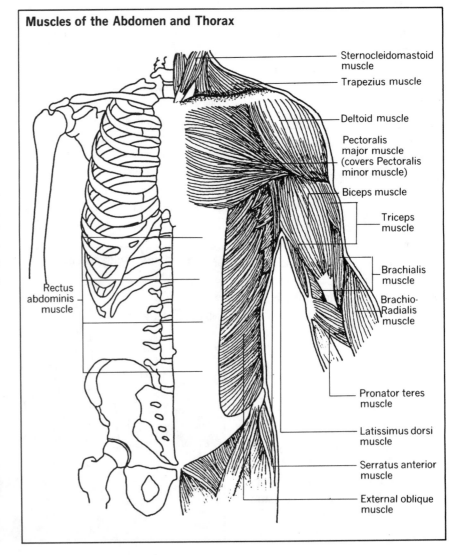

Muscles of the Abdomen and Thorax

Sternocleidomastoid muscle

Trapezius muscle

Deltoid muscle

Pectoralis major muscle (covers Pectoralis minor muscle)

Biceps muscle

Triceps muscle

Brachialis muscle

Brachio-Radialis muscle

Pronator teres muscle

Latissimus dorsi muscle

Serratus anterior muscle

External oblique muscle

Rectus abdominis muscle

digestive tract, or the contraction and dilation of the pupil of the eye, as well as countless other involuntary movements of the sense and internal organs—with the exception of the heart.

Cardiac Muscle

The third and last general type of muscle is confined to the heart area, and is called *cardiac muscle*. (Cardiac means having to do with the heart.) It is involved in the rhythmic beating and contractions of the heart, which are not under conscious control, and cardiac muscle is therefore termed involuntary.

Structure of the Muscles

Each of the three kinds of muscle shares certain structural similarities with one or both of the others. All are made up of bundles of varying numbers of hair-thin fibers. In skeletal and smooth muscles, these fibers are lined up side by side in the bundle, while in cardiac muscle the fibers tend more to crisscross over one another. Skeletal muscle and cardiac muscle are both striped, that is, they show darker and lighter bands crossing over a group of adjacent fibers, while smooth muscle lacks these distinct cross-bands.

Both involuntary muscle types, smooth and cardiac, are controlled by signals carried by the autonomic nervous system. Signals that result in movements of the skeletal muscles are carried by a different nerve network, the central nervous system. The individual fibers in a muscle bundle with a particular function all react simultaneously to a signal from the nervous system; there is no apparent time lag from fiber to fiber.

How the Skeletal Muscles Work

The great range and variety of functions served by skeletal muscles can be suggested by naming just four: the diaphragm, used in breathing; the muscles that make the eye wink; the deltoid muscle that gives the shoulder its shape; and the tongue.

As with the bones, the body tends to make its greatest demands on muscle tissue in the area of the joints and the backbone. A smoothly functioning joint requires that bone, cartilage, and muscle all be sound and able to work together effectively.

Tendons and Ligaments

We often hear the words tendon and ligament used in the description of the knee or another joint. These are actually two types of skeletal muscles, distinguished as to their function.

A *tendon* can be described as a tight cord of muscle tissue that attaches other skeletal muscle to bone. For example, the Achilles tendon running down the back of the calf, the strongest tendon in the body, connects the muscles of the calf with the bone of the heel. A *ligament* is a somewhat more elastic band of muscle fibers that attaches bone to bone.

A tendon is not always evident in the connection of muscle to bone. Various groups and shapes of muscle fibers may be similarly employed,

Muscles of the Back

- Trapezius muscle
- Infraspinatus muscle
- Deltoid muscle
- Rhomboid muscle
- Teres major muscle
- Triceps muscle
- Latissimus dorsi muscle (covers spinal erector muscle)
- External oblique muscle
- Internal oblique muscle
- Gluteus maximus muscle

Tendon

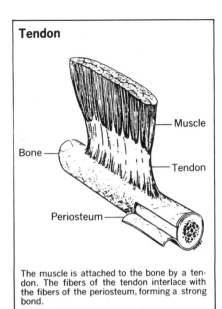

The muscle is attached to the bone by a tendon. The fibers of the tendon interlace with the fibers of the periosteum, forming a strong bond.

Muscles, Their Locations, and Exercises that Strengthen Them

Muscle	Location	Movement
Trapezius	Upper back and each side of neck	Shoulder-shrugging and upward-pulling movements
Deltoids	Shoulders	Arm raising and overhead pressing
Pectorals	Chest	Horizontal pressing and drawing arms across body
Latissimus dorsi	Wide back muscle stretching over back up to rear Deltoids	Pulling and rowing movements
Serratus	Jagged sawtooth muscles between Pectorals and lattissimus Dorsi	Pullover and Serratus leverage movements
Spinal erectors	Lower length of spinal column	Raising upper body from a bent-over position
Biceps	Front portion of upper arm	Arm bending and twisting
Forearms	Between wrist and elbow	Reverse-grip arm bending
Triceps	Back of upper arm	Pushing and straightening movements of upper arms
Rectus abdominals	Muscular area between sternum and pelvis	Sit-up, leg-raising, knee-in movements
Intercostals	Sides of waist, running diagonally to Serratus	Waist twisting
External oblique abdominals	Lower sides of waist	Waist twisting and bending
Buttocks	Muscular area covering seat	Lunging, stooping, leg raising
Leg biceps	Back of thighs	Raising lower leg to buttocks, bending forward and stretching
Frontal thighs	Front of thighs	Extending lower leg and knee bending
Calves	Lower leg between ankle and knee	Raising and lowering on toes

forming connective tissue without the formation of tendon.

Various associated tissues between or around skeletal muscles serve to reduce the wear and tear of friction in areas such as a joint, where muscle, bone, and cartilage may rub against one another. For example, the tendons that pass along the back of the hand from the wrist to the fingertips, as well as many other muscle groups throughout the body, are enclosed in lubricated sheaths. The muscle-sheathed *bursas,* lined inside with lubricating fluid, are also found in areas subject to friction, such as where a tendon passes closely over a bone.

Man's upright posture and two-legged locomotion subject the backbone to heavy stresses. It is buttressed, however, with scores of tightly packed bundles of muscle attached to either side of the spinal column.

Flexors and Extensors

Most of us probably first used the word "muscle" when, as children, we watched an older child or adult flex an arm and proudly display the bump of muscle between the crook of elbow and shoulder. This biceps muscle works together with the triceps muscle on the underside of the arm. The arm is bent at the elbow by contraction of the biceps, which makes this muscle get shorter and thicker; in this position, called *flexion,* the triceps muscle is relaxed. To return the arm to its normal straight position, called *extension,* the biceps relaxes and the triceps contracts. In this bit of muscle teamwork, the biceps, which bends the arm at the elbow joint, is called the *flexor,* while the triceps straightens the arm and is called the *extensor.* Similar flexor–extensor action can be observed at many body joints, including the fingers.

Smooth Muscle

Beginning about midway down the esophagus, layers of smooth muscle line the walls of the 25 feet of digestive tract, extending into the stomach and through the intestines. These muscles keep the stomach and intes-

Muscle Action in Forearm Movement

Biceps

Triceps

Muscles usually work in pairs to produce movement of a part of the body. Contraction of the biceps bends, or flexers, the arm. The biceps is a flexor muscle. Contraction of the triceps extends the arm. The triceps is an extensor muscle.

tinal walls continually in motion, constricting and relaxing to push food along. Smooth muscle also effects the opening and closing of important valves, called *sphincters,* along the digestive tract.

Trouble Spots

The functions and failures of the skeletal muscles are closely allied to those of the skeletal system. The same areas are vulnerable—joints and back—and the same rule holds: severe or persistent muscle pain is a cause to consult your physician.

Hernia

One type of disorder associated exclusively with a weakness or abnormality of muscle is a rupture or *hernia.* This is the protrusion of part of another organ through a gap in the protective muscle. A likely area for a hernia to appear is in the muscles lining the abdomen, although hernias may occur in any other part of the body where there is pressure against a muscle wall that is not as strong as it should be. Weight control and a sensible program of exercise—abdominal muscles being particularly liable to slackness—are good preventive measures against hernia.

All our muscles, in fact, benefit from regular exercise; but you don't have to exhaust yourself physically every day to reach and maintain the desirable plateau physicians describe as good muscle tone.

Atrophy of Muscle Tissue

Muscle tissues are likely to *atrophy* (shrink and weaken) if they are not used for too long a time. Thus, illness or injuries that cause paralysis or an extended period of immobility for the body or a part of it must be followed by a supervised program of physical therapy.   See also Ch. 8, *Diseases of the Muscles and Nervous System.*

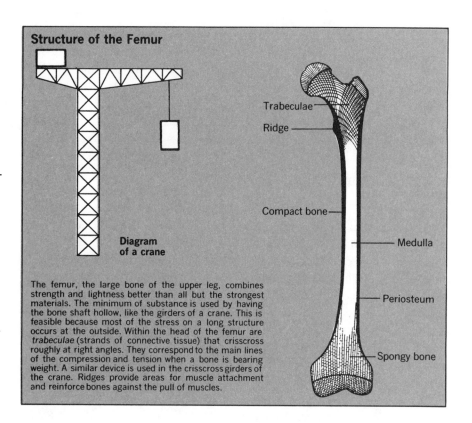

Structure of the Femur

Diagram of a crane

Trabeculae
Ridge
Compact bone
Medulla
Periosteum
Spongy bone

The femur, the large bone of the upper leg, combines strength and lightness better than all but the strongest materials. The minimum of substance is used by having the bone shaft hollow, like the girders of a crane. This is feasible because most of the stress on a long structure occurs at the outside. Within the head of the femur are *trabeculae* (strands of connective tissue) that crisscross roughly at right angles. They correspond to the main lines of the compression and tension when a bone is bearing weight. A similar device is used in the crisscross girders of the crane. Ridges provide areas for muscle attachment and reinforce bones against the pull of muscles.

Muscular Contraction

Tendon
Biceps
Triceps
Tendon
Becomes flexor
Becomes extensor

Skin, Hair, and Nails

Perhaps no other organ of the human body receives so much attention both from its owner and the eyes of others as the skin and its associated structures—hair and nails.

Vanity is hardly the issue. The simple facts are that skin is the last frontier of our internal selves, the final boundary between our inside and outside, and our principal first line of defense against the dangers of the outside world. It shows, not always clearly, evidence of some internal disorders; and it shows, often quite clearly, the evidence of external affronts—a bump, a cut, a chafe, an insect bite, or an angry reaction to the attack of germs.

In personal encounters, the unclothed portion of our skin is one of the first things other people observe, and—if we happen to have some unsightly scratch, rash, or blemish—the last thing by which we wish to be remembered. Of all our organs, the skin is the most likely candidate for a program of self-improvement.

The Organ Called Skin

It is always a little surprising to hear, for the first time, the skin referred to as a single organ. This is not to say it is a simple organ; on the contrary, it is an exceedingly complex and varied one. However, despite variations in appearance from part to part of the body, our entire outer wrapper (the more technical word is *integument*) is similarly constructed.

One might object: "But my nails and hair certainly look different from the skin on my nose!" This is perfectly true, but nails and hair are extensions of the skin, and wherever they occur are composed of similar tissues: the nail on a little toe is made of the same material as the hair.

Functions of the Skin

The skin has three main functions, and its different outward appearance on different parts of the body reflects to some extent which of these functions a certain area of skin primarily serves. The three main functions are protection (from germs or blows), temperature control (e.g., through perspiration, to aid in keeping the body's internal organs near our normal internal temperature of 98.6° F.), and perception. Nerve endings in the skin give us our sensations of touch, pain, heat, and cold. Associated with the skin's important role in temperature regulation is its function as an organ of excretion—the elimination, via perspiration, and subsequent evaporation of water and other substances. Skin is also the site of the body's natural production of vitamin D, stimulated by exposure to sunlight.

Anatomy of the Skin

Skin has three more or less distinct layers. The outermost is called the *epidermis;* the middle, the *dermis;* and the innermost, *subcutaneous* (under-skin) tissue. The epidermis may also be called *cuticle;* and the dermis either *corium* or *true skin.*

The Subcutaneous Layer

The subcutaneous layer is really a rather vague border zone between muscle and bone tissues on one side, and the dermis on the other, a kind of springy, fatty padding that gives bounce and a look of firmness to the skin above it. With age, the fatty cells of the subcutaneous layer are not continually replaced as they die, and this layer tends to thin out. The result is wrinkles, which form where the outer layers of skin lose their subcutaneous support, much like the slipcover of a cushion that has lost some of its stuffing.

Anatomy of the Skin

Approximate depth of section shown

The epidermis has been lifted to show the papillae on the dermal layer. The pattern of these papillae creates the fingerprints.

Sebaceous glands

Epidermis

Dermis

Subcutaneous tissue

Touch receptor

Capillary tufts bring blood close to surface for cooling.

Erector pili muscle causes gooseflesh.

Hair follicle

Nutrient blood vessel to hair follicle

Sweat gland

Pressure receptor nerve ending

The Dermis

The dermis is serviced by the multitude of tiny blood vessels and nerve fibers that reach it through the subcutaneous tissue. In addition, many special structures and tissues that enable the skin to perform its various functions are found in the dermis: *sebaceous* (skin oil) glands and sweat glands; minuscule muscles; and the roots of hairs encased in narrow pits called *follicles*.

The topmost layer of the dermis, interconnecting with the epidermis above it, resembles, under a microscope, nothing so much as a rugged, ridge-crossed landscape carved with valleys, caves, and tunnels. The basic forms of this microscopic terrain are cone-shaped hills called *papillae;* between 100 and 200 million of them are found in the dermis of an adult human being.

Because the dermal papillae serve as the bedrock for the surface layer of skin, the epidermis, we can understand why there is really no such thing as smooth skin; even the smoothest patch of a baby's skin appears ridged and cratered under a magnifying glass.

The distribution of papillae in the skin falls into certain distinctive patterns that are particularly conspicuous on the soles of babies' feet and on the fingertips, and give each of us our unique finger, toe, and footprints. The mathematical possibility of one person having the same fingerprints as another is thought to be about one in 25 billion. The papillae ridges on the fingertips also make it easier for us to pick up and handle such things as needles or pencils or buttons.

Finally, because there are relatively more papillae concentrated at the fingertips than on most other areas of the body, and because papillae are often associated with dense concentrations of nerve endings, the fingertips tend to be more responsive to touch sensations than other parts of the body.

The Epidermis

The bottom layer of the epidermis, its papillae fitted into the pockets of the layers of the dermis beneath it, is occupied by new young cells. These cells gradually mature and move upward. As they near the surface of the skin, they die, becoming tough, horny, lifeless tissue. This is the outmost layer of the epidermis, called the *stratum corneum* (horny layer), which we are continually shedding, usually unnoticed, as when we towel off after a bath, but sometimes very noticeably, as when we peel after a sunburn.

A suntan, incidentally, is caused by the presence of tiny grains of pigment, called *melanin,* in the bottom layers of epidermis. Sunlight stimulates the production of melanin, giving the skin a darker color. A suntan fades as the melanin granules move to the surface and are shed with dead skin cells.

Hair and Nails

Certainly the most noticeable of the specialized forms of skin are our hair and nails. What we see of them is really a dead tissue, called *keratin,* similar to the dead skin cells that are continually being shed by our bodies, but much more firmly packed together. However, hair and nails both originate in cells that are very much alive—as anyone who has plucked a group of hairs or suffered the pain of a torn-out nail knows very well. Growth occurs in this living region, with new cells pushing the dead, hard hair and nail stalks upward, then dying themselves and being replaced from below.

The bottom end or root of a hair is

Fingerprint

The pattern of ridges in a fingerprint reflects the contours of the papillae (conelike bumps) of the upper layer of the dermis, just below the epidermis.

lodged, as noted above, in a *follicle,* a hollow resembling a rounded bottle with a long, narrow neck slanting toward the skin's surface. Each follicle is supported by the little hummock of a papilla, and is serviced by tiny oil glands that lubricate the shaft (or neck) through which the hair pushes toward the surface.

The follicles of the long hairs of the scalp, groin, and armpits may be found deep in the subcutaneous layers of the skin; others are no deeper than the top layers of dermis. Attached to a follicle are microscopic muscle fibers that, if stimulated by cold or emotional factors, can contract around the follicle; the result is gooseflesh or sometimes even the sensation that our hair is standing on end.

A nail's living, growing part is found beneath the whitish half moon, or *lunula,* at its base. The lunula is sometimes obscured because a layer of epidermis (cuticle) has grown over it. Except at its very top (the part we can trim without pain), the nail is firmly attached to the ridged upper layer of the dermis, a region richly laced with tiny blood vessels.

Oil Glands

The skin's oil-producing (or *seba-*

ceous) glands are almost always associated with hair follicles, into which they seep their oils (or *sebum*). The oily substance works its way up toward the surface, lubricating both the hair and outer layers of epidermis, which need continual lubrication in order to stay soft and flexible. Also, skin oils serve as a kind of protective coat against painful drying and chapping.

Sweat Glands and Blood Vessels

While everybody is aware that the amount we perspire is related to the temperature around us, not everybody is aware that the countless tiny blood vessels in our skin—some 15 feet of them coursing beneath every square inch of skin—also react to changes in outside temperatures. Working together, and both controlled by an automatic "thermostat" in our brain, sweat glands and blood vessels have the all-important role of keeping our internal organs near their normal 98.6° Fahrenheit temperature.

The trick in maintaining an internal body temperature near normal is to conserve body heat when it is colder outside and to lose heat when it is warmer. Blood circulating near the surface of the skin is warmed (gains heat) or cooled (loses heat) according to the outside temperature.

The skin's myriad blood vessels constrict when the outside temperature is colder. This means that less blood can come into contact with the colder outside air, and therefore the overall temperature level of the blood remains warmer than if the blood vessels had not become constricted. On the other hand, when the body needs to lose heat—for example, during and after a vigorous tennis match—the skin's blood vessels dilate. This accounts for the "heat flush" or reddening of skin that light-skinned people

exhibit when very heated.

Sweat glands aid in temperature regulation by secreting moisture, which, evaporating on the skin's surface, cools the skin and therefore the blood flowing beneath it. Moisture that does not evaporate but remains as liquid on the skin or runs off in rivulets is not efficient in cooling. Humid air tends to prevent evaporation, while moving air or wind aids it. Sweat that evaporates as soon as it reaches the skin's surface usually goes unnoticed. Fresh sweat has no odor; but if it remains without evaporating, bacteria begin to give it the odor known medically as *bromhidrosis*.

There are some two million sweat glands in the skin. Each consists of a coiled, corkscrewlike tube that tunnels its way up to the surface of the skin from the dermis or from the deeper subcutaneous layer.

Potential Trouble Spots

All of us are very conscious of the condition of our skin and worry when something seems to be wrong with it. The temptations to worry too much, to overtreat, to take the advice of a well-meaning friend, to use the wrong (but heavily advertised) product are very great. Knowing about the properties of the skin and what medical knowledge has to say about skin problems can help to avoid mistakes in caring for it. See Ch. 21, *Skin and Hair*. For a discussion of adolescent skin problems, see also Ch. 3, *The Teens*.

The Nervous System and the Brain

Most of us have heard often

enough that the brain, acting as control center for a communication network we call our nervous system, is an incredible computer, weighing a mere three pounds. Its form and functions, however, are often described as being so much more intricate and complex than any existing or imagined computer that thorough knowledge of the brain seems very remote. This is certainly true. But it doesn't prevent us from knowing some general things about the brain and nervous system, or what its most significant parts are and how they work.

Basically, the nervous system has just two functions: first, getting information (impulses, signals, messages) from outside or inside the body to where it can be acted upon, usually in the brain; and secondly, feeding back information (for example, to the muscles) so that the indicated action can be taken. Thus, nerves can be divided by their function into two general types, each following a separate pathway. Those that receive information—for example, from our senses—and pass it along are called *sensory,* or *afferent* (inward-traveling). Those that relay information back, with a directive for action, are called *motor,* or *efferent* (outward-traveling).

The brain and the spinal cord can be considered as the basic unit of the *central nervous system.* All sensory and motor information comes or goes from this central core. The spinal cord is the master nerve tract (or nerve trunk) in our body and consists of millions of nerve fibers bundled together, somewhat like many small threads making up a large rope.

Like the spinal cord, all the lesser nerves, shown as single cords in a typical anatomical drawing, are made up of hundreds of thousands of individual fibers. Each fiber is part of a single nerve cell, or *neuron*. Neurons—there are 12 to 15 billion of them in our brain alone—are the basic structural units of the brain and nervous system, the tubes and transistors and circuits of which our personal computer is built.

The Brain

The appearance of the brain within the skull has been described as a huge gray walnut and a cauliflower. The inelegance of such descriptions is the least of many good reasons why we should be happy our brains are not exposed to public view.

Brain tissue—pinkish gray and white—is among the most delicate in our body, and the destruction of even a small part may mean lasting impairment or death. Its protection is vital and begins (if we are so fortunate) with a mat of hair on the top, back, and sides of our skull. Next comes the resilient layer of padding we call the scalp, and then the main line of defense—the rounded, bony helmet of skull.

The brain's armor does not stop with bone. Beneath are three strong, fibrous membranes called *meninges* that encase the brain in protective envelopes. Meninges also overlie the tissue of the spinal cord; infection or inflammation of these membranes by bacteria or viruses is called *cerebrospinal meningitis*.

Between two of the meninges is a region laced with veins and arteries and filled with *cerebrospinal fluid.* This fluid-filled space cushions the brain against sudden blows and collisions. The cerebrospinal fluid circulates not only about the brain but through the entire central nervous system. Incidentally, chemical analysis of this fluid, withdrawn by inserting a hypodermic needle between vertebrae of the spinal column (a spinal tap), can provide clues to the nature of brain and nervous system disorders.

The Cerebrum

What we usually mean by "brain" is that part of the brain called the *cerebrum*. It is the cerebrum that permits us all our distinctly human activities—thinking, speaking, reading, writing.

Only in man does the cerebrum reach such size, occupying the interior of our entire dome above the level of our eyes.

The surface of the cerebrum is wrinkled, furrowed, folded and infolded, convoluted, fissured—anything but smooth. This lavishly wrinkled outer layer of the cerebrum, about an eighth of an inch thick, is called the *cerebral cortex*. From its grayish color comes the term "gray matter" for brain tissue. There is a pattern among its wrinkles, marked out by wider, or deeper fissures, or furrows, running through the brain tissue. The most conspicuous fissure runs down the middle, front to back, dividing the cerebrum into two halves, the left hemisphere and the right hemisphere. The nerves from the left half of the body are served by the right hemisphere, and the right half of the body by the left hemisphere, so that damage to one side of the brain affects the other side of the body.

The Lobes of the Cerebrum

Smaller fissures crisscross the cerebrum and mark out various specific areas of function called *lobes*. The frontal lobes, one on the left hemisphere and one on the right in back of our eyes and extending upward behind the forehead, are perhaps the most talked about and the least understood by medical researchers. The specific functions of most other lobes in the cerebrum, such as the two occipital lobes (centers for seeing), the olfactory lobes (centers for smelling), and the temporal lobes (centers for hearing) are much better known.

The Brain Stem

The cerebrum, like a large flower obscuring part of its stalk, droops down

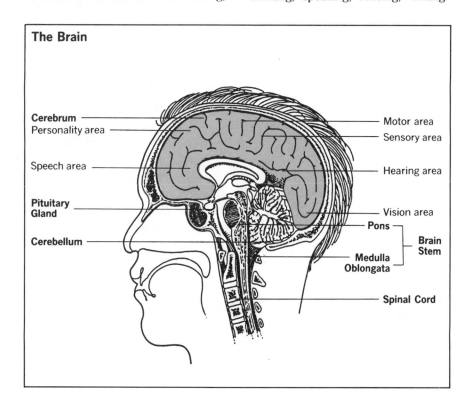

The Brain

Cerebrum
Personality area
Speech area
Pituitary Gland
Cerebellum

Motor area
Sensory area
Hearing area
Vision area
Pons
Brain Stem
Medulla Oblongata
Spinal Cord

The Brain and the Cranial Nerves

Cranial nerves

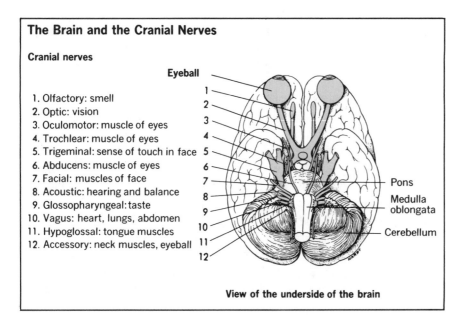

Eyeball

1. Olfactory: smell
2. Optic: vision
3. Oculomotor: muscle of eyes
4. Trochlear: muscle of eyes
5. Trigeminal: sense of touch in face
6. Abducens: muscle of eyes
7. Facial: muscles of face
8. Acoustic: hearing and balance
9. Glossopharyngeal: taste
10. Vagus: heart, lungs, abdomen
11. Hypoglossal: tongue muscles
12. Accessory: neck muscles, eyeball

Pons

Medulla oblongata

Cerebellum

View of the underside of the brain

around the *brain stem*. Thus, while the brain stem originates just about in the middle of our skull, it does not emerge completely from the folds of the cerebral hemispheres until it reaches the back of the neck. Then it soon merges into the spinal cord.

Associated with this portion of the brain—roughly speaking, between the cerebrum and the spinal cord—are centers that take care of the countless necessary details involved in just plain existing, and structures (such as the *medulla oblongata* and the *pons*) that serve also as traffic control points for the billions of nerve impulses traveling to and from the cerebrum. The largest of these "lesser brains" is the *cerebellum,* whose two hemispheres straddle the brain stem at the back of the head.

The Cerebellum

The cerebellum is the site of balance and body and muscle coordination, allowing us, for example, to "rub the tummy and pat the head" simultaneously, or tap the foot and strum a guitar, or steer a car and operate the foot pedals. Such muscle-coordinated movements, though sometimes learned only by long repetition and

practice, can become almost automatic—such as reaching for and flicking on the light switch as we move into a darkened room.

But many other activities and kinds of behavior regulated by the part of the brain below the cerebrum are more fully automatic: the control of eye movement and focusing, for example, as well as the timing of heartbeat, sleep, appetite, and metabolism; the arousal and decline of sexual drives; body temperature; the dilation and constriction of blood vessels; swallowing; and breathing. All these are mainly functions of the *autonomic nervous system,* as opposed to the more voluntary actions controlled by the *central nervous system.*

The Body's Nervous Systems

Simply speaking, the human body has only one nervous system, and that is all the nerve cells, nerve cords, nerve centers (both voluntary and involuntary) in the body. It is helpful, however, though quite arbitrary, to divide our nerves into the central and autonomic nervous systems. This division tends to obscure the countless interconnections and interplay between

the two systems. For example, where do you place the control of breathing or blinking? Such actions are automatic except when we choose to regulate them.

The Central Nervous System

The central nervous system, as noted above, includes the brain and the spinal cord. It also includes all the nerves of conscious response and voluntary action that link up with the brain and spinal cord.

Twelve pairs of *cranial nerves* originate within the brain and emerge at its base. These include the very important nerves that connect with our sense organs, nerve bundles that control the facial and neck muscles, and the *vagus* (or tenth cranial nerve) that serves the heart, lungs, stomach, intestines, esophagus, larynx, liver, kidneys, spleen, and pancreas. The vagus nerve, although anatomically part of the central nervous system, controls bodily functions that are mainly automatic.

Spinal nerves branch out from the spinal cord as it snakes its way through the vertebrae of the spinal column. All the major nerve cords that wrap around the trunk and reach the arms and hands, legs and feet, originate from spinal nerves.

The cranial nerves and the spinal nerves, together with all those nerves lying outside the confines of the brain and spinal cord, are sometimes referred to as the *peripheral nervous system.* This term can be confusing, however, because it is also used to include all the nerves of the autonomic nervous system, next discussed.

The Autonomic Nervous System

The muscles served by the central nervous system are all of one general type (striated), while the muscles served by the autonomic system are called involuntary or smooth. The autonomic nerves regulate body activity without our conscious control—for example, as we sleep. They are rather elegantly divided into two categories: *sympathetic* and *parasympathetic* nervous systems. These are distinguishable primarily by their opposite effects on the body organs. For example, impulses along parasympathetic nerve trunks dilate blood vessels, slow the heartbeat rate, and increase stomach secretions, while the sympathetic system constricts blood vessels, increases rate of heartbeat, and inhibits stomach secretions.

The Neuron—What Nerves Are Made Of

A nerve cell is a grayish blob of tissue from which protrude several short gray fibers, *dendrites,* and one longer whitish fiber, an *axon.* Both the dendrites and the axon resemble ropes with their ends splayed and frayed. Dendrites register impulses coming into the central blob of the neuron (perhaps from a neighboring neuron's axon); an axon picks up the incoming impulses and carries them away.

Both units are equally important for normal nerve functioning, but the axon is far more showy as an anatomical structure. All nerve cords are made up of the single strands of many axons, which may reach lengths of several feet. In other words, if we could stretch out certain neurons in our body—for example, those making up the sciatic nerve that runs from the small of the back to the toes—their axon "tails" would make them three or four feet long.

Myelin

A normal axon usually has a fatty coating of insulation called *myelin.* An axon severed into two pieces cannot grow together again; but if the myelin sheath is pretty much intact, a surgeon can sometimes restore nerve function by sewing the two ends together, or replace the nerve with one from another part of the body. The part of the severed axon connecting to the central portion usually remains alive in any case—which is why a person can often retain the sensation of feeling in an amputated part.

Certain serious and progressively disabling diseases involve the gradual loss (*demyelination*) of this coating, causing paralysis, numbness, or other loss of function in an organ; a demyelinated nerve fiber is not able to carry impulses to and from the brain. Two such diseases are multiple sclerosis and "Lou Gehrig's disease" (amyotrophic lateral sclerosis).

Effects of Aging

Once we reach maturity, the number of our nerve cells begins to decrease, because our bodies cannot manufacture new neurons to replace the ones that die in the normal process of living. (Other kinds of tissue are continually replenished with new cells.) This has some relation to senility, but the loss of a few million out of many billions of brain and nerve cells has

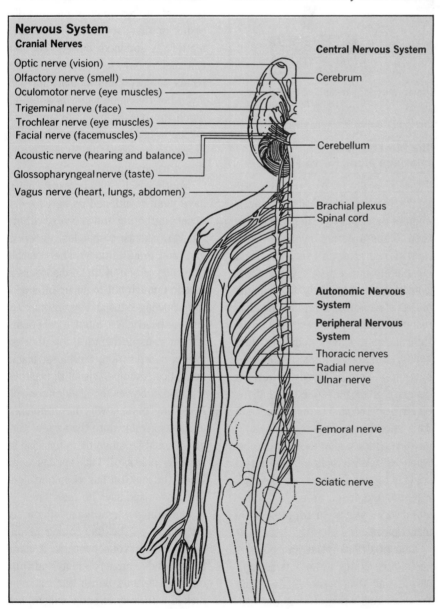

Nervous System
Cranial Nerves

Optic nerve (vision)
Olfactory nerve (smell)
Oculomotor nerve (eye muscles)
Trigeminal nerve (face)
Trochlear nerve (eye muscles)
Facial nerve (facemuscles)
Acoustic nerve (hearing and balance)
Glossopharyngeal nerve (taste)
Vagus nerve (heart, lungs, abdomen)

Central Nervous System

Cerebrum

Cerebellum

Brachial plexus
Spinal cord

Autonomic Nervous System
Peripheral Nervous System

Thoracic nerves
Radial nerve
Ulnar nerve

Femoral nerve

Sciatic nerve

THE NEURON

Sensory, or afferent ("carrying in"), neurons respond to external stimuli and conduct impulses to the central nervous system — the brain and spinal column — where the message is interpreted.

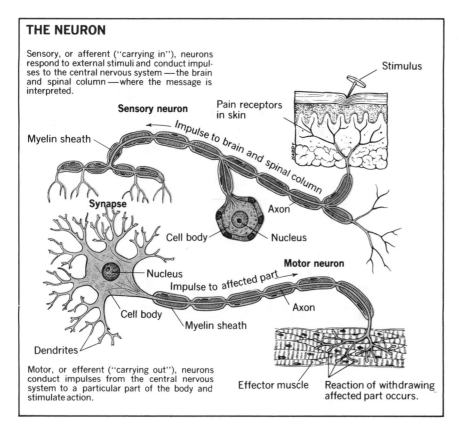

Motor, or efferent ("carrying out"), neurons conduct impulses from the central nervous system to a particular part of the body and stimulate action.

little effect on mental powers unless the losses are concentrated in one area.

Synapse, Ganglion, and Plexus

When a nerve impulse, traveling away from the neuron's central part, reaches the ends of an axon, it meets a gap that it must jump to get to the tentaclelike dendrites of the next neuron. This gap is called a *synapse.*

At certain points in the body a great many nerve cell bodies and branches are packed closely together, with a resulting profusion of interwoven axons, dendrites, and synapses. Such a concentration of nervous tissue is called a *ganglion,* or *plexus.* A blow or jolt to such an area can be extremely painful and even stupefying—affecting as it does a whole network of nerves—as anyone who has been hit in the solar plexus or learned the pressure points of karate knows.

The Movement of Impulses along Nerve Fibers

There is really no exact counterpart in the mechanical world for how an impulse moves along a nerve fiber and then jumps across a synapse to the next nerve. Nor is this movement completely understood by scientists. Suffice it to say that it is somewhat like an electrical current moving along in a chemical environment that allows the impulse to travel, in discreet little jumps, at a speed of about 200 miles per hour—quite slowly when we compare it to the speed of light or electricity: 186,000 miles per second. This speed serves us quite well in most situations, but there are times when we wish human beings' nerves could act more quickly—on the highway, for example, or when a cherished vase starts to topple off the mantelpiece.

One of the simplest and quickest kinds of reactions to an outside stimulus is one that bypasses the brain. We don't really think to pull our hand away from a piping hot radiator. This is called a *spinal reflex.* What happens is that the sensory nerve endings in the finger pick up the "too hot" impulse from the radiator; the impulse then travels to the spinal cord where it activates the motor nerve pathway back to the burned finger, carrying the message, "Jerk your finger away!"

When to Suspect Trouble

Our entire existence as human beings depends so much on the normal functioning of our brain and nervous system that any real brain or nervous disorder or disease is a very serious matter. A sprained joint or cut foot can spell doom for an animal that depends on speed and mobility for survival; but the same injury is often not much more than a painful inconvenience to us. Impairment of our brain or nervous system is far more of a threat to our survival.

Multiple sclerosis and meningitis have been mentioned as serious disorders affecting the nerves, others are Parkinsonism, shingles, encephalitis, and brain tumors. The possible presence of one of these disorders is reason enough not to shrug off any of the following signs and symptoms: recurrent headaches, intense pain of unknown cause, tremors, numbness, loss of coordination, dizziness, blackouts, tics, cramps, visual difficulties, and loss of bowel and bladder control. Also, any person who has remained unconscious for more than a few minutes should be taken to a physician as soon as possible. This applies even when the person has regained consciousness and says he feels fine.

Our complex emotions, of course, are linked to the functioning of our brain and nervous system. A mind free of undue anxiety, guilt, and frustration functions better than a mind racked with worries and conflicts, and is a much more efficient and reliable leader of the body. See also Ch. 8, *Diseases of the Muscles and Nervous System.* For a discussion of mental and emotional health, see Ch. 36.

The Circulatory System, the Heart, and Blood

When the heart stops beating—that is to say, stops pumping blood—for longer than a couple of minutes, we stop living. But the heart, fortunately, is extremely sturdy. It is also simple in construction, capable of operating at a great many different speeds, in many cases self-repairing if damaged, and probably the one continuously operating automatic pump that we could, with any confidence, expect to last 70 years or longer.

These simple facts tend to be forgotten today, in what is probably the most heart-conscious era in history. True, heart disease, along with cancer, is statistically one of today's major killers. But we should remember two circumstances: not until about 50 years ago did deaths from heart disease begin to be accurately recognized and reported; second, with longer and longer life spans, it becomes more likely that a nonstop vital organ like the heart will simply wear out. Heart transplants, open heart surgery, and artificial heart parts—often reported sensationally in the public media—have also conditioned us to think of our hearts as terribly vulnerable, rather delicate, a bit inadequate to their tasks, and quite open to improvement.

Advances in heart surgery do, indeed, hold greater promise for per-

sons whose hearts had been considered, until now, irreversibly damaged or diseased. But the great attention accorded such miracles of medicine tends to obscure the humdrum, day-in-day-out, low-key drama performed for a lifetime by a healthy, uncomplaining heart.

The Heart and Circulatory Network

Perhaps the best way to put the heart in perspective is to place it where it belongs, at the hub of the body's circulatory system. This hollow, fist-sized lump of sinewy tissue is located behind the breastbone, centered just about at the vertical midline of our chest. It is connected into a closed system of flexible tubes, called blood vessels, ranging down from finger-thick to microscopically slender, that reach into every cavern, crevice, and outpost of our body—a network of some 70,000 miles.

The heart has essentially one function—to push blood, by pumping action, through this enormous network of blood vessels. We have about six quarts of blood in our body, pumped at the rate of about five ounces every time the heart beats (normally about 72 times a minute for an adult), which we feel as our pulse. The blood circulates and recirculates through the blood vessels, pushed along by the pumping of the heart.

Arteries and Veins

The blood vessels are generally described as *arterial,* referring to the *arteries* that carry blood away from the heart; or *venous,* referring to the *veins* through which blood seeps and flows back toward the heart to be repumped. A large artery such as the *aorta* branches into smaller arteries, and these eventually into still smaller vessels called *arterioles,* and the arterioles, finally, into the smallest

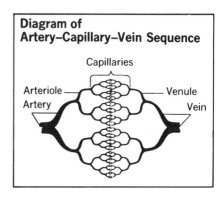

Diagram of Artery–Capillary–Vein Sequence

Capillaries

Arteriole / Artery — Venule / Vein

blood vessels, the *capillaries.* These in turn open onto other capillaries, which are the starting point for the return of blood to the heart.

The microscopic capillaries typically form a kind of cat's cradle connection, sometimes called a capillary bed, at the transition zone where arterial blood becomes venous blood. The returning blood moves from the capillaries to small veins called *venules* (the counterparts of arterioles) and through successively larger veins back to the heart.

Blood and Our Internal Fluid Environment

What makes this fairly rudimentary collection of plumbing so absolutely indispensable to life is the fluid it pumps—blood. If any part of the body—cell, tissue, or major organ—is denied circulating blood and the substances it carries with it for longer than a few minutes, that part will fail. It is the job of the heart and the blood vessels to get blood to all the body's far-flung tissues, where it both picks up and deposits substances.

Blood is really a kind of fluid tissue. About 80 percent of its volume is water, and blood's indispensable, life-sustaining power is owed in great part to its watery base, which permits it both to flow and to take up and carry materials in solution. All our tissues and organs have a kind of give-and-take arrangement with the circulating blood.

The Circulatory System

Arteries

(Carrying blood from the heart to the rest of the body)

Veins

(Carrying blood from all parts of the body toward the heart)

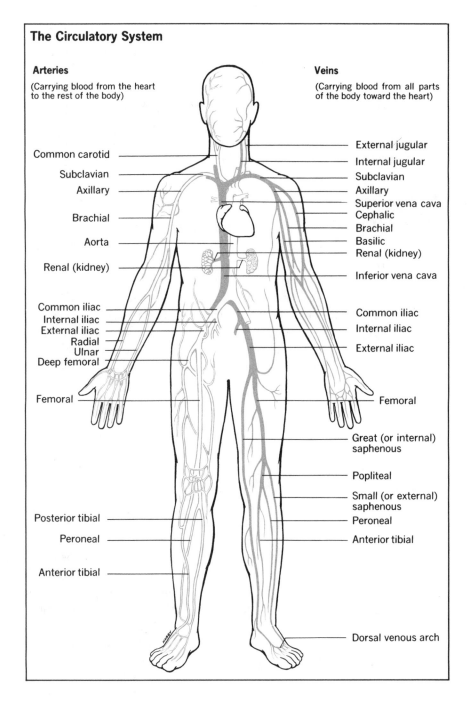

Arteries (left side):
- Common carotid
- Subclavian
- Axillary
- Brachial
- Aorta
- Renal (kidney)
- Common iliac
- Internal iliac
- External iliac
- Radial
- Ulnar
- Deep femoral
- Femoral
- Posterior tibial
- Peroneal
- Anterior tibial

Veins (right side):
- External jugular
- Internal jugular
- Subclavian
- Axillary
- Superior vena cava
- Cephalic
- Brachial
- Basilic
- Renal (kidney)
- Inferior vena cava
- Common iliac
- Internal iliac
- External iliac
- Femoral
- Great (or internal) saphenous
- Popliteal
- Small (or external) saphenous
- Peroneal
- Anterior tibial
- Dorsal venous arch

Distributor of Nutrients

Food, or more accurately the nutrient molecules needed by cells, are also transported throughout the body by the blood. In the digestive tract, food is broken down into tiny submicroscopic pieces that can pass through the tract's walls (mainly along the small intestine) and be picked up by the blood for distribution around the body.

One of the specialized, small-volume transportation jobs handled by the blood is to pick up hormones from the endocrine glands and present these chemical messengers to the organs they affect.

Composition of Blood

Blood is a distinctive and recognizable type of tissue, but this does not mean it is a stable, uniform substance with a fixed proportion of ingredients. Quite the opposite is true; its composition is ever changing in response to the demands of other body systems. Other organs are constantly pouring substances into the blood, or removing things from it. Blood in one part of the body at a given moment may be vastly different in chemical makeup from blood in another part of the body.

Despite its changing makeup, blood does have certain basic components. A sample of blood left to stand for an hour or so separates into a clear, watery fluid with a yellowish tinge and a darker, more solid clump. The clear yellow liquid is called *plasma,* and accounts for about 55 percent of the volume of normal blood. The darker clump is made up mainly of the blood's most conspicuous and populous inhabitants, the red cells that give blood its color.

Plasma

It is the plasma that enables our blood

Carrier of Oxygen

Perhaps the most critical of these give-and-take transactions occurs in the lungs; it is this transaction that if interrupted by heartbeat stoppage for more than a few minutes causes death by oxygen starvation of vital tissues. Before a unit of blood is pumped out by the heart to the body, it picks up in the lungs the oxygen that we have inhaled and which every cell in the body needs to function. The blood then transports the oxygen, delivering it to other parts of the body. By the time a given unit of blood has made a tour of the blood vessels and returned to the lungs, it has given up most of its oxygen and is laden instead with carbon dioxide, the principal waste product of living processes. The venous blood releases its carbon dioxide, to be exhaled by the lungs.

to carry out most of the transportation tasks assigned it. Being over 90 percent water, the plasma has water's property of being able to carry substances both in solution and in suspension. (A substance in solution is one, like salt, that must be removed from water by chemical or physical action, such as boiling; while a substance in suspension—such as red blood cells within whole blood in a standing test tube—separates out more readily, particularly when its watery carrier has been contained and its flow stilled.)

Red Blood Cells

Red blood cells (or *erythrocytes*) numbering in the trillions are carried in suspension by the plasma. In turn, the red blood cells carry the single most important substance needed by the body's cells—oxygen. For such an important task, the red blood cell looks hardly adequate. As it matures, this cell loses its nucleus. Lacking a nucleus, it is sometimes not even called a cell but a red blood *corpuscle*. What gives red blood cells their special oxygen-carrying ability, and also their color, is their possession of a complex iron-protein substance called *hemoglobin*.

Hemoglobin

Molecules of hemoglobin have the property of loosely combining with oxygen where it is plentiful, as in the lungs. They can then hold on to oxygen until they reach an area where oxygen has been depleted by the demands of living processes. There— usually in the fine tubes of the capillaries—hemoglobin's hold on oxygen is challenged by the demands of other cells, and the red cells give up their oxygen. The hemoglobin of red cells develops an immediate affinity for car-

bon dioxide, the waste product of cell metabolism, and the red blood cells then carry this carbon dioxide back to the lungs for exhalation.

Hemoglobin's ability to carry oxygen is not unique. Water, and therefore plasma, also have this ability. Hemoglobin's specialness lies in how much oxygen it can carry. Hemoglobin increases by more than 50 times the oxygen-carrying capacity of our blood.

White Blood Cells

White blood cells have many different shapes and sizes, all going under the general scientific name of *leukocytes*. They are typically larger than red blood cells, but far less numerous. If we accept an estimate of 25 trillion as the number of living red blood cells in our body, then the number of white blood cells might be generously estimated at around 40 billion, a ratio of one white cell to about 600–700 reds.

According to their shape, size, and other characteristics, white blood cells have been divided into various categories such as lymphocytes, monocytes, and granulocytes. But as a group these blood cells are distinguished by their common propensity for attacking foreign bodies that invade our tissues, whether these invaders be sizable splinters or microscopic bacteria. White blood cells move in force to the site of an infection, do battle with the intruding agents, and frequently strew the area with the wreckage of the encounter— a collection of dismantled alien bacteria and dead white cells, which we know as pus.

Platelets

Platelets, also called *thrombocytes,* initiate some of the first steps in the complex biochemical process that leads to the clotting of blood. They

thus help to spare us from bleeding to death from a slight injury. Platelets are the most rudimentary and diminutive of the major blood components. Like mature red blood cells, they lack nuclei, but are only one-quarter as big. By no stretch of the imagination can they be called blood cells. Rather, they are blood elements—bits of cell substance with a recognizable size and shape, circulating with the blood.

The Proportions of Blood Cells

All the several types of blood cells and subcells in a healthy body occur in proportions that, though never precisely fixed and unchanging, are recognized as having normal upper and lower limits. If a particular type of cell shows a sudden increase or decrease in population, so that its proportion relative to other blood cells shows a variation markedly outside its normal range, some infection, disease, or disorder must be suspected.

In addition to occurring in certain normal-range proportions, each type of cellular blood component has a typical shape, appearance, and set of chemical and physical properties. Variations from these norms occur in many diseases.

The analysis of blood samples (usually taken from the finger or arm) and their inspection under a microscope have proved invaluable in diagnosing illness and disease, often before a person feels any symptoms whatsoever. This is why a thorough medical checkup should always include taking a sample of your blood. It is then up to the physician to decide which of the dozens of tests should be made on your blood in the medical laboratory. One common test is a *blood count,* in which the number of a certain type of cell in a given unit of your blood can be estimated, and then compared to the normal number in the same amount of blood.

Blood Groups and Rh Factors

The identification of *blood groups* and *Rh factors* is another aspect of blood analysis. The four most common blood groups are called A, B, AB, and O, classifications based on chemical differences that may be incompatible if one group is mixed with another. Thus, it is absolutely essential before a person receives a blood transfusion to know both his own blood type and the type of the blood he is to be given. Blood group O is considered the safety for transfusion, and people with type O blood are sometimes called "universal donors." It is a wise practice to carry, along with your other important cards, a card giving your own blood type. The blood of a donor, however, is always *cross-matched* (checked for compatibility) with the blood of the person who is to receive it in order to avoid transfusion reactions.

Blood Cell Manufacture and Turnover

Most types of blood cells, both red and white, are manufactured in the red marrow of bones. The rate and quantity of total production is staggering; estimates range from one to five million red blood cells per second. This prodigious output is necessary because blood cells are disintegrating, having served their useful lives, in the same enormous numbers every second. The normal life span of a red blood cell is about four months, which means that four months from now every blood cell in your body will have died and been replaced with new cells.

The Liver As a Producer of Red Blood Cells

The red bone marrow is backed up by several other tissues that can, if called upon, turn out blood cells in quantity or serve as specialized producers of certain blood cells and blood elements. One such organ is the liver, which, before and after birth and into childhood, is a site of red blood cell production. In an emergency, such as severe internal hemorrhage, the liver sometimes reverts to its earlier function of manufacturing red cells. The liver also serves as a kind of salvage yard for the iron from dead red cells. It stores the iron for later combination into hemoglobin and passes off the rest of the red blood cell fragments as part of the bile pigments that empty into the duodenum of the small intestine.

The Spleen As a Producer of Blood Cells

Certain white blood cells, in particular the lymphocytes, are produced at a variety of locations in the body—for example, by the lymph nodes, by little clumps of tissue called *Peyer's patches* in the intestinal tract, and by the spleen.

The spleen plays a number of interesting secondary roles in blood cell production. Like the liver, it can be pressed into service as a manufacturer of red blood cells and serve as a salvage yard for iron reclaimed from worn-out red blood cells. A newborn baby is almost totally dependent on its spleen for the production of red blood cells, with a little help from the liver. In an adult, however, a damaged or diseased spleen can be surgically removed, with little or no apparent effect on the health or life span of the person, provided the patient's bone marrow is in good functioning order.

Movement of Blood Cells through the Capillaries

A blood cell must be able to slip through the microscopic, twisting and turning tunnels of the capillaries that mark the turn-about point in the blood cell's round-trip voyage from the heart. Blood cells, therefore, must be small (the point of a pin could hold dozens of red blood cells), and they must be jellylike in order to navigate the tight tortuous, capillary channels without either blocking the channel or breaking apart themselves. A red blood cell is further adapted to sneaking through the capillaries by its concave-disk shape, which allows it to bend and fold around itself. Nevertheless, so narrow are the passageways within some of the capillaries that blood cells must move through them in single file. If a substantial number of the cells are misshapen, as in sickle-cell anemia, they tend to move sluggishly or clog up the passageway—a condition that can have serious consequences. See also Ch. 9, *Diseases of the Circulatory System.*

Lymph and the Lymphatic System

Of all our body systems, perhaps the most ignored is the lymphatic system, although it forms a network throughout our body comparable to the blood vessels of our circulatory system.

Lymph is a whitish fluid that is derived from blood plasma. As plasma circulates through the body, some of it seeps through the walls of capillaries and other blood vessels. This leakage is of the utmost importance, because the leaked fluid, lymph, supplies the liquid environment around and between individual cells and tissues that is essential for their survival.

The presence of lymph requires a drainage system to keep the fluid moving. If there were no drainage system, two things could happen: the dammed-up lymph could create areas swollen with water in which cells would literally drown, or stagnant pools of lymph could become breeding

MUSCLES AND TENDONS

MUSCLES

1. Temporal
2. Mimetic muscles
3. Masseter (a muscle of mastication)
4. Infrahyoid muscles
5. Sternomastoid
6. Omohyoid
7. Deltoid
8. Pectoral muscles
9. Serratus anterior
10. External oblique
11. Rectus abdominus
12. Biceps brachii
13. Flexor digitorum superficialis (sublimis)
14. Gracilis

15. Adductor group
16. Sartorius
17. Rectus femoris
18. Quadriceps femoris
19. Vastus medialis
19a. Vastus lateralis
20. Dorsiflexors
21. Trapezius
22. Infraspinatus
23. Teres major
24. Triceps brachii
25. Latissimus dorsi
26. Rhomboideus major
27. Gluteus medius
28. Gluteus maximus

29. Digital extensors
30. Hamstring muscles
31. Gastrocnemius
32. Plantar flexors

TENDONS
33. Rectus sheath
34. Flexor retinaculum of carpal tunnel
35. Patellar tendon
36. Retinaculum of tarsal tunnel
37. Tendons of long digital extensors
38. Tendon of tibialis anterior
39. Lumbodorsal fascia
40. Fascia lata
41. Achilles   © C. S. HAMMOND & Co., N Y.

BONES
1. Skull
2. Mandible
3. Vertebrae
4. Clavicle
5. Scapula
6. Manubrium
7. Body of sternum
8. Xiphoid process
9. Ribs
10. Humerus
11. Radius
12. Ulna

BONES AND LIGAMENTS
13. Sacrum
14. Ilium
15. Coccyx
16. Femur
17. Patella
18. Tibia
19. Fibula
20. Carpals
21. Metacarpals
22. Phalanges
23. Metatarsals
24. Tarsals
25. Heel

LIGAMENTS AND JOINTS
26. Capsule of shoulder
27. Sternoclavicular
28. Capsule of elbow
29. Sacroiliac
30. Iliofemoral
31. Wrist
32. Capsule of knee
33. Ankle
34. Pubic symphysis
35. Intervertebral discs

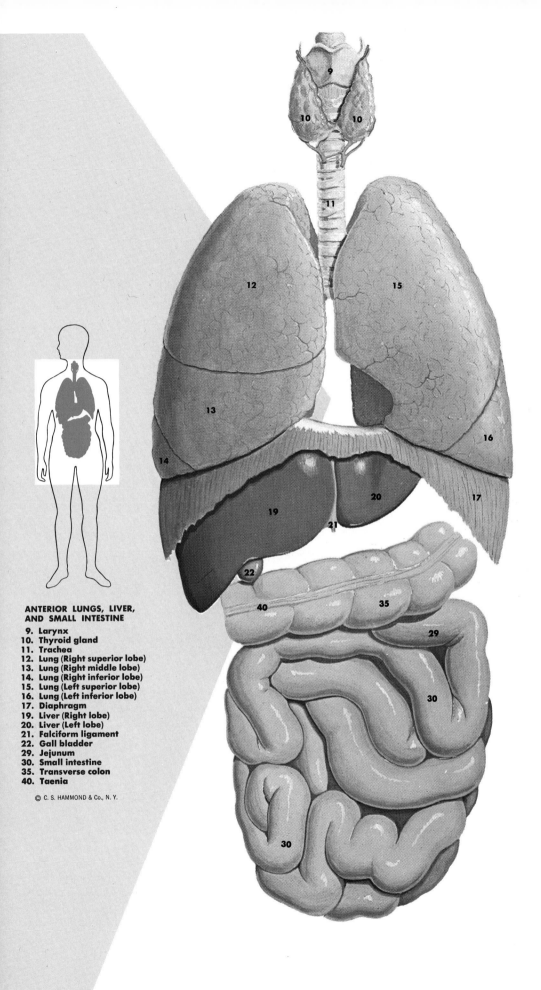

ANTERIOR LUNGS, LIVER, AND SMALL INTESTINE

9. Larynx
10. Thyroid gland
11. Trachea
12. Lung (Right superior lobe)
13. Lung (Right middle lobe)
14. Lung (Right inferior lobe)
15. Lung (Left superior lobe)
16. Lung (Left inferior lobe)
17. Diaphragm
19. Liver (Right lobe)
20. Liver (Left lobe)
21. Falciform ligament
22. Gall bladder
29. Jejunum
30. Small intestine
35. Transverse colon
40. Taenia

POSTERIOR LUNGS, LIVER, AND SMALL INTESTINE

9. Larynx
10. Thyroid gland
11. Trachea
12. Lung (Right superior lobe)
13. Lung (Right middle lobe)
14. Lung (Right inferior lobe)
15. Lung (Left superior lobe)
16. Lung (Left inferior lobe)
17. Diaphragm
18. Principal bronchi
19. Liver (Right lobe)
20. Liver (Left lobe)
21. Falciform ligament
22. Gall bladder
29. Jejunum
30. Small intestine
31. Ileum
35. Transverse colon
40. Taenia coli
41. Cystic duct
42. Portal vein
43. Hepatic artery
44. Hepatic vein

ANTERIOR CIRCULATORY SYSTEM

17. Diaphragm
23. Esophagus
37. Sigmoid colon
38. Rectum
44. Hepatic vein
49. Superior mesenteric artery
53. Common carotid artery.
54. Internal jugular vein
55. Subclavian artery
56. Subclavian vein
57. Aortic arch
58. Aorta
60. Heart
61. Pulmonary arteries
63. Superior vena cava
64. Inferior vena cava
65. Coronary arteries
66. Coeliac trunk
68. Inferior mesenteric artery
69. Renal artery
70. Renal vein
71. Common iliac artery
72. Common iliac vein
73. Femoral artery
74. Femoral vein
75. Internal iliac artery
76. Internal iliac vein
77. Kidneys (r. and l.)
78. Suprarenal glands (r. and l.)
79. Ureters (r. and l.)

POSTERIOR CIRCULATORY SYSTEM

17. Diaphragm
23. Esophagus
37. Sigmoid colon
38. Rectum
53. Common carotid artery.
54. Internal jugular vein
55. Subclavian artery
56. Subclavian vein
57. Aortic arch
58. Aorta
60. Heart
61. Pulmonary arteries
62. Pulmonary veins
63. Superior vena cava
64. Inferior vena cava
69. Renal artery
70. Renal vein
71. Common iliac artery
72. Common iliac vein
73. Femoral artery
74. Femoral vein
75. Internal iliac artery
76. Internal iliac vein
77. Kidneys (r. and l.)
79. Ureters (r. and l.)

© C. S. HAMMOND & Co., N. Y.

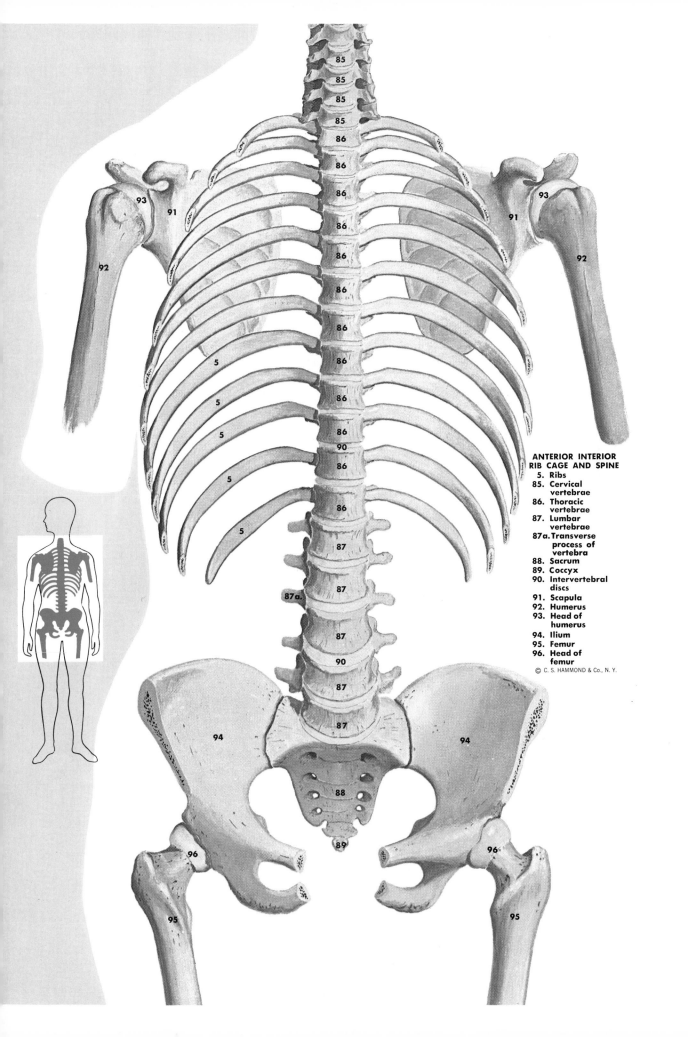

ANTERIOR INTERIOR
RIB CAGE AND SPINE
  5. Ribs
 85. Cervical
     vertebrae
 86. Thoracic
     vertebrae
 87. Lumbar
     vertebrae
87a. Transverse
     process of
     vertebra
 88. Sacrum
 89. Coccyx
 90. Intervertebral
     discs
 91. Scapula
 92. Humerus
 93. Head of
     humerus
 94. Ilium
 95. Femur
 96. Head of
     femur

**POSTERIOR RIB
CAGE AND SPINE**

5. Ribs
85. Cervical
vertebrae
86. Thoracic
vertebrae
87. Lumbar
vertebrae
88. Sacrum
89. Coccyx
91. Scapula
92. Humerus
93. Head of
humerus
94. Ilium
95. Femur
96. Head of
femur

© C. S. HAMMOND
& Co., N. Y.

**ANTERIOR CHEST
CAVITY**
1. Clavicle
2. Manubrium
3. Body of sternum
4. Xiphoid process
5. Rib
6. Floating rib
7. Cartilage
8. Anterior super-
   ior iliac spine

© C. S. HAMMOND & Co., N. Y.

**POSTERIOR
INTERIOR CHEST
CAVITY**

1. Clavicle
2. Manubrium
3. Body of sternum
4. Xiphoid process.
5. Rib
6. Floating rib
7. Cartilage
8. Anterior superior
   iliac spine

**ANTERIOR STOMACH, COLON,
AND
ORGANS OF REPRODUCTION**

23. Esophagus
24. Stomach (cardia)
25. Stomach (fundus)
26. Stomach (body)
27. Stomach (pylorus)
28. Duodenum
31. Ileum
32. Ileocolic junction
33. Caecum
34. Ascending colon
36. Descending colon
37. Sigmoid colon
39. Vermiform appendix
40. Taenia coli
45. Spleen
49. Superior mesenteric artery
50. Superior mesenteric vein
51. Pancreas (head)
52. Pancreas (tail)
80. Bladder
81. Urachus
82. Pubic symphysis
83. Inguinal ligament
100. Uterus
102. Vagina (cross section)
103. Fallopian tube
104. Ostium of fallopian tube
105. Ovary

LACTATING BREAST

97. Pectoralis major muscle
117. Areola
118. Nipple
119. Fat
120. Lactiferous (milk producing) glands and ducts
120a. Cross section of gland and duct
121. Tissue separating and supporting glandular tissue

STRUCTURE OF THE MAMMARY GLANDS

The mammary glands are composed of three major elements:
1. Their skin covering and special structures (nipple, areola).
2. The lactiferous glands or functional units of the breast.
3. The supporting structures, the connective tissue "ligaments" and the fat tissue that makes up the mass of the breast.

The breast is supported by the "suspensory ligaments." These are anchored to the sheet of connective tissue surrounding the pectoralis major muscle, and extend in a complex network separated by the fat tissue outward to the skin. The lactiferous glands are buried in the supporting tissues and empty outward onto the surface of the nipple. These glands at first are very small and clustered just beneath the nipple and areola. In pregnancy they enlarge and push downward into the mass of the breast causing it to enlarge in turn. The enlargement continues through the period of breast feeding, following which the glands gradually grow smaller and the entire breast returns to normal size.

101. Cervix
108. Myometrium
109. Endometrium
111. Placenta
113. Amniotic sac
114. Umbilical cord
116. Fetus

THE FETUS AT 3 1/2 AND 6 MONTHS

Most of the definitive development of the fetus occurs during the first 3½ months, and the remaining 5½ months is primarily concerned with gradual increase in size and maturation of organs already begun. The fetus receives all of its nourishment through the placenta and umbilical cord. There is no direct contact between fetal and maternal blood in the placenta. During its entire development, the fetus floats in a fluid (amniotic fluid) contained within a sac (the amniotic sac) attached to the placenta. This sac is in turn surrounded by the uterine cavity, the endometrium and the muscle or myometrium of the uterus.

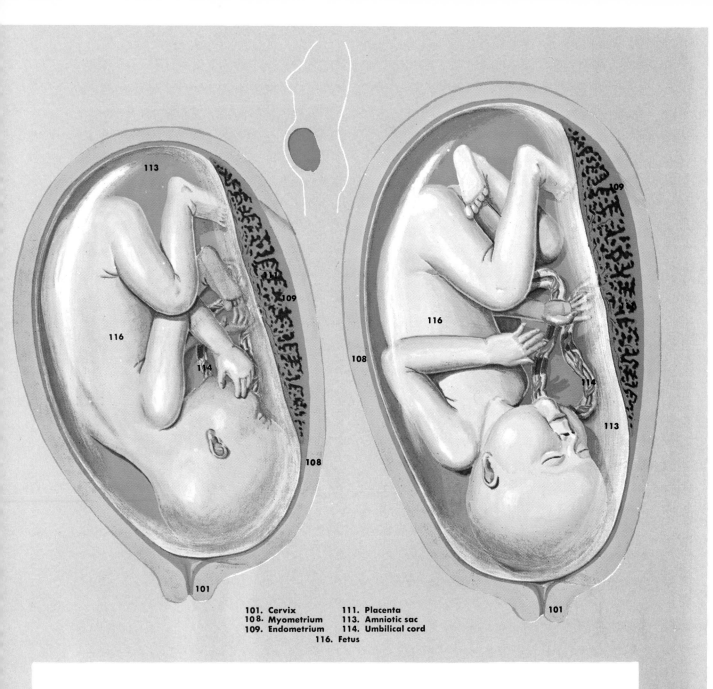

101. Cervix	111. Placenta
108. Myometrium	113. Amniotic sac
109. Endometrium	114. Umbilical cord
116. Fetus	

THE FETUS AT 8 AND 9 MONTHS

Until birth, the fetus is surrounded by the amniotic sac and fluid, and attached to the placenta by the umbilical cord. The fetus continues to increase in size and the uterus stretches to accommodate it. Usually before the eighth month the fetus assumes a head-downward position. At birth, the amniotic sac ruptures, the fluid escapes, and the child is slowly pushed out of the uterine cavity by the contractions of the myometrium. Shortly after birth of the child, the placenta is similarly expelled having been detached from the endometrium.

X-RAY OF THE HUMAN BODY
SHOWING THE
BONE STRUCTURE

grounds for infection.

As it moves through the vessels of the lymphatic system, lymph carries away from the tissues the bits and pieces of cells that have died and disintegrated, and also potentially harmful bacteria and viruses.

Lymph and Lymphocytes

Confusion often arises about the connection between the white blood cells called *lymphocytes* and the lymph itself. Lymph is not made up of lymphocytes, although it often carries

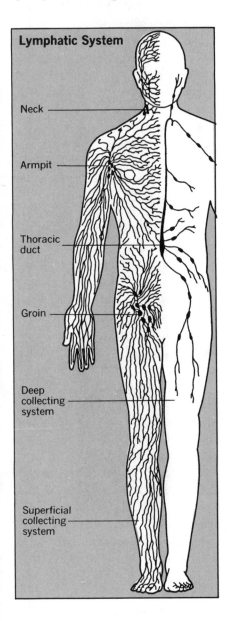

Lymphatic System

Neck

Armpit

Thoracic duct

Groin

Deep collecting system

Superficial collecting system

them; lymph is simply a watery vehicle moving through the lymphatic network. At certain points along this network, the vessels enlarge into clumpy structures called *lymph nodes* (or, misleadingly, lymph glands). Lymph nodes are major manufacturing sites for lymphocytes.

Lymph Nodes

Swollen glands are actually swollen lymph nodes, where a small army of lymphocytes is doing battle against invading bacteria or other harmful microscopic organisms. The lymph nodes, more than a hundred of them distributed around the body, serve as defense outposts against germs approaching the interior of the body. Those in the neck, groin, and armpits most frequently exhibit the pain and swelling that may accompany germ-fighting.

Circulation of Lymph

Lymph circulates without any help from the heart. From the spaces between cells, it diffuses into lymph capillaries which, like the venous capillaries, merge into larger and larger vessels moving inward toward the heart. The lymph moves—even upward from the legs and lower part of the body—because the muscles and movements of the body are constantly kneading and squeezing the lymph vessels. These vessels are equipped with valves that prevent back-flow. This is not so very different from the way venous blood makes its way back to the heart.

Eventually, master lymph vessels from the head, abdomen, and torso join in the thoracic lymph duct, which then empties into large neck veins that carry lymph and venous blood, mixed together, back to the heart.

The Heart at Work

The structure and performance of the heart, at first glance rather complicated, assume a magnificent simplicity once we observe that this pulsating knot of hollow, intertwining muscle uses only one beat to perform two distinct pumping jobs.

The heart has a right side (your right) and a left side (your left), divided by a tough wall of muscle called a *septum*. Each side has two chambers, an upper one called an *atrium* (or *auricle*), and a lower one called a *ventricle*.

How the Heart Pumps the Blood

Venous blood from the body flows into the right atrium via two large veins called the *superior vena cava* (bringing blood from the upper body) and the *inferior vena cava* (bringing blood from the lower part of the body). Where the blood enters the right atrium are valves that close when the atrium chamber is full.

Then, through a kind of trapdoor valve, blood is released from the right atrium into the right ventricle. When the right ventricle is full, and its outlet valve opens, the heart as a whole contracts—that is, pumps.

To the Lungs

The blood from the right ventricle is pumped to the lungs through the pulmonary artery to pick up oxygen. The trapdoor valve between the right atrium and ventricle has meanwhile closed, and venous blood again fills the right atrium.

Having picked up oxygen in the lungs, blood enters the left atrium through two pulmonary veins. (They are called veins despite the fact that they carry the most oxygen-rich blood, because they lead *to* the heart; just as the pulmonary artery carries the oxygen-poorest blood away from

How Blood Circulates through the Heart

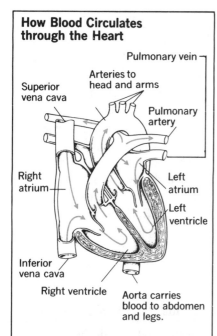

Pulmonary vein

Arteries to head and arms

Superior vena cava

Pulmonary artery

Right atrium

Left atrium

Left ventricle

Inferior vena cava

Right ventricle

Aorta carries blood to abdomen and legs.

Blood from the head and arms enters the right atrium from the superior (i.e., upper) vena cava. Blood from the torso and legs enters from the inferior (i.e., lower) vena cava. The blood, controlled by a valve, passes to the right ventricle. It is then pumped into the pulmonary artery, which divides into two vessels, one leading to each lung. After being enriched with oxygen, the blood is brought back to the left atrium via the pulmonary veins, is admitted by a valve into the left ventricle, and is pumped through the aorta to be distributed to all parts of the body.

Both atria contract at the same time, forcing blood into the ventricles. Then both ventricles contract (while the atria relax), forcing blood into the great arteries. This period of contraction is called systole, and is followed by a period of relaxation called diastole.

the heart, to the lungs.) Like the right atrium, the left atrium serves as a holding reservoir and, when full, releases its contents into the left ventricle. A valve between left atrium and ventricle closes, and the heart pumps.

To the Body

Blood surges through an opening valve of the left ventricle into the aorta, the major artery that marks the beginning of blood's circulation throughout the body. The left ventricle, because it has the job of pumping blood to the entire body rather than just to the lungs, is slightly larger and more muscular than the right ventri-

cle. It is for this reason, incidentally, that the heart is commonly considered to be on our left. The organ as a whole, as noted earlier, is located at the center of the chest.

The Heart's Own Circulatory System

Heart tissue, like that of every other organ in the body, must be continually supplied with fresh, oxygen-rich blood, and used blood must be returned to the lungs for reoxygenation. The blood inside the heart cannot serve these needs. Thus the heart has its own circulation network, called *coronary arteries* and *veins,* to nourish its muscular tissues. There are two major arteries on the surface of the heart, branching and rebranching eventually into capillaries. Coronary veins then take blood back to the right atrium.

Structure of the Heart

The musculature of the heart is called cardiac muscle because it is different in appearance from the two other major types of muscle. The heart muscle is sometimes considered as one anatomical unit, called the *myocardium.* A tough outer layer of membranous tissue, called the *pericardium,* surrounds the myocardium. Lining the internal chambers and valves of the heart, on the walls of the atria and ventricles, is a tissue called the *endocardium.*

These tissues, like any others, are subject to infections and other disorders. An infection of the endocardium by bacteria is called *bacterial endocarditis.* (Disease of the valves is also called *endocarditis,* although it is a misnomer.) An interruption of the blood supply to the heart muscle is called a *myocardial infarction,* which results in the weakening or death of the portion of the myocardium whose blood supply is blocked. Fortunately,

in many cases, other blood vessels may eventually take over the job of supplying the blood-starved area of heart muscle.

Heartbeat

The rate at which the heart beats is controlled by both the autonomic nervous system and by hormones of the endocrine system. The precise means by which the chambers and valves of the heart are made to work in perfect coordination are not fully understood. It is known, however, that the heart has one or more natural cardiac pacemakers that send electrical waves through the heart, causing the opening and closing of valves and muscular contraction, or pumping, of the ventricles near the normal adult rate of about 72 times per minute.

One particular electrical impulse (there may be others) originates in a small area in the upper part of the right atrium called the *sinus node.* Because it is definitely known that the contraction of the heart is electrically activated, tiny battery-powered devices called *artificial pacemakers* have been developed that can take the place of a natural pacemaker whose function has been impaired by heart injury or disease. Through electrodes implanted in heart tissue, such devices supply the correct beat for a defective heart. The bulk of the device is usually worn outside the body or is implanted just under the skin.

The fact that both ventricles give their push at the same time is very significant. It allows the entire heart muscle to rest between contractions—a rest period that adds up to a little more than half of a person's lifetime. Without this rest period, it is more than likely that our hearts would wear out considerably sooner than they do.

Blood Pressure

A physician's taking of blood pressure is based upon the difference between the heart's action at its period of momentary rest and at the moment of maximum work (the contraction or push). The split-second of maximum work, at the peak of the ventricles' contraction, is called the *systole*. The split-second of peak relaxation, when blood from the atria is draining into and filling up the ventricles, is called the *diastole*.

Blood pressure measures the force with which blood is passing through a major artery, such as one in the arm, and this pressure varies between a higher *systolic* pressure, corresponding to the heart's systole, and a lower *diastolic* pressure, reflecting the heart's diastole, or resting phase. The device with which a physician takes your blood pressure, called a *sphygmomanometer*, registers these

higher and lower figures in numbers equivalent to the number of millimeters the force of your arterial blood would raise a column of mercury. The higher systolic force (pressure) is given first, then the diastolic figure. For example, 125/80 is within the normal range of blood pressure. Readings that are above the normal range—and stay elevated over a period of time—indicate a person has high blood pressure, or hypertension.

Hypertension has no direct connection with nervous tension, although the two may be associated in the same person. What it does indicate is that a heart is working harder than the average heart to push blood through the system. In turn, this may indicate the presence of a circulatory problem that might eventually endanger health. See also Ch. 9, *Diseases of the Circulatory System* and Ch. 10, *Heart Disease.*

The Digestive System and the Liver

A physician once remarked that a great many people seem to spend about half their time getting food into their digestive tracts and the other half worrying about how that food is doing on its travels. The physician was exaggerating, but he made his point.

The digestive tract has essentially one purpose: to break down food, both solid and fluid, into a form that can be used by the body. The food is used as energy to fuel daily activities or to nourish the various tissues that are always in the process of wearing out and needing replacement.

A normally functioning digestive tract, dealing with a reasonable variety and quantity of food, is designed to extract the maximum benefit from what we eat. Urine and feces are the waste products—things from which our body has selected everything that is of use.

Our digestive system's efficiency and economy in getting food into our bodies, to be utilized in all our living processes, can be attributed basically to three facts.

First, although the straight-line distance from the mouth to the bottom of the trunk is only two or three feet, the distance along the intestinal tract is about 10 times as great—30 feet—a winding, twisting, looping passageway that has more than enough footage to accommodate a number of ingeniously constructed way stations, checkpoints, and traffic-control devices.

Second, from the moment food enters the mouth, it is subjected to both chemical and mechanical actions that begin to break it apart, leading eventually to its reduction to submicro-

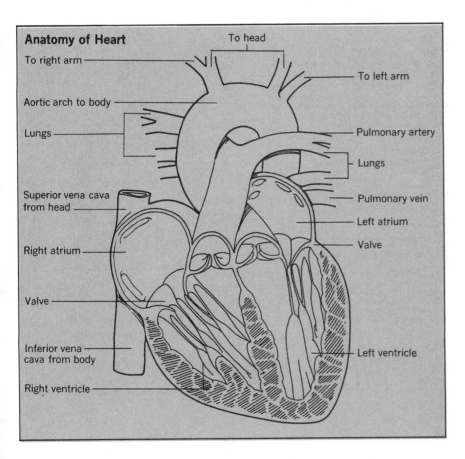

Anatomy of Heart

To right arm

To head

To left arm

Aortic arch to body

Lungs

Pulmonary artery

Lungs

Superior vena cava from head

Pulmonary vein

Left atrium

Valve

Right atrium

Valve

Inferior vena cava from body

Left ventricle

Right ventricle

scopic molecules that can be absorbed through the intestinal walls into the circulatory system.

Finally, each of the three main types of food—carbohydrates, fats, and proteins—receives special treatment that results in the body deriving maximum benefit from each.

Sensing the Right Kind of Food

Lips, eyes, and nose are generally given scant notice in discussions of the digestive process. But if we consider digestion to include selection of food and rejection of substances that might do us harm, then all three play very important roles.

The sensitive skin of our lips represents one of our first warning station that food may be harmful if taken into the mouth. It may tell us if a forkful of food is too hot or warn us of a concealed fishbone.

Our eyes, too, are important selection-rejection monitors for food. What else keeps us from sitting down to a crisp salad of poison ivy, or, less facetiously, popping a moldy piece of cake into our mouth?

As mammals' noses go, man's is a very inferior and insensitive organ. Nevertheless, we make good use of our sense of smell in the selection and enjoyment of foods. The nose adds to our enjoyment of favorite food and drink not only before they enter the mouth, but also after, because stimulation of the olfactory cells in the nasal passages combines with the stimulation of the taste cells on the tongue to produce the sensation-and-discrimination gradations of taste.

The Mouth: Saliva, Teeth, and Tongue

By the time food leaves the mouth and is pushed down into the gullet (or esophagus), it has already received a sampling of all the kinds of punishment and prodding that will be provided by the 30-foot tube that lies ahead of it. The chances are slim that any piece of food will end that journey in the same condition it started, but if it did it would have traveled those 30 tortuous feet at the rate of something less than two feet per hour. Normally, the elapsed time is between 17 and 25 hours.

As in the rest of the digestive tract, the mouth puts both chemical and mechanical apparatus to work on a bite of food. Saliva supplies the chemical action. Teeth and tongue, backed up by powerful sets of muscles, are the mashers, crushers, and prodders.

Saliva

The mere presence of food in our mouth—or even the smell, memory, or anticipation of it—sends signals to our brain, and our brain in turn sends messages back to a system of six salivary glands: one pair, called the *sublingual glands,* located under the tongue toward the front of the mouth; another pair, the *submaxillary* (or *submandibular*) glands, a bit behind and below them; and the largest, the *parotid glands,* tucked in the region where jaw meets neck behind the ear lobes.

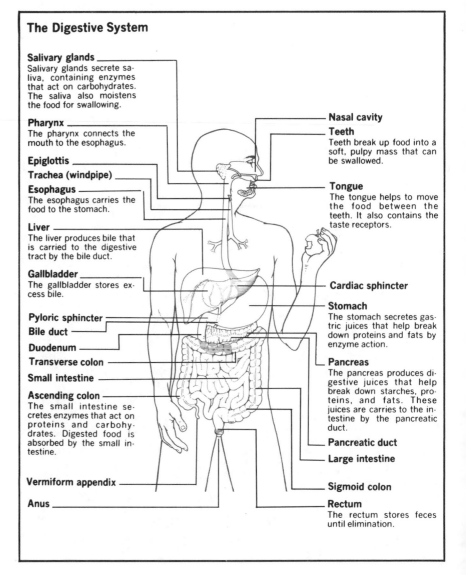

The Digestive System

Salivary glands
Salivary glands secrete saliva, containing enzymes that act on carbohydrates. The saliva also moistens the food for swallowing.

Pharynx
The pharynx connects the mouth to the esophagus.

Epiglottis

Trachea (windpipe)

Esophagus
The esophagus carries the food to the stomach.

Liver
The liver produces bile that is carried to the digestive tract by the bile duct.

Gallbladder
The gallbladder stores excess bile.

Pyloric sphincter

Bile duct

Duodenum

Transverse colon

Small intestine

Ascending colon
The small intestine secretes enzymes that act on proteins and carbohydrates. Digested food is absorbed by the small intestine.

Vermiform appendix

Anus

Nasal cavity

Teeth
Teeth break up food into a soft, pulpy mass that can be swallowed.

Tongue
The tongue helps to move the food between the teeth. It also contains the taste receptors.

Cardiac sphincter

Stomach
The stomach secretes gastric juices that help break down proteins and fats by enzyme action.

Pancreas
The pancreas produces digestive juices that help break down starches, proteins, and fats. These juices are carries to the intestine by the pancreatic duct.

Pancreatic duct

Large intestine

Sigmoid colon

Rectum
The rectum stores feces until elimination.

Salivary Glands

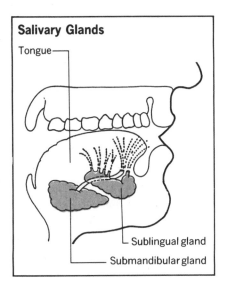

Saliva is mainly composed of water, and water alone begins to soften up food so that it can pass more smoothly down the esophagus toward encounters with more powerful chemical agents.

There is also a very special substance in saliva, an enzyme called *ptyalin,* whose specific job is to begin the breakdown of one of the toughest kinds of food our digestive system has to handle—starches. Starch is a kind of carbohydrate, the group of foods from which we principally derive energy; but in order for the body to utilize carbohydrate, it must be broken down into simpler forms, which are called simply sugars. Ptyalin, then, begins the simplification of carbohydrate starch into carbohydrate sugar.

Saliva also does a favor or two for the dominating structures of the mouth—the tongue and teeth. Without its bathing action, the tongue's taste cells could not function up to par; and because it has a mild germicidal effect in addition to a simple rinsing action, saliva helps protect our mouth and teeth from bacterial infection.

Teeth

The role of the teeth in digestion can be summed up in one word: destruc-

tion. What the wrecker's ball is to a standing building, our teeth are to a lump of solid food. They do the first, dramatic demolishing, leaving smaller fragments to be dealt with and disposed of in other ways.

Starting from the center of the mouth, we have two incisors on either side, top and bottom, followed by a canine, a couple of premolars, and three molars, the most backward of which (it never appears in some people) is the curiously named "wisdom" tooth, so called because it commonly appears as physical maturity is reached, at about 20 years of age.

Our teeth equip us for destroying chunks of food by a gamut of mechanical actions ranging from gripping and puncturing to grinding and pulverizing. The teeth in front—canines and incisors—do most of the gripping, ripping, and tearing, while the premolars and molars at the back of the jaws do the grinding.

The Tongue

The surface of the tongue is not smooth, but has a finely corrugated look and feel. This slightly sandpapery surface results from the presence of thousands of tiny papillae, little pyramid-shaped bumps. When we are young, the walls of a single papilla may contain up to 300 taste cells, or buds. As we get older, the maximum number of taste buds per papilla may decline to under 100.

There are four kinds of taste cells, distinguished by the type of taste message each sends to the brain: salty, sweet, sour, and bitter. Each of the four types is a narrow specialist in one type of taste. However, simultaneous or successive stimulation of all four types (combined almost always with information picked up by our sense of smell) can produce a tremendous variety of recognizable tastes—although perhaps not so many as some gourmets or wine-tasters might have us believe.

All four types of taste buds—salty, sweet, sour, and bitter—are found associated with papillae in all areas on the surface of the tongue; but there tend to be denser populations of one

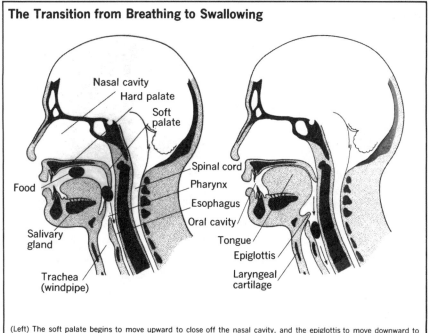

The Transition from Breathing to Swallowing

(Left) The soft palate begins to move upward to close off the nasal cavity, and the epiglottis to move downward to close off the trachea. (Right) By the time the food has passed into the esophagus, the trachea and the nasal cavity are completely shut off.

or the other kinds of taste cells in certain places. For example, salty and sweet cells predominate at the tip of the tongue and about halfway back along its sides; sour cells are more numerous all the way back along the sides; bitter buds are densest at the back of the tongue.

In addition to its tasting abilities, the tongue is a very versatile, flexible, and admirably shaped bundle of muscle. Not only can it flick out to moisten dry lips and ferret out and dislodge food particles in the oral cavity, but it also performs the first mechanical step in the all-important act of swallowing.

Swallowing

Swallow. You'll find that you feel the top of your tongue pressing up against the roof of your mouth (hard palate). You may never have thought about it consciously, but the pressing of the tongue against the hard palate prevents food from slipping to the front of your mouth—and also gives the food a good shove up and to the back of your mouth. At this point, the *soft palate* (from which the teardrop-shaped piece of tissue called the *uvula* hangs down) slips up to cover the passageway between mouth (oral cavity) and nasal cavity, nicely preventing the food from being misdirected toward your nose.

Once past the soft palate, the food is in the *pharynx,* a kind of anatomical traffic circle with two roads entering at the top, those from the mouth and nasal cavity, and two roads leading away from the bottom, the *trachea* (windpipe) and the *esophagus* or food tube.

The Epiglottis

A wedge of cartilage called the *epiglottis* protrudes from the trachea side, the side toward the front of the neck.

When we are breathing, the epiglottis is flattened up against the front wall of the pharynx, allowing free movement of air up and down the trachea. Simultaneously, the epiglottis helps to close off the entrance to the esophagus; a good part of the esophagus-closing work is done by a bundle of sinewy, elastic tissue we associate primarily with speech—the tissue of the vocal cords, otherwise known as the voice box or *larynx*. The laryngeal tissue is connected to the epiglottis above it, and supplies the epiglottis with most of its muscle for movement.

During the movement of a swallow, the larynx exerts an upward force against the epiglottis that serves to block off the trachea. At the same time, the larynx relaxes some of its pressure on the esophagus. Result: food enters the esophagus, where it is meant to go, and not the windpipe, which as we all know from having had something "go down the wrong way," produces an immediate fit of coughing.

Once we have swallowed, we lose almost completely the conscious ability to control the passage of food along the intestinal tract. Only when wastes reach the point of elimination do we begin to reassert some conscious control.

Peristalsis

The mechanical action called *peristalsis,* affected by muscles in the walls of all the organs of the gastrointestinal tract, first comes into play in the esophagus. Two layers of muscles intermesh in the intestinal walls: the inner layer encircles the esophagus in a series of rings; the outer layer stretches lengthwise along the tube. These two sets of muscles work in tandem to produce the basic action of persistalsis, called a *peristaltic wave.*

The alternative contraction and relaxation of the muscles—closing behind swallowed food and opening in front of it—combine to move both liquid and solid food (medical term, *bolus*) along the digestive tract. Gravity, in a sense, is left behind once food enters the esophagus. Because of peristalsis, we can swallow lying down or even standing on our heads; and astronauts are able to eat in near zero-gravity or under weightless conditions.

Peristalsis has another important function besides moving food through the body. The constricting and relaxing muscles serve also to knead, churn, and pummel the solid remains of the food left after our teeth have done their best.

Digestive Sphincters

If you think about it, the gastrointestinal tract has to be equipped with a number of gates that can open or shut, depending on the amount of food that is passing through. Otherwise, the food might push through so fast that little nourishment could be extracted from it: we would feel hungry one minute and glutted the next. The gastrointestinal tract is thus equipped at critical junctures with a number of muscular valves, or *sphincters,* which, usually under the direction of the autonomic nervous system, can regulate the movement of food through the digestive tube. Another function of a sphincter is to prevent backflow of partially digested food.

The muscles of a sphincter are often described as "pursestring muscles" because the way they draw together the sides of the digestive tube is roughly similar to drawing up the strings of a purse. The first of these pursestring valves occurs at the *cardia,* the opening where the esophagus meets the stomach, and is called the *cardiac sphincter,* from its location almost directly in front of the heart. (But there is no physical connection.)

Another important muscle ring is the *pyloric sphincter,* at the opening called the *pylorus,* located at the other end of the stomach, at the connection between stomach and small intestine. The release of waste from the rectum is controlled, partly voluntarily, by an *anal sphincter,* located at the *anus,* which marks the end of the tract.

The Stomach

About ten inches down the esophagus, the food we swallow must pass the cardiac sphincter. Then the food, by now fairly well diced and mashed, passes into the stomach.

Inelegant as it sounds, the stomach is best described as a rough, leather-skinned balloon. When empty, its skin shrivels around itself like a deflated balloon; but when "pumped up" by a hearty meal, the stomach becomes a plump, J-shaped bag about a foot long and six inches wide, holding about two quarts of food and drink.

The Passage of Food through the Stomach

Although its food-processing function tends to get more attention, the stomach's role as a storage reservoir is equally important. A moderate, well-rounded meal with a good blend of carbohydrates, proteins, and fats takes usually a minimum of three hours to pass out of the pyloric sphincter into the small intestine—more if the meal is heavy in fats and rich foods. Thus, a meal that might take us 15 minutes to eat, may take up to 20 times as long to pass from the stomach into the small intestine. This decelerating of food's rate of passage has two very significant re-

sults: first, it allows time for the food-processing activities within the stomach; and second, it releases food (in a mushy form called *chyme*) in small, well-spaced amounts that can be efficiently handled by the small intestine.

Although the stomach is not an absolutely essential organ—a person can live a full life with part or even all of it removed—it is a tremendous convenience. Without a stomach, frequent, carefully selected, well-chewed small feedings rather than "three square meals a day" are necessary so as not to overburden the small intestine, which can handle only a small quantity of food, well-mashed, at one time. If too much food goes directly to the small intestine, only so much nourishment (carbohydrates, proteins, fats) per meal can be supplied to the body, with the result that we would be weak from hunger after going a few hours without eating.

It will come as no surprise to know that the food processing done in the stomach is both mechanical and chemical. The three layers of crisscrossing muscles in the stomach walls are rarely still. They contract and relax continually, squeezing, pummeling, and mixing the stomach's contents into chyme. So active and relentless is the stomach's muscular activity that it actually "chews up" pieces of food that have been swallowed too hastily.

Stomach Chemicals

The various chemicals found in the stomach are produced and secreted into the stomach cavity by some 40 million gland cells that line the interior stomach walls. The constant wiggling and jouncing of the stomach helps to mix these chemicals thoroughly into the food. Each of the chemicals is secreted by a special type of cell and has a specific function. They include the digestive enzymes pepsin, rennin, and lipase; hydrochloric acid; and wa-

tery mucus.

A look at the special assignments of rennin, pepsin, hydrochloric acid, and mucus—and how they interact with and depend upon one another—provides a good glimpse into the elegant and complex chemical events that occur when the stomach encounters a swallow of food.

Rennin and Pepsin

Rennin, well known to cheesemakers, has essentially one task: to turn milk

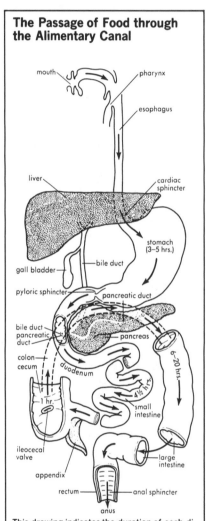

The Passage of Food through the Alimentary Canal

mouth — pharynx
esophagus
liver — cardiac sphincter
bile duct
stomach (3–5 hrs.)
gall bladder
pyloric sphincter — pancreatic duct
bile duct — pancreatic duct
pancreas
colon
cecum — duodenum
6–20 hrs.
4½ hrs.
1 hr.
small intestine
ileocecal valve
large intestine
appendix
rectum — anal sphincter
anus

This drawing indicates the duration of each digestive process. Food enters the mouth and is passed through the pharynx and esophagus into the stomach, where it is partly digested. The small intestine completes digestion and absorbs digested food. The large intestine absorbs excess water. Indigestible residue collects in the rectum for later disposal.

into milk curds. But the curds are not ready to pass on to the small intestine until they are further dismantled by *pepsin*. Pepsin has other duties as well: one of them is to begin the breakdown of proteins. But pepsin can only begin to split up protein foods after they have been worked on by *hydrochloric acid.*

Hydrochloric Acid

Hydrochloric acid is a corrosive substance and, except in very dilute strengths, could quite literally eat away the lining of the stomach. (This is apparently what happens in cases of gastric ulcers.) Mucus secretions, with the help of fluids in the food itself, dilute the hydrochloric acid to a point where (in a normal stomach) it is rendered harmless. Even so, the normal, healthy condition inside our stomach is slightly acid. The slight acidity of the stomach serves to inhibit the growth of organisms such as bacteria.

The Small Intestine

By the time food-turned-chyme gets through the pyloric sphincter, it has already traveled about two-and-a-half feet: about 6 inches from lips to epiglottis; 10 or 12 inches down the esophagus; and about a foot through the stomach. But at this point it has actually traveled less than one-tenth of the gastrointestinal (GI) tract, and the longest stretch lies just ahead: the 20-plus feet of the small intestine, so named because of its relatively small one-to-two inch diameter. The preparation of food particles to pass through the walls of the GI tract is completed in the small intestine—almost completed, in fact, before the chyme has traveled the first foot of the small intestine. By the time it leaves the small intestine, chyme has

given up virtually all its nutrients. In other words, the process called *absorption* or *assimilation* has taken place: the nutrients have left the GI tract for other parts of the body via the circulating blood and lymph. What passes on to the large intestine is principally waste and water.

The small intestine is somewhat arbitrarily divided into three sections: the *duodenum,* the *jejunum,* and the *ileum.*

The Duodenum

Within this horseshoe loop, eight to ten inches long and about two inches in diameter, more chemical interactions are concentrated than in any other section of the GI tract. One of the first jobs in the duodenum is to neutralize the acidity of the chyme. The final steps of digestion, and the absorption of food through the intestinal lining, proceed best in a slightly alkaline environment.

The alkaline juices needed to neutralize the acidity of the chyme come mainly from the liver in the form of bile. Bile produced by the liver but not needed immediately in the duodenum is stored in concentrated form in the gallbladder, a pouchlike, three-inch-long organ. On signal from the autonomic nervous system, the membranous muscular walls of the gallbladder contract, squeezing concentrated, highly alkaline bile into a short duct that leads to the duodenum. Bile components are indispensable for the digestion and absorption of stubborn fatty materials.

Through a duct from the pancreas, a host of pancreatic enzymes, capable of splitting apart large, tough molecules of carbohydrate, protein, and fat, enters the duodenum. These digestive enzymes manufactured by the pancreas are the most powerful in the GI tract.

What triggers the production of

bile and pancreatic juice for the duodenum? Apparently, it is a two-step process involving hormones. When the stomach walls secrete hydrochloric acid on the arrival of food, hormones are released; they travel to the liver and pancreas with instructions to step up their production of digestive juices.

Still other strong enzymes are secreted by the walls of the duodenum and join the bile and pancreatic enzymes in the duodenum.

Thus, in the not quite foot-long tube of the duodenum, the final breakdown of food—digestion—reaches a dramatic climax. The nutrients in the food eaten some hours ago have almost all been reduced to molecules small enough to be absorbed through the intestinal walls into the bloodstream. Carbohydrates are reduced to simpler sugars; proteins to amino acids; and fats to fatty acids and glycerol.

Some absorption of these nutrients occurs in the duodenum, but the far greater proportion takes place in the next two, longer sections of the small intestine: the eight- to ten-foot jejunum and the twelve-foot ileum. Likewise, some oversize food molecules that get past the duodenum may be digested further along in their passage through the small intestine.

The Jejunum

As peristalsis pushes the nutrient broth out of the duodenum and into the first reaches of the jejunum, a gradual change in the appearance of the intestinal lining is evident. Greater and greater number of *villi*—microscopic, hairlike structures—sprout from the already bumpy walls of the intestinal lining into the GI tube.

The Villi

The villi (singular, *villus*) have the primary responsibility for absorbing amino acids (from protein), sugars (from carbohydrates), and fatty acids and glycerol (from fats) from the digested contents of the small intestine, and starting them on their way to other parts of the body. What the villi do not remove from the chyme—such as the cellulose fragments of fruits and vegetables—passes on to the large intestine in a thin, watery soup almost completely lacking in nutritional value.

Gland cells near the bottom of a villus secrete various enzymes, mucus, and other substances that perform digestive "mop-up operations" along the whole length of the small intestine.

The Ileum

In this third and final 12-foot section of the small intestine, villi line the walls in such profusion that the intestinal lining resembles, under moderate magnification, nothing so much as a plush, velvety carpet. The greatest numbers of the estimated five or six million villi in the small intestine are found along the lining of the ileum, making it the primary absorption site of the GI tract.

Also adding to the ileum's absorption efficiency is its gradually narrowing diameter (just one inch at its junction with the large intestine), which helps to keep the chyme always in close contact with the swishing villi. The end of the ileum is marked by the *ileocecal valve,* beyond which lies the first bulge of the large intestine, the *cecum.*

Principally because of vigorous peristaltic contractions and relaxations, the walls of the small intestine are always moving like the walls within some spasmodically flexing, nightmarish tunnel. Attached to the intestinal walls, the villi, too, are always in restless motion: waving and thrashing, protracting and retracting, even growing thinner or fatter.

Although the entire distance through the small intestine, from the pyloric sphincter to the ileocecal valve at the junction with the large intestine, is only a bit over 20 feet, the villi give the small intestine's internal lining a relatively gigantic surface area—over 100 square feet. This is about five times the surface area of our body's skin. Of course, the greatly enlarged surface area gives the small intestine lining that much more space in which to absorb nutrients.

The small intestine is supported in the abdomen by a fan-shaped web of tissues called the *mesentery.* Attached at the back of the abdomen, the mesentery connects to the small intestine at various points, and yet allows it some freedom to squirm and sway— much like the V network of ropes that attaches either end of a hammock to a tree. Nerve fibers and blood vessels also reach the small intestine via the mesentery.

The Liver, Gallbladder, and Pancreas

These three organs all share a common function—sending digestive substances to the duodenum—although, except in the case of the gallbladder, it is not their only function. Lying outside the GI tract proper, they nevertheless are indispensable in the processes of digestion and absorption. Digestive fluids from all three converge like tributaries of a river at the common bile duct, and their flow from there into the duodenum is controlled by a sphincter muscle-ring separating the duodenum and common bile duct.

From the liver, bile drips into the *hepatic duct,* which soon meets the *cystic duct* arriving from the gallbladder. Converging, they form one duct, the *common bile duct,* which meets the *pancreatic duct,* carrying enzymatic fluid from the pancreas. Like a smaller river meeting a larger one, the pancreatic duct loses its own name at this confluence and becomes part of the common bile duct, which empties on demand into the duodenum. When the sphincter of the bile duct is closed, bile from the liver is forced to back up into the cystic duct, and eventually into the gallbladder. There it is stored and concentrated until needed, when it flows back down the cystic duct.

The Liver

Four pounds of highly efficient chemical-processing tissues, the liver is the largest solid organ in the body. You can locate it by placing your left hand over your right, lowermost ribs; your hand then just about covers the area of the liver. More than any other organ, the liver enables our bodies to benefit from the food we eat. Without it, digestion would be impossible, and the conversion of food into living cells and energy practically nonexistent. Insofar as they affect our body's handling of food—all the many processes that go by the collective name of nutrition—the liver's functions can be roughly divided into those that break down food molecules and those that build up or reconstitute these nutrients into a form that the body can use or store efficiently.

Breaking Down Food Molecules

Bile, as we have seen, assists in the destruction of large food molecules in the small intestine, enabling absorption of nutrients by the villi. Bile acts to increase alkalinity, breaking down big fat molecules; stimulates peristalsis; and prevents food from putrefying within the digestive tract. Unusable portions of the bile, destined to be eliminated as waste, include excess cholesterol, fats, and various components of dead disintegrated cells. Pigments from dead cells in bile give feces its normal, dark, yellow-brown color. Other cell fragments in bile, especially iron from disintegrated red blood cells, are reclaimed from the intestines and eventually make their way via the bloodstream to other parts of the body, where they are built into new cells.

Reconstituting Nutrients

Oddly enough, the liver rebuilds some of the proteins and carbohydrates that the bile has just so effectively helped to break down in the digestive tract. But this is really not so strange as it sounds. The types of proteins and carbohydrates that can be used by man for cell-rebuilding and energy are usually somewhat different in fine structure from those in food. Thus, the liver receives the basic building blocks of proteins and carbohydrates—amino acids and sugars— and with them builds up molecules and cells that can be utilized by the human body. The amino acids and sugars reach the liver through the *portal vein,* which is the great collection tube for nutrient-carrying blood returning from capillaries along the stomach and small intestine.

Glycogen and Glucose

In the liver, sugars from the small intestine are converted into a special substance called *glycogen;* amino acids are made available as needed for building new cells to replace the cells that are always naturally dying in a healthy normal body. Glycogen, simply speaking, is the liver's solution to a difficult space and storage problem. The form of carbohydrate the body can use best is a sugar called *glucose,*

but the liver isn't large enough to store the necessary amount of glucose. The answer is glycogen, a tidy, compact sugar molecule that the liver can store in great quantities. When a call comes from any part of the body for glucose, the liver quickly converts some glycogen to glucose and releases it into the bloodstream. By this mechanism, healthy blood sugar levels are maintained.

The liver also builds up human fats from fatty acids and glycerol, packs them off to storage, then reverses the process when necessary by breaking down body fats into forms that can serve as fuel to be burned by the body for energy.

Other Functions

In addition to its functions closely related to digestion and nutrition, the liver also serves as a storehouse and processor of vitamins and minerals— it is, in fact, the manufacturer of vitamin A. It can remove many toxic substances from the blood and render their poisons harmless. It picks up spent red blood cells from the circulation and dismantles them; and it continually manufactures new blood elements.

The liver is also a manufacturing site for *cholesterol,* a substance belonging to the class of body chemicals called steroids. Above-normal levels of cholesterol in the blood have been linked to hardening of the arteries and heart disease; but cholesterol in the proper amounts is needed by almost every tissue in the body. Some brain and spinal tissues, for example, have cholesterol as one of their main structural components.

With all these vital chemical activities and more, the liver might be expected to be a most delicate and fragile organ. In a sense it is: minor liver damage from one cause or another is thought to be fairly common. But

what saves our lives (and us) is that we have a great deal more of it than we need for a normal healthy life. Before symptoms of a liver deficiency appear, more than 50 percent of the liver cells may be destroyed. Furthermore, the liver has a great capacity for regeneration, rebuilding diseased tissues with new liver cells.

The Gallbladder

Bile stored in the gallbladder is much more concentrated and thicker than bile that is fresh from the liver. This allows the three-inch gallbladder to store a great deal of bile components. But the thickening process can also create problems in the form of extremely painful gallstones, which are dried, crystallized bile. Fortunately, the entire gallbladder can be removed with little or no lasting ill effect. All that is missing is a small storage sac for bile.

The Pancreas

This manufacturer of powerful digestive enzymes, only six inches long, resembles a branchlet heavily laden with ripe berries. Its important role in digestion is often overshadowed by the fact that it also manufactures the hormone *insulin.* The pancreas cells that manufacture digestive enzymes are completely different from those that manufacture insulin. The latter are grouped into little clusters called the *islets of Langerhans,* which are discussed under *The Endocrine Glands* in this chapter.

The Large Intestine

The large intestine, also called the large bowel, is shaped like a great, lumpy, drooping question mark— arching, from its beginning at the ileocecal valve, over the folds of the small intestine, then curving down and descending past more coiled small intestine to the anus, which marks the end of the GI tract. From ileocecal valve to anus, the large intestine is five to six feet in length.

The junction between the ileum and the *cecum,* the first section of the large intestine, occurs very low in the abdomen, normally on the right-hand side. The cecum is a bowl-like receptacle at the bottom of the colon, the longest section of the large intestine.

Just below the entrance of the ileum, a dead-end tube dangles down from the cecum. This is the *appendix vermiformis* (Latin, "worm-shaped appendage") commonly known as the appendix. Three to six inches long and one-third inch in diameter, the appendix may get jammed with stray pieces of solid food, become infected, swell, and rupture, spewing infection into the abdominal cavity. This is why early diagnosis of *appendicitis* and removal (*appendectomy*) are critically important.

Sections of the Colon

The colon is divided into three sections by pronounced *flexures,* or bends, where the colon makes almost right-angle changes of direction. Above the bowl of the cecum, the *ascending colon* rises almost vertically for about a foot and a half.

Then there is a flexure in the colon, after which the *transverse colon* travels horizontally for a couple of feet along a line at navel height. At another flexure, the colon turns vertically down again, giving the name of *descending colon* to this approximately two feet of large intestine. At the end of the descending colon, the large intestine executes an S-shaped curve, the *sigmoid flexure,* after which the remaining several inches of large intestine are known as the *rectum.*

Some people confuse the terms rectum and anus: the rectum refers specifically to the last section of the large intestinal tube, between sigmoid flexure and the anal sphincters, while the anus refers only to the opening controlled by the outlet valves of the large intestine. These valves consist of two ringlike voluntary muscles called anal sphincters.

Any solid materials that pass into the large intestine through the ileocecal valve (which prevents backflow into the small intestine) are usually indigestible, such as cellulose, or substances that have been broken down in the body and blood in the normal process of cell death and renewal, such as some bile components. But what the cecum mainly receives is water.

Functions of the Large Intestine

The principal activity of the large intestine—other than as a channel for elimination of body wastes—is as a temporary storage area for water, which is then reabsorbed into the circulation through the walls of the colon. Villi are absent in the large intestine, and peristalsis is much less vigorous than in the small intestine.

As water is absorbed, the contents of the large intestine turn from a watery soup into the semisolid feces. Meanwhile, bacteria—which colonize the normal colon in countless millions—have begun to work on and decompose the remaining solid materials. These bacteria do no harm as long as they remain inside the large intestine, and the eliminated feces is heavily populated with them. Nerve endings in the large intestine signal the brain that it is time for a bowel movement.

The Peritoneum

Lining the entire abdominal cavity, as well as the digestive and other abdominal organs, is a thin, tough, lubricated membrane called the *peritoneum.* In addition to protecting and supporting the abdominal organs, the peritoneum permits these organs to slip and slide against each other without any harm from friction. The peritoneum also contains blood and lymph vessels that serve the digestive organs. See Ch. 11, *Diseases of the Digestive System.*

The Respiratory System and the Lungs

The heart, by its construction and shape, tells us a great deal about the lungs and respiration.

Interaction between Heart and Lungs

The heart is divided vertically by a wall called a septum into right (your right) and left parts. The right part is smaller than the left: its muscles only have to pump blood a few inches to the lungs, while the muscles of the left half have to pump blood to the whole body.

The function of the right half of our heart is to receive oxygen-poor blood from the veins of the body. Venous blood empties into the top-right chamber, or right atrium, of the heart, and the right ventricle pumps that oxygen-poor blood (via the pulmonary artery) to the lungs, where the blood, passing through minute capillaries, picks up oxygen.

From the lungs, the oxygen-rich blood flows back into the heart's left atrium via the pulmonary veins; and from the left atrium, the oxygen-rich blood drains into the left ventricle,

Interaction between Heart and Lungs

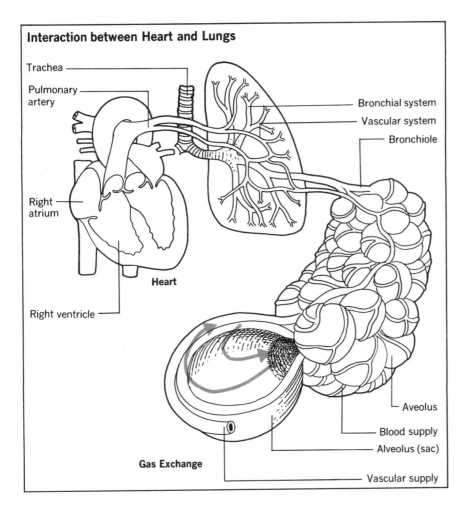

Trachea
Pulmonary artery
Right atrium
Heart
Right ventricle

Bronchial system
Vascular system
Bronchiole

Aveolus
Blood supply
Alveolus (sac)
Vascular supply

Gas Exchange

from whence it is pumped via the aorta to the body.

The blood pumped to the lungs by the right ventricle is oxygen-poor blood; it has given up its oxygen to the cells that need it around the body. But this "used blood" is rich in something else—carbon dioxide. As the body's cells have taken oxygen, they have given up carbon dioxide to the circulating blood. For both oxygen and carbon dioxide, the "carrier" has been *hemoglobin,* a complex iron-protein substance that is part of our red blood cells.

Capillaries and Alveoli

The pulmonary artery carrying this lung-bound blood soon branches into smaller and smaller vessels, and eventually into microscopic capillaries that reach into every crook and crev-

ice of the lungs.

In the lungs, the walls of the capillaries touch the walls of equally microscopic structures called *alveoli* (singular, *alveolus*). The alveoli are the smallest air sacs of the lungs. These tiny, expandable air cells are the destination of every breath of air we take. Estimates of the total number of alveoli in both our lungs vary between 300 million and a billion—in any case, we normally have several hundred million of them.

Carbon Dioxide and Oxygen Exchange

Where they meet, the membranous walls of both a capillary and an alveolus are both about as thin as any living tissue can be—a thickness that is only the width of one cell. Under such

conditions, the carbon dioxide carried by the hemoglobin in our blood to the lungs diffuses (as tiny gaseous "bubbles") across both the wall of a capillary and the wall of an alveolus.

Once inside the sac of the alveolus, carbon dioxide is ready to be exhaled from the body by "breathing out." One indication of just how well this system works is the fact that the air we exhale has roughly 100 times more carbon dioxide than the air we breathe in.

At the same time that hemoglobin dumps carbon dioxide at the interface of the capillary and alveolus walls, it picks up the oxygen made available from inhaled fresh air that has reached the alveoli. The molecular oxygen bubbles cross the membranes in the same way—but in the opposite direction—as the carbon dioxide.

Hemoglobin in the capillaries picks up the oxygen and carries it via veins leading away from the lungs, to the left atrium of the heart.

Essential Role of Moisture

The alveolar membranes are supplied with a thin film of moisture that is absolutely indispensable to the exchange of gases in the lungs. As in so many of our body's reactions, our evolutionary descent from water-dwelling ancestors is revealed by the wet environment demanded if our lungs are to supply our body with oxygen.

The Alveoli

Bronchiole
Pulmonary artery
Pulmonary vein
Cross section of alveolus
Capillaries on alveolus

The branches of the pulmonary tree terminate in the alveoli, grapelike clusters of air sacs covered by capillaries, where the gaseous exchange occurs.

Respiration at the One-Cell Level

Oxygen molecules, then, are carried to the body's cells by the hemoglobin of the arterial blood pumped by the heart's left ventricle. But how does a cell take oxygen from the blood and use it?

Exchange of Gases

The transfer of oxygen from blood to cell is accomplished in much the same way as the exhanges that take place in the lungs. The circulating arterial blood has a surplus of oxygen; the cells have a surplus of carbon dioxide. When the oxygen-rich blood reaches the finest capillaries, only the very thinnest membranous walls (of cell and capillary) separate it from the carbon-dioxide-rich cells. As in the lungs, both these gases (dissolved in water) diffuse through these thinnest of membranes: the oxygen into the cell, the carbon dioxide into the blood for eventual deposit in the alveoli, and exhalation.

Within the cell, the oxygen is needed so that food, the body's fuel, can be burned to produce energy. At the cellular level, the most convenient and common food is a fairly simple carbohydrate molecule called glucose.

Conversion of Carbohydrates into Energy

Energy is locked into a carbohydrate molecule such as glucose in the form of chemical bonds between its atoms. If one of these bonds is broken—say, a bond holding together a carbon and a hydrogen atom—a bit of pent-up energy is released as if, in a stalemated tug of war. the rope suddenly broke and both teams went hurtling off a few feet in opposite directions. This is precisely the effect of respiration within a cell: the cell "breaks the ropes" holding together a carbo-

hydrate molecule. The result is the release of energy—either as body heat or to power other activities within the cell.

It is useful—but a somewhat misleading oversimplification—to consider cellular respiration as a type of burning, or combustion. When a typical cell burns food, a carbohydrate molecule (glucose) together with molecules of oxygen are changed into carbon dioxide and water. During this change, chemical energy is released—energy that has been trapped, as we have seen, in the carbohydrate molecule. That complex, energy-rich molecule has been dismantled into the simpler molecules of carbon dioxide (CO_2) and water (H_2O). Oxygen is necessary here just as it is in fiery combustion. But the energy released here, instead of rushing out as heat and flame, is used to power the living activities of the cell.

This description of cellular respiration is all right in principle, but the trouble is this: if it all happened at once—if carbohydrate was so abruptly dismantled, split up at one stroke to water and carbon dioxide—such a great amount of energy would be released that the cell would simply burn itself up. As one biologist has said, the cell would be in exactly the same position as a wood furnace built of wood.

What protects the cell is its army of enzymes. These remarkable protein molecules combine briefly with energy-containing food molecules, causing them to break down bit by bit, so that energy is released gradually rather than all at once.

Carbon Dioxide— Precious Waste

In most of our minds, oxygen tends to be the hero of respiration and car-

bon dioxide the villain or at least the undesirable waste gas. This isn't really a fair picture. While it is true that too much carbon dioxide would act as a poison in our body, it is also true that we must always have a certain amount of the gas dissolved in our tissues. If we did not, two potentially fatal events could occur. First, our blood chemistry, especially its delicate acid-alkali balance, would get completely out of control. Second—and something of a paradox—the body's whole automatic system of regulating breathing would be knocked out.

It is the level of carbon dioxide in the bloodstream that controls our breathing. This level is continuously being monitored by the autonomic nervous system, specifically by the lower brain's "breathing center" in the medulla at the top of the spinal cord. When the level of carbon dioxide in our body goes above a certain level, signals from the medulla force us to breathe. Almost everybody has played, "How long can you hold your breath?" and knows that, past a certain point, it becomes impossible *not* to breathe. When you are holding your breath, the unexhaled carbon dioxide rapidly builds up in your system until the breathing center is besieged with signals that say "Breathe!" And you do.

Our Big Breathing Muscle: The Diaphragm

What gets air into and out of our lungs? The answer may seem as obvious as breathing in and out. But except for those rare instances when we consciously regulate our breathing pattern—which physicians call "force breathing"—we do not decide when to inhale and when to exhale. And even when we do force-breathe, it is not primarily the action of opening the

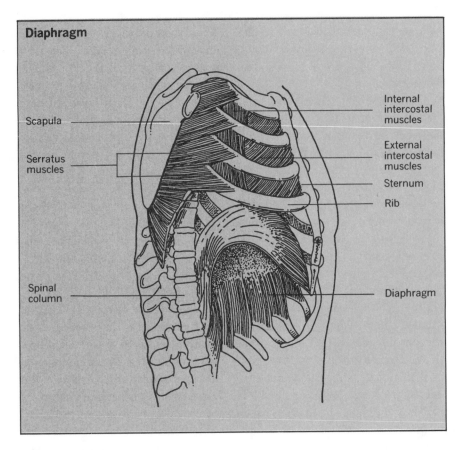

Diaphragm

- Scapula
- Serratus muscles
- Spinal column
- Internal intercostal muscles
- External intercostal muscles
- Sternum
- Rib
- Diaphragm

mouth and gulping in air, then blowing it out, that gets air down the windpipe and into the alveoli of the lungs. The main work of inhaling and exhaling is done by the contraction and relaxation of the big helmet-shaped muscle on which the lungs rest and which marks the "floor" of the chest or thoracic cavity and the "ceiling" of the abdominal cavity. This muscle is the *diaphragm.*

It is the diaphragm that causes the lungs to swell and fill with fresh air, then partially collapse to expel used gases. The muscles and tendons of the sinewy diaphragm are attached at the back to the spinal column, at the front to the breastbone (*sternum*), and at the lower sides to the lower ribs.

The diaphragm contracts and relaxes on orders from the brain's breathing center, orders that are carried along the pathways of the autonomic nervous system. When the medulla sends messages to the breathing muscles to contract, the diaphragm is pulled downward, enlarging the space filled by the lungs. This creates a temporary partial vacuum, into which air rushes, inflating and expanding the lungs. When the diaphragm relaxes, the lung space is reduced, pushing air out.

Other Breathing Muscles

The diaphragm muscle's leading role in breathing is supported by several other muscles that play minor parts. Among these are the *intercostal muscles* between the ribs that give the rib cage a slight push upward and outward, enlarging the thoracic cavity, and the *serratus muscles,* which are mainly muscular sheaths along the ribs, to which other muscles are attached.

The Trachea and the Lungs

The right lung (your right) is somewhat bigger than the left. The lungs hang in the chest attached to the windpipe or *trachea.*

The Trachea

The trachea itself branches off at the back of the throat, or *pharynx,* where the epiglottis prevents food from entering the trachea and channels swallowed food along its proper route, the esophagus. The top part of the trachea forms the voice box or *larynx,* made up of vocal cords—actually two flaps of cartilage, muscle, and membranous tissue that protrude into the windpipe—whose vibrations in response to air exhaled from the lungs give us our voice.

Below the larynx, the trachea descends five or six inches to a spot just about directly behind your breastbone, where the first of many thousands of branchings into *bronchi, bronchioles,* and alveoli occurs. C-shaped rings of cartilage give the trachea both support and flexibility. Running your finger down the front of your neck, you can feel the bumps made by the cartilage rings.

Above the base of the trachea in midchest the lungs arch on either side like giant butterfly wings, then fall to fill out the bottom of each side of the thoracic cavity.

The Pleural Membranes

Both lungs are encased in moist, clinging, tissue-thin membrane called the *pleura,* which also lines the inside of the thoracic cavity where it comes into contact with the pleural coating of the lungs. The slippery pleural membranes hold tightly to each other, because there is an air lock or vacuum between them, but at the same time are free to slide over each other. The principle is the same as that illustrated by moistening the surfaces of two pieces of plate glass and placing the moistened surfaces together: the two pieces of glass will slide over each other but will resist being pried apart, because a partial vacuum exists between them.

The Pleural Cavity

The vacuum space between the pleura of the lung and the pleura of the thoracic cavity—although it is normally not a space at all—is called the *pleural cavity.* Each lung has its own pleural membrane: that of one lung does not interconnect with the other, so that one pleura may be injured without affecting the other.

It is extremely fortunate for us that the pleural linings both stick fast and can slide along each other's surfaces. Although the lungs are virtually without muscle, they are extremely elastic and in their natural condition are stretched fairly taut, held to the sides of the thoracic cavity by the suction of the pleura.

Collapsed Lung

Should this suction be broken and the pleural linings pull apart, the lung would shrink up like a deflated balloon. Such a condition, caused by the rush of outside air into the pleural cavity, is known medically as *pneumothorax* and causes a lung collapse. Violent injuries such as gun and stab wounds, various lung diseases, and obstructions of the breathing tubes can cause a lung or portion of a lung to collapse.

In the surgical procedure called *artificial pneumothorax,* a physician deliberately injects air between the pleural linings to collapse a portion of a lung. This is done to rest a lung in severe diseases such as tuberculosis, or to control heavy bleeding within the thoracic cavity.

Pleurisy

The intense chest pains called *pleurisy* are caused by inflammation of the pleura. The pleural linings lose their slipperiness and the increased friction stimulates pain receptors in the pleural lining of the chest. There are, however, no pain receptors in the lungs' pleural linings nor in the lungs themselves: this is why pain is not an early warning signal of lung cancer.

The Bronchi

Just behind the breastbone and just in front of the heart, the trachea divides into the right bronchus and the left bronchus, leading respectively to the right and left lungs. These are the primary two *bronchi* or *bronchial tubes.* Each is the main trunk of a bronchial tree that serves its respective lung.

Soon after leaving the trachea, each bronchus branches repeatedly into smaller tubes called *bronchioles,* which in turn branch into alveolar ducts, which terminate finally with the hundreds of millions of microscopic air sacs called alveoli, discussed at the beginning of this section. The alveoli are the site of the all-important exchange of carbon dioxide and oxygen.

Lobes and Segments

The larger right lung has three distinctive sections, or *lobes*—upper, middle, and lower. The left lung has only an upper and lower lobe. The lobes themselves are divided into smaller segments. Medically, these lobes and segments are important because they are somewhat independent of each other and can be damaged or removed surgically, as in operations for lung cancer, usually without damaging the function of adjacent, healthy segments or lobes.

The fact that a lung segment, lobe, or even an entire lung can be removed implies that we have plenty of reserve lung tissue, and this is indeed the case. When we are at rest, we use only about one-tenth of our total lung capacity. The total surface area exposed within our lungs to outside air is, amazingly, 600 square feet. This compares to a mere 20 square feet of skin surface. To appreciate the incredibly intricate, lacelike finery of the lungs' structure, we need only know that those 600 square feet of surface area are contained within two organs that together weigh only two-and-a-half pounds.

Oxygen Requirements

How much air do we breathe, and how much oxygen do we absorb into our body from the air? A normal, moderately active person breathes in and out (a complete respiration or breath cycle) about 18 times a minute; that is, the diaphragm contracts and relaxes 18 times a minute, or something over 25,000 times every day. At about four-fifths of a pint of air per breath cycle, this means that we inhale and exhale about 20,000 pints, or 10,000 quarts, or 2,500 gallons of air every day.

Only a very small proportion of this volume is oxygen that finds its way into our bloodstream: about a pint every minute in normal, quiet breathing, a little over 1,400 pints, or 700 quarts, or 175 gallons of oxygen every day. The amount of oxygen our lungs are capable of delivering to our body, however, varies tremendously: during sleep a person may need only a half-pint of oxygen per minute, half the average, while the lungs of a hard-driving athlete striving to break the mile record can deliver up to five quarts to the bloodstream—ten times the average.

At any given time, there are about two quarts of oxygen circulating in our blood. This is why a stoppage of breathing has an upper time limit of about four minutes before it causes irreversible damage or death. With our body needing about a pint of oxygen every minute for normal functioning, we have about four minutes before we use up the oxygen dissolved in our blood and other tissues.

Pollution Control— Filters, Cleaners, and Traps

Air pollution being what it is these days, it is fortunate that we have several natural devices that serve to filter out and wash away most of the impurities in the air we inhale.

Air gets into the lungs from outside about equally well via the nose or mouth. The mouth offers the advantage of getting more air in at a faster rate—absolutely a must if we have to push our body physically. But the nose has more and better equipment for cleaning air before it reaches the trachea. Via the mouth, air must only pass over a few mucous membranes and the tonsils, which can collect only so many germs and impurities.

Nose Filter System

Air taken in through the nose, however, first meets the "guard hairs" (*vibrissae*) of the nostrils, and then must circulate through the nasal cavity, a kind of cavern framed by elaborate scroll-shaped bones called *turbinates,* and lined with mucus-secreting membranes and waving, hair-like fibers called *cilia.* Foreign particles are caught by the cilia and carried away by the mucus, which drains slowly down the back of the throat.

It would be nice to be able to ascribe an important function to the eight *paranasal sinuses,* four on either side of the nose: the headache and discomfort of sinusitis might then be more bearable. But these "holes in the head" seem to exist simply to cause us trouble; for example—swell-

ing to close the nasal air passages, making it impossible to breathe, as recommended, through the nose.

Filter System beyond the Nose

The cleansing and filtering action started in the nose and mouth does not stop there, but is repeated wherever air travels along the air passages of the lungs. Cilia project inward from the walls of even the tiniest bronchioles of the lungs, and impurities are carried from the alveoli on films of mucus that move ever back toward the trachea for expulsion—as when we cough. See also Ch. 12, *Diseases of the Respiratory System* and Ch. 13, *Lung Disease.*

The Endocrine Glands

Technically speaking, a gland is any cell or organ in our bodies that secretes some substance. In this broad sense, our liver is a gland, because one of its many functions is to secrete bile. So too, is the placenta that encloses a developing baby and supplies it with chemicals that assure normal growth. Even the brain has been shown by modern research to secrete special substances. But lymph glands are not considered true glands and are more correctly called lymph nodes.

Physicians divide the glands into two categories. *Endocrine glands* are also known as *ductless glands,* because they release their secretions directly into the bloodstream. *Exocrine glands,* by contrast, usually release their substances through a duct or tube. Exocrine glands include the sebaceous and sweat glands of the skin; the mammary or milk glands; the mu-

cous glands, some of which moisten the digestive and respiratory tract; and the salivary glands, whose secretions soften food after it enters the mouth. The pancreas has both an endocrine and an exocrine function and structure.

Role of the Endocrine Glands

The *endocrine glands* have the all-important role of regulating our body's internal chemistry. The substances they secrete are complex compounds called *hormones,* or chemical messengers.

Together with the brain and nerves, the system of endocrine glands controls the body's activities. The nervous system, however, is tuned for rapid responses, enabling the body to make speedy adjustments to changing circumstances, internal and external. The endocrine glands, with some exceptions, like the adrenal, are more concerned with the body's reactions over a longer period of time—from season to season, as it were. They regulate such processes as growth, levels of metabolism, fertility, and pregnancy.

For a group of tissues that exercise awesome power over our body's well-being, the endocrine glands are surprisingly small and inconspicuous—all of them together would weigh less than half a pound. Nor are they placed with any particular prominence in our body. They tend to be little lumps of tissue attached to or tucked behind grander bodily structures. Their power comes from the hormones they release into the bloodstream.

Scientists have discovered the exact chemical makeup of a number of these complex substances, have extracted several in pure form from living tissue, and have succeeded in making a few synthetically in the lab-

Endocrine Glands

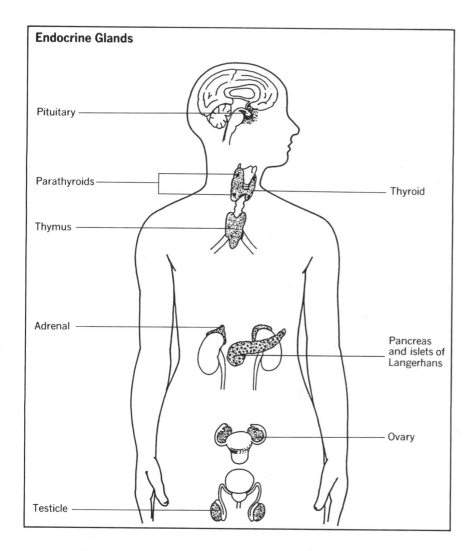

Pituitary

Parathyroids

Thymus

Adrenal

Testicle

Thyroid

Pancreas
and islets of
Langerhans

Ovary

The Posterior Lobe and the Hypothalamus

The posterior lobe, so far as is known, does not make any of its own hormones, but serves as a storehouse for two hormones manufactured by the *hypothalamus,* located in the brain's cerebellum. The hypothalamus, apart from having a role in controlling the body's autonomic nervous system, also functions as an endocrine gland, secreting its own hormones, and as a connecting link between the brain's cerebral cortex and the pituitary gland.

The posterior lobe of the pituitary releases the two hormones it receives from the hypothalamus, called *vasopressin* and *oxytocin,* into the bloodstream. Vasopressin plays a role in the fluid balance of the body; oxytocin is thought to pace the onset and progress of labor during childbirth.

The Anterior Lobe

The anterior lobe secretes no less than six known hormones, five of which act as stimulators of hormone production by other endocrine glands. The sixth, identified as *somatotrophin*

oratory. This avenue of research, called *endocrinology,* has enabled physicians to treat persons suffering from certain endocrine gland disorders.

Hormones have been aptly described as chemical messengers. Their action, while still not completely understood, is that of catalysts. This means that the presence of a hormone (the name comes from a Greek word meaning "arouse to activity"), even in very small quantities, can affect the rate at which a chemical change occurs or otherwise stimulate a reaction, and without itself being affected. The hormone is a promoter, either of a positive or negative sort; it speeds up a process or slows it down.

The endocrine glands form an interdependent family. The functioning

or malfunctioning of one can affect all the others.

The Pituitary—Master Gland

The *pituitary* is often called the master gland because the hormones it secretes play an active part in controlling the activities of all the other endocrine glands. This impressive power is wielded from two little bumps at the base of the brain, about midway between the ears at eye level. The two parts, or lobes, are connected by a tiny bridge of tissue, the three structures together being about the size of a small acorn. The lobe lying toward the front of the head is the *anterior lobe;* the one at the back, the *posterior lobe.* Each lobe is really an independent gland in itself, with its own quite distinct activities.

The Pituitary Gland

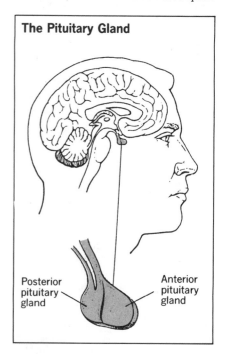

Posterior
pituitary
gland

Anterior
pituitary
gland

in medical textbooks, is more popularly known as the *growth-stimulating hormone* or simply as the growth hormone. It controls the rate of growth and multiplication of all the cells and tissues in our bodies—muscle, bone, and all our specialized organs.

Gigantism

In rare instances, during childhood, the pituitary releases too much or too little somatotrophin. If too much is secreted, the result is an overstimulation of growth processes, causing a disorder known as *gigantism.* Victims of this disorder have been known to grow nine feet tall and weigh 500 pounds.

Dwarfism

If too little somatotrophin is secreted, *dwarfism* results. This pituitary-type dwarf, of which Tom Thumb was one, is different from a dwarf suffering from a disorder of the thyroid (another endocrine gland, discussed below). The pituitary dwarf is usually well proportioned despite a miniature size, while the thyroid dwarf typically has short, deformed limbs.

Neither pituitary gigantism nor dwarfism affects basic intelligence. If oversecretion of somatotrophin occurs after full size has been reached—as, for example, because of a tumor affecting the pituitary, the condition known as *acromegaly* occurs. The bones enlarge abnormally, especially those of the hands, feet, and face.

Anterior Pituitary Hormones

Of the five anterior pituitary hormones that regulate other endocrine glands, one affects the adrenal glands, one the thyroid, and the remaining three the sex glands or gonads (the

Pituitary Gland

Vasopressin

Oxytocin

Posterior lobe

ACTH
TSH
FSH
LTH
FSH
LH

Anterior lobe

testicles in men and the ovaries in women). Each is identified by a set of initials derived from its full name, as follows:

- *ACTH,* the *a*drenocorticotrophic *h*ormone, affects the production of hormones by the outer "bark" of the adrenal glands, called the *adrenal cortex.*

- *TSH,* the *t*hyroid-*s*timulating *h*ormone, also known as *thyrotrophin,* causes the thyroid gland to step up production of its hormone, *thyroxin.*

- *FSH,* the *f*ollicle-*s*timulating *h*ormone, spurs production in women of estrogen, a sex hormone produced by the ovaries; and in men, of sperm by the testicles. Follicle here refers to the *Graafian follicles* in the ovary, which contain developing female egg cells whose

growth is also stimulated by FSH. Graafian follicles have approximate counterparts in the male—tiny pouches (seminal vesicles) on either side of the prostate gland that store mature sperm cells.

- *LH,* the *l*uteinizing *h*ormone, transforms a Graafian follicle, after the follicle has released a ripened egg cell, into a kind of tissue called *corpus luteum.* The corpus luteum, in turn, produces *progesterone,* a hormone that prepares the mucous membrane lining the uterus (the endometrium) to receive a fertilized egg.

- *LTH,* the *l*actogenic *h*ormone, or *luteotrophin,* stimulates the mother's mammary glands to produce milk; LTH also joins with LH in promoting the production of progesterone by the sex glands.

The last three hormones mentioned—follicle-stimulating, luteinizing, and lactogenic—are sometimes called the *gonadotrophic* hormones because they all stimulate activity of the gonads.

The Adrenal Glands

Resting like skull caps on the top of both kidneys are the two identical *adrenal glands.* Each has two distinct parts, secreting different hormones.

Adrenaline

The central internal portion of an adrenal gland is called the *medulla.* Its most potent contribution to our body is the hormone *adrenaline* (also called *epinephrine*). This is the hormone that, almost instantaneously, pours into our bloodstream when we face a situation that calls for extraordinary physical reaction—or keeps us going past what we think to be our normal

Adrenal Glands

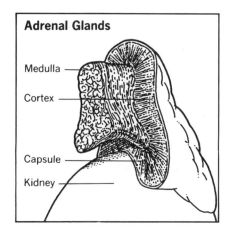

Medulla

Cortex

Capsule

Kidney

limit of endurance.

A surge of adrenaline into the bloodstream stimulates our body to a whole array of alarm reactions—accelerating the conversion of stored foods into quick energy; raising the blood pressure; speeding up breathing; dilating the pupils of the eyes for more sensitive vision; and constricting the blood vessels, making them less vulnerable to bleeding.

Adrenaline provides a good example of the interdependence of the endocrine system. Its production stimulates the secretion of ACTH by the pituitary gland. And ACTH, as noted above, causes the adrenal cortex to accelerate production of its hormones. Some of these adrenal cortex hormones enable the body to call up the reserves of energy it does not normally need. For example, body proteins are not usually a source of quick energy, but in an emergency situation, the adrenal cortex hormones can convert them to energy-rich sugar compounds.

The Corticoids

There are some 30 different hormones, called the *corticoids*, manufactured in the adrenal cortex—the outer layer of the adrenal. A few of these influence male and female sexual characteristics, supplementing the hormones produced in the gonads. The others fall into two general cat-

egories: those that affect the body's metabolism (rate of energy use), and those that regulate the composition of blood and internal fluids. Without the latter hormones, for example, the kidneys could not maintain the water–salt balance that provides the most suitable environment for our cells and tissues at any given time.

Corticoids also influence the formation of antibodies against viruses, bacteria, and other disease-causing agents.

Extracts or laboratory preparations of corticoids, such as the well-known cortisone compounds, were found in the 1950s to be almost "miracle" medicines. They work dramatically to reduce pain, especially around joints, and hasten the healing of skin inflammations. Prolonged use, however, can cause serious side effects.

The Islets of Langerhans

Strewn at random throughout the pancreas are hundreds of thousands of tiny clusters of cells. Each of them, when seen under a powerful microscope, forms an "islet" of its own, similar to the other distinct islets, but markedly different from the pan-

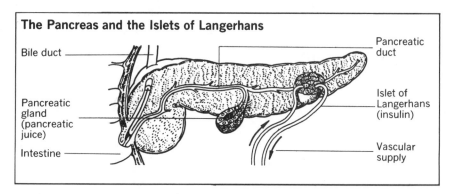

The Pancreas and the Islets of Langerhans

Bile duct

Pancreatic gland (pancreatic juice)

Intestine

Pancreatic duct

Islet of Langerhans (insulin)

Vascular supply

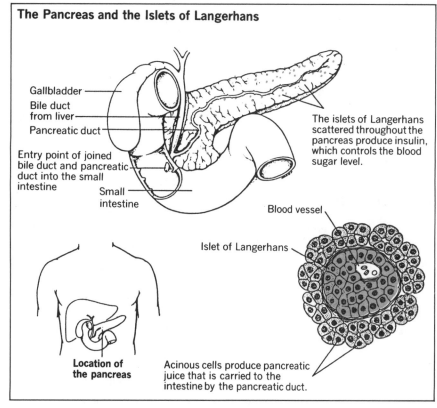

The Pancreas and the Islets of Langerhans

Gallbladder

Bile duct from liver

Pancreatic duct

Entry point of joined bile duct and pancreatic duct into the small intestine

Small intestine

The islets of Langerhans scattered throughout the pancreas produce insulin, which controls the blood sugar level.

Blood vessel

Islet of Langerhans

Acinous cells produce pancreatic juice that is carried to the intestine by the pancreatic duct.

Location of the pancreas

creatic tissue surrounding it. These are the *islets of Langerhans,* named after the German scientist who first reported their existence in 1869. Each of these little cell clumps—up to two million or more of them—is a microscopic endocrine gland.

They secrete the hormone *insulin,* and the disease that occurs if they are not functioning properly is *diabetes mellitus.*

Actually, the islets of Langerhans produce not only insulin, but also a related hormone called *glucagon.* Both regulate the amount of sugar (glucose) that is present in the bloodstream and the rate at which it is used by the body's cells and tissues. Glucose supplies the energy for life and living processes.

When insulin and glucagon are not in sufficient supply, the cells' ability to absorb and use blood sugar is restricted, and much of the sugar passes unutilized out of the body in urine. Because the body's ability to obtain energy from food is one of the very foundations of life, diabetes calls for the most careful treatment.

One of the great advances of twentieth century medicine has been the pharmaceutical manufacture of insulin and its wide availability to diabetics. With regulated doses of insulin, a diabetic can now lead a normal life. See Ch. 15, *Diabetes Mellitus* for a full discussion of this disease.

The Thyroid Gland

The *thyroid gland* folds around the front and either side of the trachea (windpipe), at the base of the neck, just below the larynx. It resembles a somewhat large, stocky butterfly facing downward toward the chest.

Thyroxin

The thyroid hormone, *thyroxin,* is a complex protein-type chemical con-

Thyroid Gland

Thyroid cartilage

Parathyroid

Thyroid

Trachea

taining, along with various other elements, a large percentage of iodine. Like a number of other hormones manufactured by the endocrine glands, thyroxin affects various steps in the body's metabolism—in particular, the rate at which our cells and tissues use inhaled oxygen to burn the food we eat.

Hypothyroidism

A thyroid that is not producing enough thyroxin tends to make a person feel drowsy and sluggish, put on weight (even though his appetite is poor), and in general make his everyday activities tiresome and wearying. This condition is called *hypothyroidism.*

Hyperthyroidism

Its opposite—caused by too much secretion of thyroxin—is *hyyperthyroidism.* A hyperthyroid person is jumpy, restless, and may eat hugely without gaining weight. The difference between the two extremes can be compared to environments regulated by two different thermostats, one set too high and the other set too low.

Although a normally functioning thyroid plays a significant part in making a person feel well, physicians to-

day are less willing than in former years to blame a defective thyroid alone for listlessness or jittery nerves. Thirty or forty years ago it was quite fashionable to prescribe thyroid pills (containing thyroid extract) almost as readily as vitamins or aspirin; but subsequent medical research, revealing the interdependence of many glands and other body systems, made thyroxin's reign as a cure-all a short one.

Of course, where physical discomfort or lethargy can be traced to an underfunctioning thyroid, thyroxin remains an invaluable medicine.

Goiter

One disorder of the thyroid gland—the sometimes massive swelling called *goiter*—is the direct result of a lack of iodine in the diet. The normal thyroid gland, in effect, collects iodine from the bloodstream, which is then synthesized into the chemical makeup of thyroxin. Lacking iodine, the thyroid gland enlarges, creating a goiter. The abnormal growth will stop if iodine is reintroduced into the person's diet. This is the reason why most commercial table salt is iodized—that is, a harmless bit of iodine compound has been added to it.

The Parathyroid Glands

Four small glands, each about the size of a small pea, cling to the base of the thyroid gland, two on each of the thyroid's lobes curving back of the trachea. These are the *parathyroids,* whose main role is to control the level of calcium—as well as other elements needed in carefully regulated amounts by the body—in the bloodstream and tissues. The parathyroids secrete two hormones: *parathormone* when blood calcium is too low; *calcitonin* when the calcium level is too high. These hormones work by controlling the interchange of calcium between bones and blood.

The most common symptom of defective parathyroids is *tetany*—a chronic or acute case of muscle spasms, which can be controlled by administration of synthetic parathyroidlike chemicals or concentrated vitamin D preparations.

The Gonads

The *gonads* refer to both the two male testicles and the two female ovaries.

There are four hormones secreted by the gonads: the female sex hormones, *estrogen* and *progesterone;* and the male hormones, *testosterone* and *androsterone*. Each sex merely has a predominance of one or the other pair of hormones. Men have some of the female hormones, and women some of the male hormones.

In both sexes, puberty is signaled by the release of the gonadotrophic hormones (or *gonadotrophins*) of the pituitary gland. These stimulate the production of sex hormones by the sex glands and the subsequent appearance of secondary sexual characteristics. In men, these include the enlargement of testicles and penis, growth of facial, axillary (armpit) and pubic hair, and enlargement of the larynx, resulting in deepening of the voice. Pubescent women also experi-

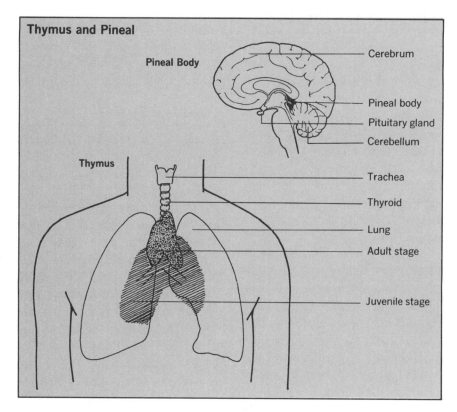

Thymus and Pineal

Pineal Body

Cerebrum
Pineal body
Pituitary gland
Cerebellum

Thymus

Trachea
Thyroid
Lung
Adult stage

Juvenile stage

ence pubic and axillary hair growth, in addition to breast growth and changes in the genital tract that give it child-bearing capability.

Estrogen and progesterone control the cyclic changes within the uterus that involve the development, ripening, and discharge of the egg (ovulation) to be fertilized; the preparation of the lining of the uterus to receive a fertilized egg; and this lining's subsequent dismantling—all the complex biochemical events that occur as part of every woman's menstrual cycle.

The Thymus and Pineal Glands

These are the least known of the endocrine family; in fact, physicians do not know the function of one of them—the *pineal*—and are not even agreed that it is an endocrine gland. Situated near the hypothalamus, at the base of the brain, this tiny, pinecone-shaped body has follicles that suggest a glandular function and some calcium-containing bits that medical researchers have descriptively dubbed "brain sand."

The *thymus*, only slightly better understood, has the intriguing characteristic of shrinking in size as a person grows up. It is located in the middle of the chest, about midway between the base of the neck and the breast line. There is some evidence that the secretions of the thymus play a role in the body's natural immunity defenses. See also Ch. 14, *Diseases of the Endocrine Glands*.

The Gonads

Sperm

Egg
Corpus luteum
Primary follicle
Mature follicle
Stroma

Ovary

Ductus deferens
Epididymis

Seminiferous tubules

Testis

The Sense Organs

Once upon a time, a grade-school teacher would ask, "How many senses do we have?" And his pupils would confidently chorus back, "Five!" People who displayed a knack for predicting future events, or whose quick reactions seemed to give them a jump over most everybody else, were credited with having a "sixth sense."

Scientists now recognize about twice that number—12 or 13 or more. Man, of course, has not grown a number of new senses in addition to the traditional five: sight, hearing, touch, smell, and taste. What has happened is that scientists have discovered many more specific kinds of sense receptor cells. For example, whereas touch was formerly thought of as just one sense, it has now been divided into no less than five different senses, each having its own special kind of receptor cell in the skin.

We can talk with a little more justification of the five sense organs, the five anatomical structures we associate with our senses—the eyes, ears, nose, tongue, and skin. But here, too, it does seem to be oversimplifying things to thus equate the nose—having only a tiny patch of olfactory (sense of smell) receptor cells—with the marvelously complex arrangement of sensing structures that make up the eye. Moreover, the other sense organs are not nearly so specialized as the eye. For example, a good case could be made for the nose being more valuable as an air purifier than as an organ of smell, or for the tongue being more valuable as an aid in digestion than as a source of the taste sensation.

Suppose we accept the proposition that pain is one of the senses of the skin; how then do we explain a pain from inside our bodies—say, a stomachache or a deep muscle pain? The answer, of course, is that there are pain receptors in many other places besides the skin.

What Is a Sense?

A sense is a nerve pathway, one end of which (the receptor end) responds in a certain way to a certain condition affecting our bodies, and whose other end reaches to a part of our brain that informs our conscious mind of what has happened or is happening. A sense is thus distinguished from the body's countless other nerve pathways by the fact that our brain *consciously* registers its impulses, although the impulses themselves are no different from those of the autonomic nervous system.

While remaining aware of the limitations of the traditional list of five sense organs, let us now analyze what they can do and how they operate:

- The eye (vision): Nerve impulses to the brain are stimulated by light waves, from which the brain forms visual images.

- The ears (hearing): Nerve impulses to the brain are stimulated by sound waves, out of which the brain forms meaningful noise, such as speech. Deep within the ear, also, are structures that give us balance.

- The nose (olfaction): Nerve impulses to the brain are stimulated by airborne chemical substances, moistened within the nasal cavity, from which the brain elicits distinctive smells.

- The tongue (taste): Nerve impulses to the brain are stimulated (in presence of water) by chemical substances in food, from which the brain forms sensations of sweet, salty, sour, bitter, or combinations of these tastes.

- Skin (touch): Nerve impulses to the brain are stimulated by the presence of outside physical forces and changes in the physical environment, including varying temperatures, which the brain registers as feelings of contact, pressure, cold, heat, and pain. (Some medical texts add traction, as when the skin is pulled or pinched, as well as the sensation of tickle.)

The Eye

Rather than take a name-by-name anatomical tour of the eye, let's instead take just three programmed tours of the eye to explore:

- the transformation of light energy into vision;

- focusing, or how the structure of the eye prepares light for transformation into vision; and

- the supporting structures and service units of the eye.

Transforming Light Energy into Vision

If you could look through the opening in the front of your eye (the *pupil*), and see to the very back surface of your eye (as if you could see through the needle valve opening to the inside skin of a basketball), you would see your own *retina*. On your retina are located all the sense receptor cells that enable us to see. There are none anywhere else in the body.

Rods and Cones

A good argument can be made that man's vision is really *two* senses. For on the paper-thin retina are two quite anatomically distinct sense receptors (nerve endings) named, for their appearance under high magnification, *cones* and *rods*. The cones are concentrated at a tiny spot on the retina called the *fovea*.

If the focusing machinery of the eye (cornea, lens, etc.) is working just right, light rays from the outside have their sharpest focus on the fovea. Surrounding the fovea is a yellowish area called the *macula lutea* (Latin, "yellow spot"). Together, the fovea and macula lutea make a circle not much bigger than the head of a pin.

All our seeing of colors and fine details is accomplished by the cones of the fovea and the macula lutea. Beyond the yellowish circumference of the macula lutea, there are fewer and fewer cones: rods become the dominant structures on the retina. It has been estimated that there are something less than 10 million cones on the retina of each eye, but more than 10 times as many rods—100 million of them or more.

Although the tight circle of cones in each eye gives man his ability to do close, detailed work (including reading) and to discriminate colors, the cones are virtually useless in detecting objects that are a bit off center from our direct focus, and furthermore operate only in good lighting conditions or in response to bright light sources.

The rods compensate for the specialized limits of the cones. They take over completely in dim light, and also give us the ability to detect peripheral objects and movements—"out of the corner of the eye." Because the rods are not sensitive to colors, our seeing at night is almost completely in black-and-white.

You can give yourself an interesting demonstration of the interacting functions of your own cones and rods if you walk from bright, sunny daylight into a dimly lit theater. In the bright light, your cones have been picking out sharp images and colors. But once

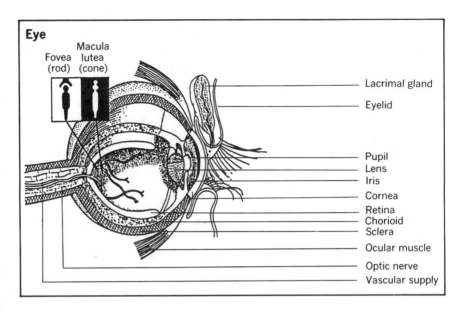

Eye

Fovea (rod) — Macula lutea (cone) — Lacrimal gland — Eyelid — Pupil — Lens — Iris — Cornea — Retina — Chorioid — Sclera — Ocular muscle — Optic nerve — Vascular supply

in dimness, the cones become inoperative. For a few moments, in fact, you may see almost nothing at all.

Visual Purple

The momentary interval after the cones stop working but before the rods begin to function is explained by a curious pigment present in the eye called *visual purple*. This substance is manufactured constantly by the rods, and must be present for the rods to respond to dim light—but it is destroyed when exposed to bright light. Thus, after entering a darkened room, it takes a few moments for visual purple to build up in the retina.

One of the principal constituents of visual purple is vitamin A, which is why this vitamin (present in carrots and other yellow produce) is said to increase our capacity to see in the dark.

The Optic Nerve

Every nerve ending is part of a larger unit, a neuron or nerve cell, and the sense receptors called rods and cones are no exception. Like all nerve cells, each rod and cone sports a long nerve fiber or *axon* leading away from the site of reception. In each eye, fibers serving the hundred-million-plus rods and cones all converge at a certain

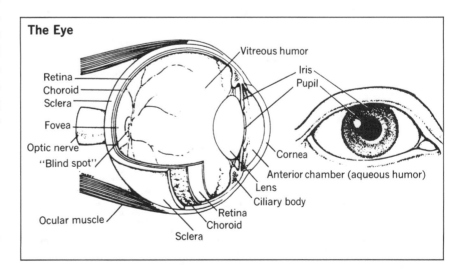

The Eye

Retina — Choroid — Sclera — Fovea — Optic nerve — "Blind spot" — Ocular muscle — Vitreous humor — Iris — Pupil — Cornea — Anterior chamber (aqueous humor) — Lens — Ciliary body — Retina — Choroid — Sclera spot just behind the retina, forming the *optic nerve*. There are no rods and cones at the point where the optic nerve exits from behind the retina at the back of the eyeball: that is why everybody has a "blind spot" at that point. An image passing through that spot completely disappears.

From the retina, both optic nerves set a course almost directly through the middle of the brain. Right and left optic nerves converge, their individual fibers partially intertwining a short distance behind the eyes. Then this joint optic nerve trunk proceeds toward the rear of the head, where the *occipital lobes,* the brain's "centers for seeing," are located. Just before reaching the occipital lobes, the optic nerve splits again into thousands of smaller nerve bundles (called *visual radiations*) that disappear into the visual cortex or "outer bark" of the occipital lobes. Only at this point are the bits of light energy that have stimulated our rods and cones transformed into images that our brain can "see."

Focusing and Light Control

Lacking the structures of the retina and their connection to the brain via the optic nerve, we could not see. Lacking reasonably normal functioning of the cornea, lens, and iris, we do not see well.

Good vision depends upon the eye being able to bend incoming light rays in such a way that the image being observed falls directly on the retina—in other words, upon proper focusing. The bending or *refraction* of light rays is the joint work of two curves, transparent slivers of specialized tissue through which light passes on its way to the retina. These are the *cornea* and the *lens*. Broadly speaking, the degree of curvature and thickness of these two structures determines whether we see well or poorly, are nearsighted or farsighted.

The Cornea and Lens

The cornea, which does the major light-bending, has a virtually fixed curvature and thickness. The lens puts the finishing touches on the focusing. Its thickness and curvature are adjustable—more or less without our conscious awareness—depending on whether we wish to focus on something nearer or farther away. The lens is made thicker or thinner, a process called *accommodation,* by the relaxing and contracting of tiny, attached *ciliary muscles*. Normally, these muscles do not have to work at all if we are looking at objects more than 20 feet away: but they often are overworked by a great deal of close work.

The Pupil and Iris

Effective focusing in various light conditions also depends upon the diameter of the hole through which light enters the eye. This hole is the *pupil*. Its diameter is controlled automatically—wider in dim light, narrower in bright light—by the muscles of the surrounding *iris*. The iris muscle contains pigment that gives our eyes color (brown, blue, green, etc.). The pupil, opening into the dark interior chamber of the eye, is black. A fully dilated (widened) pupil, as would occur in the dimmest light, illuminates over 15 times more retinal surface than the tiny "pinhole" pupil of an eye exposed to very bright light.

Structural Support and Protection of Eye

Two outer layers protect the eye. The tough outermost layer is the *sclera,* the white of the eye. Underlying the sclera is another layer, the *choroid,* which contains numerous tiny blood vessels that service the sclera and other structures on the eyeball. Both sclera and choroid have concentric openings that allow for the hole of the pupil. The cornea is really a specialized extension of the sclera,

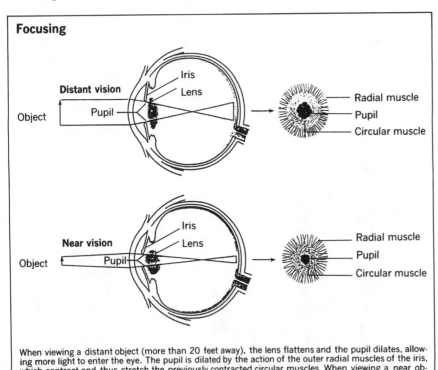

Focusing

Distant vision — Object — Pupil — Iris — Lens — Radial muscle — Pupil — Circular muscle

Near vision — Object — Pupil — Iris — Lens — Radial muscle — Pupil — Circular muscle

When viewing a distant object (more than 20 feet away), the lens flattens and the pupil dilates, allowing more light to enter the eye. The pupil is dilated by the action of the outer radial muscles of the iris, which contract and thus stretch the previously contracted circular muscles. When viewing a near object, the lens becomes more oval and the pupil contracts as more light enters the eye. This prevents overstimulation of the retina. The pupil is reduced in size by the contraction of the inner circular muscles, which serve to stretch the previously contracted radial muscles.

Muscles of the Eye

Superior muscle

Inferior muscle

Lateral muscle

Medial muscle

Eyelid muscle

Oblique muscles

and the iris of the choroid.

Two trapped reservoirs of fluid within the eye are important in maintaining the eye's shape as well as the frictionless operation of its moving parts. These two reservoirs contain fluids called the *aqueous humor* and *vitreous humor*. The tiny space between the cornea and lens, corresponding to the pupil, is called the anterior chamber and is filled with the clear, watery, aqueous humor. The larger interior space behind the lens is called the posterior chamber, and is filled with the vitreous humor.

Muscles for Movement of Eye

In addition to the tiny muscles within the eye that control the opening of the pupil and the shape of the lens, we also have a number of elegant muscles that control the movements of each eyeball, and make both eyeballs move together in unison.

The movements of each eyeball are affected by six muscles attached to its top, bottom, and sides. The teamwork between these muscles—some contracting while others relax—allows the eye to move from side to side, up and down, and at all intermediate angles (obliquely). One of our eyes is always a dominant or leading eye; that is, its movements are always followed by the other eye.

Our protective eyelids, of course, are controlled by opening and closing muscles that lie outside the eye proper. These muscles can function both voluntarily and involuntarily.

Lubrication and Hygiene of Eye

Without the moisture provided by tears, our eyeball would scrape excruciatingly on the inside lining (*conjunctiva*) of the eyelid. In addition to lubrication, tears also have a cleansing action, not only because they supply water for washing and rinsing but also because they contain a mild germicide called *lysozyme* that kills bacteria and other potentially harmful microbes.

Ciliary Muscle Contraction

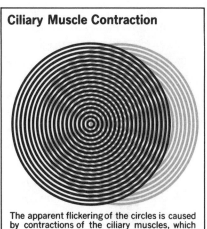

The apparent flickering of the circles is caused by contractions of the ciliary muscles, which control the accommodation (or change in thickness) of the lens for accurate focusing of objects at a variety of distances.

Tears are produced by the *lacrimal glands* above the eyeball, just under the eyebrow, a bit further toward the temple side than the nose side. They are discharged from several short ducts and spread over the surface of the eyeball by blinking. The *conjunctival sac* at the bottom inner (nose) side of the eye—visible in the mirror as a pinkish flap of tissue—serves as a collecting pool for tears; from there, they drain down a duct into the nasal cavity. This is why somebody who is crying also snuffles and must blow his nose.

There is another tiny drainage network in the eye, located at the interconnection of the cornea and iris, which serves to keep the fluid pressure of the space filled by the aqueous humor within normal limits. Drainage of this area is through microscopic conduits called the *canals of Schlemm*. Improper drainage can cause build-up of pressure, such as occurs in glaucoma, and impairment or loss of vision.

The Ear

Within the tunnels and chambers of the ear lie the two special types of sense receptors that give us, respectively, the sense of hearing and the sense of balance.

The Outer Ear

The *outer ear* includes that rather oddly shaped and folded piece of flesh and cartilage from which earrings are hung, and more important, the external *auditory canal*, a tunnel leading from the ear's opening to the *tympanic membrane*, or *eardrum*.

The Middle Ear

The *middle ear* includes the inner surface of the eardrum and the three

Ear

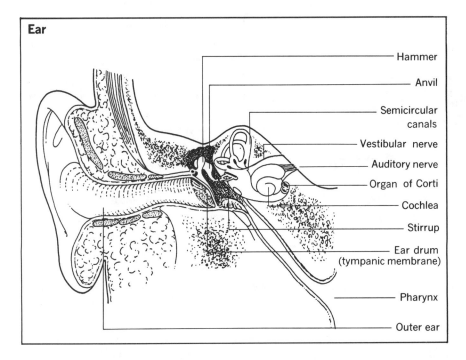

- Hammer
- Anvil
- Semicircular canals
- Vestibular nerve
- Auditory nerve
- Organ of Corti
- Cochlea
- Stirrup
- Ear drum (tympanic membrane)
- Pharynx
- Outer ear

tiny, bony *ossicles,* named long ago for their shape (apparently by some blacksmithing anatomist), *the hammer, the anvil,* and *the stirrup;* or in Latin: *the malleus, the incus,* and *the stapes.* These bones respond to the vibrations in the air that are the basis of sound, vibrate themselves, and transmit their vibrations to the inner ear, where the sense receptors for hearing are located, and the *auditory* (or *acoustic*) *nerve* to the brain begins.

The middle ear is connected to the back of the throat (pharynx) by the Eustachian tube. This tunnel between throat and middle ear makes the pressure on the inside of the eardrum, via the mouth, the same as the pressure of the atmosphere on the outside of the eardrum. (Thus yawning helps to equalize pressure.) Without it, or if the Eustachian tube becomes clogged, the taut membrane of the eardrum would always be in imminent danger of bursting.

The Inner Ear

The chambers of the *inner ear* are completely filled with fluid, which is jostled by the ossicles "knocking" on a thin membrane called the oval window, separating the middle from the inner ear. Another flexible membrane, the round window, serves to restrict the motion of the inner ear fluid when the movement is too stormy.

Organ of Hearing

Within the inner ear is a bony structure coiled like a snail shell about the size of a pea. This is the *cochlea,* the actual Latin word for snail or snail shell. Following the internal spiral of the cochlea is the *organ of Corti,* the true sense receptors for hearing.

The organ of Corti is made up of thousands of specialized nerve endings that are the individual sense receptors for sound. These are in the form of tiny hairs projecting up from the internal membrane lining the cochlea; they wave like stalks of underwater plants in response to the oscillating currents of the inner ear fluid. There are some 20,000 of these hairs within the cochlea, responsive to almost as many degrees of movement of the fluid. These thousands of nerve endings merge at the core of the

cochlea and exit from its floor as the nerve bundle of the *auditory nerve.*

Organ of Balance

The organ of balance, or equilibrium, is also behind the oval window that marks the beginning of the inner ear. The principal structure consists of three fluid-filled *semicircular canals* arranged, like the wheels of a gyroscope spinning on a perfectly flat plane or surface, at right angles to each other. When we are in a normal, upright position, the fluid in the canals is also in its normal resting state. But when we begin to tilt or turn or wobble, the fluid runs one way or another in one or more of the canals. This fluid movement is picked up by crested, hairlike nerve endings lining the inside of the canals and relayed as nerve impulses along the *vestibular nerve* to the brain. Then, the brain sends messages to the muscles that can restore our equilibrium.

The Semicircular Canals

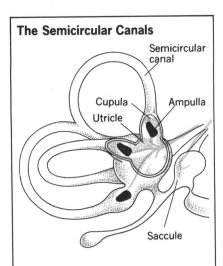

- Semicircular canal
- Cupula
- Ampulla
- Utricle
- Saccule

The semicircular canals are swollen at their bases into three ampullae in which receptors are located. When the head moves or accelerates, the fluid within the canals (endolymph), tends to move slower than the head, and the cupula is displaced. This is communicated to the hairlike nerve receptors. Soon the endolymph catches up to the head movement and the cupula returns to its normal position. When movement stops, the endolymph continues to move, the cupula is again displaced, and the nerve receptors are activated until the endolymph ceases to move.

The Ear and the Perception of Sound

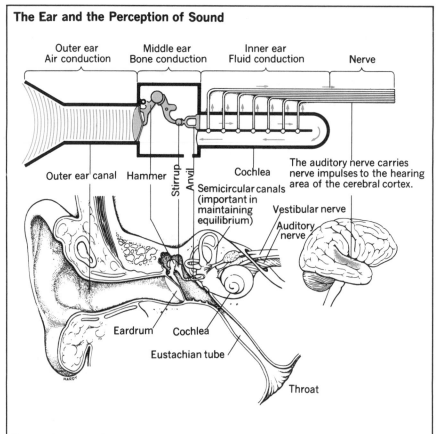

The sound waves are funneled through the outer ear canal to the eardrum. The vibrating eardrum sets into motion the three bones of the middle ear. The bones terminate in an opening in the fluid-filled cochlea. The vibrating bones set the fluid in motion. This stimulates nerve endings, which unite to become the auditory nerve. The nerve impulses are carried to the hearing area in the cerebral cortex.

The term *labyrinth* is sometimes used to refer collectively to the cochlea, semicircular canals and associated structures of the inner ear. The space or cavity within the labyrinth is called the *vestibule,* which gives its name to the vestibular nerve.

How We Hear

Just as our eye has certain special equipment—its focusing apparatus—to prepare light for the retina, so our ear has special equipment to prepare vibrations for reception by the organ of Corti.

This equipment consists of structures that amplify the vibrations reaching the ear, or, more rarely, damping (decreasing) the vibrations caused by very loud or very close occurrences.

Sound waves are really vibrations in the air that reach the eardrum at the narrow end of the funnel-shaped auditory canal. These vibrations set the membrane of the eardrum vibrating ever so slightly. Behind the eardrum, the first ossicle encountered is the hammer, which is attached to the eardrum by a projection descriptively called the hammer-handle.

From the eardrum, vibrations travel up the handle and set the hammer vibrating. The hammer, in turn, sets the anvil vibrating; and the anvil, the stirrup. The stirrup then knocks like an impatient caller on the oval window of the inner ear, and the then vibrating oval window stirs the fluids within the cochlea. This chain of events can account for a tremendous amplification of vibrations—so that we are literally able to "hear a pin drop."

Tiny muscles in the middle ear relax or tighten the eardrum and adjust to changing volumes of sound. For example, a muscle connecting the stirrup and the eardrum relaxes when the stirrup is vibrating violently in the presence of very loud noises. A lax eardrum is less likely to rupture and transmits fewer vibrations to the delicate mechanisms of the middle and inner ear than a taut one. Thus we have to some degree built-in, automatic protection against the assaults of noise pollution—but not nearly enough, according to physicians who are convinced that more and more cases of deafness are caused by the incessant battering of the modern world against our eardrums. Human eardrums are not made to withstand the sound of jet planes taking off, for example.

The Nose and Tongue

The sense receptors on the tongue and within the nasal cavity work very closely together to give us our sense of taste. These five kinds of receptors—the olfactory cell in the nose and the four special cells or taste buds on the tongue for discriminating salty, sweet, sour, and bitter tastes—also have a functional similarity. All are chemical detectors, and all require moisture in order to function. In the nose, airborne substances must first be moistened by mucus (from the olfactory glands) before they can stimulate olfactory cells. In the mouth, the saliva does the wetting.

The general number and distribution of the four types of taste receptors are described earlier in this chapter under "The Digestive System and the Liver." These nerve endings, numbering in the hundreds of thousands, merge into two nerve bundles traveling away from the tongue to the

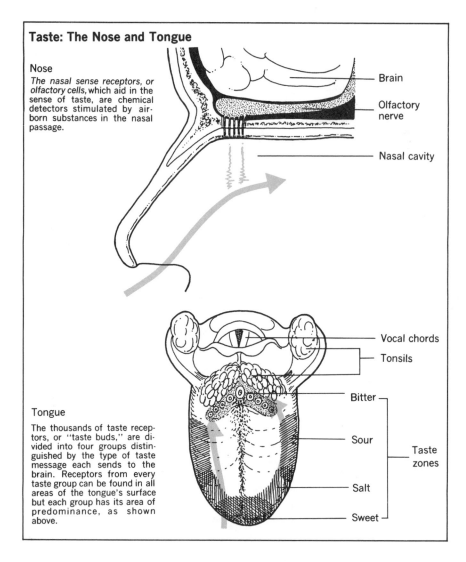

Taste: The Nose and Tongue

Nose
The nasal sense receptors, or olfactory cells, which aid in the sense of taste, are chemical detectors stimulated by air-born substances in the nasal passage.

Brain

Olfactory nerve

Nasal cavity

Tongue
The thousands of taste receptors, or "taste buds," are divided into four groups distinguished by the type of taste message each sends to the brain. Receptors from every taste group can be found in all areas of the tongue's surface but each group has its area of predominance, as shown above.

Vocal chords

Tonsils

Bitter

Sour

Taste zones

Salt

Sweet

brain's "taste center." The receptors toward the rear of the tongue collect into the *glossopharyngeal nerve;* those at the front and middle are directed along the *lingual nerve.*

Our smell receptors are clustered in an area about a half-inch wide on ceiling of the nasal cavity. This is called, appropriately enough, the smell patch. The nerve endings pass upward through the sievelike *ethmoid bone,* separating the nasal cavity from the brain, and connect to the olfactory bulb, which is the "nose end" of the *olfactory nerve.* At the other end of the olfactory nerve is the "nose brain" or *rhinencephalon*—a tiny part of the cerebrum in man, but quite large in dogs and other mammals whose sense of smell is keener than man's.

Although man's sense of smell is probably his least used sense, it still has a quite remarkable sensitivity. With it we can detect some chemicals in concentrations as diluted as one part in 30 billion—for example, the active ingredient in skunk spray. Also, man's ability to smell smoke and to detect gas leaks and other warning scents has prevented many a tragedy.

Skin

The sensations stimulated by the various types of sense receptors in the skin are described at the outset of this section. It is worth noting, however, at the end of our tour of the sense organs that the senses associated

with the skin are really in a class by themselves. Perhaps the most telling indication of their unique place in the hierarchy of senses is the fact that practically our entire central nervous system is given over to handling the impulses transmitted by these receptors. See also Ch. 16, *Diseases of the Eye and Ear.*

The Urinogenital System and the Kidneys

In large part our good health depends on the quality of the body's internal environment. There is a kind of ecological principle at work within us—if one chain threatens to break, one system becomes polluted, one balance is tilted, then the whole environment is in imminent danger of collapsing. The major responsibility for keeping our internal environment clean and unclogged lies with our two kidneys. They are the filters and purifiers of body fluids: the body's pollution-control stations, its recycling plants, and its waste-disposal units.

The Kidneys

The kidneys are located just behind our abdominal cavity on either side of the spinal cord, their tops usually tucked just under the bottommost rib. Each of our kidneys is four to five inches long and weighs about half a pound. The right kidney is normally placed a bit below the left, to accommodate the bulky liver lying also on the right side above it. Neither kidney is fixed rigidly; both can shift position slightly. Lying outside the muscular sheath of the abdominal cavity, the kidneys are more vulnerable than most internal organs to outside blows, but good protection against all but the severest jolts is afforded by surrounding fatty cushions, the big back muscles, and the bone and musculature associated with the spinal column.

As it has with the lungs, the liver, and most other vital organs, nature has supplied us with a large reserve capacity of kidney tissue—a life-giving overabundance in the event of kidney disease or injury. Indeed, normal function of only one-half of one kidney can sustain a person's life.

The kidney's task of purifying our internal environment—that is, our circulating blood—is really a double task. Each kidney must purify the blood that passes through it, sending back into circulation only "clean blood"; and it must dispose of the impurities it has taken from the blood. The latter is accomplished by the urine draining down a tube, or *ureter*, leading from each of the two kidneys

to one common urinary *bladder*. Urine is discharged from the bladder down another tube called the *urethra* to the external opening for urination.

How the Kidneys Process Body Fluids

Blood is brought to the kidney by a renal artery, is treated in the kidney's unique microscopic structures, and exists via the renal vein. (*Renal* means associated with the kidneys.) The sheer volume of blood processed by both our kidneys is prodigious: between 400 and 500 gallons are processed every day.

Internal Structure

Within each kidney are over a million microscopic units called *nephrons*. The nephron is the basic functional unit of the kidney—a little kidney in itself—and is really a superbly engi-

neered and coordinated arrangement of many smaller structures, all working together.

Blood arriving at the kidney from the renal artery is quickly channeled into finer and finer vessels, until finally it flows into a kind of cat's cradle or "ball of wool" structure called a *glomerulus* (composed of intertwining, microscopic vessels called glomerular capillaries). The entire structure of the nephron is built around the microscopic glomerulus (Latin, "tiny ball"). Surrounding the glomerulus, like a hand lightly cupping a ball of wool, is another structure called *Bowman's capsule*. Fluid and dissolved materials filter out of the blood from the glomerular capillaries through the membranes into Bowman's capsule.

Substances in Bowman's Capsule

The fluids and dissolved materials filtering into Bowman's capsule are by no means all wastes and impurities. In fact, some of the substances must soon be reclaimed. Among the waste substances captured by Bowman's capsule and destined for excretion in urine are various nitrogen salts and other waste products of cellular metabolism, as well as actual or potential poisons that have entered or accumulated in the bloodstream. Nonwaste substances include needed sugars and salts, and water.

Reclaiming Essential Substances

Before we leave the glomerulus altogether behind, it should be noted that like any capillary bed, this small ball of blood vessels has not only an inflow from the renal artery but also outflow vessels leading eventually back to the renal vein.

From the cupped lips of Bowman's capsule, fluid and dissolved substances from the blood trickle into a single tube called a kidney *tubule*. The

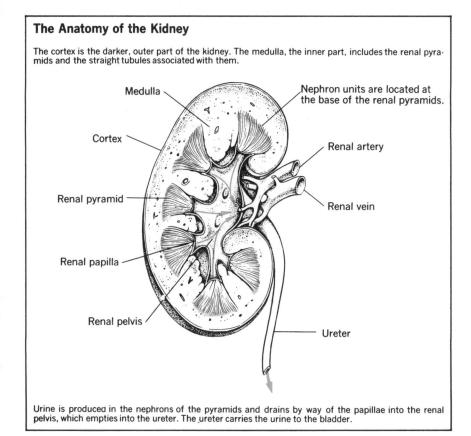

The Anatomy of the Kidney

The cortex is the darker, outer part of the kidney. The medulla, the inner part, includes the renal pyramids and the straight tubules associated with them.

Medulla

Cortex

Renal pyramid

Renal papilla

Renal pelvis

Nephron units are located at the base of the renal pyramids.

Renal artery

Renal vein

Ureter

Urine is produced in the nephrons of the pyramids and drains by way of the papillae into the renal pelvis, which empties into the ureter. The ureter carries the urine to the bladder.

The Nephron

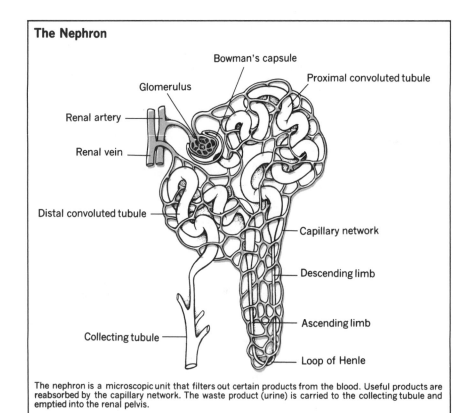

The nephron is a microscopic unit that filters out certain products from the blood. Useful products are reabsorbed by the capillary network. The waste product (urine) is carried to the collecting tubule and emptied into the renal pelvis.

outflow vessels from the glomerulus wind closely over and around the tubule, forming a capillary network around it. By this means the non-waste substances are reclaimed and returned to refresh the blood moving away from the nephron.

The tubule itself makes many twists and turns—including one hairpin turn so stunning that it has its own medical name—*Henle's loop.* So much twisting and turning gives the tubule a great deal more surface area than a simple, straight tube would have within the same space, thus increasing the amount of water and dissolved substances that can be recaptured by the encircling capillaries.

If there were no recapturing system in the kidneys, death would probably result from dehydration. Even if that could be avoided, the loss of essential salts and other substances would prove fatal in a short time.

The arithmetic of the situation goes something like this: every day, an estimated 42 gallons of fluid filter out of the glomeruli and into the two kidneys' approximately two and a half million tubules. Dissolved in this 42 gallons—representing about three times the body's weight—are about two-and-a-half pounds of common salt, just one of the many substances in the fluid that our body needs in sufficient amounts. The loss of either water or common salt at a rapid rate would prove fatal in a matter of hours.

But so efficient is the tubule-capillary recapturing system that only an average of less than two quarts of fluid, containing just one-third ounce of salt, pass daily out of the kidneys into the ureter and are excreted as urine. In other words, over 99 percent of both the water and common salt removed from the blood at Bowman's capsules is returned to the blood.

The Kidneys and Blood Pressure

A surprising insight into the critical role played by our kidneys in almost every body function is provided by the relation of blood pressure to kidney function. The blood in the glomerular capillaries must be at higher pressure than the fluid around them, so that the fluid and its dissolved substances can push through the capillary membranes toward Bowman's capsule. If blood pressure in the body falls too low (severe *hypotension*) the formation of urine ceases.

On the other hand, if a portion of the kidney is suffering from anemia due to some disorder, kidney cells secrete *pressor hormones,* which serve to elevate the blood pressure. Thus high blood pressure (*hypertension*) may be a sign of kidney disorder.

The Urinary Tract

From the ends of the million or so tubules in each kidney, urine drains into larger and larger collecting basins (called *calyces,* singular *calyx*) which drain in turn into the kidney's master urine reservoir, the *kidney pelvis.* Then, drop by drop, urine slides down each ureter to the urinary bladder.

Urine is held in the bladder by the contraction of two muscle rings, or *sphincters,* one located just inside the bladder before it meets the urethra, and the other encircling the urethra itself. When about a half-pint has accumulated, nerves convey the urge to urinate to the brain, and the person voluntarily causes the sphincters to relax, emptying the bladder. (In exceptional circumstances, the elastic-walled bladder can hold two or three quarts of urine.) Up to the point where the bladder drains, the male and female urinary tracts are very similar, but after the bladder, any similarity stops.

Female Urethra

The female's urethra, normally about

The Female Urinary System

- Kidney
- Ureter
- Bladder
- Urethra

The Male Urinary System

- Kidney
- Ureter
- Bladder
- Prostate gland
- Urethra

one and a half inches long, is not much more than a short channel by which urine is eliminated from the bladder. Its very shortness often gives it an undesired significance, because it represents an easy upward invasion route for bacteria and other infection-causing microbes from the outside. Acute and painful inflammations of the urethra (*urethritis*) and bladder (*cystitis*) are thus common in women. These lower urinary tract infections, however, can usually be halted before spreading further up the urinary tract by the administration of any of several antimicrobial drugs. See Ch. 25, *Women's Health* for more information on these disorders.

Male Urethra

In contrast to the female, the male's urethra is involved with reproductive functions. So closely connected are the male's lower urinary tract and genital organs that his urethra (from bladder to the outside) is properly called the urinogenital (or genitouri-

nary) tract. This is the reason why the medical specialty known as *urology* deals with both the urinary and genital apparatus of men; but with only the urinary tract of women. The urologist's specialty does not extend to the female genital and childbearing organs, which are the concern of the

gynecologist and *obstetrician.*

However, all the distinctly male sex glands and organs are linked more or less directly into the eight- or nine-inch length of the male urethra.

The Genitals

The Female Reproductive System

As indicated above, the urinary and genital systems of women are dealt with by two different medical specialties. For this reason, the female genitals are discussed elsewhere. For a description and illustration of the female reproductive system, see Ch. 3, *The Teens.* For a description of infections of the female reproductive tract, see Ch. 25, *Women's Health.*

The Male Reproductive System

From its emergence below the bladder, the male urethra serves as a conduit for all the male sexual secretions.

Prostate Gland

Directly below the bladder outlet, the

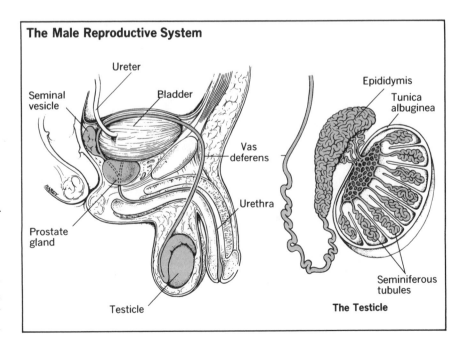

The Male Reproductive System

- Ureter
- Seminal vesicle
- Bladder
- Vas deferens
- Urethra
- Prostate gland
- Testicle

- Epididymis
- Tunica albuginea
- Seminiferous tubules

The Testicle

prostate gland completely enwraps the urethra. The prostate secretes substances into the urethra through ejaculatory ducts; these substances are essential in keeping alive the spermatozoa that arrive from their manufacturing sites in the *testicles* (or *testes*).

Testicles

The two testicles hang down within a wrinkled bag of skin called the *scrotum*. Although the vulnerable position of the testicles remains something of an evolutionary mystery, one clue is that the optimum production of spermatozoa takes place at a temperature some degrees lower than the normal internal body temperature.

Spermatozoa produced in the testicles travel upward toward the urethra through a seminal duct or tube called the *vas deferens* (one from each testicle). (These are the ducts, incidentally, that are tied and cut in the male sterilization procedure known as a vasectomy.) The sperm cells are then stored, until ejaculation, in little reservoirs called *seminal vesicles* which are situated on either side of the urethra in the area just above the prostate gland.

The portion of the male urethra from the bladder to where it emerges from the encircling prostate, having received the emission of both the prostate and the testicles, is called the prostatic or posterior urethra. The remainder, mainly consisting of the conduit running down the middle of the shaft of the penis, ending in the external opening called the *meatus,* is known as the anterior urethra. See also Ch. 17, *Diseases of the Urinogenital System.*

2

The First Dozen Years

Birth, Infancy, and Maturation

Before the Baby Arrives

When a husband and wife decide to have a baby they should both undergo complete physical examinations. This will make it possible to detect and treat abnormalities like diabetes and anemia that might affect the future pregnancy. A pregnant woman should have periodic checkups so that her physician can observe both her progress and that of the growing fetus. Such observation will help to assure a pregnancy and delivery that are free from troublesome complications.

What the Newborn Baby Looks Like

At birth the baby's skin is wrinkled or scaly, and may be covered by a cheesy substance called *vernix caseosa*. During the first two weeks the skin will become quite dry to the touch. The skin of white newborns is red, and sometimes turns yellow during the first few days. Black newborns often are not as dark as they might be later. Their skin becomes just as yellow as that of white babies, but the change is more difficult to observe.

The newborn's head is large in proportion to the rest of its body. The genitals too may seem large, especially in girls. Newborn girls may have

swollen genitalia that is a result of *edema* (fluid in the tissues, causing puffiness), but the swelling is usually present for only a few days after birth.

The eyes, slate blue in color, can open and react to light, but are unable to focus. Noises produce a *startle response*, a complex involuntary reaction marked by a sudden, jerky, arm and leg movement. The newborn cries a great deal, sucks, and may sneeze.

The infant's stomach may look rather large and protuberant, and, of course, it has the stump of the umbilical cord dangling from it. The umbilical cord has been cut and tied near the navel, and will eventually fall off.

If you feel the front and back of the baby's head, you will notice one or two soft spots, called the *anterior* and *posterior fontanelles*. The posterior fontanelle usually closes at the baby's second month of life, and the anterior at 18 months or earlier.

You also may feel many different ridges in the baby's head. These are the borders of the different skull bones, which fuse as the baby gets older. They are present so that the skull can grow as the baby's brain and head continue to grow.

Soon after birth, you may detect a

swelling on the baby's head just under the scalp. This is called *caput succedaneum*. It is nothing to worry about, as it dissolves a day or two after birth. Occasionally, another swelling known as *cephalhematoma* may also be present. This, too, disappears, within a few weeks.

The baby's weight will, of course, vary. Most full-term babies weigh between six and eight pounds. Babies of diabetic mothers are often heavier, and may weigh up to twelve pounds.

Some Advice to New Mothers

Unless the new father and mother are really prepared to change some of the conditioned patterns of their relationship, both can be in for a very difficult time. The father suddenly finds himself taking second place in his wife's attentions and affection. The new mother is tired physically and mentally. In-laws and other relatives may infringe on the couple's privacy and interfere with their right to make their own decisions. The new mother may find it hard to reconcile her maternal instinct with her desires as a woman and wife.

All of these problems can be minimized if the mother follows a few commonsense guidelines:

● The new baby is a shared responsibility. Do not shut your husband out of the experience of parenthood. Let him learn to feed the baby, diaper her, hold her, get acquainted with her. Make your husband feel just as important to the baby as you are, and just as important to you as he was before the baby was born.

● Arrange for some kind of assistance in your home, and don't wait until the day you bring the baby home to do it. Plan ahead. You will be physically and emotionally tired after childbirth, no matter how marvelous you may feel when you leave the hospital. During the hospital stay the baby was cared for by a trained staff. At home the burden will fall mainly on you, unless you take steps to get help. If you cannot get your mother or another relative to stay with you, engage a housekeeper or some other trained person. The investment will pay off for you, the baby, and your husband.

● If it is at all possible, arrange to have a separate area for the baby. It is best for a baby not to be kept in the parents' room. Parents must have privacy. If you do not have a bedroom for the baby, section off some spot where you can put a crib and a dressing table to hold the supplies you will need when you feed, change, bathe, and dress her.

● Don't make the baby the focus of attention 24 hours a day. If she fidgets and fusses at times, try not to get nervous. Don't run to her at every whimper so long as you know she has been fed, is dry, and nothing is really wrong. Relax. The baby will be very sensitive to your emotional responses, particularly when you hold her. Through your physical contact you will develop a kind of communication with your baby which she will sense when you pick her up or feed her.

● As important as it is for you and your husband to avoid overhandling the baby, it is more important that family and friends be made to follow a "hands off" policy except at your discretion. A new baby should not be subjected to excessive stimulation. For example, you

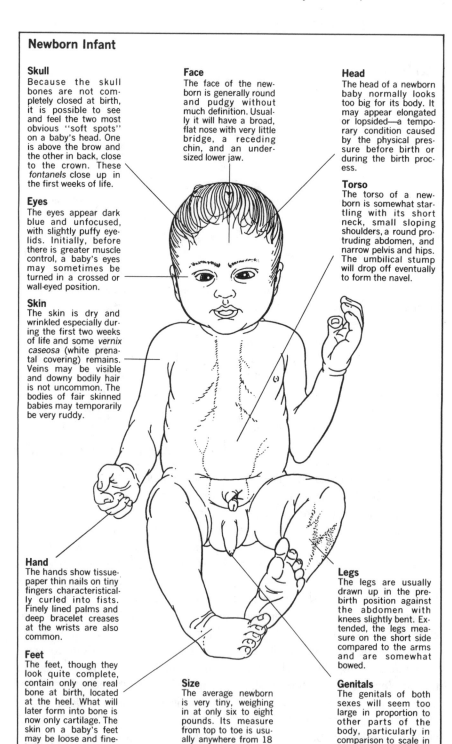

Newborn Infant

Skull
Because the skull bones are not completely closed at birth, it is possible to see and feel the two most obvious "soft spots" on a baby's head. One is above the brow and the other in back, close to the crown. These *fontanels* close up in the first weeks of life.

Eyes
The eyes appear dark blue and unfocused, with slightly puffy eyelids. Initially, before there is greater muscle control, a baby's eyes may sometimes be turned in a crossed or wall-eyed position.

Skin
The skin is dry and wrinkled especially during the first two weeks of life and some *vernix caseosa* (white prenatal covering) remains. Veins may be visible and downy bodily hair is not uncommon. The bodies of fair skinned babies may temporarily be very ruddy.

Hand
The hands show tissue-paper thin nails on tiny fingers characteristically curled into fists. Finely lined palms and deep bracelet creases at the wrists are also common.

Feet
The feet, though they look quite complete, contain only one real bone at birth, located at the heel. What will later form into bone is now only cartilage. The skin on a baby's feet may be loose and finely lined.

Face
The face of the newborn is generally round and pudgy without much definition. Usually it will have a broad, flat nose with very little bridge, a receding chin, and an undersized lower jaw.

Size
The average newborn is very tiny, weighing in at only six to eight pounds. Its measure from top to toe is usually anywhere from 18 inches to 21 inches.

Head
The head of a newborn baby normally looks too big for its body. It may appear elongated or lopsided—a temporary condition caused by the physical pressure before birth or during the birth process.

Torso
The torso of a newborn is somewhat startling with its short neck, small sloping shoulders, a round protruding abdomen, and narrow pelvis and hips. The umbilical stump will drop off eventually to form the navel.

Legs
The legs are usually drawn up in the pre-birth position against the abdomen with knees slightly bent. Extended, the legs measure on the short side compared to the arms and are somewhat bowed.

Genitals
The genitals of both sexes will seem too large in proportion to other parts of the body, particularly in comparison to scale in the adult.

may notice that if you pick her up and put her back in her crib, and then let someone else hold her a few minutes later, the baby may cry. If you slam a door, the baby's body reacts in the startle reflex, the involuntary reaction previously described. A baby needs a quiet, organized home, free from the kind of upsetting distraction that comes from being surrounded and fussed over by too many people. You and your husband must decide when you want the baby to have visitors and how those visitors are to behave. You must do this even if it causes hurt feelings among your friends and relatives. When the baby is a little older there will be time enough for friends and relatives to admire and play with her.

Feeding the Baby

One of the first questions a mother-to-be must ask herself is how she will feed her baby.

Breast-feeding is certainly the simplest method, and many women believe that a both mother and child get more emotional satisfaction from it than from bottle-feeding. It is also, obviously, less expensive.

Breast-Feeding

Almost any healthy woman who wants to breast-feed her baby can do so. All she needs is the desire and motivation. No special preparation is necessary except, perhaps, some stimulation of the breasts, as prescribed by her physician during pregnancy.

On the other hand, a variety of different factors might necessitate a change from breast to bottle-feeding. Although breast-feeding may be discontinued at any time, some mothers may feel a sense of failure or frustration at being unable to continue having

the intimate relationship that so many other mothers enjoy. No harm will come to the baby by being switched to a formula. Once started on a formula, however, it may be difficult to go back to breast-feeding on a regular basis. For a while, at least, the mother will have to stimulate her breasts artificially to increase their milk-producing capacity.

The First Few Days

When a mother first starts to breast-feed, she may be worried that she won't have sufficient milk for the baby. Her breasts are just beginning to fill up with a creamy, yellowish substance called *colostrum*. Transitional and then regular breast milk will not come in for three to five days or longer. Colostrum contains more protein and less fat than breast milk. Secretions of colostrum are small, but during this time the baby does not need very much fluid, and the colostrum will give her adequate nutrition.

Actually, it is important that the milk does not fill the breasts right away because engorgement would be so severe that the baby would not be able to suck well or strongly enough to empty them. During engorgement, the mother's breasts feel extremely tender and full. A good nursing brassiere will lift and support the breasts and alleviate the tender sensation during the one- or-two day period of the engorgement.

Some Advice to Nursing Mothers

If you do not have enough milk for the first few days, don't worry about it. Let the baby suck on your nipples for three, five, or even ten minutes. Don't keep her on your breasts for twenty or thirty minutes right from the beginning. Start with three minutes the first day, five minutes the

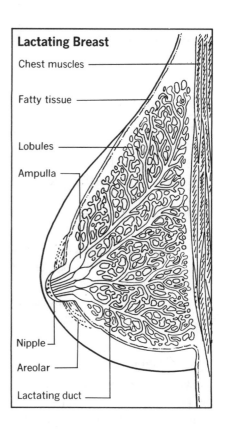

Lactating Breast

Chest muscles

Fatty tissue

Lobules

Ampulla

Nipple

Areolar

Lactating duct

second, and so on until you work up to fifteen or twenty minutes. In this way you will toughen your nipples so that your breasts will become accustomed to the baby's sucking. A bland cream may be used to massage the nipple area, particularly if the nipples become sore or cracked.

Be sure to use both breasts. By emptying the breasts, milk production is stimulated; thus an adequate milk supply is dependent upon using both breasts. To avoid any soreness or tenderness, use one breast longer than the other during each nursing period.

Let us assume, for example, that at the first feeding of the day you nurse the baby on the left breast for a long period, then on the right for a short period. During the next feeding the right breast will become the first one on which the baby nurses (for the long period), and the left will be nursed second (for the short period). After a few weeks you should be nursing the baby on the first breast for twenty minutes and on the other for ten minutes.

The Feeding Schedule

Depending on how often the baby wants to feed, you will be wise to adhere to a modified demand schedule. Don't watch the clock and feed the baby every four hours on the dot. You might feed at approximately every fourth hour, which means that you could start a second feeding early—at a three-hour interval—or late—at a five-hour interval. And, needless to say, never wake your baby up at night. She will awaken you.

Bottle-feeding

New parents have a choice between prepackaged formulas and the homemade variety. Either provides the same basic nutritional requirements.

The basic homemade formula for newborns consists of evaporated milk, water, and sugar or one of the sugar derivatives. Twice as much water as evaporated milk is used with one to two tablespoons of sweetening. A similar formula can be made with whole milk in somewhat different proportions. As the baby gets older, the formula will be changed from time to time by your physician.

If one formula does not agree with the baby, it will not help to put her on a similar formula; its ingredients are likely to be virtually the same. You must switch to a radically different formula, such as one containing no milk at all or no carbohydrates. It is up to your physician to advise you which modified formula to try.

As to how much formula should be given at each feeding, let the baby decide. If she is satisfied with two-and-a-half ounces, she is probably getting enough. If she wants up to four-and-a-half ounces, give it to her. The amount is not important as long as

your physician feels the baby is in good health.

A final thing to remember about feeding is this: whether you use breast or bottle, you must give your baby the love, warmth, and body contact that she needs. As you feed her, you are not only providing nutritional nourishment for her growing body but giving her emotional and mental food for her developing personality.

The First Six Months

It is extremely important that the baby have regular health supervision. Your baby's physician—whether pediatrician or general practitioner—will check the baby's height and weight on each visit, and make certain she is growing and gaining at a satisfactory rate. Often, the first sign of illness in a baby is a change in her height and weight pattern.

Although no two children develop at the same rate, it is possible to make certain generalizations about their development. See the charts in this chapter showing the growth rates for boys and girls.

By two months a baby often holds her head up when she lies on her stomach or when she is being held up. She recognizes large objects, and she knows her bottle or feeding position. She can probably smile.

Sometime during the second or third month, your physician will start a series of injections against diphtheria, whooping cough, and tetanus (called *DTP*), as well as oral immunizing agents against polio—the *Sabin vaccine*. See the chart in the "Alphabetic Guide to Child Care" under "Immunization" later in this chapter.

The Three-Month Mark

By three months most babies are eating some solids specially processed

for babies—fruits, cereals, vegetables, meats—in addition to having formula. They may, of course, still be entirely on breast milk. Your physician will also suggest the use of vitamin supplements, in the form of drops, which can be added to the baby's milk or solid food. All babies need vitamins A, C, and D. Occasionally, vitamin B is also prescribed. If fluorides are not present in your drinking water, they are often added to the baby's vitamins to retard tooth decay.

At Four Months

By four months the baby will look at moving objects. Do not be surprised if her eyes cross. This is a normal condition during early infancy, and may even persist for a year.

At about this time, the baby may also learn to turn over from front to back—an important milestone. Some babies may have developed bald or flat places on the back of the head from lying more or less in one position. At about this time the condition should begin to disappear.

The Second Six Months

At six months most babies smile when they are brought to the physician's office. At one year of age a visit to the physician is more likely to produce tears and screams. The friendly, sociable attitude of the six-month-old gives way to one in which strangers are shunned or mistrusted, and everyone other than mother may qualify as a stranger.

By the sixth month the baby may roll over when placed on her back. She may learn to crawl, sit, pull herself up, and even stand. By a year she may start to walk, although walking unaided does not often occur so soon.

At this stage the baby is full of life and activity. She won't lie still when you change her diaper, and often needs distraction. She cries if you put her down or leave her alone. Unless you are firm and resist running to her first whimper, you may set the stage for spoiling her as she gets older. Of course, if she continues to cry for any considerable length of time—not more than half an hour—make sure there is nothing wrong with her besides her displeasure at your not appearing like a genie because she screams or fusses.

Other Changes

Other changes occur at this age. Where before she had been a good sleeper, she may now not want to go to sleep or she may awaken at night. Let her know that you are nearby, but don't make a habit of playing with her in the middle of the night—not if you value your sleep.

If you should notice, as many parents do at about this time, that your baby seems to be left-handed, do not try to make her right-handed. Each of us inherits a preference for one hand or the other, and it is harmful to try to change it. In any case, you are not likely to know for sure which hand your child prefers until the second year of her life.

In this second six-month period, the baby will probably take some of her milk from a cup. Don't be surprised if she takes juices out of a cup but insists on taking milk from a bottle. If she tries to hold the bottle or cup herself, let her. Of course, it may be wise to keep a mop handy at first, but after few months her skills will improve. In any case, nonbreakable cups are recommended.

Diet and Teeth

The baby's diet is soon expanded to include pureed baby foods. You might even want to try the somewhat lumpier junior foods; as more of her teeth erupt, the baby will enjoy lumpier food more and more. Teething biscuits can be added to the diet, too. By the time she is one year old she will usually have six teeth (incisors), although, because no two children are alike, she may have none at all. By the end of the first year she will have lost some of her appetite, and her rapid weight gain will cease. This is entirely natural in a period when the outside world is taking more and more interest.

As she starts to move around she wants to investigate everything. Keep dangerous objects—detergents, poisons, and medicines, especially baby aspirin—out of her reach. Tell her "no" to emphasize the seriousness of certain prohibitions. She should understand what "no" means by the time she is one-year-old, and will also probably respond to other simple commands.

It is essential that your baby's health supervision be continued without interruption. During the second six months of life she will complete her protection against diphtheria, whooping cough, tetanus (DTP), and polio (Sabin), and be tested for exposure to tuberculosis (the tuberculin test).

Behavioral Development during Infancy

During a child's first year she needs a warm and loving emotional environment in the home. It is during this time that a child establishes what psychiatrists and psychologists call basic trust. That is, she learns to be a trusting individual who feels that her important needs—those of being cared for, fed, and comforted—will be met by other human beings, initially by her mother.

Emotional Needs

Such activities as holding and cuddling the infant, talking to her, and playing with her in an affectionate, relaxed way are important for her emotional growth. Experiments with animals have shown that if the infant animal does not get sufficient cuddling and physical contact from its mother during its early development, it is unable to perform adequately as an adult later in life. It has also been shown that infants growing up in an environment lacking warm, loving, close physical and emotional contact with a mother or a mother-substitute often fail to thrive and may even die.

Fondling and Sucking

During the first year, most of an infant's satisfactions and gratifications are through the skin's perception of being touched—through physical contact with her mother and other caring adults—and through the mouth, especially sucking. Infants have a great need to suck even when they are not hungry, and this sucking should be both allowed and encouraged.

Parents frequently worry that if they respond to a baby's crying by picking her up they will spoil her, and the baby will cry often in order to get attention. In general, it could be said that during its first year an infant cannot be spoiled. When an infant cries she usually does so because she is uncomfortable, hungry, sick, or needs some physical attention.

Social Responses

As she matures, one of a child's tasks is to begin to see herself as separate from the world around her. During early infancy, the infant does not see herself as an individual who is separate from her mother, from other adults, and from the rest of the world. But, gradually, some time within the first year of life, this feeling of separateness and individuality begins to emerge in the developing infant.

One of the important and gratifying events in the early months of a child's life is the smiling responses. For the first time the infant can respond in a social way to other human beings. It is often at this time that the infant's mother and father begin to think of her as a real person and an individual. Thus the smile could be considered one of the infant's first social communications.

Suspicion of Strangers

Somewhere around the age of eight months, an infant who has in the past without complaint allowed anyone to pick her up begins to distinguish her mother from other individuals. When picked up by another the infant usually cries, acts frightened, and, in general, looks unhappy. This response indicates that she can now tell her mother and other individuals apart—an important and normal step in an infant's development.

Fear of Separation

Some time later, usually around the age of one year, the infant begins to become fearful upon separation from her mother. When her mother walks out of the room or leaves the baby with a sitter, the child may respond with crying, fear, and anger. This again indicates that the infant can now tell her mother from strangers and does not like being separated from her. Although the response is normal and usually subsides within three to four months, parents should learn to leave the child in the hands of a competent sitter, and walk out without guilt or anger. The child must learn that separations are temporary and that parents do return.

The Second Year: The Toddler Stage

It is during the second year of a child's life that begins to develop independence and separateness from his mother. Beginning with his growing ability to walk, usually some time early in the second year (age 12 to 16 months), an infant starts to explore the world around him more actively. He experiments with greater and greater distances and increasing independence from his mother.

Toward the end of the second year, children frequently become quite independent, trying to do many things for themselves, and resenting their parents or other well-meaning adults doing things for them. Even if the child is not yet capable of performing the tasks he attempts, he should be encouraged in these early moves toward independence. It is also during the second year that speech begins to develop, with the child's first words usually being "ma ma," "da da," "milk," and the ever-present "no."

Developing Relationships with Mother and Father

It is in this phase of the child's life that he develops a real relationship with his mother. In most homes, mother is the loving, warm, secure comforter in his life, the giver of rewards and disciplinarian of his activities, the center of his life. During this period it is imperative that the child's father spend as much time with his son or daughter as possible, so that the child begins to recognize the difference between his relationship to his mother and father.

In some cases the father, because of the demands of business, may find it impossible to spend enough time with his family. This is an unfortunate fact, but one that can be dealt with positively, because it is the quality of the time a father spends with his child rather than the quantity that is most important.

Testing Himself and the World around Him

The toddler is insatiably curious. He wants to explore and investigate everything. Take him outdoors as much as possible. Let him meet children of his own age so that he can play and learn the beginnings of social contact.

Physically, the toddler tries to do many things apart from walking, running, and climbing—including quite a few things that he can't do. He is easily frustrated and may have a short attention span. (Girls are better than boys in this respect.) Don't be impatient with your toddler; don't punish him for his clumsiness. He has a great many experiences ahead of him, and many skills to learn and develop.

You can now expect a negative reaction to your control. Obviously, you must set limits on your child's behavior—on what is acceptable and what is not, while still giving him the freedom to express his emotions and energies in vigorous physical play.

Make the rules easy to understand so that the child will not become confused about what is expected of him. And do not set up impossible standards.

The Third Year

The third year is extremely important. Children are usually toilet trained, show marked growth in their language abilities, and demonstrate a continuing and growing independence.

Negativism

From two to about three and perhaps beyond, a child is extremely negative.

When asked to do anything or when asked about anything, he often responds by saying, "No, no, no, no, no." This saying of the word "no" on the slightest provocation indicates a child's wish to become separate and independent from parents, to do what he wants to do when he wants to do it, and to be free from the control of others.

The child's desire for independence can be respected and encouraged by parents within limits, but this does not mean that a parent must give in to a child on every issue. A parent should try to determine what is really important and not make an issue over petty matters that can best be handled with relaxed good humor.

Language Development and Play

A rapid spurt in language development takes place at this time. A child may increase his vocabulary from about 50 words at the beginning of the third year to an almost countless vocabulary at the end of the third year. It is during this year, too, that children first show marked interest in imaginative play activities. Play, including making up stories, using toy trucks and cars, blocks, dolls, and toy furniture, is vital activity for children and should be encouraged by parents. It is through play that children express their feelings, often feelings that cannot be expressed in ordinary ways. The child also experiences what it feels like to be an adult by playing the role of physician, fire fighter, police officer, teacher, mother or father. In addition, during play children discharge tensions and learn to use their muscles and bodies.

Exploring the Body

From very early infancy, all children show a strong interest in their own and in other's bodies. During infancy this takes the form of playing with his own or his mother's body. A baby puts his fingers in his own mouth, in his mother's mouth, ears, eyes, and pats her on the tummy or on the breast. An infant also explores and touches his own body, including the genital region. This interest is normal and need not be discouraged.

Dental Development

The roots of all 20 primary teeth are complete at the child's third year of life. These teeth, which began erupting between 6 and 7 months of age, are called the *central incisors*. The primary teeth, the last of which usually fall out between the eleventh and thirteenth year, are smaller and whiter than the permanent teeth, of which there are 32. The first permanent tooth erupts between 7 and 8 years of age, while the last, the third molars, or *wisdom teeth*, erupt between the seventeenth and twenty-first year.

The Preschooler

This is the age when many children go to school for part of the day and begin learning how to get along with other children in play and in organized activities. They also begin to meet adults other than their parents.

First Separation from Mother

During the ages of three and four, the preschooler develops increasing interest in the world around him, in children his own age, and in himself. One of the key problems that the preschooler has to deal with is his impending separation from his mother when he becomes old enough to go to school. This can often be made less painful by arranging for the child to spend at first short and then increasingly longer periods of time away from his mother. By using baby-sitters both in the evening and during the day, by later having the child spend three or more half-days a week at a preschool, and lastly by enrolling him in kindergarten for either all day or half a day, five days a week, the mother can ease the child's adjustment to the world outside the home.

Although his first nearly full-time separation from mother is difficult for the child, it may be difficult for the mother as well. Mothers often feel that this initial separation from their child will eventually lead to their child's growing up and leaving home. Parents are often nostalgic and somewhat regretful about their children's first going off full time to school. The child's fearful anticipation of a strange situation can be eased by a mother's anticpating school with the child, talking with him about it and reassuring him regarding his fears of abandonment or separation.

Differences between Boys and Girls

A word might be mentioned here concerning differences between boys and girls. At the age of five most girls are ready to attend kindergarten; they can sit in their seats for long periods of time, pay attention to a teacher, and be interested in a task. Boys, because of their somewhat slower rate of maturity, are often less ready than girls for coping with a classroom situation at the age of five.

A child of five grows at a slower rate than in earlier years, but his body is nonetheless changing. The protruding abdomen and knock-knees of the toddler begin to disappear.

Television

Students of the medium suggest that television offers some worthwhile programs for the young child. At the same time, the experts warn that television watching can, over time, become addictive. A basically passive experience, it may also decrease the quality of family life and raise early obstacles to literacy and learning.

The parent's main task, insofar as television watching is concerned, is to find ways to use "the tube" to help the child develop. Parents can, for example, turn on programs that their child enjoys, that do not frighten or overexcite, and that the toddler can learn from. The television should not be used as an "electronic baby-sitter"; as much as possible, parents should watch when their child does. If a child is 18 months old or older the experts say parents should select the special programs they want their child to see. Television should not, finally, be used as a reward for being good. Such an approach can suggest the TV is more important than interesting games and other worthwhile activities.

Personal Hygiene

Good habits of cleanliness should be established. The child should know that hand-washing before meals is essential even when the hands look clean. He will learn this only if he sees parents do it. As he gets older he should select his own clean clothing and know that dirty clothing should be washed. A daily routine of washing or bathing should be set up, and the child should be encouraged to observe it.

School-Age Children: Parent–Child Relationships

Beginning around the age of four, boys show a decided preference for their mothers. A boy may, for example, tell his mother that when he grows up he would like to marry her

and kick father out of the house. At times he may even suggest that he would work to support her and that life would be much nicer if daddy were not around.

This interest in his mother is often expressed in what may be thought of as sexual ways. That is, the child of this age enjoys his mother's affection, including kissing, hugging, and close bodily contact. This wish to have mother all to himself and to have father out of the picture is called the *Oedipal complex* by psychiatrists and psychologists, after the ancient Greek tragedy, *Oedipus Rex*, in which Oedipus kills his father and marries a woman whom he later discovers to be his mother.

At about this same age, similar emotional developments take place in a girl. She will likely be somewhat seductive, coy, and coquettish with her father, and may talk about marrying father (or a man like father) and having mother out of the picture. This phase of emotional attachment between a girl and her father is called the *Electra complex* after the Greek play, *Electra*.

At these times, both the girl and the boy have a strong, although not always conscious, wish to displace the parent of the same sex and have the opposite-sexed parent all to themselves. Strong conflicts disturb children in this phase of development, for they also realize that they love and need the same-sexed parent to instruct them, to guide them, to provide for them, and to love them.

Identification

Both males and females eventually resolve these conflicts by abandoning their so-called sexual attachment to the opposite-sexed parent, forming a closer attachment to the same-sexed parent and trying to be like that parent. This is not a conscious decision,

but one that a child makes without realizing it. This process of *identification* with the parent of the same sex starts very early, perhaps as early as the second year, and continues through adolescence, but it is especially noticable from five to ten.

Much of the energy that had previously been utilized in loving the parent of the opposite sex is now spent in loving the parent of the same sex. The boy follows father around, wants to do whatever he does, and holds as his greatest ambition to be exactly like father when he grows up—even to marrying a woman like the one father did.

The girl during this same period spends the energy that was once expended in love for her father in an attempt to learn to be like mother and perhaps eventually to marry a man resembling in some way her father. This, however, does not mean that children do not continue to love the opposite-sexed parent; it means only that their primary attachment during these years is to the same-sexed parent. It is this process of identification with the same-sexed parent that facilitates the chief task of the school-age child from 5 or 6 to 11: the task of learning.

Six Years to Adolescence

The years from 6 to 11 have generally been regarded as quiet years as far as emotional development is concerned. Many of the tasks of earlier childhood have been completed, and the relatively stormy years of adolescence have not yet begun. A child's interests begin to turn more and more away from his family and to other children his own age, usually children of the same sex. At this stage, a child's interest in learning is broad and intense.

During this period children begin to be more and more individualistic. Some are solitary, others sociable; some are athletic, others not. One likes only other children, another prefers the company of adults. Some children have imaginary fears that disappear with age or when the fears are discussed with an adult who can explain how or why they originated.

Curiosity about Sex

The child's earlier curiosity about naked people may change to a concern about being clothed and being with people who are clothed. Questions about sex should be answered simply and truthfully.

Adolescence

Adolescence arrives anywhere from 9 to 14 years of age. A girl usually enters adolescence at 10, a boy at about 12. Adolescence lasts through the teens.

In female children, there is growth of the breasts and nipples; the pelvis matures, and the external genitalia develop. Axillary (underarm) and pubic hair appear. On the average, girls have their first menstrual period around age thirteen, but it can occur between 10 and 16 years of age. Be sure to explain menstruation to your daughter before the beginning of adolescence.

In male children, the penis and testes develop. Facial, axillary, and pubic hair appear. The voice begins to deepen.

In both boys and girls, there is a rapid growth in height and weight which is related to sexual development. In general the average height of the adolescent is double what is was at age two. See Ch. 3, *The Teens.*

Alphabetic Guide to Child Care

The following Guide is an alphabetically arranged list of articles dealing with many of the problems that confront parents. It includes articles on physical disorders and ailments of childhood; behavioral and emotional problems; and on situations that occur normally in the life of almost every child which may cause tension or distress for parents, child, or both. It is hoped that having information about such normal developmental tensions will help to minimize them.

A note on the cross-references: Where a particular subject is covered elsewhere within this Guide, the reference is printed in small capital letters. (For example: See also TONSILLITIS.) References to sections in other chapters are printed in italic type along with the chapter number. (For example: See "Tonsils and Adenoids" in Ch. 20, *Surgery*.)

Accidents

All children have accidents and injure themselves. Some do more frequently or more seriously than others. Parents should treat the ones that are minor and seek immediate medical attention for ones that are major. The parents' response to an injury can greatly determine the child's response to it. Calm, responsible behavior will keep the child calmer, even in a serious accident.

For minor injuries such as cuts and bruises, treatment can be completed at home. Cuts and scrapes should be washed thoroughly with warm (not hot) water and 3 percent hydrogen peroxide. A skin disinfectant can be applied, only if the cut is not deep. A bandage should be applied during the day to keep dirt out. The cut should be left uncovered when possible, though, to allow it to dry and heal. Once the cut or scrape has scabbed over, a bandage need not be used, unless the scab is damaged or tears off.

Sprains, unless very minor, are difficult to treat at home. It is not likely that a parent can determine the damage to muscle tissue. Sprains can be more painful than breaks and can inflict severe damage to ligaments and tendons. X rays are usually required to determine the damage done to the limb.

Minor sprains that show slight swelling or discoloration of the skin can be treated by applying ice to the injured area as soon as possible after the accident. Keep the limb elevated for ten to twenty minutes with the ice pack on the injured joint. Have the child avoid using the limb for a while. Once movement can be made without serious pain, warm water soaks or baths will help reduce swelling. If pain persists for more than 24 hours, consult a physician.

Bruises are caused by bleeding under the surface of the skin with no cut to the surface of the skin. Black eyes are bruises under the eye tissue. Minor bruises can be treated with cold water or ice packs to the area hurt. (Eyes should receive only water packs, ice against the eye is not recommended.) As the bruise fades a purple or yellow tint to the skin will remain for a few days or so as the body removes the last of the dried blood from the bruised tissue. Bruises can take several days to fade and heal. If it takes longer, a doctor should be consulted.

Head injuries in children are also common. A sharp blow to the head, or a fall, can trigger vomiting in a child. This, in itself, is not a danger signal. Danger signals are:

- Both pupils in eyes not dilated equally.
- Eyes do not move together when following something.
- Child sleeps immediately, or is hard to waken during a nap. Any child should be awakened every three hours to check, for 24 hours after the accident.
- More than one episode of vomiting.
- Any sign of mental disorder—speech or movement difficulties, dazed focus or attention, or any type of non-response.
- Increasing headache.
- Blood or fluid from nose or ears. If any one of these symptoms appear, contact the local hospital emergency facilities immediately.

For more information, see Ch. 35, *Medical Emergencies,* and "The Emergency Room" in Ch. 20, *Surgery.*

Adenoidectomy

See "Tonsils and Adenoids" in Ch. 20, *Surgery.*

Adenoids, Swollen

The adenoids are clusters of lymph tissue located behind the soft palate where the nasal passages join the throat. Along with the tonsils and lymphoid tissues elsewhere in the body, the adenoids are involved in warding off infection. When they themselves become inflamed because of bacterial or viral invasion, they become swollen. Swelling may also occur because of allergy.

Swollen adenoids may block the air passages sufficiently to cause mouth breathing, which in turn will not only give the child an "adenoidal" look, but will lead to more frequent upper respiratory infection, as well as to eventual malformation of the lower jawbone. Chronic swelling may also block the eustachian tube, causing pain in

the ear and increasing the possibility of ear infection as well as of intermittent hearing loss. The child's physician can keep track of the severity of such symptoms during periodic checkups and can evaluate the need for surgery. See also TONSILLITIS. For a description of adenoidectomy, see "Tonsils and Adenoids" in Ch. 20, *Surgery.*

Adopted Children

No matter what their individual differences about child rearing, all specialists agree that an adopted child should be told that she was adopted. It doesn't matter that the adoptive parents have come to feel that the child is completely their own. Biologically, she isn't, and it is her human right to find this out not from a neighbor or schoolmate but from the people she trusts as her parents. The fact of her adoption should be talked about naturally in the child's presence even before she can understand what it means. If she is being raised in a loving atmosphere and feels secure in the acceptance of her adoptive parents, she isn't likely to be upset by the reality of her situation.

When the child becomes curious about the circumstances of her adoption, or if she wants to know about her "real" mother and father, she should be given no more—and no less—information than the adoption agency provided originally.

A widow or divorcee who remarries when her children are still very young may be faced with the possibility that her second husband wants to legally adopt the offspring of her first marriage. Far-reaching consequences are involved in such a decision, and it should not be undertaken lightly. The problem should be discussed with a lawyer who can present the facts in a detached way so that the decision will

cause the least anguish and fewest unpleasant consequences.

Aggressiveness

In the rough and tumble of play, some puppies are obviously more aggressive than others, and one of them is clearly determined to be top dog. The same is true of children, especially in any society where energy and enterprise are rewarded.

Aggressive tendencies are natural; the form they take is up to the civilizing efforts of the parents. It is they who have the responsibility of helping a child understand that bullying and bossiness are unacceptable. It seems that because of inheritance, body build, or temperament, some youngsters, whether male or female, are more clearly aggressive than others. It is especially for such children that healthy outlets must be provided for aggression—in the form of toys and playground activities when they are little, and in suitable physical and intellectual endeavors when they get older.

Guilt Feelings

Making a child feel guilty about the strength of his aggressive feelings or thwarting them constantly won't wipe out or destroy the feelings; they'll simply be turned inward, or take the form of nail-biting, or express themselves in some sneaky and antisocial way. Parents who are upset by children's play that simulates violence and who disapprove of toy guns should make their feelings clear without making the youngster feel like a monster because he enjoys them. Aggressiveness that expresses itself in violence and bloodshed—as it so often does in Westerns and in TV programs—should not be the day-in-day-out entertainment to which children are exposed no matter what the parental feelings are.

Boy/Girl Differences

As for a boy who doesn't seem aggressive enough to suit a parent's idea of what a boy should be, or a girl who seems too aggressive to conform to family notions about what "feminine" is all about: these stereotypes are being reexamined and discarded by many people because they are too confining and too rigid to permit the full development of a child's personality. It's no disgrace for a boy to cry, and it should be a source of pride to have a daughter who's determined to be the best math student in the fourth grade.

Allergies

See NUTRITION, and Ch. 24, *Allergies and Hypersensitivities*.

Anger

Anger is a feeling that everyone is familiar with. There are moments when even the most controlled and civilized adult experiences the kind of anger that might become blind rage. A child whose bike has been stolen has a right to her anger; a child whose baby brother has broken a valuable doll is justifiably angry. Some youngsters seem to be angry all the time because they feel they're always being pushed around by adults. (Many adults are always angry because they feel they're being pushed around by other adults.) Almost continuous anger seems especially common among some children of six, seven, and eight. Their theme song is "It isn't fair" and they get to be known as injustice-collectors, angry at their friends, siblings, teachers.

Means of Expressing Anger

When parents know that a child's anger comes from a healthy feeling of outrage or because of confusion, they should allow the anger to be expressed—in words or tears. But it does have to be made clear that smashing things in a fit of rage or having a tantrum is unacceptable. A child at the mercy of powerful feelings of rage can be frightened by them and should be helped to understand and control them. It's also a comfort to children to know that grown-ups get terribly angry from time to time, but that part of growing up consists in being able to handle one's feelings and in learning how to express them in the right way at the right time. Thus, a father who is in a rage with his boss will find ways of letting him know that he feels an injustice has been done rather than swallow his anger at work and let it out against his wife or children as soon as he comes home.

Animal Bites

See "Animal Bites" in Ch. 35, *Medical Emergencies*.

Anxiety

Children become chronically anxious when their parents constantly criticize them for failing to measure up to some unachievable standard of perfection. Likewise, parents become anxious about being parents when they criticize themselves for failing to measure up to some unachievable standard of perfection.

Anxiety is one of the most widespread and most debilitating stresses from which people of all ages suffer in the United States, chiefly because many Americans have been victimized by the notion that everybody can be everything. Thus, a parent will expect a little child to be good, bright, neat, polite, aggressive enough to complete adequately but not so aggressive that the other children don't like him, relaxed and cheerful at the same time that he's supposed to do all his chores and the homework and remember to be nice to his baby-sister. What child burdened with such expectations isn't going to feel anxious about fulfilling them so that he can gain his parents' love and approval?

Parents may waste emotional energy feeling anxious because they think they're inadequate mothers or fathers, perhaps because they lose their tempers from time to time or because they're often too tired to play with their toddler and stick him in the playpen just to keep him out of trouble. A child will also be made chronically anxious if he's always being threatened with punishment, or if he's made to feel that he's bad when he's trying to be good but doesn't know how. The way to keep anxiety at a minimum is to have achievable goals. Is the child healthy, moderately well-behaved, cheerful, and inspiring no complaints from his teachers? Are you as a parent helping him to be healthy, moderately well-behaved, cheerful, and cause no trouble at school? If pressure on the child is small, and he still seems anxious, counseling may be considered.

Asthma

Asthma, also known as *bronchial asthma*, is a respiratory disturbance in which breathing becomes difficult and labored and is accompanied by a wheezing sound. It is a chronic disorder in which the bronchial tubes suddenly contract or go into spasm, thus cutting off the passage of air from the windpipe to the lungs. Spasms are accompanied by secretion of mucus into the air passages and a swelling of the bronchial tubes, causing the intake and outflow of air to be further obstructed. The disorder may be triggered by a variety of factors; in children it is associated chiefly with allergy and emotional stress. In some cases, asthma may accompany a bacterial or viral infection of the nose or throat.

The Asthma Attack

It can be very frightening to witness a child's first asthma attack, because judging from the sounds and the effort involved in breathing, the child seems to be suffocating. Call the child's pediatrician promptly. Until the physician can be consulted for emergency treatment, parents should try to be calm and reassuring. Immediate symptoms can be alleviated by prescribed medicines given orally or by injection, or by placing the child in a moist environment, such as in the bathroom with the shower turned on (but not *in* the shower). Otherwise, the child should be kept in bed in a humidified room. The condition itself should be carefully assessed by the physician to decide whether desensitization to a particular food or pollen is necessary, whether a pet has to be given away, or whether the child's emotional needs are being neglected. Chronic asthma should not go untreated because frequent and acute attacks can affect general health. Medicines now available can sometimes prevent acute attacks if taken daily by inhalation when one is well.

Autism

See under MENTAL ILLNESS.

Baby-sitters

Families who can always count on a grandparent or an older child to look after the little ones in their absence are spared the complications and expense of hiring baby-sitters. How-

ever, many parents must rely on their own resources, especially when both parents work. In such situations the sitter has become an indispensable adjunct of the family.

Instruction in Baby-sitting

All aspects of the sitter's responsibilities and privileges should be covered. Does the sitter do the dinner dishes? May local phone calls be made? May the refrigerator be raided? The potential employees should be encouraged to ask all the questions they feel uncertain about. Instructions should include a list of hourly rates with all variants: base rate per hour; increase in rate after midnight; increase per number of children to be looked after, and so on.

Cooperative Sitting

For families who want to get out occasionally but can't afford the extra expense of a sitter, a cooperative parents' pool is a good solution. Each month, one participating parent is responsible for keeping track of who had been sitting for whom, how many hours are owed and how many have been "paid for" and so on. The advantage of this arrangement is that mothers or fathers sit for each others' children and no money changes hands. If such a cooperative pool is worked out, remember that the more accurately the records of time asked for and given are kept, and the more businesslike the arrangements, the longer the system will work and the less friction there will be. Each group should decide for itself what the maximum number of participants should be, and as the group becomes too large to function efficiently, it can split into two separate pools.

Provide for Emergencies

Parents should always leave clear and explicit instructions about possible emergencies with baby-sitters and if possible should leave a telephone number where they can be reached. As the children become opinionated about hired sitters, their wishes should be taken into account. When your own youngsters begin to be hired as sitters themselves, you should keep track of where they're working and when they'll be escorted home. Meet the family for whom they will be sitting, *before* the first sitting.

Beds

Infants should not be left on a full size bed to nap. Because the mattress does not fit snugly against the frame or the wall, a child risks becoming wedged between the mattress and the solid object and suffocating. Crib mattresses are designed to fit tightly against the frame, avoiding the risk of suffocation. To further protect an infant from suffocation, he should not be given a pillow while napping or sleeping. An infant who rolls over and is unable to lift his head may suffocate in the pillow.

Bedtime

From babyhood on, the routine of bedtime should be as relaxed as possible for both parent and child. Little babies love to be chanted to (even off-key) or talked to in a gentle tone of voice (even though they don't understand the words) or rocked a bit in their crib. Some little ones seem to resist and fight falling asleep: they fuss and whimper, and then, as though they had been bewitched in the middle of a cry—off they go, all of a sudden. Toddlers may want to hear the same story every night for months, or may cling to the bedtime bottle for quite a while after they've begun to use a cup in the daytime.

Keeping things peaceful at bedtime doesn't mean giving in to the child's pressures or whims. It generally involves keeping one's voice calm, pleasant, and firm: "It's bedtime, and you tell me which story to read to you tonight." The youngster who keeps calling out after having been tucked in—for water, for a last hug, for a last question, for a last trip to the bathroom—isn't determined to make a nuisance of herself; she's just a little scared and wants to make absolutely sure that you're still there. If the family tradition calls for prayers at bedtime, the tone should be cheerful. No child can be expected to relish, "And if I die before I wake I pray the Lord my soul to take" as an accompaniment to sleep.

In a crowded family where siblings share a bedroom, compromises have to be made about the bedtime hour: the younger ones may stay up a little later than they otherwise would, and the older ones may go to bed a little earlier—but they have the pleasure of each other's company. Adjustments in the bedtime hour should be made from time to time not because of a child's wheedling, but because you decide that the occasion calls for it.

Bedwetting

See "Bedwetting" in Ch. 17, *Disease of the Urinogenital System.*

Behavior Problems

See AGGRESSIVENESS, ANGER, DELINQUENCY, DESTRUCTIVENESS, DISHONESTY, DISOBEDIENCE.

Birthmarks

See "Pigment Disorders and Birthmarks" in Ch. 21, *Skin and Hair.*

Biting

Some children learn that their strongest weapon when angry is their teeth. They may bite siblings, friends, and occasionally parents. Because of the enormous risk of infection from the bite, and because it can inflict extreme pain to the person bitten, biting should be strongly discouraged by any child.

Blindness

See DISABLED CHILD.

Booster Shots

See IMMUNIZATION.

Boredom

Babies are usually too hungry or too sleepy—or too cranky—to be bored. Toddlers have so much to investigate around the house that boredom is not likely to be one of their problems. As a child gets older and complains about having nothing to do, you might get him involved in a household chore by saying, "Let's . . ." rather than "Why don't you" or "How would you like to." "Let's tidy the cans on the pantry shelf" or "Let's make some cookies" can make a three-year-old feel useful and interested.

Rainy Days

If you're too busy for a cooperative effort and there's a long rainy day ahead, provide for it in advance by keeping a "boredom box" in the closet and renewing its contents from time to time: wrappings saved from gifts; bits of material; boxes of various sizes; discarded magazines to be cut up; old clothes for dress-up activities, and the like.

Coping with Boredom Can be Productive

A child who is never allowed to be bored because his parents or older siblings feel that they have to entertain him or play with him is deprived of the possibility of calling on his own resources and learning how to amuse himself. The fact that an only child may have to live through stretches of boredom often contributes to his exploring his own abilities in a creative way. Sometimes just asking a child to "Tell *me* a story" can work wonders. Some parents solve the recurrent problem of boredom by organizing informal play groups of three or four children; others find a nursery school the best solution.

Convalescence

An older child who is recovering from an illness that has kept him out of school and isolated him from his friends may require some special project to work on in addition to catching up on his homework. A period of protracted convalescence is a good time to introduce a new hobby or craft such as model-making or clay sculpture that may solve the boredom problem for years to come.

Brain Damage

Brain damage refers to an organic defect of the brain—that is, tissue destruction—caused by an injury to the nervous system occurring before, during, or after birth. Such injury can be caused by toxic chemicals as well as by physical trauma. It can result in any of a variety of neurological disorders, such as cerebral palsy or other impairment of motor coordination, mental retardation, convulsive seizures, hyperkinesis, or perceptual difficulties.

Minimal Brain Damage

Minimal brain damage (or, more formally, *minimal brain dysfunction*) refers to a condition of some children who suffer from a motor or perceptual impairment that may affect their ability to learn or use language, interfere with memory, or make it difficult for them to control their attention. Some learning disabilities are attributed to minimal brain damage. See also DYSLEXIA.

Brothers and Sisters

Rivalry and jealousy and bickering are inevitable among brothers and sisters; companionship, a helping hand, and good times together are part of the picture too. Parents can keep resentments and quarrels at a minimum by not playing one child off against the other or by refraining from holding up one child as an example of virtue to another. In an atmosphere of equal recognition, brothers and sisters will love and respect each other most of the time and fight only occasionally. Special privileges granted on the basis of such distinctions as "Well, he's the oldest" or "She's the youngest" or exceptions made because "He's a boy" or "She's only a girl" can cause resentments that last a lifetime.

Burns

See "Burns" in Ch. 35, *Medical Emergencies.*

Camps

There seems to be no end to the diversity of camps available for summer enrollment. Most urban and suburban communities have day camps in which children may be accepted for certain minimum periods. They range from expensive groups that offer sightsee-ing trips, swimming instruction, and other special attractions to groups that cost very little and function more or less like day-care centers. "Sleepaway" camps run by organizations such as the Scouts and the 4-H Clubs are comparatively cheap and will register a child for a week rather than for a month or for the entire summer. Camps subsidized by community funds or private endowment are available for urban children from poor families.

Special Camps

The proliferation of special camps has been a blessing to the parents of handicapped children: those with diabetes, muscular dystrophy, learning disabilities, obesity, and other problems need no longer be deprived of a camping experience with their peers. In many cases, particularly for overweight youngsters, the summer experience can be a major health contribution.

In general, an effort should be made to choose a camp that suits the tastes and temperament of the child. A youngster who hates competitive sports is likely to have a miserable time in a camp that emphasizes team spirit. He may enjoy a place that offers lots of nature study, hiking, and animal care. A child eager to improve his swimming should go to a camp with better-than-average water sport facilities rather than one that concentrates on arts and crafts and offers only a nearby pond for all water activities. Information about camps that have official standing can be obtained by writing to The American Camping Association, 5000 State Rd., 67 N, Martinsdale, IN 46151.

Cancer

Rare as it may be and affecting only one child in about 7,000 each year, cancer still claims the lives of more children between the ages of one and fourteen than any other single disease. Among the cancers that more commonly affect children in their early years are the following: *acute lymphocytic leukemia,* in which white blood cells proliferate in the bone marrow in such great quantities that they disrupt normal blood production; *neuroblastoma,* which may occur in any part of the body but characteristically involves a tumorous growth in the sympathetic nerve tissues of the adrenal glands; *brain* or *spinal cord tumor; Hodgkin's disease,* or cancer of the lymph nodes; *Wilms' tumor,* a rare kidney cancer that accounts for about one-fifth of all childhood cancers; *retinoblastoma,* an eye tumor that is probably hereditary and is most frequently encountered in children under four; and *bone cancer* that may attack the long bones of the forearm and leg during the growing years. Many of these cancers can now be arrested, and some can be cured if symptoms are detected early enough. See Ch. 18, *Cancer,* for further information about cancer.

Early Symptoms

Early detection is best accomplished by calling to a physician's attention any of these symptoms that last for more than a few days: continued crying or pain for which there appears to be no explanation; intermittent nausea and vomiting; the development of lumps or swellings in or on any part of the child's body; stumbling or walking unsteadily; a loss of appetite and general lassitude; any marked change in bowel or bladder habits; any unexplained discharge of blood, whether in the stool or urine, or in heavy nosebleeds, or any marked slowness of bleeding to stop after an injury.

Celiac Disease

Celiac disease, officially known as *malabsorption syndrome*, is the designation for a group of congenital enzyme deficiencies in which certain nutriments are not properly absorbed from the intestinal tract. *Celiac* means having to do with the abdomen. Celiac disease is characterized by frothy, bulky, and foul-smelling stools containing undigested fats. Diarrhea may alternate with constipation, the child has severe stomach cramps, and the abdomen becomes conspicuously bloated. If the disease is untreated, anemia results, and the child's growth is impaired. Early symptoms should be brought to a physician's attention so that a correct diagnosis can be made based on laboratory investigation of the stools. Treatment consists of a special, gluten-free diet under a physician's continuing supervision. *Gluten* is a protein component of wheat and rye; special breads, cookies, etc., must therefore be used. If the diet is strictly adhered to, full recovery can be expected although it may take over a year.

Cerebral Palsy

Cerebral palsy is the general term for a group of abnormal conditions commonly associated with a brain disorder that causes the loss or impairment of muscle control. Approximately one child in about 7,000 suffers from some degree of this disability. Damage to the nervous system that results in cerebral palsy may have occurred before birth, during delivery, or in rare cases, as a consequence of accident, injury, or severe illness during infancy or childhood. Because symptoms vary widely, each individual case is assessed for proper treatment by a team of therapists under the supervision of a specialist, usually a pediatrician. One of the most important aspects of treatment involves parental understanding of the fact that it is essential that they help the child to help himself as much as possible. Guiding the youngster towards self-acceptance and independence requires the patience, persistence, and resourcefulness of the entire family, and may require a certain amount of group therapy and counseling. For a discussion of symptoms and treatment, see "Cerebral Palsy" in Ch. 8, *Diseases of the Muscles and Nervous System*.

Cheating

See DISHONESTY.

Checkups

Medical and dental checkups are essential to everyone's health, but they are especially important for the growing child. An infant should be examined by a physician every month for the first six months, and less frequently after that. The pediatrician usually recommends a schedule for immunization and future checkups. If possible, parents should try to maintain continuity with the same physician so that when an illness occurs, the child sees the physician as an old friend rather than a threatening stranger. Continuity also gives the physician a total picture of the child in sickness and in health and enables him to diagnose variations from the normal with more accuracy. Parents who cannot afford the services of a private physician can be assured of good infant and child care at a local child-health station or at the well-baby clinic of a nearby hospital. Between checkups, it's a good idea for parents to keep a running list of questions or problems they would like to discuss with the doctor at the next visit.

Chicken Pox

Chicken pox cannot be prevented at this time. It does \not usually cause any severe complications in a child, but it can be serious in an adult. It is highly infectious and spreads rapidly.

Chicken pox is caused by a virus. Its incubation period is two to three weeks. Symptoms include those of the common cold, a fever, general malaise, and a rash.

The rash, which may be either mild or severe, is different from that produced by measles or by rubella. The measles rash is red and blotchy. Chicken pox has bunches of blisters close together. These blisters are filled with fluid, and there is a reddened area around each lesion. As new blisters appear, the older ones become encrusted. The rash may affect the mouth, nose, ears, vagina, penis, or scrotum. In an older child the symptoms may be more severe than in a younger one, and may be accompanied by headache and vomiting.

Treatment

The only way to treat chicken pox is symptomatically. The rash is very itchy, and an affected child must be prevented from scratching. Otherwise, he may develop a secondary infection and be left pitted and scarred.

Treatment involves the use of lotions, such as Calamine, applied locally to the pox to relieve the itching. If the child is old enough, it's a good idea to let him paint it on himself. Your physician may also prescribe medicine to be taken orally to help the child stop scratching the blisters. In a few days, the rash clears up, the lesions dry, and the crusts fall off.

Child Abuse and Neglect

Child abuse and neglect have been defined in various ways.

In 1962, Dr. C. Henry Kempe, chief pediatrician at the University of Colorado Medical Center, coined the term *battered child syndrome*. According to Dr. Kempe's definition, the victim of battering is "any child who [has] received *nonaccidental* injury or injuries as a result of acts or omissions on the part of his parents or guardians." Under the Child Abuse Prevention and Treatment Act (Public Law 93-247), passed by Congress in 1974 and amended in 1978, child abuse and neglect are defined as

> the physical or mental injury, sexual abuse or exploitation, negligent treatment, or maltreatment of a child under the age of 18 by a person who is responsible for the child's welfare under circumstances which indicate that the child's health or welfare is harmed or threatened thereby.

Abuse and neglect clearly take many forms. *Physical abuse* may involve punching, scalding, suffocating, headcracking, and stomping. *Sexual abuse* can mean intercourse, incest, rape, sodomy, or impairing of a minor's morals (see SEXUAL ABUSE). *Physical neglect* occurs when parents or parent surrogates fail to provide the essentials of a normal life. These include food, clothing, shelter, care, and supervision. Under *emotional abuse or neglect* authorities include parental failure to provide love and proper direction, parental rejection, and deprivation of mothering.

Incidence

Figures on the incidence of child abuse and neglect are difficult to confirm. Many such cases are never reported. At least one agency, the National Center on Child Abuse and Neglect, a federal agency, has concluded that more than one million children are maltreated each year. Another estimate indicates that some 3,000 children die annually in New York City alone as a result of physical abuse.

Most of the abuse victims are three years old or younger. Some authorities believe that the cases of neglect are far more numerous than those of actual abuse.

Control

Approaches to control of the problem of child abuse and neglect have been both legislative and social. Laws passed by all 50 states require physicians and other professionals to report suspected cases of child abuse. In increasing numbers the states also require reports from nurses, teachers, counselors, social workers, clergymen, law enforcement officers, attorneys, and coroners. Some states provide for penalties, including fines up to $1,000 or prison sentences of as much as one year, for persons mandated to report but failing to do so.

Control measures have focused in addition on the rehabilitation of abusive parents and protection of abused children. The National Center on Child Abuse and Neglect, established in 1974 as part of the Children's Bureau of the federal Office of Child Development, receives funding that makes possible protective services for the short-term care of endangered children outside the home. The Center also provides counseling for parents, foster-care payments, and other services.

On the principle that the abusive parent must be treated if child abuse and neglect are to be controlled, various organizations have instituted parent-oriented programs. Parents Anonymous sponsors therapy sessions in which abusive parents can meet to help themselves and each other. "Helplines" operating in many communities offer aid and counseling to parents who have abused a child but are afraid to contact a social service or other agency. A number of other agencies and groups provide emergency, counseling, outreach, and related services to parents or parent surrogates. Some helplines have workers available to visit homes in life-threatening situations.

Other groups and agencies take a multidisciplinary approach. Alliance, a division of Catholic Charities, brings together existing community agencies that work together in teams to treat child abuse and neglect cases. Hospital-based treatment programs may include a physician, nurse, social worker, and consulting psychiatrist. Lay therapists may visit homes under other programs, and "foster grandparents" over 65 years of age may be recruited to care for battered children who have been hospitalized.

Sources of Help

Persons seeking help or advice on abused and neglected children can look in their communities' yellow pages under the heading "Social Services Organizations." A number of organizations that offer assistance are listed in the SEXUAL ABUSE section. Others include:

- Parents Anonymous, 1733 South Sepulveda, Ste. 270, Los Angeles, CA 90045; 213/410-9732.

- American Association for Protecting Children (a division of the American Humane Association), 9725 E. Hampden Ave., Denver, CO 80231; 303/695-0811.

- Parents without Partners, 8807 Colesville Rd., Silver Springs, MD 20910; 301/588-9354.

- Parents United, P.O. Box 952, San Jose, CA 95108; 408/279-1957.

Cholesterol

Cholesterol poses two types of problems in children. The first is a lack of cholesterol in children whose parents have kept them from infancy on low cholesterol diets. Parents should keep in mind that the body requires some cholesterol to function correctly and that the protein derived from meat and eggs is almost essential to growing bodies. Children who are not fed meat, dairy products, or eggs need to have the protein, amino acids, and other nutrients replaced by either pills or a very well balanced diet. Certain vitamins cannot be found in a vegetarian diet, such as one type of vitamin B. Children on restrictive low-fat, low-cholesterol diets can suffer growth failure and malnutrition unless the diet is supervised by a doctor.

The second problem is an extremely elevated cholesterol level. Although general testing of children for high cholesterol is not recommended, one statistic that proved reliable in spotting 9 out of 10 children with raised levels was the amount of television watched. Children who watched two or more hours of television a day were more likely to have cholesterol levels exceeding 200 mg. More importantly, less than half of those children who had raised levels and watched two hours of television came from families who had a history of high cholesterol. This means that these children are not from high-risk families, but they still manage to increase their cholesterol because of their eating patterns and lack of exercise in their daily routine. The flag that points to the problem is excessive TV viewing. Snacking while watching TV, and not exercising, are the suspected culprits.

Circumcision

Circumcision is a surgical procedure in which the foreskin, or *prepuce*, that covers the cone-shaped tip of the male infant's penis is removed. The Book of Genesis speaks of circumcision as a religious rite. Once relatively common in the United States, the procedure has become more rare. The American Academy of Pediatrics has stated that "routine circumcision of the newborn infant lacks medical justification."

Usually performed a few days after birth, the procedure takes only a few minutes and can be done in various ways. A scalpel may be used, for example. Possible complications include excessive bleeding, infection, and urinary obstruction resulting from contraction of the skin at the base of the foreskin. But complications are infrequent.

The parents of the newborn male infant should decide whether to have their son circumcised or not. They may first consult their obstetrician or pediatrician. Most decisions are made on the basis of family, religious, or cultural traditions. Many family health insurance policies today provide no coverage for the procedure.

Cleft Palate and Cleft Lip

A *cleft palate* is a split in the roof of the mouth sometimes extending to the lip and into the nose. The split is caused by the failure of the two sides of the face to unite properly during prenatal development. The condition occurs in about 1 out of 1,000 births and is sometimes associated with a foot or spine deformity. It is in no way related to mental retardation.

An infant born with a cleft palate cannot suck properly unless a special device, called an *obturator*, is inserted into the split to close it against the flow of air. Where this is undesirable, feeding may be done with a spoon or a dropper.

Because the condition eventually causes speech distortion, it should be corrected at about 18 months of age, before the child begins to talk. The surgery consists of reconstructing the tissue. Sometimes, even at this early age, the child may need some corrective speech therapy following the operation.

If the split occurs only in the lip, commonly called a *harelip*, surgery may be recommended when the infant weighs about 15 pounds, usually at the age of 12 to 15 months. When the operation is performed this early, there is no danger of speech impairment, and the result is only a thin scar.

Clothing

Standards have been set up the U.S. government for infants' and children's sleepwear to be flame retardant or flame resistant. Even flame retardant material, though, will burn when fire is held against the cloth. The difference is that when the flame is removed, the retardant material ceases to burn. Nontreated material will continue to burn and fuel further flames.

Until recently this meant that sleepwear for small children had to be non-natural fibers. Synthetic material could be coated so that it would not continue to burn after the flame was removed. Cotton does continue to burn and increases the likelihood of serious injuries to a child in case of fire. However, recent improvements in chemical treatment of cotton has provided the clothing industry with flame retardant cotton. Check clothing labels to see if the cotton is treated. If it is not labeled as flame retardant or resistent, it should not be considered for sleepwear.

Labeling should be checked on all clothing to be used as sleepwear.

Many manufacturers produce clothing for infants that looks like sleepwear but is labeled daywear or playwear to avoid the need for flame retardant treatment of the cloth. If the clothing is not marked flame retardant, or is not specifically labeled as sleepwear, it should not be used to clothe a sleeping child.

Clubfoot

Clubfoot is a bone deformity characterized by an inturning or outturning of the foot. An orthopedist must put the clubfoot and part of the leg into a cast to correct the condition. If casting does not cure the abnormality, orthopedic surgery may be necessary.

Occasionally, a benign and easily correctable condition involving a child's legs may have been produced by the position the baby was in while still in the uterus.

The mother can help to correct the condition by daily passive exercises of the baby's feet. She does this by turning the feet correctly for a few minutes every day. To maintain the corrected position, the application of plaster is sometimes necessary. Such a procedure requires the attention of an orthopedic surgeon.

Colic

During the first three or four months, many babies have occasional attacks of *colic*, a general term applied to infantile digestive discomfort. After feeding, the baby may cry out in pain and draw up her arms and legs. Her abdomen may feel hard. Apart from making sure the baby is as comfortable as can be, there's not much that can be done for colic. You must try not to let the baby's crying make you a nervous wreck, for your nervousness will be communicated to the baby, which will only create a vicious circle of increasing tension. Usually

colic tapers off at about the third month. If the baby's colic attacks are very frequent or persistent, consult your pediatrician.

Color Blindness

Color blindness is a genetic inability to distinguish between certain colors, most commonly between red and green. This defect, which is characteristically male, is inherited through the mother. That is, a woman whose father was color blind can pass the trait to her son without herself suffering the defect. About 8 million people in the United States have the red/green form of color blindness which can neither be cured nor corrected. Many of them are scarcely aware of their deficiency. Parents who suspect that their child may have this minor disability can arrange for simple testing.

Common Cold

By recent count, there are about 150 different viruses that cause common cold symptoms, and because not a single one of them can be treated effectively by medicines, coping with a cold seems to be part of the human condition. Parents who are sniveling, sneezing, and coughing should ask the physician what precautions to take when handling the baby.

Young children with stuffy noses and breathing difficulties should be kept indoors, near a humidifier or steam kettle if the air is especially dry. Nose drops should not be given unless the physician says so. Older children may not want to miss school because of a cold. If they do go, they should be given lots of liquid when they get home and steered in the direction of an afternoon nap. Colds in and of themselves are unavoidable and not serious, but the proper pre-

cautions should be taken to prevent complications, such as an ear infection or a sore throat.

Competitiveness

See AGGRESSIVENESS.

Conscience

See GUILT AND CONSCIENCE.

Constipation

Parents who are anxious about the frequency of their own bowel movements or who are excessively refined in their attitudes towards defecation are pretty sure to transmit these feelings to their children unless they make some effort not to. Concerns of this kind are one sure way of constipating a child. Actually, if a child is eating a proper diet, getting enough exercise, and drinking a sufficiency of liquids, constipation is not likely to be a problem.

Frequency of Bowel Movements

Not everyone has a bowel movement every day. On the other hand, some people routinely have more than one movement a day. There is considerable variation among normal patterns of bowel movements. This should be borne in mind before parents conclude that their child is constipated. Children need to be assured that they are not necessarily abnormal if they deviate from the one-a-day pattern.

However, any abrupt change in the normal pattern of bowel movements should be noted, and if it persists contact a physician. Frequent small movements can be a sign of constipation.

A youngster on a light diet because of illness, or one who is dehydrated because of a fever, may suffer from mild constipation that will clear up when he recovers. If constipation becomes chronic, don't resort to enemas or laxatives on your own; discuss the problem with your physician who will want to check on other symptoms that might indicate an intestinal disorder.

Cradle Cap

This condition is marked by yellowish crusts on the baby's scalp. It is usually harmless, and can be taken care of by regular shampooing. Occasionally, a special soap as well as a very fine comb may be helpful.

Crib Death

See SUDDEN INFANT DEATH SYNDROME.

Crossed Eyes (Strabismus)

Do not be alarmed if your baby's eyes do not focus. Crossed eyes are a common condition that usually corrects itself somewhere between the ages of six and twelve months. If crossing of the eyes persists after one year, an ophthalmologist (eye specialist) should evaluate the baby's vision.

If a real problem does develop, one eye—or each eye alternately—may cross, turn outward, or focus below or above the other. Frequently the reason for "turning" is that there is a larger refractive error in one eye than in the other. Eyeglasses will often correct this condition.

Occasionally, eye muscle weakness is the cause of crossed eyes. This is most often true of premature children. The weakness of some muscles causes overaction of other muscles.

Eyeglasses will often prevent the need for eye surgery. Sometimes, however, surgery will be necessary to straighten the eyes. Either before or after surgery the eyes may need further attention in the form of eye drops, a patch to cover one eye, or glasses.

Croup

Croup, a most harassing and terrifying experience for new parents, is a spasm of the windpipe or trachea, especially involving the larynx. When such a spasm occurs, an affected child has great trouble in breathing and produces a cough that sounds like the bark of a dog. In some cases, the child can't breathe at all.

An attack of croup is an emergency. The younger the child, the more dangerous it is. You must get the baby's airway open. The best thing to do is to take the child into the bathroom, shut the door, and turn on the hot water of the shower full force, or of the bathtub and sink if you don't have a shower. The idea is to fill the room with hot steam in order to loosen the mucus plug in the baby's trachea, thus enabling him to cough up the mucus.

Get to your physician as soon as possible so that more effective treatment can begin. If the croup is viral in origin, antibiotics may not help; but when the infection is caused by bacteria, your physician will put the child on one of the antimicrobial agents. If your child is subject to croup, it is a good idea to invest in a hot or cold air vaporizer and use it whenever he has congestion resulting from a cold.

In a really severe emergency, when the windpipe closes completely, a *tracheostomy* must be performed so that the throat can be opened and an airway inserted. A tracheostomy should be performed in a hospital, but if for some reason it is performed elsewhere, the child should be hospitalized as quickly as possible.

Curiosity

If we weren't born curious, we'd never learn a thing. Even before a child can walk and talk, curiosity motivates a good part of her behavior: putting things into her mouth, poking at things, pointing at people, and as the natural urge to speak becomes stronger, holding things up or bringing them to mother or father in order to find out what they're called.

Respecting Curiosity

A parent who respects the child's curiosity will be attentive to it and satisfy it as part of the ongoing learning experience. It doesn't take any extra time when a toddler is sitting in your lap to say the words for the parts of your face (and hers) as she touches them, or the words for her articles of clothing as she tries to help put them on. Dealing with the "why" stage of curiosity is more complicated, especially because in many instances, the child is asking "Why?" for the sheer joy and sense of power of being able to do so.

Many parents who don't know anything about mechanics or astronomy have developed a sense of security by heading for the children's shelves at the local library and reading the simplest books on the subject that interest their preschool children so that they can answer some of their questions. Of course, no one can answer all the questions that a child might ask during an average day. Some should be answered by mother, some by father, and some will have to wait. There's no harm in telling a four-year-old child who wants to know why the wind makes a whistling sound that she'll find out about such things when she goes to school. That's a much better answer than "Don't ask so many questions." Questions should always be listened to even if the answers aren't readily available.

As the child reaches the age of eight and can do a certain amount of reading, it's a good idea to invest in a fairly simple encyclopedia. With such a source of information available, it's possible to respond to some questions with "Let's go find the answer together."

Each family must decide for itself where the line is to be drawn between legitimate curiosity and unacceptable snoopiness or nosiness as children get older and become interested in such matters as how rich the neighbors are, or "What were you and mommy fighting about when I was falling asleep last night?"

Cystic Fibrosis

Cystic fibrosis is an inherited disease in which the child cannot handle the normal secretions of the respiratory tract. There is a lack of ciliary action—the beating movement by the hairs of the cells lining the bronchial tubes of the lungs. Thick mucus collects at the base of the lungs, obstructing the smaller air passages and causing labored breathing and chronic cough.

Respiratory Complications

Bacteria multiply in the accumulated lung secretions, predisposing the patient to chronic bronchitis and other respiratory infections, such as pneumonia. Lung tissue changes can result eventually in severe, permanent damage to the lungs.

Digestive Complications

The abnormally thick, viscous mucus produced by the cystic fibrosis patient tends to obstruct the ducts or openings of the mucus-secreting glands. When such mucus obstructs the pancreas, it interferes with its ability to supply important digestive enzymes to the intestinal tract, thus leading to poor digestion and malabsorption of a number of important nutrients. A child with cystic fibrosis may therefore be poorly nourished in spite of an adequate diet.

Other Complications

Tissue changes in the lungs can restrict blood flow to the heart, leading to increased blood pressure and chronic heart strain. Loss of large amounts of salt through malfunctioning sweat glands can become a very serious problem for youngsters in hot weather, causing dehydration and heat exhaustion. Laboratory tests usually find an abnormally high concentration of salt in the sweat of cystic fibrosis patients. (Indeed, the skin of a cystic fibrosis patient is apt to taste salty.) Some tissues may show three times the normal concentration of sodium and twice the normal levels of potassium.

Treatment

There is no known cure for cystic fibrosis. Treatment includes the use of humidifiers and inhalation medication in the form of aerosols to loosen secretions. Another method used is *postural drainage*—lying facedown with the head lower than the feet to let gravity help loosen secretions. Antibiotics are used to control infections; special diets with reduced fat intake and added nutrients are prescribed to compensate for abnormal digestive function. Other medical techniques are utilized in individual cases to maintain normal heart and lung function.

The discovery of the defective gene involved in triggering cystic fibrosis is expected to improve diagnostic testing for the genetic disorder. The subsequent discovery of the cell malfunction that blocks the making of a protein will also enable scientists to improve treatment of the disease with aerosol inhalers and with mucus-thinning medication. Several drugs are being tested with success on patients.

Once considered strictly a disease of early childhood, an increasing number of cases of cystic fibrosis have been detected in recent years among adolescents and adults. Symptoms of the disease, including respiratory difficulty with chronic coughing, may resemble those of an allergic reaction.

How the Disease Is Inherited

Cystic fibrosis is transmitted to a child only when both parents are carriers of the trait. When only one parent carries the trait, however, some of the children can become carriers. Through marriage with other carriers, they may then become the parents of a child afflicted with the disorder.

Information on new treatment techniques, the location of treatment centers, and genetic counseling may be obtained from the national headquarters of the Cystic Fibrosis Foundation, 6931 Arlington Rd., Ste. 200, Bethesda, MD 20814.

Daydreaming

See FANTASIES.

Deafness

Major advances have been made in recent years in educating and socializing incurably deaf children who are normal in all other ways. Starting with a proper assessment of the child's degree of deafness at the earliest possible time and the fitting of a hearing aid are two crucial considerations. The child's instruction in lipreading and the use of her own vocal equipment are professionally supervised, and the rest of the family is very much involved in the whole process. Nowadays an important advance in speech therapy is the use of a feedback system that make it possible for the youngster to be self-corrective. Parents seeking information about special schools and services, summer camps, and other facilities can write to the following agencies: Alexander Graham Bell Association for the Deaf, 3417 Volta Place, N.W., Washington, D.C. 20007; American Speech-Language-Hearing Association, 10801 Rockville Pike, Rockville, MD 20852. See also HEARING.

Death

Some children's first experience of death is the loss of a grandparent; others may have to confront the fact of death for the first time when a beloved pet dies. A child wants to know where people or animals go when they die. Parents should be as honest as possible in answering such questions and tell their offspring what they themselves truly believe. Those parents who believe that there is life after death should say so; those who do not should say that they do not. Whatever one's beliefs, there are better ways to phrase them than "Grandma is in heaven watching you" or "People who are naughty go to hell when they die."

Death of a Parent

A child who has to cope with the death of a parent may be so disoriented that his behavior will seem odd to the adults around him. He may pretend that the death never happened; others may protect themselves from the shock by burying their feelings and never talking about the dead parent. Still others may feel rage at hav-

ing been abandoned. Many youngsters are overwhelmed by guilt, feeling that in some magic way they caused the death because from time to time they secretly wished it. In cases where the bereft child cannot cope with the loss, it may be advisable to provide some help in the form of psychiatric therapy.

Delinquency

Juvenile delinquents are minors who are guilty of breaking the law or who are engaged in associations and activities considered harmful to children's morals, such as running errands for gamblers, acting as a lookout during a robbery, or sniffing glue for kicks. Swiping a candy bar or a comic book at the age of ten doesn't define a child as a hardened delinquent, but where such behavior becomes chronic, it's a sign that something is wrong that needs to be corrected. With the guidance of a therapist, it may turn out that the child alone is not entirely responsible for his delinquent tendencies. See also DESTRUCTIVENESS, DISHONESTY, DISOBEDIENCE.

Dental Care

The proper attitude toward dental care is best instilled not by lectures or warnings, but by example. Parents who themselves go regularly to the dentist for checkups, who take care of their teeth by keeping them clean with routine brushing and the use of dental floss, can do more for their child's dental health than those who depend on stern warnings to shape the attitudes of their children. Parents can hardly expect their offspring to be heroic about dental visits when they themselves scarcely ever go unless they have a toothache.

Start Early

Dental care can begin by having the toddler accompany the parent to the dentist so that his baby teeth can be inspected and he can be given a special toothbrush of his own with instructions about how to use it. In communities where the water supply is not fluoridated, the dentist may recommend an ongoing program of fluoride application to the teeth themselves. Some families find that a pediatric dentist who specializes in children's dentistry can deal with a frightened or anxious child more expertly than the family dentist. Other families use the services of the dental clinics that are part of the dental schools of large universities.

No matter who is in charge of the family's dental health, it is important that professional attention is given to the child's dental development at every stage: fillings for decay in the first teeth, routine cleanings and checkups, and preventive orthodontics where advisable. Another aspect of dental care involves keeping the consumption of sweets to a minimum, and making sure that the child's daily diet contains the proper nutrients for building healthy teeth. See also ORTHODONTICS. For full discussion, see Ch. 22, *Teeth and Gums*.

Destructiveness

"It was an accident!" is a common cry when a child destroys a valuable object because of carelessness. And it probably was an accident. Parents who don't want precious bric-a-brac or other delicate possessions broken had better put them out of the reach of curious and clumsy little fingers. Young children should not be punished because their toys always seem to be destroyed; better to give them playthings that are sturdy and comparatively indestructible.

The child who is destructive unwittingly should not be spoken to in the same way as one would speak to a boy who willfully breaks his sister's doll or a girl who spitefully tears her brother's model-making manual. Destructiveness born of anger ("I was so furious, I smashed a dish") may happen rarely, but when it does, it should be commented on as an unsuitable way of dealing with the problem that caused the anger in the first place. When destructiveness gets out of hand or involves group activities amounting to vandalism, parental action should be taken with the guidance of a professional counselor.

Developmental Disability

Any disability that interferes with a child's normal development is a *developmental disability*. The term has been used more specifically, however, to refer to mental retardation, cerebral palsy, epilepsy, and autism.

Diabetes

No one knows why some children develop diabetes. Diabetes is a noncontagious disease that results from the body's inability to produce enough insulin for the normal metabolism of sugar. The diabetic child is thus improperly nourished because the sugar that should be incorporated into the tissues is excreted in the urine. Finding sugar in the urine facilitates early diagnosis. Also, because this disorder causes a disturbance in the metabolism of fat, there is an increase of fat in the blood, detectable in a routine blood count. Juvenile onset diabetes can be more volatile that adult onset diabetes. Control is usually though injectable insulin.

Insulin treatment has undergone some improvements in the past few years. Human insulin is now readily available; beef-pork insulin was common in usage before. There is less likely to be an allergic reaction to human insulin produced through genetic reproduction. Also, doses can be adjusted to the individual though the mix of fast-acting and slow-acting preparations.

Early Signs

Parents who are themselves diabetic will be alert to any symptoms in their offspring. The disease occurs more frequently in children where there is a family history of diabetes. However, because the disorder may occur in children where there is no previous family history of diabetes, alertness to the following signs is advisable: an abnormally frequent need to urinate; an excessive desire for fluids; itching of the genitals; general listlessness; frequent boils and carbuncles; slow healing of cuts and bruises.

If a diagnosis of diabetes is made by the physician, the child may be hospitalized for a few days for a series of definitive tests, and all the members of the family will be educated in the best way to supervise the child's diet and daily routine so that serious complications can be avoided. Professional guidance is also available to ensure that the youngster's emotional adjustment is a healthy one. For a full discussion see Ch. 15, *Diabetes Mellitus*.

Diaper Rash

See RASHES.

Diapers

Some controversy has built up in the past few years over which is more ecologically sound—cloth diapers or paper diapers. Paper diapers in landfills take more than one hundred years to deteriorate. If the plastic lining is removed, it is believed that the paper will deteriorate only weeks faster than the diaper left intact. Effective recycling of paper diapers does not yet exist, and it may be years before the material can be sanitized to the point of recyclability.

Cloth diapers, on the other hand, require strong soaps and chemicals to clean. To insure the sterility and whiteness of the cloth, bleach and harsh detergents are used. These go into the water supply and affect the plant and animal life. The energy used for hot water to wash the diapers also adds to the environmental cost.

Many parents try to use paper diapers only while traveling or in places where having a soiled diaper to carry or clean would be extremely inconvenient. This infrequent use of paper diapers allows for the occasional convenience of the throwaway while reducing paper waste.

Some parents believe that cloth diapers cause more diaper rash; other parents believe that the sealed paper diaper causes more diaper rash. The biggest cause of diaper rash is excessive moisture against the baby's skin, which can be avoided by frequent diaper changes, for whatever diaper used. Excessive use of powders and creams can also increase the problem because of the pasty substance that forms when these encounter moisture.

Diarrhea

Diarrhea, or loose and watery bowel movements, is common in babies because they are more sensitive to certain intestinal germs than older children. They may also be reacting to a change in their formula or to the roughage in a newly introduced fruit or vegetable. In older children, diarrhea may occur not only as a symptom of bacterial or viral infection, or because of food poisoning, but also as an allergic response, or because of overexcitement or anxiety.

Diarrhea in an infant should always be brought to a doctor's attention if it continues for more than 24 hours. The same holds true for an older child, especially when there are also symptoms of cramps, fever, or aches and pains in the joints. Persistent diarrhea from any cause, because it can lead to serious dehydration especially in infants, requires prompt medical attention.

Diphtheria

Diphtheria is a severe and contagious bacterial infection, often fatal if untreated. Once one of the most threatening of all childhood diseases, there are now fewer than 1,000 cases a year in the United States because of widespread and effective immunization.

The first symptoms—fever, headache, nausea, and sore throat—may be confused with the onset of other disorders. However, there is a manifestation of diphtheria that is uniquely its own: patches of grayish yellow membrane form in the throat and grow together into one large membrane that interferes with swallowing and breathing. The diphtheria bacteria also produce a powerful toxin that can eventually cause irreversible damage to the heart and nerves. Diagnosis is usually verified by laboratory identification of the bacteria in a throat culture.

If diphtheria does occur, it is best treated in a hospital. The prompt prescription of antitoxin serum and antibiotics results in recovery in practically all cases. See IMMUNIZATION.

Disabled Child

Whether a handicap is hereditary or acquired, mental or physical, temporary or permanent, it is always a condition that prevents a child from participating fully on an equal footing in the activities of her own age group. But how fully she can participate and her attitude toward her disability are usually a reflection of the attitudes of her parents, teachers, and the community. Of primary importance is an assessment at the earliest possible age of the extent to which the handicap can be decreased or corrected.

Exactly how deaf is the deaf child? Can surgery repair a rheumatic heart? Is a defect of vision operable? Is the child with cerebral palsy mentally retarded or is the seeming mental malfunction a reversible effect of the physical condition? Parents should investigate all the available services offered by voluntary organizations and community groups that might help them and their child. See Ch. 36, *Voluntary Health Agencies*.

One promising development in recent years is the attempt to integrate handicapped children, whenever possible, into the mainstream of education rather than segregate them in special classes. School systems in various parts of the United States are placing deaf, blind, physically disabled, and emotionally disturbed youngsters into classrooms with their nonhandicapped peers and providing them with essential supportive services at various times during the school day. The experience of dealing with nonhandicapped children will provide them with a more realistic preparation for their adult lives.

Discrimination

See PREJUDICE.

Dishonesty

Nobody is honest about everything all the time, and that goes for children as well as adults. It's unrealistic to expect a child never to lie about anything.

Little children like to make things up and can't be held strictly accountable for some of their tall stories when they're still at an age at which fact and fantasy are not clearly distinguished. A colorful exaggeration needn't call for an accusation of lying. It's better to respond with, "That's an interesting story," or "You're just imagining."

Lying and Punishment

As youngsters get older, they should feel secure enough to tell the truth about having been naughty, knowing that although they may be punished, they will get approval for having told the truth. Children shouldn't be so fearful of their parents that dishonesty is their only protection against a beating.

Cheating

Children who are pressured beyond their ability to perform are the ones likeliest to cheat; so are those for whom winning has been held up constantly as a transcendent value. A child who has been caught cheating at school is usually punished by the authorities. If the incident is discussed at home, the parents might reexamine their values before adding to the child's burdens. A youngster who cheats regularly at games will suffer the natural punishment of exclusion by his peers.

Stealing

Young children who embark on group enterprises of stealing "for fun"—whether it's taking candy from the corner market or shoplifting from a department store—needn't be viewed as case-hardened criminals unless the stealing becomes habitual.

A nine-year-old who swipes a candy bar once or twice and regrets it belongs in a different category from one who is hired as a lookout for older delinquents. Children usually have respect for other people's property when they have property of their own that they value and don't want anyone else to take.

Disobedience

Father gets a parking ticket because he forgot about alternate sides of the street on Wednesdays; mother has a whipped cream dessert in spite of her physician's orders not to. Are mother and father disobedient? When Junior comes home from the playground at five instead of obeying orders to come home at four, is his disobedience any worse than theirs? Genuine forgetfulness, negligence, or occasional breaking of a rule is only human. Willful chronic disobedience is another matter.

Some children with a strong urge toward independence may test out many parental rules by disobeying them on purpose. A child who has been ordered not to spend any time with another child because the families are feuding, may, by flouting the order, be telling his parents that he has a right to choose his own friends. Where disobedience affects a youngster's health or safety or morals, it's time for parental action, not necessarily in the form of punishment, but in taking stock of the situation to find out why the child won't obey.

Divorced Parents

See "Separation and Divorce" in Ch. 5, *The Middle Years.*

Dreams and Nightmares

Children go through periods of having "bad dreams" or nightmares that wake them up in the middle of the night in a state of terror and bewilderment. It won't do to say, "It's just a dream." To a young child who is just beginning to grasp the difference between what's real and what isn't, nightmare can be extremely threatening. If the child wants to describe the dream after she collects herself, she should be allowed to do so even at 3:00 A.M. She may amplify and exaggerate a little bit, but that's only to let you know that she's been very brave through it all. Parental patience is called for; with a certain amount of reassurance, the child can usually be led back to bed and to sleep.

Youngsters whose sleep is regularly interrupted by nightmares or who are in the grip of the same nightmare may be feeling anxious about a daytime activity or may be feeling guilty about some undiscovered naughtiness. A tactful chat can sometimes reveal what the trouble is so that it can be disposed of during waking hours.

Night Terrors

Some children may have occasional nightmares—often called *night terrors*—in which they scream or tremble in terror. They may sit up in bed while still asleep, or even walk around. Their terror is certainly real, but the parents should remember that the cause of it is purely imaginary. Accordingly, they have no reason to be alarmed; in spite of the child's appearance, she is not in any danger, and no drastic action is called for.

Simply comfort the child, who frequently will be disoriented and confused in a half-awake state, until she can go back to sleep. She will probably have no recollection of the episode the next morning.

If night terrors occur only occasionally, there is no cause for concern, although it might be a good idea to check on the television shows your child is watching before bedtime. If there is a great deal of tension in the household, that could be a contributing cause. If night terrors are persistent or frequent, however, a physician should be consulted. See also SLEEPWALKING.

Dyslexia

Dyslexia is a condition in which an otherwise average or intelligent child suffers from a complex of motor-perceptual disabilities that interfere with the orderly processing and acquisition of language. The disability that results in an inhibition of symbol recognition essential for learning how to read, write, and spell is thought to originate in some form of brain circuitry malfunction that may have been caused by injury or by genetic defect. Recent researchers have established some connection between dyslexia and a faulty pathway between the lower brain—the cerebellum—and the inner ear, causing the dyslexic child to suffer from a mild and permanent form of motion sickness that interferes with learning.

Symptoms

The symptoms of dyslexia vary considerably and may include: garbled or disordered development of speech during the early years; an inability to learn the relationship between sounds and symbols for purposes of reading aloud; an inability to learn how to spell or how to organize written expression; confusion about serial order, as in naming the days of the week or in number concepts; unusual difficulty in doing simple repetitive tasks.

If a parent suspects that a child is suffering from dyslexia, a diagnosis should be made on the basis of tests administered by trained professionals. The child's pediatrician or the school guidance counselor should be consulted about where such tests are best given and assessed. Should the child be diagnosed as dyslexic, an appropriate remedial program or an accredited special school can help surmount some of the learning difficulties.

Earache

Earache is one of the most common complaints of childhood.

As Secondary Infection

Earache is often attributable to bacterial infection of the middle ear and should be treated promptly by a physician. Because the eustachian tube that connects the back of the throat with the middle ear is shorter and wider in a child than in an adult, it affords easier entry to bacteria. Infections of the ear may thus occur as the result of a sore throat or a postnasal drip. Infectious mucus from the nose is often forced into the middle ear by way of the eustachian tube because young children are inclined to sniff it back rather than to blow it out. And when a child is mastering the technique of noseblowing, he should be told that neither one nor both of the nostrils should be pressed closed in the process. Rather, both nostrils should be blown out gently at the same time, and with the mouth open. If gentle blowing doesn't clear the nostrils, the nose should be wiped as necessary.

Recognizing Earache in an Infant

Earache in an infant may be combined with fever and the kind of crying associated with sharp pain. A toddler may indicate the source of discomfort by pulling at the earlobe. Until the pediatrician can prescribe proper medication, discomfort can be relieved by applying a heating pad to the involved ear and giving the child a non-aspirin pain reliever.

Other Causes

Earache may also accompany teething or tooth infection, or it may be the result of pressure caused by water that has been trapped in the ear after swimming or bathing. In small children, an earache may be a sign that the youngster has stuffed a bean or a tiny plastic object so far into his ear that it won't come out as easily as it went in. If you suspect such an occurrence, avoid poking and prodding in an attempt to remove the object. The child should be taken to a physician or to a hospital so that the object can be removed with the proper instruments and the ear examined and treated for possible injury.

Consequences of Neglect of Earache

An earache should always be brought to a physician's attention without delay because untreated middle ear infections can lead to irreversible hearing loss. The leading cause of mild hearing loss in toddlers is believed to be *serous otitis media*, or serous infection of the middle ear. This condition is specifically an inflammation of the middle ear with an accumulation of fluid behind the eardrum. When the condition is chronic or improperly treated during the first three years, it may impair hearing permanently and as a consequence lead to a failure to develop normal language skills. Occasionally the physician may have to make a small opening in the eardrum to drain the fluid, a procedure known as a *myringotomy*. Tubes may be inserted to drain the ear. The small tubes will eventually pop out themselves. Other treatments may include surgery on the eustachian to expand constricted areas and allow drainage through the auditory tube. The isthmus of the auditory tube is the narrowest point in the canal and may close during swelling or inflammation. See also HEARING.

Eczema

See under RASHES.

Education

See SCHOOL.

Epilepsy

Epilepsy in childhood most commonly takes the form of petit mal or psychomotor episodes.

Petit Mal Seizures

Petit mal episodes are characterized by brief lapses of consciousness, sometimes occurring many times a day. The child does not fall down but simply stops what he is doing and may appear to stare absently.

Psychomotor Seizures

Psychomotor episodes are characterized by the performance of some activity during a brief lapse of consciousness. The child may walk around in circles, or sit down and get up in a purposeless way. During this type of seizure the child may babble nonsensically or chant the same word over and over. Such an attack may last no more than a few minutes, and when the child recovers he is likely to have no memory of its occurrence.

In many instances, parents who expect a certain amount of bizarre behavior from their youngsters may not realize that a form of epilepsy is the cause. Should such incidents occur frequently, they should be called to the attention of the physician who may think it advisable to have the child examined by a neurologist.

A parent witnessing a *grand mal* or convulsive epileptic seizure for the first time may be unduly alarmed and take measures that may harm the child rather than help. For a description of emergency measures during a grand mal seizure, see Ch. 35, *Medical Emergencies.* For a full discussion of epilepsy, see Ch. 8, *Diseases of the Muscles and Nervous System.*

Exercise

Some children seem to sit around a great deal; others are on the move from morning until bedtime. A youngster might be listless or lethargic because there's something the matter that needs to be investigated by a physician. This type of sitting around is quite different from playing with dolls for hours at a time or looking at picture books instead of running around. A young child who really cannot sit still at all may have a problem that needs diagnosing by a physician, too. Practically all children are found between these extremes.

Exercise as a Developmental Need

Toddlers must be allowed to get the exercise necessary for the development of their bodies. They shouldn't be confined in a playpen for most of the day. Three- and four-year-olds who don't go to a nursery school and have no play equipment in their backyard (if they have a backyard), should be taken whenever possible to a local park or playground that has swings, slides, seesaws, jungle gyms, or other devices that are safely designed and installed. Most schools have some kind of supervised gym activity or a free time for yard play, and if they don't, they should. If this sched-

uled exercise is insufficient for a nine- or ten-year-old, inquiries can be made about athletic facilities at a local YMCA, settlement house, church, or fraternal organization.

Choice of Activities

As children get a little older, they should be permitted to choose the exercise that appeals to them unless there's a good reason for its being forbidden. A girl who wants to join a sandlot baseball team shouldn't be forced to go to a ballet class, and a boy inspired by the dancing he's seen on TV shouldn't be discouraged if the family can afford the lessons. Exercise needn't be synonymous with competition unless the youngster wants it to be. See also "Physical Fitness" in Ch. 3, *The Teens.*

Eyeglasses

Now that infants and youngsters have periodic eye checkups with their physicians, and regular tests are given to all students, more children are wearing glasses than in former years. In addition to *strabismus* (crossed eyes), the three major eye problems encountered in children are *myopia* (nearsightedness), *hyperopia* (farsightedness), and *astigmatism.*

Myopia

The *myopic* or nearsighted child cannot see distant objects well but can see close objects clearly. A very young child so afflicted may stumble and fall easily. An older child attending school may make errors in copying because she has difficulty in making out the words and figures written on the chalkboard. She may be called a behavior problem or may even be said to be mentally retarded. Most cases of myopia can be helped with glasses.

Hyperopia

The *hyperopic* (also called *hypermetropic*) or farsighted eye is shorter from front to rear than the normal eye, and if not corrected will often hinder close work like reading. When a farsighted child reads she often complains of blurring of the printed page, sleepiness, and headache. Farsightedness is often associated with crossed eyes and is usually correctable with glasses.

Astigmatism

In *astigmatism* or distorted vision, there is an uneven curvature of the cornea or lens surface of the eye. This condition causes some light rays to focus further back than others and produces a blurred, distorted image on the retina.

Either a farsighted or nearsighted eye can be *astigmatic;* the abnormality can usually be corrected by properly prescribed eyeglasses.

Fantasies

Every normal child has fantasies, some highly pleasurable, some fearful and frightening. Young children sometimes have a hard time sorting out what they imagine from what's real; this may be especially true when a nightmare interferes with sleep. Many children quite consciously say, "Let's pretend" or "Let's make believe" when they embark on a dress-up activity; others simply and straightforwardly act out their fantasies by playing games of violence with toy guns. An only child may create a fantasy companion with whom she has conversations; a child who is encouraged to draw may give shape to her fantasies in pictures that mean a lot to her but not much to anyone else.

Daydreaming

Some children infuriate their energetic parents by sitting around and daydreaming (with one sock on and one off) instead of doing their chores. Whatever form fantasies may take, they are an inevitable part of growing up and should be respected, unless they become the equivalent of a narcotic escape from reality rather than a means of enriching it. When a child's fantasy life appears to be turning into a substitute for his real one, the time has come to consult a psychiatric authority.

Fears and Phobias

Babies are fearful about being dropped, and they're frightened by a sudden loud noise. (You *can* make babies cry by saying, "Boo!" When they get older and catch on, they'll think it's fun to be scared.) Toddlers are taught to be afraid of a hot stove, and as children get a little older, they develop night fears that become bad dreams. Many parents transmit, deliberately or unknowingly, some of their fears to their children: fear of dogs, or thunder and lightning, or infection by germs.

Only a thin line separates sensible caution from anxiety. Where a threat of punishment is involved, an anxiety may develop that can last a lifetime. Parents should control the impulse to say such things as, "Don't eat that, it's going to make you sick" or "Don't climb so high, you're going to fall" or "Don't play in the mud; the germs will make you sick." Or, worse yet, "If you do that, the bogey man will get you" or "God will punish you."

Phobias

If fears are often legitimate and usually outgrown through reassuring experiences, phobias are deep-seated unconquerable fears. Many adults suffer from them; two of the most common are *claustrophobia*, the fear of being in an enclosed place, and *acrophobia*, the fear of heights. *Phobia* is a clinical term and shouldn't be used to describe a youngster's aversion to school at a particular time, or his apprehension about elevators and escalators. If parental reassurance can help a child overcome fears of this type, they need not be classed as phobias.

Fever

As every parent knows, babies can run very high fevers. In itself, a rectal temperature of 103° F or 104° F is not necessarily cause for alarm. (Normal rectal temperature is about ½° F to 1° F higher than the oral norm of 98.6° F.) Of course, you should take the immediate step of calling your pediatrician to find out what's causing the fever.

If a baby's fever goes over 104° F, the infant may experience convulsions. To avoid this possibility, he may be bathed with cool water or with equal parts of water and alcohol. (The alcohol is not necessary.) If convulsions do occur, protect the baby from injuring himself by seeing that his head and body don't strike anything hard. The convulsion, though frightening, is usually brief and ends of its own accord. Get in touch with your physician without delay.

Although the mechanism that results in fever is not precisely understood, the elevation in temperature is almost always a sign that the child's normal body processes are being disturbed. A child old enough to talk can let you know that his throat is sore or that he has an earache.

Possible Causes

Fever is often the sign of the onset of an infectious disease such as measles or influenza; it usually accompanies severe sunburn; it may be a warning that the infection of a local cut is spreading through the rest of the body. When it comes suddenly and rises quickly, along with cramps or diarrhea, it may indicate a gastrointestinal infection or food poisoning. No matter what a child's age, if temperature by mouth rises above 101° F, a physician should be informed of the fever and accompanying symptoms.

Treatment

Until a diagnosis is made and treatment prescribed, the feverish youngster should be put to bed and kept on a diet of light foods and lots of liquids. If the elevated temperature is combined with stiff neck, aching joints, or headache, nonaspirin medication can be given for relief according to dose instructions indicated.

Fluoridation

Although it has been unequivocally established that fluoridated drinking water is the best safeguard against tooth decay, many parts of the United States continue to resist this public health measure, thus placing a special burden on the parents of preschool children. Families in such communities are strongly urged to consult their dentist or the closest dental clinic connected with a university's college of dentistry for advice on the appropriate measures to be taken to protect their children's teeth. A consultation of this nature is advisable as soon as the baby shows signs of teething, because the fluoride treatments should begin as early as possible.

In many areas where the water supply remains unfluoridated, programs in the public schools supply youngsters with fluoride tablets every day. Although this method of applying the chemical is less effective than its availability in the drinking water, it is a step in the right direction. Concerned parents can make an effort to initiate such programs where none exists by contacting state public health officials.

Foot Care

Unless the child's pediatrician indicates the need for corrective or orthopedic shoes, parents need have little concern for pigeon toes or bowed legs or flat feet. If a shoe salesman suggests remedial footwear, his suggestions should be discussed with a physician before complying with them. A good general rule to follow about the fit of shoes is that they should be about three-quarters of an inch longer than the foot itself. For a child whose feet have a tendency to perspire heavily, sweat socks made of cotton or wool are to be preferred to those made of synthetics. Blisters that form on the instep, heel, or any other part of the foot because of ill-fitting footwear must be treated promptly to avoid serious infection.

Friends

Everyone needs friends. Some children need only one; others seem to enjoy having several. A three-year-old who is just beginning to learn about sharing may be more relaxed playing with just one other child; a ten-year-old may like the hurly-burly of a group of friends to get together with when school is out.

Parents Please Stay Out

Parents should try to steer clear of squabbles between children. One day, Nancy and Harriet are best friends, the next, bitter enemies, because of some real or imagined outrage. Left to their own devices, the children will probably patch things up. If parents get involved, the situation gets magnified out of all proportion. It's not unusual in such situations for the two sets of parents to stop speaking to each other and the two little girls to go back to being best friends again.

Keeping Bad Company

What's to be done about "unsuitable" friends? Some parents may think a particular child is unacceptable because she's too aggressive or too foul-mouthed. If your child seems fond of her nonetheless, voice your opinions, but don't forbid the youngster from coming to the house. Any attempt to break up the friendship is likely to be resisted until your child learns from experience that your judgment was the right one. Children who are discouraged from bringing their friends home because they make a mess or make too much noise are actually deprived of feeling at home in their own house.

Friendships between girls and boys may begin in nursery school and continue for years afterward. Although the tone of the friendship may change, the closeness can be very valuable if it doesn't exclude other relationships.

Frostbite

See Ch. 35, *Medical Emergencies*.

Guilt and Conscience

Children often feel as guilty about bad thoughts as they do about bad deeds. After being angry, a child may feel as badly about having had a fleeting wish to hurt his mother as he would have felt had he actually hurt her. A child should be helped to understand that his thoughts are his own, that his thoughts cannot harm anybody, and that he will not be punished for his thoughts. He should understand that it is only actions of certain kinds that cannot be allowed and that will result in a reprimand or punishment. In other words, a child should not be made to feel guilty for angry or aggressive thoughts toward other members of his family, but only for angry and aggressive acts.

A parent might say to a child, "I understand that you really disliked your brother when you hit him, in fact, even hated him and would have liked to hurt him. It's okay for you to be angry with him, but I am not going to let you hurt him." A clear distinction should be made between hostile feelings and hostile behavior.

Headaches

Children get headaches just as adults do. The difficulty in diagnosing and treating them comes from the different symptoms that children experience. It is believed that up to 10 percent of preadolescents suffer from migraine headaches.

Symptoms of headaches in children include aggression, agitation, vomiting, nausea, visual problems, insomnia, and profuse sweating. Causes are the same as they are in adults: tension, stress, eye strain, migraine, or emotional or physical problems. For a child experiencing frequent or severe headaches, a physician should be consulted to eliminate the possibility of an underlying physical disorder, such as near or farsightedness. Once the doctor has determined that no physical disorder exists, treatment of the psychological cause should be considered. Undue pressure from home or the school can create as much stress on a child as an adult experiences in the workplace.

Medication of children should be taken only under the supervision of a qualified doctor. Children respond to certain medications much differently than adults, and care must be taken in administering the types and quantities of drugs. Also treatment of any child with aspirin should be supervised because of the risk of Reye's Syndrome.

Diagnosis and treatment of children with headaches is difficult. Parents should continue to seek treatment for their children until they are satisfied that the problem has been addressed and is being remedied.

Health Records

It may seem somewhat troublesome to keep orderly health records for every member of the family, but the accumulated information can be extremely helpful if it can be supplied at a moment's notice to a physician or a hospital. Chronologically arranged facts can also provide the material eventually needed by summer camps and school applications and insurance policies.

A notebook containing essential data about past illnesses, accidents, allergies, surgery, and other facts can be extraordinarily helpful and time-saving in supplying a physician with a medical history that simplifies diagnosis and treatment. Such a notebook should have separate sections for immunizations and booster shots and their dates; annual weight and height progress; illnesses with dates and special notations; accidents with dates and any permanent consequences; hospitalization and reason;

individual problems relating to allergies, hearing, vision, speech, and the like. Visits to physician and dentist should be recorded, and the blood type entered in a conspicuous place. If possible, parents should also provide a summary at the back of the notebook of their own major illnesses, disabilities, and surgical history.

Hearing

Approximately half of all adult hearing problems are thought to have originated in childhood. About five out of every hundred children reveal some hearing disability when screening tests are given. Total deafness among children is uncommon, and where it does exist, its symptoms become manifest to parents and physicians alike during infancy.

Partial Hearing Loss

Partial hearing disability, on the other hand, is common, and is likely to be overlooked until it may be too late to correct its consequences.

A physician begins to suspect a hearing problem when the mother of a young baby tells him that the child does not react to her voice, to noises, or to other auditory stimuli. As the child gets older, he may not speak properly. Because he has never heard speech, he cannot imitate its sound and may fail to develop normal language skills. Sometimes these children, like visually handicapped children, are mistakenly called mentally retarded or are classified as suffering from hyperkinesis or brain dysfunction. Often the undetected hearing disability stemmed from a middle ear infection that was treated inadequately or not treated at all.

Language Problems

A hearing loss of 15 decibels is considered sufficiently large to produce language problems for a very young child, causing a major handicap in the acquisition of language skills. Specialists therefore recommend that parents ask that their physician test a baby's hearing, especially during and after an ear infection. If a compensatory hearing aid is necessary, the baby should be supplied with one immediately. Speech will not develop normally—that is, the language function of the brain will be impaired—unless the essential sounds of language can be perceived during the first two years of life.

Just as glasses or surgery can help eye problems, simple hearing aids, the surgical removal of excessive lymphoid tissue blocking the eustachian tube, or special instruction in lip reading can often help a hearing problem and open up a new world for the child afflicted with a hearing disability.

Heart Disease

See RHEUMATIC FEVER. See also "Congenital Heart Disease" in Ch. 10, *Heart Disease*.

Hernia

A *hernia* is a condition in which part of an organ protrudes through a weak spot or other abnormal opening in the wall of a body cavity. There are three types of hernias that may occur in children.

Umbilical Hernia

The most common is an *umbilical hernia*, in which there is a protrusion of some of the contents of the abdomen through an opening in the abdominal wall at the navel where the umbilical cord was attached. When the baby cries or strains, the protrusion becomes more obvious, and when the baby is at rest, the bulge recedes. An umbilical hernia usually disappears by the time a child reaches the second year. Because it represents no danger to any of the body functions, the condition need be no cause for concern. It is very common in non-Caucasian children.

Inguinal Hernia

The second most common type of hernia in childhood is known as an *indirect inguinal hernia*, occurring frequently in boys. At birth it may have the appearance of a marble located under the skin at the groin. In time, it may descend into the scrotum that encloses the testicles. This type of hernia is usually corrected by simple surgery that repairs the weakened musculature. The weak muscles are often present on both sides.

Hiatus Hernia

Another congenital hernia is known as a *hiatus hernia* (or *diaphragmatic hernia*) in which part of the stomach protrudes upward through the part of the esophagus that opens into the diaphragm. In some cases, this structural defect is self-healing. Surgical correction is advised only if the hernia interferes with respiration. See also Ch. 11, *Diseases of the Digestive System*.

Hospitalization

Most children at some time in their first 15 years of life require at least one hospitalization, ranging in time from a few days to many months. This can be a frightening experience and may leave permanent emotional scars on a child. Parents can do many things to make the experience less harmful.

Growth Rates in Boys*

*Adapted from National Center for Health Statistics *NCHS Growth Charts,* 1976. Monthly Vital Statistics Report. Vol. 25, No. 3, Supp. (HRA) 76-1120. Health Resources Administration, Rockville, Maryland, June, 1976. Data from The Fels Research Institute, Yellow Springs, Ohio. © 1976 Ross Laboratories

These charts indicate the rate of growth of boys and girls from birth to 36 months in the United States. In each chart the upper gray area indicates the range of growth in height from the 5th to 95th percentile, and the lower gray area indicates a similar range in weight. (If a boy or girl is in the 95th percentile in height, 95% of all other boys and girls are not as tall as he or she. If someone is in the 50th percentile in weight, half of other children weigh more and half weigh less. If one is in the 25th percentile

Preparing the child for the hospital stay may be the most important task for the parent. There are many books available for different age groups on going to the hospital. Authorities generally agree that parents should:

● Try to answer all the questions the child asks. If you have no answer, try to find one.

● Be as honest as possible. The child will want to know why he or she

Growth Rates in Girls*

*Adapted from National Center for Health Statistics *NCHS Growth Charts,* 1976. Monthly Vital Statistics Report. Vol. 25, No. 3, Supp. (HRA) 76-1120. Health Resources Administration, Rockville, Maryland, June, 1976. Data from The Fels Research Institute, Yellow Springs, Ohio. © 1976 Ross Laboratories

of weight, 75% of other children weigh more and 25% weigh less. Thus, the percentile indicates how your child compares in height or weight with other children of the same sex and age in the United States.) Height, indicated at the left-hand side of each chart, is shown in inches and in centimeters. Weight, indicated at the right-hand side of each chart, is shown in kilograms and in pounds. The bottom and top lines of each chart indicate age in months.

has to go to the hospital, what will be done there, how long it will take, and whether it will hurt.

- Be reassuring. The child should know that he or she will receive

good care and that the hospital visit will be temporary.

- Explain what the hospital is and what it is like—with wheeled carts, people in uniform, and so on.

- Using sheets as gowns, role-play to make it clear that under the gowns will be helping people.

- Let the child know when they will be in the hospital and how long they will stay.

Most hospitals today try to work with parents to make the child feel at home and to allay the child's fears. Many hospitals offer rooms so that parents can "room in"—and stay near the young patient. A playroom may be available. Hospital staff members may hold parent-nurse sessions to introduce mothers and fathers to the hospital's schedule, locations of facilities, and other details. Parents of a child who has to be hospitalized can, by learning as much as possible and co-operating with the staff, help alleviate a child's natural fears of separation, of mutilation, and of the strange new situation.

Fear of Separation

Hospitalization for an operation or an illness affects different children at different stages of their development in different ways. Very young children may be particularly worried about separations from their mothers. Parents can help with this fear by assuring the child that separation will not be permanent.

If at all possible, the child's mother or another member of the family should stay with the child during much of the hospital stay. During an extended hospitalization, of course, this may become difficult or impossible. Barring accidents, children should always be forewarned of a hospitalization; if they are not, they may feel they were deceived by their parents and lose trust in them.

Fear of Mutilation

Children of about 4 to 10 or 11 may be more worried about possible damage or mutilation of their bodies than about separations from their families. They often have fears that parts of their bodies may be cut out or that in some way they may be permanently harmed. They may feel that when they come back from the hospital they will not be the same as they were when they went in. Matter-of-fact reassurance by the parents can be most helpful in alleviating these fears.

Fear of the Strange

Both younger children and older children aged 10, 11, or 12 may fear the new or strange, such as the anesthetic that goes with an operation. The child should be allowed to talk out fears. Simple explanations usually help. A child can, for example, understand that when you get sick taking medicine can sometimes make you better. At other times an operation, or surgery, is the only thing that will help. In the hospital, physicians or nurses may have to make tests to find out what is wrong. One such test is the X ray, which is simply a "picture" of a part of the child's body.

The parent can prepare the child for the operating room and for the operation. Everything in this special place, for example, must be kept perfectly clean, so nurses and physicians wear long-sleeved gowns. They also wash carefully before the operation begins. They wear sterile gloves so that they can touch patients without passing on germs. They also wear masks, shoe coverings, and caps. They may make a small opening in the patient's skin so that they can take out or get rid of whatever is making the child sick. The physicians and nurses use stitches, or sutures, to pull the skin edges together and allow healing to begin. Some stitches may be under the skin; these simply melt, or dissolve, by themselves.

A dressing may be placed over the part of the child's body that was opened up. These pieces of soft cloth protect the skin opening and keep out germs. When the dressing comes off, a white scar may remain. The scar will not open up and it will not hurt. It will be a sign that the child was sick, got well, and came home.

Hostility

See ANGER.

Hyaline Membrane Disease

Hyaline membrane disease, now technically called the *respiratory distress syndrome*, is a disorder that affects approximately 50,000 newborn babies each year, and until recently was fatal for about half of them. The disorder occurs especially among premature infants, those born by caesarian section, and those with diabetic mothers. In premature infants, the immaturity of the lungs may result in a collapse of the air space within the lungs themselves when the first breath is exhaled. Each new breath then becomes a greater struggle, and with the spread of lung collapse, exhaustion and asphyxiation may occur.

A treatment known as *continuous positive airway pressure* is now being successfully used in many of the special hospital units equipped for newborns with disabilities. The therapy involves a pressure chamber that forces high-oxygen air into the lungs and keeps these air spaces open. The method has already prevented thousands of infant deaths. Newborns who need this assistance acquire the ability to breathe normally in about a week.

Hyperkinesis

Hyperkinesis is a behavioral disorder diagnosed in a large number of schoolchildren—more often boys than girls—who are unable to concentrate and who are overactive and excitable. These characteristics cause them to become disruptive in the classroom as well as disturbing to their families. There are indications that this disorder manifests itself in infancy, when the physician might describe an excessively fretful and restless baby as *hypertonic*, and prescribe medication to calm him down.

For reasons not yet understood, it has been found that the symptoms of hyperkinesis often respond to antidepressants or stimulants, and as a result, a significant number of otherwise unmanageable youngsters are being treated medically. Although the medication enables them to conform to classroom situations, it may have the negative effect of appetite loss; to avoid sleep difficulties, the medication is never given in the evening.

Hyperkinesis appears to run in families, although there is some evidence that imperceptible brain damage may be one of its causes. Parents of a clinically hyperkinetic child—not one who is simply rambunctious—should seek advice about proper treatment from the psychiatric and neurological staffs of the nearest teaching hospital or from specialists recommended by the family physician.

Imagination

See FANTASIES.

Immunization

Recently developed vaccines against measles, mumps, and rubella (German measles) should eventually wipe out these diseases in the same way that smallpox has been eliminated practically everywhere in the world. Routine immunization follows a schedule of shots administered with minor variations by most pediatricians and child care clinics. Severe reactions are rare, but should they occur, they should be reported to the physician promptly.

Keeping Records

Records should be kept of the child's immunization history so that booster shots can be given at proper intervals. Because families move from one place to another, changing physicians as they relocate, it saves a great deal of time and trouble if immunization data is written down rather than committed to memory. See HEALTH RECORDS.

DTP Injections

DTP stands for diphtheria, tetanus, and pertussis (or whooping cough). DTP injections are usually given in the muscles of the mid-thigh or upper arm, at intervals of one month, sometimes longer. To prevent fever or other severe reactions, the two- to five-month-old baby should receive one grain of baby aspirin within a few hours after the injection. If she nevertheless develops fever or has other severe reactions, your physician may have to give lower doses, and therefore give more than three injections. Very rarely is a severe reaction reported with smaller doses of the vaccine. If there is such a reaction, no further injections of pertussis vaccine will be given.

Occasionally, redness or a lump appears at the site of the injection. This is a local reaction. It is harmless and will disappear within a few weeks. If it does not, consult your physician.

It is recommended that a booster or recall shot be given at one-and-a-half and at three years of age. Another recall injection of only TD (tetanus-diphtheria toxoid) is given at six years and at twelve years.

DTP Reactions

Adverse reactions to the DTP vaccine have been reported in a few cases. The reactions ranged from permanent neurological damage to such mild symptoms as persistent crying and unusual sleepiness. Crying may be high-pitched and may continue as long as three hours or more. Sleepiness may resemble a shocklike state. Some children may run temperatures of 105° F or higher. In cases of suspected adverse reactions to DTP or any other vaccine, a pediatrician or family physician should be called immediately.

Parents may want to discuss their children's medical histories with their family physicians or pediatricians before taking a child in for an inocculaton. The American Academy of Pediatrics suggests that children with personal histories of convulsions or allergic reactions to DTP or other vaccines should not be given the DTP vaccine. The same is true of children born prematurely.

Independence

Many parents feel that the most memorable moment in a child's progress towards independence comes when he takes his first steps alone. Upright and walking! Most children accomplish this by going independently from the secure arms of one adult to the waiting arms of another.

Recommended Schedule for Active Immunization of Normal Infants and Children		
Recommended Age	**Vaccine**[a]	**Comments**
2 months	DTP, OPV	Can be initiated earlier in areas of high incidence
4 months	DTP, OPV	2-month interval desired for OPV to avoid interference
6 months	DTP	OPV optional for areas where polio might be imported (e.g., some areas of southwestern United States)
12 months	TB test	May be given simultaneously with MMR at 15 months (see text)
15 months	Measles, Mumps, Rubella; DPT, OPV	MMR preferred
24 months	Hemophilus b polysaccharide vaccine	
24 months	Hemophilus b	Hemophilus b polysaccharide vaccine for Hemophilus influenza type b
4–6 years[b]	DTP, OPV	

[a] DTP—diphtheria and tetanus toxoids with pertussis vaccine. OPV—oral, attenuated poliovirus vaccine contains poliovirus types 1, 2, and 3. Tuberculin test—mantoux (intradermal PPD) preferred. Frequency of tests depends on local epidemiology. The Committee recommends annual or biennial testing unless local circumstances dictate less frequent or no testing (see tuberculosis for complete discussion). MMR—live measles, mumps, and rubella viruses in a combined vaccine (see text for discussion of single vaccines versus combination). Td—adult tetanus toxoid (full dose) and diphtheria toxoid (reduced dose) combination.

[b] Up to the seventh birthday.

As youngsters move toward greater independence, they will do so with confidence if they can start out from a secure foundation of rules and limits, and return to the security of acceptance and understanding should they come to grief.

The Toddler Stage

The toddler relishes the independence of being able to explore the house or the playground but he won't go very far before he returns to check in with the person in charge of him so that he can start out all over again. He voices his independence, too: "no" to naps; "no" to outings; "no" to a bath. This is the phase during which parents must be wary of asking "Would you like to" or "Do you want to" instead of just proceeding with the business at hand. Patience is required for the self-assertive fumblings and clumsy efforts at self-feeding and putting clothes on. Assistance should be subtle and tactful, not hurried and bossy: "Baby do, daddy help," is the general idea.

School Age

As the child moves into the larger arena of school and friendships, "I'm not a baby any more" may become a complaint if he wants more freedom than he's permitted to have. At this stage, he begins to learn that responsibility goes hand-in-hand with freedom and independence. Old enough to ride the bike farther and farther from home means taking on the responsibility of keeping it in good repair and obeying all the traffic rules.

Influenza

See "The Common Cold, Influenza, and Other Viral Infections" in Ch. 12, *Diseases of the Respiratory System.*

Insect Stings and Bites

When a child is bitten or stung by an insect, he often complains about the pain or the itching, but with the application of a lotion or salve to relieve discomfort and a bandage to prevent infection, the incident is soon forgotten. There are times, however, when a sting or a bite may require emergency treatment.

It has been estimated that about four children out of every 1,000 have serious allergic reactions to the sting of a hornet, wasp, bee, yellow jacket, or the fire ant. A child who has sustained multiple stings, or whose body, tongue, or face begins to swell because of a single sting should be taken to the hospital immediately. Tests can clearly distinguish between those children who are highly sensitive to stings and those who are not.

Preventive Measures

A physician should be consulted about the advisability of testing youngsters who are going off to camp for the first time or who are planning long hikes. Rather than curtail the activities of a child who turns out to have an acute sensitivity, it may make sense to plan a series of desensitization treatments against the particular venom. For children who are very allergic to insect stings, an emergency kit containing adrenaline is now available and should always be carried.

Mosquitoes

Every effort should be made to eradicate mosquitoes by eliminating their breeding places. A mosquito bite can be a serious threat to a child's health because these insects transmit several diseases. Where mosquitoes are a problem, infants and children should be protected against them by screens, netting, and the application of repellents.

Ticks

Families that travel and those that have pets should guard against the possibility of infection by disease-bearing ticks. A species of tick known as *Ixodes dammini* can transmit an illness called Lyme disease while another common tick may carry Rocky Mountain spotted fever.

Rashes may appear as symptoms of infection by either tick. The Lyme disease rash may be circular and hot to the touch. It may have a diameter as wide as 28 inches. Untreated in either children or adults, Lyme disease may trigger chills, fever, general feelings of malaise, fatigue, and attacks of arthritis that may last weeks or months to years. Heart and nerve abnormalities may appear. Penicillin is used to bring Lyme disease under control in pregnant women and children.

Less prevalent than Lyme disease, Rocky Mountain spotted fever usually produces a rash on the soles of the feet and the palms of the hands. Prompt medical attention is essential to prevent possible complications. See ROCKY MOUNTAIN SPOTTED FEVER and LYME DISEASE under RASHES.

Intelligence and IQ

Intelligence is a quality, not a quantity. It therefore cannot be measured as precisely as height or weight; nor can it be exemplified as definitely as mechanical skill or athletic ability or musical talent. Although child development authorities and educators may disagree about how to assess intelligence, they generally agree on the following premise: no matter what is inherited and what is instilled by experience, children function best in later life if their earliest years of nurture bring out and develop their inborn capacities.

Encouragement and Enrichment

Beginning with proper prenatal diet and care, a healthy baby is born, and from then on, her intellectual capacities are shaped by experience. Loving and attentive parents give her the self-confidence to explore and learn. She is encouraged to express herself in language. She is exposed to a variety of experiences that will stimulate her curiosity and interest: plants, drawing materials, pets, picture books, outings to the beach. Her efforts to use her intelligence by asking questions are respected and encouraged rather than minimized and ignored.

IQ Tests

Once a child gets to school her capabilities may or may not be measured by a standard IQ test. Such tests, which have been abandoned in some states, assess specific areas of intelligence and are graded according to a statistical norm. Newer techniques for measuring intelligence are designed to compensate for a cultural bias that some authorities believe exists in the standard tests.

Jealousy

See BROTHERS AND SISTERS, NEW BABY.

Kidney Diseases

For a discussion of kidney diseases, see Ch. 17, *Diseases of the Urinogenital System*, and Ch. 18, *Cancer*.

Learning

See CURIOSITY, INTELLIGENCE AND IQ, READING, SCHOOL.

Lead Poisoning

Lead poisoning in children is usually associated with the ingestion of paint and plaster flakes containing high levels of lead. This is a problem in city slums where old buildings are being leveled, or in cases where youngsters manage to gnaw on repainted cribs and other furniture originally covered with lead-base paint. In homes being renovated, the dust from removal of lead paint can cause an increase in lead levels in the blood.

Lead poisoning is a serious danger to the health of approximately half a million children in the United States. Irreversible brain damage and anemia can occur if the condition becomes chronic; convulsions and death may occur in an acute case. To lessen such hazards, legislation now requires new cars to use only lead-free gasoline.

Learning Disability

A child with a learning disability is one who, though otherwise normal, cannot acquire certain skills or assimilate certain kinds of knowledge at the same rate as most other children. Obviously, almost every child lags behind her peers at one time or another in certain subjects; but the difficulties of a learning disabled child are far more severe. A 16-year-old who suffers from a learning disability may, for example, be capable only of third- or fourth-grade math while functioning at her own grade level in other subjects. Some learning disabilities are attributed to minimal brain damage, but in most cases the cause is unknown. See also DYSLEXIA.

Leukemia

See CANCER.

Lying

See DISHONESTY.

Malnutrition

Poor nutrition or undernourishment can occur not only as a result of a faulty diet, but also because a child may have a metabolic defect that prevents her body from making proper use of a particular essential nutrient. Temporary malnutrition may also accompany a long illness in which the child's appetite wanes.

Although malnutrition is usually associated with poverty and child neglect, it can also occur because of ignorance, carelessness, or fanaticism. Children have been found to be malnourished by parents following a macrobiotic diet or a faddish type of vegetarianism. Using vitamins as a substitute for food can also cause certain types of undernourishment.

Older children, especially girls approaching puberty, may embark on starvation diets in an attempt to ward off inevitable body changes and end up seriously malnourished. The general signs of malnutrition are increasing physical weakness, vague and unfocused behavior, as well as the particular symptoms associated with anemia and vitamin deficiencies. See also Ch. 27, *Nutrition and Weight Control*.

Measles

Measles is by far the most dangerous of the common childhood diseases because of its possible complications, such as meningitis, encephalitis, and severe secondary staphylococcus infection. Fortunately, widespread protection is available in the live measles vaccine, which should be given to every child over one year of age.

Symptoms

Measles, a highly contagious disease caused by a virus, has an incubation period of one to two weeks. The most noticeable symptom is the rash that begins on the head and face within a few days after the onset of the disease, and gradually erupts all over the body, blending into big red patches. Other symptoms include fever up to 104° F or higher, a severe cough, sore throat, stuffy nose, inflammation of the *conjunctiva* (the mucous membrane on the inner part of the eyelid and extending over the front of the eyeball), sensitivity of the eyes to light, enlarged lymph nodes, and a generalized sick feeling.

Any child who has contracted measles should be seen by a physician and watched carefully for possible complications. Moreover, if he is of school age, the school should be promptly notified. This, of course, is true for any contagious disease.

Treatment

Measles can be treated only symptomatically. During the incubation period, an injection of gamma globulin will lessen the severity of the disease, or occasionally prevent it. If there are other children at home besides the affected one, they should also receive gamma globulin injections. Antibiotics are of no help unless there is a secondary bacterial infection.

It is now suspected that vaccinations given in the United States and Canada during the 1960s and 1970s were not triggering permanent immunity to measles. Anyone who has been vaccinated during that period should consult his or her physician about reimmunization. The number of cases, including adult cases, of measles has risen dramatically. This is partly because of the need for revaccination in adults; it is also because many parents are not having their children immunized. Measles can be fatal and vaccination can protect against needless deaths from this preventable disease.

All parents should make certain that their children are vaccinated against this potentially serious disease. See IMMUNIZATION.

Medication

New parents can save themselves time and trouble by getting into the habit of writing down a physician's instructions about medication when the child requires it. Although dosages are usually clearly indicated on labels prepared by the pharmacist according to the prescription, the physician may add comments about how or when to change the dosage.

How to Give Medicines to Children

As for administering medication, a calm and assured approach and a minimum of fuss are more effective than wheedling and urging. A very young child may need to be distracted by cheerful conversation as the spoon goes into her mouth; an older child can be given some factual information about the medication and what it will do. No matter what the youngster's age, parents should never trick or fool her about what she's being given, nor should candied medicine be used under any circumstances. Setting up this type of confusion in a young mind can lead to an overdose of "candy" serious enough to require emergency hospitalization.

Overusing Medication

As a child gets older, she will become increasingly conscious of the medication her parents take. Families that are constantly swallowing one or another kind of pill—diet pills, sleeping pills, tranquilizers—might give some thought to their attitude towards drugs and how these attitudes are affecting their children. Generally, it's a good idea to refrain from medicating a child unless the pediatrician recommends it.

Old Medicines

Once the illness for which a particular medication has been prescribed is definitely over, the remains of the bottle or the leftover capsules should be flushed down the toilet. Old, outdated pills can be dangerous. For safety's sake, parents should review the contents of the medicine cabinet on a regular basis and get rid of any medications left over from a previous illness. Basic medications that are essential for occasional emergencies should be reviewed for continuing effectiveness. Some of these might have a limited shelf life and be completely ineffective should they be needed.

Meningitis

Meningitis is an inflammation of the *meninges*, the thin membranes that cover the spinal cord and the brain. The inflammation, which may be caused by a virus or by bacteria, is more common among children than adults, and may occur in epidemics. This is especially true if the infectious agent is meningococcal (*meningococcal meningitis*), because the meningococcal bacteria are also found in the throat and are transmitted by coughing, sneezing, and talking. This type occurs mostly in young adults. Another type of meningitis that commonly occurs among young children during the spring and summer is caused by such organisms as the mumps virus and the coxsackievirus.

Symptoms

Whatever the cause, the symptoms are generally the same: headache, fever, vomiting, and stiff neck. If untreated, the child may go into delirium and convulsions. Drowsiness and blurred vision may also occur, and if the disease develops in an infant, the pressure on the brain caused by the inflamed meninges will create a bulge on the soft spot (fontanelle) of the baby's head. No time should be lost in calling the physician about any of these symptoms.

Meningitis was almost always fatal before the availability of antibiotics, and although it is no longer the threat it once was, it must be treated promptly if irreversible consequences are to be avoided.

Mental Illness

Behind the search for the causes and treatment of mental illness in children is the current research in the relationship between that mysterious entity called the mind and that palpable physical organism called the brain. Parents of children diagnosed as mentally ill are themselves caught up in this distinction, often preferring to call their youngsters "emotionally disturbed." It is now estimated that about one-and-a-half million youngsters under 18 require some kind of treatment for mental illness, and this figure does not include the one million children diagnosed as hyperkinetic. The two most serious forms of childhood mental illness are autism and schizophrenia.

Autism

The term "early infantile autism" was coined in the 1940s to describe babies and young children who show unpredictable deviations in development. Some never learn to speak; others refuse to look anyone directly in the eye. Autistic children may have one or two extraordinary skills and be incapable of remembering their own names. In spite of a tendency on the part of a few specialists to ascribe autism to a rejecting mother's refusal to love the infant, most authorities now describe this mysterious disorder as an organic condition caused by neurological rather than by psychological abnormalities. The same conclusions are more or less being reached about schizophrenia.

Schizophrenia

In schizophrenia, a child is likely to exhibit any of the following symptoms: confused speech and thinking; lack of emotional responsiveness; withdrawal into fantasy; and, occasionally, hallucinations. There are indications that genetic inheritance plays some role in this disorder, and that environmental influences are also involved.

Studies suggest that symptoms originate in abnormalities of brain chemistry that may be corrected by the proper medication. Over the past twenty years, many special schools, both day schools and residential ones, have been established for training autistic and schizophrenic children. The most successful enlist the cooperation of parents as cotherapists. The National Society for Children and Adults with Autism was organized to initiate schools, offer counseling to parents, and foster research. The Society operates a National Information and Referral Service that can be addressed at 1234 Massachusetts Ave., NW,

Ste. 1017, Washington, DC 20005. See also HYPERKINESIS.

Mental Retardation

An estimated six million people in the United States are in some degree mentally retarded—almost three percent of the population. Mental retardation occurs among all nationalities, races, and religions, and among the children of those in the highest social and economic groups as well as the lowest.

What Is Mental Retardation?

Mental retardation is a developmental disability in which the individual's rate of development as a child is consistently slower than average. Learning cannot be acquired at the usual rate, and the child encounters difficulties in social adjustment.

Degrees of Mental Retardation

Mentally retarded children (and adults) are classified into four categories depending upon the degree of retardation.

Mildly retarded children—those with IQs roughly between 50 and 70—belong to by far the largest category; nearly 90 percent of all retarded people fall into this group. IQ scores by themselves can be misleading, but they are a convenient guide to probable learning and development patterns if understood properly—that is, simply as one of the criteria by which the degree of a child's disability can be estimated. The retardation of mildly retarded children is usually not apparent until they are of school age. With special educational help, such children can achieve satisfying progress in school and, as adults, will be capable with proper training of handling any of a wide variety of regular jobs. They may be indistinguishable from nonretarded people and can be expected to take their places in the life of their community.

Moderately retarded children— those with IQs somewhat below 50— belong to a group that comprises about 6 percent of all retarded people in the United States. The retardation of these children is usually apparent before they begin school, often during the child's first year, in the form of delayed developmental landmarks— for example, late sitting, late standing, late walking, and delayed talking. Many children with Down's syndrome (Mongolism) fall into this group. These children require a more sheltered environment than the mildly retarded, but can be trained as adults to do productive, satisfying work.

Severely and profoundly retarded children often have other handicaps, such as impaired motor coordination or defective vision or hearing. The great majority of these children can be taught to care for their basic needs, and many can do useful work under supervision.

Causes

There are numerous causes of mental retardation. Some cases are specifically caused by congenital factors (conditions existing at or before birth). Among these are the following: deprivation of oxygen to the brain of a baby during the birth process; the mother's contraction of rubella (German measles) during the first three months of pregnancy; complications resulting from Rh factor blood incompatibility between mother and baby; a grossly inadequate prenatal diet of the mother; syphilis; hydrocephalus (accumulation of spinal fluid in the brain); or any other pressure or injury to the brain of the fetus.

Some forms of retardation result from hereditary factors, the genetic makeup of the parents. Down's syndrome and phenylketonuria (PKU) fall in this category.

Mental retardation can also occur as a result of disease. Inflammation of the brain is a possible complication of measles—now wholly preventable by the administration of the measles vaccine. Other causes are brain injuries that result from a severe blow to the head, as from a fall. Some of these injuries are deliberately inflicted, usually by parents. (See CHILD ABUSE AND NEGLECT.) Among environmental hazards, lead and mercury poisoning are of particular importance. Lead-based paint chips have been eaten by unattended children. (See LEAD POISONING.)

If retardation is suspected by parents, medical advice should be sought immediately and a thorough evaluation of the child conducted. Some types of retardation can be greatly benefited by medical and educational treatment. It should be emphasized that all retarded children can learn and that many can be helped to the extent that they can become productive citizens. Parents would like further information about mental retardation or who are in need of counseling should write to the Association for Retarded Citizens, P.O. Box 6109, Arlington, TX 76005. See also DISABLED CHILD.

Money

Money may not be the root of all evil, but it certainly is the cause of a lot of family quarrels. To communicate to children the value of money and how to use it, spend it, save it, borrow it, lend it, and earn it, parents should try to clarify their own attitudes and settle their own differences.

Young children hear money talked about all the time: "We can't afford it," "That's a bargain," "That's a waste of money." What does it all mean to a preschooler?

The Weekly Allowance

The best way for a child to get first-hand experience in dealing with "I need" and "I want" in terms of cash on hand is to give her a weekly allowance. There isn't any point in doing this until she has mastered addition and subtraction. If the prospect of getting an allowance is motivation for improving her number skills at school, so much the better. The amount of the allowance should be calculated in terms of what it's supposed to cover. These details should be spelled out so that there's no confusion about who is responsible for paying for what. As the child gets older, the amount is adjusted for increasing needs—social occasions such as a ten-year-old might enjoy when she and her friends stop for an ice-cream cone on the way home from school.

Saving

If the family feels that a child should be required to save part of her allowance, a piggy bank and a brief talk about the virtues of saving are essential. Some children get so anxious about money that they turn into misers. When this occurs, it may be advisable to point out that the money is not meant to be hoarded but to be spent on needs and treats. Children who receive birthday or other special presents in the form of money from relatives can open a bank account and learn about interest accrual. Although the money is rightfully theirs, they might be encouraged to consult the family before they spend it all on a passing enthusiasm.

Mumps

Mumps, a mild disorder in most children, is caused by a virus and has an incubation period of from two to three weeks. The most familiar symptom is swollen glands involving the jaw. The glands usually affected are the *parotid glands*—large salivary glands below and slightly in front of the ear—although other glands may be affected, too. Other symptoms include fever and a general sick feeling. No rash is present. Mumps lasts about five days; then the swelling disappears.

In an adolescent boy, the disease sometimes causes an inflammation of the testes (called *orchitis*) and may be very painful. In addition, if it involves both testes, there is a possibility—fortunately only a very slight one—that sterility will result.

In older children mumps occasionally produces the complication called *mumps meningoencephalitis*. The signs of this more serious disease are headache, fever, and extreme debilitation. Finally, there may be an inflammation of the pancreas, which can cause severe abdominal pain and vomiting.

Because mumps is now preventable, every boy and girl should be given the mumps vaccine. Boys should be given the vaccine before puberty.

Muscular Dystrophy

See Ch. 8, *Diseases of the Muscles and Nervous System*.

Nausea and Vomiting

Nausea, the signal that vomiting may occur, is often described as feeling sick to the stomach. The feeling is experienced when irritated nerve endings in the stomach and elsewhere send messages to the vomiting reflex in the brain. When the nerve irritation is acute, vomiting occurs.

Physical Causes

Although nausea and vomiting are usually associated with a child's upset stomach or the sudden onset of a high fever and an acute infection, many youngsters feel nauseated and throw up because of motion sickness in a car or plane, or as the result of severe pain occasioned by a bad fall or other accident. A physician should always be consulted when nausea and vomiting are accompanied by fever, cramps, or diarrhea. For the child who feels sick in a moving vehicle, the physician can prescribe suitable medication. For a youngster who has swallowed a toxic substance, vomiting must often be induced. See Ch. 35, *Medical Emergencies*, for further information on poisoning.

Emotional Stress

Chronic nausea may result from emotional stress. A child who doesn't want to go to school because of some threatening situation, or who is always too anxious before a test because of pressures to do well, or who is fearful about some athletic challenge but ashamed to admit it—children under these pressures are likely to develop symptoms of nausea. However, instead of dismissing the recurrence of nausea and vomiting as typical of an oversensitive child, parents should try to find out the source of the problem and, if necessary, arrange some family therapy sessions with the child.

Nervous Habits

Nervous habits both express and release inner tension, and because growing up isn't an easy process, it's inevitable that most children have one or another way of dealing with their fears, anxieties, and emotional pressures. There's no point in parental scolding or ridicule or punishment, because any of these approaches simply adds yet another pressure to those that exist already. After all, most adults have nervous habits too—whether it's smoking, or picking at a cuticle, or tooth-grinding—and no amount of nagging is likely to put a stop to any of them.

Some nervous habits can be unhealthy, and some can be socially unacceptable but essentially harmless. All are unconscious, and most eventually disappear with age. Among the habits that may need looking into in order to decide that they have no basis in a physical disorder are squinting and throat-clearing. Hair-twirling and foot-shaking can be entirely ignored. Nail-biting may persist for years, or it may yield to vanity or the comments of friends.

Thumb-sucking, abandoned at two, may recur at three because of the arrival of a new baby or because of the stresses of going to nursery school. Many school-age children continue to suck their thumbs when they're going to sleep. There's no need to worry about this habit unless the dentist notices the beginning of an orthodontic problem, in which case, the dentist and not you should discuss it with the child. Nose-picking in public is almost always abandoned when a child enters school. If a big fuss has been made about it, he may continue the habit at home as a gesture of defiance—or because it really is unconscious. When done in private, it's completely harmless.

Masturbation bothers many parents more than it should. In and of itself, there's no harm in it, but as a chronic expression of anxiety, it might be dealt with tactfully and indirectly by trying to get to the source of the tension rather than by punishing or humiliating the child.

New Baby

It's a good idea for parents to talk about the anticipated arrival of a new baby with their child or children before the pregnancy is really obvious. Conversations can be casual, and questions should be answered simply and factually. If any basic changes are to be made—especially if a child is to be shifted to a bed so that the new arrival can have the crib—this transition should be accomplished before the infant appears. Adults should refrain from asking such questions as "Would you like a little brother or a little sister?" or "Isn't it wonderful that there's going to be a new baby in the family?" Preparations made in advance of going to the hospital should, if possible, consider whether the child would prefer to stay at home or with a relative during mother's absence. When the baby is brought home and well-wishers arrive with presents, it's comforting for the first-born to sit in mother's or daddy's lap while visitors coo over the infant in the crib. Thoughtful baby-present givers will always include a little present for the baby's older siblings, too. Parents should do their best to make baby's big brother or sister feel that the new baby is his or hers no less than mother's or father's. See also BROTHERS AND SISTERS.

Nightmares

See DREAMS AND NIGHTMARES.

Night Terrors

See DREAMS AND NIGHTMARES.

Nosebleeds

Children are likely to have nosebleeds more often than adults, and they are usually no cause for alarm. A blood vessel near the nostril may be injured by energetic noseblowing, the presence of a foreign object, or by an accidental blow or an intentional wallop.

Apply Pressure

A minor nosebleed is most effectively stopped by applying pressure over the bleeding area. A child old enough to follow instructions should be told to sit down, hold the head slightly forward, and compress the soft portion of the nose between thumb and forefinger, maintaining the pressure for about five minutes and breathing through the mouth. Application of an ice pack to the outside of the nose is usually helpful. Fingers should be withdrawn very slowly in order not to disturb the clot that should have formed.

Packing the Nostril

If this method doesn't stop the bleeding, a small twist of sterile cotton can be inserted gently into the nostril so that some of it protrudes. Light pressure should be applied once again for five minutes and the cotton allowed to remain in place for a while. Should the bleeding continue in spite of these measures, the child should be taken to a hospital emergency clinic.

Nutrition

Children's nutritional requirements are not the same as adults. Although that may seem like an obvious statement, the fact is many parents do not take it into account when planning meals.

Infants are incapable of digesting many products. Introduction of new food to an infant should be done one item at a time. If the baby has an allergic reaction, the parent then knows what it is in response to. If the baby has eaten two or three new items, it isn't possible to tell without another feeding which one the child is allergic to.

Children can outgrow some intolerances to food. A baby that could not properly digest citrus fruit may be able to handle it well a few months or years later. Some allergies, though, get worse with each exposure. Common food allergies and intolerances include nuts, berries, milk, eggs, and fish.

Children do not require the same quantity of food as an adult. Small children will eat less at a meal, but may need to eat more frequently during the day. Their stomach holds less so they get hungry more frequently.

Children also do not require the same quantity of minerals and vitamins as adults. Childrens' vitamins are available but should not be used to replace a healthy diet. Good eating habits in children establishes a pattern that they are likely to follow for the rest of their lives. Also, children should not become adapted to the idea of taking a pill every day.

Several studies show that children who are obese can diet effectively and that they are more likely to keep the weight off than adults are. Overweight children who diet for a period even as short as 10 weeks are less obese than overweight children who never diet at all. One study demonstrated that dieting in childhood does not completely prevent obesity but it does limit the amount of weight gain to less than half that gained by those who never dieted as children.

Weight is an extremely sensitive subject to children. Adolescents in particular are susceptible to negative self-images based on weight, and to criticism by others. Disorders related to eating are covered in *The Teens* under Anorexia and Bulimia.

Weight gain can commonly be traced to the amount of television a child watches. Obesity and television viewing are related through two habits. The first is that for every hour the child is plopped in front of a television is an hour the child is not playing and exercising. The other is that television watching is usually accompanied by snacking on high-fat, high-salt or sugar pre-processed food.

Orthodontics

Orthodontics is the branch of dentistry that specializes in the correction of *malocclusion* (an improper alignment of the upper and lower teeth at the point where they meet) or to irregularity of tooth positioning. Emphasis is now being placed on the prevention of malocclusion before it can occur. General practitioners of dentistry, *pedodontists* (specialists in children's dentistry), and orthodontists now believe that the need for expensive, time-consuming, and emotionally unsettling orthodontics can sometimes be avoided by beginning treatment as early as the age of four.

The positioning of the permanent teeth is the result not only of inheritance, but of other variables, such as lip-biting and thumb-sucking. Premature loss or partial disintegration of primary teeth also has a strong influence on whether the permanent teeth will be properly positioned.

Preventive Orthodontics

By the time the child is five, an X ray will show exactly how all the permanent teeth are situated in the gums. In some cases, it may be possible to guide these teeth as they erupt. If potential overcrowding and eventual crookedness are indicated, some baby teeth may be pulled to make room for the permanent ones. Normal positioning may also be accomplished by establishing a different balance of muscular forces.

Corrective Appliances

Corrective orthodontics uses many different types of appliances for the repositioning of permanent teeth, all of which operate on the same principle of applying pressure to the bone. Widening the arch of the upper jaw, for example, is accomplished by the use of a screw appliance fixed to the upper teeth so that the two halves of the hard palate are slightly separated along the middle suture, permitting new bone to fill in the space. Specialists point out that a bonus of this orthodontic correction is increased respiratory ease for youngsters who were formerly mouth-breathers.

Parents who have been advised by the family dentist that an orthodontic consultation is advisable for a child, and who are concerned about the eventual economic burden that prolonged treatment might represent, should get a second opinion from the clinical staff of a dental school associated with a university. See also DENTAL CARE.

Pacifiers

Some parents can't stand the sound of a baby's crying; others can't stand the sight of a baby sucking on a pacifier. Whatever the preference, what the baby needs during the early months is satisfaction for the sucking impulse. For most babies, this need seems to taper off at about six months; with those babies in whom the need remains strong, the thumb seems to be a convenient substitute for the pacifier. Whatever decision is arrived at between you and your physician, the important thing to keep in mind is that the pacifier is no substitute for holding and cuddling the baby when she wants comforting, and that sometimes a parent is more dependent on a pacifier than the baby is.

If pacifiers are used regularly, more than one should be available, and they should be inspected periodically to make sure that bits and pieces of rubber haven't been chewed so loose that they may be swallowed and lodge in the windpipe.

Pets

Rural children usually have their own pet animals even if the animals aren't allowed in the house. Suburban families are likely to own a dog that's a pet as well as a discouragement to prowlers. It's the city child who may have to wage a persistent campaign before his parents capitulate to the idea of a pet. Yet even the smallest apartment can accommodate a pet bird or a small fish tank; a cat and a litter box won't cause extra crowding. Of course, dogs offer the greatest companionship but also impose the greatest responsibility; they do have to be housebroken and walked in all weathers at least twice a day. If a child brings a stray animal home, the dog or cat must be checked by a vet before it becomes a household member. Once a youngster can read, the acquisition of a pet hamster or a guinea pig or a pair of gerbils will provide the incentive for trips to the library for books on care and feeding.

Choosing a Dog

When a dog is to be the choice, it's often cheaper and more satisfactory to select one from the litter of a healthy dog you know than to buy one in a pet shop or from a commercial kennel. The Anti-Cruelty and other animal shelters can provide pets at little or no charge to families. The breed chosen should be suitable in terms of size, temperament, and cost of feeding. Relative advantages and disadvantages should be checked out at the library by the child whose responsibility the pet will be.

For an only child, a pet animal is almost a must, not only for companionship, but so that there's a being in the house who's smaller and more helpless than she is. In families where allergies are a problem, the physician should be consulted about the type of pet that will cause the least discomfort to a vulnerable member of the household.

Pica

Pica is the technical term for an abnormal desire to eat substances that are not fit for food, such as clay, earth, plaster and the like. This tendency is not to be confused with the tendency of babies and toddlers to put unsuitable things into their mouth. Pica is habitual and compulsive, and may result in serious disabilities. Because the phenomenon is especially conspicuous among poor and neglected children, some authorities associate it with nutritional deficiency, others with unsatisfied emotional needs. Signs of pica should be brought to the attention of a physician or a social service agency that can provide guidance on how the child's circumstances should be altered even if the total environment cannot be changed. See also LEAD POISONING.

Pills

See MEDICATION.

Pinworms or Threadworms

See Ch. 11, *Diseases of the Digestive System*.

PKU

PKU stands for *phenylketonuria*, an inherited metabolic defect. Approximately one baby in 10,000 is born with this disease, in which the body is incapable of producing certain enzymes that are essential for the metabolic conversion of the amino acid phenylalanine. The disorder causes the amino acid and some of its by-products to accumulate in the blood-stream to a dangerous degree. If the condition goes undetected and untreated, irreversible brain damage and mental retardation are the result.

PKU babies are characteristically blond and blue-eyed, with sensitive skin and faulty muscle coordination. In many parts of the United States, state laws require that three days after birth, all babies be given the blood test that detects the presence of PKU so that treatment can begin at once if necessary. Supervised treatment usually continues for several years, and in some communities is available at special therapy centers. Parents or prospective parents who would like to find out whether any member of the family is a carrier of the recessive gene that transmits the PKU disorder can arrange for diagnostic testing and genetic counseling based on the results.

Play

See FANTASIES, TOYS, SAFETY.

Pneumonia

See "Pneumonia" in Ch. 12, *Diseases of the Respiratory System*.

Poison Ivy, Oak, and Sumac Rashes

Poison ivy and poison oak are two plants readily found across the United States. Poison sumac is found in marshes in the southern and eastern states. Children frequently come in contact with the plants while playing, hiking, or camping. The oils from the surface of the plant brush against the skin and usually, within hours, a itchy painful rash appears on the skin.

If contact with poisonous plants is suspected, the first thing one should do is wash the area of skin thoroughly with soap and water as soon after exposure as possible. Removing the poisonous oils can eliminate or reduce the inflammation. Care should be taken not to spread the oils from the infected skin to other skin. Particular care should be given to not touch or rub your eyes after contact with one of these plants. You should also be cautious of rubbing your eyes after scratching infected or exposed skin.

The rash is an itchy red group of small blisters. Cold water dressings can help reduce the itching. Use clean cotton cloth soaked in a solution of one teaspoon of salt per pint of water. Antihistamine medication can help reduce the itching and rash. If the rash persists, becomes infected, is severe, or covers a large part of the child's body, consult a physician immediately.

Poisons and Poisoning

Every year, hundreds of thousands of children swallow some poisonous substance—in too many cases with fatal results—because of parental carelessness, or because the child hasn't been given clear and unequivocal instructions about the difference between "candy" and medicine. Poisoning because of the ingestion of sugar-coated aspirin is a continuing problem; iron-containing multiple vitamins that seem to be a gourmet treat to some children also present a problem because iron in excess doses is a stomach irritant.

Safety Measures

Toddlers can do themselves damage because they're curious about everything, and their sense of taste isn't all that discriminating. Thus it's an absolute necessity to see that all household cleansers and strong chemicals are kept on high shelves rather than on the floor. Many bottles containing medicines come with safety caps that presumably cannot be opened by children—for instance, because pressure must be applied—but can be opened by adults. The experience of many parents, however, is that whereas their children can often open such caps, *they* frequently have a great deal of difficulty. Suffice it to say that the perfect childproof bottle cap has yet to be designed.

Because it's practically impossible for anyone except an expert to know what substances are poisonous to children in what amounts, or which seeds of which plants are harmful if swallowed, many authorities feel strongly that parents should immediately call the closest Poison Control Center for first-aid information rather than try to cope with antidotes or emetics on their own. The Centers are available by phone on a 24-hour-a-day basis. See Ch. 31, *Medical Emergencies*, to find the Poison Control Center nearest you. Make a note of the telephone number and make sure it's available to baby-sitters as well as to all responsible family members.

Poliomyelitis

Until the Salk vaccine was developed in the 1950s, there was no protection against polio (or, as it was then popularly called, *infantile paralysis*). The disease caused paralysis of the extremities and could cause death by paralyzing the muscles used in breathing.

The Salk vaccine utilizes doses of killed virus and is given by injection. Although it is still widely used in many parts of the world, in the United States the Sabin live virus vaccine, which is given orally, has virtually supplanted it. Repeated series of booster shots are unnecessary because the immunity persists for years.

It is advisable that a child receive three doses of the Sabin vaccine, six to eight weeks apart, starting at about the age of two months. One method employs *trivalent* vaccine, in which each dose contains three kinds of vaccine—to give protection against three strains of polio. Three separate doses are necessary, however, to insure full protection. The other method employs *monovalent* vaccines, in which each dose insures protection against a different type of polio.

Posture

"Stand up straight" is an order that many parents issue to their children with the regularity of drill sergeants. Actually, most youngsters tend to slump and have a potbellied look until they're about nine years old. This inelegant posture is not necessarily the sign of any disorder.

Youngsters who are regularly checked by a physician and given a good bill of health are not in any danger of developing a permanent curvature of the spine because they slouch. However, certain kinds of chronically poor posture may be an expression of some disorder that should be checked. Among these are flat feet, nearsightedness or astigmatism, or a hearing loss.

Emotional problems may also be expressed in a child's bearing. Anxiety can lead to carrying one shoulder higher than the other as if warding off a blow. Shyness or insecurity may cause a hangdog stance. For pubescent girls, embarrassment about burgeoning breasts may result in a round-shouldered slump. Some of these causes of poor posture should be discussed with a physician; others may be temporary and shouldn't be turned into major problems by incessant and unproductive nagging. A better corrective is participation in a dancing class or an exercise class. Sports such as ice-skating and bicycle-riding are good posture correctives, too.

Prejudice

The A student (female) who avoids studying mathematics because "girls aren't supposed to be good in math" and the black boy who goes out for the track team even though he'd rather be in the science club "because blacks are better at sports than at brainwork" have unconsciously accepted the prejudiced views of other people about them. What a waste for themselves and society!

Children who are raised in an atmosphere of contempt for and fear and mistrust of Catholics, Jews, Italians, blacks, women, men, are likely to spend the better part of their lives alternating between apprehension and arrogance. It's difficult to believe that adults can have a prejudice such as, "All Orientals are sneaky," which is supposed to describe millions of human beings, or "She's only a girl," which makes a judgment about one-half of the human race.

Being the Object of Discrimination

Parents who have themselves been discriminated against have to prepare their children for the reality of discrimination and how to cope with it. A child raised in an atmosphere of love and respect will have enough self-esteem to refuse to accept anyone else's false notions about him.

Privacy

Every child has a right to a certain amount of privacy even when he's very young. If, for instance, a parent or older child doesn't allow anyone into the bathroom when he's using it, a four- or five-year-old should be given the same option. When children share the same room, or even the same furniture, each one should have a drawer of his own and a shelf of his own for his things. Respecting his private property will lead him to respect other people's. A youngster does like the privacy of playing with his friends without having a parent hovering around all the time, and he certainly doesn't want anyone listening in on his phone conversations by the time he's nine or ten.

Parents have a right to privacy, too! Children should be led to understand—pleasantly but firmly—that some adult conversations are private and not meant for their ears. They should also be taught that when an older member of the family is behind a closed door, it's rude to barge in without knocking.

Puberty

See Ch. 3, *The Teens*.

Punishment

Severe physical punishment should be avoided. Ideally, punishment should be carried out because it has an instructional value for the child rather than because it helps a parent relieve his or her feelings of anger or frustration. Severe physical punishments— for example, the use of sticks, belts, or hard blows to the body—are extremely frightening and may even be permanently injurious to the child. They are also illegal actions, constituting child abuse. Frequently, this kind of discipline can evoke even further anger on the part of the child and lead to further misbehavior.

Duration

Punishments should not be long and drawn out, but should be as immediate as possible and last only a reasonable length of time. For example, withdrawal of television privileges for a month for a seven-year-old's misbehavior would be excessively long, because at the end of the month it would be difficult for her to remember what she had done that was wrong. Excessively long punishments are also difficult to enforce. If possible, a punishment should be related to the misbehavior for which the child is receiving the punishment.

Immediacy

Punishment "when father gets home" or a day later frequently has little meaning for the child and is unlikely to help her stop misbehaving. Rewards for good behavior should also be immediate; affection and approval for most children are often more powerful rewards than candy and money.

Rashes

Rashes of one kind or another are among the most common occurrences of childhood. Whether it's the discomfort of diaper rash soon after birth, the childhood markings of chicken pox, or a case of poison ivy, most skin eruptions aren't too serious and are usually of brief duration.

The First Six Months

Skin rashes are especially common during the first six months. They may result from overheating or overdressing, or to the use of detergents, powders, perfumes, and oils which cause *contact dermatitis*. In addition, certain foods may make the baby break out in facial rashes. Prolonged contact with wet diapers causes *diaper rash*, from the ammonia produced by urine.

Skin rashes can usually be prevented or controlled by:

- Control of temperature
- Proper clothing
- Avoidance of irritating perfumes, powders, and detergents in laundering baby clothes
- Avoidance, in certain circumstances, of milk or other foods, as suggested by your physician
- Avoidance of rubber pants over diapers
- Applications of ointments to rashy areas

If a disturbing skin condition persists or gets worse, your physician will check for special infections like impetigo or fungus, and, should they exist, recommend proper treatment. During the early years, most children develop the characteristic rashes of the contagious childhood diseases, and at these times, a physician's care is usually essential for the prevention of complications.

Eczema

Some children suffer from intermittent eczema that has a tendency to run in families. Eczema can be extremely uncomfortable, because the more it itches, the more it is scratched, and the more it's scratched, the more it itches. This cycle may be triggered by an allergy to a particular food or pollen; it may be a contact dermatitis caused by a particular fabric, or it might flare up because of emotional tension created by family arguments or anxiety about schoolwork. Eczema should be treated by the family physician who may be able to discover its source and prevent further attacks.

Other Allergic Rashes

Other rashes that are essentially allergic in origin are those resulting from contact with poison ivy, oak, or sumac. For information about these and other skin conditions, including hives, see "Disorders of the Skin," in Ch. 21, *Skin and Hair*.

The discomfort of many rashes can be eased by ointments or salves. Plain cornstarch is helpful for prickly heat. Rashes that are bacterial in origin, such as impetigo, or parasitic, have to be treated by a physician with antibiotic or fungicidal preparations.

Roseola

Among the more common rashes of early childhood is the one known as *roseola infantum*. It is believed to be caused by a virus. It begins with a high fever that subsides in a few days. There are no other specific signs of illness, and the end of the disorder— when the fever is usually gone—is signaled by the appearance of a body rash of red spots that disappear overnight. The one aspect of roseola that requires medical attention is the fever. Because high temperature can produce convulsions in infants and babies, efforts should be made to reduce it by sponging and nonaspirin medication. Antibiotics are not indicated unless there's some sign of a secondary infection.

Pityriasis Rosea

A long-lasting rash thought to be viral in origin is *pityriasis rosea*, easily identifiable because the onset of this infection is preceded by one large raised red scaly eruption known as the herald patch. The rash itself appears symmetrically and in clusters on the trunk, arms, and legs, and in some children on the hands and feet as well as the face. Unfortunately, this rash may last for more than a month. There is no treatment for it, and, although it leaves without a trace and almost never recurs, it can cause severe itching that should be eased with a salve or ointment. Soap is very irritating and should be avoided.

Rocky Mountain Spotted Fever

Among the diseases caused by organisms known as rickettsiae and transmitted to people by the animal ticks that are infected with them is *Rocky Mountain spotted fever*, also called *tick fever*. In addition to rising temperature, headache, nausea, and malaise, this disease produces a characteristic rash that starts on the ankles, lower legs, and wrists, and then spreads to the rest of the body. Children who wander about in the woods during the summer or whose pets run loose in tick-infested areas should be watched for the presence of a tick on the skin and the ensuing rash. Rocky Mountain spotted fever is a serious disease against which youngsters should be protected by wearing the proper clothing.

Lyme Disease

A rash may be the first visible symptom of Lyme disease, which had been reported in 34 American states by the late 1980s. Caused by a tick-carried bacterium, the disease can produce symptoms similar to those of arthritis, multiple sclerosis, and heart disease. The initial rash can extend over an area 28 inches across. Antibiotics including tetracycline and penicillin may be used in treatment. The risk of infection may be reduced by frequent inspections of skin areas and prompt removal of the pinhead-sized ticks. If not embedded, ticks can be brushed off; if embedded, they can be lifted out with a tweezers. The skin should be washed carefully with an antiseptic such as rubbing alcohol.

Reading

Children who see their parents reading or who've heard an older sibling say, "Don't interrupt me when I'm reading" are much more likely to want to learn how to read than those who have never seen an older person absorbed in a book or magazine.

Reading Difficulties

No matter how much the world changes, the child who can't read easily is handicapped. Where a true reading problem exists, parents should confer with the school about a practical solution. If a learning disability appears to be the explanation, tutoring or a special class may be essential. See DYSLEXIA.

Reading for Information

Many youngsters who don't see the point in reading for pleasure when there are so many other things they'd prefer to do may dash off to the library if they want information about horses or sailing ships or sewing. Families who would like their youngsters to read more than they do have the responsibility of providing a quiet corner, a decent reading light, and an occasional hour of uninterrupted leisure and privacy. Parents who object to their ten-year-old daughter's habit of "always having her nose in a book" instead of "getting some fresh air and exercise" should withhold their criticism unless the physician recommends a change in the child's activities.

Retardation

See MENTAL RETARDATION.

Reye's Syndrome

Reye's Syndrome is a childhood disease that affects the nervous system and the liver and can result in death. The symptoms normally occur after the child has suffered from the flu or a respiratory illness. The symptoms include vomiting, rash, and disorientation or confusion. If not immediately treated, seizures, respiratory arrest, and coma follow shortly. There is no cure but the dangerous manifestations of the disease can be treated to avoid complications, permanent damage, or death.

The syndrome is believed to be linked to treating the child with aspirin or aspirin-containing medication during the initial illness. Cases of Reye's Syndrome have decreased sharply since 1980, with the increase in public awareness of the link between the disease and the use of aspirin for children.

Given the risk of Reye's Syndrome, it is highly recommended that parents avoid aspirin for children during any illness with fever, flu, diarrhea, or respiratory symptoms. If symptoms persist or if aspirin was given just before the onset of symptoms, please notify a physician. Reye's Syndrome is diagnosed symptomatically.

Rheumatic Fever

Once called growing pains, rheumatic fever is actually a disease of the connective tissues, a secondary manifestation of a primary infection by streptococcus bacteria of the throat or tonsils. Its chief symptoms are pains and tenderness in the joints and sore throat.

Rheumatic fever may be mild enough to escape attention or it may be disabling for a period of months. The insidious aspect of the disease is that it may damage the child's heart in such a way that tissue is permanently scarred and function is impaired in the form of a heart murmur. Acuteness of symptoms varies. Any time from a week to a month after the occurrence of strep throat, the child may complain of feeling tired and achy. Fever usually accompanies the fatigue, and pains in the joints may precede swelling and the development of nodules under the skin in the areas of the wrists, elbows, knees, and vertebrae. The pediatrician can usually detect an abnormal heart finding. The sooner treatment begins, however, the less likely the risk of permanent heart damage.

Close supervision of the affected child may be essential over a long period. Antibiotics, aspirin, hormones (cortisone), and other medicines control the course of the disease and protect the child from its potentially disabling effects. See also "Rheumatic Fever and Rheumatic Heart Disease" in Ch. 10, *Heart Diseases*.

Roseola Infantum

See under RASHES.

Rubella (German Measles)

Rubella was once thought of as a benign disease. Then it was discovered that it could have serious consequences if it were contracted by a woman during the first three months of her pregnancy. The virus that causes rubella is transmitted from the infected woman to her unborn baby, and has been linked to birth defects of the heart, eye, ear, and liver, and to mental retardation.

In addition, a baby who has been exposed to the disease in utero may infect others even though he himself is not affected by it and shows no symptoms. (In fact, most babies are immune to rubella during their first year.) The rubella virus is highly contagious and spreads rapidly.

Rubella has been on the increase in recent years, largely due to the number of young adults who have never been vaccinated. Although it can be a mild illness, it can also cause severe birth defects if contracted by a pregnant woman. Because of the risk of miscarriage and birth defects, pregnant women are advised against getting the immunization during the course of their pregnancy. Anyone who suspects that they or their children were not vaccinated should seek immunization immediately.

The incubation period for rubella is two to three weeks. Symptoms include earache, swollen glands behind the ears, a low-grade fever, and a usually mild, blotchy rash that erupts over the body but lasts only a few days.

Runaways

In growing numbers children and youth ran away from home in the early and middle 1980s. The runaways left home for various reasons. Some were escaping physical or sexual abuse while many others had severe long-term psychological and other problems. A smaller percentage faced temporary or less severe home or school difficulties. Other reasons include "status criminal offense problems"—minor violations of the law that would not be violations at all if committed by an adult—and "poor communication" with parents. Truancy is an example of a status offense. Many children who leave home are not technically "runaways." Professionals call these children *throwaways* because they have in fact been thrown out of the parents' home.

Social service professionals believe many young persons leave home to escape from "dysfunctional families." In such families, parental separation or divorce, poverty, unemployment, and high mobility have, separately or in combination, made the home ineffective as a nurturing environment. The young person may become labeled as a "failure" or "troublemaker"; and a lack of warmth may characterize parent–child relations. In other cases delinquency among a youngster's friends may exert a powerful influence.

The runaways represent diverse age and economic groups. They come from a variety of racial backgrounds. A large proportion are in the 15 to 16 age group. But runaways range in age from 10 or younger to 18.

Parents faced with the fact that a child has run away have to make difficult choices. The child who stays away overnight or for two or more nights has usually not traveled more than 10 miles from home. He or she is usually staying with friends. Only about one in five ventures more than 50 miles from home. The parent or parents of a runaway, considering such facts and not wishing simply to wait, can:

- Look for the youngster themselves. Recommended by many social workers as a logical first step, such a search may involve calls to relatives or the child's friends, checks on favorite haunts, and "driving around" in areas that the young person knows and frequents.

- Report the runaway to police. A "first impulse" alternative, calling the police may not be in the child's best interest. For one thing, the police, especially in large cities, are swamped with such reports. Parental searches actually succeed in finding runaways more frequently than police do. As a second consideration, once reported to police the youngster may be drawn into the juvenile-justice system. In some states, that could result in incarceration with adult offenders or delinquent juveniles. Other states provide that a runaway cannot be held—or cannot be held more than a brief, specified period.

- Contact a local branch of the National Network of Runaway and Youth Services. A private, nonprofit organization with more than 500 community-based shelter programs, the Network serves runaway, homeless, and other "problem" young people. It offers shelter and hotline services 24 hours a day, seven days a week. While not a search operation, the Network also provides crisis and long-term individual and family counseling, outreach, advocacy, referrals for medical, legal, and mental health assistance, and followup services.

- Contact the National Communications System. Supported by the U.S. Department of Health and Human Services, the system operates a nationwide toll-free telephone hotline. Services provided center on referral and crisis intervention aid.

Some national or local services have been established primarily to help runaways obtain clothing, shelter, and food. These organizations also try to mediate between parents and children and to bring families together. Three such groups operate the Runaway Hotline (800/231-6946), the National Runaway Switchboard (800/621-4000), and the National Center for Missing and Exploited Children (800/843-5678).

What happens after a child returns home may determine whether he or she will run away again. Family counselors suggest that parents remain calm. No matter how stressful the runaway incident may have been, parents should try to accept their child as a person. Many runaways, counselors say, are "testing the waters," or experimenting, or seeking a sense of self and identity. If the family can discuss what has happened, the problems that caused the young person to run away may be resolved.

In difficult situations, counseling may be necessary. More and more parents are turning also to inpatient psychiatric services. Usually, these parents have tried other solutions before turning to psychiatry. Contributing to the trend toward hospitalization and professional treatment is the increasing availability of insurance to cover the expected costs.

Safety

See "Accident Prevention" in Ch. 36, *Voluntary Health Agencies*.

Scarlet Fever

Scarlet fever used to be a disease that everyone dreaded. It is highly contagious, and can result in severe after-effects like rheumatic fever, or the kidney disease known as nephritis.

It is now known that scarlet fever is simply a streptococcal infection—a strain of a specific organism that also causes a diffuse red rash. It can be dealt with quite simply by your physician, the usual treatment being a ten-day course of penicillin, which cures the streptococcal infection and prevents most complications.

Schizophrenia

See under MENTAL ILLNESS.

School

In the United States, an elementary school is a place where children are taught not only how to read, write, handle numbers, and correlate sets of facts, they are also taught how to get along with children different from themselves, how to express themselves creatively, and how to become responsible citizens of a democratic society. If the reality of education falls short of these goals, parents are supposed to exert influence on the proper authorities to see that they are in fact accomplished.

Nursery School

For a child, leaving the protection of the family if only for a half-day in a nearby nursery school is a big step forward. The step is likely to be taken with eagerness if parents present the school as a pleasurable place to be, and not as a dumping ground for a youngster who's in the way of a new baby or a working mother.

Elementary School

The elementary grades represent a major change in many different ways, but most importantly because new authority figures begin to displace parents as the source of all wisdom. Adults and older siblings can help a child make a happy and productive adjustment to school by talking about it with interest and respect. Wherever possible, one or another parent should be present at parent-teacher meetings and participate in the activities of the child's group, such as class trips, visiting days, and the like.

Homework

When youngsters come home with school assignments that they find baffling, parents should feel free to ask the teacher for clearer instructions. If the child is at fault through inattention or ignorance, it might be pointed out to her that whether or not she gets a good education depends on how hard she's ready to work and not how efficiently the teacher can spoon-feed her.

Private Schools

Some families feel that the local public school is not the best place for their children to learn during the lower grades. Alternative private schools, whether denominational, discriminatory, or for gifted children, may have advantages that are less apparent to the child than to the parents, especially if attendance isolates the youngster from her friends in the neighborhood.

Staying Home from School

It's not unusual for a child to avoid going to school once in a while by saying she's sick. She may actually need a rest from the routine every few months. This is quite different from truly getting sick at the thought of facing school. A child who is nauseated in the morning, or who throws up, or who has a stomachache at breakfast, is probably experiencing feelings of anger, resentment, or anxiety beyond her ability to cope with them. Whatever it is in the school situation that's worrying her, she should be given the opportunity to talk about what's going on and the reassurance that efforts will be made to help straighten things out.

For children with disabilities, special facilities are often provided within the structure of the local school so that they can spend at least part of their day with their own age group.

Sex Education

Children need and deserve to have access to correct information about sexual functioning. If there is a natural openness in a family about questions of all types, children first start asking questions about sex when they are three or four; it is then that parents can begin describing sexual functioning to their children.

Questions about Body Parts

The first questions about sex usually have to do with the functioning of body parts. For example, children want to know where urine comes from, what happens to food when they eat it, where feces come from, and where babies come from. Explanations should be given in a straightforward, unembarrassed manner. Children should not be overloaded with information that they do not understand, but parents should be willing to answer questions to the best of their ability.

With older children, particularly 11- and 12-year-olds, it is often helpful for sexual questions to be answered by the parent of the same sex. Reading a book on sexual development together with the child can be a good experience for both parent and child. Parents frequently wonder if sex education may not lead children to engage in experimentation. Most of the evidence on this question indicates that children are more likely to experiment sexually when they are ignorant than when their questions about sex are reasonably and accurately answered.

Sexual Abuse and Incest

Of all the forms of child abuse (see CHILD ABUSE), sexual abuse, including incest, is the most common. Estimates of the number of sexual assaults on children in the United States range as high as five million annually. As many as 80 percent of these assaults occur within families. In many cases the adults reside outside the family but are closely acquainted with their victims.

Child sexual abuse takes many forms. While tens of thousands of children and young people are sexually attacked or molested, thousands of others are filmed, photographed, or otherwise exploited for the private recreational purposes of abusers. An estimated 50,000 children disappear annually; most of them are never found. Experts say many of these lost children are forced into a kind of sex-slavery, becoming victims of the "kiddie porn" (child pornography) trade. Within the home, sexual abuse may include rape, inappropriate fondling, exhibitionism, sexual intercourse, sodomy, and other acts.

Who are the victims of child sexual abuse? They are both males and females; they range in age from a few months to 16 years or older. The mean age at which a child experiences sexual abuse is nine. The victims represent all socioeconomic groups, all races, all geographic regions.

Protecting Your Children

Parents have the delicate task of maintaining a loving, touching family relationship while also teaching their child or children to recognize and reject "bad touches." Parents do not want to instill in their child fear, hysteria, or paranoia. But they should want their child to know how to escape or avoid abuse within or outside

---

Safety Tips for Parents

1. Know your children's friends.
2. Never leave your child unattended.
3. Be involved in your child's activities.
4. Listen when your child tells you he or she does not want to be with someone.
5. Pay attention when someone shows greater than normal interest in your child.
6. Have your child fingerprinted and know where to locate dental records.
7. Be sensitive to changes in your child's behavior or attitudes.
8. Take a photograph of your child each year (4 times each year if under age 2).
9. Be prepared to describe your children accurately—including clothing, visible identifying marks, or special characteristics.
10. Develop a set procedure should you and your child become separated while away from home.
11. Do not buy items that visibly display your child's name.
12. Be sure your child's school or day-care center will not release your child to anyone other than you or someone you officially designate.
13. Instruct the school to contact you immediately if your child is absent or if someone other than you arrives to pick up him or her without advance notice from you.

---

the home. Without dwelling on the details of what *could* happen, show what a bad touch involves—generally, a pinch, hard slap, or a touch in a body area normally covered by a bathing suit. One exception, of course, is a physician's examination. Parental approval makes such an examination acceptable.

Children can and should learn to say "no" to an adult, psychologists tell us. Having said "no," whether the

---

would-be abuser is a friend, relative, or stranger, your child should leave the scene quickly. Then he or she should report the incident to a parent. "Be sure to emphasize that if someone asks them not to tell that they should immediately tell," advises one authority. Parents should make it clear that they will not be mad if they receive such a report.

Parents need to instruct children periodically in the ways to respond appropriately to abusers' approaches. But then they have to listen if the child wants to talk. Children have to be sure both of the parents' love and their willingness to pay attention.

Symptoms to Watch For

A child encountering molestation or sexual abuse of any kind is undergoing an emotionally stressful experience. But the young person may be too shy to reveal what has happened. If a parent suspects that a son or daughter has been molested, one authority suggests, asking directly if anything has happened.

What symptoms might cause suspicion? As published in "Child Protection Alert," a publication of the American Christian Voice Foundation, there are at least 25 symptoms that you should watch for:

1. Explicit (sometimes bizarre) sexual knowledge
2. Precocious sexually related experimentation or speech
3. Toilet training relapses
4. Smearing of feces or urine
5. Gagging and unexplained vomiting
6. Speech problems
7. Regressive behavior
8. Masturbation

9. Withdrawal from normal human contact

10. Stomach and head pains

11. Bedwetting

12. Suicidal depression and/or self-destructive tendencies

13. Excessive fear of selected individuals or locations

14. Loss of appetite

15. Unexplained bruises or injuries in genital areas

16. Blood spotting or unexplained substances on underwear

17. Abrupt or radical behavioral or attitude changes

18. Lack of self-esteem or self-worth

19. Ulcers, colitis, anorexia, or other stress related disorders

20. Alcohol or drug abuse

21. Frequent nightmares

22. Excessive passivity

23. Vaginal or urinary tract infections

24. Infections of the mouth, gums, or throat. (Be vigilant for venereal diseases of the anus or throat. Incidences are no longer uncommon in children.)

25. Unexplained gifts, extra money, or the presence of pornography in your child's possession

Sources of Help

Where does a parent seek help once it's certain that molestation or abuse has occurred? The recommended first stage is to notify the police or local rape crisis center, or (where incest is the crime) the state child protection agency. To avoid adding to your child's stress, parents should *not* confront the offender while the child is present. Make sure the young victim has a complete physical examination if only to reassure the boy or girl that no permanent physical damage has been done. Depending on need, you may also want to ensure that the child gets counseling. Resource centers that provide diverse kinds of aid include:

- CHILD HELP National Child Abuse hotline: 800/422-4453

- Child Find hotline: 800/A-WAY-OUT for mediation; 800/I-AM-LOST for abducted children children or people identifying missing or abducted children.

- National Center for Missing and Exploited Children: 800/843-5678 or 202/634-9821

- The Adam Walsh Child Resource Center: 305/475-4848

- National Crime Information Center (F.B.I.): 202/324-2311

- National Runaway Switchboard: 800/621-4000

Sibling Rivalry

See BROTHERS AND SISTERS, NEW BABY.

Sickle-cell Anemia

See Ch. 9, *Diseases of the Circulatory System*.

Sisters and Brothers

See BROTHERS AND SISTERS.

Sleep

See BEDTIME, DREAMS AND NIGHTMARES, SLEEPWALKING.

Sleepwalking

Sleepwalking may be distressing to the parent who witnesses it, but it usually does the child no harm. If the child seems to be about to do something dangerous, it's a good idea to wake her up with a few reassuring remarks and guide her back to bed. In most sleepwalking incidents, the child goes back to bed by herself and gets up the next day without the slightest recollection of her nighttime prowl. Parents shouldn't tease or scold or make the child feel peculiar about walking in her sleep. It can be ignored unless it continues over a long period, and then it might be mentioned to your physician.

Smallpox

Smallpox has been eradicated everywhere in the world. Vaccination against smallpox has therefore been discontinued in the United States.

Smoking

Young children who see older children in the family or at home smoking cigarettes are going to equate smoking with being grown up even if their parents don't smoke. A ten-year-old who sneaks off to experiment with a cigarette shouldn't be treated like a criminal, but he should be told that he is harming himself. Parents who smoke and wish they didn't should concentrate on their own efforts to stop and hope that their offspring get the message. In any event, it might help to emphasize how hard it is to stop smoking once one has acquired the habit.

Sore Throat

"It hurts when I swallow" is a common complaint of childhood. It may be connected with a cold or tonsillitis, but if there is tenderness at the sides of the neck and a rise in temperature, the physician should be called promptly so that tests can be made to see whether the child has strep throat. Often a throat culture is necessary. A streptococcus throat infection that is undiagnosed and untreated can have serious consequences. See also STREP THROAT, TONSILLITIS.

Speech Impediments

Among the more common speech defects are *lisping* (the substitution of *th* for *s* and *z* sounds); *lallation* (the inability to pronounce *l* or *r* correctly), and stuttering. Although many children do outgrow their speech disabilities, a considerable number do not.

Therapy

Corrective therapy should be undertaken without too much delay. There have been many advances in the techniques used by speech pathologists, including the audiovisual devices and feed-back systems that promote self-correction. A list of certified speech pathologists can be obtained from the American Speech-Language-Hearing Association, 10801 Rockville Pike, Rockville, MD 20852. See also STUTTERING.

Stealing

See DISHONESTY.

Stepchildren

See Ch. 5, *The Middle Years*. See also ADOPTED CHILDREN.

Stomachache

A wide variety of disorders begins with some kind of abdominal pain, but in most cases, a stomachache is temporary and unaccompanied by any other symptoms. Digestive upsets are frequent in infancy, becoming rarer as the baby approaches the fourth month. See COLIC.

After the baby's first year, a stomachache may signal the onset of a cold or some other infection. The physician should be called if any of the following conditions occurs:

- When the stomach pain is accompanied by fever, vomiting, or diarrhea

- If moderate pain lasts for a considerable time—several hours, for example

- If the pain is obviously acute—the child is doubled over

- If the location off the pain shifts from one place to another

Never give a child a laxative or an enema except on a physician's orders.

A youngster who complains regularly of stomachaches without any other symptoms, and who might also complain of headaches or constipation shouldn't be dismissed as a worrier. The problem should be discussed with your physician so that an investigation can be made of possible causes. In many cases, constipation is the source of stomach pain. When the constipation is cleared up, the stomach pains cease.

Stomach pain may also be of psychosomatic origin, in children as well as in adults. If the pain cannot be explained after a physical examination and tests have been made, parents should consider how they can lighten some of the stresses and tensions in the child's life.

Strabismus

See CROSSED EYES.

Strep Throat

Streptococcal infections, commonly called strep throat, are caused by bacteria that inflame and infect the tissues in the throat. Symptoms include sore throat, swollen glands, redness or blotchy white spots on the throat and tonsils. Severe throat pain may occur for three to four days of the two-week run of the illness. Strep infections should be treated immediately after diagnosis by a physician with antibiotics such as erythromycin or penicillin.

Strep throat poses several risks to the health of both the adult and child sufferer. If left untreated, strep bacteria may produce the toxin that triggers scarlet fever, which also requires treatment with penicillin.

Strep can also lead to rheumatic fever. Rheumatic fever can develop into rheumatic heart disease, leaving the child with a heart murmur. Also treated with penicillin, the disease leaves little damage if caught and treated early.

The last serious problem to arise from a strep infection is relatively new. There a new strep type produces the same symptoms as toxic shock syndrome. The rare form of streptococcus causes low blood pressure, rash, high fever, and rapid organ and blood destruction. It ends in death in 20 percent of the cases. It affects children and adults. Due to the rapid onset of serious and deadly symptoms, it is essential that medical treatment be sought immediately if you or your child suffers any one of the signs of this disease.

Stuttering

Stuttering, or stammering, is a speech dysfunction where the words are spoken with hesitation, repetition, prolongation, or stumbling on one or more syllable of a word. Parents should bear in mind, though, that many children stutter when they are learning to speak. At this stage it is not a permanent problem, and the child will usually outgrow it as ease with language increases.

For a child who continues to show hesitation in speech after the age of four or five, the parents should consider getting professional guidance of a physician, speech therapist, or counselor as recommended by the child's pediatrician. The speech problem may be related to cerebellar disease or a neuromuscular defect or a problem with the voice box. There is also some research being done on hearing problems with stutterers. Some patients respond well to speech therapy when the sound of their voice is played back on a delay through earphones. The slight delay allows them to speak without hesitation. Why this works is not fully understood.

Stuttering can also be related to emotional or psychological problems. Stress from early childhood speech impairment may create a psychological block to speaking. Other problems may enter into the reason for stuttering. It is not uncommon for there to be both emotional and physical reasons for stuttering.

For more information, please call the toll-free hotline for the National Center for Stuttering at 800/221-2483. They will provide information and guidance to parents.

Sudden Infant Death Syndrome

Sudden Infant Death Syndrome, sometimes referred to as SIDS and generally known as *crib death*, claims about 10,000 babies every year. It is the chief single cause of fatalities in infants, usually occurring between the ages of one month and six months. Although there are a number of plausible theories being investigated, its cause remains unknown. In some cases, autopsies indicate a hidden infection or an unsuspected abnormality, but in 80 percent of the deaths, no obvious explanation can be found. One cause appears to be an inherited heart irregularity, and another is respiratory distress, discussed under HYALINE MEMBRANE DISEASE. Improved hospital facilities for the care of premature babies who are considered to be at higher risk than those born at full term, as well as prenatal tests and ultrasonic alarm systems that monitor breathing are expected to reduce the number of SIDS victims.

Parents of infant SIDS victims often suffer intensely, apart from their natural grief, from feelings of guilt, as if they were somehow careless or negligent. They must be reassured that they could not possibly have foreseen the susceptibility of their child to this affliction and that there is therefore no way they could have averted its tragic result. They will have suffered enough without the wholly unwarranted feeling that they were somehow responsible.

Swallowed Objects

Babies in a crib or playpen can certainly be depended on to put anything within reach into their mouths, so it's a good idea to make sure that surfaces are cleared of anything that would cause a crisis if it were swallowed. Plastic toys and rattles should be inspected for loose parts. Pins, buttons, and small change should be kept in drawers. It's no serious matter if a child swallows a cherry stone or a plum pit or a small button, because these are not likely to cause problems in their passage through the digestive system. They will be disposed of in regular bowel movements.

Emergencies

Emergencies occur when the object is stuck in the windpipe or when it goes into the bronchial passage. If it is in the windpipe and isn't coughed up right away, use the first aid maneuver for "Obstruction in the Windpipe," Ch. 35, *Medical Emergencies* without delay. If is doesn't work the first time, do it again—and again. You must clear the windpipe. If all efforts fail, rush the child to a hospital.

Swearing

Sooner or later most children learn swear words, either from hearing their parents use them or from their peers. Young children may use curse words without knowing what they mean or without appreciating how offensive they may be.

Nowadays it is virtually impossible for children to avoid hearing words in everyday use that were strictly taboo when their parents were growing up. However jolting it may be to hear foul words issuing from their angelic-looking children, parents should be neither surprised nor unduly upset if this happens occasionally, especially if they themselves use curse words. They might well point out to the child, however, that many people object strongly to such language, and if they want to be treated courteously by adults, they had better watch their language.

Swimming

Every child should learn to swim, and the earlier the better. Families fortunate enough to have their own large pools can accomplish this in their own backyards; others may spend summers near a suitable body of water.

Although there's nothing like the ocean for water play, it's not a good place to try to teach a small child how to swim. There are too many extraneous hazards, such as undertow, waves, and unexpected depths. Many communities have outdoor public pools; most large cities have indoor and outdoor pools where professional instruction is available. Even when a child can swim moderately well, she should not be allowed to do so alone, and she shouldn't be allowed to go out in a boat by herself either. Rubber floats, rafts, and the like shouldn't be made available to youngsters until they can swim. A nonswimmer depending on such a device is in trouble if it should drift away from her in deep water.

Talking

The ability to speak is part of the human heritage. How soon and how clearly a child begins to do so depends on several factors. First and foremost is the ability to hear.

Hearing and Speech

Any illness or infection in infancy that has caused even a small hearing loss will interfere with the baby's perception of sounds. This in turn will prevent the normal development of those parts of the brain that govern the imitative aspect of speech.

A Stimulating Environment

How much attention and stimulation the baby gets from his environment and the people around him will have a great effect on how much he tries to say and the age at which he begins to say it. Being listened to and automatically corrected instead of being ignored or teased is the indispensable feedback process that enriches the learning of language. The clarity of the child's speech depends to a large extent on the examples before him; what his ears hear his brain will order

his vocal equipment to imitate. Parents who want a child to outgrow baby talk should avoid responding to the baby in kind. Normal adult speech should become the norm toward which the child is constantly striving. See also HEARING, SPEECH IMPEDIMENTS, SWEARING.

Tantrums

See ANGER.

Tay-Sachs Disease

Tay-Sachs disease is an inherited disorder of the nervous system. It causes degeneration of the nerves, starting after six months of age. Infant development through pregnancy and the first six months is normal, but the disease can be detected through genetic testing. The first symptoms to appear are subtle, becoming more obvious with motor deterioration. They include a slowing of development, loss of vision, and eventually convulsions. A cherry-red spot develops on the retina of the eye. The child will lose the motor coordination that he already had, and will deteriorate to the point where he will be unable to lift his head. The child will not normally survive past the age of four.

Tay-Sachs is found with higher prevalence among the following populations: Ashkenazi Jews, Eastern European Jews, and French Canadians. Testing is recommended to anyone from these populations, and testing is also recommended for all Jews to determine if one is a carrier of the disease.

Tay-Sachs is a form of cerebral sphingolipidosis. It is the infantile onset of the disorder. The others are Jansky-Bielschowsky disease (early juvenile), Spielmeyer-Vogt and Batten-Mayou disease (late juvenile), and Kufs' disease (adult onset).

Symptoms are similar and include blindness within two years of the onset of the disorder.

Teething

Babies of four to six months drool a great deal and put their fingers in their mouth. These habits, and the telltale small bumps you may detect on the baby's gums, are the signs of teething. But they don't necessarily mean that the first tooth is about to erupt. That may not happen until he is nearly one year old, although it usually happens earlier.

Teething may or may not be painful. If the baby does fret, medication is available to alleviate the pain. (A little whisky rubbed on the gums is a home remedy that often helps.)

Tetanus

Tetanus (also called *lockjaw* because it causes spasms of the jaw) can occur at any age as the result of contamination of a simple wound. The causative organism is usually found in soil, street dust, or feces.

The disease is preventable by immunization. The triple vaccine DTP should be started at two to three months of age. See also IMMUNIZATION.

When a child suffers a puncture wound, dog bite, or other wound that may be contaminated, ask your physician to give the child a booster dose of tetanus toxoid if she has not had a shot within one year.

Tick Fever

See "Rocky Mountain Spotted Fever" under RASHES.

Toilet Training

During the toddler stage parents begin to teach their child how to control his bowel and urinary functions.

When to Start

A simple question parents always ask is, "How do I know when my child is ready to be toilet trained?"

Generally, children do not have muscular control over their bowel movements and urination until about the age of two, so attempting to toilet-train a child much before this is usually wasted effort. If it is accomplished, the result is usually a training of the parents rather than of the infant. Toilet training should usually take place some time between the age of two and three and one-half.

A child is emotionally ready when he understands what is meant by toilet training and is willing to perform toilet functions without expressing fear of them. This may occur at any age, but is perhaps most apt to start between the ages of 18 and 24 months. With a first child it is usually later than with a second or third child, because the first child has no siblings to emulate. But a first child should be trained, usually, by the time he is three. Training the child to stay dry through the long night hours may take even longer.

Resistance to Toilet Training

Early toilet training—training that is begun during a child's first year—may work, but as a child develops and asserts his personality and independence, he will resent any insistence on manipulating the control of his bodily functions. He may get even by refusing to empty his bowels when put on the potty. Worse yet, if another baby has entered the scene, the early-trained child may develop constipation, or may revert to wetting and having bowel movements in his training pants.

When you feel the child is ready for training, establish the fact that going to the bathroom is a normal part of daily life. If the child expresses fear, don't struggle with him. Don't fight about it. Take him right off the potty and let him know that you are not concerned or displeased. A genuine complication can arise if the child connects his fear of toilet functions with your displeasure at his failures.

Training can usually be facilitated by praise from the parents for putting the bowel movement and the urine in the proper place, rather than by punishment. Excessive punishment or the threat of it usually results in anger on the child's part and increasing stubbornness and resistances to toilet training. Praise immediately following the proper performance of the act is far more effective in encouraging compliance with the parents' goals.

Tonsillectomy

See "Tonsils and Adenoids" in Ch. 20, *Surgery*.

Tonsillitis

The tonsils are two masses of soft spongy tissue that are partly embedded in the mucous membrane of the back of the throat. Bacterial or viral infection of this tissue is known as tonsillitis. It used to be considered advisable to remove the tonsils if they became enlarged—which they normally do in the process of filtering out mild infections.

Nowadays, an occasional bout of tonsillitis isn't considered sufficient reason for surgical removal of the tonsils, especially because they're likely to be less prone to infection as the child gets older. However, even a mild case of tonsillitis should be called to a physician's attention. Acute symptoms such as swollen tonsils, sudden high fever, swollen neck glands, and severe pain when swallowing must be treated promptly since they might be an indication of a strep throat. The proper antibiotics are always effective in controlling this infection so that it doesn't turn into rheumatic fever or involve the kidneys. Tonsillitis caused by a virus usually responds to aspirin, bed rest, and a soft diet. See also ADENOIDS. For a description of tonsillectomy, see "Tonsils and Adenoids" in Ch. 20, *Surgery*.

Toy Safety

Toys come with a recommended age of use. It is important that parents heed the information. Some toys are unsuitable for certain ages, not only because of an inability to use it correctly, but because there may be pieces of the toy that are harmful. These are just a few examples of toys that can be safe at one age and not another; games may have small pieces can be swallowed by little children; electrical toys should only be handled by children old enough to understand the danger. Toys hanging in the crib should not be used by infants old enough to pull themselves up to a standing position because they may strangle on cords and strings of the toy. It should be noted that it is not always the case that only younger children should avoid older children's toys. Toys that are safe for younger children may tip, break, or pinch with the increased size and weight of an older child.

Not all toys come with recommendations or fulfill the safety standards set up by the U.S. government. Cheap imitations may not meet the rigid standards of the more established companies' toys. Several hundred toys are recalled each year, and more may have not yet been tested. It is important that a parent take responsibility for evaluating the safety of any toy to be given to a youngster.

For detailed and important information on age recommendations for toys

(*Which Toy for Which Child*) and for a listing of products recommended for their reliability and safety, please write to U.S. Consumer Product Safety Commission, Washington, DC 20207 or call 1-800-638-CPSC. *The ABC's of Toys and Play* is also a worthwhile publication on how to select toys for children. It is published by Toy Manufacturers of America, Inc., 200 Fifth Avenue, New York, NY 10010.

Tuberculosis

See Ch. 12, *Diseases of the Respiratory System*.

Twins and Triplets

Multiple births may be *identical*—that is, the result of the splitting of a single egg fertilized by a single sperm—or they may be *fraternal*, which means that they developed from different eggs fertilized by different sperm. Most multiple births are fraternal; except for their birthdays, most twins and triplets are no more alike than other brothers and sisters of the same family.

Although there is no ready explanation for the occurrence of multiple births, the tendency is thought to be genetically determined through the mother. Twins occur about once in every 86 births, triplets once in every 8,000. Multiple births can be anticipated by a physician at least a month before delivery. They usually arrive about two weeks early, and if they give any indications of prematurity, they receive special hospital attention.

Urinary Infections

Urinary infections of either viral or bacterial origin are more common among girls than boys, especially during the preschool years. Such an in-fection is sometimes the explanation for a fever unaccompanied by other symptoms. Any inflammation that creates a burning sensation during urination should be cultured and treated promptly because it can spread from the bladder to the kidneys and create a major problem.

Girls can be spared frequent infection if tactful suggestions are made at an early age about their toilet routines. Fecal matter is high in bacterial content, so little girls should learn to wipe their bottoms from front to back. This procedure reduces the possibility of contaminating the urethra after a bowel movement.

Vaporizer

A vaporizer is a device similar to a humidifier that moistens the air with steam and thus alleviates some of the discomfort of respiratory congestion. During the winter months when heated interiors are likely to be especially dry and when colds are more common, children and grown-ups can benefit from moist air that keeps the throat and nasal and bronchial passages from feeling like sandpaper. Medication shouldn't be added to a vaporizer except at the physician's recommendation. If the device is used near a child's bed throughout the night, it should be placed on a surface high enough to prevent bumping into it accidentally should the child wake up in the middle of the night to go to the bathroom.

Vomiting

See NAUSEA AND VOMITING.

Warts

See Ch. 21, *Skin and Hair*.

Water Beds

Because of the softness and the motion of a waterbed, infants up to *at least* twelve months of age should never be left unattended on a waterbed. Infants left even briefly on a waterbed have suffocated. The risks are that the infant will become trapped between the mattress and the frame or wall, or become wedged between a sleeping adult and the mattress, or sink face first into the mattress and be unable to push himself up. Several infant deaths originally attributed to SIDS are now considered suffocation due to a waterbed. At least 24 infants have died while left to nap on the parents' waterbed in the last decade.

Whooping Cough

Whooping cough (also called *pertussis*), like diphtheria a bacterial disease, occurs more frequently than diphtheria because immunity to it wears off, especially in the older child in whom the disease may appear as a severe bronchitis.

Whooping cough can be very serious in young babies because it can cause them to choke and be unable to catch their breath. If your child does contract whooping cough, call your physician immediately. He or she may give a specific drug against the organism that causes the disease as well as a specific antitoxin against the poison that the bacillus releases.

It is advisable to immunize children against whooping cough as early as possible. The effective triple vaccine known as DTP provides immunization not only against whooping cough, but against diphtheria and tetanus as well.

Worms and Parasites

See Ch. 11, *Diseases of the Digestive System*.

3

The Teens

Puberty and Growth

The bridge between childhood and adulthood is a period of growth and change called puberty. There seems to be no standard pattern for the physical changes of puberty. Two boys of the same age who have been nearly identical throughout childhood may appear to set off along entirely different paths of physical development as they enter the teenage years. One may quickly shoot up to a height of five feet eight inches within a couple of years while his companion lags for a while at preteen size, then begins growing into a six-footer. One may develop a heavy beard in his early high-school years while the other boy will have no use for a razor until he is in college. However, both boys are normal youngsters, and each will eventually attain all of the physical attributes of adulthood.

Similarly, one girl may begin menstruating in her 11th year while a classmate will not experience her first menstruation until she is 16. One girl may need a bra while still in grammar school but her friend will fret about a small bustline for many years. But both girls can look forward to normal womanhood. Each has an individual pattern of development, and if there

is any rule of thumb about puberty it is that each youngster has his or her own time schedule for the transformation into a mature man or woman.

Puberty: Changes in Girls

The physical changes that occur in the female body during puberty probably are more dramatic than those associated with a boy progressing into manhood. One definite milestone for the girl is her first *menstruation*, commonly regarded as the first sign of puberty. Actually, the first menstruation, known as the *menarche*, is only one of several signs of puberty, along with the slimming of the waist, gradual broadening of the hips, the development of breasts, the appearance of hair about the genitals and in the armpits, and a change in the rate of growth.

The Menarche

The age at which a girl first experiences menstruation generally varies over a period of ten years and depends upon the structural development of the youngster, her physical

condition, the environment, and hereditary factors. Menarche can occur as early as the age of 7, and most physicians would not be overly concerned if a girl did not begin to menstruate until she was approaching 17. The age range of 9 to 16 usually is considered normal. The median age for the start of menstruation is around 13½ years, which means that 50 percent of all females are younger than 13 years and 6 months when they reach the menarche, and half are on the older side of that age when they first menstruate. In general, the pubertal experiences of a girl follow a pattern like that of her mother and sisters; if the mother began menstruating at an early age, the chances are that her daughters will also.

If the girl has not reached the menarche by the age of 18, she should be examined by a *gynecologist*, a physician who specializes in problems related to the female reproductive system. A medical examination also should be arranged for any girl who experiences menstruation before she reaches the age of eight or nine years.

When menarche occurs on the early side of childhood, the condition

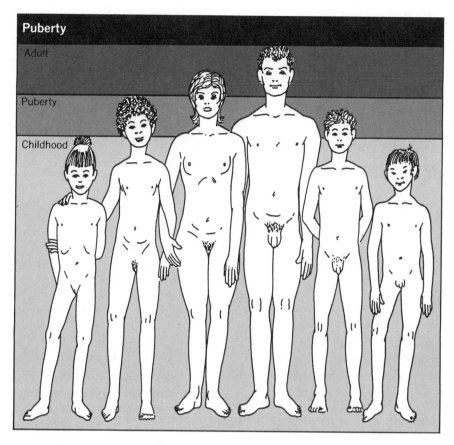

Puberty

Adult

Puberty

Childhood

is sometimes called *precocious puberty*. The child may suddenly begin menstruating before her mother has told her what to expect, a situation that can prove embarrassing to both child and parents. It may first be detected by a teacher at school; occasionally, a young girl may be aware of bleeding from the vagina but because of fear or false modesty does not report the event to her mother or teacher. For this reason, parents should be alert for changes associated with early puberty and be prepared to explain the facts of life to their children. Also, in the case of precocious puberty, parents should arrange for medical consultation to be certain the bleeding actually is the result of first menstruation and not the effects of an injury or tumor.

Growth Spurt before Menarche

During the year or two preceding the menarche there is a growth spurt of

two or three inches. This is because of the hormone changes of puberty. The *hormones* are chemical messengers secreted by glands in various parts of the body and carried rapidly through the bloodstream to organs or other glands where they trigger reactions. The spurt in growth preceding menarche results from the secretion of a growth hormone that is produced by the pituitary gland, and androgen, a hormone secreted by the adrenal glands. They produce rapid growth of the bones and muscles during puberty. The girl who is first among her classmates to menstruate often is larger than those who are of the same age but have not yet reached the menarche.

From numerous research studies of the menarche, it has been learned that poor nutrition and psychological stress sometimes delay the onset of menstruation, that girls reared in cities tend to menstruate earlier, and that climate is a factor, although both

tropical and arctic climates seem to be related to early menarche. The first menstrual periods also are likely to occur during the school year, September to June, rather than during the summer vacation.

The First Menstrual Cycles

The first menstrual cycles tend to be very irregular and have been known to be as short as 7 days and as long as 37 weeks. Even when regularity becomes established, the adolescent menstrual cycle usually is longer than the average for adult women. The typical menstrual cycle of a young girl may be about 33 days, compared to an average of 28 days for an adult woman. About three years elapse before the menstrual cycles become regular. In the meantime, irregular menstrual patterns can be considered as normal for girls during puberty.

The first menstrual cycles also are *anovulatory*. In other words, the young girl's ovaries have not matured sufficiently to produce an *ovum*, or egg cell, that can be fertilized by the sperm of a male. There are, of course, the exceptions that make newspaper headlines when a little girl gives birth to a baby. But anovulatory menstruation generally is the rule for the first few months after the menarche.

Delayed Puberty

Delayed puberty probably causes as much anguish as precocious puberty. The last girl in a group of childhood chums to develop breasts and experience the menarche may feel more self-conscious than the first girl in the class to menstruate. If the signs that usually precede menarche have not appeared by the age of 17 or 18, a medical examination should be considered, even though the girl may be a late-late-bloomer at the other end of the spectrum from the 7- or 8-year-old child who has menstruated.

The absence of menstruation after a girl is 18 can be the result of a wide variety of factors. The cause sometimes can be as simple as an *imperforate hymen,* a membrane that blocks the opening of the vagina. It can be the result of a congenital malformation of the reproductive organs, such as imperfect development of the ovaries. Accidents, exposure to carbon monoxide gas, or diseases like rheumatic fever or encephalitis in earlier years can result in brain damage that would inhibit the start of menstruation. The relationship between emotional upset and delayed menarche was vividly demonstrated during World War II when some girls who suffered psychological traumas also experienced very late signs of puberty.

Preparing Your Daughter for Menstruation

A mother's main responsibility is to convince her daughter at the beginning of puberty that menstruation is a perfectly normal body function. The mother should explain the proper use of sanitary napkins or tampons and encourage her daughter to keep records of her menstrual periods on a calendar.

The mother also should explain that menstruation usually is not a valid reason to stay in bed or avoid school or work. The girl should be advised that bathing and swimming should not be postponed because of menstruation. There are many old wives' tales about menstruation that are not true. But there may be some truth to stories that loss of menstrual blood can be weakening, particularly if the girl's diet does not replace the body stores of iron which may be lowered during menstrual flow. Iron is a key element of the red blood cell, and if iron-rich

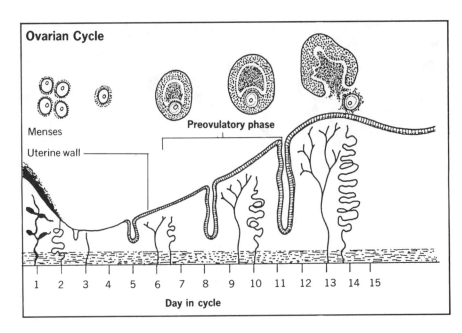

Ovarian Cycle

Menses

Uterine wall

Preovulatory phase

Day in cycle

foods are not included in the meals of women during their years of menstruation they can eventually suffer a form of iron-deficiency anemia.

Hormone Activity: Becoming a Woman

Although the sex hormones are the key to what makes girls grow into women and boys into men, both sexes appear to receive secretions of male and female sex hormones in approximately equal amounts for about the first ten years of life. But as puberty approaches, the adrenal glands of girls seem to increase production of a female sex hormone, *estrogen.* Meanwhile, a nerve center in the hypothalamus area of the brain stimulates the pituitary gland, the master gland of the body, to secrete another kind of hormone, *gonadotropin.* Gonadotropin in turn activates a *follicle-stimulating hormone* that causes a maturation of the ovaries, which are part of the original equipment girls are born with but which remain dormant until the start of puberty.

During the second decade of life, the hormone activity stimulates the development of body tissues that not only grow in size but give a girl more

womanly contours. However, the fully mature contours of a woman usually do not appear until after the ovaries are functioning and still another female sex hormone, *progesterone,* has been introduced in the system. The ovaries, uterus, Fallopian tubes, and vagina gradually mature as the menarche draws near.

Puberty: Changes in Boys

The appearance of male sexual characteristics during puberty is also influenced by hormonal changes. But the manifestation of male puberty is somewhat more subtle. The pituitary gland in a boy also secretes a gonadotropic hormone that stimulates maturation of *gonads.* In the male, the gonads are the *testicles,* the source of *sperm.* But whereas maturation of the ovaries in females leads to the menarche, there is no obvious sign in the boy that *spermatozoa* are being produced.

However, the secondary sexual characteristics, such as the growth of a beard and pubic hair, the spurt of growth of bones and muscles, the increase in size of the sex organs, and the deepening of the voice, are all in-

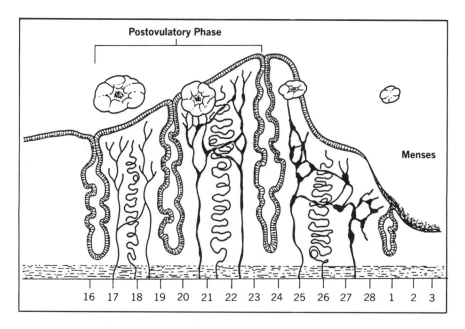

Postovulatory Phase

Menses

16 17 18 19 20 21 22 23 24 25 26 27 28 1 2 3

dications of puberty. The changes in a boy's characteristics during puberty are usually spread over a period of two years, beginning with an increase in the size of the penis and testicles and reaching completion with the production of spermatozoa in the testicles. During the two-year period there usually is a noticeable increase in the chest size of a boy, with the broad shoulders of manhood appearing during the peak of bone and muscle growth. Generally, the appearance of pubic and facial hair, as well as hair in the armpits, follows the growth of the shoulder and chest area and precedes the change in voice.

The Testicles

The testicles are contained in a walnut-size sac of skin called the *scrotum*. It is held outside the body by a design of nature in order to maintain a temperature for spermatozoa production that is less than internal body temperature. Muscle fibers in the scrotum hold the testicles closer to the body for warmth in cold weather and relax to allow the sperm-producing organ to be farther away from the body when surrounding temperatures are warm.

In some cases, one or both testicles do not descend from the abdomen during the male child's early years. The result is that the undescended testicle or testicles will not produce sperm. An *incompletely descended testicle* always lies somewhere along the normal path to the scrotum. An *ectopic* testicle has deviated from that path and lies somewhere near the inguinal canal, at the junction of the thigh and the lower part of the abdomen. In a third departure from normal

development, a *retractile testicle* has stopped short of the scrotum. It can be manipulated into the normal position or may descend to that position at puberty.

The danger of malignant change—of tumor development—usually warrants surgical removal of the incompletely descended and the ectopic testicle. A testicle trapped in the inguinal region may become inflamed because of the pressure of larger body parts in the area. In some cases, physicians are able to assist the descent into the scrotum through administration of hormones or by surgery. At some point during puberty, a medical examination should include a check on the condition of the testes.

Genital Size

Many boys are as sensitive about the size of their genitals as girls are about breast size. In the case of an empty scrotum because of undescended testicles, it is possible to have the scrotum injected with silicone plastic for cosmetic or psychological reasons so the sac appears less flaccid or larger. The size of the penis may become the

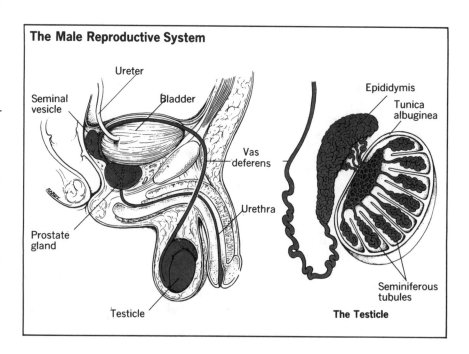

The Male Reproductive System

Ureter

Seminal vesicle

Bladder

Epididymis

Tunica albuginea

Vas deferens

Urethra

Prostate gland

Seminiferous tubules

Testicle

The Testicle

subject of discussion in the school shower room. If a boy appears sensitive about the subject, he should be assured that there is a wide variation in normal sizes and that like ears, noses, and other body parts the dimensions have little to do with function.

Nocturnal Emission

Another cause for concern by adolescent boys is the *nocturnal emission.* The nocturnal emission, sometimes called a *wet dream,* is the automatic expulsion of *semen* through the penis while the young man is asleep. The semen is secreted by the *prostate gland,* the *seminal vesicle,* and other glands that open into the *urethra.* The opalescent white fluid carries spermatozoa during intercourse and if the young male does not engage in sexual intercourse or does not masturbate, the semen simply accumulates until it overflows during a nocturnal emission. It is a harmless, normal occurrence.

Bone Growth

As the growth spurt subsides in the late teens, the *cartilage plates,* or *epiphyses,* in the long bones of the body close. Until the growth plates become filled in with calcium deposits, each long bone is in effect three bones—a central shaft separated from the ends by the cartilage growth plates. The growth plates are not completely replaced by bone until a female is about 20 and a male 23 years old. But the rate of growth begins to taper off as sexual maturity is achieved. After that, young women tend to retain fatty tissue and young men gain in muscle mass. It is a time to begin weight watching so that the hazards of obese adult life can be avoided. But the ravenous appetites developed

during the period of rapid body growth and intense physical activity can easily evolve into bad eating habits during the teen years.

Skin and Hair Problems

Hereditary influences may determine many of the physical and psychological traits that an individual first becomes aware of in the teen years. Because of the various crossovers of the 23 sets of *chromosomes* and the nearly infinite combinations of *genes,* it is not always easy to predict how a child is going to appear as a young adult. But some features, such as hair color and eye color, usually can be identified with one or both parents; other traits may seem to be those of uncles, aunts, or grandparents. Heredity and hormones frequently are involved in the distribution of hair on the body and the oiliness of the skin, both of which can cause concern to teenagers who are plagued by an overabundance or lack of these cosmetic traits. An example of hereditary influences on hair patterns can be seen in early baldness. A receding hairline is not a trait of the parents but rather an influence of the genetic makeup of a grandparent—the trait skips a generation.

Removal of Excess Hair

While not much can be done about baldness that is hereditary, there are ways of handling the problems of excess hair. If a woman has excess hair on her face, arms, and legs, it can be removed by shaving, with wax, by electrolysis, or depilatories. Shaving is the most direct but not always the most satisfactory method of hair removal because it is intended only as a temporary measure. An alternate shortcut is bleaching with diluted hydrogen peroxide; the hair is still there

but it is not as noticeable. Another method involves the use of hot wax spread on the skin and allowed to harden. When it is removed quickly, the hair is pulled away.

Depilatories are chemicals that destroy the hair at the skin line. Both hot wax and depilatories have longer-lasting effects than shaving, but they must be repeated at intervals of several weeks.

Depilatories, too, can produce unpleasant allergenic reactions. The only permanent method of removing excess hair is *electrolysis,* which is a time-consuming technique. Each hair root has to be burned out individually with an electric current. Electrolysis is recommended only for small areas and because of the time and expense involved would not be feasible for removing excess hair from regions other than the face.

Acne

There is some evidence that *acne* is partly hereditary. But it is such a common problem among teenagers— it has been estimated that up to 90 percent of all youngsters endure some degree of acne—that it must have been inherited from a mutual ancestor like Adam or Eve. In fact, one of the deterrents to effective control of the skin disorder is that acne is so common that it is neglected by many youngsters. Waiting to outgrow acne can be a serious mistake, because the pimples, blemishes, blackheads, and boils that make life miserable for so many teenagers can be eliminated or considerably reduced. They can also cause scarring. A physician should be consulted in cases of severe or especially persistent acne.

Overactive Oil Glands

Acne is not a serious threat to the life of a youngster, but it can be seriously disfiguring at a time of life when most young people are sensitive about their appearance. It can occur at any time from puberty into early adulthood, and it is caused by poor adjustment of the skin to secretions of sebaceous glands. The imbalance resulting from hormones in the bloodstream will correct itself eventually. But to prevent permanent scarring, a program of simple skin care must be followed faithfully.

Acne is caused by overly-active oil glands in the skin. When the oil glands become clogged, blackheads and pimples appear. The color of blackhead is not caused by dirt but rather by a chemical change in the secretions of the oil glands. To treat acne, a person should wash the skin to clear the plugged pores and oil glands. This is done by keeping the skin dry enough to peel away soiled layers and remove dirt from the pores. Most topical medications seek to keep the skin sufficiently dry to enhance peeling.

Skin Care

The face should be washed several times a day with warm water and mild soap. It should be dried thoroughly and gently with a clean towel. Careless handling of blemishes, such as squeezing blackheads, and picking at pimples and scabs can result in scarring. Teenagers also should avoid touching their faces. If the condition of the skin is worse than a few mild blemishes, a dermatologist will be able to prescribe topical medication, antibiotics, or hormones to treat the problem. Treatment often takes several months before there is noticeable improvement.

Other Precautions

Young women should not use cold creams or cosmetics unless they have been approved by a physician. Young

men who shave must be careful to avoid cutting pimples. A physician also should be consulted about how diet can help control acne. Although the skin disorder is not a dietary disease, there is some evidence that certain foods tend to aggravate it. However, there is a lack of agreement among physicians as to whether chocolate, carbonated beverages, nuts, sweets, and other specific snack items may be the culprits. And there always is the possibility that because each youngster develops along an individual path, a food item that causes one teenager's face to break out with blemishes will not affect a sibling or classmate in the same way.

Diet

It is no surprise that many American teenagers have poor eating habits. A survey by the Food and Nutrition Board of the National Research Council recently showed that 40 percent of boys between 13 and 19 years of age and 60 percent of the girls in the same age group subsisted on diets that were substandard. Generally, the young people surveyed had abandoned the healthy eating habits of their families. They habitually skipped breakfast and failed to make up the nutritional loss during other meals.

There are several reasons for this phenomenon. Perhaps the most prominent reason is that teens are anxious to break away from their home. They therefore rebel against any form of convention or parental advice. The popularity of fast food institutions and snack shops is a also great contributor to the problem. Such places have become frequent hangouts for teenagers after school and on weekend evenings. With social gatherings in these surroundings, teenagers begin to develop poor eating habits. Frequently, they fill themselves

up with non-nutritive foods and have no appetite later for balanced meals. At home, teenagers are great snack-eaters, and much snacking occurs while they are watching television. The combination of inactive television-watching and munching on junk foods leads to an unhealthy physical condition in teenagers.

Calories and Nutrition

A calorie is a unit of energy, and the human body requires a certain amount of energy each day in order to sustain life and continue normal physical activity. The amount of caloric intake varies according to the individual. Much of it depends on physical activity, size, and metabolic rate.

Calories in themselves are not bad. However, excessive intake of calories can lead to severe weight and health problems. Often the problem is not calories but the consumption of "empty calories" or non-nutritive foods. For instance, an unhealthy snack of a soda (100 calories) and French fries (roughly 450 calories) adds up to 550 "empty" calories. Conversely, a glass of skim milk (80 calories) and an apple (60 calories) is a healthy snack that adds up to only 140 calories.

To maintain the proper balance between foods consumed and energy used in work and play, a teenager must regulate his or her caloric intake. Much of the regulation occurs naturally. For example, when a person eats a lot, he or she is not hungry for a longer period of time than usual. Often, people crave foods that have been lacking in their diet. Thus, without conscious effort, most people are able to limit their consumption of foods to normal levels.

Nonetheless, it is important for teenagers to learn healthy eating habits and be aware of the potential of gaining weight. It is the awareness that is important for teenagers, not the strict regulation of body weight and caloric intake. Regularly checking one's weight on a scale is not a good idea. It will only foster unhealthy obsessions in teenagers who will worry about the loss or gain of a single pound. This can lead to skewed images of a teenager's physique and perhaps serious eating disorders. It is more important that a teenager monitor weight through the fit of his or her clothing.

Calcium and Phosphorus

Among the important minerals in teenage diets are calcium and phosphorus. Milk is the most easily available source of calcium and phosphorus, which are required for the development of strong bones during the period of life in which the body is still growing. Calcium also is required for the effective contraction of muscle tissues and is vital for normal heart function. The recommended daily intake of milk for teenagers is four eight-ounce glasses. It can be served as fluid whole milk, as skim milk, buttermilk, evaporated milk, or as nonfat dry milk. Cheese or ice cream can be substituted for part of the fluid milk allowance. One cup of ice cream is equivalent in calcium to one-half cup of milk. A one-inch cube of cheddar cheese is equal to two-thirds of a cup of milk, which also is equivalent in calcium to one cup, or eight ounces, of cottage cheese. Cream cheese can be substituted for milk in a two-to-one ratio; that is, two ounces of cream cheese are equal to one ounce of milk.

Iron

Iron is needed for the formation of *hemoglobin,* the substance that gives red blood cells their red coloration and is responsible for the transport of oxygen and carbon dioxide in the bloodstream. Hemoglobin has such an affinity for oxygen that without it humans would require 60 times as much blood to transport oxygen from the lungs to tissues throughout the body. Studies indicate that girls are five times as likely to need additional supplies of iron in their diets because of blood loss through menstruation. Recommended sources of iron are liver, heart, kidney, liver sausage, meat, shellfish, egg yolk, dark molasses, bread, beans and other legumes. If basic food lists seem drab and boring, the teenager might think of the iron sources in terms of a peanut butter sandwich or two hamburgers; either choice would provide the daily iron needs for a girl. Other minerals that are important to a teenager's diet include the following:

- Sulfur is needed by the body for hair, skin, nails, and cartilage, and is available by eating nearly any protein-rich foods.

- Iodine is needed for normal thyroid control of body metabolism and is supplied in the form of iodized table salt.

- Potassium is a tonic for the nervous system and the muscles and is available in adequate amounts in most kinds of meats, as well as bananas, orange juice, and milk.

- Magnesium collaborates chemically with calcium and phosphorus for normal muscle and nerve function, and is found in most forms of protein.

Note: Many of these nutrients are readily available in a normal diet. In most cases, it is not necessary to supplement a teenager's diet with these minerals. Children and teens should not rely on vitamin pills to make up for an unhealthy diet. It is better to eat nutritionally.

Weight Problems

Teens who are seriously overweight or who are contemplating radical weight reduction programs should be examined by a physician. Otherwise, unfair comparisons with other persons of the same age and height may lead to wrong conclusions about the need to gain or lose weight. The weight–height standards are based on averages, and there are many youngsters who are above or below the average but quite healthy and normal.

Another reason for a medical exam is to check the possibility of disease as the cause of the weight problem. The exam will also indicate whether the youngster has some other disorder that could be aggravated by a sudden weight loss.

Achieving optimum weight is only one step toward proper physical conditioning. A youngster who has been able to avoid physical activity by living in an elevator apartment, riding a bus to school, and watching TV after school hours instead of working or playing could be right on the button as far as weight for his age and height are concerned, but his muscular development and heart and lung capacity could be at the same time at a very low ebb.

Anorexia Nervosa

One of the most common eating disorders is anorexia nervosa, which occurs most often in teenage girls. It is a psychological disorder that in extreme cases results in death. The victims starve themselves in an exaggerated attempt to lose weight.

The most obvious trait is excessive and unnatural thinness. When anorexics become critically thin, they develop downy hair, called lanugo. Other symptoms include obsession with exercise and "healthy" eating habits, emphasis on self-control and discipline, high achievement in school, alternative periods of strict fasting and binging, and rituals surrounding food preparation and eating.

Anorexics may weigh themselves several times a day and avoid eating when they are hungry. Most, according to experts, are usually preoccupied with their appearance or bodily "image" as a result of personality or ego problems and social insecurities. Anorexics frequently suffer from amenorrhea–cessation or delay of menstruation. Amenorrhea can have serious physical consequences.

Treatment of anorexia nervosa involves psychiatric counseling and, sometimes, hospitalization to ensure weight gain.

Bulimia

When binges become "gorge and purge" sessions—stretches of overeating followed by self-induced vomiting—the condition is called bulimia. Purging can involve vomiting, using laxatives, or taking diuretics. Bulimia may exist in conjunction with anorexia nervosa or it may afflict people who are of normal size or are slightly overweight. Like anorexics, most bulimics are female, who perceive themselves as larger and fatter than they really are. Studies have shown that 11 percent of high school females and 10 percent of female college students suffer from anorexia nervosa and/or bulimia.

Much of the problem stems from a poor self-image, some social insecurities, and a lack of self-control. Treatment involves psychiatric counseling. Physical damages may include a ruptured esophagus, dental caries, and hypoglycemia. For more information, or guidance to resources in your community, please contact the National Association of Anorexia Nervosa and Associated Disorders, Box 7, Highland Park, IL 60035; 312/831–3438.

Physical Fitness

It is important for young people to understand the major benefits of daily exercise. Good physical conditioning is as important as weight control during the teen years. While not everybody can be an athletic champion, almost anyone can improve his or her heart, lungs, and muscles. All that is required is time, discipline, determination, and patience. Teenagers are advised to join school athletic teams or exercise independently after school. Walking to school rather than driving is another means of getting exercise.

Exercise Goals

One of the goals of physical conditioning for teenagers is to tone and develop muscles. Muscles that are exercised regularly will grow in size and strength. Those that are not will atrophy (shrink in size).

Exercise allows for an increase in the number of individual muscle fibers as well as an increase in the number of blood capillaries that supply the muscle tissue with nutritive substances. Consequently, the muscles become more efficient and more toned.

In addition to muscle development, physical conditioning should include optimum cardiopulmonary fitness. The increase in heart activity and oxygen consumption is the basis for aerobic workouts. Aerobic means, literally, "with oxygen." Aerobic training involves maintaining a steady rate of physical activity so that the heart, lungs, and muscles work together at a level that is more demanding than a body's state of rest. Jogging, running, and rapid walking are common examples of aerobic training.

Exercise Precautions

The individual goals should be kept within sensible limits to avoid injury or impaired health. Overexertion can cause dizziness, nausea, and hyperventilation. Teenagers should avoid excessive exercise during severely hot and humid weather. To avoid dehydration, drink plenty of water before and after exercising.

Choosing Proper Equipment

When exercising, it is essential that a teenager use proper athletic gear to avoid injuries. The knees are one of the most vulnerable body parts. As such, a teenager must be fitted with high-quality athletic shoes, which should be replaced as soon as they wear out. A podiatrist can provide insoles for proper foot balance for pavement or grass field. Protective gear, such as a mouth piece, shin guard, or riding helmet, is also important.

The Use of Steroids

In recent years, a substantial number of male teenagers have been abusing steroids in the hopes of developing bulky muscles. While this nonmedical use of anabolic steroids is illegal, its use is rampant.

There are considerable risks involved with taking steroids at such a young age. Adverse physical effects include stunted growth, acne, vomiting, and, for boys, enhanced breast development. In girls, side effects may be the development of permanent facial hair and deepened voices. For all users, there is a risk of long-term dependence or addiction to the drug. The psychological effects are equally serious. They include irritability, violent behavior, depression, mania, psychosis, and in some cases suicide.

Care of the teeth

During the teen years, careful supervision by the dentist and cooperation from the teenager are especially necessary. The poor eating habits of many teenagers are reflected in their cavity rate, which is usually higher during adolescence than in later life.

If a young person is conscientious about oral care, he can avoid not only a high cavity rate, but also bad breath and the unpleasant appearance of food particles left on the teeth. These problems are really caused by the same thing—*dental plaque.* For more information on this subject, see Ch. 22, *The Teeth and Gums.*

Need for Frequent Checkups

During the adolescent period, the dentist will often recommend more frequent checkups than in the past. Small cavities are treated before they become deeper and infect the pulp, the inner chamber of the tooth, containing nerves and blood vessels. Should the pulp become infected, the tooth must have special treatment, usually a root canal process, or be extracted.

The dentist also treats tooth decay, or *caries,* more popularly known as cavities, to prevent their spread. While they are not thought to be contagious, cavities begin as a break in the tooth surface, which later enlarges. Food debris can become lodged in the cavity, be attacked by bacteria, and cause a cavity on the next tooth. The only way to avoid such a problem is to have the affected tooth treated immediately.

Front teeth often decay for the first time during this period. They are restored with a silicate or plastic filling close in color to the tooth rather than silver or gold, which would be unattractive. Unfortunately, these materials are not permanent and will need to be replaced in time. As a result, neglect of diet and oral cleanliness by an adolescent may mean that

he may need many replacement fillings in the same cavity over his lifetime.

Orthodontic Treatment

The development and growth of teeth is completed during the adolescent period. When oral growth is improper, the adolescent needs treatment by an *orthodontist,* a dental specialist who treats abnormalities of the bite and alignment of teeth and jaws. Correction of such conditions as buck teeth, which mar a person's appearance, is a major reason for orthodontic treatment. But there are also major health reasons for orthodontic care. If teeth, for example, come together improperly, efficient chewing of food is impossible. The digestive system is strained because chunks of improperly chewed food pass through it. Orthodontic treatment will, therefore, result in lifelong better health and appearance. For more information, see Ch. 22, *The Teeth and Gums.*

Stimulants and Alcohol

Initial exposure to caffeine, tobacco, drugs, and alcohol usually occurs during adolescence. Teenagers should be fully educated regarding their physical effects and potential danger. They should learn how to use them, if at all, sensibly and in moderation, and to resist peer-group pressures.

Caffeine

Caffeine, which is naturally present in coffee and tea and is used in many carbonated beverages and medications, stimulates the central nervous system to overcome fatigue and drowsiness. It also affects a part of the nervous system that controls respiration so that more oxygen is

pumped through the lungs. In large amounts, caffeine can increase the pulse rate, but there are few long-range effects because the substance is broken down by the body tissues within a few hours and excreted. Because of the action of caffeine in stimulating an increased intake of oxygen, it sometimes is used to combat the effects of such nervous system depressants as alcohol.

Nicotine

Nicotine is one of nearly 200 substances in tobacco. It affects the human physiology by stimulating the adrenal glands to increase the flow of adrenaline. The blood vessels become constricted and the skin temperature drops, producing effects not unlike exposure to cold temperatures. When comparatively large amounts of nicotine are absorbed by the body, the pulse becomes rapid and the smoker has symptoms of dizziness, faintness, and sometimes nausea and diarrhea. The release of adrenaline, triggered by nicotine, will produce temporary relief from fatigue by increasing the flow of sugar in the blood. However, the effect is transient, and the feeling of fatigue will return again after the increased blood sugar has been expended.

Other Properties of Tobacco

The nicotine in tobacco can be absorbed simply by contact with the mucous membranes of the mouth; the tobacco does not have to be smoked to get the nicotine effects. Burning tobacco produces a myriad of substances found in the smoke of many plant materials when they are dried and burned. More than 50 different compounds are known to occur in concentrations of one microgram or more in each puff of tobacco smoke. Again, laboratory tests have demonstrated that the substances in burning tobacco do not have to be inhaled; most of the chemical compounds can be absorbed through the mucous membranes while a puff of smoke is held in the mouth for a few seconds. At least ten of the substances in tobacco smoke have been shown to produce cancer in animals. Other chemicals in tobacco tars are known as *cocarcinogens;* although they do not produce cancer themselves, they react with other substances to produce cancers.

Smoking and Disease

The relationship among tobacco smoking and cancer, heart disease, and emphysema-bronchitis is well established, even if some of the cause and effect links are missing. Large-scale studies of the death rates of smokers and nonsmokers have been carried on for more than 20 years. One group, consisting of nearly a quarter-million war veterans, yielded results indicating that smokers are from 10 to 16 times as likely to die of lung cancer as nonsmokers. (The higher ratio is for heavy smokers.) Similar results have been obtained from studies of smokers and nonsmokers with heart disease and lung ailments.

Buerger's Disease

One of the possible, although rare, effects of smoking is the aggravation of symptoms of a particularly insidious circulatory disorder known as *Buerger's disease.* As noted above, one of the effects of nicotine is a drop in skin temperatures. Smoking a single cigarette can cause the temperature of the fingers and toes to drop as much as 15 degrees Fahrenheit; the average is a little more than a 5-degree drop. The temperature change re-

sults from constriction of the blood vessels at the extremities. Blood clots may develop in the vessels that have been constricted, cutting off the flow of blood to the tissues of the area. When there is numbness or pain in the extremities, the condition should receive swift medical attention to prevent serious consequences.

Carbon Monoxide Accumulation

Another little publicized effect of smoking is the accumulation of carbon monoxide in the blood. Carbon monoxide is one of the lethal gases emitted in automobile exhaust. It is also produced by burning plant materials such as tobacco. It is a dangerous gas because of its strong affinity for the hemoglobin of red blood cells. Unlike oxygen and carbon dioxide, which become temporarily attached, then released, from the hemoglobin molecule, carbon monoxide becomes permanently locked into the red blood cell chemistry so that the cells are no longer effective for their normal function of transporting oxygen to the body tissues. With the oxygen-carrying capacity of part of the red blood cells wiped out, brain cells and other tissues suffer a mild oxygen starvation and the results are a form of intoxication.

A strong whiff of carbon monoxide can be fatal. Smokers, of course, do not get that much of the substance into their blood, but they do pick up enough carbon monoxide to render up to eight percent of their red blood cells ineffective. Experiments at Indiana University show that pack-a-day smokers have the same level of carbon monoxide in their blood as subjects who inhale an atmosphere of one-fourth of one percent carbon monoxide. That level of carbon monoxide increases the shortness of breath during exercise by approxi-

mately 15 percent, and, the study shows, about three weeks of abstinence from smoking are required to permit the oxygen-carrying capacity of the blood to return to normal. It is the carbon monoxide of burning plant materials that produces most of the "high" associated with the smoking of many substances.

Alcohol

Alcohol usually is not considered a potentially dangerous drug because it is easily available at cocktail lounges and liquor stores and is served generously at parties. Alcohol has been used by man for thousands of years, at times as a sedative and anesthetic, and when used in moderation has the effect of a mild tranquilizer and appetite stimulant. But when consumed in excess amounts, alcoholic beverages can produce both psychological and physical dependence. It can produce illusions of being a pick-me-up, but studies indicate that this is due to a letdown of inhibitions and the weakening of some functions of the central nervous system, particularly in the cerebral cortex.

Parents and teachers share an important responsibility to educate young people about the use and misuse of alcohol. Like marihuana, the effects of alcohol on human beings are not thoroughly understood. Some users develop a tissue tolerance for alcohol so that their body tissues require increasing amounts. When alcohol is withdrawn from such users, they develop tremors, convulsions, and even hallucinations. However, there are many varied reactions to the use of alcohol, and an individual may react differently to alcoholic drinks at different times. See Ch. 29, *Substance Abuse.*

Drugs

During the 1960s there was an alarming increase in drug use among teen-agers—a problem that deservedly received nationwide attention. Education concerning the hazards and occasional tragedies accompanying drug use is imperative.

Marihuana

Marihuana affects the central nervous system, including the brain, after it enters the bloodstream. According to some researchers, the substance accumulates in the liver. Some of the effects of marihuana are not unlike those of tobacco. The rate of the heartbeat is increased, body temperature drops, and blood sugar levels are altered. The drug user also feels dehydrated, the appetite is stimulated, coordination of movements becomes difficult, there are feelings of drowsiness or unsteadiness, and the eyes may become reddish. Taken in higher strengths, marihuana can cause hallucinations or distortions of perception.

Varying Effects

Scientists are uncertain about the pathways of the drug in the central nervous system and its effects on other body systems. The drug's effects seem to vary widely, not only among individual users but also according to the social setting and the amount and strength of the marihuana used. The effects, which usually begin within 15 minutes after the smoke is inhaled and may continue for several hours, vary from depression to excitement and talkativeness. Some users claim to experience time distortions and errors in distance perception. But others sharing the same marihuana cigarette may experience no effects at all.

Although marihuana is not addictive, in that users do not develop a physical dependence upon the substance and withdrawal of the drug produces no ill effects, there are dangerous results from the use of marihuana. Marihuana users find it hard to make decisions that require clear thinking, some users develop psychotic reactions or an emotional disorder called "acute marihuana panic," and there is some evidence that the active ingredient is transmitted by expectant mothers to their unborn children.

Hallucinogens

Marihuana sometimes is described as a *hallucinogen* because of visual hallucinations, illusions, and delusions reported by users after they have inhaled the smoke from a large number of "joints" or "sticks" of the drug. But marihuana should not be confused with the true hallucinogenic drugs such as *mescaline* and *LSD* (lysergic acid diethylamide) which are known by doctors as *psychomimetic* drugs because they mimic psychoses.

LSD and Mescaline

LSD and mescaline have marked effects on perception and thought processes. Teenagers usually become involved with the use of LSD because they are curious about its effects; they may have heard about its purported "mind-bending" properties and expect to gain great personal insights from its use. Instead of great insight, however, the user finds anxiety, depression, confusion, and frightening hallucinations. The use of LSD is complicated by the reappearance of hallucinations after the individual has quit using the drug; the very possibility of repeated hallucinations causes a sense of terror.

Morphine and Heroin

Besides the hallucinogenic drugs, there are *opium* derivatives, *morphine* and *heroin*. Morphine is one of the most effective pain relievers known and is one of the most valuable drugs available to the physician. Morphine and heroin depress the body systems to produce drowsiness, sleep, and a reduction in physical activity. They are true narcotics, and their appeal is in their ability to produce a sense of euphoria by reducing the individual's sensitivity to both psychological and physical stimuli.

Addictive Properties

A great danger lies in the ability of the body tissues to develop a physical dependence on morphine and its derivative cousin, heroin. The degree to which heroin's "desirable" effects are felt depends in part on how the user takes it. *Sniffing* is the mildest form of abuse, followed by *skin-popping*—subcutaneous injection—and then by *mainlining*—injecting directly into a vein, which is the method used by almost all those dependent on heroin.

The body adjusts to the level of the first doses so that increasingly larger injections of the drug are required to produce the same feelings of euphoria. The ability of the body to adjust to the increasingly larger doses is called *tolerance*. And with tolerance goes *physical dependence*, which means that when heroin or morphine is withdrawn from the user he experiences a violent sickness marked by tremors, sweating and chills, vomiting and diarrhea, and sharp abdominal pains. Another shot of heroin or morphine temporarily ends the withdrawal symptoms. But the user, now dependent upon the drug, must continue regular doses or face another bout of the withdrawal sickness. Heroin has no value as a medicine and is available only through illicit channels at a high price. The heroin addict usually is unable to hold a job because of effects of the drug and often turns to crime in order to finance his daily supply of the narcotic.

Shortened Life Span

The health of a narcotics addict declines so that his life span is shortened by 15 to 20 years. He usually is in continual trouble with the law because of the severe penalties for illegal possession of narcotics. If he sells narcotics, as many heroin addicts are driven to do to get enough money to support their habit, the punishment is even more severe.

Amphetamines and Barbiturates

Other commonly abused drugs are *amphetamines,* also known as *uppers* or *pep pills,* and *barbiturates,* sometimes called *downers* or *goof balls.* Amphetamines are used by physicians to curb the appetite when weight reduction of patients is needed and to relieve mild cases of depression. However, some physicians doubt that amphetamines should be used as a weight-control medication because of the risks involved; other experts have questioned whether the drugs are actually effective for that purpose.

Amphetamines stimulate the heart rate, increase the blood pressure, cause rapid breathing, dilate the pupils of the eyes, and produce other effects such as dryness of the mouth, sweating, headache, and diarrhea. Ordinarily, amphetamines are swallowed as tablets, but a more extreme form of amphetamine abuse involves the injection of the drug, usually Methedrine, directly into the vein.

Dangers of Amphetamines

The danger in the use of amphetamines is that they induce a person to do things beyond his physical endurance, cause mental disorders that require hospitalization, and, in large doses, can result in death. Although they do not produce the kind of physical dependence observed in the use of narcotics, amphetamine withdrawal for a heavy user can result in a deep and suicidal depression.

Barbiturates

Barbiturates are sedatives used by physicians to treat high blood pressure, epilepsy, and insomnia, and to relax patients being prepared for surgery. They slow the heart rate and breathing, lower blood pressure, and mildly depress the action of nerves and muscles.

Dangers of Barbiturates

Barbiturates are highly dangerous when taken without medical advice. They distort perception and slow down reaction and response time, contributing to the chances of accidents. Barbiturates are a leading cause of accidental poison deaths because they make the mind foggy and the user forgets how many pills he has taken, thus leading to overdosage. They also cause physical dependence with withdrawal symptoms that range from cramps and nausea to convulsions and death. See also Ch. 29, *Substance Abuse.*

Adolescent Suicide

Suicides among teenage boys and girls increased greatly in number during the middle 1980s. Health experts termed the phenomenon an "epidemic of self-destruction." In some areas suicides or suicide attempts took place in clusters. Often, groups of close friends were involved. In some cases of cluster suicides or attempts, it appeared that a suicidal attitude was contagious.

Suicide became the second leading cause of death among adolescents. In the nearly 30 years beginning in the late 1950s, the suicide rate among teenagers tripled. Preadolescents also began to take their own lives more frequently: public health personnel reported suicides among children as young as three.

Risk Factors

As educators, social workers, psychiatrists, and others became involved in community efforts to prevent teenage suicides, a number of "risk factors"—signs of an intent to take one's life—were isolated. Changes in a teenager's behavior, whether in peer relationships, school activities, or academic performance, were said to be primary indicators. So were emotional shifts, particularly toward anger or irritability. Depression and withdrawal, experts said, might accompany the emotional changes. Sadness, changes in eating and sleeping habits, and preoccupation with death were other signs.

Young people considering suicide showed other symptoms. Many reported headaches, stomachaches, and other ailments. Some talked about taking their own lives. A young person who had lost a close friend through suicide was at unusual risk, according to studies. Family histories of suicide and parental depression were cited as indirectly contributing factors.

Parent Involvement

For parents concerned about the possibility of a child's or teen's suicide, such clues are only clues. The parent still has the task of trying to resolve the potential suicide. Authorities make the following suggestions.

Act at Once

Where a preadolescent or adolescent gives clear signals—usually risk factors appearing in combination—that suicide might be contemplated, parents should seek help immediately. Local suicide hotlines or suicide prevention centers should be contacted; counseling may have to be started.

School Help

Many schools cooperate in efforts to prevent suicides. The schools may sponsor group meetings at which students talk out their feelings about suicide, and such meetings may be appropriate as a first or second step. A representative of the community crisis or prevention center normally takes part in such meetings. Many schools have special counselors, psychologists, and others who can serve as direct lines to sources of help.

Out-of-School Contacts

Group meetings provide all teenage participants with the names and locations of out-of-school contact persons who may be able to help them in a crisis. Most crisis agencies operate 24 hours a day, seven days a week, providing aid during the "danger hours" between late afternoon and midnight. Parents may want also to contact clergy, trusted friends or relatives, or others.

Peer Support

Where possible, peer support should be mobilized in the effort to prevent a suicide. Many young people, especially the friends of a depressed or otherwise suicidal teenager, can help—and will do so rather than hear later that a suicide has taken place. But parents should, according to experts, remember that a youngster

with high status among his or her peers may influence those peers. Committing suicide, the high-status young person may convince others that "life isn't worth it." Surviving boy- or girlfriends are especially at risk.

Social and Sexual Maturation

The Prospect of Adulthood

As a youngster passes from childhood into adolescence, it is the psychological adjustments rather than the physical changes that are most likely to produce difficulties. The emotional problems, of course, are related to the hormonal activity of the developing body. However, the conflicts that frequently are upsetting to both the adolescent and other members of his family are the result of adjustments that must be made between the young person and the society in which he must live.

In our own culture, the teenager must continually adjust to a complex set of rules and regulations. He frequently may feel that he must accept the responsibilities of adulthood before he is entitled to the privileges of being treated as an adult. Childhood is only a step behind, but he has learned to suppress or ignore childhood relationships. He can easily forget the point of view of children and even resent the ability of his parents to recall the "cute" incidents of his earlier years. At the same time, he may be startled by the suggestion that within a few short years he and his teenage friends will face the selection of a career, marriage, establishment of a home, and a lifetime of responsibili-

ties he may feel ill-prepared to assume.

Future Outlook for Teenagers

While a teenager may feel competent enough to handle adult responsibilities and decisions, he or she may have misgivings about what the future holds. Fear and uncertainty of the unknown can cause anxiety in teenagers, though they may not express it. They are aware that the choices they make—what college or vocational school they select, what profession they choose, who they marry, where they decide to live—can affect their entire lives.

An abundance of educational opportunities and careers choices is available for any teenager. It is the parents' responsibility to expose teenagers to all of the options and to guide them toward attainable goals. Parents should recognize a teen's strengths and weakness and direct him or her to the most appropriate educational institution or profession. Career and college guidance counselors at high school are very helpful.

In the past few decades, the outlook for males and females have become nearly identical. There are virtually no educational or professional barriers that separate men and women. There are male nurses and female doctors, husbands who stay at home and wives who work.

The career options and lifestyles that teenagers may select are seemingly endless. Traditional social conventions are changing. Many marriages occur after both spouses have established careers, allowing for arrangements that were not possible for many parents of current teenagers. Given the professional opportunities for women, many families are dual-income, or, in some cases, the men choose to stay at home. Much of this depends on the economic needs of a particular family, but the options are there for nearly any kind of work situation and lifestyle. Such instances of role-reversal and dual-income families have provided a new and promising outlook for teenagers.

Advanced Education

The educational requirements for current jobs place an added strain on the pace of growing up. Many teenagers must have some vague professional goals in order to choose the proper means of attaining them. This primarily includes an appropriate education. All professions require a certain level of education and expertise. While much of the experience is learned on the job, many professions require college degrees and even graduate degrees. In many blue-collar professions, training is essential. It can be obtained through vocational schools, apprenticeships, or training programs.

Need for Independence

Adolescence is a time when a child slowly develops into an adult. With physical changes come psychological changes as well. As such, a teenager wants to be treated like an adult, not a child. These demands are often manifested in rebellious actions and disdainful remarks.

In a desire to act independently, a teenager may exhibit reclusive behavior in order to avoid contact with parents. He or she may be reluctant to divulge information. Sneaking out of the house is a common gesture. These are distinct attempts to dodge unsolicited advice from parents who are only too anxious to give it.

Parents should not be offended by these actions, rather they should allow their child to explore the world independently. Such an education will make them more confident and well-

adjusted as adults. Teenagers who are not allowed much freedom are often more difficult to control and can cause more damage out of spite.

Conflicts between Parent and Teenager

Some conflicts between the generations are avoidable. The parents may be protective and slow to cut the apron strings because they love their children and want to prevent them from becoming involved in unhappy situations. The teenager resents the overprotective actions of the parents, regarding them as evidence that they do not trust their own children.

A keystone in the training for adulthood is the concept that being an adult entails more than just privileges and the authority to make decisions; along with decision-making goes a responsibility to the family and society for the consequences of one's decisions and actions.

Few parents, of course, would refuse to bail out a teenage son or daughter in real trouble. And even when a youngster is rebellious enough to leave home, he should know that the door will always be open to him when he decides to return. Again, limiting the options available to a teenager can lead to a snowballing of bad decisions and resulting complications.

In many cases, the conflicts between parents and teenagers derive from the illusion that a younger child has more freedom of choice. A small child may actually seem to have a freer choice of friends he can bring into his home and the games he can play with them. But there are always limitations to a child's choices, and parents are more understanding of the bad choices by attributing mistakes to the fact that "he's only a child."

Older youngsters become involved

in situations in which the decisions are more important. A boy and girl at the age of five can "play house" together in an atmosphere of innocence. However, the same boy and girl could hardly suggest to their parents that they intended to play house at the age of 15. If the boy and girl, although next-door neighbors, are of different social or ethnic backgrounds, they may become aware of parental prejudices in addition to new rules of propriety as they grow into their teenage years.

Decisions of the teen years can involve the use of tobacco, alcohol, owning an automobile, handling of money, overnight trips with friends, association with friends who use drugs illegally, and relationships with members of the opposite sex. The consequences of all alternatives should be outlined for the adolescent.

Search for Identity

Part of the youngster's struggle for independence will involve what sometimes is described as a search for identity. A child accepts without much questioning that he is a member of a certain family and lives in a certain neighborhood. But as he grows older, he becomes aware of his status in the family as well as the status of his family in society. A seven-year-old could not care less about the background of his family or that of his second-grade friends. As he becomes a teenager he learns that such subjects may be matters of concern to parents and their circle of friends. He may imitate the attitudes of his family or disregard them, perhaps inviting criticism that he is rebellious.

More important to the youngster, however, is a growing concern about his position and role in life and where it may lead. He is still in the so-called formative years and is sensitive to countless influences in the world about him. Teenagers become concerned with approaching education and career decisions. It is natural for them to identify with older members in the family, teachers, and celebrities.

Need for Privacy

For the teenage girl, party invitations, dances, and diaries are important and an increasing amount of privacy is required. Even if she must share a room with a sister, there should be a part of the room that is her territory. She should have personal belongings that are not shared by a parent or sibling. If she has her own room, everything in the room probably will be regarded as her property. Even her mother should respect her privacy by knocking on the door and getting permission to enter her private world.

Although sometimes less sensitive about such matters, boys also are likely to insist on a certain amount of privacy as they grow older. They may share a room with a brother but they need trunks or other containers with locks in which they can keep personal possessions. Proof that such desire for privacy is not a passing fad for young men is found in their adult compulsion for private offices and a den or workshop area at home.

Contacts with Older Friends

Young teenagers, through part-time jobs as babysitters or errand boys, usually come in contact with young adults outside the family circle for the first time. The young adults may accept the teenagers as peers, which is flattering to the youngsters, who may in turn admire and imitate the young adults. If the teenager has been able to identify closely with his family's sense of propriety, the contacts can be a good social experience. But if the youngster has not been able to identify effectively with his parents and family members, he may be vulnerable to misguiding influences. Because of the urge for adult status, the teenager may find a premature outlet for testing his abilities to live the adult life in the company of young adults. He (or she) can absorb a lot of information—and misinformation—about sex, alcohol, drugs, and other subjects.

Teenagers certainly should not be cautioned against contacts with all young adults, but they should also have a reliable older person aside from their parents with whom they can discuss matters they would not discuss with a mother or father. The alternate adult might be a clergyman, the family physician, a teacher, or even a favorite aunt or uncle. Such an arrangement provides the youngster with a means of learning a bit more about life in an independent manner and from a different point of view than could be obtained within his own immediate family circle.

Relationships with the Opposite Sex

First teenage contacts with the opposite sex tend to be awkward and sometimes embarrassing despite the best efforts and intentions of parents. The meetings may be at school dances or movie dates, perhaps in the presence of a chaperon who is a teacher or parent.

Overcoming Insecurity

Some youngsters will feel more secure than others in social gatherings; those who feel insecure may not participate at all when such opportunities first arise. As the youngsters grow older, however, they find that more and more of their friends are dating or going to dances or parties to meet members of the opposite sex.

Some boys or girls who feel insecure may find that they are more gregarious or less ill-at-ease if they fortify themselves with a couple of drinks of an alcoholic beverage, or with drugs, before they join their friends. Youngsters who feel the need for stimulants or depressants in order to enjoy parties usually can be helped with psychological counseling to overcome their fears of inadequacy.

Young people should be assured that getting together at parties of mixed sexes is a natural thing to do. It has been going on for generations and although an individual youngster may feel ill-at-ease at his first few dances or parties, he probably will survive. As the boy or girl attends more parties the chances increase that he or she will meet a person of the opposite sex who is particularly attractive. If the feeling is mutual, the acquaintanceship may develop into more or less steady dating.

Going Steady

Steady dating, which leads to a formal engagement and marriage in many cases, should not be encouraged at an early age or before a young person has had an opportunity to date a number of prospective partners. At the same time, it should not be discouraged to the point of producing a rebellious reaction. As was pointed out earlier, some girls admit going steady with a boy for no other reason than to demonstrate their independence of judgment.

Controlling the Sexual Impulse

Teenagers who spend a lot of time together at parties, in their homes, or at recreational meetings such as beach outings are likely to be physically attracted to each other. It may begin with kissing, dancing, holding hands, or simply a natural urge to neck or pet. In more primitive societies, the couple might simply indulge in sexual intercourse without any concern for the possible consequences. But in our own society, young people are expected to control their natural urges.

Influence of the Mass Media

Complicating sincere efforts of a teenager to make the right decisions in relations with the opposite sex is the constant exposure of youngsters to movies, magazine articles, books, and other media suggesting that sexual relations between unmarried couples are not only acceptable but a common practice. Compared to the image of young love as displayed in movie promotion advertising, a teenage boy and girl may believe that a few ardent hugs and kisses in a secluded spot may be as innocent as making a plate of fudge together in the girl's kitchen.

Some girls, but not all, are as easily aroused as boys by close bodily contact with the opposite sex. Physical contact for most boys arouses sexual desire, partly because of the physiological makeup of the male.

The Sex Drive in Boys

Males are so constituted that during periods of abstinence from intercourse, their sperm builds up. During periods of sperm buildup, the male sex drive increases in strength. There are no standards or averages for the male sex drive; instead there is a wide variety of sexual appetites and abilities.

A girl who cuddles too closely to a boy may trigger a response she did not expect and may not want. Depending upon the boy and the status of his sex drive at that time, he might accept the girl's approaches as a suggestion that she is willing to have intercourse or is at least interested in petting. If the girl is simply being friendly, the results can be embarrassing to one or both of the youngsters. If the boy is the type who likes to discuss the details of his dates with friends, the girl may discover a sudden and unwelcome change in attitude by other boys of the group.

Walking hand-in-hand, or with an arm around the waist, and kissing that is not too passionate, usually are acceptable ways for young teenagers to display affection. And there are activities such as hiking or bicycle riding that afford a boy and girl a chance to be together and apart from the rest of the world. There also are picnics, ball games, movies, and concerts that permit togetherness without setting the stage for hard-to-control sexual impulses.

Masturbation

Another manifestation of the natural sex drives of young persons is masturbation. Discouraged by the rules and standards of society from fulfilling sex urges in the same manner as married couples, teenagers discover they can find sexual satisfaction in masturbation. Despite the stories that warn of physical or mental decay for youngsters who masturbate, the practice is not harmful unless the parents make an issue of it.

If there are dangers in masturbation, they are likely to be the isolation and loneliness associated with the practice and the confusion and anxiety that can result if the young person feels guilty or is punished or criticized for masturbating. Masturbation is such a natural reaction that most youngsters discover it by themselves even if the subject is never discussed by friends or family members. But for many young people, masturbation may violate religious or other beliefs or values. These youngsters may want to discuss the practice with a physician, understanding clergy, or some other trusted person.

Sex Education

Because boys and girls in their teens may be capable of producing children and are known to have strong sexual urges, they should be provided with authoritative information about human reproduction and birth control. It is up to the parents to make decisions regarding the proper sources of such information, how much information should be given, and at what age.

One of the reasons for the popularity of sex education in the schools is that teachers can get the parents off the hook by explaining the facts of life to youngsters. However, by forfeiting their prerogative to explain sex and human reproduction to their own children, parents must depend upon the teacher to make an acceptable presentation to the youngsters. The likely alternative is that youngsters will obtain a considerable amount of misinformation from friends and acquaintances at street-corner seminars or by experimentation.

In the days when the majority of the population lived on farms or near rural areas, children learned a few things about sex and reproduction simply by working with farm animals. They learned that cats produced kittens, dogs produced puppies, cows produced calves, and so on. This on-the-job type of sex education also provided farm youngsters with a smattering of genetics, because cross-breeding strains of animals frequently had economic consequences. It was not too difficult for the rural youngsters to relate their barnyard education to human experience.

Children enrolled in sex education

classes in the urban areas of America today receive similar information—dogs have puppies, cats have kittens, etc.—by watching movies and reading books. However, the lessons may be superficial or incomplete, depending upon the teacher and the prescribed curriculum. For example, the children in one eastern school were taught that the baby develops in the mother's abdomen, which led some youngsters to believe the baby lived in the mother's stomach until born. "Why isn't the baby digested by the stomach acid?" asked one confused girl. And when asked how the baby gets out when it's time to be born, the teacher told the students that such questions should be answered by their parents. The point here is that parents should establish some rapport with their children to be sure they are learning a practical set of facts about adult love, sex, and reproduction, including the possible emotional and physical consequences of premarital sexual intercourse.

Although parents may find it difficult or embarrassing to explain the facts of life to their own children, it is one of the most important contributions that can be made to a maturing youngster. At the present time, at least one out of six teenage girls in the United States will have an unwanted pregnancy. Obviously, thousands of parents and teachers are not providing adequate instruction in sex education subjects.

The Male Reproductive System

Any instruction in the facts of life should begin by use of the proper names for the body parts involved. In the male, the external sex organs are the *penis* and the *testicles,* or *testes.* The penis contains a tiny tube, the *urethra,* through which urine is eliminated. Much of the fleshy part of the

penis is composed of spongy tissue. When the penis is stimulated sexually, the spongy areas become filled with blood, which makes the penis larger and firm, a condition called an *erection.* The testicles contain male *sperm cells,* also called *spermatozoa.*

The sperm travel up tubules inside the abdomen to a storage organ, or reservoir, the *seminal vesicle.* The sperm storage area also contains a thick white fluid called *semen* that is secreted by glands that open into the urethra. One of the glands, the *prostate,* serves partly as a control valve to prevent urine from mixing with the semen, since both are discharged through the urethra. The semen, containing millions of sperm, empties periodically in a more or less automatic action, being squeezed out of the seminal vesicle by pulsating contractions. The contractions and ejection of semen are called *ejaculation.* During the sex act, or *intercourse,* with a female, the semen is ejaculated into the woman's vagina.

The Female Reproductive System

The *vagina* is the proper name for the tubular female sex organ. At the end of the vagina is an opening, called the *cervix,* which leads into the *uterus.* The uterus, or *womb,* is shaped somewhat like an upside-down pear. When a baby develops within the mother's abdomen, it grows inside the uterus. The uterus also is the source of the bloody discharge that occurs periodically during the fertile years of women. When the blood is discharged it is called *menstruation,* or the menstrual period. The menstrual blood passes out through the vagina, which stretches to become the *birth canal* when a baby is being born. The urethra of a female empties outside the vagina.

The Menstrual Cycle and Conception

Unlike the male reproductive organs, which produce perhaps millions of spermatozoa each day, the female reproductive system ordinarily releases only one germ cell, called an *ovum* or egg, at a time. An ovum is released at an average frequency of once every 28 days. It should always be remembered that the 28-day figure is only an average; the actual time may vary considerably for reasons that are only partly known. The cycles are more likely to be irregular for teenage girls than for mature women. An ovum is released from one of the two *ovaries,* or sex glands, comparable in function to the male testicles, located on either side of the uterus. The ovum, or egg, is transported from the ovary to the uterus through a *Fallopian tube.*

If the ovum encounters male sperm during its passage from the ovary to the uterus, there is a good chance that fertilization, or *conception,* will occur through a union of a spermatozoon and the egg. The fertilized ovum, called a *zygote,* soon divides into a cluster of human tissue cells that become the embryo of a baby. For further information about pregnancy, see under Ch. 4, *The Beginning of a Family.*

During the time that the egg is maturing in the ovary and passing into the uterus after its release, the membrane lining of the uterus becomes thicker because it accumulates blood and nutrients. If the ovum is fertilized, it finds a spot in the membrane where it becomes attached and develops rapidly into an embryo, gaining its nourishment from the blood and nutrient-enriched lining of the uterus. If the ovum is not fertilized, it passes through the uterus, and the blood-rich membrane sloughs off. The blood and some of the cells of the membrane become the discharged material of menstruation. The unfertilized ovum could pass through undetected because it is nearly microscopic.

After menstruation has begun, the female reproductive cycle starts over again. The lining of the uterus once more builds up its supply of blood and nutrients to support a fertilized ovum. Ordinarily, the next ovum will be released about 14 days after a menstrual period begins. If a female does not have intercourse, or avoids intercourse during the time the ovum is released, or in some other manner is able to prevent sperm from reaching an ovum, she will not become pregnant but will experience a menstrual period at intervals that average around 28 days.

When fertilization of an ovum occurs, menstruation ceases and no further egg cells are released until the outcome of the pregnancy has been determined. In other words, the cycles of ovulation and menstruation start anew after the baby is born or the pregnancy has been terminated.

Contraception

The first rule of birth control is that no method is guaranteed to be 100 percent effective. Sexual intercourse nearly always is accompanied by some risk of pregnancy, and the teenagers who try to beat the odds should be willing to take the responsibility for the results. Teenagers should be provided with the basic facts of birth control as soon as they are capable of producing children themselves. But the emphasis should be on the relative unreliability of the techniques which do not require a visit to a physician's office. Many birth controldevices and substances can bepurchased without a physician's prescription. But if young men and women were aware of their chances of effecting a pregnancy while using

such methods, they probably would have second thoughts about taking the risk. See Ch. 4, *The Beginning of a Family,* for a full discussion of birth control methods.

Venereal Disease

Equally important in the education of teenagers is a knowledge of the hazards of venereal disease. A poster prepared for a New York campaign against venereal disease carried the words "If your son is old enough to shave, he's old enough to get syphilis." The American Social Health Association estimates that 300,000 teenagers each year become infected with one or more forms of venereal disease. Most insidious has been the recent increase in gonorrhea, partly because girls who carry the infection may show no symptoms. A girl may have a slight but seemingly unimportant vaginal discharge. She may not be aware that she has gonorrhea until she is contacted by health officials after her boyfriend has reported to a physician for treatment. For more information on venereal disease, see Ch. 17, *Diseases of the Urinogenital System.*

Two reasons for the rising incidence of gonorrhea after it was once thought to be virtually eliminated by antibiotics are that condoms, once used as a mechanical barrier by males, have become less popular since teenage girls have obtained the use of oral contraceptives, and that new strains of the bacteria are resistant to the antibiotics. Some boys delay treatment when they realize they are infected with VD; they believe it makes them appear "tough" to be able to go without medical treatment even when it endangers their health. Because of rebelliousness, youngsters may have a venereal disease

and either refuse to tell their parents or boast about it, depending upon which approach they think will make them appear independent.

It is a bitter irony for many parents to realize that their children might carry the spirit of independence and privacy into areas that could endanger their health, for untreated syphilis can result in blindness, insanity, and heart disease. Such grave consequences can be avoided in most cases by establishing effective channels of communication between parents and teenagers, or between teenagers and another responsible adult.

The Generation Gap

Despite the attention devoted in recent years to the so-called generation gap, the gap is nothing new to the process of evolving from childhood to adulthood. Every generation has had its generation gap—a period in which the fledgling adult tests his ability to make his own way in the world. In previous eras youngsters were considered old enough to take on an adult role when they were big enough physically. A boy left home to become a farm hand or a factory apprentice. A girl would leave home to become a live-in maid with another family. Sometimes the generation gap was masked by great social upheavals such as a war or a wave of emigration. The fictional hero of many romantic stories was a young man who left home to make his own way in the world, discovering in the process a girl who wanted to be rescued from her environment. With a few jet-age variations the adolescent boys and girls of today experience the same emotional struggles as nature develops their minds and bodies toward becoming another generation of adults.

4

The Beginning of a Family

Family Planning

When and How to Plan

Planning a family basically means figuring out when you want children, how many you want, and how long you choose to wait between pregnancies. It is always recommended that you discuss these things before marriage. It is going to be a major sticking point in a relationship if you want four children and your partner's idea of family is a parakeet.

When to have a family is also important. If you are in your twenties or early thirties and wish to have children, you have several years for doing so. If you are in your late thirties or older, having children may be an immediate priority. This is true for both men and women. Although most men are physically capable of fathering children throughout their lives, they should be young enough to participate actively in the raising of the children. If you father a child when you are 51 years old, you will be 72 when the child graduates from college. This is something to consider when you make the decision to become a parent.

Any plan should leave room for flexibility. Priorities and situations may change during the course of a relationship. Both partners should be aware of this possibility and be flexible to the shifting situations.

Almost no couple expects problems with fertility or conception when they plan a family. Yet approximately 10 percent of all couples have enough difficulty conceiving that they require fertility testing or treatment.

For those whom infertility is not an issue, planning pregnancies involves decisions about birth control and spacing of pregnancies.

Timing Between Pregnancies

The minimum time a couple should leave between pregnancies is set by the period of time the baby is breastfed. Breastfeeding and pregnancy tax the mother's and the fetus's health. It is recommended that any mother who is breastfeeding a child, and is pregnant, wean the child.

For the recovery of the physical health of the mother, two years is the average recommended wait. This puts the children almost three years apart in age.

The length of time between children should take into consideration the age and health of the parents, the number of children the couple wants, and the difficulty they have in conceiving. For a couple that suffers through a miscarriage for every successful pregnancy, a long wait may not be recommended. It should also be noted here, though, that a good gynecologist/obstetrician will be able to recommend what is in the mother's best health interest in spacing of pregnancies. For any couple that experiences difficulties with pregnancies, a doctor's advice on their particular situation should be the primary source of information.

Once physical considerations are understood, it becomes a matter of personal priority for the parents. Some parents prefer to wait until one child is in school, or at least out of diapers, before having another child. Having two toddlers can be quite trying on a parent's energy and patience. For first-time parents, having children close in age may help in arranging the parents' schedule around the children. The problems of arranging for day care may only be extended a year or two if the children are close in age. For children five years apart, working parents have at least one child in day care for ten years. For more discussion on child care and day care, see the end of this chapter.

Conception

Once you decide that you would like to have a child, planning the pregnancy involves two basic schedules. The first is deciding when you want the child to arrive. This includes deciding when pregnancy would be convenient. The second is discovering when fertility occurs each month in the woman's cycle.

When to Get Pregnant

In deciding when the best time of the year to have a baby arrive, several things should be taken into account. If you plan on taking time off from work for the child, you should consider the work you do and when a break in the work load would prove easiest to pull away. If you are a teacher, summer months may provide an ideal time for birth. If you can schedule delivery in June, the baby will be almost three months old before you start back to school in the fall. For others, a sabbatical or independent project may be timed to coincide with periods at home.

Weather may also help you decide when you wish to get pregnant. Buying winter clothing for the last stage of pregnancy can be costly. Getting a winter coat, and sweaters, and longjohns to fit during the eighth and ninth month of pregnancy may require buying clothes you won't ever wear again. Getting summer dresses and cotton pants for the last trimester of the pregnancy may be cheaper. Some women, however, cannot bear the thought of being eight months pregnant in the August heat.

Holiday schedules are also important. Some children love having birthdays around Christmas and Hanukkah. Other children hate it, feeling that their birthdays are overlooked in the festivities of the season. Preholiday births may allow a family to see distant relatives without taking an added trip across the country. For parents who work, holiday births may allow them to spend vacation time with their newborn.

Each family works on a slightly different schedule than the next. Their needs and what works best for them have to be determined on an individual basis. Even within that family, schedules may shift between the birth of one child and the next. Planning can help ease the burden of time off and child care that may be essential to making a family work.

How to Get Pregnant

Once you have decided on starting or continuing a family, planning the pregnancy involves calculating the fertile period in the menstrual cycle. For some parents, this requires no effort at all. Some women get pregnant immediately after stopping birth control. For others, months of timing ovulation may be required for successful conception.

The best method to figure out an ovulation cycle is to work with your physician. There are some things you can do in advance to help, though. Write down the starting and ending date of your period, for several months. If anything significant happens during the month that may have changed the cycle, such as an illness, note it in your calendar.

Your physician can give your specific information on physical characteristics and signs of ovulation that you should watch for. Basal body temperature fluctuates just before ovulation. If you chart your temperature every day at the same time, usually first thing in the morning, you should notice a slight change in the body temperature approximately two weeks before your period. The rise in temperature of about .4 to .8 degrees Fahrenheit appears normally within 24 hours of ovulation. It should last a few days and then the temperature should return to a normal level.

Some women do not get a sharp increase in temperature. It may be more subtle, more gradual, or even may drop in temperature slightly. It is important that you chart more than a couple months to get a better general view of your own body's rhythm.

Checking the viscosity of mucous production can also give some signs of ovulation. Cervical mucous production becomes more transparent and more elastic as ovulation occurs. There are also physical characteristic changes that can be noted under a microscope.

By establishing and keeping a calendar for these changes, a woman should be able to, with the help of her obstetrician or gynecologist, determine when she is fertile. If, after several months of intercourse during periods of fertility, the couple still has not conceived, the physician will recommend testing for egg and sperm production.

The Menstrual Cycle

The menstrual cycle runs, on average, every 28 days. As many women have cycles longer than 28 days as have cycles shorter than 28 days. Some women's cycles are not always the same length. Cycles may vary each month, with no true regularity. Some may alter between two lengths. For example, a woman may have a cycle that is 28 days, followed by a cycle of 30 days. She may then repeat the pattern. For women who have extremely irregular cycles, birth control pills can help regulate their menstrual flow. When they stop taking the pill,

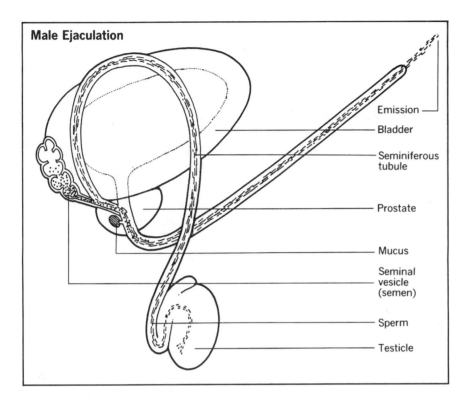

Male Ejaculation

- Emission
- Bladder
- Seminiferous tubule
- Prostate
- Mucus
- Seminal vesicle (semen)
- Sperm
- Testicle

though, they may return to their previous irregularity.

Some women have lower abdominal pain midway through their cycle that accompanies ovulation. Called *mittelschmerz*, the pain can vary from a dull ache lasting hours to a sharp pain that only lasts minutes. The pain is believed to be caused by the release of the ovum from the ovary.

A new cycle is marked from the first day of menstruation. On the first day after menstruation stops, the body's hormonal levels are at their lowest for estrogen and progesterone. The uterine lining is at its thinnest. As the level of estrogen rises the blood-lined wall of the uterus builds. The wall prepares for the embedding of a fertilized egg. For the average cycle (28 days) the wall continues to build for two weeks.

While this is occurring, at least one egg is developing in an ovary. The ovary that develops the egg may alternate from left side to right. How this is controlled by the body's hormonal system is not yet understood. After approximately two weeks, the

body releases luteinizing hormone (LH), triggering the release of the ripe egg from the ovary.

The egg travels down the fallopian tube. This may take from one to five days. While the egg is in the fallopian tube, the body continues to prepare the uterine wall for implantation of a fertilized egg.

If intercourse takes place during this period of time, the egg and the sperm meet up in the fallopian tube. One sperm will penetrate the egg wall and the egg immediately produces a

barrier that prevents a second sperm from penetrating. The fertilized egg, called the blastula during that stage of development, continues to travel down the fallopian tube to the uterus.

If the egg implants on the tube wall, or lodges against something and cannot continue on to the uterus, it will continue growing in the fallopian tube. It will only take a matter of days for the embryo to outgrow the size of the tube. Spots of blood will be the first sign of an *ectopic pregnancy*, or a pregnancy that develops outside the uterus. The accompanying pain will continue to get worse until treatment is sought. After a few days of spotting and pain the fallopian tube will rupture, producing tremendous pain and blood flow. This is an extreme emergency and medical attention should be sought immediately.

If the embryo successfully makes the journey to the uterine lining, it will usually implant against the blood-filled wall. The embryo will develop a cord attachment to the wall, establishing the placental link between the mother and the embryo. Through this cord flows the blood that will keep the embryo alive and nourish its development.

Some eggs will not successfully lodge against the wall. They may pass undetected with the menstrual blood. They may also temporarily lodge

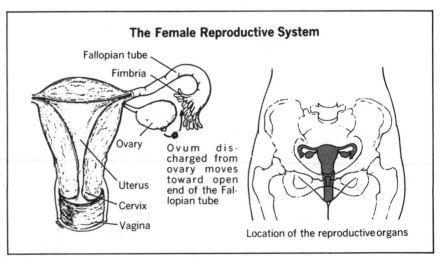

The Female Reproductive System

- Fallopian tube
- Fimbria
- Ovary
- Uterus
- Cervix
- Vagina

Ovum discharged from ovary moves toward open end of the Fallopian tube

Location of the reproductive organs

against the wall, delaying menstruation, but then be dispelled by the body. One in ten pregnancies is estimated to end in some form of miscarriage. See the section on Miscarriage, in this chapter, for more information.

If the embryo successfully attaches, it will usually continue to develop normally through to completion of pregnancy. The presence of the embryo triggers hormonal signals that shut off the menstrual cycle. This prevents further development of eggs in the ovaries, keeps the uterine lining intact, and seals the cervix to prevent infection and allow amniotic fluid to fill the uterus.

If the egg is unfertilized during its passage through the fallopian tube, it will either pass into the uterus and then wash out with the menstrual blood or will deteriorate before leaving the body.

Approximately a week past ovulation the ovary will trigger an increase in progesterone production. This, in turn, will cause the deterioration of the uterine wall's blood lining. The deterioration takes about four days before menstruation begins.

Menstruation is the passing of the blood from the uterine wall. The blood is shed, on average, two weeks after the day of ovulation. Menstruation lasts from three to seven days. The flow of blood will vary during the course of menstruation, with the heaviest flow occurring early on after onset.

Extremely heavy periods, called *menorrhagia,* may occasionally occur during one's lifetime. If it is a persistent problem, consult with your gynecologist. *Dysmenorrhea* is the technical term for periods with cramps. As anyone who has had cramps can testify, they can be quite painful. There are several medications that can be taken to ease or relieve the pain of cramping with menstruation. Most require a physician's prescription.

Some over-the-counter medications, such as ibuprofen, can also help. Cramps are the accompanying contractions of the uterus that force the lining to be shed. Many women stop having dysmenorrhea after the birth of their first child. Other women who previously had no problem suffer from cramps after childbirth. Birth control pills can also eliminate or reduce menstrual pain.

Birth Control

Spacing of pregnancies can be controlled by birth control. Several options are available to couples who wish to prevent pregnancy either permanently or temporarily. Temporary measures mean that, once the method of control is stopped, the woman can become pregnant. Permanent birth control is almost always surgically achieved and it involves cutting or removing part or all of the reproductive system. Once a permanent surgical procedure has been done, it is extremely difficult or impossible to reverse. For that reason, it is rarely performed on patients who have never had children.

In the discussion of different types of birth control, a failure rate is given. The failure rate is determined by the number of people who conscientiously use the birth control and still get pregnant. The rate is per year, not per use. So if one person in one hundred has a failure, that means that one woman in hundred gets pregnant during one year of use.

Oral Contraceptives

The birth control pill comes in various types. The main ingredient in all of them is synthetic estrogen. Synthetic estrogen has two common types: mestranol and estradiol. The quantity of estrogen in a pill can vary from .03

milligram to .1 milligram for the average dosage. The pill will also contain synthetic progestogen, of which there are several types. Commonly used progestogens are norgestrel, norethindrone, and ethynodiol diacetate. Levels of progestogen can vary from .15 milligram to 2 milligrams.

The two hormones work in combination to prevent ovulation. Pills with the hormones are taken every day for 21 days. Some pill packages come with seven extra pills containing inactive ingredients. The cycle is 28 days, so the schedule will either be 21 days on pills, 7 days off, or 21 days on hormone pills, and 7 days on placebos (pills with no effect). The reason doctors prescribe the 21/7 set of pills is that the patient is less likely to forget a pill if one is taken every day without exception.

After the 21st pill with hormones is taken, the level of estrogen drops as the placebo (or no pill) is used. After 24 to 48 hours, the menstrual cycle will begin. It will usually be lighter in flow and take fewer days than previous periods. The pill may also eliminate cramping.

The effectiveness rating of the pill is less than one pregnancy for 100 women (a year) for pill doses of .35 milligrams or higher of estrogen. For pill doses of less than .35 milligrams of estrogen, there is a very slightly higher pregnancy rate.

Some women experience side effects with oral contraceptive pills. Side effects may be minor, from headaches to weight gain, or they may be major, from blood clots to strokes. The increase in risk is directly affected by the patient's age and smoking habits. Women over the age of 35 or smokers increase the risk of heart attack, stroke, and blood clots considerably by taking the pill. The pill does not have any linkage to uterine cancer, cervical cancer, or breast cancer. If a woman already has breast cancer, taking the pill is not recommended because it may stimulate tumor growth, but it is not linked to beginning cancerous development.

Oral contraceptives can only be obtained through prescription by a licensed physician. The physician will determine the dosage the woman takes, and will usually start on the lightest effective dosage. Dosage is insufficient if the woman experiences bleeding during the 21 day cycle, heavy menstrual flow, or other unusual symptoms. Consult with your prescribing physician if you experience problems. Occasionally switching from one type of synthetic estrogen to another, without increasing dosage, can remedy a problem.

Once on the pill, women who decide to get pregnant should stop taking the pill. Restarting ovulation may take a few months so it may be a while before the woman becomes pregnant. *It is not dangerous* for a woman to become pregnant immediately after stopping oral contraceptives. It is not a major health concern if pill taking overlaps pregnancy slightly. It may cause some problems if pill-taking continues past the first trimester.

There is no medical reason for stopping the use of oral contraceptives if there are no side effects. It was once believed that a woman should cease pill taking for a period of months, either every year or every ten years. Neither has proved to be of medical benefit.

The Mini-Pill

The mini-pill is the nickname of the progestin-only oral contraceptive. For women who run higher health risks by taking estrogen, the progestin pill may be an alternative. The risk of pregnancy is at least 1 percent higher than for the combination pill, and missing a day increases the likelihood of unwanted pregnancy (a higher risk than missing a combination pill). The risk of ectopic pregnancy (the fetus develops outside the uterus, usually in the fallopian tube) is also greater. Ectopic pregnancy can be an extremely painful, serious complication with the risk of sterility to at least one fallopian tube. Any woman on the mini-pill who suffers from lower stomach pain should be tested immediately for a possible ectopic pregnancy.

IUDs

Intrauterine devices (IUDs) are small metal pieces inserted semi-permanently into the woman's uterus. Barring complications they remain in place for one to two years. One type sold in the United States is a form called the Copper T. It is made of copper and is t-shaped, measuring less than 1 inch in length. The other is a double s-shape. Two small threads descend from the tail of the device, through the cervix into the vagina. These threads are used to check position of the IUD and to withdraw the IUD after the prescribed period of time.

IUDs are recommended only for women who have already had one successful delivery, are active in a mutually monogamous relationship, and who do not plan on getting pregnant for a few years. The device is inserted at the doctor's office after verification that the woman is not pregnant, has no current pelvic infection or disease, and has never had an ectopic pregnancy.

Because of the problematic history of the IUD, most of the devices were taken off the market. The Dalkon Shield was associated with a number of serious problems and triggered numerous lawsuits against the company. Since then, research and testing of IUDs has improved. However, there are still serious potential complications from using an IUD, so a woman who gets one is required by the IUD manufacturer to sign a Patient Consent, after the side effects have been explained by her doctor. The side effects are too numerous to list here, but the major ones are septic or spontaneous abortion, perforation of the uterus or cervix, ectopic pregnancy, or fetal damage during pregnancy. Common minor complaints are cramping, heavy menstrual flow, anemia, or amenorrhea (no period).

Pregnancy rates for IUDs vary from less than 1 pregnancy for 100 women using the device, to 8 pregnancies per 100. Individual devices have varying rates and their effectiveness is also determined by the size of the woman's uterus. The larger the uterine cavity, the less likely she will conceive while using the IUD. Some women accidently expel the IUD; this occurs less frequently with the large size IUDs inserted into larger width uteruses.

Condoms

Condoms are rubber or natural material sheaths that fit over the glans and shaft of the penis. Natural material condoms are usually made from sheep intestinal tissue and will protect against unwanted pregnancy but may allow the AIDS virus to pass through. For this reason, rubber condoms are preferred for both protection against pregnancy and disease.

Several types of condoms are available to the general public. They are purchased without a prescription at a drug store, pharmacy, or other general merchandise shop. They come with or without lubrication on the rubber, and with or without a reservoir tip. The reservoir tip is intended to hold the semen after ejaculation.

Similar to the male-worn condom is the female-worn condom—a rubber sheath inserted into the vagina. The physical appearance of the female-condom is a tube, with a sealed ring at the top. The plastic ring, similar to a diaphragm ring, fits against the cervix at the top of the vagina. Attached to the diaphragm-like ring is the long, round sheath of rubber. The sheath covers the entire vaginal wall and the end of the sheath (another, larger ring) remains outside the body around the vaginal opening.

Condoms, even without the use of a spermicide, have a low failure rate. When used correctly, the rate is 2 pregnancies for every 100 users. In actuality, the pregnancy rate is closer to 10 percent, since the condom is frequently used incorrectly. One of the more common errors is placing the tip of the condom too close to the glans of the penis, leaving no room for the semen after ejaculation. Other reasons are tearing or mispositioning of the condom during intercourse, although this is extremely rare. Another, more common problem is the use of petroleum jelly for lubrication. Petroleum products deteriorate rubber material. Only water-based lubricants should be used. Also, the penis should be withdrawn while still erect, to insure that the condom remains in place throughout intercourse. Correct storage of the condom, away from heating sources, helps keep the condom in good condition.

Condoms, when used with spermicides, have an even lower failure rate, at less than 1 percent. Spermicide foams and creams kill any sperm that may pass beyond the condom barrier. Spermicides also help protect against venereal disease. Condoms, and condoms with spermicides, offer the best protection against contracting a venereal disease during intercourse.

Spermicides

Spermicides come in creams, foams, and jellies. They may be inserted into the vagina with a plastic applicator, or by suppository or tablet. The spermicide should surround the cervix. The specific requirements vary from type to type, but usually the spermicide must be applied within 30 minutes before intercourse. It must be reapplied for each episode of intercourse. The spermicide should remain in place for at least eight hours after intercourse.

Spermicides are most commonly used with diaphragms, condoms, or other barrier methods of birth control. On their own, spermicides have an estimated failure rate of 15 percent. The two most common ingredients in spermicides are nonoxynol and oxtoxynol. The percentage of the spermicide in the cream, jelly, or foam will vary from 1 percent to more than 12 percent. Some people may have allergic responses to the higher percentage spermicides, but the higher concentrations are more effective in preventing pregnancy.

Diaphragms and Other Barriers

Barrier methods of birth control work by placing a physical barrier, usually of rubber, over the cervical opening to the uterus. The barrier remains in place for at least several hours after intercourse to prevent sperm from entering into the uterus. Barriers are used in conjunction with spermicidal creams, foams, or jellies to enhance protection against sperm passage.

The single-most common form of barrier is the diaphragm. The diaphragm is prescribed by a physician after sizing a women for the dimensions of the diaphragm. If a woman loses or gains more than ten pounds, or becomes pregnant, she should be checked to see if the diaphragm size has to be changed.

The rim of the diaphragm is coated with a spermicidal agent and then is put in place before intercourse. Another application of spermicide is required for each episode of intercourse. The diaphragm should be removed 24 hours after the last episode of intercourse and should be washed thoroughly before reuse.

The failure rate for diaphragms when used with spermicides is 3 percent, when used correctly. The difficulty in using a diaphragm is that positioning of the diaphragm and correct size of the diaphragm are all essential to the success rate. The percentage of failure of different brands of diaphragms, combined with experience of the woman in using it and whether she has had children, can increase the failure rate to as high as 20 percent.

Cervical caps are smaller types of rubber barriers. They are currently unavailable in the United States, except for those women participating in the initial pre-FDA studies on their effectiveness. One of the reasons they are not currently marketed in the U.S. is because the failure rate can be extremely high on them, as high as 44 percent.

A contraceptive sponge is also available as a barrier method. The contraceptive sponge works something like a diaphragm, but is thrown out after use. The sponge is moistened before placement against the cervix, and it releases spermicides for 24 hours after intercourse. It must be removed after 24 hours. The failure rate is almost 18 per 100 users for women who have never had children. It becomes much higher with women who have had children, at 28 percent failure.

Natural Birth Control Methods

Natural birth control is called that when it requires no outside preven tion method for pregnancy. Natural methods include rhythm method, withdrawal, and abstinence.

Rhythm method involves determining the woman's ovulation cycle and avoiding intercourse during the days before and after ovulation. Ovulation occurs *on average* fourteen days before the next period. This is only reliable for a woman who has an exact 28 day cycle with the normal ovulation timing. Many women ovulate earlier or later in the menstrual cycle, and many cycles are longer or shorter than 28 days. To determine ovulation, vaginal body temperature can be charted and physical characteristics of vaginal secretions can be monitored for changes over a period of several months to determine regularity and time of ovulation. If a couple chooses to use rhythm method for birth control, it is recommended that you consult with a doctor for specific details of monitoring temperature and secretions patterns. It is a relatively complex procedure and requires a great deal of commitment by both partners to make this effective. Rhythm method has as high as a 20 percent failure rate when used correctly. It is much higher when used by couples inexperienced in monitoring ovulation.

Withdrawal method refers to the withdrawal of the penis prior to ejaculation, during intercourse. The risk in this method is that preejaculative liquids can contain enough sperm to impregnate a woman. Also, semen on the exterior of the vagina, or the labia, can also travel back into the uterine cavity and fertilize an egg. Timing on withdrawal is essential and should be done prior to any ejaculation. Because of this, withdrawal is often considered an inadequate form of birth control. It can be emotionally and physically dissatisfying. It also has an exceedingly high failure rate, estimated between 20 and 40 percent.

This is only slightly better than no birth control at all.

Abstinence is the decision to not engage in intercourse. It is the only method of birth control that is 100 percent effective. For individuals who are not involved in mutually monogamous relationships, it is the most effective method of preventing AIDS and other sexually transmitted diseases.

Permanent Birth Control

Permanent birth control is obtained surgically. It is usually nonreversible. Surgical sterilization is available to both women and men.

Tubal Ligation

Tubal ligation is the surgical blocking of the fallopian tubes. The fallopian tubes transport the egg from the ovary to the uterus. By blocking the path that the egg travels, the egg is no longer capable of making contact with the sperm. Tubal ligation is done by cutting, tying, banding, cauterizing, or removing a section of each tube so the path is no longer continuous. Depending on the surgical method used to block the tube, the ability to reverse the procedure (should you decide later to have children) may be nearly impossible. Also depending on the method used to tie off the tubes, the number of women who become pregnant after a tubal ligation is, at the highest, 2 in 1000.

Tubal ligation can be done immediately following childbirth, if the doctor is briefed on the decision well in advance of the delivery. It can also be done by scheduled surgery at any time. Fifteen percent of all women over the age of 45 have elected to have a tubal ligation.

Hysterectomy

Hysterectomy is the removal of the uterus and, perhaps, the cervix. This procedure is completely irreversible. Chances of pregnancy following the procedure are none.

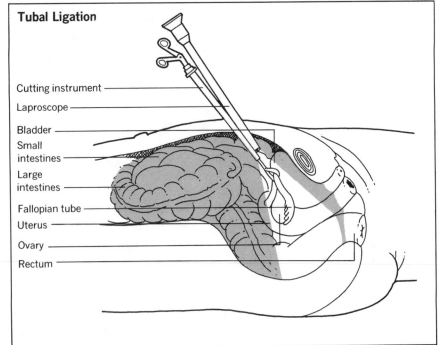

Tubal Ligation

Cutting instrument
Laproscope
Bladder
Small intestines
Large intestines
Fallopian tube
Uterus
Ovary
Rectum

A *subtotal hysterectomy* is the removal of the uterus, leaving the cervix, fallopian tubes, and ovaries in place. A *total hysterectomy* is the removal of the cervix as well as the uterus. *Oophorectomy* and *ovariectomy* are both used to describe the surgical removal of one or both of the ovaries. *Ovariohysterectomy* is the removal of the ovaries, fallopian tubes, and uterus. The quantity of tissue removed will be determined by the patient and the doctor, based on the reasons for the operation. For removal of cancerous tissue, all the organs may need to be removed. For sterilization, only a subtotal hysterectomy may be necessary.

Hysterectomies have become increasingly used to correct problems that may be remedied by medication, or which may be temporary in nature and not warrant surgery. To recommend a hysterectomy solely for birth control is unusual. It should only be done in cases where tubal ligation is not sufficient in correcting problems, or where some underlying physical problems require surgery. Although hysterectomies are common, they are still considered major surgery and should be approached as such, by both the doctor and the patient. Recoveries can take six weeks or longer.

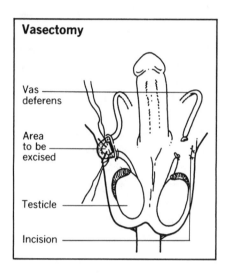

Vasectomy

Vas deferens

Area to be excised

Testicle

Incision

Vasectomy

Vasectomy is sterilization of the male by cutting the vas deferens, the tubes that transport the sperm. The surgery is normally performed in the doctor's office with local anesthesia. Incisions are made either on each side of the scrotum or on the center midline of the scrotum. The tubes are then cut, and tied or cauterized on each end. Pain following the procedure is usually responsive to non-aspirin painkillers. Heavy lifting or strenuous exercise should be avoided for a week.

Vasovasotomy is the surgical procedure that attempts to reconnect the vas deferens after a vasectomy. This operation is done for men wishing to reverse the surgical sterilization. Success at this procedure can vary from 30 to 75 percent, depending on the type of initial sterilization procedures, and on the skill of the surgeon in reconnection of the tubes.

Infertility

Infertility can stem from numerous problems. It is estimated that as high as one in ten couples cannot conceive a child. There are an estimated 1.8 million women in the United States who are classified as infertile, which is about 5 percent of the female adult population of reproductive years.

Infertility can stem from the male reproductive system about 40 percent of the time, the female system about 40 percent of the time. But it also is a combination of problems shared by both partners a majority of the time.

A couple is considered for fertility testing after a prolonged period of time in which they have actively been trying to conceive and have been unable. A prolonged period of time should be considered at least several months, and probably one year. After that, you should consult with your doctor about the need to test for fertility problems.

Blockage of the Fallopian Tubes

Thirty percent of the women who are infertile suffer from blockage of both of the fallopian tubes. Blockage can stem from scar tissue that develops from surgery, injury, diseases such as pelvic inflammatory disease (PID), or birth defects. Abnormal tissue growth from ailments such as endometriosis can block the passageway with excess tissue growth. Some of these blockages can be treated surgically; others are irreparable and the women will not be able to conceive naturally.

Hysterosalpingography

This is a long name for the X-ray technique that is used to check for defects and blockage in the fallopian tubes and uterus. (Hystero refers to the uterus, salpingo for the fallopian tube, and graphy for the X-ray technique.) A radiopaque dye is injected into the uterus and fallopian tubes. Then an X ray is made to check for unusual formations and blockages that may be obstructing the path of the egg to the uterus. Two X rays will be taken; one on the day of the dye insertion, and one 24 hours later.

Transcervical Balloon Tuboplasty (TBT)

One of the surgical techniques used to unblock damaged fallopian tubes is called transcervical balloon tuboplasty (TBT). A deflated balloon at the end of a flexible guiding tube is inserted into the fallopian tube and inflated. As angioplasty works on blocked arteries, the tuboplasty works by inflating in the area that is restricted, forcing the tube open. The inflation is done several times to force the scar tissue open and clear the passageway. The surgery is done through outpatient care, which means that it can be performed without a costly overnight stay at a hospital. It is shown to be effective for more than half of the women deemed treatable for fallopian tube blockage.

Treatment of Uterine Disorders

Several problems can arise from uterine dysfunction or disease. Tumors, polyps, and endometrial growth can prevent implantation of fertilized eggs in the uterine lining. There are several surgical procedures, mostly done in the doctor's office, that can correct the problems. *Dilation and curettage (D and C), endometrial biopsy,* and *endometrial curettage* are procedures that allow the physician to remove unusual growths from the cervix and uterine walls.

Hormonal Deficiencies

Hormones regulate the development and release of the ovum from the ovary and prepare the uterine wall for reception of the fertilized egg. Low levels of certain hormones can disrupt any one of the numerous stages of the menstrual cycle. Hormonal problems affect one third of all infertile women.

Anovulatory cycles are menstrual cycles in which no egg is released. *Amenorrhea* is when there is no menstruation, with or without ovulation. *Inadequate endometrium* is when the lining of the uterus is not sufficient for the fertilized egg to lodge on. All of these conditions can be treated with synthetic hormones. Many couples are able to conceive after hormonal treatment. The physician determines the hormone levels through a series of exams. Urine testing, mucous testing, and biopsies will give the different hormone levels for the various hormones required for successful fertilization.

Sperm Count and Formation

The single largest contributing factor to male infertility is sperm count or formation. Testing of sperm involves three studies: count, motility, and morphology.

Sperm Count

The number of sperm present in a single ejaculation should be at least 20 million in one milliliter. For a full determination of sperm count before a male is diagnosed as infertile, testing should be performed more than once. *Oligospermia* is the reduced count of sperm; *azoospermia* is the complete absence of sperm.

Several factors influence sperm production. Alcohol consumption, drug use, and restrictive clothing all reduce sperm count. Blocked ducts in the epididymis or in the vas deferens can also reduce the number of sperm present during ejaculation. Low hormone levels may reduce sperm count. Methods for reversing or correcting low sperm count problem can range from the simple—elimination of affecting factors such as alcohol—to the difficult—surgical reparation of the vas deferens to remove blockage.

Sperm Motility

Motility is the ability of the sperm to travel through the fluid present. A normal score for sperm motility is that two hours after ejaculation, 50 percent of the sperm are still actively swimming. If the sperm die unusually quickly, it is less likely that one will make the passage through the female cervix and uterus and meet up with the egg in the fallopian tube.

Sperm Morphology

The structure of the sperm (morphology) is a small oval body with a whiplike tail that is used to propel the sperm through the uterus. The tip of the sperm body has a cap with enzymes that deteriorate the protective coating on the ovum when the two press together. Sperm that is misshapen, or missing a tail or the enzyme cap, will not be able to successfully penetrate an ovum. In a morphology test, at least 60 percent of the sperm should be normally structured.

Motility and morphology problems present barriers to natural fertilization. With new techniques, *in-vitro fertilization* can take place, barring other complications with the sperm. Some men are able to successfully impregnate their spouses without surgical intervention, despite deficient sperm; others may require extensive intervention.

Immunological Problems

In some partners, the female will develop an immunological response to the male's semen. This means that her immune system attacks the sperm, responding the same way it would to an invasion by a virus. The immune system destroys the sperm before it can reach the ovum. Why this occurs is unknown, but the response fades if exposure to the sperm is eliminated. The treatment for immunological attacks is eliminating intercourse or using condoms for several months until the female's immune system shuts off the mechanism that responds to the sperm.

Alternative Forms of Conception

There have been a number of breakthroughs in conception for couples who experience difficulty in beginning a pregnancy. There are methods for overcoming problems in sperm production, egg production, fertilization, and immune compatibility. For couples wishing to have a biological child related to both parents, one parent, or neither parent but carried by the female, these are the current methods of fertilization.

IVF

In-vitro fertilization (IVF) is the method of conception where the egg is fertilized by the sperm in a glass dish. Several eggs are removed, surgically and non-surgically, from the female. The sperm are concentrated and added to the dish to fertilize the eggs. One or two days later, a couple fertilized eggs are reinserted into the female to impregnate her. More that one are usually implanted because not all will be viable. The remaining fertilized eggs can be frozen for future implantation into the biological parent. The eggs can be donated to parents who do not have the reproductive capability to produce eggs and semen or who have genetic disorders that they do not want to pass on. The success rate for impregnation is not high; about 11 to 15 percent.

GIFT

Gamete intrafallopian transfer (GIFT) is similar to IVF in the first stage. Eggs are removed from the female and placed in a dish with sperm. The difference between IVF and GIFT is that the eggs and sperm are then immediately reinserted into the female's fallopian tube before or while the eggs are being fertilized. This allows the process to resemble more closely the natural process of conception. Fertilization of the egg should take place in the fallopian tube where the eggs and sperm are deposited and then the gamete (fertilized egg) can travel the path to the uterus as it would naturally. The success rate of GIFT is around 17 percent. This rate is expected to improve as GIFT is practiced more frequently.

ZIFT

Zygote intrafallopian transfer follows the same procedure as GIFT except that the eggs and sperm are kept together for eighteen hours before reinsertion. Fertilized eggs are then reinserted into the fallopian tubes where they should make the journey to the uterine lining as they would in natural conception.

Artificial Insemination

Artificial insemination is the oldest of the methods used to circumvent infertility problems. The method involves nonsurgical insertion of sperm into the vagina or uterus. This can be done to provide more concentrated sperm count from the father, or provide sperm from a donor if the father is infertile. This is mainly successful on women who are not experiencing infertility problems themselves.

Surrogacy

For women who are unable to carry a fetus to term in a pregnancy, one of the alternatives is to have another women carry the fetus. Depending on the physical problems of the parents, the surrogate mother may carry a donor egg or the egg of the infertile mother. The egg may be fertilized by a donor or by the father. In some cases the surrogate provides the egg and undergoes one of the procedures above with the father's sperm. Surrogates have been relatives, friends, or hired women whom the couple does not know. The legal involvement is complicated for surrogacy and requires serious consideration before undertaking this arrangement.

Pregnancy

Once you have conceived, the baby has nine months of growth and change to prepare itself for the outside world. There are numerous physiological changes to the mother as the baby grows inside her, and many emotional changes and discoveries for both parents.

As soon as a women realizes she may be pregnant, she should schedule an appointment with a gynecologist/obstetrician. The doctor will perform a blood test that can confirm the mother's pregnancy status. Once a women finds that she is pregnant and decides to proceed with the pregnancy, her doctor will schedule her for monthly exams, through the 28th week of pregnancy. Then she may see her doctor every other week from the 30th week to the 36th. After the 36th week of pregnancy, she should be seen every week until delivery. Delivery should occur before the 42nd week.

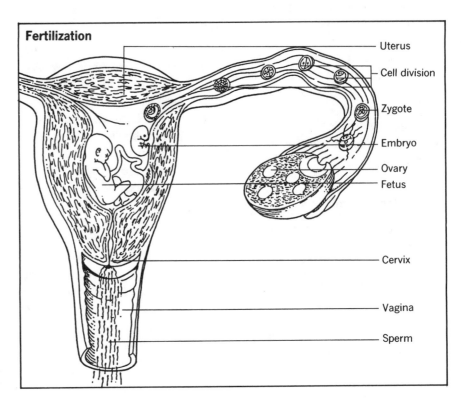

Fertilization — Uterus, Cell division, Zygote, Embryo, Ovary, Fetus, Cervix, Vagina, Sperm

First Trimester

The first three months of pregnancy take the embryo from a single free-floating cell to a formed two-inch recognizable fetus. The mother's breasts enlarge to prepare for the production of milk. The uterus increases in size to make room for the growing fetus and the surrounding liquid, called *the amnion*. The placenta forms to process the mother's blood and carry nutrients and water to the fetus. The umbilical cord is the connection between the mother and her child. Through this cord the nutrients travel to the baby and waste material travels back to be processed out by the mother's system.

Because of the direct link between the mother's blood and the baby's blood, the mother must be diligent about the foods and drugs she ingests. Many chemicals can pass through the placenta; some will do irreparable harm to the forming baby. Alcohol, caffeine, chemicals from cigarette smoke, and some medications will pass through the placenta and have been shown to harm the developing fetus. In large quantities, they can cause brain damage, deformity, or death. Any medication should be approved by the pregnant woman's obstetrician before use.

The first examination should be to confirm your pregnancy and run an initial screening for health problems and general health history. A complete physical will either be done then or at a following appointment.

At your first visit with your obstetrician, after you know you are pregnant, your doctor should give you information on what to expect.

Morning Sickness

During the second and third months of pregnancy, usually, morning sickness may plague the expectant mother. With the raised hormone levels, and the increased pressure on the internal organs from the growing uterus, the stomach can become easily upset. Morning sickness usually occurs during the first hours after awakening, and can start immediately upon rising.

Although the mechanism of morning sickness is not understood, it is believed that the combination of having gone all night without food and the pressure on the stomach from lying down create the nausea. Munching on crackers and dry toast before arising and continuing to snack through the day will help. Some women experience morning sickness throughout the day; others never experience it. Morning sickness can range from slight nausea to regular vomiting and increased inability to hold down food.

Frequent Urination

As the uterus grows it puts pressure on the surrounding organs. This pressure will shift during the pregnancy from the bladder to the intestines, then to the lungs, as the size of the uterus expands. During the first trimester the main pressure occurs on the bladder, creating the need for the pregnant woman to urinate more frequently. It may cause her to awaken at night to use the bathroom.

Fatigue

Many women experience fatigue during the first trimester of pregnancy. Some women will also continue to experience fatigue throughout the pregnancy. Others experience a respite from being tired during the second trimester. Some of the fatigue may come from restless sleep or interrupted sleep caused by changes in the mother's body. It also stems from the shift of energy to the developing fetus, taxing the mother's body. This new draw of energy requires an increased intake of food by the mother to compensate for the increased need. Despite the fact that the mother may not look pregnant, her nutritional needs increase immediately upon becoming pregnant.

Second Trimester

It is usually sometime during the fourth month that a woman starts "showing." This means that the stomach becomes slightly, but visibly, distended with the growth of the fetus. This may not be noticeable when the woman is fully clothed.

By the end of the second trimester, the pregnant woman will probably have felt the baby move. The baby will begin by rolling and moving about in the amnion surrounding it. It eventually fills the space to keep from moving extensively, but arm and leg jabs will become more apparent and more vigorous as the baby grows. The baby will double in size during the second trimester, getting to an average length of 13 inches by the end of the sixth month. All of the organs and all of the features are in place and developing.

Constipation

The pressure of the growing uterus will shift slowly from the bladder to the intestines. This will relieve the need to urinate as frequently as before, but there will be increased difficulty with bowel movements because of the added pressure. This will result in constipation for some pregnant women.

Varicose Veins

With increased body weight concentrated in the pelvic area, some women experience problems with varicose veins. Leg veins are under increased pressure and may bulge into visible bubbles on the surface of the skin. This may be caused by weakened venal (vein) walls, expanded blood volume, and decreased tension in the muscles. By using aids such as support panty hose and avoiding prolonged standing, the pregnant woman can alleviate some of the problems. Her physician can guide her to other methods of avoiding or exacerbating the problem.

Breathlessness

Breathlessness can start in the second trimester, triggered by hormonal changes that affect the capillaries in the lungs. It will continue into the last trimester because the uterus will push up on the diaphragm, the muscle that controls lung expansion.

Third Trimester

The baby continues to grow, adding fat cells and filling out. The eyes, ears, and mouth are all functioning. The lungs are beginning to expand and contract, taking in amniotic fluid in preparation for breathing air. During the eighth or early ninth month, the baby will rotate into a head down position to prepare for descent through the birth canal. By the ninth month the baby is too big in the womb to make large movements. The sensations the mother feels are the baby jabbing and poking with arms and legs.

Depending on the status of lung development and on the emergency care available, a baby born during the third trimester can survive. The lungs are ill-equipped to deal with the intake of oxygen, but new treatments are available to help the child survive.

Contractions

Some women experience mild uterine contractions throughout the second and third trimester of pregnancy; others only experience contractions toward the end of the third trimester. These contractions can be thirty seconds to several minutes in duration. They usually start at the top of the uterus and the woman experiences a tightening sensation that moves down the uterus to the pelvic floor. The contractions should not be extremely painful, and if they become uncomfortable, changing position or lying down may relieve them. The contractions, known as *Braxton Hicks contractions*, are preparing the uterine muscles for delivery. The contractions may be difficult to distinguish from true labor toward the end of the pregnancy. False alarms, where the expectant mother thinks labor has begun, are caused by this. Lying down should alleviate Braxton Hicks contractions, but not true labor.

Fatigue

As in the first trimester, fatigue can become a daily obstacle. The pregnant woman's body is carrying a large weight and large drain on her energy system. As the baby gets closer to delivery, the amount of energy required increases, increasing the likelihood that the mother will tire easier.

Awkwardness

Falling, tripping, dropping things, and general inability to get into and out of chairs and cars is a normal part of pregnancy. The shift in a woman's center of gravity can occur rapidly during the last trimester, giving her little time to adjust. Moving and stepping over things becomes more difficult as the woman's line of vision with her feet and the ground becomes blocked. Her added weight can make some movements more difficult. And the swelling that comes from general edema can make handling small objects more cumbersome. All of these problems disappear after delivery.

Edema

General swelling of the extremities, the hands and feet particularly, is a normal aspect of pregnancy. About 75 percent of pregnant women experience some swelling from retention of fluids. It is usually helpful to *increase* water intake to alleviate some of the swelling. Increased fluids help the body flush out excess liquids. Talk to your doctor if swelling becomes a problem. *Pre-eclampsia* and *toxemia* occur in a small percentage of women, where swelling is extreme and life threatening if not treated. Your doctor will monitor for pre-eclampsia by checking your blood pressure, weight gain, and degree of swelling.

Breathing Difficulties

As the size of the baby grows, the baby and the uterus will push on the diaphragm muscle that controls breathing. This added pressure keeps the woman from deep breathing and can be painful. Also the baby may temporarily lodge a foot against her ribs or diaphragm, causing sharp pains. During the last two weeks or so, the baby will drop into the pelvic girdle and the pressure will be relieved on the diaphragm. This is called *lightening*. (Note: Shortness of breath, rapid and shallow breathing and/or rapid pulse should be reported immediately to a doctor.)

Prenatal Diagnosis and Tests

During your pregnancy, you will undergo a few or many of the following examinations. Depending on your health and potential health risks, these tests may be performed more than once; some may be done each month. Other tests may be added. Each provides you and the physician with information about your health and the health of the developing baby. Prenatal care increases the chances of having a healthy baby tremendously. Less than 2 percent of the women who see their obstetrician regularly after the second month of pregnancy have an underweight baby.

Home Pregnancy Tests

Home pregnancy tests can now be purchased in almost any pharmacy or drugstore. The prices range from $5.00 to more than $20.00. All the tests work on the same principle—they test for the presence of the hormone Human Chorionic Gonadotropin (HCG), which is present at high levels during pregnancy. A chemical in the home testing kit will change colors when HCG is present. The tests are 99 percent accurate in labs, but probably around 95 percent accurate in home use, where circumstances are not as controlled. A false-negative test will register if the HCG levels are not high enough yet. A false-positive reading may occur if you have unusually high HCG readings or another chemical which mimics HCG in the test. If you have not had your period and you suspect that you may be pregnant, it is advisable to have a doctor's test regardless of the results of the home kit. You should seek medical advice as soon as possible.

Blood tests

Blood is tested during your first examination to determine if you are pregnant. Either during the same examination or at a follow-up examination, blood is tested for the following: anemia; infectious diseases, including sexually transmitted diseases and AIDS; immunities to childhood diseases, especially German measles; and diabetes. Sometime before delivery blood will be checked again for diabetes, sexually transmitted diseases, and hepatitis.

Rh Compatibility Test

Rh is the part of the blood type that labels the blood positive or negative. The only time this poses a problem is when the mother is Rh negative and the father is Rh positive and the offspring develops Rh positive blood. This used to pose serious threat to the pregnancy, but can now be treated adequately with drugs.

Urine tests

The physician will check your urine, probably at each visit, for sugar (diabetes), protein (toxemia), bacteria (infection), and perhaps drug use.

Pelvic Exams

Pelvic exams are done throughout pregnancy to check the position of the fetus and the status of the vaginal walls and the cervix. As you approach delivery, the cervix muscle will *efface* and *dilate*, meaning that the walls will thin and the cervical opening will increase. During your early visits to the doctor, a pap smear will be performed to check for infections and unusual growths on the cervix. Other smear tests will be done for diseases such as chlamydia. These tests may be repeated late in pregnancy.

Ultrasound

By using sound waves to reflect off the fetus in the uterus, the doctor is able to determine the size, position, and occasionally the sex of the forming baby. Ultrasound can be performed anytime after about the fifth week of pregnancy. Your physician will let you know what scheduling is used in his or her office. Some obstetricians perform ultrasound to get an accurate date on the pregnancy by the size of the fetus; others may wait to do one reading later to determine general position and health.

Ultrasonography is performed *transabdominally* (across the stomach) or *transvaginally* (through the vagina). If the ultrasound is done transabdominally, then the woman must drink plenty of fluids beforehand to fill the bladder. This allows the bladder to push the uterus up for better positioning as well as provide an obvious sighting for the bladder so it is not misidentified.

Amniocentesis

To determine the genetic makeup of the developing baby, a small portion of the amniotic fluid can be drawn out of the womb to pick up floating cells, which contain the baby's genetic information. This allows the doctor and the pregnant woman the opportunity to screen for different inheritable diseases. Amniocentesis is usually performed on higher risk patients during the fourth or fifth month of pregnancy. Armed with the information provided, the parents can choose to carry the baby to term, abort the fetus, or have intrauterine surgery performed to remedy problems with the fetus.

The fluid is drawn out by a syringe that is inserted into the woman's naval to the level of the uterus. Using ultrasound to avoid the placenta and the fetus, the needle draws up fluid.

This procedure runs about a one in one hundred risk of causing amniotic leaking, and a one in two hundred risk of infection. The risk of triggering spontaneous abortion is even lower.

Chorionic Villus Sampling (CVS)

A newer procedure than the amniocentesis, the CVS samples the tissue that forms between the interior uterine wall and the beginning placenta. The needle-like tube is inserted either through the vagina or the stomach and guided by ultrasound to the chorionic villus. This testing procedure is usually performed during the third month of pregnancy.

The benefits of the test are that it can be performed earlier in the pregnancy, and a determination to discontinue the pregnancy poses less risk to the woman when decided during the

Abnormal Presentations during Delivery

Breech

Buttocks presentation

Retroflexed uterus

Abnormal Shoulder-arm presentation

first trimester. Amniocentesis can only be done after the start of the second trimester. The risk is that, because it is a newer procedure, the spontaneous abortion rate following CVS is higher than the rate for amniocentesis. As doctors become more practiced with the procedure it is believed the rate will even out.

Fetal Monitoring

External and internal monitoring of the fetus are done to check on the heart rate and stress of the fetus. External monitoring involves registering the heartbeat via ultrasound readings and, if needed, a pressure gauge to measure contractions.

Internal monitoring is done only during delivery and if some level of distress is suspected or likely in the fetus. The monitoring electrode is placed on the baby's scalp through the opening in the cervix. This can only be done after dilation has started. A catheter that measures pressure can also be inserted into the uterus to measure contraction pressure. Both of these units can be connected to the monitor reader by cord or by radio wave.

Monitoring is now a regular procedure during delivery. It allows the doctors to check on the health of the baby and provides an early warning if the baby is in distress. It should be set up so that it does not interfere at all with the birthing process.

Apgar Test Score

When the baby is born, you will probably be given an Apgar score that refers to the general health of the baby. The scores range from 0 to 10 and are based on five criteria: skin color and

Birth Sequence

Dilated cervix
During the first stage of labor the cervix dilates to form a passageway into the vagina, the birth canal. Contractions of the uterus may occur at intervals of approximately 5 to 15 minutes, with brief periods of rest in between, which permit oxygen to flow to the fetus.

Ruptured amniotic sac
Ruptured amniotic sac ordinarily signals the onset of the second and generally shorter stage of labor. Contractions during this stage occur in more frequent succession and are more intense. The so-called *bag of waters*, which contains the amniotic fluid, is ordinarily discharged during a strong contraction but may even rupture before labor begins.

Delivery
As the fetus moves into the lower pelvic region the mother naturally experiences a conscious impulse to bear down and help its entry into the world. She may feel a few moments of increased pressure or pain as the infant's head gradually appears and is followed by the rest of its body.

Placental stage
Placental stage is the third stage of labor and is characterized by the expulsion from the womb of the placenta, or *afterbirth*, to which the baby is connected by the umbilical cord. This cord is not cut until all the placental blood has pulsed into the baby's body.

appearance, heart rate, respiratory effort, muscle tone, and reflex responses. Stillborns rate a zero with no pulse, blue skin, and no response system; extremely healthy babies can score a 10 with good coloration, good crying, and strong pulse and muscular activity.

Birthing

There are three basic stages to birthing: labor, delivery, and placental delivery. The average length of birthing is 14 hours for the first birth and 8 hours for births after that. This is only an average though. Some women will experience mild true contractions for 24 hours before significant dilation begins. Some women have labors that last an hour or less. Although it may seem ideal for women who have experienced extremely long labors to have a 20 minute birthing process, there are risks with short labors. The most likely thing with short labors is that you won't get to the hospital on time. Since no one knows when labor will begin or how long it will last, it is extremely important for every woman who is pregnant to have a good understanding of what happens during birthing and what to do as soon as labor begins.

Labor

Labor is marked with the beginning of regular contractions of the uterus. In some women this will be similar to the Braxton Hicks contractions they have been experiencing during the days preceding labor. For others the true labor contractions will be much harder and much more severe in pressure and duration.

Latent Phase

During the initiation of labor the contractions will be some distance in time apart—up to a half hour. Contractions may be regularly spaced or may come irregularly. Because of the possible differences in pressure and duration, some women do not recognize the early stages of labor.

Contractions should come more rapidly, eventually getting to a pace of every five minutes. The contractions are slowly opening the cervix (dilatation) and thinning the cervical muscle (effacement) to allow for the passage of the baby into the vaginal canal. The muscle will eventually thin and open to 10 centimeters during the last part of labor.

Call your doctor when you know labor has begun. Most doctors recommend that women wait out this period at home. Talk to your doctor about what activities are recommended and what should be avoided during this phase. Since the latent phase of labor can last up to one full day, resting is important.

Active Phase

The contractions come more rapidly, last longer, and are stronger in pressure. The contractions force the cervical muscle to dilatation of 7 centimeters. If the amniotic sac did not break during the latent phase, it will break now. The attending physician may choose to break the sac to help the baby's head to *crown*. Crowning occurs when the baby's head moves into the pelvic bone region and becomes visible through the vaginal canal. The act of crowning will normally break the amniotic sac if it has not already ruptured.

By the active phase you should be attended by your health care person. Contractions will reduce to every two or three minutes and may last one full minute. If the attending physician decides that the vaginal canal is not wide enough to accommodate the size of the baby's head, he or she may decide to perform an *episiotomy*. This procedure involves a small incision in the

tissue between the vagina and the anus or off to the side of the vagina. The majority of first births have this procedure; about half the women who have given birth before have an episiotomy again.

Transitional Phase

This can be the most difficult part of the birthing process because it comes at the end of the hard work of labor. The extremely strong contractions are still two to three minutes apart but are now lasting over a minute. The contractions have peaks in pressure that are much stronger than previous contractions. The cervix dilates to a full 10 centimeters, usually in less than an hour. This is the point where breathing exercises learned in birthing classes will come in handy. You may be too anxious, annoyed, or fatigued to consider them though. The coach is there to help with this. At the end of the transition the baby's head forces through the canal and the largest width of the head passes the cervical opening.

Delivery

At this point you can start to push. The point from the end of transition to the actual delivery of the baby should be less than one hour and in some women can take less than fifteen minutes. The baby will usually descend head first with the head facing the back of the mother's body. Other possible positions include the baby facing front, the baby descending feet or butt first (breech delivery) or an arm or leg descending first. All fetal positions except head first, face back, may require medical intervention.

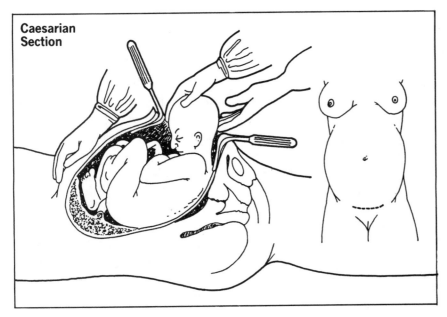

Caesarian Section

Placental Delivery

The last part of the birthing process is the delivery of the placenta. The delivery of the placenta usually follows the birth of the baby by less than one hour. It can occur within five minutes or it may take some time. Nursing the baby during this period helps because the stimulation of the nipples causes uterine contractions that help separate the placenta from the uterine wall, arrest bleeding, and shrink the size of the uterus. The placenta should be delivered in one solid piece.

It is during this time that any tears or surgical cuts will be repaired by the doctor. The episiotomy will be stitched.

Caesarian Sections

In some cases the mother is not able to deliver a baby through the vaginal canal. This can be due to several possible circumstances. If the baby is in one of several breech positions, such as arm or leg descended, the doctor may elect to perform a caesarian instead of attempting to shift the baby for vaginal delivery. If the baby's head is too large to pass through the pelvic girdle bones, or if the pelvic opening is too small to accommodate even a normal size infant, caesarian section will be performed. Also, if the mother does not dilate entirely or if the contractions are not adequate to push the baby into the birth canal, a caesarian will be performed.

In all these circumstances, caesarians are performed to avoid undue stress on the fetus and the mother during the birthing process. The uterus will only be able to provide life support to the infant for a few days after labor has begun. As the physical status of the placenta deteriorates, the loss of oxygen-rich blood will harm the fetus. The pressure from continued contractions will also eventually stress the fetus. Vaginal walls and the cervical muscle will swell from the extended pressure of contractions. It becomes essential to the health of both the mother and the child that labor not continue for too long.

A caesarian section begins with a local anesthesia to the mother that numbs the belly region. An incision is made after anesthesia that opens a small section of the stomach (usually right above the pubic hair). A second incision is made into the uterine wall.

If amniotic fluid remains in the uterus, it will be suctioned away with the same type of tube the dentist uses. The baby is then lifted from the uterus either by hand or by forceps. The umbilical cord is clipped. The placenta may be delivered through the surgical opening. Then both layers of the incision are stitched closed (frequently with metal or plastic clips).

Birthing Places

There are several alternatives for where you can have your baby delivered. Check with your community and your attending physician to see what is available and review what you are comfortable with.

Hospitals

Some hospitals offer a variety of options to the traditional sterile delivery rooms that were common for women over the past forty years. They may have private patient rooms where the mother can decide who attends the birth. All the equipment that will be needed is in the room. The baby may still sleep in the nursery, but will be brought to the mother for feeding.

Birthing Room

Birthing rooms are a step away from private patient rooms. The room is equipped for most emergencies, except caesarians. The father and others can be present throughout the delivery. The atmosphere in the room is designed to be homey and comfortable. For most of the labor the woman will remain on a traditional bed. The bed can then be broken down into a birthing bed for the final stage of labor and delivery. The baby will most probably remain in the room with the mother during her recovery.

Home Delivery

Not usually recommended for first-time pregnancies, the home delivery is just that—delivering the baby in your home. Your attending medical personnel will be there for assistance, but except in emergencies, the full labor and delivery will take place in the home. Screening for this is intensive, because there is little that can be done in emergencies except to take the woman to the hospital in an ambulance.

Birthing Assistants

Along with the choices one can make on where to give birth, one also has choices for who will assist.

Obstetricians

Traditional medical practitioners, obstetricians, are fully trained medical doctors who specialize in pregnancy and birth. They usually assist in deliveries in the hospital, either in delivery rooms or birthing rooms. There may be some in your community, though, who will perform home births.

Nurse Practitioners

Nurse practitioners have several years of medical training although there are procedures that a doctor can perform that a nurse practitioner cannot. The nurse practitioner specializing in birthing will be able to assist in all deliveries, with an attending physician for caesarian sections.

Although arrangements vary from clinic to clinic, there is usually one obstetrician on staff with several nurse practitioners. It is likely that you would only see the doctor once or twice during the course of your pregnancy. The nurse practitioner would be able to handle most of your concerns.

Midwives

Certified midwives may also hold nursing degrees, although this is not a requirement in all states. They will assist in all deliveries, but, like the nurse practitioner, cannot perform caesarian sections. They are trained for all aspects of pregnancy and delivery.

Complications of Pregnancy

Occasionally something goes wrong during pregnancy or childbirth. This may be some problem that can be treated either with medication or surgically. There are some problems, though, that cannot be remedied. In some cases, the mother may lose the fetus.

Miscarriage

When the body rejects the embryo or developing fetus for whatever reason, this is considered a miscarriage or *spontaneous abortion*. There are numerous reasons why a miscarriage may take place. A shift in hormone level, a defect in the embryo, or another factor that interferes with the normal development of the fetus.

Early Miscarriage

Occurring in the first trimester of pregnancy, early miscarriage may be as frequent as one in ten pregnancies. Many miscarriages go undetected because the woman may not realize she has conceived and the body sheds the developing egg before any signs of pregnancy occur. In most of these miscarriages, it is believed that the egg would not have survived to delivery because of physiological defects. Other reasons may include inadequate hormonal development of the uterine lining and a faulty immune reaction to the embryo.

Symptoms

Symptoms of early miscarriage include cramps from the uterine area, not unlike menstrual cramps. This is caused by the uterine contractions that force the lining to be shed. Heavy bleeding accompanies or follows the cramping when the lining is expelled. The bleeding may also be present without accompanying pain. Light bleeding that persists for a few days or more can also signal an impending spontaneous abortion. With any of these symptoms, the attending physician should be contacted immediately.

Upon examination the doctor will determine if the cervix has become dilated—a sign of miscarriage. The physician will guide you through treatment that follows a miscarriage, or will help to arrest the symptoms if a miscarriage has not yet taken place.

Late Miscarriage

Occurring during the second or early third trimester, late miscarriages are physically more difficult to endure. (Psychologically both early and late miscarriages can be difficult if the woman has prepared for the upcoming baby.) Late miscarriages can be caused by trauma, insufficient uterine or cervical capability, or exposure to chemical or drug substances that trigger a miscarriage.

Symptoms

Bleeding, a pink discharge, a brown discharge, or cramping may precede a late term miscarriage. Some women will experience uterine contractions and spotting without it signaling difficulty with the pregnancy. However, any changes in the mother's condition or any experience of the symptoms above should be discussed with the attending physician immediately.

The mother will be examined by the attending medical person to see if the cervix has begun to dilate. If a miscarriage has begun, several steps may be used to prevent it continuing. Continual bed rest, hospitalization, and surgery are just a few of the possible remedies, depending on the reasons for the threat of miscarriage. If the miscarriage does occur, the doctor will try to determine the reasons for it to prevent a reoccurrence in subsequent pregnancies.

Late miscarriages will follow the stages of labor in some women, once miscarriage has become inevitable. The woman will have to expel the fetus and the uterine lining, along with the placenta. A dilatation and curettage (D & C) may be required to clean the uterus after a miscarriage to ensure that no infection sets in. Once the doctor determines that the uterus is sound, and that the reason for miscarriage has been remedied (if possible) then a new pregnancy may begin.

Stillbirths

A baby delivered after about the 20th week of pregnancy will be diagnosed as a stillbirth instead of a miscarriage.

Symptoms

Following the pattern of the late miscarriage, stillbirths can be late miscarriages or they can be full deliveries. The fetus may have already died *in utero* or may die during the labor and delivery. Many of the reasons that apply to late miscarriage also apply here. Other reasons for stillbirths can include deterioration of the uterus, umbilical strangulation, infection of the amnion or uterine lining, or other physiological defects.

Abortions

Different than a spontaneous abortion, an *induced abortion* is when the doctor ends the pregnancy medically. This can occur for several reasons. The woman may elect to have the pregnancy terminated. This is legal through the first trimester in all states, and through the second trimester in some states. If the fetus threatens the life of the mother or has died *in utero*, the pregnancy can be terminated at any point.

There are several methods of inducing an abortion. All involve opening the cervical muscle to remove the fetus. This requires local anesthesia in a first trimester abortion, and can require general anesthesia after the first trimester. Performed in a doctor's office or in the hospital, the medical procedure is considered less risky than birthing. If performed by unqualified personnel or in unsanitary conditions, the risks increase greatly. When the tissue from the pregnancy remains after an abortion, infection can set in. It is therefore extremely important that competent medical personnel be sought to perform abortions.

During the first trimester a D & C can be used to remove the embryo. The uterus can also be aspirated by vacuum. This is a method that removes all the embryonic tissue at once. Second trimester abortions usually involve a chemical injected into the uterus that triggers the body to expel the fetus and induce labor. A pill, RU 486, has been introduced in Europe that triggers spontaneous abortion. It is still being tested for use in the United States.

Genetic Disorders

There are 4,300 genetic defects that can be passed on to offspring. Of those 4,300 there are about 600 that are common enough to be tested for in couples where the risk is considered high. It is estimated that three percent of all births are to children carrying a genetic defect. These can range from mild disorders such as night blindness to serious and life threatening disorders such as Tay-Sachs and sickle cell anemia. If one grandparent or immediate family member carries a known genetic disorder, the attending physician may recommend genetic testing and counseling. Even if abortion is not considered by the parents, genetic testing will allow the parents to prepare for any eventuality.

Child Care

Bringing the Baby Home

Once the child is born, the mother will spend a couple days to a couple weeks in the hospital, depending on her condition after delivery. Caesarian deliveries can keep a woman in the hospital for several days to assist in recovery from the surgery.

Preparation for the baby should be made before delivery, if at all possible. This includes preparing the baby's sleeping area, buying clothes, diapers, and other essentials for the baby. It has been considered by some to invite bad luck to purchase and set up a baby's room before the birth. Others may worry about how they would handle coming home to a nursery if the baby did not survive or was required to remain at the hospital for some time.

Some parents find that, if they did lose the child, disassembling the nursery helped in the mourning process. It may be more difficult for parents to come home to a house where there are no signs of the infant, than to return to a nursery where they have to confront their loss.

In most circumstances, though, the parents return home from the birthing process with baby in hand. It is more than likely that the new mother will be tired from the hard work of delivery. The father will also have been functioning with little sleep if he assisted in delivery and is helping with the feeding and care of the newborn. So having the nursery set up with essentials is one way of assuring that the new family is not adding to the increased demand in their time with this new member.

Essentials in the nursery should include: diapers (cloth, disposable, or both) t-shirts in more than one size, a washtub, a car seat, a crib with a mattress that fits snugly against the sides, blankets, a bunting suit and clothing appropriate to the season, soft terry towels and washcloths, flame resistant pajamas, and a chair for the parent to sit in during feedings. Other items to consider are: a baby monitor that lets you hear the baby when you are in another room, a nightlight, a little music box or recorder that plays lullabies, bottles for feeding, a bottle warmer, pacifiers, clips to hold the pacifier to the baby's clothes, a mobile that hangs over the crib, a stroller, a baby carrier (sling or backpack), a diaper bag, baby oil, powder, shampoo, hypoallergenic soap, and other assorted toiletries. Some of these you may receive as gifts; others you will no doubt want to supply yourselves.

It is important when purchasing items such as carriers, cribs, car seats, and other equipment where safety plays a major role, that you consult with consumer guides, professional recommendations, and that you contact the U.S. Consumer Product Safety Commission, Washington D.C. 20207, (800) 638-2772 to find out if any complaints are registered on the products you are considering. It is worth your baby's safety to take the time to research the things that your baby will spend so much time using. You cannot determine quality by price and, remember, the manufacturer isn't going to put warnings about defects on products they sell.

When buying clothes for the baby, keep in mind that many babies are born bigger than the newborn size of clothing. There is no guarantee for your baby's size, so you should be equipped with several sizes of clothing in case you come home with a big baby. You don't want a nine pound baby and a roomful of six-pound size t-shirts.

Post-Partum Depression

It is estimated that 50 percent of all women suffer from some form of the blues when returning home with their baby. This can be caused by several things. There is a let-down that comes from having an event that you have prepared months for be over. This can be accompanied by the fact that the pregnant woman is the center of attention until the baby comes. Then the baby is the center of attention.

Frequently, well-meaning friends will bring gifts over addressed and wrapped for the parents and enclose baby stuff. This is fine, except that upon receiving the thirteenth baby outfit, the mother may begin to feel left out. She and the baby are separate beings and the occasional gift to the new mother, for her own use, is a welcome change.

The physical fatigue that comes with birthing, nursing, and caring for a child that has to be fed night and day can also lead to exhaustion and depression.

Some parents take several weeks to bond with their babies. The baby may feel like a stranger when the parent (not just the mother) holds him. The baby, for all practical purposes, *is* a stranger. You are just getting to know his wants, needs, and desires. Each baby is unique in the way he wants to be held, in what the different types of crying mean, and how he responds in general to life around him.

Even experienced parents must get used to this new being and his new personality. This takes time. So the sensation that you are not madly in love with or attuned to the child is neither unusual nor incomprehensible. The feelings will develop as you become more comfortable with your baby.

The feelings of inadequacy that arise from all of these potential sources of depression may increase the depression. You may feel like an inadequate or deficient parent because you are not as good a parent as you expected. The ability to be a parent takes time and learning. You should allow adequate time to develop the skills that make you comfortable with your new baby.

If, after several weeks, you still have feelings of depression and inadequacy, talk to your doctor about counseling. It may be a passing problem or it may be tied to other aspects of your life. A good counselor should be able to help you sort everything out and get to the root of your insecurity with your baby. But, again, allow yourself a normal amount of time to adjust without brow-beating yourself about it.

Both fathers and mothers can suffer from post-partum depression. It is important that the new parents communicate with each other about their feelings and their needs. Chances are that the other parent will not only understand what you are feeling, but will be experiencing some of the same feelings as well.

Other methods of handling this period can include talking with other parents about the new stresses that accompany parenthood. Support groups, new parent groups, and other such gatherings may already exist in your community. If not, try to start one, provided it doesn't add a major burden on your time.

If you miss some aspect of your life before baby, such as going out, then make some effort to treat yourself to such an occasion. Talk with friends and keep from isolating yourself if you feel a need to share company. If, however, the problem is too much company and no private time, then feel free to establish visiting hours, as you would have in a hospital when someone else is watching out for your health and well-being.

Serious post-partum depression

Severe post-partum depression that requires immediate counseling has the same symptoms that require immediate counseling even without a baby. The symptoms include: suicidal thoughts, violent urges (particularly directed inward or toward the baby), chronic insomnia, extreme lethargy, loss of appetite, complete inability to function, and general sense of despair. Any of these symptoms should be discussed thoroughly with your physician and/or a counselor as soon as possible.

After the Birth: Physical Changes

The mother's body will take several weeks to get back to something resembling the pre-pregnancy state. Weight gain, uterine expansion, and breastfeeding all change the body and take some time to undo.

Weight gain

Depending on how much weight the mother has gained during the course of the pregnancy, it can take several weeks to several months to get back down to her pre-pregnancy size. If you have gained the recommended 20 to 25 pounds during pregnancy, it will take about two months to lose the extra weight if you don't diet. If you are breastfeeding, dieting should only be done under strict supervision of your doctor.

The uterus will remain distended for several weeks following delivery. Breastfeeding helps reduce the size of the uterus because a hormone (oxytocin) that increases uterine contractions is released during breastfeeding.

Extra water is maintained in the mother's body during the pregnancy, and this water takes some time to eliminate. The extra fluids will be eliminated from the mother through frequent urination and heavy sweating. It is important that the new mother continue to replenish her fluids despite this apparent flood of liquids leaving her body. Increased intake may help increase the speed with which the body eliminates the unneeded fluids.

The body will also pick up extra weight in the breasts if the mother continues to breastfeed. For mothers who are bottlefeeding, it will take several days for the breasts to reduce in size.

Exercising to help tone and shape the pelvic, stomach, and thigh muscles, is a good method of speeding your return to your usual size. Talk with your physician for post-partum exercises that will not tax your muscles but will help build back up and firm them.

Lochia

For several days following a delivery, whether vaginal or caesarian, the body will excrete through the vagina a discharge that will shift from dark brown to yellowish-white. This discharge is the product of the body shedding the last particles of blood and fluids from the uterus.

Warning signs that are not part of the normal discharge include: bright red blood after about the fourth day, heavy bleeding that requires pad changes of more than one an hour (at any time following delivery), foul smelling discharge, heavily clotted blood, or an absence of discharge during the first two weeks following delivery. Other symptoms to watch for include: lower abdominal pain after the second day and/or lower abdominal swelling. *All of these symptoms require immediate consultation of your doctor.*

Perineal pain

With or without an episiotomy, the perineal area is normally sore following vaginal deliveries. The head of the baby has pushed against the muscles and the muscles are likely to be bruised. Talk to your physician about methods of alleviating soreness if the pain moves beyond irritating. For mild pain try soaking baths, sitting on inner tubes or cushions, lying on your side instead of sitting up, and continuing with Kegel exercises to alleviate some of the discomfort.

Fever

Puerperal fever is a sign of infection following delivery. Although it is extremely uncommon now (it was once a major killer of post-partum women) any fever that lasts for more than a few hours, or which gets over 100 degrees, should be reported immediately to your doctor. It may be just a virus or from the changes taking place for breastfeeding, but your doctor should be notified of any fever during the first month you are home.

General fears and concerns

Most parents have some fears and concerns surrounding the birth of their baby and the general routine that is required once the baby is home. Other concerns are around the various changes and symptoms that both the mother and the baby go through following birth. Some may involve simple things like dry skin; some may be more disconcerting, like rashes and red patches. If you cannot find any answers in your stock of books on pregnancy and babies, or if you are really concerned, you should not hesitate to call your doctor. If he or she feels that you need guidance and are panicky, then request some good books to help you understand what to expect. In any case, no concerned and caring doctor will object to a new parent needing reassurance about the mother's and the baby's health. It is better to ask questions and find out that there is nothing to worry about than to not ask questions and leave a potentially serious problem ignored.

Child Care and Day Care

Once you have a child, you make a choice about how that child is to be cared for during the years before school. The majority of families in the United States can no longer afford to have one parent stay home to raise a child. This means that, for at least part of the week, the child will be cared for by someone other than a parent.

Most parents have caretakers either come to their home or they drop the child off at the caretaker's place. The child will be there three to eight hours a day. Some children are in child care for up to twelve hours, depending on the parents' schedule.

For children with only one primary caretaker, and this counts for more than one quarter of American children, time in day care is essentially the same amount of time as the average adult full-time employee. The quality of the care is as influential on the child's upbringing as the quality of the parental care received during nonwork hours. Because of this, child care selection is extremely important to the safety and well-being of any child entrusted to someone else.

Child Care in the Home

Nannies, au pairs, child care workers, and babysitters, are the names for people who come to, or live in, the homes of the child for whom they care. The arrangements can range from one caretaker to one child, to one caretaker for two or three families' small children. The ability of the parents to pay for child care determines the type of care selected.

Few families can afford the salary and the living space required of the live-in nanny. For those who can, the nanny provides a registered, reliable, trained caretaker who will supervise the child for as many years as the parents deem necessary. Au pairs are much the same type of worker, except they usually do not have educational training for child care. They tend to be younger workers, less likely to stay for more than a year or two in the same position. Many au pairs are foreign students seeking a chance to live abroad for a while.

Child care workers and babysitters may come to take care of the child during assigned hours. They may live somewhere else and their work hours are scheduled for regular work patterns. They may work for one family, or a few families may pool together resources and use one caretaker for several children. One child care worker should care for no more than four or five children at a time, to provide the best safety and education for the children.

When hiring someone to come watch your children in your home, several things should be considered. The most important is to check the personal history of whomever is being considered. This now means going beyond personal recommendations. Check for police records, work papers, history of employment, and any other documentation that the person can provide to show stability, reliability, honesty, and integrity *while working with children*. In most situations, the caretaker will be unsupervised while working with your small children. Children's versions of events may not fully explain events you should know about, or may exaggerate problems with the caretaker that are not important. You have to have complete faith that this person is delivering the service you expect in a manner that meets with your full approval. If you have the opportunity to observe at least one full day of activity under the care of the worker, you should take it. This gives you a sample of how your child will spend important hours of his development. It also allows you to watch how a worker deals with the frustrations and problems that come up every day when dealing with youngsters.

Child Care Centers and Programs

Many states are now requiring registration of child care centers. Even for individuals who run informal-style child care in their own home, licensing may be required. The state will set up rules of how much space is needed per child, how many staff employees per child, what kind and variety of food is to be served, what activities are allowed, and what type of insurance is needed to cover for accidents while at the center. Check to see if your state has a licensing program,

and what the licensing requirements are. If your state does have such a program, you should only use licensed facilities for your child. If there is no mandatory licensing, find out if there is a voluntary licensing program for day care. You should check references thoroughly for programs that have no governmental inspection. Even with licensing, you want to ask the same types of questions that the licensor asks:

- How many staff per student?

- With whom is a sick staff member replaced?

- What food is provided for the children?

- What activities are provided for?

- What instruction and education is the child given?

- What are the age ranges of the children enrolled?

- How many children does the facility accommodate?

- How many children per classroom or room?

- Are any activities off the center grounds? Is permission obtained in advance to take the child off the grounds?

- What is the policy for sick children? Are they allowed in the classroom? If a child is brought to the center, obviously sick, what procedures are followed by the day care staff?

- If a child gets sick or injured while at day care, what procedures are followed?

- What is the policy of allowing children to leave with someone other than a parent? Is advance notice required? Is the parent the only acceptable guardian to be picking up a child? (Although it may seem initially that you would only want a

parent picking a child up, you may wish to carpool, or have a babysitter or a relative pick up a child. You want to make absolutely sure, though, that the child cannot leave with anyone who walks in and asks to take the child home.)

- What are their hours? What are their pickup times? If you are late, what do they do with the child?

- What is the discipline policy of the center? (This is of fundamental importance that the policies be explained in advance of enrollment.)

- Do they expel children? For what reasons?

Look around the facilities. Are they clean, well kept, and brightly lit? Are there appropriate ranges and types of toys for your child's age? Are there any safety violations or potentially dangerous aspects to the room's design (such as an open staircase without guardgates).

Attend the facilities while day care is in session. Observe the interaction of the children to see if they are well cared for, occupied in a manner you find suitable, and playing or interacting positively. Get references from parents whose children are the same age as yours and are currently using the day care program.

Once you have enrolled in the program, continue to monitor the classroom atmosphere. Occasionally drop by early before picking a child up to watch the activities. Continue to talk to other parents who have children in the same program. And, above all, continue to talk to and listen to your child about how he has spent his day.

Day care can be one of the most influential and rewarding experiences for a child. Your child will learn to interact with other adults, and perhaps other children, depending on the type of care you select. It will provide him or her with early educational experience that will be the foundation of the entire learning experience. If it is a positive experience from the start, it is likely that your child will continue to enjoy learning throughout his or her lifetime.

5

The Middle Years

Maintaining good health over the years is far simpler, less expensive, and more comfortable than restoring health that has become poor. Because some diseases cannot be cured after they are contracted, it is only logical to try to prevent all possible health problems. The techniques of modern preventive medicine are available to Americans of every age.

All people are not beautiful or handsome, but nearly everyone can have the kind of attractiveness and vitality that comes from good health. The health of an individual depends upon the kind of body he inherits and the care he gives it. Good health can be thought of as a state of social, physical, and mental well-being, a goal virtually everybody can attain—if the responsibility for maintaining one's own health, with occasional help from the health experts, is accepted.

Keeping Fit

Physical Changes

Physically, middle age should be a pleasant plateau—a time to look back on a vigorous youth, enjoy an active present, and prepare for a ripe old age.

Middle age should not be measured by chronological age but by biological age, the condition of various parts of the body. You might say that the middle-aged body is like a car that has been driven a certain number of miles. It should be well broken in and running smoothly, but with plenty of reserve power for emergencies, and lots of mileage left.

Biological age should be measured by the state of the heart, arteries, and other essential organs, the length of life and comparative health of parents and grandparents, temperament and outlook on life, and outward appearance. The way you have fed or treated yourself is important. Eating the wrong kinds of food, being overweight, smoking too much, or worrying too much can add years to biological age.

However, no one should be surprised if he is not in quite the shape he was when he was 25 or 30 years old. At age 40 to 50 it is perfectly normal to have only 80 percent of the maximum breathing capacity, 85 percent of the resting cardiac output, 95 percent of the total body water, and 96 percent of the basal metabolic rate. These factors, however, should not slow anyone down very much.

There is one difference, though, that can be anticipated in middle age. Reaction time and decision-making processes may be a bit slower. This is because the nervous system is one of the most vulnerable to aging. The cells of the central nervous system begin to die early in life and are not replaced, while other organs are still growing and producing new cells. Specific response to input is delayed because it takes a greater length of time for an impulse to travel across the connections linking nerve fibers.

Thus, though you may function as usual under normal conditions, you may find it a little harder to respond to physical or emotional stress. However, if you have followed a sound health maintenance program, including good nutrition, enough mental and physical exercise and rest, and moderate living habits, you should respond to unusual physiological or emotional stress quite adequately.

The Importance of Checkups

Physical disabilities associated with

chronic disease increase sharply with age, starting with the middle years. While more than half (54 percent) of the 86 million persons who have one or more chronic conditions are under age 45, the prevalence of disability from illness is greatest in the 45 and older age group. Of those under 45 who have chronic conditions, only 14 percent are limited in activity as compared with almost 30 percent of the 45 to 64 age group. And only 1 percent of those under 45 with chronic illness are completely disabled, as compared with 4 percent in the 45 to 64 age group.

These figures suggest that it is wise to have an annual checkup so that any disease process or condition can be nipped in the bud. Further evidence of the value of medical checkups comes from the Aetna Life Insurance Company, which compared two groups of policyholders over a five-year period. Those who did not have checkups and health counseling had a death rate 44 percent higher than the group who did. Regular checkups will not only help prolong life, they will also help you to live it more comfortably.

Here are some other good reasons for having a physical checkup:

- If an organ has been attacked by serious disease in youth, it may deteriorate at an early adult age.

- Heredity may play an important role in determining the speed at which various organs age. If your parents and grandparents had arteriosclerosis, there is a chance you might develop this condition in your middle years.

- Your environment (smog, poor climate, etc.) might affect the rate at which your body ages, particularly the skin.

- Individual stresses and strains or abuses or overuse (of alcohol, for example) may create a health problem in middle age.

- The endocrine glands (pituitary, thyroid, parathyroids, adrenals, ovaries, testicles) play important roles in aging. Serious disease of one or more of these glands may lead to premature aging of an organ dependent upon its secretions.

- At middle age you are more likely to be beset by emotional strains at work or at home that could make you an early candidate for heart disease, arteriosclerosis, and other degenerative disorders.

- The earlier a chronic disease is detected, the better the chance that it can be arrested before permanent damage is done. This is especially true in the case of glaucoma, diabetes, heart disease, cancer of the lung or breast or other cancers—all of which could have their onset in middle age.

To help detect disease and other debilitating conditions, many physicians utilize automated medical screening, which combines medical history with selected physiological measurements and laboratory tests to give the physician a complete health profile of the patient. This profile should indicate the probability of any chronic condition, which the physician could then pinpoint with more thorough tests.

Also, annual checkups enable the physician to observe changes taking place over a period of time. For example, he is able to observe gradually changing blood chemistry levels or a progressive increase in eye pressure that could signal the onset of disease.

Don't Try To Be Your Own Physician

A panel of medical specialists from the University of California at Los Angeles recently found that many men of 40 years and older were dosing themselves with unnecessary pills and "conserving" their energy by increasing bed rest to the point that it actually became enervating.

These physicians point out that increasing dependence on pills can be harmful as well as expensive. Laxatives are a good example of a popular commercial medicine taken unnecessarily by large numbers of people. Perhaps only one person in 100,000 may have an actual motor disability of the bowels, and most constipation can be easily corrected through proper foods and exercise, without resorting to laxatives. Also, taking vitamin pills or avoiding all high-cholesterol foods is unnecessary—unless recommended by a physician.

But, most important, "conserving" energy through prolonged bed rest or avoiding exercise can be fatal. The panel members pointed out that before age 40, a person exercises to improve his performance, but that after age 40 he exercises to improve his chances of survival.

Physical Fitness and Exercise

In middle age most of us stop performing most forms of exercise other than those that we enjoy doing. In other words, we find it easier to bend an elbow than lift weights. This is unfortunate, because in middle age most of us need regular exercise to maintain both mental and physical fitness and to increase endurance, strength, and agility.

As noted earlier, in middle age there is some decrease in breathing capacity, cardiac output, and metabolic rate; yet exercise can improve these functions. The more often the normal heart and circulatory system are required to move blood to active regions of the body through exercise or movement, the more efficient they become. Protracted exercise also improves the work of the lungs by increasing their ability to expand more fully, take in more air, and utilize a greater proportion of the oxygen in the inhaled air.

While exercise alone cannot eliminate obesity, it can help prevent it by improving digestion and bowel movements and by burning up excess calories. Exercise can also make you feel, look, and think better. Some traditional formal exercises, however, like touching the toes while keeping your knees stiff, or doing deep knee bends, are potentially harmful in middle age; they put too much stress on weak parts of the back and legs.

Despite protests about not having enough time, everyone has time to exercise, particularly if it is worked into the daily routine—for example, walking instead of riding to the train, office, store, or bus stop. You might find you'll get there faster, especially in traffic-clogged metropolitan areas, and you'll save money as well. More important, those minutes of "stolen" exercise accrue over the years in the form of improved health.

Sports and Games

If you don't like formal exercise, you can get exercise informally—through a favorite sport, whether it be golf, tennis, swimming, jogging, skiing, cycling, or whatever. Many sports and games are stop-and-go activities that do not provide helpful, rhythmic exercise, but here's how you can make them more beneficial.

Golf

Instead of riding in a golf cart between shots, walk—in fact, stride vigorously, lifting your head and chest. And don't make golf a cut-throat competition or business pursuit. Relax and enjoy it—count your blessings rather than your bogeys.

Tennis

Like golf, tennis can be a cut-throat competitive sport or a pleasant pursuit. If it's played with muscles tied in knots from nervous tension, it will not provide any fun or healthful exercise. Also, players over 30 are well-advised to play more doubles than singles and to avoid exhausting themselves in the heat of competition.

Swimming

Along with fast walking and jogging, swimming is one of the best all-around exercises. When swimming, most of the muscles are exercised and lung capacity and cardiac output are improved. The exercise potential can be increased by doing pull-ups with the diving board or ladder and by bobbing up and down in the water.

Jogging

This popular sport can be combined with walking, done in a group or alone, either outdoors or indoors, and alternated with other exercises. Moreover, it doesn't require any special equipment and has been recognized by fitness experts as one of the best exercises for the heart and circulation. However, it is wise to get your physician's advice and approval before embarking on a jogging program.

Skiing

Skiing is healthful as well as fun. You can get in shape for skiing and improve your ability by jogging and by practicing some of the techniques needed in skiing—such as the rhythmic left-right-left-right twist of foot, knee, and leg in short turns. To do this exercise, stand up straight with your feet quite close together and flex your knees forward so that the weight goes onto the balls of the feet. Now, arms apart for balance, twist your feet and knees to the left without twisting your upper body. As you do this, try the modified half-bends of the traversing position that all ski schools teach. Then reverse the position to the right, and keep repeating.

Other Sports

Other worthwhile sports for healthful exercise include badminton, bicycling, canoeing, rowing, table tennis, skating, and squash. However, they should be sustained for at least 30 minutes at a time, ideally four times a week, and should be combined with supplemental exercises.

A Word of Warning

Everyone should beware of becoming a weekend athlete and punishing himself with an overdose of exercise or sports only on weekends. It makes as much sense as stuffing yourself on weekends and starving the rest of the week. It's far more sensible—and healthful—to engage in sports activities for an hour or so at a time on a daily basis.

Exercises

Participating in sports activities is not the only way to keep fit. Special exercises can help reduce tension and build muscles. For instance, one way to relax is to do rhythmic exercises, particularly for the trunk, that help to improve circulation. You can also try exercises that will relieve tense muscles and improve breathing. The exercises described below were developed by Dr. Josephine L. Rathbone of Columbia University.

Breathing to Relax

Lie on your back on the floor with knees bent and feet resting on the floor. Take a deep breath, letting both the abdominal wall and chest rise. Hold the air for a few seconds, then expel it through your mouth with a gasp. Repeat four or five times at regular intervals.

For Tense Arms

Standing erectly, swing both arms forward, then to the side, letting them drop during the swings so that your hands brush your thighs with each motion. Keep your shoulders low. Repeat a few times. Then, sit on the edge of a chair and clench one hand tightly. Swing your arm vigorously in large circles, keeping your hand clenched. Then repeat with other arm.

For Tense Legs

Sit on the edge of a table with lower legs hanging free. Then, alternately, swing them backward and forward. Try to keep your legs moving in rhythm.

For Stomach Tension

Kneel with your feet under your hips and swing your trunk down to one side and around, sweeping your arms in a wide circle, coming up again on the opposite side. Or stand with your hips supported against the wall, feet apart and a few inches from the wall. Bend your body forward, arms drooping, and let your body sway from side to side, with your arms and head loose.

Relaxing at Work or Home

Relieve tension while sitting by holding the spine erect, shoulders low. Turn your head so that the chin touches first one collarbone, then the other. Move slowly and rhythmically.

Yoga

You can also relax and become revitalized through various Yoga exercises. Courses are taught at many recreational centers. Some of the exercises require only a minimum of time, and can be done not only before and after the workday but in the office during the lunch hour.

Isometrics

Isometric exercises—pitting one muscle against another without moving—can also be practiced at odd moments. These exercises should, however, be done only by healthy persons, and not by anyone with a cardiac problem. To strengthen arm and shoulder muscles through isometrics, put the fist of one hand against the palm of the other and push without moving. Or push up with your arms from a chair or the edge of a table. Strengthen arm and neck muscles by grasping the back of the neck with laced fingers and pulling forward—again, without movement.

All of the above exercises and sports can put you on the road to physical fitness. Just remember, whatever form of exercise or sport you choose, make it fun and do not strain yourself unduly.

Rest and Sleep

Rest and sleep adequate for one's personal needs are another vital component of good health and good appearance. They also influence human relationships and mental alertness. Scientists believe that during sleep the body replaces tissue cells and eliminates waste products created by fatigue at a faster rate than when awake.

Sleep also rests the heart and blood system, because heart muscle contractions and blood pressure are slower then. Excessive fatigue from lack of sleep increases susceptibility to a number of ailments, including the common cold. If an individual gets an adequate amount of sleep (usually seven to eight hours for an adult), he will feel ready to meet the day's activities. If not, his memory may not be sharp, and he may be irritable because his nervous system has had inadequate rest.

A quiet, dark, ventilated room, a fairly firm mattress, and performance of a moderate amount of exercise during the day will aid sleep. When worry, frustration, or anxiety make it difficult to sleep, a conscious attempt to relax will help. Sedatives or sleeping pills should not be taken unless they are prescribed or recommended by a physician.

Personal Hygiene

Disease germs can enter the body only in a limited number of ways. One of the major ways is through the skin. The skin is a protective covering which, when broken, can admit harmful bacteria or viruses easily.

Simple precautions are very effective. The hands come into contact with disease germs more than any other part of the body. Therefore, they should be washed whenever they are dirty, prior to preparing food or eating, and after using the lavatory.

The rest of the body must also be kept clean, because adequate bodily cleanliness will remove substances that, by irritating the skin, make it more susceptible to infection. Bathing also improves the muscle tone of the skin. Hair should also be washed frequently enough to prevent accumulation of dust and dead skin cells.

Openings in the body are also paths by which disease germs can enter the body. The nose and ears should be carefully cleaned only with something soft, for instance, a cotton swab. Genital orifices should be kept clean by frequent bathing. Any unusual discharge from a body opening should be promptly reported to a physician. The problem can then be treated at its earliest stage—the easiest time to solve the problem.

Personal hygiene includes care of the nails. They should always be kept clean and fairly short. Hangnails can be avoided by gently pushing back the cuticle with a towel after washing the hands.

Care of the Feet

"My feet are killing me!" is a complaint heard more frequently in middle age, especially from women. The devil in this case usually takes the shape of fashionable shoes, where the foot is frequently squeezed into shapes and positions it was never designed to tolerate. Particularly unhealthy for the foot was the formerly fashionable spike heel and pointed toe.

Any heel two inches or higher will force the full weight of the body onto the smaller bones in the front of the foot and squeeze the toes into the forepart of the shoes. This hurts the arch, causes calluses on the sole of the foot, and can lead to various bone deformities.

The major solution to this problem is to buy good shoes that really fit. The shoes should be moderately broad across the instep, have a straight inner border, and a moder-

ately low heel. To fit properly, shoes should extend one-half inch to three-fourths inch beyond the longest toe.

Avoid wearing shoes that have no support; also, avoid wearing high heels for long periods of time. Extremely high heels worn constantly force the foot forward and upset body balance. Changing heel height several times a day will rest the feet and give the muscles in the back of the legs a chance to return to their normal position. It's highly desirable to wear different shoes each day, or at least alternate two pairs. This gives the shoes a chance to dry out completely. Dust shoes with a mild powder when removed.

Shoes should not be bought in the morning. They should be tried on near the end of the day, when the feet have broadened from standing and walking, and tightness or rubbing can be more easily detected.

As to hosiery, socks and stockings should extend a half-inch beyond the longest toe. Stretch socks are fine in many cases, but plain wool or cotton socks help if your feet perspire a lot.

Foot Exercises

Exercise your feet by trying these simple steps recommended by leading podiatrists:

- Extend the toes and flex rapidly for a minute or two. Rotate the feet in circles at the ankles. Try picking up a marble or pencil with your toes; this will give them agility and strength.

- Stand on a book with your toes extended over the edge. Then curl your toes down as far as possible, grasping the cover.

- After an unusually active day, refresh the feet with an alcohol rub. Follow this with a foot massage, squeezing the feet between your

hands. When you are tired, rest with your feet up. Try lying down for about a half-hour with your feet higher than your head, using pillows to prop up your legs.

- Walk barefoot on uneven sandy beaches and thick grass. This limbers up the feet and makes the toes work. Walking anywhere is one of the best exercises for the feet if you learn to walk properly and cultivate good posture. Keep toes pointed ahead, and lift rather than push the foot, letting it come down flat on the ground, placing little weight on the heel. Your toes will come alive, and your feet will become more active.

Foot Ailments

Doing foot exercises is particularly important in middle age, because the foot is especially vulnerable to the following problems.

Bunions

A bunion is a thickening and swelling of the big joint of the big toe, forcing it toward the other toes. There is also a protuberance on the inner side of the foot. Unless treated, this condition usually gets progressively worse. Surgery is not always necessary or successful. Often, special shoes to fit the deformed foot must be worn.

Stiff Toe

People suffering from this problem find that the big joint of the big toe becomes painful and stiff, possibly due to a major accident or repeated minor trauma. This condition usually corrects itself if the joint is protected for a few weeks, usually by a small steel plate within the sole of the shoe.

Hammer Toe

This clawlike deformity is usually

caused by cramping the toes with too small shoes. The pressure can be eased with padding and, in some cases, the deformity can be corrected by surgery.

Ingrown Toenail

Cutting the nail short and wearing shoes that are too tight are major causes of ingrown toenails; the edge of the nail of the toe—usually the big toe—is forced into the soft outer tissues. In some cases the tissues can be peeled back after soaking the foot in hot water, and the offending part of the nail can be removed. To prevent ingrown toenails, the nails should be kept carefully trimmed and cut straight across the nail rather than trimmed into curves at the corners. For severe or chronic cases of ingrown toenails it is best to seek professional treatment.

Morton's Toe

This is the common name for a form of *metatarsalgia,* a painful inflammation of a sheath of small nerves that pass between the toes near the ball of the foot. The ailment is most likely to occur in an area between the third and fourth toe, counting from the large toe, and usually is due to irritation produced by pressure that makes the toes rub against each other. In most instances, the pressure results from wearing improperly fitted shoes, shoes with pointed toes, or high heel shoes, which restrict normal flexing of the metatarsals (the bones at the base of the toes) while walking.

Temporary relief usually is possible through removal of the shoes and massaging of the toes, or by application of moist, warm heat to the afflicted area. In cases of very severe pain, a doctor may inject a local anes-

thetic into the foot. Additional relief sometimes can be obtained by wearing metatarsal arch supports in the shoes. However, continued irritation of the nerves can result in the growth of a tumor that may require surgical removal.

Care of the Teeth

An attractive smile is often the first thing that one notices about others. In addition to creating an attractive appearance, healthy teeth and gums are a basic requirement for good overall health. The dentist should be visited at whatever intervals he recommends, usually every six months.

Neglect of oral hygiene and the forgoing of dental checkups are commonplace in the middle years. An often-heard excuse is that the eventual loss of teeth is inevitable. Years ago, loss of teeth really was unavoidable. Today, however, thanks to modern dental practices, it is possible for nearly everyone to enjoy the benefits of natural teeth for a lifetime.

Problems of Aging

When the human body reaches middle age, a number conditions that are the result of advancing years begin to make themselves felt. These include wrinkling of the skin, baldness, varicose veins, and the body's decreased ability to deal with nicotine, caffeine, alcohol, and excess calories.

Skin

The skin usually starts to show its age in the mid to late 30s. At that time it starts to lose its elasticity and flexibility, and becomes somewhat thinner. Little lines—not yet wrinkles—start to show up, usually crow's feet around the eyes.

Wrinkling takes place at different times with different people, and sometimes in different areas of the skin. Heredity may play a part.

Treatment for Wrinkles

While wrinkles do not hurt, many people want to do something about them. Experienced physicians and dermatologists have a number of techniques for removing or minimizing wrinkles. One accepted method is *dermabrasion,* or planing of the skin. The physician sprays on a local anesthetic, then scrapes the skin with a motor-driven wire brush or some other abrasive tool. The treatment usually takes one session, and no hospital stay is required. There will be some swelling and scab formation, but this should clear up in a week to ten days.

Another method is called *cryotherapy,* in which the physician freezes the skin with carbon dioxide. This induces peeling, which improves the appearance of flat acne scars and shallow wrinkles.

The use of retinoic acid, or Retin-A™, for the treatment of wrinkles has become popular in recent years. Retinoic acid was originally used for the treatment of acne and has not yet been studied for long-term use for wrinkles. The effect is temporary on wrinkles and skin will return to original condition after discontinued use. Some side effects include heightened sensitivity to sunlight and skin irritation or rash.

Skin Texture Change

Besides wrinkling, the skin has a tendency in some people to become thinner, leathery, and darkened as they move towards the 40s and 50s. This effect can be minimized if the skin is toned up with cold cream and other emollients that provide the moisture and oil the skin needs. Also, overexposure to the sun—one of the prime agers of the skin—should be avoided.

In fact, most physicians feel that the sun is a lethal agent, and that exposing the face to too much sun is like putting it in a hot oven. Many say that the sun destroys some inherent good qualities of facial skin, and ruins any chance of improving the appearance through cosmetic surgery.

Cosmetic Surgery

Cosmetic surgery for both men and women is becoming increasingly popular and sophisticated. Cosmetic surgery procedures include *rhinoplasty* (nose); *facial plasty* or *rhytidoplasty* (face lift); *blepharoplasty* (upper eyelids and bags under the eyes); breast augmentation and reduction; as well as the dermabrasion and other methods mentioned earlier. See "Plastic and Cosmetic Surgery" in Ch. 20, *Surgery*.

Baldness

The problem of baldness has its roots in ancient history. Men were worried about baldness 4,000 years ago. But until recently, medical opinion agreed largely with the statement by Dr. Eugene Van Scott, head of the Dermatology Service of the National Cancer Institute: "Baldness is caused by three factors: Sex, age, and heredity. And we can't do a thing about any of these."

Other causes of male baldness include infections, systemic diseases, drugs that have a toxic effect, mechanical stress, friction, and radiation. Diet does not usually affect baldness, but chronic starvation or vitamin deficiencies can contribute to dryness, lack of luster, and hair loss. Also, ex-

cessive intake of vitamin A can cause hair loss.

In women, loss of hair is quite common toward the end of pregnancy, after delivery, and during menopause. A hysterectomy, crash dieting, severe emotional stress, high fever, a major illness such as thyroid disease or diabetes, certain allergies, and the use of systemic drugs such as steroids and amphetamines—all can produce hair loss.

There are two common types of baldness in men: male pattern baldness (*alopecia*) and patchy baldness (*alopecia areata*). The latter is more common in women.

Male Baldness

Male pattern baldness may begin as early as the early 20s or 30s. Hair falls out from the crown until a fringe of hair remains at the sides and along the back of the head. At the onset, a bald spot may appear on the crown of the head; balding spots in other areas may merge to form the fringe pattern.

In patchy baldness, hair may fall out suddenly in patches. In this case, hair usually returns after going through three growth periods. The new hair may be thinner than the original hair. Although patchy baldness is self-limiting and often self-curing, therapy is indicated for some patients. The therapy may consist of injections of soluble steroid suspensions directly into the scalp. Regrowth may begin in three to four weeks, but remains localized at the sites of injections.

Hair transplants remain the most dependable way to grow new hair—especially in men with male pattern baldness. The process involves cut-

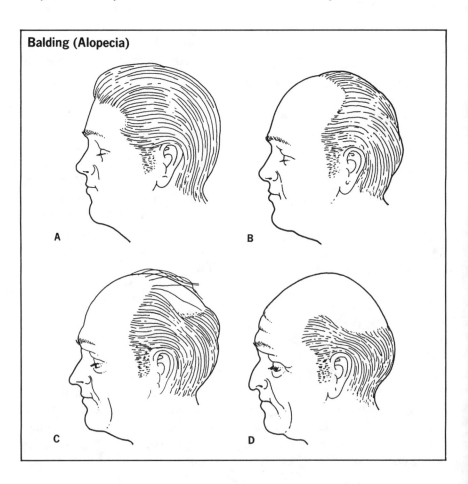

Balding (Alopecia)

A   B

C   D

ting out *punch grafts,* small patches or plugs of hair and follicle-bearing tissue, from the back or sides of the head. The grafts are immediately inserted into recipient incisions that are slightly smaller than the plugs. In a two- or three-hour session a physician can transplant 60 to 80 plugs of hair. Adequate coverage of a balding crown usually requires 200 to 400 plugs.

Female Baldness

The hair on the crown of a woman's head may thin out, but women seldom become bald as men do. Progesterone, administered in careful, dose-regulated treatments, has been used successfully by some dermatologists. The progesterone is applied to the scalp as a cream or ointment.

Drug Treatments

Other forms of therapy have come into experimental use for both men and women. Many of them involve the use of drugs. In one treatment carefully monitored doses of cortisone are injected into the scalp. In another, the drug psoralen may either be applied to the scalp directly or taken internally. A combination of drugs including 8-methoxypsoralen and inosiplex may be used in conjunction with ultraviolet irradiation.

Most acclaimed of all the new drug therapies is minoxidil, a derivative of the blood pressure-reducing drug Loniten. Physicians simply order Loniten reformulated as a topical solution. Thicker than water, the minoxidil has been used generally by prescription as a gel. Visible improvement is never guaranteed, and in most cases results can take from four months to a year.

Minoxidil must be prescribed by a physician and requires medical monitoring about every four months. It must be used indefinitely to maintain new hair growth. Early findings suggest that the drug works best on men who have not been bald for a long time. Some dermatologists believe that patients with minoxidil-generated growths of hair can gradually, over time, switch to low-dose, modified use patterns.

Excess Hair

For some middle-aged women, the problem is too much hair in the wrong place, instead of too little. Excess hair can grow on the face, chest, arms, and legs. In some instances, unwanted hair may be a sign of an endocrine disorder that can be detected by a physician. In other cases, it can be caused by chronic irritation, such as prolonged use of a cast, bandage, or hot-water bottle; it can also be due to excess exposure to the sun, iodine or mercury irritation, or localized rubbing.

Excess hair can be bleached, shaved, tweezed, waxed, or removed by chemical depilatories and electrolysis. Only electrolysis is permanent. See "Hair Removal" in Ch. 21, *Skin and Hair.*

Varicose Veins

Another complaint of middle-aged men and women is *varicose veins.* About half the women over 50 years of age have these enlarged veins with damaged valves in their thighs and calves.

Varicose veins can occur in various parts of the body. They are, however, most common in the legs.

Varicose veins are usually caused by years of downward pressure on the veins, causing the valves to break down. This often happens to people who must stand for many hours at a time. The large, bluish irregularities are plainly visible beneath the skin of

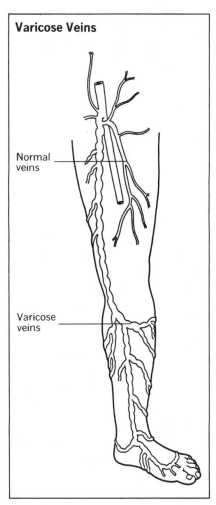

Varicose Veins

Normal veins

Varicose veins

the thighs and calves, and they cause a heavy dragging sensation in the legs and a general feeling of tiredness and lack of energy.

Treatment

In most instances, the best treatment involves surgery to tie off the main veins and remove all superficial veins that lend themselves to this procedure (called *stripping*). In other cases, varicose veins can be relieved by wearing elastic stockings or compression bandages.

Varicose veins that remain untreated can cause *varicose ulcers,* which usually form on the inner side of the leg above the ankle. Treatment calls for prolonged bed rest, warm applications, and surgical ligation and stripping of the varicose veins responsible for the ulcers. Thus, it is wise to consult a physician if varicose veins appear.

Menopause

The permanent end of a woman's menstrual cycle is called *menopause*. The duration of time it takes for the body to change over to a non-menstruating hormonal structure varies. It may be as short as a year; some women may experience menopausal signs and occasional periods for up to ten years.

The average age bracket for menopause is between 40 and 50 years of age. However, about 12 percent of women reach menopause between ages 36 and 40; 15 percent between 51 and 55; and 6 percent either earlier than 40 or later than 55. What this basically means is that menopause can normally occur anywhere between 36 and 56 years of age.

The *premenopausal period* is the period of time before frequently irregular menstruation or cessation of menstruation. The body begins to undergo changes that may go unnoticed. Ovulation may be irregular and skip menstrual cycles. The estrogen and progesterone levels may lower.

Signs that accompany the premenopausal period include increasing or lessening menstrual flow, skipped or shortened periods, and occasional irregularly timed menstruation.

The *perimenopausal period* is the onset of noticeable changes. The menstrual cycle may abruptly cease, or become unpredictable and irregular. Hormone levels of estrogen and progesterone continue to decline. Egg production becomes increasingly irregular or ceases entirely. Egg production may or may not correspond to menstrual flow. A woman can continue ovulating without having a pe-

riod, or may have periods without ovulation.

The most familiar signs of menopause occur during the perimenopausal period. These occurrences should be considered "signs" and not "symptoms" since they do not represent anything going wrong. They are not a sign of illness.

The one sign that everyone is aware of is the "hot flash." Referred to as flashes or flushes, this is a rapid increase in blood vessel dilation at the surface of the skin. The skin temperature can rise between four to eight degrees. The internal body temperature may drop with the increase of the surface temperature. A common hot flash pattern is a sudden feeling of extreme warmth, occasionally accompanied by heavy sweating, and chills following, as the internal body temperature cools. For some women, flashes occur daily; for others they may only occur once every several weeks. Some menopausal women never experience them. Many women experience flashes but are not disturbed by them.

Hot flashes at night, which produce heavy sweating and chills, are sometimes referred to as "night sweats." They may just be nighttime flashes. They can, though, lead to loss of sleep and thereby trigger fatigue, irritability, and insomnia. Problems with sleep should be discussed with your physician.

Dressing for fluctuations in body temperature may help reduce some undesirable side effects. Wear layers of clothing so when you are warm you can take off the top layer. The top layers are available, then, if you get cold later. It is commonly feared by some women that others can tell when one is experiencing a hot flash. This is rarely true; the usual physical response is a slight blush that goes unnoticed by others. Reassurance by friends can help relieve anxiety.

Other signs of menopause that may be problematic or startling when they occur include flooding. This is the sudden onset of a very heavy menstrual flow. It can occur without warning and normal amounts of menstrual protection may not be adequate. As with the hot flashes, this may never happen, or it may happen extremely infrequently, or it may be a recurrent problem. It is, however, usually only a problem in terms of hygiene and embarrassment. Flooding alone is not normally a symptom of an underlying problem. If there is no underlying disease, no surgery or treatment is required for this. If you are distressed by flooding and need reassurance, or *if it is accompanied by pain* please see a physician.

Vaginal changes that occur during menopause can include a thinning of the vaginal wall. This is normally associated with the reduction of estrogen production. The vagina will produce less lubrication and hold less moisture. The signs of this may include perceived dryness, itching, irritation from walking, and pain or discomfort during intercourse. Because the loss of lubrication may be the underlying cause, using douches and feminine hygiene sprays are not recommended. A water-based lubricant, such as K-Y Jelly™, is recommended for discomfort, particularly with intercourse. You should avoid oil-based lubricants, such as Vaseline™, as they are more difficult for the body to absorb and may create problems with infection.

Mood swings are also commonly cited as a sign of menopause. They may accompany the hormonal swings of the early stages of menopause or they may occur later. Many women do not have noticeable mood change at all.

The change of mood may be sudden or may be slow. Depression has been noted by some women, with its passing as the body adapts to the new hormonal levels. Knowing that it is caused by hormonal changes may help some women adjust to temporary shifts in mood. Debilitating or distressing changes should always be discussed with your doctor.

The *post-menopausal period* is the rest of one's life after menopause. The menstrual cycle has ceased entirely. The production of eggs has stopped. The body's production of estrogen and progesterone is very low. The body is back to a stable, predictable physical pattern.

Hysterectomies and Hormonal Supplements

When problems arise with the reproductive organs, or the body's response to the fluctuation in hormone production, there are a few methods of alleviating the problems.

Hysterectomy, the surgical removal of the uterus, and oophorectomy, the surgical removal of the ovaries, are medical procedures done to alleviate major medical problems or remove cancerous tissue. Cancer of the uterus, ovaries, or cervix are frequently treated with removal of the cancerous and surrounding tissue. Hemorrhaging that has not responded to hormonal or other surgical techniques (such as a dilation and curettage—D&C) may be corrected with a hysterectomy.

Other problems that can be alleviated surgically are noncancerous fibroid growths, endometriosis (the uterine tissue invades other tissues), and physical impairment or deterioration of the uterus or ovaries, as is the case with collapse of the uterus through the cervix.

There are several types of hysterectomies, differing in how much of the sexual reproduction system is removed.

A *subtotal hysterectomy* is the removal of the uterus, leaving the cervix, fallopian tubes, and the ovaries in place. A *total hysterectomy* is the removal of the cervix as well as the uterus. *Oophorectomy* and *ovariectomy* are both used to describe the surgical removal of one or both of the ovaries. *Ovariohysterectomy* is the removal of the ovaries, fallopian tubes, and uterus. The quantity of tissue removed will be determined by the patient and the doctor, based on the reasons for the operation. For removal of cancerous tissue, all organs may need to be removed. For sterilization, only a subtotal hysterectomy may be necessary.

Although hysterectomies are common, they are still considered major surgery and should be approached as such, by both the doctor and the patient. Recoveries can take six weeks or longer.

A physician may prescribe estrogen and progesterone supplemental pills to reduce or eliminate some of the adverse physical reactions to menopause. Hormonal treatment may reduce or eliminate hot flashes and vaginal wall thinning and drying. It can reduce heavy menstrual bleeding. However, hormone therapy increases a woman's risk for heart disease and strokes. It is also believed to increase the risk of breast cancer. The risks and benefits should be explained by and discussed with your physician before starting any treatment.

Male Sexuality and Aging

Most men are capable of having intercourse, and fathering children, throughout their lives. Aging can reduce some physical capacity in sexual performance, but the vast majority of men remain sexually capable through old age.

Physical problems that can be encountered, however, involve testicular failure and testicular cancer.

Testicular cancer is relatively rare, affecting less than 2 percent of the adult male population with cancer. Symptom include include a noticeable lump in the the testicle, swelling, and some alteration in the consistency of the affected testicle. The symptoms may also include dull aching from the lower abdomen, groin or scrotum. Men are now recommended to do monthly physical check for lumps, as women are recommended to do self-breast exams. The reason is that testicular cancer, when caught early, has a very high survival rate. If left unchecked until the yearly physical, the cancer has a chance to spread.

Testicular failure is when the body shuts off the functions of the testes. This may be caused by hormonal deficiency and can be cured through hormonal replacement therapy. Since hormonal therapy can lead to prostate problems, it is recommended that a physician closely monitor any medication for testicular failure.

Vasectomy

Vasectomy is the sterilization of the male by cutting the vas deferens, the tubes that transport the sperm. The surgery is normally performed in the doctor's office with local anesthesia. Incisions are made on each side of the scrotum or on the center of the scrotum. The tubes are then cut, and tied or cauterized on each end.

Vasovasotomy is the surgical procedure that attempts to reconnect the vas deferens after a vasectomy. This operation is done for men wishing to reverse the surgical sterilization. Success at this procedure can vary from 30 to 75 percent, depending on the type of initial sterilization procedures, and the skill of the surgeon in reconnection of the tubes.

Drugs, Chemicals, and Alcohol

Most substances consumed in excess cause temporary problems at the least, and permanent damage to your health at the worst. One of the problems with excess is that as you age, you are able to tolerate less. Most people recognize that, as they grow older, they are less able to handle the rigors of exercise and stress. It is not expected, though, that they will tolerate less the effects of cigarettes, alcohol, and chemicals such as caffeine.

There are two basic risks that come from indulgence of these substances. One is from long-term use; the other is from individual instances of overindulgence.

- With the continued use of a substance such as nicotine over a long period of time, the cumulative effects on the body begin to take a toll. The body removes the substance less rapidly from the system. The delicate tissues of the kidneys, liver, lungs, or other vital organs may become damaged or destroyed from processing what the body basically responds to as a poison. The risk is that you will become one of those to suffer the consequences of long-term use. Some of the damage may be reversed if the habit is broken. Other effects may be permanent, risking scarred tissue, destruction of the organ, and, eventually, death.

- Binging in drinking, or taking drugs, always runs the risk of an overdose—forcing major trauma to the body and, perhaps, resulting in death. Binging on cigarettes, food, and caffeine may not result in such an immediate and dramatic response, but the short-term damage can also be substantial to the body. As you age, your body will tolerate such abuses less and less well.

Nicotine

Nicotine is thought to get into the system through the membranes of the mouth and related areas. Thus, a person who holds an unlighted cigar in his mouth may absorb nicotine.

While a little nicotine is not harmful, most steady smokers absorb too much nicotine for their own good. Lung cancer kills over 142,000 persons a year. Lung cancer only had a 13% survival rate, for living five years after diagnosis and treatment. Also, cigarette smoking is believed to be a primary cause of *emphysema* (a disease that decreases efficiency of the lungs) which kills over 15,000 persons a year. Approximately 100,000 cigarette smokers die from heart attacks each year.

In their book *Vigor for Men Over 30*, the authors, Drs. Warren R. Guild, Stuart Cowan, and Samm Baker, suggest these tips on giving up smoking:

- *Try a program of enjoyable physical activity.* They suggest that if the urge to smoke becomes overpowering, the smoker should take a brisk walk, do a set of invigorating exercises at home or in the office, or engage in an enjoyable sport.

- *Don't use antismoking drugs or other nostrums without a physician's advice.* Such devices may do more harm than good. Your physician is the one who can advise you on the best way to cut down on smoking, and he can help you cope with any withdrawal symptoms such as nervousness, dizziness, or insomnia.

- *Don't try to cut down on too many things at the same time.* Concentrate on cutting down on your smoking, and relax about cutting down on diet and drinking, too. One reduction at a time is best.

- *You've got to quit completely.* Like the alcoholic, you've got to say, "This is my *last* cigarette"—and mean it.

- *Quit when there's a major break in your routine.* The recovery from an operation or illness is a good time to stop. After you have established the habit of *not* smoking, make that habit a part of your daily life.

- *Try something different to throw desire off the track.* Take a shower—you can't light a match under water. Also, you can't hold a cigarette if you're playing table tennis or practicing your golf swing.

Caffeine

Laboratory studies show that caffeine appears to work on the central nervous system: fatigue and drowsiness fade while mental activities quicken. But too much caffeine can produce headaches, irritability, and confusion.

Although tea leaves contain almost twice as much caffeine as an equal weight of coffee, smaller amounts of tea are used to make a cup of tea, thus lessening the per-cup intake rate. Cola and chocolate also contain caffeine. Although these drinks are not addictive, abstaining from them is no easy matter, as anyone who has tried to give up coffee drinking can attest.

Ordinarily, drinking a few cups of coffee or other caffeine beverage is not harmful—unless your physician tells you to cut down. But if you find that you need a caffeine beverage to keep going, you might be better off taking a rest instead.

Alcohol

Many physicians feel that a person's capacity to handle liquor diminishes after age 40, and that alcohol intake should be cut down after this age.

Also, some people seem to develop an allergic reaction to alcohol—an allergy that can be fatal. One physician described the extra dry martini as "the quick blow to the back of the neck."

Drinking too much and too fast can jar the whole system. It tends to make the drinker nervous and on edge instead of providing calming relief from tensions. The hard-pressed executive is especially vulnerable to the quick, fast drink he takes to provide instant relaxation when he is fatigued.

"The key to the real value of alcohol is intelligent drinking," says Dr. Harry J. Johnson, of the Life Extension Institute. Dr. Johnson says that he sometimes recommends a drink or two before dinner, which he says is the best time to indulge. However, Dr. Johnson suggests a tall, well-diluted highball taken in a peaceful, quiet setting.

How to Avoid Drinking

If you find that drinking is a problem at business luncheons, conventions, and cocktail parties, Dr. Warren R. Guild recommends the following commonsense ways to pass up drinks:

- Say "no thanks" if you do not like the taste or effect of alcohol. Order a juice or nonalcoholic beverage just to have something to sip. Actually, many more jobs and clients have been lost through drinking too much than by not drinking at all.

- Wait for others to order drinks. If someone else refuses a drink, you can decline too. Or, you could say, "I'm not having one but you go ahead." This usually sets the pace for drinking.

- Instead of a powerhouse martini, try vermouth on the rocks, beer, wine, or a well-diluted highball.

- Use dieting as a reason to cut down or out on drinking. You have a good excuse—a drink has 100 or more calories.

- Make arrangements with your favorite restaurant or bar to serve you "your usual." You could make this a nonalcoholic drink.

Remember that alcohol definitely decreases your ability to concentrate, absorb, or produce thoughts or ideas. After drinking you will not be as efficient at writing, drawing, handling objects, or driving. If the level of alcohol in your blood exceeds 0.05 percent—which, depending on weight, is approximately the equivalent of two ounces of hard liquor or two bottles of beer at one session—*you are not a safe driver.*

Treating a Hangover

What if you do drink too much and have a hangover? Is there anything you can do about it? Dr. Harold T. Hyman, formerly of the Columbia University College of Physicians and Surgeons, recommends calling a physician if the case is particularly bad. You should keep in mind that alcohol is toxic, and can be deadly in large quantities. It is not unheard of to have people die of alcohol poisoning, when they have ingested too much alcohol in one evening. Blacking out, passing out, and vomiting are all signs of severe overindulgence and should not be treated lightly.

Less acute sufferers should, on awakening after a binge, take warmed fluids (tea, consommé, clam broth). As soon as your stomach feels in shape, eat warm, soft foods at frequent intervals—poached egg, milk toast, pureed soup, mashed potatoes. Despite your craving for cold, carbonated fluids, avoid them; they may cause stomach cramps.

To prevent a hangover as you drink, Dr. Guild recommends taking *fructose.* Fructose, or *levulose,* is a crystalline sugar, the sweetest of the sugars. It increases the rate at which the body metabolizes and eliminates alcohol. It seems to work best when the alcohol is combined with something naturally high in fructose, as the tomato juice in a Bloody Mary, for example. Or just sip tomato juice between drinks.

Looking for quick panaceas in the medicine cabinet to cure a hangover or any other condition seems to become increasingly popular after age 40. Panaceas are all right up to a point, but indiscriminate self-treatment can do a great deal of harm, because it may mask a more serious illness or may prevent a condition from clearing up if left alone. In drinking, as in eating, the key is moderation.

Proper diet

Proper diet is an important contribution an individual can make to his good health, because foods build body tissues and provide energy for the body to work. Adequate diet planning is not difficult. The basic rules of good nutrition must be learned. See Ch. 27, *Nutrition and Weight Control,* for a full treatment of diet and nutrition. Applying these rules to a daily diet will take only a few minutes of planning when the menu is decided upon, and will reap enormous rewards in good health and appearance. The hardest part of planning a balanced diet is to avoid selecting food solely on the basis of taste or convenience and ignoring nutritional value.

Vitamins

Eating a proper, balanced diet will fulfill vitamin and other nutritional requirements. Therefore, there is no need for a healthy person who eats nutritious foods to take vitamin pills. Vitamins and other food supplements should be taken only on the advice of a physician or dentist. If a person decides he is deficient in some dietary element and purchases a patent medicine to treat the problem, he may only make it worse. It is rare to find someone deficient in only one element, and by trying to treat himself, he may delay seeking the advice of a physician.

Breakfast

Many Americans neglect breakfast, an important contribution to good diet. Studies prove that men, women, and children need an adequate breakfast. A good breakfast can provide a start in obtaining the day's vitamin and mineral requirements. It is also a help to dieters and those trying to maintain a stable weight, since those who have eaten a good breakfast are able to avoid mid-morning snacks such as sweet rolls, cakes, and the like, which are usually high in carbohydrates and calories.

Weight and Health

Overweight is one of the biggest deterrents to successful middle age, and is also one of the greatest threats to health and longevity. As one physician said, "Consider how few really obese persons you see over 60 years of age." Unfortunately, in middle age most of us maintain the eating habits of our youth while we cut down on our exercise. The result: added weight that acts as a deterrent to our physical well-being.

The overweight person is more likely to develop arthritis, diabetes, heart disease, high blood pressure, kidney trouble, and many other disabling or fatal disorders.

As reported in *Nation's Business,* "If you are overweight by 10 percent, your chances of surviving the next 20 years are 15 percent less than if you had ideal weight; if you are 20 percent overweight, your chances are 25 percent less; if you are 30 percent overweight, 45 percent less." In other words, the odds are against the overweight.

If you do not know what your ideal weight should be, a physician can tell you. To check yourself, try the "pinch" test. Take a pinch of skin on your upper arm just below the shoulder. If more than a half-inch separates your fingers, you are too fat. Try the same test on your stomach when you're standing erect. And, of course, your mirror can reveal the tell-tale signs of middle-age fat—the double chin, sagging belly, flabby arms and legs.

Good Eating Habits

Is there any magic way to reduce? The only sure way is to *eat less,* and to continue this practice all the time. It will not help if you go on a crash diet and then resume your normal eating habits. And while exercise will help control weight and burn up excess calories, probably the best exercise is to push yourself away from the table before you've overeaten.

Calories do count, and usually the caloric intake of a person in the 40- to 55-year age bracket should be about one-third less than that of a person between ages 25 and 40. Again, your physician or a good calorie-counter can help you determine what to eat and how much.

Here are some additional tips from nutritionists to help you lose weight:

- *Cut down on quantity.* Eat just enough to satisfy your appetite— not as much as you can. Even low-calorie foods will add weight if you eat enough of them.

- *Eat less more often.* Spread your food intake over several meals or snacks. Some hospitals have been experimenting with five meals a day, spreading the recommended total food intake over two full meals a day (brunch and dinner) and three snacks (continental breakfast, afternoon snack, and evening). They find that the stomach handles small amounts of food better, that metabolism keeps working at a good pace all day, and that blood sugar levels (your energy reserve) do not drop between meals.

- *Avoid high-calorie foods.* Cut out breads, rolls, jellies, jams, sauces, gravies, dressings, creams, and rich desserts. These are the villains that add calories and are not as rich in nutrients.

- *Look for natural flavors.* Cultivate an interest in the natural flavor of what you eat. Try vegetables without butter, coffee and tea without cream and sugar. You might want to substitute a squeeze of lemon on your vegetables or noncaloric sweeteners in your beverages.

- *Serve only just enough.* Keep portions small and put serving dishes with leftovers out of sight. Taking seconds is often just a habit. Cultivate the idea of just one serving, and you will find it satisfies the appetite. Another idea: serve meals on smaller plates. the portion will look big if only in relationship to the size of the plate.

In order to maintain a healthy body and a youthful appearance while dieting, you must make sure you eat the necessary proteins and nutrients.

This can be done by selecting foods from the four basic food groups. See Ch. 27, *Nutrition and Weight Control.*

As a panel of experts on middle age said in a recent interview: "Two factors are vital to successful middle age: physical activity and a variety of interests. Move around but don't rush around. Keep an open mind and a closed refrigerator. Remember that variety is more than the spice of life—it's the wellspring of life. The person who pursues a variety of activities will usually stay fit long after middle age."

Living Life
to the Fullest

No wise man ever wished to be younger. —JONATHAN SWIFT

Staying young is looked on by most of the rest of the world as a peculiarly American obsession. This obsession is certainly fostered and exploited by the advertising industry, but its causes have to be looked for elsewhere.

In many countries, it is the old who are venerated for their wisdom and authority. This point of view is likely to prevail in societies that stay the same or that enjoyed their greatest glories in the past.

America is another matter. Because of its history, it is literally a young country. It is also a nation built on the idea of progress and hope in the future. And to whom does the future belong if not to youth?

Keeping up with change is unfortunately identified by too many people with how they look rather than how they think or feel. To be young in heart and spirit has very little to do with wearing the latest style in clothes—no matter how unbecom-

ing—or learning the latest dances. Maintaining an open mind receptive to new ideas, keeping the capacity for pleasure in the details of daily living, refusing to be overwhelmed by essentially unimportant irritations can make the middle years more joyful for any family.

A Critical Time

Nowadays, the average American can expect to reach the age of 70. Thus, for most people, the middle years begin during the late 30s. Ideally, these are the years of personal fulfillment accompanied by a feeling of pride in accomplishment, a deeper knowledge of one's strengths and limitations, and a growing understanding and tolerance of other people's ideas and behavior.

Emotional Pressures

In many families, however, the pleasures of maturity often go hand in hand with increased pressures. It's no simple matter for the typical husband and wife in their 40s to maintain emotional health while handling worries about money, aging parents, anxiety about willful teenagers, tensions caused by marital friction, and feelings of depression about getting older. To some people, the problems of the middle years are so burdensome that instead of dealing with them realistically—by eliminating some, by compromising in the solution of others—they escape into excessive drinking or into sexual infidelity. It doesn't take much thought to realize that those escapes do nothing except introduce new problems.

Physical Symptoms
of Emotional Problems

For others, deep-seated conflicts that come to a head during the middle

years may be expressed in chronic physical symptoms. Many physicians in the past intuitively understood the relationship between emotional and physical health, but it is only in recent years that medical science has proved that feelings of tension, anxiety, suppressed anger, and frustration are often the direct cause of ulcers, sexual impotence, high blood pressure, and heart attacks, not to mention sleeplessness and headaches.

Of course, there are no magic formulas that guarantee the achievement of emotional well-being at any time of life. Nor does any sensible person expect to find a perfect solution to any human problem. However, it is possible to come to grips with specific difficulties and deal with them in ways that can reduce stress and safeguard emotional health.

Sexuality during
the Middle Years

In spite of the so-called sexual revolution and all its accompanying publicity, it is still very difficult for most people to sort out their attitudes towards sexual activity. It is a subject that continues to be clouded by feelings of guilt and anxiety, surrounded by taboos, and saddled with misinformation. For each individual, the subject is additionally complicated by personal concepts of love and morality.

Many people were shocked when the Kinsey reports on male and female sexual behavior appeared. More recently, militant efforts have been made in various communities to prevent the schools from including sex education in their courses of study. Yet marriage counselors, family physicians, ministers, and all other specialists in human relations can attest to the amount of human misery caused by ignorance about sex—all the way from the ignorance that results in a 15-year-old's unwanted pregnancy to the ignorance of a 50-year-old man about his wife's sexual needs.

Sexuality After Menopause

Sexual relations between partners can continue throughout the life of the marriage. There is no reason that a person cannot remain sexually active, barring medical complications, for one's entire life.

Sexual function will change with aging. It takes longer for a man to obtain an erection and it takes longer to achieve orgasm for both partners. Women may suffer from thinning and drying of the vaginal walls following menopause, but the difficulties that this may cause are easily remedied. Lubricants that are water-based (unlike petroleum jelly, which is oil-based) can be used to replace natural lubricants. If it takes longer to arouse one partner, then set aside a little more time for romance.

It may be easier for the couple to enjoy lovemaking in the morning, after a good night's rest, rather than the end of the evening when they both may be tired. Since it is likely that there will be no children in the house to interrupt, couples may find that there is a renewed interest in sex, because of a new-found freedom that comes with having grown children and having no fear of pregnancy.

There are circumstances, though, that may arrive that hinder or block sexual relations. These are discussed in brief here.

Problems with Sexual Activity

Occasional problems with sexual drive or capabilities are normal. Most people will experience some fluctuation during their lifetime. If a problem persists beyond a few weeks, or if any pain is associated with sexual intercourse, you should consult with your doctor. Although the causes may be psychological, it is best that you do not draw this conclusion without speaking with a medical expert first. Some of the problems that may be experienced follow.

Impotence

Impotence is defined as a lack of adequate erection to complete intercourse. This can be experienced on a temporary basis because of fatigue, overindulgence in alcohol or drugs, stress, or other factors that physically affect the system. It can be experienced on a more long-term basis and still not be physiological in origin.

Some of the psychological causes for impotence include: resentment, hostility, and anger at one's spouse; stress and anxiety from any aspect of one's life; and fear of sexual inadequacy and impotence. This last point is important because the fear of impotence can bring on impotence. If one experience of impotence triggers fear, the cycle of fear and inability to perform can prolong recovery. It is important to remember that over half the cases of impotence are psychologically based and are cured once the cause is resolved.

Physiological reasons for impotence usually involve the blood flow and the nerve response to the penis. In diabetics, the combination of nerve loss and restricted blood flow can reduce sexual capacity. With some men, artery blockage restricts the flow of blood to the penis. Surgery may be able to remedy some causes of impotence. Your doctor can advise you on any specific problems you encounter.

New Treatments

Where other approaches fail, the impotent male can either undergo a test for erectability or try one of the new treatments currently available. Conducted during sleep, the tests provide evidence indicating that impotence in any given case has physical or psychological causes. Physical causes may include such diseases as diabetes; some drugs or medication, including those used to treat high blood pressure; and alcohol abuse, hardening of the arteries, or testosterone or thyroid hormone deficiencies.

These tests have shown that physical causes underlie impotence in nearly half of all cases. As a result much research has been conducted into physical "cures." All of the tests operate on the accepted medical principle that "normal" men have approximately five erections during every sleep period. In what is called the *stamp test*, a strip of stamps is wrapped around the penis before the subject retires for the night. Fitted snugly around the shaft of the penis, the strip tears along one of the perforated edges if the subject experiences an erection while sleeping.

Two other tests are more reliable. In one, a *snap gauge band* made of elastic fabric and Velcro is wrapped around the penis; the band has three snaps designed to open at various stages of penile rigidity. A third test utilizes a *Nocturnal Penile Tumescence Monitor* to tell exactly when erections occur, with what rigidity, and for how long. Two circular elastic silicone bands are attached to the penis; sensor wires connect the bands to an apparatus like an electrocardiograph machine.

Of the prosthetic devices used to "cure" impotence, three can be implanted in the penis in operations that take one to three hours under local anesthetic. The simplest utilizes two semirigid rods that keep the penis permanently erect. A second implanted type, made of flexible, plastic-covered metal wire, also maintains the penis in a constantly erect state but can be bent into an erect or downward position. A third type works hydraulically to pump the penis into a naturally erect state. Two expandable metal tubes implanted in the penis function with an attached tiny pump in the scrotum and a water reservoir placed behind the muscles of the lower abdomen. Pressure on the pump causes the penis to erect; valves make possible penile relaxation.

Disinterest

Disinterest, which was referred to as frigidity in women, can be experienced by both women and men. It may be traced to hostility or resentment toward the partner, lack of adequate satisfaction during intercourse, other psychological impediments, or physical problems. Some medications can reduce libido; depression may also reduce the sex drive. Consult with your physician to eliminate physical reasons, and follow up with therapy if no physical ailments are suspected.

Self-Image Problems

If you do not believe yourself to be physically appealing, it is likely that you will regard a partner with suspicion and hostility if he or she finds you physically appealing. You may be willing to perceive insult and ill-intent where none is meant if you do not believe yourself to be a desirable partner.

Self-image is one of the most important aspects of sexuality. The belief that one is too old, too fat, too thin, too wrinkly, too whatever can be a huge obstacle to a satisfying life. Self-image is estimated to be a problem for half of the male population and the majority of the female population. One cannot change the view others have of beauty, but one can improve a self-image. This may require counseling, but is worth it in the long-run, since the ability to be happy rests with the ability to be happy with oneself.

Sexual Activity and Disability

Disabilities, whether the result of genetics, disease, accident, or aging, need not be a complete barrier to sexual satisfaction. Most disabilities allow some form of sexual gratification and with an understanding partner, this can be worked out. Counseling and training may be needed to develop the emotional support and understanding necessary to achieve a fulfilling relationship with your partner, but if both are willing participants in the learning process, this can be achieved. Talk with your physician or a therapist specializing in disabilities about your situation. If they cannot provide guidance, they should be able to direct you to someone who can.

Coping With Retirement

For more people, retirement makes up several years of their lives. As the average age of men and women extend into the seventies, the number of years one spends in retirement increases. These years can be spent with a fulfilling and exciting lifestyle, or they can pass slowly, with little to look forward to. It is important that people consider their retirement before they get to it. If they have not done so and find themselves at retirement age, it is important that they set goals and prioritize how they want the days to be spent.

Preparation for Retirement

The single biggest concern to most retirees is finance. With Social Security under constant scrutiny by the government, it is important that everyone consider what money they have coming in from sources other than the Social Security program.

Start planning for your retirement by figuring out *exactly* what money you will have coming in, and when, for your retirement. Questions you will need to investigate include:

- What are you and your spouse's pension benefits from work?
- How are these benefits affected by the death of the spouse, before and after retirement age?
- What are you scheduled to receive from Social Security?
- What are your savings and other benefits worth?
- What other sources of income will be available to you after retirement?

You should fill in the *Request for Earnings and Benefit Statement* form SSA-7004 every three years to insure that the government records of your earnings are accurate. They are only obliged to correct your records for the previous three years. This also keeps you informed of what you are entitled to for your income credits. The form is available through all Social Security offices.

You should also be aware that the age of retirement for Social Security is no longer strictly held at 65 years of age. For people born between 1954 and 1960, the age is 66. For those born in 1960 and after, the age is 67. There is a reduction of payments related to your age, if you retire early.

Once you have figured out what money you have coming in, you need to do a budget for what you will be spending after retirement. This is tricky since inflation and property-cost fluctuations can be hard to predict. However, it is better to guess than to just ignore this step.

You need to figure out basic expenses, and then extra expenses and perks. If you would love to sail around the world, don't just assume you can't do it. Calculate it into your retirement needs and see if you can save enough now with investments to allow for your dreams.

Basic expenses should include as a minimum:

- Property and income taxes
- House repairs, rent, and other living quarter expenses
- Medical insurance and expenses
- Food, clothing, and day-to-day purchases
- Expenses remaining for children (college, etc.)
- Emergency income for nursing homes, catastrophic illness or other incapacitating problems
- General entertainment and activity costs

Once these are down on paper, discuss what your goals and ambitions are for the years ahead. Budget in those expenses. Some possibilities include, but certainly are not limited to:

- returning to school
- traveling
- pursuing a hobby
- moving to another climate
- starting another career or business

Assume that you will live to at least 95. This way you likely to have enough for the majority of your retirement. You are better off overpredicting, rather than underpredicting, your age at death.

Calculate your expenses for the total of the thirty years. You can set inflation at 5% or higher, or use a guide to retirement earnings. Then figure out what you will have as income when you retire. If you have enough saved, and enough pension to provide for all your needs, then you are set for retirement. If not, you need to calculate what you have still to save.

There are several guides available for a more exact method of predicting costs and savings. The American Association of Retired Persons (AARP) can guide you to sources. Their address is: 601 E Street, NW, Washington DC, 20049; phone (202) 434-2277.

When to Retire

Once you have figured out your financial needs and earnings for retirement, you can estimate how many years you have saved for, and how many years you still need to work to gain enough income to provide for retirement. If you can afford early retirement, and you have activities that would fulfill you, it should be considered as an option. If you find that you have to continue working beyond the time you had assumed for retirement, you may be able to manage with less hours or a job with less pressure without influencing your pension.

Beyond Retirement

Once you have the finances figured out for your retirement (or if you have retired), you need to figure out how you are going to spend your time. These years can be the most rewarding and exciting of your life. There are literally hundreds of ways for you to spend your time. If you are thoughtful about your retirement planning, you may find that you still don't have enough time in the day to do everything that you want.

Volunteer Work

Volunteer work can be one of the most rewarding ways to spend your time. Depending on your community, there will be a variety of places that are happy to train and utilize volunteers in different positions. Depending on your personal needs, volunteer positions can range from basic tasks—such as greeting visitors, assisting patients in reading, or escorting people—to jobs that resemble working positions, such as accounting, staff management, and teaching. You can select what you want to do with the level of effort you are interested in putting in. You can do more than one volunteer position to fill different needs. You may want to work one or two days with children, and then take on a more pressured, or less pressured, position elsewhere for another day of activity. You should research and ask around about the organizations that take volunteers. Most arts organizations, museums, zoos, hospitals, schools, day care centers, and nonprofit organizations rely on their volunteers for many jobs.

Community Activism

You may be interested in pursuing your volunteer work in another arena entirely. Political and social activism is based on volunteer support. That support is both financial- and assistance-based. You are in a position, once you retire, to take your expertise to an organization that fights for the positions you support and believe in. If no organization exists in the area you want to dedicate your time, then start one. Chances are good that if you are interested in something, others are out there who are also interested. This resolves two potential problems in retirement: activity and social contact. you will meet people with similar interests by participating in community organizations.

Home Management

Once you have retired, you will probably be spending a few more hours, at least, in your home. This is when the dripping faucet, the faded carpet, and the stained walls will become more annoying. Do not take on more repair work than you can do physically or afford financially. Plan repairs and redecorating to accommodate your time and your budget. Overhauling your home may be a goal, but it should be planned as such and not decided on one afternoon. The stress of remodeling and renovating should be taken into account with your physical health.

Leaving the Children and Children Leaving

One of the major turning points in many lives is when the children grow up and leave the house. Children will usually move out of their parents houses, for at least part of the year, between the ages of 18 and 21. The majority of children are permanently out of the house by the time they are 22.

For many families, this shift from being a full-time caregiver to a child to a parent of independent adults is a difficult one. Regardless of the continued contact through visits and calls, the separation of living space may be difficult for the parent to adjust to. It may also be difficult for the child to adjust to; transition to adulthood can be rocky.

Once the children are off on their own, the parent may find him- or herself with a sense of loss, lack of purpose, or anxiety. All of this may be attributed to the last child moving out, or it may be to a combination of events, such as a child leaving and a sixtieth birthday. If you or your spouse experience any prolonged or severe bouts of depression, it is important to consult with a therapist, even if you are sure you recognize the source of the depression. Recovering from the depression is what you should be working toward.

Many parents, however, find the empty home an enjoyable change. After adapting to the new patterns of living without children, they find that the respite from caring for others can be exhilarating. For some parents, this may be the first time in two decades where their days are completely their own to decide. It provides the opportunity to put oneself first. Although there may be some residual guilt about self-indulgence, it should pass quickly. This is the opportunity to nurture and care for yourself and your spouse as you have cared for your children. And, as any parent will attest, your children will continue to provide you with parenting concerns for the rest of your life.

The biggest consideration you should focus on during this transition is your emotional and mental state. As with any major life change, the period of transition will create stress, mood changes, and susceptibility to depression. If you experience any of the warning signs of depression (suicidal or violent thoughts, inertia, or chronic insomnia are some of the signs), please contact your physician or therapist.

Separation and Divorce

Marriage in this country is based on the highly personal concept of love rather than on such traditional foundations as a property merger between two families or an arrangement determined by the friendship of the young people's parents. It is often assumed, therefore, that if mutual love is the basis for embarking on a marriage, its absence is a valid reason for dissolving it, either by legal separation or divorce.

The idea of divorce is not particularly modern; in practically every time and place where a form of marriage has existed, so has some form of divorce, with reasons ranging from excessive wife-beating to failure to deliver a piece of land mentioned in the marriage contract.

The High Rate of Divorce

What is new is the high rate of divorce. Figures now indicate that in the United States as a whole, approximately one in every four marriages is terminated by legal arrangement. However, these figures by no means indicate that the family as an institution is on the way out, because a constantly increasing number of people who get divorced get married again.

There are many reasons for the growing rate of separation and divorce:

- Over the last 50 years, a continually increasing percentage of the population has been getting married.

- Although the trend toward earlier marriages has leveled off in recent years, a significant number of people still marry at earlier ages than was common in the past. (The number of divorces is highest among the poorly educated group who marry under the age of 21.)

- The legal requirements for separation and divorce are less rigid than formerly.

- With increasing independence and earning capacity, women are less frightened of the prospect of heading a family.

- The poorer groups in the population, in which desertion was a common practice, are more often obtaining divorces.

Contrary to popular belief, there are more divorces among the poor than among the rich, and more among the less well-educated than among the educated. Also, most divorces occur before the fifth year of marriage.

Telling the Truth to Children

Most people with children who are contemplating a breakup of their marriage generally make every effort to seek professional guidance that might help them iron out their differences. When these efforts fail and steps are taken to arrange for a separation or divorce, it is far healthier for parents to be honest with each other and with their children than to construct elaborate explanations based on lies.

A teenager who is given the real reason for a divorce is less likely to have something to brood about than

one who is told lies that he can see through. If the real reason for a divorce is that the parents have tried their best to get along with each other but find it impossible, the child who is in his teens or older can certainly understand this. If the marriage is coming to an end because the husband or wife wants to marry someone else, the explanation to the child should avoid assigning blame. When the rejected parent tries to enlist the child's sympathy by blackening the character of the parent who is supposedly the cause of the divorce, results are almost always unpleasant. Under no circumstances and no matter what his age should a child be called on to take the side of either parent or to act as a judge.

Nor should children be told any more about the circumstances of the breakup of a marriage than they really want to know. Young people have a healthy way of protecting themselves from information they would find hurtful, and if they ask few questions, they need be told only the facts they are prepared to cope with. Of course, as they grow older and live through their own problems, they will form their own view of what really happened between their parents.

After the Separation

Traditionally, in separation and divorce proceedings, the children have remained in the custody of the mother, with financial support arrangements and visiting rights spelled out for the father. Although an increasing number of fathers have been awarded custody of their children in recent years, it is still commonly the mother who must face the problems of single parenthood after divorce. Although teenage children may need some extra attention for a while, there is no need for a mother to make

a martyr of herself, nor should she feel guilty when she begins to consider remarrying.

The father should be completely reliable in his visiting arrangements, and if he has remarried, should try to establish good relationships between the offspring of his former marriage and his new family.

Losing a Spouse

As you and your spouse get older, you should begin to prepare for the fact that one of you will probably survive the other. This can be the most difficult challenge you face. Having a spouse or a child die can be the most strenuous and difficult parts of life. It can occur at any time during adulthood. Widows and widowers are not just people in their 70s and 80s. One can lose a spouse at 21 or 41 and experience the same sense of loss and confusion.

Depending on the preparations made before the spouse dies, the concerns of the surviving spouse may range from mourning and adjusting to single life to attempting to arrange financial support, dividing inheritance, and struggling to sort through all the legal and financial matters that may be left by the deceased.

Preparing a will is one of the things you can do in preparation for your own and your spouse's death. You cannot assume that everything will be easily handled if you die and your spouse is surviving. Wills provide some legal assistance to the surviving spouse to sort through finances during the difficult times that follow the spouse's death.

It is important for anyone, of any age, to maintain a strong support group of friends and family. Without this, any change in one's life will be confronted alone. With a strong group of supporters, almost any tragedy can be weathered. Meeting people and making friends can be a difficult thing to do. By joining clubs, support groups, and organizations, you are reaching out to people with similar backgrounds or interests. It is likely that you will be able to establish some contacts through such activities. You and your spouse may wish to pursue this together, or you may each seek out friends of your own interest. If you have relocated or do not, for whatever reason, have a circle of friends you can turn to, it is important to establish one. It makes the transition to widowhood easier if your support group is in place.

If you have already lost a spouse and have not prepared for it, you can still seek out a support group in your community. This may be found in churches and synagogues, community centers, and in local organizations. As explained before, it is important to watch for any warning signs of serious depression and seek professional counseling immediately if any are experienced.

Loss of a Parent

The loss of a parent may affect your family when you or your partner lose a parent, or when you lose a spouse and your children have lost a parent.

It is important to work through the mourning period. Some people respond to death by attempting to plow through the time, as if unscathed by the event. Others shut down entirely and refuse consolation or assistance in coping. Neither response may be in the best interest of the mourner.

Coping with death is a personal experience. Each individual will respond uniquely to a loss of a family member. And each individual may respond differently to different losses. Mourning one's parent will be different than mourning one's spouse. It is important for everyone to remember this when adjusting to a death in the family.

The mourning period can range from several days to several months. There is no correct period of time to spend in mourning. If you are not comfortable with the amount of time you are taking to get over the loss, then feel free to speak to someone about it. But there is no rule of thumb for how long you should spend mourning.

Any inability to function through day-to-day activities, such as eating, sleeping, bathing, grocery shopping, or other mundane events, should be taken as a sign of serious depression and not part of general mourning. You may not feel like socializing, but you should still have the energy to take good hygienic care of yourself. As always, any behavior that is threatening to life and health should be referred to professional counseling immediately. You should watch for such signs in yourself, your parents and your children after experiencing any family member's death.

6

The Later Years

Aging
and What To Do About It

Growing older could mean growing healthier. In many ways you are as old as you think and feel. Consider these points:

- No disease results just from the passage of years.

- We age piecemeal—each organ separately rather than uniformly.

- In retirement you have less daily stress and strain, and you have more time to take care of yourself.

What, then, makes a person think and feel old?

The Aging Process

Physically, we mature at about 25 to 30, when the body reaches maximum size and strength. Then, body tissues and cells are constantly being rebuilt and renewed. Nutrition, rest, exercise, and stress influence the length of time that the body can maintain a balance between the wearing down and rebuilding of body tissues. When more cells die than can be reproduced, they are replaced by a fibrous, inert substance called *colagen*. The living process slows down to compensate, and we begin aging; strength and ability start to decline.

But this happens at various intervals. For instance, vision is sharpest at age 25; the eye loses its ability to make rapid adjustments in focus after age 40. Hearing is sharpest at about age 10, then diminishes as you grow older. Sensitivity to taste and smell lessens after age 60.

The decline in strength and muscle ability is long and gradual; there are even gratifying plateaus. At age 50, a man still has about four-fifths of the muscle strength he had when he was 25.

Although physical abilities may decline, mental abilities may actually improve during the middle years, and memory and the ability to learn can remain keen. Dr. Alfred Schwartz, dean of education at Drake University, was asked: "Can a 70-year-old man in reasonably good health learn as rapidly as a 17- year-old boy?" Dr. Schwartz answered:

Indeed he can—provided he's in the habit of learning. The fact that some older people today are not active intellectually is no reflection on their ability to learn. There is ample proof that learning ability does not automatically decline with age.

Regardless of what you may have heard, organic brain damage affects less than one percent of those over age 65.

But in thinking about physical change, remember that this is just one aspect of aging. Age is determined by emotional and intellectual maturity as well as by chronological years.

Can a person do anything to retard aging?

Most *gerontologists* feel that the reason more people don't live longer is that they are not willing to follow a regimen of diet, exercise, rest, recreation—coupled with the exclusion of various excesses. And while there isn't anything you can do to set back the clock, you can keep in good health by making sure to have regular physical examinations, sufficient exercise, adequate rest, nutritious food, and a positive mental attitude.

A Positive Mental Attitude

Mark Twain once said: "Whatever a

man's age he can reduce it several years by putting a bright-colored flower in his buttonhole." A lively, fresh outlook is essential for enjoyable living at any age. Most physicians believe there is a direct connection between one's state of mind and physical health. This is especially true when you are faced with the challenges of retirement. Plato said: "He who is of a calm and happy nature will hardly feel the pressure of age, but to him who is of an opposite disposition, youth and age are equally a burden."

Experts in the field of aging have found that most older people can relieve transitory depression by a deliberate shift of thought or by physical activity. If you look upon retirement as an opportunity to take better care of yourself and to pursue old and new interests, you'll go a long way toward better health.

The Annual Checkup

For peace of mind and to maintain and improve your health, make it a habit to see your physician at least once a year. To remind themselves, many people make an appointment on their birthday. An annual checkup is especially important in later years and should not be put off or neglected.

During a routine checkup, the physician pays special attention to enlarged lymph nodes of the neck, armpits, and groin, and the front of the neck. He also checks the condition of veins and arteries and looks at your knees and arches—which are of particular importance to older people.

He makes tests for arteriosclerosis, high blood pressure, diabetes, brain tumors, and other diseases. He can feel and tap your body to check your lungs, liver, and spleen, and he can take electrocardiographs to detect changes in your heart. Simple tests can note bladder and kidney conditions.

In addition, the physician usually asks about personal habits—smoking, drinking, eating. He also wants to know about any unusual symptoms you might have. Be completely frank with your physician, answer his questions as directly as possible, and give all information that might be helpful.

When explaining the nature of your ailment or symptom, tell him what part of the body is involved, what changes are associated with the symptoms, and whether symptoms occurred after a change of diet or medicine. Tell him about any previous experiences with this condition and what treatments you might have had.

It is extremely important to tell your physician about any pills you are taking—including aspirin, tranquilizers, and sleeping tablets. Even the most common drug can affect the potency of medication he might prescribe.

After he has taken your case history and after he has all the reports from your tests, the physician will want to talk with you, explain his findings, and perhaps make some recommendations. Take his advice; don't try to be your own physician.

If you have questions, don't be afraid to ask them. Have him explain the nature of your ailment, how long it may take for relief or cure, how the therapy or medication is expected to work, and the possible impact on your everyday activities.

Hopefully, by following his advice you'll stay healthy and well. However, if you are at home and feel ill, call your physician if:

- Your symptoms are so severe you can't endure them.

- Apparent minor symptoms persist without explainable cause.

- You are in doubt.

For more information, see "The Physical Examination" in Ch. 26, *Physicians and Diagnostic Procedures.*

Oral Health

It is especially important in later years to have regular dental checkups. After age 50, over half of the American people have some form of *periodontal disease*, and at age 65 nearly all persons have this disease.

Brushing teeth and gums regularly is a defense against periodontal disease. Use dental floss to remove all food particles and plaque from areas between the teeth, especially after each meal. See "Periodontal Disease" in Ch. 22, *The Teeth and Gums*, for more information on this subject.

Dentures

If you do lose some teeth, they should be replaced with bridges or partial or full dentures, because the cheeks and lips will otherwise sag and wrinkle and make you look older than you really are. Chewing ability and the clarity of speech are also impaired if missing teeth are not replaced. See "Dentures" in Ch. 22, *The Teeth and Gums.*

Diet and Health

Just what are your food requirements as you grow older? Basically you need the same essential nutrients that you have always needed, except that you face special problems. You need to:

- Select food more carefully to eat adequate proteins, vitamins, and minerals—while cutting down on calories.

- Get the most nutritious food for the least money and make the most of what you buy.

- Avoid bad eating habits—make mealtime a pleasure rather than a chore.

- Learn new techniques to stretch meals, use leftovers, and substitute lower-priced items with the same nutritional value for higher-priced foods. In other words, learn how to shop well.

Basic Requirements

How can you get the essential nutrients every day? A good rule is first to eat recommended servings from the Basic Four Food Groups (see below) established by the National Research Council. Then, eat other foods that you like, as long as they do not go over the recommended daily caloric intake. The average man in the 55-to-75-year age group should consume 2,200 calories a day; the average woman in the same age group, 1,600 calories a day. This is a drop of between 500 and 600 calories a day from what was needed at age 25. As you grow older, your physical activity decreases and your metabolism slows, causing body fats to build up at a much higher rate and making you more prone to hardening of the arteries and certain heart conditions.

Here are the Basic Four Food Groups:

Meat Group

Two or more servings from this group of foods are recommended daily. A serving is two to three ounces of cooked meat, fish, or poultry; two eggs; occasionally one cup of cooked dry beans or peas; one-half cup peanut butter; or one cup cottage cheese.

Dairy Foods

Dairy food requirements may be satisfied by two cups of milk or its equivalent in cheese, ice cream, etc. A one and one-third ounce slice of cheddar-type cheese or one scant pint of ice cream is equivalent to one cup of milk. Imitation ice cream or ice milk where vegetable fat has been substituted for butterfat has just as much protein.

Vegetables and Fruit

The daily vegetable and fruit requirement consists of four or more servings. A serving is one-half cup. Include one serving of citrus fruit each day and dark green or deep yellow vegetables every other day.

Bread and Cereal Group

Each day have four or more servings of whole grain, enriched, or restored products such as breads, cereals, rice, hominy grits, noodles, or macaroni. One serving is a slice of bread; one-half to three-fourths cup cooked cereal, pasta, or rice; one medium potato.

Use other foods such as sweets, baked goods, or desserts to complete meals and treat the sweet tooth. But remember to count calories. Nutritionists have found that skinny animals live longer than fat ones, and this seems to be true of people, too.

Beware of food fads and so-called health foods unless these are recommended by your physician. Also, do not buy vitamins and mineral tablets unless prescribed. When you obtain vitamins from food, your body uses the amount necessary to maintain proper health, appetite, and resistance to infection. Your body promptly eliminates excesses of vitamin C and the B complex, and stores an excess of vitamins A and D in your liver and other body organs. It may take up to seven years of practically complete deprivation for a previously healthy adult to show signs of a vitamin deficiency.

Some older people may go on low-fat diets because of fear of cholesterol caused by talk and advertisements for unsaturated fats. Get a physician's recommendation before curtailing your fat intake—too little fat and dairy products can be as harmful as too much.

Also, unless prescribed, do not take iron tonics or pills. Usually you'll get adequate iron intake if you eat meat, eggs, vegetables, and enriched cereals regularly. Adding more iron to a normal diet may even be harmful.

Eating Habits

If you find that mealtime is a chore rather than a pleasure, try these tips to enhance your meals:

- Try a two-meal-a-day schedule. Have a late breakfast and early dinner when you are really hungry. But be sure to get your Basic Four requirements in these two meals.

- Drink a glass of water as soon as you wake up to promote good digestion, weight control, and bowel movements.

- Try a walk or light exercise to stimulate appetite and to regulate body processes. Moderate exercise also will help regulate weight because it burns up calories.

- You might sip glass of wine before dinner. Recent research shows wine is very useful to older people in improving appetite and digestion. Port, a light sherry, and vermouth with a dash of soda are good appetite stimulators.

- Make meals interesting by including some food of distinctive flavor to contrast with a mild-flavored food; something crisp for contrast with softer foods, even if it is only a pickle or a lettuce leaf; some brightly colored food for eye appeal.

- Pep up your food with a judicious use of herbs and spices or flavor-enhancers like wine, bottled sauces, fruit juices, and peels.

- If some food causes you distress, eliminate it and substitute something else of equal nutritive value. Green salad may include too much roughage for the intestinal tract; ham or bacon may be supplying your body with too much salt, which increases water retention. Or you may be drinking too much coffee, tea, or soft drinks.

- Be realistic about your chewing ability. Food swallowed whole may be causing digestive problems. If your teeth are not as good as they were or if you are wearing dentures, try cubing, chopping, or grinding foods that are difficult to chew. Let your knife or meat grinder do part of the work.

- Try a different atmosphere or different setting for your meals. Use candlelight, music, and your best linen on occasion. Move outdoors when the weather is good; eat your lunch in the park and dinner on the patio.

- Occasionally invite a friend or relative to dine with you. It's surprising what stimulating conversation and an exchange of ideas can do to boost your mood and appetite.

- Try a new recipe or a new food. Thanks to modern transportation, foods are available in larger cities from many areas and other countries. Eat eggplant or okra, avocado or artichoke, gooseberry jam, or garbanzo beans in a salad. And why not have a papaya with lemon juice for breakfast?

Cooking Hints

Try these ideas for preparing food more easily; they are especially useful if you have only a single gas or electric burner:

- Combine your vegetables and meat—or some other protein food—in a single pot or pan. You can cook many hot, nourishing meals of this kind: Irish stew, braised liver or pot roast with vegetables, ham-and-vegetable chowder or fish chowder, a New England boiled dinner.

- Combine leftovers to make a one-dish meal. Leftover meat combines beautifully with vegetables, macaroni, or rice. Add a cheese or tomato sauce or a simple white sauce and heat in a baking dish. Chopped tomatoes or green onions or chives will give extra flavor and color to the dish.

- Round out one-dish meals with a crisp salad topped with cut strips of leftover cooked meat or poultry or another raw food, bread, a beverage, and perhaps a dessert.

- Mix leftover cooked vegetables with raw fresh ones, such as chopped celery, cucumber slices, tomatoes, green pepper, shredded cabbage, to make an interesting salad.

- Cream vegetables, meat, fish, or chicken. Or serve them with a tasty sauce. Use canned tomato or mushroom soup for a quick and easy sauce. If the dish is a bit skimpy, a hard-boiled egg may stretch it to serving size.

- Add a bit of relish, snappy cheese, or diced cucumber to a cooked dressing for meat or vegetable salad.

- If you cook a potato, an ear of corn, or some other vegetable in the bottom of a double boiler, you can use the top to warm rolls, heat leftover meat in gravy, or heat such foods as creamed eggs or fish.

The Value of Exercise

As you grow older, exercise can help you look, feel, and work better. Various organs and systems of the body, particularly the digestive process, are stimulated through activity, and, as a result, work more effectively.

You can improve your posture through exercise that tones supporting muscles. This not only improves appearance but can decrease the frequency of lower-back pain and disability.

Here are some other benefits of exercise: it can increase your ability to relax and tolerate fatigue; it improves muscle tone; reduces fat deposits; increases working capacity of the lungs; improves kidney and liver functions; increases volume of blood, hemoglobin, and red blood cells, leading to improved utilization of oxygen and iron.

Also, physically active people are less likely to experience a heart attack or other forms of cardiovascular disease than sedentary people. Moreover, an active person who does suffer a coronary attack will probably have a less severe form. The Public Health Service studied 5,000 adults in Framingham, Mass., for more than a decade. When any member of the group suffered a heart attack, his physical activity was reviewed. It was found that more inactive people suffered more fatal heart attacks than active members.

Walking for Exercise

Exercise need not be something you *must* do but rather something you *enjoy* doing. One of the most practical and enjoyable exercises is walking. Charles Dickens said:

Walk and be happy, walk and be healthy. The best of all ways to lengthen our days is to walk, steadily and with a purpose. The wandering man knows of certain ancients, far gone in years, who have staved off infirmities and dissolution by earnest walking—hale fellows close upon eighty and ninety, but brisk as boys.

The benefits of walking were revealed in a recent Health Insurance Plan study of 110,000 people in New York City. Those who had heart attacks were divided into two groups— walkers and nonwalkers. The first four weeks of illness were reviewed for both groups. At the end of the time 41 percent of the nonwalkers were dead, while only 23 percent of the walkers were. When all physical activity was considered, 57 percent of the inactive had died compared to only 16 percent of those who had some form of exercise.

Walking is as natural to the human body as breathing. It is a muscular symphony; all the foot, leg, and hip muscles and much of the back musculature are involved. The abdominal muscles tend to contract and support their share of the weight, and the diaphragm and rib muscles increase their action. There is automatic action of the arm and shoulder muscles; the shoulder and neck muscles get play as the head is held erect; the eye muscles are exercised as you look about you.

Other Types of Exercise

Swimming and bicycling exercise most of the muscles, and gardening is highly recommended. The fresh air is beneficial, the bending, squatting, and countless other movements exercise most parts of the body.

Surprisingly, most games do not provide good exercise. According to a physical fitness research laboratory at the University of Illinois, the trouble with most games is that the action

is intermittent—starting and stopping—a burst of energy and then a wait. The bowler swings a ball for two and one-half seconds and gets about one minute of actual muscular work per game. Golf is a succession of pause, swing, walk—or, more often, a ride to the next pause, swing, and so on. Also, you spend a lot of time standing and waiting for the party ahead and for your partners. Tennis gives one more exercise but it too involves a great deal of starting and stopping, as does handball. No game has the essential, tension-releasing pattern of continuous, vigorous, rhythmic motion found in such activities as walking, running, or jogging.

For formal exercises, you could join a gym, but you might find your enthusiasm waning after a few weeks. You could also exercise at home; there are many excellent books on exercise that provide programs for you to follow at home on a daily basis.

But everyone's exercise capacity varies. It is best to discuss any new exercise program with your physician, especially if you have some illness or are out of practice. Then select an exercise which is pleasant for you and suitable to your condition.

It is most important always to warm up before any strenuous exercise. The U.S. Administration on Aging's booklet, *The Fitness Challenge in the Later Years*, states:

> The enthusiast who tackles a keep-fit program too fast and too strenuously soon gives up in discomfort, if not in injury. A warm-up period should be performed by starting lightly with a continuous rhythmical activity such as walking and gradually increasing the intensity until your pulse rate, breathing, and body temperature are elevated. It's also desirable to do some easy stretching, pulling, and rotating exercises during the warm-up period.

The booklet outlines an excellent program—*red* (easiest), *white* (next), and *blue* (the most sustained and dif-

ficult). Each program is "designed to give a balanced workout utilizing all major muscle groups."

A Word of Caution

You may be exercising too strenuously if the following happens:

- Your heart does not stop pounding within 10 minutes after the exercise.

- You cannot catch your breath 10 minutes after the exercise.

- You are shaky for more than 30 minutes afterwards.

- You can't sleep well afterwards.

- Your fatigue (not muscle soreness) continues into the next day.

Sensible, moderate exercise geared to your own physical capacity can help to give you a sense of all-around well-being. As Dr. Ernest Simonson, associate professor of physiological hygiene at the University of Minnesota Medical School, has said:

> Those who exercise regularly never fail to mention that it makes them feel better in every way. It's common logic if one feels better, his attitude towards others will be more congenial. When one is in a cordial, happy frame of mind, he will likely make wiser decisions, and his world in general will look better.

Weight Control

Importantly, both diet and exercise affect the individual's ability to control his weight (see Ch. 27, *Nutrition and Weight Control*; "Weight Problems" in Ch. 23, *Aches, Pains, Nuisances, Worries*; and Ch. 37, *Physical Fitness*). Healthy habits in both areas provide a complete answer for many older persons. For others, some additional effort is required.

The same diet rules that help the older person feel well and function adequately will make weight control simpler. But persons beyond middle age who have weight problems should make extra efforts to bring their weight down. Extra pounds of fat only make it harder for the vital organs to function; excess poundage also forces the heart to work harder. A variety of diets may be used to bring your weight back to where it should be. But the calorie-counter program may suffice for most persons.

Exercise provides the second key to weight control. Many physicians feel that older persons of both sexes should walk at least a mile daily. Other exercises acclaimed by physicians include golf, gardening, working on or around the house, and similar activities. Some other basic rules regarding exercise and diet should be noted:

- Avoid junk, or high carbohydrate, food where possible.

- Make certain you are eating foods that provide enough protein.

- Eat to assuage hunger, not to drive away boredom.

- Remember that appetite usually decreases with age, and act accordingly.

- Avoid vitamins unless they are prescribed by your physician, and use them accordingly.

- Try every day to eat foods in the four basic groups.

- Keep moving; walk daily—to the store, post office, church, around the block.

- If you exercise already, do it regularly; a little exercise daily is better than a lot on weekends.

- If you don't exercise but are thinking of starting a program of workouts of some kind, start slowly and build up—following your physician's recommendations.

- If stress gives you problems, find ways to relax without eating or drinking; consider light exercises, yoga, meditation, breathing exercises, or some other method.

Skin Problems

As a person grows older, his skin begins to wrinkle; oil and sweat glands slow down, causing the skin to become dry. Also, the skin may lack the elasticity and tone of normal skin, and this might cause changes in facial contours.

However, the skin, like other parts of the body, tends to age according to various factors. Among prime agers of the skin are exposure to sunlight and weather; the sailor and chronic sunbather may have older-looking skin than their years. Also, hereditary and racial factors influence skin age.

Itching

The skin often itches as one grows older. Itching usually stems from external irritations or internal diseases. External irritations may be more severe in winter because of lack of humidity and because the skin oil does not spread properly. Too many baths or wearing wool garments could also cause itching. You can correct this by cutting down on bathing, maintaining correct temperature and humidity, and applying skin creams.

If itching does not clear up in about two weeks, the trouble may be due to any of a number of internal diseases, some of them serious. Thus, it is wise to see your physician if itching persists.

Skin Cancer

Skin cancer can be easily diagnosed and treated. The two most common types are *basal cell* and *squamous cell*.

The basal cell type begins with a small fleshy *nodule*, usually on the face. It may take several months to reach one-half to one inch in diameter. In about a year it begins to ulcerate and bleed. Then it forms a crust, which it sheds at intervals, leaving another ulcer. If you notice anything like this, see your physician. He can usually remove the ulcer by a local operation.

Squamous cell cancer is often aided by smoking and exposure to the sun. The lesions may appear on the lips, mouth, and genitalia, and they tend to spread and increase in size. Horny growths in exposed areas—face, ears, neck, and scalp—may be forerunners of squamous cell cancer. Again, your physician can treat or operate effectively. See also Ch. 18, *Cancer.*

Vitiligo

Vitiligo, loss of pigment, is not caused by a disease, but it could be a hereditary problem. The affected area of skin has patches of whiteness throughout, but these can be masked by cosmetics.

Senile Purpura

Sometimes the skin develops *senile purpura* as one grows older. The characteristic hemorrhages of this condition usually appear on the extremities, and the purple color gradually fades and leaves mottled areas of yellow-brown. Generally, the skin is thin, fragile, and transparent in appearance.

Stasis Dermatitis

Sometimes in association with such conditions as varicose veins, the skin may develop *stasis dermatitis*, an acute, chronic condition of the leg, associated with swelling, scaling of the skin, and in some cases, ulcer formation. It may exist for years with or without ulceration.

If any of the above conditions develop, it is wise to consult your physician rather than try to treat yourself.

Other Skin Conditions

Other skin conditions that may develop in the later years may include an increase in coarse hairs on exposed places such as the upper lip or chin. The downy hairs in the ears and nose become thicker and more apparent, and the eyebrows may become bushy. Graying hair is popularly associated with aging, but its onset often depends upon genetic factors and varies so much that it cannot be used as a reliable measure of age.

The earlobes may elongate as you grow older and the nails may become coarse and thickened or thinner and brittle.

Relieving Skin Conditions

As mentioned earlier, you can use some creams to relieve dryness and scaliness in older skin. The best of such creams are the water-in-oil emulsions (cold creams) such as Petrolatum Rose Water Ointment USP XVI, or oil-in-water emulsions such as Hydrophilic Ointment USP XVI. Wrinkle creams will not help much, but some conditions may be masked by regular cosmetic items such as powder, rouge, mascara, hair dyes, etc.

Sunscreens may aid in preventing acute and chronic overexposure to the sun's rays.

Various types of surgery may be performed to correct older skin con-

ditions, but they won't work for everyone. Among some of the more common types of surgery are plastic surgery, dermabrasion (skin planning), chemosurgery (chemical cautery), cryosurgery (freezing of the skin), and electrosurgery (employing electricity). See "Plastic and Cosmetic Surgery" in Ch. 20, *Surgery*.

Hearing Loss

About three out of ten persons over age 65 have some hearing loss; at age 70 to 80 this percentage increases greatly.

Causes

While some hearing loss can be blamed on bad listening habits (tuning out people and conversation a person does not want to hear), the two major causes are conduction loss and nerve defects. A person with conduction loss hears high-pitched sounds best; a person with nerve impairment hears low sounds best. A combination of the two is called mixed hearing loss.

Conduction loss can be caused by excessive ear wax, diseases of the ear, disturbances of the eardrum, or abnormalities inside the ear. It can also be caused by *otosclerosis*, a bony growth over the window to the inner ear. Most of these conditions can be treated by an ear doctor (*otologist*). He can remove wax from the ear, repair or replace eardrums, remove bony growths, and loosen or remove fixed ear bones.

Nerve defects (sensorineural hearing loss) may be another story. They are caused by wear and tear on the ear, disease, certain drugs, and blows and skull fractures, and usually cause permanent damage that cannot be helped by surgery or medical treatment.

Some persons complain about ringing in the ears (*tinnitus*) that may start without warning and vary in intensity and quality. What causes tinnitus in one person may not cause it in another, but often it is caused by wax in the ear, middle ear infection, arteriosclerosis, or certain drugs.

Hearing Aids

In most cases a hearing loss can be helped with a hearing aid or surgery. But if you think you have a hearing problem your first task is to see your physician. If your problem is not medically treatable, and if your physician believes a hearing aid will help you, you should see a dispensing audiologist. The American Speech-Language-Hearing Association, 10801 Rockville Pike, Rockville, MD 20852, will supply a directory of certified practitioners on request. If you have trouble finding an audiologist, an experienced hearing-aid dealer may be able to advise you on the device best suited to your needs. The National Hearing Aid Help Line (800/ 521-5247), a service of the National Hearing Aid Society, provides lists of dealers certified as dispensing audiologists.

A hearing test at a hearing aid clinic may be your next stop. Here trained audiologists will scientifically measure your hearing and assist you in trying on different kinds of aids. The audiologists do not sell hearing aids, but can tell you what kind is best for you. Basically, there are four basic kinds of aids:

- Body types that operate with a cord running to the receiver mold in the ear from a miniature microphone carried in a pocket, pinned to the clothing, or worn in a special carrier. These devices are about one to one and one-half inches long and weigh about two ounces. They are more suitable for profound or severe hearing loss.

- Behind-the-ear types that weigh only about one-half of an ounce and fit behind the ear. A plastic tube leads from the microphone, amplifier, and receiver to the earmold that fits in the ear.

- Hearing aids that fit inside the ear canal and weigh about one-sixth of an ounce. This model is hardly visible and has become the most popular among hearing aid wearers.

- A type that fits in the outer ear.

A fifth kind of hearing aid, one that is built into eyeglasses, has a very limited use.

Buying a Hearing Aid

No single hearing aid is ideal for every hard-of-hearing person. Thus testing is essential if you are to find the right aid (which is why you should not buy one through the mail). You may want to bring a friend or relative when you are being fitted. A familiar voice serves as a yardstick to help you judge which aid is best. Some things to consider are the quality of the sound, the aid's ability to help you understand speech in both noisy and quiet places, comfort, ease of use, and price—including the earmold and the expected costs of upkeep.

It takes time to get used to a hearing aid. An aid amplifies all sounds—wanted and unwanted. It also changes most sounds, giving them an "electronic" character. Voices may sound unnatural and tinny. Normal noises may be harsh and grating. But special circuiting in many of today's aids limits the sound level reaching the eardrum. These *automatic gain controls* prevent discomfort but may distort speech. A still newer approach is to use filters to screen out background noises.

In addition to greatly reducing the sizes of many hearing aids, technological advances are expanding the usefulness of hearing aids continually. Noise blockers filter out sounds that do not fit with speech patterns. Tiny microphones reduce the buzzing noises picked up by some older hearing aid models. Treble and bass dials give the wearer a way to adjust sound quality to background noises. With the dials the wearer can also make adjustments to the hearing fluctuations resulting from bodily changes.

If you do not want to wear a hearing aid, or cannot adjust to one, you can try lip reading or speech reading. Each involves watching the lips and vocal chords to determine what another person is saying.

Talking to the Hard-of-Hearing

If you are talking to someone who has some hearing difficulty, he'll understand you better if you speak slowly and distinctly and use the lower range of your voice. Face him when you speak; let him see the movements of your lips. It also helps to point to visible objects.

Above all, don't shout. In fact, raising your voice sometimes pitches it into a higher frequency which a hard-of-hearing person may find difficult to understand.

Other Health Problems

The following health problems might also confront an older person. (Many of these conditions are discussed at greater length elsewhere in the book; in such cases, cross-references are supplied for your convenience at the end of the section.)

Heart Disease

The heart is the strongest, toughest muscle in the body. It is like an engine that could run 70 years or more without an overhaul. The heart has a complete maintenance and repair system, enabling many heart disease victims to continue long and useful lives.

While heart disease is not necessarily a product of aging, some heart and blood vessel problems become more acute as one grows older.

The following symptoms do not necessarily indicate heart disease, but it is wise to see a physician if you notice any of them:

- Shortness of breath

- A feeling of tightness in the chest or pain directly related to exertion or excitement

- Swelling of the feet and ankles

- Unusual fatigue

There is much that physicians can do to prevent heart conditions or to relieve them once present. But there is much that you can do to help yourself:

- Weight:
  Extra pounds of fat mean more work for the heart.

- Diet:
  The rules of sound nutrition apply to proper heart care.

- Smoking:
  Heavy cigarette smokers suffer three times as many heart attacks as do pipe or cigar smokers. Nonsmokers are safest.

- Exercise:
  Exercise improves the pumping action of the heart as well as circulation, digestion, and general health.

Worry

Worry increases tension and elevates blood pressure. Try to cultivate a philosophical approach to the daily ups and downs. See Ch. 10, *Heart Disease*.

Strokes

Strokes are not hopeless; even severely paralyzed patients may make remarkable progress. A *stroke* occurs when the blood supply to a part of the brain tissue is cut off and, as a result, the nerve cells in that part of the brain can't function. When this happens, the part of the body controlled by these nerve cells can't function either.

Whenever the blood supply is cut off from an area, small neighboring arteries get larger and take over part of the work of the damaged artery. In this way nerve cells that have been temporarily put out of order may recover, and that part of the body affected by the stroke may eventually improve or even return to normal.

Once a stroke has occurred, a sound rehabilitation program can help the patient resume as many normal activities as possible. This program can be worked out in cooperation with the physician, patient, family, and local organizations. See Ch. 9, *Diseases of the Circulatory System*.

Arthritis

There are two main types of arthritis: *rheumatoid arthritis* and *osteoarthritis*.

Rheumatoid arthritis—which can cause pain and swelling in joints, nerves, muscles, tendons, blood vessels, and connective tissue in the whole body—can strike at any age, but it occurs mainly in the 25-to-40-year age group. The exact cause of rheumatoid arthritis is unknown.

Osteoarthritis is a degenerative joint disease that affects almost everyone who lives long enough; it is a product of normal wear and tear on the joints over the years. Poor posture and obesity are contributing causes, as are heredity and trauma.

Osteoarthritis is usually mild, and it seldom cripples. Pain is generally moderate. Unlike rheumatoid arthritis, which is inflammatory, spreads from joint to joint, and affects the whole body, osteoarthritis confines its attack locally to individual joints. Rarely is inflammation a problem.

Osteoarthritis is likely to develop in any joint that has been required to take a lot of punishment or abuse: the knee or hip joints of someone who is overweight; joints injured in an accident; joints injured or overused in sports; joints subjected to unusual stresses and strains in work or play; joints with hidden defects that were present at birth.

There is no specific cure for arthritis, but the pain and swelling can be controlled. In other than acute cases, common aspirin has proved the safest and most popular medication.

Adequate rest for both the body and the affected joint is a fundamental treatment. Heat, controlled exercise, hydrotherapy, and massage are all effective if done under a physician's supervision. See "Arthritis and Other Joint Diseases" in Ch. 7, *Diseases of the Skeletal System*.

Cancer

Cancer strikes at any age, but it does strike more frequently in the later years. Many factors are believed to contribute to cancer; frictional and chemical irritations like cigarette smoking, irritation of the skin and mouth (such as poor dentures), exposure to the sun, X rays, or radioactive elements. Common sites are the lips, mouth, stomach, intestines, rectum, liver, pancreas, lungs, breast, kidney, bladder, skin, uterus, and prostate.

Early detection and prompt treatment are the best protection against cancer. If any of the following seven danger signals lasts longer than two weeks, be sure to get a checkup.

- Unusual bleeding or discharge
- A lump or thickening in the breast or elsewhere
- A sore that does not heal
- Change in bowel or bladder habits
- Hoarseness or cough
- Indigestion or difficulty in swallowing
- Change in wart or mole

Great strides have been made in treating cancer through surgery, radiotherapy, and chemotherapy. See Ch. 18, *Cancer*. For cancers affecting women only, see "Cancers of the Reproductive System" and "Cancer of the Breast" in Ch. 25, *Women's Health*.

The Eyes

The eye does age. After age 40, failing vision is usually caused by natural hardening of the lens, making it difficult to see close objects. However, failing vision may also be the first symptom of a serious bodily disorder, or of glaucoma or of a cataract, which requires a physician's immediate attention.

Both glaucoma and cataract can be treated effectively. About 90 percent of glaucoma cases can be checked with eye drops and about 95 percent of cataracts can be removed by a painless operation.

Other diseases that may develop in later years affect the blood vessels of the eye. A common condition is *senile macula degeneration* which causes a blind spot to appear when the victim looks directly at something. The exact cause of senile macula degeneration is not known. See under Ch. 16, *Diseases of the Eye and Ear.*

Diabetes

Most likely candidates for diabetes are overweight persons past 40, particularly those who have a hereditary history of diabetes, and especially older women.

The exact cause of diabetes is not known, but it is a functional disorder in which the body cannot handle certain foods—mainly sugars and starches. Symptoms include increased thirst, constant hunger, frequent urination, loss of weight, itching, easy tiring, changes in vision, and slow healing of cuts and scratches.

Treatment and control consist of planned diet, exercise, and, in many cases, insulin shots or oral medication. Well-controlled diabetics can lead active lives. See Ch. 15, *Diabetes Mellitus.*

Constipation

There is no truth in the notion that a daily bowel movement is necessary for good health. A movement every day or twice a day may be all right for one person; for another every three or four days may be enough.

The two most common causes of chronic constipation are physical inactivity and poor food and water habits. Ironically, constipation may be caused by swallowing a cathartic nightly to induce a bowel movement. The habit eventually leads to chronic constipation because normal bowel movement ceases and bowel evacuation depends on using a cathartic.

To maintain proper bowel movement, try the following:

- Drink eight to ten glasses of water a day. Take two glasses of water on an empty stomach as soon as you get up.

- Drink more fruit juices and eat more dried and fresh fruits.

- Get at least one-half hour of moderate exercise daily. Walking, for example, is excellent, particularly if you relax while you walk.

- Give yourself enough time for normal bowel movement and set up a regular time for evacuation.

- If you are constipated, consult your physician to make sure it is simple and functional. See under Ch. 23, *Aches, Pains, Nuisances, Worries.*

Back Problems

As we grow older, the back muscles—weakened by inactivity, poor posture, and almost unavoidable wear and tear—start to complain.

Other causes of back problems are muscle and joint strain, changes in the spine, psychological tension, and internal diseases. Here are some tips to help avoid backache:

- Learn to lift correctly. Use your leg muscles, which are stronger than back muscles, by placing your feet closer to the base of the object, bending your knees outward, and pushing up with your legs.

- Avoid subjecting your back to any sudden, erratic motion.

- Try to improve your posture when sitting and walking.

- Sleep on a firm bed; a bed board may be helpful.

- Get regular exercise of a type that stimulates all your muscles rather than just a few.

- If you sit for a long period, get up and stretch occasionally.

- Beware of excess weight. Extra weight on the abdomen pulls on the vertebrae at the small of the back, increasing the spine's normal curve and causing pain.

- Try never to become overfatigued or exhausted, either physically or mentally. Emotional pressure, from work or personal problems, causes muscle tension. See "Backaches" in Ch. 23, *Aches, Pains, Nuisances, Worries.*

Because the feet are farthest away from the heart's blood supply, they are often the first areas affected by circulatory diseases. Also, arthritis and diabetes might first show up in the feet.

Warning signs include continued cramping of the calf muscles, pain in the arch and toes, and unusually cold feet—especially if accompanied by a bluish skin. Brittle or thickened toenails or burning, tingling, and numbness may also signal a circulatory disease.

Foot ulcers may be one of the first signs of diabetes. Some *bunions*—swollen, tender, red joints—are caused by arthritis. Swelling around the feet and ankles suggests a possible kidney disorder.

If you have these symptoms, go to a *podiatrist* (a foot doctor) or to your own physician. They are trained to recognize these symptoms.

Most older people, however, suffer from minor aches and pains in the feet that are caused by poor foot care or abuse. See "The Vulnerable Extremeties" in Ch. 23, *Aches, Pains, Nuisances, Worries.*

Care of the Feet

To prevent these problems, treat yourself to daily foot care. Dry your feet thoroughly and gently after bathing and inspect the skin for abrasion, rough spots, or cracks. Dry carefully between the toes. If the skin is dry or scaly, lubricate it with lanolin or olive oil. Next, apply a medicated foot powder recommended by your podiatrist or physician over the entire foot, especially between the toes, as a preventive measure against athlete's foot.

When you cut your nails, do it with a strong light and be careful to cut straight across the nail to prevent ingrown toenails. Avoid the use of strong medications containing salicylate and strong antiseptics like iodine, carbolic acid, lysol, or bleach. Harsh chemicals that attack toughened skin can irritate normal tissue and cause infection. Avoid using hot water bottles, electric pads, or any form of extreme heat or cold. Diabetics should visit a podiatrist regularly.

The Prostate

Men over 50 may have an enlarged *prostate*. (This is not caused by sexual excesses or venereal disease.) The exact cause is not known, but it's estimated that some type of enlarged prostate is present in about 10 percent of 40-year-olds and 80 percent of 80-year-olds.

The prostate is a rubbery mass of glands and muscle tissue about the size and shape of a horse chestnut. It is wrapped around the urethra and base of the bladder at the point where they join. The prostate functions as part of a man's sexual apparatus, providing a fluid that transports and nourishes the spermatozoa.

Symptoms of an enlarged prostate include difficulty in urination. There might be an initial blocking of the urine, or the stream may lack force. You may feel that you can't empty the bladder, and you may have urgent needs to urinate. You may have pain or blood in the urine from straining.

If you have any of these symptoms, your physician can easily check for enlarged prostate by a simple rec-

tal examination. If he discovers an enlargement, he can usually treat it in early stages with simple massage. But if it has progressed too far, he may have to operate.

An operation is usually performed through the urethra or by an incision in the lower abdomen. The choice depends upon the individual problems of the patient and the judgment of the surgeon. In either case, the patient usually recovers completely in a short time.

A rectal examination can also discover early stages of cancer of the prostate, which is not uncommon in men over 40. Some 20 percent of men over 60 have this condition, and it is most common in men over 70.

Unfortunately, this disease does not manifest itself early, so it is important that men over 40 have the diagnostic rectal examination. If the disease is detected early and treated— usually by surgery, hormonal therapy, and possibly radiation—the cure rate is very high. If found late, the cure rate is low.

When treatment is by surgery, the entire prostate and upper urethra may be removed. In some cases, the disease may be retarded or relieved by treatment with female hormones. (The male hormone is known to hasten prostate cancer.)

In both enlargement and cancer of the prostate, early detection is vital to a successful cure. That is why it is important to have a rectal examination. See also "Cancer of the Prostate" in Ch. 18, *Cancer*.

Alzheimer's Disease

Alzheimer's disease is a group of brain disorders marked by progressive deterioration and affects both memory and reasoning abilities. Victims of Alzheimer's, which is a form of dementia, or mental deterioration (see "Dementia" in Ch. 8, *Diseases of*

the Muscles and Nervous System), undergo various behavioral changes. These include an inability to concentrate, anxiety, irritability, agitation, withdrawal, and petulance. Persons suffering from Alzheimer's may wander about and lose their way. They may have temper tantrums and engage in obsessional behavior, such as repeatedly washing dishes. Time and place disorientation may be accompanied by delusions and depression. In the later stages of the disease, sufferers often lose bladder and bowel control.

Diagnosing Alzheimer's in its early stages is difficult despite its numerous symptoms. Laboratory tests that could identify the disorder do not exist. Adding to the problems of diagnosis, various other disorders have similar symptoms. The best medical alternative, a complete physical examination, generally includes a review of any drugs or medications the patient has been taking as well as standard laboratory tests. The latter help to rule out other diseases or disorders that may be treatable. A clinical evaluation can include a CT (computed tomography) scan, an EEG (electroencephalogram), and assessment of evidence from family members and the patient regarding the latter's (or patient's) mental state.

Even when diagnosed with relative certainty, Alzheimer's disease cannot be cured. But some symptoms, including depression and delusions, can be treated. The effect is to slow the progress of the disorder. Where Parkinson's disease or heart problems accompany Alzheimer's, treatment can focus on alleviation of those conditions.

Theories regarding the causes of Alzheimer's abound. Because it is known that the disease leads to severe atrophy and distortion of the cerebral cortex, researchers have explored both genetic and physiological theories. On the genetic side, studies have indicated that persons with relatives who had or have Alzheimer's face three or four times the normal risks of becoming victims. On the physiological side, Alzheimer's patients have been shown to lack adequate supplies of *choline acetyltransferase* (CAT), a neurotransmitter, or chemical, that enables brain signals to travel from one cell to another. Such findings, it is hoped, will lead eventually to cures.

Meeting the Challenge of Leisure

Leisure Activities

In ten years of retirement, you will have the leisure time equivalent of working 40 hours a week for 21 years. You cannot fish this time away and you cannot rest it away. Whatever you do for long must have meaning—must satisfy some basic need and want. Certain needs remain constant throughout life:

- Security—good health, income, and a recognized role in society

- Recognition—as an individual with your own abilities and personality

- Belonging—as a member of a family, social group, and community

- Self-expression—by developing abilities and talents in new areas and at new levels

- Adventure—new experiences, new sights, and new knowledge

There are many activities that can satisfy these basic needs and wants to keep you mentally and physically in top shape.

Travel

Travel satisfies your need for adventure in many ways. If you travel off-season at bargain rates, you'll find that time truly is money. Most travel problems stem from rushing to meet a schedule. Making every minute count on a fast-paced European tour can be expensive and exhausting. For the same transatlantic fare, you can spend a full year in Europe at one-third the daily cost of a three-week vacation.

Wherever you travel, it isn't enough just to sightsee. Try to center your travel around an interest or a hobby. You can take art or music tours—tours that stress education, night life, culture, or special interests. You can travel on your own or with a group. But whatever you do, participate; don't just observe.

Doing things instead of just observing adds new dimensions to the pleasure of going places. For people who participate, travel means the adventure of enjoying exciting new places, people, and experiences. To help plan your trip, write to the government tourist offices of foreign countries (ask your library for addresses); to the National Park Service, Washington, DC; and to state or local chambers of commerce (no street addresses necessary).

Gardening

Gardening satisfies one's need for self-expression in many ways. Being outside in the fresh air and planting living things can bring satisfaction and peace of mind.

Gardening is a many-faceted hobby that offers many challenges. You can go into plant breeding, growing for resale, introducing new plants, collecting the rare and unusual, plant selecting, or simply cultivating what you find personally appealing and satisfying.

Your local library or bookstore has many books on the subject. There are local and national garden clubs that you can join to learn about your hobby and to meet other people who are interested in gardening. Write the Government Printing Office, Washington, DC 20401, for help and advice. In addition, state extension directors at state colleges and universities, county agricultural agents, and local plant nurseries can give expert advice and information.

Reading

Reading offers excitement, adventure, pursuit of knowledge, and an introduction to new people and places. Your local library is the best place to launch a reading program—and you may be surprised to find that it offers more than books. Most libraries have art and music departments, audiovisual services (films and microfilm copies), foreign language departments, periodical rooms (newspapers and magazines), writing classes, genealogy workshops, and special courses of general interest.

Hobbies

A hobby can be any physical or mental activity that gives you happiness, relaxation, and satisfaction. It should not be just a time killer—it should offer some tangible reward. Also, it should have continuity, not be too expensive, and not make undue demands on time and energy. Perhaps you would prefer a series of hobbies, some serious and some just for fun. They can be related to your work or completely unrelated. In any event, a hobby should be something you've always wanted to do.

Before selecting a hobby, consider these points:

- Do you like to do things alone? Consider arts, crafts, reading, sewing, fishing—activities that are not dependent on others, although you can enjoy them with others.

- Do you like groups? Seek hobbies that include other people—organizational, sport, game, or craft activities.

- Do you like to play to win? Try your luck in competitive or team games that stress winning.

- Do you have to be an expert? Too many of us are afraid to try new activities because we hate to fail or look clumsy. But be fair; judge your efforts in light of your past experience and present progress; do not compare yourself to someone who's been at it longer than you.

- Do you put a price tag on everything? Many people will not engage in an activity if it costs too much. Yet, many hobbies fail because they're tried on a shoestring without adequate equipment. Also, some people do not want to do anything unless it brings in money. If so, perhaps you should look for something that's an offshoot of the work or business you know best.

Creative Crafts

Creative crafts are difficult for most of us because we are conservative, afraid to make mistakes, sensitive because of buried and almost forgotten blunders. Yet creativity is essential to life. Without it we don't live fully; through creative skills we refurbish old interests and develop new ones.

Most of us are happiest with creative crafts that do not require intricate work or fine detail and that are not too demanding physically. Some crafts best suited to retirement years include weaving, rug making, sewing, ceramic work, knitting, plastic molding, woodwork, leathercraft, and lapidary.

You can learn these and other crafts and also market your products through senior centers, adult education classes, and senior craft centers.

Volunteer Work

Through community service and volunteer work, thousands are not only helping others but are serving themselves. Such activities keep time from hanging heavy, give purpose to retirement, and in some cases may lead to paying jobs and a second career.

Participating in community activities is not difficult. In some communities a call to the city clerk is enough to get started. In others, a letter to the mayor will bring faster results. In larger cities, call the Volunteer Bureau in your area; this is a United Fund agency that acts as a clearing house for volunteer jobs.

If you wish to have the type of volunteer job that leads to a second career, you might consider doing work for one of the government programs utilizing the skills of older people. All of these programs have been assembled under the umbrella of one organization called ACTION. For additional information about any of the following programs, write to ACTION, Washington, DC 20525.

- The Foster Grandparent Program hires low-income men and women over 60 to give love and attention to institutionalized and other needy children.

- The Peace Corps is seeking the skills of retirees. However, you must be skilled in some trade or profession, pass a tough physical examination, and complete a rigorous orientation and training program. For information, write to ACTION, Washington, DC 20525, and request a copy of *Older Volunteers in the Peace Corps*. It lists specific skills needed in the Peace Corps.

- Other programs within ACTION include the Retired Senior Volunteer Program, the Service Corps of Retired Executives, the Active Corps of Executives, and VISTA (Volunteer in Service to America). Many of the workers in these programs are paid.

There are other volunteer jobs that may not pay a salary, but do fill a basic need by allowing you to pass along your skills and ideals to younger people. You can do this through the Boy Scouts, Girl Scouts, Boys Clubs of America, YMCAs and YWCAs, hospitals, schools for the handicapped and mentally retarded, and many other organizations.

Continuing Social and Intellectual Activities

The one organ we can depend upon in old age is the brain. At 80, a person can learn at approximately the same speed he could when he was 12 years old. But like any organ, the brain must be kept active and alert by constant use.

One of the best ways to exercise the brain is through some process of continuing education. This does not have to mean going back to school or taking formal classes. Continuing education can take the form of participating in discussions in senior centers, "Y's," town meetings, or study courses. You can find out about educational opportunities and possibilities by contacting local, state, or national offices of education; state employment offices; the information service of your Community Council or Health and Welfare Federation; the Adult Education section of the U.S. Office of Education, Washington, DC 20202; the National Education Association, 1201 Sixteenth Street, NW, Washington, DC 20036; the State Commission on Aging (write to your state capital).

Your local library may have some suggestions (and perhaps offers some classes), and your local "Y" is probably offering some programs.

The federal government continues to be a prime source of educational literature. Each year the government prints about 50 million books, pamphlets, brochures, reports, and guidebooks on everything from astrology to zoology. For a free price list of specified subjects, write to the Superintendent of Documents, Government Printing Office, Washington, DC 20401.

Formal and informal learning situations can help you keep pace with change and the future. Continuing education prepares you to live contentedly with a free, independent spirit and mind—while providing you with the means for improved social integration, participation, and satisfaction.

Sexual Attitude and Activity in the Aged

We have come far since the Victorian era when talk about sex was taboo. Now science is taking a candid look at sex in the later years and is exploding old myths as well as exploring new truths. Such enlightenment can help reduce any remaining guilt in this area.

After Age 60

In one study to determine the pattern of sexual behavior after 60, researchers at Duke University quizzed 250 people aged 60 to 93 about their sexual activities. Of the 149 who were married, 81 reported they were still sexually active; even in the single group, 7 of the 101 questioned reported "some sexual activity."

Dr. Gustave Newman, who conducted the study, reported 10 percent of the couples over 60 as having sexual relations more than once a week, though couples over 75 unanimously reported less activity.

"No age is an automatic cut-off point for sex," claims the late Dr. Isadore Rubin in his study, *Sexual Life After Sixty*. "But," he continues,

sexuality cannot flourish in a climate where rejection of aging as a worthwhile stage of life leads inevitably to self-rejection by many older persons . . . the men and women who "act old" in their sexual activity before their bodies have really called a halt become sexually old long before their time.

Physiological and Psychological Changes and Sex

Postmenopausal women may experience painful intercourse due to a decrease in vaginal lubrication. This problem is easily remedied with the use of nonpetroleum-based vaginal creams or jellies.

Many women take a renewed interest in sex after menopause. Dr. William H. Masters and Mrs. Virginia E. Johnson in their study *Human Sexual Response* credit the tendency of many women to experience a second honeymoon in the early 50s to the fact that they no longer have to worry about pregnancy and usually have resolved most of the problems of raising a family.

On the other hand, they tell us:

Deprived of normal sexual outlets, women exhaust themselves physically in conscious or unconscious efforts to dissipate their accumulated and frequently unrecognized sexual tensions. Many demonstrate their basic insecurities by casting themselves unreservedly into their religion, the business world, volunteer social work, or overzealous mothering of their mature children or grandchildren.

While some women become more responsive as they grow older, Masters and Johnson point out, "There is no question that the human male's responsiveness wanes as he ages."

Men may experience less sexual urgency, delayed or partial erection, and less defined ejaculations because the body's secretion of the male hormone testosterone decreases with age and the conduction of nerve impulses is less rapid. Also, arteries in the penis are less able to maintain the blood pressure necessary for a full erection.

Another common concern for older men is impotence, that is, diminished or no sexual response. Nearly everyone experiences impotence from time to time, often from such routine problems as fatigue, stress, or illness. The incidence of impotence, however, definitely increases with age. (By age 65, 30 percent of men report chronic impotence; by age 75, 55 percent do.)

Impotence has been linked to such problems as diabetes, Parkinson's disease, liver or kidney disease, and lower back problems. Other causes are certain medications, excessive alcohol consumption, drug abuse, and smoking. Most cases of impotence, however, can be traced to psychological problems such as anxiety, depression, or marital problems. About 80 percent of these cases can still be overcome with psychotherapy.

Sexual dysfunction in women is often called *frigidity* and implies a *cold* woman who cannot become excited sexually. As with men, there are both organic and psychological causes which can often be treated.

Although sex for most healthy men and women over 60 may not be quite the same as it was for them in their 20s, that does not mean it cannot be good, or even better. A change in attitudes and expectations about sex may have surprising results. Couples may find new enjoyment in reducing the pace of lovemaking and exploring different ways of giving each other pleasure besides intercourse.

Health Concerns

For those not so healthy older men and women, especially most of those who have suffered heart attacks, there is no reason for them not to have sex. After a heart attack most are able to resume sexual activity within a few months, although patients with angina pectoris may be advised to proceed cautiously.

According to Dr. Philip Reichert, former executive secretary of the American College of Cardiology:

> We must get rid of the notion that every heart patient lives under an overhanging sword and that he faces the constant threat of sudden death. The congenial married couple, accustomed to each other and whose technique is habituated through many years of companionship, can achieve sexual satisfaction without too great an expenditure of body energy or too severe a strain upon the heart. . . .

Hypertension sufferers may sometimes indulge in a restricted form of sexual activity with medical supervision. And modern therapy and surgical methods can often prevent or delay impotence caused by prostate disease or diabetes.

Where any health problem is involved, it is best to analyze your sex needs and those of your partner; consult with your physician and partner as to how you can both attain satisfaction without harm to your health; see your physician regularly and report

accurately distress symptoms and the conditions causing them.

Recent research has dispelled other long-held ideas about sex, too—among them the myth that masturbation is childish and harmful to health. Moreover, Rubin points out: "All studies of older persons have shown that autoerotic activity, while not as common as in the younger years, is far more prevalent in later years than most of us have imagined."

Dr. Lester W. Dearborn, marriage consultant, in pointing out the role masturbation plays in the lives of the single or widowed, comments:

> It is to be hoped that those interested in the field of geriatrics will . . . encourage the aging to accept masturbation as a perfectly valid outlet when there is a need and other means of gratification are not available.

Cellular Therapy and Hormone Treatment

To keep older people vigorous and active, some researchers have experimented with *cellular therapy* as a means of retarding aging. Dr. Paul Niehans, a Swiss physician, introduced the idea of cellular therapy in the 1930s with his theory that organs begin to deteriorate in old age when the body fails to replace the cells that compose it. He prescribed a treatment whereby a person is injected with cells from healthy embryonic animal organs. (He used sheep, pigs, and calves.) He believed that the animal cells from a particular organ would migrate to the same organ in the aging body and reactivate it. Thus, kidney troubles could be cured with cells from an embryonic animal kidney. Although such notables as Sir Winston Churchill, Pope Pius XII, Somerset Maugham, and Dr. Konrad Adenauer submitted to it, cellular therapy is not widely accepted in the

United States today as an effective agent against aging.

More to the point, most researchers feel, are the current experiments with hormones. Hormones help women through the tension of menopause and are used to treat impotence and loss of sexual desire. However, some studies have linked estrogen hormone therapy statistically with uterine cancer. For this reason and because of side effects, hormones face many years of testing before they will be used extensively to retard aging.

Mental Outlook

Good health plus a romantic outlook promote sex appeal at any age. Showing affection, whether sexually or not, keep you sparkling and lively no matter what your age.

A good wholesome attitude toward life, a hearty sense of humor, a sympathetic interest in other people—all help make up the indefinable something that makes us appealing to the opposite sex. Cleanliness, neat suitable apparel, and good posture all add to the image we create of ourselves in other people's minds. So do the manners we reflect in the courtesies we show the people around us—the thoughtful little things we do for them, our reactions to the things they do for us.

If you're a woman over 65 who is looking for companionship, you'll probably find a good personality uplift will get you farther than a face or bust lift. If you're a man who is hoping to find feminine companionship, you will probably find a good spiritual overhaul more image-enhancing than dyeing your hair. Also, a good night's sleep is the best aphrodisiac.

The Right Housing

Selecting retirement housing is like

selecting a spouse; there are many possibilities, but few that are right.

Ideally, the right housing should take care of you rather than requiring you to take care of it. It should give you shelter, security, and privacy; allow you freedom; and keep you near friends, relatives, and a grocer who delivers.

To Move or Not to Move

What is the right housing for you—the one that you are in or some other place? The answer to this question depends upon the state of your pocketbook and the state of your health.

Advantages of Moving

Right now you might be in good health, but this could change. Would stairs become a problem? Could you keep up the house and garden? Would you want more adequate heat? Older people are more comfortable when the temperature is over 75° F. You might also need better lighting in several rooms.

If you are retired, you might find that you cannot keep up expenses on the old house. You might find that your larger, older house does not suit the reduced size of your family or your need for work or recreation. You could probably save money by living in a smaller place that requires less upkeep. You could also arrange to move nearer children and grandchildren, or into an area where you could find new opportunities for work and recreational activities.

Advantages of Staying Put

But by staying in your home you would remain in familiar surroundings and near old friends. You could maintain your comfortable routine and remain independent as long as possible. If you have unused space, you could move into the first floor and shut off the second floor to save on heat and maintenance. Or you could convert part of the house into apartments.

Where to Live?

Many older persons fulfill ambitions of long standing by moving to warmer climates after retirement. The question whether such a move should be undertaken should be considered with other questions relating to housing.

Moving to a different climate makes sense for many reasons. Many elderly persons feel threatened or restricted by cold winters and their usual accompaniments—snow, sleet, and high winds. Having more leisure time, older persons feel that warmer temperatures will make it possible to take part in more activities for more hours of the day than if they "stay put." Some persons move so that they can live closer to friends who have already moved—or to children or other relatives. Some move to play golf or tennis outdoors the year around.

An individual or couple considering a move to a warmer climate should look at a number of basic considerations. A key one relates to the cost of living in the new area or state. Living on incomes that may have been substantially reduced by retirement, older persons without special preferences may select that state that offers the cheapest living. Studies indicated in 1979 that the "10 best states to retire to" from a personal-financial point of view were, in order:

1. Utah, because of lower energy costs, growing job opportunities, moderate living costs. A drawback: Utah may have extremely cold winters.

2. Louisiana, because of cheap living costs—about 10 percent lower than other states—and low real estate taxes.

3. South Carolina, for the same reasons. A drawback: physician shortages in some communities.

4. Nevada, because of new housing, jobs, no state income or inheritance taxes, and average living costs.

5. Texas, with moderate housing costs away from major cities, and normal, if rising, living costs.

6. New Mexico, where energy costs are low, jobs are increasing in number, and cheap housing is plentiful.

7. Alabama, the cheapest and lowest as regards costs of living. Drawbacks: few new jobs, medical care lacking in some areas.

8. Arizona, because of good, relatively inexpensive housing, warm climate, good medical care. Drawbacks: rising living costs, high taxes.

9. Florida, with a warm climate, no income tax, good medical services. Drawbacks: living costs high in coastal areas; property taxes rising.

10. Georgia, because of mild climate, low living costs. Drawbacks: slow growth in jobs, locally poor medical services.

"Retirement to the sun" entails many other decisions. States like New Mexico offer a wide range of sites, from urban to desert, from high mountains to empty plains. Some of the states with favorable tax laws and cheap living costs have little to offer in the way of cultural attractions. Other states may lack recreational activities.

Psychological Trauma

Moving 100 or 1,000 or 2,000 miles to live in a warmer climate obviously involves some pain of separation and loss. The psychological trauma occasioned by a departure from old friends and familiar surroundings has caused major problems for some older persons. For that reason, the psychological challenge should be given deep consideration *before* any move is made.

How to alleviate the trauma of leaving the familiar for the unfamiliar? Some persons spend a year in the new locale, return home, and *then* make up their minds to move or not to move. Others, including those who cannot afford such trial living, at least visit the target region to "get a feel" for it and its way of life. Whatever your situation, the wisdom of considering at least five factors cannot be disputed:

- In the new home under the sun, will you be able to entertain family, including children and grandchildren, and in that way to minimize the pain of separation?

- Are friends or relatives already located in the new area—and can you live near them (not *with* them, if possible)?

- Will you be able to swing into enough new activities to eliminate any possibility that you might feel useless, wasted, or frustrated?

- Can you maintain your old, or a decent, standard of living once you have moved?

- Can you stand the first 9 to 12 months in the new home without climbing the walls? Studies have shown that those who can last out a year or more will very likely adjust and continue to enjoy life.

Requirements of Retirement Housing

Whatever you plan to do, your retirement housing should be located near or be easily accessible to shops and recreation centers by public transportation. To make living arrangements more pleasant, individual housing units should contain at least 400 square feet, and there should be two or more rooms.

The new dwelling unit should be equal to or better than the housing you have been used to in the past. It should be suitable for comfortable living in both health and sickness—easily adaptable to convalescent needs with either two bedrooms or a bedroom and sleeping alcove.

In addition, retirement housing should incorporate the following:

- All rooms on one floor, and that floor reached by few, if any, steps

- No thresholds or tripping hazards

- Nonslip surfaces in hallways, bedrooms, and kitchens

- Handrails by all steps and inclines

- Adequate illumination in halls, near steps, and in other potentially hazardous areas

- Fully automatic central heating

- Doors and halls wide enough to accommodate a wheelchair

Public Housing

If you decide to move and to rent instead of buying, consider public housing projects. These projects are available to single men and women 62 or older, as well as to families whose head is 62 or older or has a spouse at least 62. Local housing authorities build, purchase, or lease the units and set entrance requirements and maximum income limits. Rents are comparatively low.

The Housing and Urban Development Agency also makes loans for nonprofit (and profit) sponsors that will build housing for senior citizens with moderate or higher incomes.

Retirement Hotels and Communities

You might also consider retirement hotels, which are especially numerous in Florida, California, and Texas. These hotels are usually refurbished former resorts that provide room and board at a fixed monthly rent.

Retirement communities offer housing of various types, usually apartments, cooperatives, and individual units. It usually costs about $450 a month or more to cover mortgage payments, living, and maintenance expenses.

Would you like retirement community living? It's usually the life for people who like people and who enjoy being active. For those who don't, it can be a bit tiring. Some couples do not like the closeness and activity found in a retirement community and prefer living in a less social environment.

Lifetime Care Facilities

In contrast to the emphasis on independent living in retirement communities, many projects sponsored by church, union, and fraternal organizations stress lifetime care (room, board, and medical care for life), with fees based on actuarial tables of life expectancy at age of entry. Housing alone costs from $10,000 to $30,000, depending upon age and type of living accommodation, *plus* a monthly charge of around $250 per person to cover meals, medical care (exclusive of Medicare), maintenance, and other expenses. In many cases, lifetime care for a couple could cost around $90,000.

Cooperatives and Condominiums

In addition to lifetime care facilities,

many church, fraternal, and union groups offer other types of housing. In the case of church-sponsored housing, residence usually is not restricted to members of the sponsoring faith.

Some of these units are operated as *cooperatives;* others as *condominiums.* The major difference in the two is that condominium owners have titles to their units, while cooperative residents are stockholders in the cooperative association with occupancy rights to specific units. Condominium owners pay their own taxes; cooperative residents pay taxes in their monthly charges.

Mobile Homes

You might also want to consider a mobile home. A suitable one must be at least 10 feet wide and 50 feet long.

What is it like to live in a mobile-home park? Certainly, there is a closeness in these parks that you would not have in a normal neighborhood. Typically, the mobile home is placed on a lot 25 to 30 feet wide and 75 feet deep. This means that you could have 12 families within a radius of 100 feet.

Residents visit back and forth and hold frequent picnics, barbecues, and other social activities. This would not be the way of life for someone who did not enjoy group activities.

Be Realistic

To find out what type of housing is best for you, look around the area to see where you want to live. Each community is different, shaped by the people who live there. Talk to the residents and do some serious thinking before you move, not forgetting to carefully consider your financial position in regard to the new locale. Try to be realistic; don't expect to find the perfect climate for health and happiness. The nearest thing to it would be

a place that encourages outdoor life, is neither too hot nor too cold, has a relative humidity of around 55 percent, and enough variety in weather, with frequent but moderate weather changes, to be interesting and not too monotonous.

If you have any doubts about the location as far as health is concerned, check with your physician.

When Faced with Ill Health

How can you help yourself or others when faced with a serious or terminal illness?

Alvin I. Goldfarb, M.D., former consultant on Services for the Aged, New York State Department of Mental Hygiene, notes the importance of self-esteem, self-confidence, sense of purpose, and well-being to a person who is seriously ill or dying. Supported by the idea, "I've led a good and full life," older people can face a serious or terminal illness with dignity. Sometimes this acceptance may be almost an unspoken and tacit understanding between the aging and society to help the separation process along.

When a person is terminally ill, the chances are that he is not in severe pain. With the increasing supply of pain-relieving drugs and the possibility of sedation, very few elderly patients suffer greatly with pain. While a fear of death probably exists in most people, when death is actually encountered the fear is seldom overwhelming, even though it may deeply affect others directly involved with the dying patient.

Most patients are at least aware of the possibility of dying soon; those with lingering conditions are particularly adept at self-diagnosis. But more often, they notice a change in social relationships with friends, family, and medical personnel.

Patient–physician relationships can be vital in helping the seriously ill patient retain peace of mind. It is the physician's responsibility to give compassion and recognize fear, even when it is hidden. Likewise, he should respond to a patient's hidden wish to discuss his illness. Of course, there is no set formula for communicating with seriously ill patients. Each individual needs a different approach, and most physicians are sensitive to this.

Many physicians report that death, except in unusual cases, is not accompanied by physical pain. Rather, there is often a sense of well-being and spiritual exaltation. Physicians think this feeling is caused by the anesthetic action of carbon dioxide on the central nervous system and by the effect of toxic substances. Ernest Hemingway wrote, "The pang of death, a famous doctor once told me, is often less than that of a toothache."

Stages of Death

According to physicians, people die in stages—rapidly or slowly, depending on circumstances. First comes *clinical death*, when respiration and heartbeat cease. The brain dies as it is deprived of oxygen and circulating blood, and *biological death* occurs.

Life can be restored in the moments between clinical death and brain death if circulation and respiration are continued through the use of medical devices that stimulate the heart and lungs.

After the brain ceases to function, cellular death begins. Life is not considered to be completely lost until the brain stops functioning. It is possible for surgeons to remove viable organs after biological death for transplant or other use.

Many clergymen and physicians insist that we need more honest communication about death, as such communication is probably the single most useful measure to avoid unnecessary suffering. Sound knowledge never made anyone afraid. And although death will probably always remain essentially a mystery, scientists will continue to search for a better understanding of its nature. By such means they may learn a great deal more about life.

The Autopsy

Family members adjusting to the death of a loved one may face the question of whether or not an autopsy should be performed. More and more, medical experts are underscoring the need for an autopsy as a means of confirming the cause of death. The postmortem examination may also "provide a reasonable context for accepting death," according to Daniel W. McKeel, director of autopsy pathology at Washington University School of Medicine. From a family and genetic point of view, the autopsy may reveal information about specific conditions or medical problems in the deceased that survivors can use to guide their own health practices and concerns.

Contrary to some reports, the autopsy need not delay funeral arrangements or disfigure the body so as to require a closed casket. Autopsies are generally mandatory in homicide, suicide, burn deaths, deaths resulting from on-the-job injuries, operating room deaths, and questionable or unwitnessed deaths.

7

Diseases of the Skeletal System

The bones and joints of the human body, although designed to withstand a great deal of stress, are subject to a variety of disorders that can affect people of all ages. Some skeletal deformities are the result of congenital defects, and can be treated by physical therapy or surgery with varying degrees of success. Arthritis and related joint diseases, caused by wear and tear over the years, probably affect more people than any other skeletal disorder.

Man's erect posture makes the spine especially vulnerable to problems of alignment, often causing considerable pain. Bone tissue can also be invaded by tumors and by infections of the bone marrow. Also, stress to bones and joints can cause fractures or dislocations, which require prompt medical treatment to prevent deformity or loss of mobility.

Congenital Defects

As the fetus develops in the womb, its bony skeleton first appears as soft cartilage, which hardens into bone before birth. The calcium content of the mother's diet aids the fetus in bone formation and in the development of the normal human skeleton. Thus the basic skeletal structure of an individual is formed before his birth. In some instances, the bones of the fetus develop abnormally, and such defects are usually noticeable soon after delivery.

The causes of skeletal birth defects are not always known. Some may result from hereditary factors; others have been traced to the mother's exposure to X rays, radiation, chemicals, drugs, or to disease during pregnancy. Among the more common birth defects are extra fingers, toes, or ribs, or missing fingers, hands, toes, feet, or limbs. Sections of the spine may be fused together, often without causing serious problems later in life, although some fused joints can hinder the motion of limbs. The sections of the skull may unite prematurely, retarding the growth of the brain.

Defects of the Skull, Face, and Jaw

Various malformations of the skull, face, and jaw can appear at birth or soon after. They include *macrocephaly* (enlarged head) and *microcephaly* (very small head). Microcephaly is caused by the premature fusion of the cranial sutures in early childhood. If brain growth increases very rapidly during the first six months of life in infants whose skulls have fused prematurely, the brain cannot expand sufficiently within the rigid skull, and mental retardation results. Surgery is used to widen the sutures to permit normal brain development.

Cleft lip and *cleft palate* are common facial deformities and are visible at birth. These are longitudinal openings in the upper lip and palate. They result from failure of the area to unite in the normal manner during embryonic stages of pregnancy. They should be corrected at an early age. If surgery is performed in infancy there is a good chance that the child will mature with little or no physical evidence of the affliction and with no psychological damage as a result of it. See "Cleft Palate and Cleft Lip" in Ch. 2, *The First Dozen Years*, for further information.

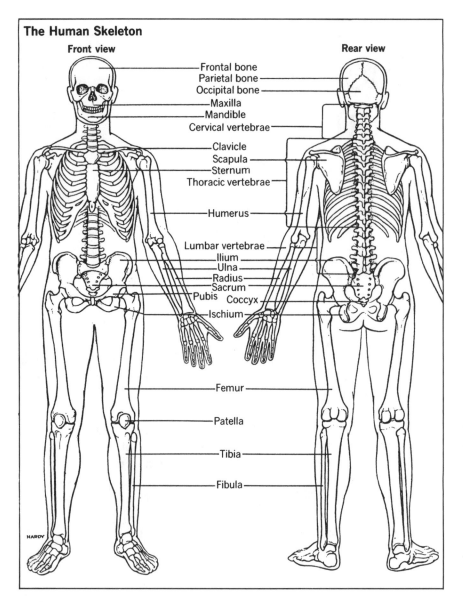

The Human Skeleton

Front view   Rear view

Frontal bone
Parietal bone
Occipital bone
Maxilla
Mandible
Cervical vertebrae

Clavicle
Scapula
Sternum
Thoracic vertebrae

Humerus

Lumbar vertebrae
Ilium
Ulna
Radius
Sacrum
Pubis   Coccyx
Ischium

Femur

Patella

Tibia

Fibula

Defects of the Rib Cage

Every normal human being has 12 pairs of ribs attached to the spine, but some people are born with extra ribs on one or both sides.

Although such extra ribs are usually harmless, one that projects into the neck can damage nerves and the artery located in that area. In adults extra neck ribs may cause shooting pains down the arms, general periodic numbness in the arms and hands, weak wrist pulse, and possible diminished blood supply to the forearm. Surgery may be required to remove the rib and thereby relieve the pres-sure on the nerves or artery. Minor symptoms are treated by physio-therapy.

Congenital absence of one or more ribs is not uncommon. An individual may be born with some ribs fused to-gether. Neither condition creates any serious threat to health.

Congenital Dislocation of the Hip

Dislocation of the hip is the most com-mon congenital problem of the pelvic area. It is found more often in girls than in boys in a five to one ratio. Babies born from a breech presenta-tion, buttocks first, are more likely to develop this abnormality than those delivered head first. The condition may be the result of inherited char-acteristics.

Clinical examination of infants, es-pecially breech-born girls, may reveal early signs of congenital hip disloca-tion, with the affected hip appearing shorter than the normal side. If the condition is not diagnosed before the infant is ready to walk, the child may begin walking later than is normal. The child may develop a limp and an unsteady gait, with one leg shorter than the other.

Early diagnosis of this condition is important, followed by immediate re-duction and immobilization by means of a plaster cast or by applying trac-tion. Permanent deformity, disloca-tion, uneven pelvis, retarded walking, limping, and unsteady gait are possi-ble complications if this condition re-mains untreated. Surgery is some-times required.

Arthritis and Other Joint Diseases

Arthritis is probably the most common of all disabling diseases, at least in the temperate areas of the world. It has been estimated that 10 percent of the population suffers from one of the many forms of arthritis. In the United States alone, more than 13 million persons each year seek professional medical care for arthritis. Of this number, some three million must restrict their daily activities, and about 750,000 are so disabled by ar-thritis that they are unable to attend school, work, or even handle common household tasks.

Arthritis apparently is not associ-ated with any stage of civilization; it has been diagnosed in the skeletons of prehistoric humans. There is even evidence that arthritic diseases afflict a variety of animals, including the dinosaurs that inhabited the earth more than 100 million years ago. Arthritis caused pain and suffering to such famous personages as Goethe, Henry VI, Charlemagne, and Alexander the Great.

Arthritis and *rheumatism* are terms sometimes used interchangeably by the layman to describe any abnormal condition of the joints, muscles, or related tissues. Many rheumatic or arthritic diseases have popular names, such as "housemaid's knee," "baseball finger," or "weaver's bottom." Physicians usually prefer to apply the term *arthritis* to disorders of the joints, especially joint disorders accompanied by inflammation. More than 75 different diseases of the joints have been identified; they are classified according to their specific signs, symptoms, and probable causes. The list includes bursitis, gout, and tendinitis in addition to the major disorders, rheumatoid arthritis and osteoarthritis.

Rheumatoid arthritis and osteoarthritis are examples of two types of arthritic ailment that are quite different diseases. Rheumatoid arthritis usually develops from unknown causes before the age of 45 and is marked by a nonspecific inflammation of the joints of the extremities; the inflammation is accompanied by changes in substances found in the blood. A victim of rheumatoid arthritis may develop limb deformities within a short period of time. Osteoarthritis, on the other hand, is most likely to produce symptoms after the age of 45. Here the cause is simply wear and tear on the cartilage cushions of the joints, mainly weight-bearing ones such as the hips and knees. Both kinds of joint disorders afflict millions of persons with painful and disabling symptoms.

Osteoarthritis

The most common form of arthritis is *osteoarthritis*, which is also known by the terms *hypertrophic arthritis* and *degenerative joint disease*. It can be said quite accurately that if you live long enough you will experience osteoarthritis. In fact, osteoarthritis is most common in areas of the world where people have the greatest longevity. The first signs of osteoarthritis may appear on X-ray pictures of persons in their 30s and 40s, even though they have not yet felt pain in the weight-bearing joints, the hips and knees, where discomfort usually appears first. Studies show that nearly everybody has at least the beginning signs or symptoms of osteoarthritis after they reach their 50s. It affects both men and women, although women may not experience symptoms until after they have reached the menopause.

Causes

A somewhat simplified explanation of the cause of osteoarthritis is this: the joints between the bones of a young person are cushioned and lubricated by cartilage pads and smooth lining membranes; normal wear and tear on

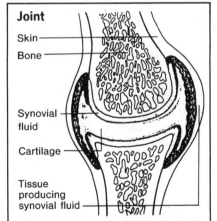

Joint

Skin

Bone

Synovial fluid

Cartilage

Tissue producing synovial fluid

All of the body's joints allow movement of the bones through this combination of ball and socket contours. Cartilage allows the bones to move without scraping or catching. Synovial fluid helps reduce friction in the movement.

the joints during a lifetime of activity gradually erodes the protective layers between the bones. In addition, the bones may develop small growths at the joints, a factor that aggravates the situation. There is evidence that heredity plays a role in the development of these bone growths, which are ten times more likely to occur in women than in men.

While hips and knees are among the most likely targets of osteoarthritis, the disease also can involve the hands, the shoulders, or back. Weight-bearing joints are commonly involved when the patient is overweight and spends a great deal of time standing or walking.

Symptoms

Except for the descriptions of aches and pains by victims of osteoarthritis and X-ray examination of the joints, a physician frequently has little information to go on in making a diagnosis of this disease. In some cases, there may be enlargement of the joint and some tenderness. But few cases are marked by the excessive warmth, for example, associated with rheumatoid arthritis. There are no laboratory tests that can distinguish the disorder from other rheumatic or arthritic diseases.

Osteoarthritis seldom causes the degree of discomfort experienced by patients afflicted by rheumatoid arthritis; the disease is not as disabling for most patients, and even the stiffness associated with osteoarthritis is milder, usually lasting only a few minutes when activity is attempted, while the stiffness of rheumatoid arthritis may continue for hours.

Arthritis of the Hip

Although most cases of osteoarthritis are not seriously disabling, arthritis of

Hip Disorders

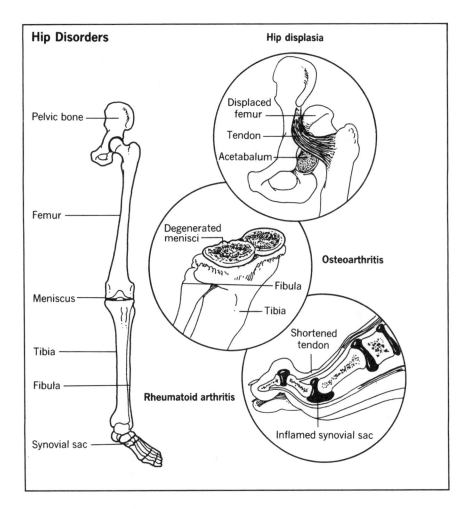

Hip displasia

Displaced femur
Tendon
Acetabalum

Degenerated menisci

Osteoarthritis

Fibula
Tibia

Shortened tendon

Rheumatoid arthritis

Inflamed synovial sac

Pelvic bone
Femur
Meniscus
Tibia
Fibula
Synovial sac

the hip is a prominent cause of disability in older persons. It produces pain in the hips, the inner thigh, the groin, and very often in the knee. Walking, climbing steps, sitting, and bending become very painful, because the joint is destroyed by degeneration of bone and cartilage. Stress and strain on the hip joint further aggravate the condition, which becomes worse with advancing age.

Surgery to replace the head of the femur or the entire hip joint with metal or plastic parts has brought relief from pain and restored mobility to some patients suffering from severe arthritis of the hip.

Small children sometimes suffer from transient arthritis of the hip, of unknown cause, manifested by pain, limitation of hip movement, and impeded walking. Because the condition usually disappears within six weeks, the only treatment is bed rest. Transient arthritis must not be mistaken for the more serious pyrogenic hip arthritis of children and adults, marked by high fever.

Spinal Arthritis

The aging process is the prinicipal cause of spinal arthritis. Other contributing factors are disk lesions and injury. Spinal arthritis causes pronounced bone degeneration and disability. The sufferer experiences severe back pain radiating to the thighs as a result of interference of the nerve roots from *osteophytes*, or spurs, formed in the joints. In mild cases, physical therapy may be the only treatment required.

Treatment of Osteoarthritis

For most patients, osteoarthritis is not likely to be crippling or disabling. The effects generally are not more serious than stiffness of the involved joints, with occasional discomfort and some pain. When weight-bearing joints are involved, the basic remedies are weight control and adequate rest for the areas affected. In some instances, the patient may have to learn new postural adjustments; symptoms often appear in another joint after the first has been affected because the patient tends to favor the joint that first caused pain and shifts weight or muscle stress to the second joint.

Physical therapy and corrective exercises are helpful. A physician may recommend the use of aspirin or another analgesic for the pain. Steroid drugs may be injected into an injured joint, but usually only for temporary relief. Surgery is sometimes recommended for removal of troublesome bone spurs or to correct a serious problem in a weight-bearing joint, where a metal cup or other device may be inserted as part of an artificial joint.

Rheumatoid Arthritis

Rheumatoid arthritis occurs at a much earlier age than osteoarthritis, appearing at any time from infancy to old age, but most commonly afflicting persons between the ages of 20 and 35. Women are three times as likely to be victims of rheumatoid arthritis as are men, although men seem to lose that advantage after the age of 50. All races seem to be equally vulnerable. Recent studies also suggest that two common beliefs about rheumatoid arthritis probably are untrue. The facts show that the disease is not hereditary and that it is not more prevalent in cold, damp climates.

Symptoms

Rheumatoid arthritis can begin as part of an acute illness, with high fever and intense inflammation of the joints, or it can develop insidiously with little or no discomfort except for fatigue, loss of appetite, weight loss, and perhaps a mild fever. Sometime later the victim becomes aware of aches and pains in the joints and muscles and seeks medical attention. Frequently, deformities develop before the patient realizes that rheumatoid arthritis may be the cause of swollen joints, pain, redness, or excessive warmth about the affected area.

The inflammation of a joint caused by rheumatoid arthritis may continue for weeks or it may last for a period of years. During inflammation, tendons become shortened and muscles lose their normal balance. The result is the deformity of joints commonly associated with rheumatoid arthritis, such as a swan-neck shape in the fingers. Muscular weakness develops and there is a loss of grip strength in the hands when that area is affected. Patients may be unable to make a tight fist.

A common symptom of rheumatoid arthritis is a stiffness that develops during periods of rest but gradually disappears when activity resumes. After a night's sleep, the stiffness may persist for a half hour or much longer. The stiffness may result, at least in part, from the muscular weakness that accompanies the disease.

Although the effects of rheumatoid arthritis are most commonly observed in the hands or feet of patients, other body joints such as the elbows, shoulders, knees, hips, ankles, spine, and even the jawbones may be involved. It is possible for all of a patient's joints to be involved, and the involvement often is symmetrical; that is, both hands will develop the symptoms at the same time and in the same pattern.

Probable Causes

The exact cause of rheumatoid arthritis is unknown, although a variety of factors have been associated with the onset of the disease. Emotional upsets, tuberculosis, venereal disease, psoriasis, and rheumatic fever are among conditions associated with the beginnings of the disease. Various viruses and other microorganisms have been isolated from the inflamed tissues of patients, but medical researchers have been unable to prove that any of the infectious agents is the cause. Efforts have also been made to transmit rheumatoid arthritis from a known victim to a normal volunteer by transfusions and injections of substances found in the victim's tissues, but without success in tracing the causative factor.

Treatment

The symptoms of rheumatoid arthritis intensify or abate spontaneously and unpredictably. Available methods of treatment do not cure the disease but relieve the symptoms so that the pain is reduced and some normal movement is facilitated. Proper nutrition, heat, rest, and exercise are also helpful. A number of drugs can reduce the inflammation of the joints, but they may have undesirable toxic side effects. Accordingly, before any drug therapy is embarked upon, the patient should seek the advice of a physician specializing in arthritic disorders.

Aspirin

The most common drug used to treat all kinds of arthritis is aspirin; it is also the most economical. Occasional side effects, such as irritation of ulcers or other gastrointestinal upsets, as well as buzzing in the ears, can result from aspirin use, especially in massive doses; such complications can some-

times be avoided by the use of specially coated aspirin tablets. The size of the dose usually is started at a minimum level and gradually increased until the physician finds a level that is most helpful to the patient but does not result in serious side effects.

Several other types of medication have been tried as alternatives to aspirin. One of the newer drugs, *indomethacin*, is about as effective as aspirin, but when taken in large doses it also seems to cause side effects, including nausea, heartburn, and headache.

Sulindac, a nonsteroidal antiinflammatory drug (NSAI), made its appearance on the U.S. market in the late 1970s. Under the trade name Clinoril, sulindac came into wide use in the treatment of a variety of arthritic disorders. These included osteoarthritis, rheumatoid arthritis, gouty arthritis, and painful shoulder.

Sulindac both relieves pain and reduces fever while attacking inflammations. In those respects it resembles other antiarthritis drugs such as fenoprofen (trade name: Nalfon), naproxen (trade name: Naprosyn), and tolmetin (trade name: Tolectin). Sulindac can be ingested on a twice-daily basis; but in use it was found to have adverse side effects, some of them serious. For example, some patients reported abdominal pains, nausea, and constipation. Diarrhea can also occur. Some side effects involved the central nervous system, and included dizziness, drowsiness, and headache.

Among other drugs used to treat arthritis, DMSO (dimethylsulfoxide) attracted widespread attention in the early 1980s. Research indicated that DMSO might have value as an antiarthritic agent. The Arthritis Foundation of the United States indicated, however, that DMSO might serve as "a short-term analgesic for pain due to limited conditions." A liquid that arthritis sufferers rubbed on their skin,

DMSO was reported to have such negative side effects as skin rashes and halitosis.

Many other drugs promising relief for victims of arthritis have made their appearance in recent years. For example, penicillamine (trade name: Cuprimine) was found to help patients with rheumatoid arthritis. Experiments with many other drugs—including aclofenac, flurbiprofen, and proquazone—are under way.

Steroids

The cortisone-type (steroid) drugs have proven effective in controlling severe cases of rheumatoid arthritis. They can be given orally or injected directly into the affected joints. However, these drugs generate a number of undesirable side effects, and withdrawal often results in a severe recurrence of the original symptoms. Thus, steroid drug therapy is a long-term process that can make the patient totally dependent on the medication. Some physicians are reluctant to inject steroid drugs into the joints because the effect is temporary and there is a danger of introducing infection by repeated use of the needle. In addition, some patients do not seem to respond to the steroid drugs and X-ray studies of the joints may show progressive destruction of the tissues despite the medications.

Rest

Bed rest is recommended for acute cases and up to 10 hours of sleep per day is advised for mild cases of rheumatoid arthritis. The patient also should take rest periods during the day whenever possible, reducing fatigue and stress on the affected joints. As in severe cases of osteoarthritis, the patient should try to adjust his daily work habits to avoid strain on weight-bearing joints.

Exercise

Patients tend to avoid moving arthritic joints because of pain and stiffness. Exercise of an arthritic joint, however, helps prevent the adjoining muscles from shrinking and weakening. A program of physiotherapy—including hot packs and exercise—can be extremely helpful.

The exercise program should carry the joints through their normal range of movement. Exercises should be performed every day but not carried to the point of fatigue. In addition to exercises intended to prevent limitation of normal joint movement, isometric-type exercises should be used to maintain or increase muscle power in other parts of the body that might otherwise be neglected because of limited activity by the patient.

Posture

The patient should be encouraged to maintain proper posture as much as possible, through correct positioning of the body when standing, sitting, or reclining in bed. A sheet of thick plywood may be used under a mattress to prevent it from sagging. Chairs should be firm with straight backs. Pillows should be avoided whenever possible.

Crutches, canes, leg braces, and other devices may be needed by the patient in advanced stages of rheumatoid arthritis. In some cases, orthopedic surgery is recommended to help reconstruct the limbs and joints as a part of rehabilitation.

Heat

Massages or vibrating equipment are not recommended as part of the therapy for rheumatoid arthritis patients. Heat in the form of hot baths, hot compresses, or heating pads, however, may be helpful. Paraffin baths are particularly helpful in treating hands or wrists.

Diet

While osteoarthritis patients are advised to lose as much weight as possible, rheumatoid arthritis patients tend to suffer from weight loss and nutritional deficiencies. Part of the cause may be a loss of appetite that is a characteristic of the disease and part may be the gastrointestinal problems that frequently accompany the disorder and that may be aggravated by the medications prescribed. Some physicians advise that rheumatoid arthritis patients include adequate amounts of protein and calcium in their diets as a preventive measure against a loss of bone tissue.

Juvenile Rheumatoid Arthritis

A form of arthritis quite similar to adult rheumatoid arthritis afflicts some children before the age of 16. Called *juvenile rheumatoid arthritis* or *Still's disease*, it includes a set of symptoms that nevertheless differentiate it from adult rheumatoid arthritis. In addition to the rheumatoid joint symptoms, the patient may have a high fever, rash, pleurisy, and enlargement of the spleen. The onset of the disease may appear in the form of an unexplained childhood rash and fever, with arthritic symptoms developing as much as several weeks later. A possible complication is an eye inflammation that can lead to blindness if untreated.

Treatment

Juvenile rheumatoid arthritis is treated with aspirin or steroid drugs, or both, along with other kinds of therapy used for the adult version of rheumatoid arthritis. Steroid therapy is often more effective against rheumatoid arthritis in children than in adults. There may be a complete remission of the disease or the patient may experience rheumatoid symptoms into adult life.

Ankylosing Spondylitis

A kind of arthritis that affects the spine, causing a fusion of the joints, is known as *ankylosing spondylitis*. About 90 percent of the patients are young adult males. There is some evidence that it may be a hereditary disease.

Like other forms of arthritis, ankylosing spondylitis is insidious in its start. The patient may complain of a backache, usually in the lumbar area of the back. Some victims of the disease have claimed they were without pain but felt muscle spasms and perhaps tenderness along the lower part of the spine. Then stiffness and loss of motion spread rapidly over the back.

Along with fusion of the spine, the ligament along the spine calcifies like a bone. X-ray photographs of the spinal column may show the backbone to resemble a length of bamboo. A complication is that the spine is bent and chest expansion is limited by the fusion so that normal breathing is impaired.

Treatment of the disease consists of physical therapy and exercises to prevent or limit deformity and the use of aspirin or other drugs to reduce pain.

Gout

Gout is an arthritic disease associated with an abnormality of body chemistry. There is an excessive accumulation of uric acid in the blood resulting from the chemical abnormality, and the uric acid, in the form of sharp urate crystals, may accumulate in the joints, where they cause an inflammation with symptoms like those of arthritis. A frequent target of the u-rate crystals is the great toe, which is why gout patients occasionally are pictured as sitting in a chair with one foot propped upon a pillow.

Primary Gout

There are two forms of gout, primary gout and secondary gout. Primary gout is presumed to be linked to a hereditary defect in metabolism and afflicts mostly men, although women may experience the disease after menopause. The painful inflammation may develop overnight following an injury or illness or after a change in eating habits. The patient may suddenly feel feverish and unable to move because of the tenderness of the affected joint, which becomes painfully swollen and red.

Although the great toe is a common site for the appearance of gout, it also may develop in the ankle, knee, wrist, hand, elbow, or another joint. Only one joint may be affected, or several joints might be involved at the same time or in sequence. The painful attack usually subsides within a week or so but it may return to the same joint or another joint after an absence of a few years. The inflammation subsides even if it is not treated, but untreated gout may eventually result in deformity or loss of use of the affected joint. During periods between attacks the patient may show no signs of the disease except for high blood serum levels of uric acid and the appearance of *tophi*, or *urate* (a salt or uric acid) deposits, visible in X-ray photographs of the joints.

Secondary Gout

Secondary gout is related to a failure of the kidneys to excrete uric acid products or a variety of diseases that are characterized by overproduction of certain types of body cells. Failure of the kidneys to filter out urates can, in turn, be caused by various drugs, including aspirin and diuretics. Gout symptoms can also be caused by efforts to lose weight rapidly through a starvation diet, because this speeds up the breakdown of stored body fats. Among diseases that may precipitate an attack of secondary gout are Hodgkin's disease, psoriasis, and some forms of leukemia.

Chronic Gouty Arthritis

A form of arthritis called *chronic gouty arthritis* is associated with patients who have abnormal levels of uric acid in their blood. While they may or may not be plagued by attacks of acute joint pain, the urate deposits apparently cause a certain amount of stiffness and soreness in various joints, especially during periods of stormy weather or falling barometric pressure. The tophi or urate crystals may spread to soft tissues of the body, such as bursae, the cartilage of the ear, and tendon sheaths. More than ten percent of gout patients eventually develop kidney stones formed from urate deposits in the kidney.

Treatment of Gout

Because gout was traditionally associated with certain meats that are rich in chemicals called *purines*, special diets were once a routine part of the treatment. In recent years, there has been less emphasis placed on maintaining a low-purine diet for gout patients. This change in therapy is mainly the result of the relatively good success in maintaining proper uric-acid levels in gout patients with medications. However, adequate fluid intake is still recommended to prevent development of urate kidney stones.

Infectious Arthritic Agents

There are at least 12 types of arthritis

and rheumatism that are associated with infections involving bacteria, viruses, fungi, or other organisms. One of these diseases is known as *pyrogenic arthritis*. The arthritis-causing organisms infect a joint and induce pain and fever and limitation of joint movement by muscle spasm and swelling. Treatment includes bed rest and antibiotics. If untreated, destruction of the joints is possible.

Gonococcal Arthritis

This disease is transmitted by the gonococcal bacteria associated with venereal disease. As in the venereal disease itself, the arthritic effects are more likely to be treated at an early stage in men than in women because men are more likely to develop obvious infections of the urethra and thus seek medication from a physician. In females, the initial infection is likely to go unrecognized and untreated by antibiotics. The infection, meanwhile, may spread to body joints and produce acute attacks of arthritis. The symptoms tend to appear first in the wrists and finger joints; there may also be skin lesions that occur temporarily in areas near the joints.

Tuberculous Arthritis

As the name suggests, this disease is associated with tuberculosis and can be serious, leading to the destruction of involved joints. The infection spreads to the joints from other areas of the body. The early symptoms include pain, tenderness, or muscle spasm. In children and young adults the infection tends to settle in the spinal joints. If there is an absence of pain, the disease may go unnoticed until changes in posture or gait are observed. If untreated, the disease may progress toward spinal deformity. When detected early in the course of the disease, treatment with anti-

tuberculosis drugs and physical therapy may control the disorder. In some cases, surgery may be required.

Rubella Arthritis

This form of arthritis derives from an infection involving the rubella virus. The arthritis symptoms may appear shortly after a rash appears, or they may be delayed until after the rash has faded. The onset of the arthritis effects may be accompanied by fever and a general feeling of illness; pain and swelling are most likely to occur in the small joints of the wrists, knees, or ankles. The physician usually advises aspirin for the pain while it lasts, usually about a week. Eventually all signs and symptoms may subside without joint destruction.

Bacteria That Cause Arthritis

A type of bacteria that causes spinal meningitis also may cause symptoms of arthritis. The pain usually is not severe and may be limited to a few body joints. Antibiotics are administered to control the infection, although this form of the disease does not respond as rapidly to the medication as some of the other versions of arthritis caused by infection.

Several other kinds of bacteria may invade the joints and precipitate or aggravate arthritic symptoms. They include the increasingly common strains of bacteria that have become resistant to control by antibiotics. Patients who are being treated with steroid drugs or those whose resistance to infection has been lowered by disease are among the most vulnerable victims.

Fungal Arthritis

While fungal infections are relatively rare causes of arthritis, there are at least four kinds of fungus that have been identified as the responsible or-

ganisms in joint inflammations. The fungus seems to be carried by the bloodstream to the area of the joint where it causes an inflammation in the tissues surrounding the bony structures. The infection usually can be treated with special antibiotic remedies that destroy fungal organisms, but surgery is occasionally necessary to ensure eradication of the source of the inflammation.

Psoriatic Arthropathy

Arthritis also may be associated with psoriasis (a chronic skin condition marked by bright red patches and scaling) in a disease known as *psoriatic arthropathy*. This variation of the disease is marked by a deep pitting of the nails along with a chronic arthritic condition. The disease may be mild or very destructive and the sacroiliac region of the spine may be involved. The uric acid levels associated with gout frequently are elevated in patients with psoriasis, so gout symptoms also can appear. Unfortunately, one of the medications commonly used in the treatment of rheumatoid arthritis and gout, chloroquine, cannot be used as therapy for psoriatic arthropathy symptoms because the drug aggravates the psoriasis. Otherwise, the treatment is quite similar to that used for rheumatoid arthritis—analgesics such as aspirin and steroid drugs. In severe cases, methotrexate may be administered to control both the joint and skin symptoms.

Other Arthritic Diseases

Two kinds of arthritis once associated with venereal diseases are no longer considered a hazard of intimate contact. One is syphilis-caused arthritis, which is a possible problem but actually quite rare because of improved control of syphilis. The second is *Rei-*

ter's syndrome, a form of arthritis in which there is also involvement of urethritis, or inflammation of the urethra, and conjunctivitis, an inflammation of the eye. The disease also may be accompanied by skin lesions and a fever, pain in the heels, and a urethral discharge. Perhaps because Reiter's syndrome seems to affect young men and symptoms may be similar to those of gonococcal arthritis, it was once assumed that this form of arthritis was a kind of venereal disease. However, there is a lack of evidence that the disease is transmitted by sexual contact.

Rheumatic Fever

This generalized inflammatory disease, which affects the entire body with pain and swelling of the joints, sometimes is classified as a form of arthritis. Rheumatic fever usually follows a sore throat or tonsillitis caused by streptococcus bacteria; however, the disease is not regarded as a streptococcal infection by itself. A common effect of rheumatic fever is a scarring of the heart valves due to inflammation of that tissue. The heart valve damage is permanent. The streptococcal infection itself can be controlled by antibiotic medications. For further information, see "Rheumatic Fever and Rheumatic Heart Disease" in Ch. 10, *Heart Disease.*

Bursitis

The *bursa* is a fluid-filled sac located in the muscle near most joints. The fluid lubricates the joint, thereby providing smooth joint movement. Infection or injury may cause inflammation of the bursa. This condition is known as *bursitis* and can be very painful. The most commonly affected joints are the shoulder, knee, and hip.

Calcium deposits in the shoulder

tendon or calcification of the bursa (*calcific bursitis*) leads to more painful shoulder problems. This may be similar to *interstitial calcinosis,* a condition in which calcium deposits are found in the skin and subcutaneous tissues of children. Recovery from calcific bursitis is achieved by medical care, minor surgery, and resting the inflamed joint. Radiation treatments can sometimes speed the recovery process.

Living with Joint Diseases

The control of arthritis requires skilled medical supervision over extended periods of time. The causes of the major forms of arthritis are still unknown, although various theories have been formulated to explain it based on metabolic, biochemical, and microscopic tissue studies. Despite years of intensive research, it has not been possible to isolate a microorganism that is generally agreed to be a cause of rheumatoid arthritis. Viruses have been implicated in a number of arthritic diseases and may be a cause of rheumatoid arthritis; the evidence remains elusive, however, and the vi-

rus theory will remain a theory until the specific causative organism has been isolated and tested.

Whatever the mystery surrounding the causes of osteoarthritis and rheumatoid arthritis, severe crippling can be prevented in 70 percent of the cases if the patient seeks medical care early in the disease and receives proper medical treatment. The course of the disease varies from patient to patient and in many cases is confined to a few joints, causing little or no impairment of function. Commonly, however, there is a tendency toward relapse or continued inflammation.

The arthritis patient needs to develop a sense of coexistence with the disease, a tolerant attitude toward the problems of possible pain or disability without surrendering to arthritis. Millions of people have learned to live with arthritis and have found that it is possible to work, travel, raise families, and enjoy many of the recreational activities pursued by people not afflicted by the disease.

Joint Replacement

Over the years, various methods of

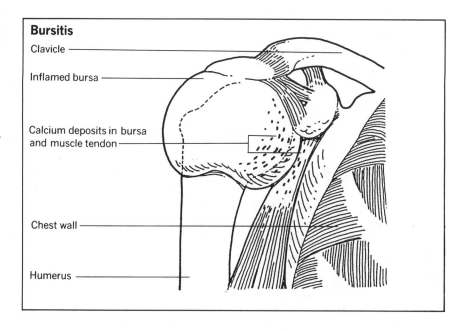

Bursitis

Clavicle

Inflamed bursa

Calcium deposits in bursa and muscle tendon

Chest wall

Humerus

Joint Replacement (Hip)

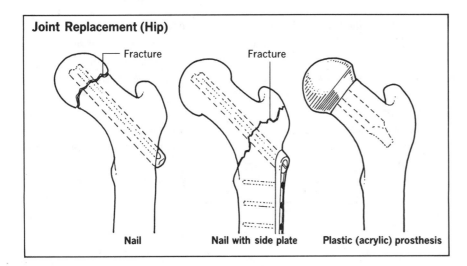

Fracture

Fracture

Nail

Nail with side plate

Plastic (acrylic) prosthesis

replacing joints have evolved. Like artificial hips, artificial knee, elbow, ankle, shoulder, toe, and finger joints are becoming more and more common. Technically known as arthroplasty, joint replacement both relieves pain, including the pain of arthritis, and improves function.

Materials used in joint replacement operations include metal, plastic, and ceramic components. Because of the tasks they perform in bodily movement, hip, knee, and ankle arthroplasties are undertaken much more often than those involving other parts. Developments in knee replacement surgery include a "cementless knee" that has a porous surface of chrome cobalt beads; aided by the beads, the patient's bone cells grow right into the knee replacement.

In each type of operation, the surgeon faces special problems. The elbow, for example, is not a simple hinge or joint but has three sections. Each involves one of the three arm bones that meet at that point: the humerus, the radius, and the ulna.

Surgical joint replacement techniques are continually evolving. In all cases, the patient faces some risks. Patients are also told usually that joint replacements do not really cure arthritis or osteoarthritis even though they normally relieve pain.

Defects and Diseases of the Spine

Spinal Curve Deformities

When looked at from the side, the normal human spine follows a shallow S-shaped curve. If there is an exaggerated forward curvature of the spine, that condition is described as a *lordosis*. This type of spinal curvature is uncommon except in late pregnancy, and is caused by hip deformity or a defect in posture.

Kyphosis

Kyphosis is an exaggerated backward spinal curvature characterized by a humpback appearance. A person with this disorder develops an abnormal-looking thorax (or chest) due to the hump in the back and may sometimes find it difficult to lie on his back. The condition is brought on by untreated fractures of a vertebral body, a spinal tumor, osteoporosis, or spinal tuberculosis. If the principal cause is diagnosed and treated, recovery is possible.

Scoliosis

Scoliosis is a lateral curvature of the central part of the spine and appears mostly in children from birth and young adults up to age 15. Early diagnosis and proper orthopedic care are important. If scoliosis appears in early adulthood, the prognosis is better than if the disease starts in infancy. Growth of the curvature ends

Vertebral Column

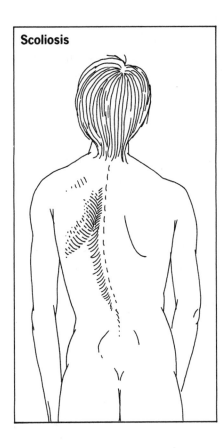

Scoliosis

when the individual's skeletal development ceases.

Scoliosis creates an ugly spinal deformity, and this is usually the only symptom. Sometimes there may be an acute attack of sciatica. Treatment of scoliotic children requires hospitalization. In simple cases, a cast is applied from the chest to the waist to reduce the curvature. Fusion of the vertebral bodies with bone grafting to maintain the fusion may be necessary.

Spinal Tuberculosis

Chronic pulmonary tuberculosis can spread to the skeletal system, including the vertebral column. Spinal tuberculosis, also known as *Pott's disease*, affects one or more vertebrae in children and young adults. It is currently a relatively rare disease.

The diseased vertebrae may collapse because of the pressure from the vertebrae above, resulting in a humpback deformity and possible paralysis of the lower limbs. The usual symptoms are back pain, stiffness, and limited movement. Antibiotics are administered to combat and cure the infection.

Spinal Infections

Fever-inducing microorganisms may reach the spine via the blood and lymph channels, resulting in spinal osteomyelitis or a general inflammation of the vertebrae. This results in bone destruction, pressure on the spinal cord, and paralysis of the legs. Successful treatment includes bed rest, drug therapy, and sometimes a body jacket (for immobilization) made from plaster of Paris.

Tumors

The spinal column is affected by both malignant and benign tumors. They can either destroy the bony makeup of the affected vertebra, apply pressure to the spinal cord with resultant paralysis, or interfere with the nerve roots.

Spinal tumors are generally destructive. Some, like *meningiomas* and *neurofibromas*, result in lack of control over bowel and bladder function in addition to the loss of functioning of the lower extremities. Malignant tumors of the spinal column may originate from cancer of the prostate, uterus, bladder, lungs, or breast.

The symptoms of spinal tumors are pain, deformity, weakness, and lower limb paralysis. Diagnosis requires careful study of the subjective symptoms, as well as special tests and radiological examinations. Treatment may involve radiation therapy and chemotherapy; some tumors can be surgically removed. In many instances, the patient may be given analgesics to relieve the pain.

Back Pain and Its Causes

Most adults have experienced some form of back pain. Back pain is a serious physical impairment in persons of all ages, but it occurs more frequently in older persons.

Lumbago and Sciatica

Lumbago refers to general pain in the lower back. Technically, it is not a disease but a symptom that is accentuated by bending, lifting, turning, coughing, or stooping. Pain from neu-

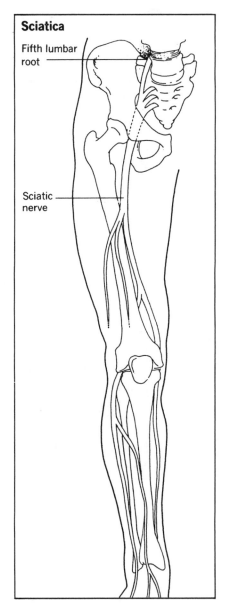

Sciatica

Fifth lumbar root

Sciatic nerve

ritis of the sciatic nerve adds to one's misery, with pain shooting down the legs. This form of back pain is commonly known as *sciatica*, and, like lumbago, can be considered a symptom of some other condition. Treatment depends on the underlying cause of both.

Slipped and Herniating Disks

Between each two vertebrae is a fibro-cartilaginous disk that acts as a cushion. These disks are subjected to strain with every movement of the body, especially in the erect position. Increased pressure may cause a disk to protrude or herniate into the vertebral canal, causing what is referred to as a *slipped disk*. This condition can also be brought on by injury, degeneration caused by aging, unaccustomed physical activity, or heavy lifting.

The herniating disk presses against nerves in the area, resulting in low back pain, sciatica, and in some instances, disabling muscle spasm. Back rest and a surgical corset may help milder forms of slipped disk by allowing natural healing to take place. Treatment may also include bed rest with intermittent traction to the legs for several weeks. Spinal fusion may be required in severe cases.

A severely herniated disk can be surgically removed to relieve pain and other symptoms. Disk removal is followed by fusion of the vertebral bodies on both sides of the removed disk. Fusion is accomplished by bridging the vertebral space with a bone graft. For a fuller description of surgical repair of a slipped disk, see under "Orthopedic Surgery" in Ch. 20, *Surgery*.

Spondylolisthesis

A forward displacement of one vertebral body over another results in a painful condition known as *spondylolisthesis*. In mild cases there may be no symptoms at all. But in more advanced forms, there is severe low back pain when in the erect position and on bending, with the pain radiating to the legs. The displaced vertebra interferes with nerve roots in that area.

Mild cases require no treatment. Severe cases may require fusion of the vertebral segments with bone grafting; less severe symptoms can be relieved by a specially fitted corset.

Muscle Spasms and Strained Ligaments

Lack of physical exercise and unaccustomed bending can cause acute backache from undue muscle strain. Backache from strain on the ligaments is not uncommon in women following childbirth. The symptoms are similar to general low back pain. Physiotherapy with moist heat and massage helps restore muscular tone and relieve the pain. Muscle-relaxing drugs are sometimes prescribed.

Sacroiliac Pain

The *sacroiliac* joints in the lower back, where the *iliac* (hipbone) joins the sacrum, are a common location for osteoarthritic changes, rheumatoid arthritis, tuberculosis, and ankylosing spondylitis. The most common site of pain is in the lower lumbar region, radiating to the thighs and legs. X-ray diagnosis helps to pinpoint the cause of this particular form of back pain.

Herniated Disk

Spinal cord

Spinal column (vertebra)

Herniated disk pressing against cord

Intervertebral disk

Lumbar region

Other Disorders of the Skeletal System

Because bone consists of living cells, it is constantly changing as old cells die and new cells take their places. Any systemic disease during the growing period may temporarily halt the growth of long bones. As the aging process continues, dead bone cells are not replaced as consistently as in earlier life. The bony skeleton thus loses some of its calcium content, a process known as *decalcification* or *bone atrophy*, and the bones become fragile.

Pelvis and Hip Disorders

The hip joint presents most of the problems in the pelvic area. Symptoms may appear in early infancy in the form of congenital hip dislocation, in older children as tuberculous and transient arthritis, as slipped epiphysis in young adults (discussed below), and as osteoarthritis in adults and the aged. Early diagnosis of these conditions is very important in reducing the possibility of permanent deformity.

Diagnosis is achieved by physical examinations for signs of abnormal joint stability and mobility, postural changes, unstable and painful hip movement, fixed joint deformity, and pain in the lower back. Measurement of both lower limbs may indicate the presence of abnormal hip structure. X-ray examination of the pelvic area and both hips aids in diagnosis, as does blood analysis, which may yield evidence of early signs of gouty or arthritic conditions.

Slipped Epiphysis

This condition occurs in late child-hood, between the ages of 9 and 18. The head of the *femur*, or thighbone, slips from its normal position, affecting one or both hips. The individual feels pain in the hip and knee, has limitation in joint movement, and walks with a limp. Usually there is evidence of endocrine disturbances.

Legg-Perthes' Disease

This is an inflammatory condition of unknown origin involving the bone and cartilage of the femoral head. It is found mostly in children between 4 and 12 years old and usually affects one hip. The symptoms are thigh and groin pain, joint movement limitation, and a walking impediment.

Successful treatment requires extended hospitalization with weight traction applied to the diseased hip and limitation of body weight on the affected side. Untreated Legg-Perthes' disease leads to permanent hip joint deformity and possible osteoarthritis around middle age.

Coxa Vara

This hip deformity is caused by a misshapen femur and causes shortening of the leg on the affected side; as a result, the person walks with a limp. The condition may be related to bone softening brought on by rickets, poorly joined fractures of the hip, or congenital malformation of the hip joint. Some cases may require surgical correction.

Any attack of persistent unexplained hip pains, limitation of movement, and walking impediments should be referred to the family physician for further investigation. Early diagnosis is crucial in controlling and eradicating many of the crippling diseases of the pelvic area.

Other Bone Disorders

Osteoporosis

This metabolic disorder is marked by porousness and fragility of the bones. When the condition is associated with old age, it is called *senile osteoporosis*. While the exact cause of the disorder is unknown, most physicians believe that calcium deficiencies—or inadequate calcium intake—may be a primary cause. Other contributing causes may be protein deficiency and a lack of the sex hormones androgen and estrogen. Postmenopausal women experience a dramatic decrease in the production of estrogen, which maintains bone strength. Because of its link with estrogen, osteoporosis is quite common among postmenopausal women.

Researchers stress the need for

Osteoporosis

Demineralization

both good diet and exercise as means of arresting or preventing osteoporosis. Calcium, estrogen, and vitamin D supplements may also help. A calcium-rich diet should include low-fat milk and cheeses; yogurt and ice cream; red kidney, lima, and soybeans; fish; watermelon, oranges, raisins, and strawberries; Brazil and other nuts; and green, leafy vegetables.

New methods of diagnosis have made possible earlier detection of osteoporosis. Three noninvasive methods include *absorptiometry*, measuring bone loss in the wrist and foot; *dual-photon absorptiometry*, a similar technique that indicates degrees of bone loss in the spine and hip; and an application of the CT scan that also measures loss of spinal bone. Blood tests, today the subject of research, may provide a means of very early detection. Once bone loss has been found to be too rapid, physicians can suggest ways to slow the rate of loss before fractures occur.

Osteogenesis Imperfecta

During the formation and development of bones, a process called *osteogenesis*, the bones may grow long and thin but not to the required width, becoming brittle so that they fracture easily. This condition is known as *osteogenesis imperfecta*. The individual may grow out of the condition in the middle twenties after suffering numerous fractures while growing up. A child thus afflicted cannot participate in games or other strenuous activities.

Paget's Disease

Paget's disease is characterized by a softening of the bones followed by an abnormal thickening of the bones. Its cause is unknown, and it manifests itself after the age of 30. It may cause

pain in the thighs, knees, or legs, as well as backache, headache, and general fatigue. Symptoms include deafness, deformity of the pelvis, spine, and skull, and bowed legs. Although there is no known cure, Paget's disease is not usually fatal, but is eventually disabling.

Osteomyelitis

Osteomyelitis is an inflammation of the bone caused by fever-inducing bacteria or mold organisms. The invading microorganisms usually reach the bone through the bloodstream after entering the body through a wound or ulcer; the infection also can begin through a compound fracture or during surgery. The staphylococcus germ is most frequently the causative agent, and the most frequent site is the shaft of a long bone of a child. In adults, osteomyelitis usually occurs in the pelvis or spinal column.

Symptoms

Symptoms are fever, chills, and pain, with nausea and vomiting, especially in younger patients. There also may be muscle spasms around the affected bone. The infected bone usually is sensitive to the touch but X rays may reveal no abnormality during the early stages. Redness and swelling sometimes appear in tissues above the inflamed bone, and as the disease progresses the patient may find that simply moving the affected limb is painful. The infection can involve a joint, producing misleading symptoms of arthritis.

Causes

Examination by a physician usually reveals signs of a recent wound, ulceration, or similar lesion that may have been accompanied by pus from the invading bacteria. Laboratory tests of

the blood usually will show an abnormal number of white cells and the presence of the infectious microorganism. Signs of anemia also may be found.

Treatment

Treatment may include the use of antibiotics for a period of several weeks. In difficult cases, surgery may be required to drain abscesses or to remove dead bone tissue. Before the advent of antibiotic drugs, osteomyelitis could be a fatal disease; early and proper treatment with modern medications has virtually eliminated that risk.

Diet and Bone Disorders

A proper diet is necessary to maintain the health of the skeletal system. The body's retention of the bone-building minerals, phosphorus and calcium, depends on vitamin D, which is manufactured in the human skin through the action of the sun's ultraviolet radiation.

Rickets

An insufficient supply of vitamin D and a lack of exposure to sunlight leads to a vitamin deficiency disease known as *rickets*. It can occur in infants and small children who live in northern latitudes and thus are not exposed to sufficient sunlight to permit their body to manufacture vitamin D. Rickets slows growth and causes bent and distorted bones and bandy legs. Symptoms first appear between the age of six months and the end of the first year. If rickets is recognized in time, it can be cured by a diet containing adequate vitamin D and by exposure to sunlight. If the disease is unchecked, the bones may develop permanent curves.

Bone Tumors

Benign and malignant tumors can occur in bone and bone marrow, although these growths are far less common than tumors of the body's soft tissues. Children and adolescents are more susceptible to bone tumors than adults. Since X rays cannot show whether a bone tumor is benign or malignant, surgical biopsy of the affected tissue is necessary in all cases.

Benign Tumors

These tumors usually take the form of an overgrowth of bone tissue, often near a joint, with many cysts or hollow spaces in the affected tissue. These growths often cause pathological fractures, in which a bone breaks for no apparent reason. Swelling, pain, and limited mobility in the joint nearest the tumor are the most common symptoms. Treatment consists of surgical removal of the tumor, after which the surrounding bone gradually repairs itself as it does after a fracture.

Malignant Tumors

Bone cancers may be primary (originating in the bone tissue itself) or caused by metastasis of cancer cells from a site elsewhere in the body. The most common types of primary bone cancer are *osteogenic sarcoma*, a rapidly growing form of cancer that often spreads into nearby muscles; *chondrosarcoma*, which begins in cartilage at the end of a bone; and *Ewing's sarcoma*, a highly malignant cancer of the shafts of the long bones in children.

Bone cancer of the extremities is treated by amputation of the affected limb, followed by radiation therapy. If treatment is begun early enough and all the cancerous tissue is removed, the prognosis for survival is favorable.

Injury to Bones and Joints: Fractures and Dislocations

Bones can be broken or displaced when the body is subjected to a violent impact or when a limb is suddenly wrenched out of its normal position. Auto and bicycle accidents and accidents in and around the home account for many such injuries. See Ch. 31, *Medical Emergencies*, for information on accidents and how to provide treatment.

A *fracture* is a break in a bone as a result of injury or pathological weakness. Tumors, for example, can destroy bones to such an extent that a spontaneous fracture occurs due to pathological weakness. Osteoporosis can also cause such fractures.

A *dislocation* is a displacement of any part, especially a bone. During this process the joint-capsule ligaments and muscle may be torn. The displaced bones must be reset by a bone specialist in their original position and immobilized until healing is complete. If this is not done, there is every possibility that the unhealed muscles will not provide the necessary support, thereby causing chronic spontaneous dislocation.

Injury (*trauma*) to bones and joints should not be dismissed lightly, especially if pain persists. If untreated, fractures and dislocations may heal with the bones out of alignment. Permanent deformity and joint degeneration are two possible complications.

Crush injuries, such as those occurring in some industrial and automobile accidents, may result in the clogging or blockage of blood vessels that supply blood to an extremity. When this happens, tissues below the blockage may die, and wounds do not heal because of lack of oxygenated blood and nutrition. If the fractures and wounds are not properly treated, *gangrene*, or the death of soft tissues, can sometimes result, requiring amputation just above the site of blockage and at a location that will make the healing process possible.

Kinds of Fractures

Incomplete fractures are those that do

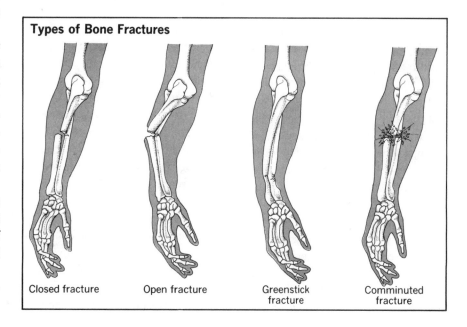

Types of Bone Fractures

Closed fracture   Open fracture   Greenstick fracture   Comminuted fracture not destroy the continuity of the bone. In a *complete fracture*, the bone is completely broken across. A *simple* or *closed fracture* is one in which the fragments are held together under the surface of the skin by the muscles and soft tissues. In a *compound* or *open fracture* one or both fragments pierce the skin, resulting in an open wound. In some cases the bony fragments can be seen protruding through the skin.

Comminuted fractures are the result of crushed bones. Several fragments appear at the trauma site. *Greenstick fractures* occur when one side of the bone is broken and the other bent. This type of fracture is more common in long bones, especially the forearms, clavicle, and legs of young children. *Stress fractures*, tiny cracks in the bone, can occur in the bones of the foot or leg of athletes who put these bones under repeated stress, such as ballet dancers and long-distance runners.

Healing of Fractures

When a bone breaks, new bone cells called *callus* are laid down at the ends of the fracture to unite the fragments. This is the beginning of the healing process, the speed of which is dependent on the nature of the fracture.

Simple, incomplete, and greenstick fractures heal readily. Rest is usually sufficient to heal stress fractures. However, compound fractures have wounds and fragments to complicate the healing process. Cleaning and suturing the wound and administering antibiotics reduce the chance of infection and promote healing.

Comminuted fractures may have to be disimpacted and all fragments reset, usually by an orthopedic or general surgeon. Some very serious fractures of the extremities may require surgical insertion of metallic pins, nails, plates, wires, or screws to hold

the fragments in proper position, thereby promoting rapid healing with minimal deformity. Such devices must be made from corrosion-free and rustproof metals because they may remain in the body for a few months or throughout the person's lifetime.

Age and the Healing Process

The age of the fracture victim determines the speed of healing. In healthy, normal children, broken bones mend quickly because a rapid bone-cell manufacturing process is constantly in progress during the growth of the child. This is further advanced by proper diet, including daily intake of milk and milk products to provide the calcium required to build healthy bones.

In young adults, new bone cells do not develop as rapidly as in the growing child, but under normal circumstances, this will not present problems with the healing of fractures. Fractures in the aged heal slowly or not at all, depending on the age and health of the individual.

Treatment of Fractures

Correction of a fracture or dislocation is called *reduction* and is usually performed by an orthopedic surgeon. Bones that are merely cracked do not require reduction; they heal with the aid of immobilization. More serious fractures require manipulation, pressure, and sometimes, as mentioned above, wires, pins, nails, and screws, to bring the fragments together so that they can unite.

Healing of fractures and dislocations following reduction requires proper immobilization, which also reduces pain by preventing movement of the fragments. Immobilization is usually accomplished by the use of splints or plaster casts or by applying

(Top) A metal plate is fastened with screws to secure a fractured bone in the arm (the radius). The enlarged portion shown in cross section is also shown as it appears in the patient's arm. *(Bottom)* A steel rod has been driven through the center of the femur of the leg to hold the jagged ends of the fractured bone in proper alignment. Such appliances are sometimes left in place indefinitely when there are no adverse reactions.

traction. Traction subjects the fractured member to a pulling force by means of a special apparatus, such as a system of weights and pulleys.

After a fracture or dislocation is reduced and immobilized in a cast, the injury is X-rayed to ensure that the immobilized reduction will heal without deformity. If the reduction is not satisfactory, the cast is removed, the fragments are remanipulated to provide better reduction, and a new cast or bandage is applied. Periodic X-ray rechecks help the physician ascertain the degree of new bone formation as the healing continues. Casts are also checked to make sure there is not excess swelling of tissues and compression of blood vessels in the area.

How long a cast must remain depends on the extent of the injury and the rapidity of healing. A broken wrist may heal in four to six weeks while a fractured tibia may require four months of immobilization in a plaster cast.

Fracture of the Pelvis

Pelvic injuries are most often caused by falls in the home or on slippery streets and by industrial or automobile accidents.

The pelvis bears the entire weight of the body from the waist up and must bear the stress of general body motion during daily activity. The bony architecture of the pelvis does not readily permit the use of a plaster cast to immobilize a fracture. Consequently, fractures of the pelvis require bed rest for at least three weeks, depending on the nature of the injury and the age of the patient.

Simple fractures in children and young adults heal readily with complete bed rest and proper home care. Among the aged, the creation of new bone cells occurs more slowly, and this complicates the management of serious pelvic fractures in people over 65. Prolonged inactivity from extensive bed rest presents other health hazards for the aged, such as sluggish digestion and respiratory or vascular complications.

Fracture of the Hip

Falls are a major cause of hip fractures—the most common type of pelvic injury. Intense pain with limitation of hip movement and external rotation of the lower leg are indications of a hip fracture. When this occurs, a physician should be contacted immediately. The patient should be placed flat in bed until medical advice has been obtained. Proper diagnosis requires X-ray examinations.

Patients with hip fractures must be hospitalized. Although a hip fracture may be treated with traction, this method requires months of bed rest and is rarely used. The best method for treating such fractures is to nail the hip together with a metallic pin. The operation is performed by a surgeon, usually an orthopedist, who uses X-ray examinations during surgery to ascertain that the pin is in the correct position. Some hip fractures may also require a metallic plate screwed to the bone to help immobilize the fracture.

After plates and pins have been inserted, the patient can be out of bed within a day. This speeds recovery and prevents the complications of prolonged bed rest. Hip nails are usually left in the patient, depending on the nature of the fracture and the patient's age. Recuperation includes periodic medical checkups and X-ray examinations.

Hip Replacement

In recent years the technique of total hip replacement has become well advanced. The technique can be used where the hip joint has been injured or severely weakened by disease.

Called *total prosthetic replacement of the hip*, the operation involves removal of the upper portion of the large leg bone, the femur, and of the ball-like joint that holds it in the hip socket. A substitute piece shaped like the removed section of bone is attached to the femur. Care has to be taken during the operation to make certain the new part is firmly attached—by embedding the replacement part in the shaft of the bone. In addition, the surgeon tries not to destroy or damage the muscles and other tissues surrounding the hip. The replacement part is usually made of metal; a commonly used material is a durable cobalt-chromium alloy that produces no painful reactions in surrounding bones and tissues.

With modern techniques, hip replacement surgery can restore most patients to virtually normal levels of functioning. The implanted parts can carry weight and stand the strains of everyday use. Metal screws and a grouting agent (mortar of plastic cement or other material) help to join the metal implant to the leg bone. Patients may begin to walk one to three days after surgery. While they can later play golf or other nonstrenuous games, they are usually told to avoid more demanding activities, such as tennis or handball, because of the danger that they might fall and injure the replacement hip.

Some patients have had successful hip replacement surgery on both their right and left sides. Later they were able to function with good mobility and without pain.

Pubic Fracture

Pubic fractures can cause ruptures of the bladder with urine leaking into the pelvic cavity. Routine urinalysis for the presence of blood cells is always necessary in cases of pelvic fractures. Surgical repair of the bladder may be required.

Skull Injury

Although the skull is very thick, it is not invulnerable. Head injuries can result from sports or playground accidents, falls, automobile or industrial accidents, or sharp blows to the head. Head injuries can cause linear or hairline skull fractures, depressed skull fractures (dents), brain injury due to fracture fragments or foreign bodies piercing the brain (as in the case of a bullet wound), or *concussion* with or without bone damage. The effects of concussion can show up as dizziness, nausea, irritability, the tendency to sleep deeply or lose consciousness, a weak pulse, and slowed respiration.

Any of these injuries can cause blood vessels to rupture and bleed. The resulting blood clots form what is known as a *subdural hematoma*, which may cause increased pressure on the brain. Patients with a subdural hematoma feel dizzy, slip slowly into unconsciousness, and may die unless immediate hospital care is available. Usually half of the body on the opposite side of the clot becomes paralyzed.

A depressed fracture can also apply pressure on the brain at the area of the depression. Surgery is required to relieve the pressure.

No skull injury should be treated lightly. A child may hit his head in a playground or in the backyard and conceal this from his parents, or a baby-sitter may be afraid of losing her job if she reports such a fall. An alcoholic may slip on the street and strike his head on the sidewalk. Anyone who suffers a blow to the head or who falls on his head should be observed carefully for possible later complications. If such incidents are followed by vomiting, drowsiness, and headaches, immediate medical attention should be sought.

Facial Injury

A blow to the eye may fracture the upper or lower borders of the eye socket. It can also cause what is commonly known as a black eye, the blue-black appearance of which results from bleeding under the skin. The swelling can be reduced by applying an ice pack to the area.

Fractures of the facial bones, jaw, and nose result from a direct blow to these areas. The impact may rupture blood vessels and cause facial deformity. Dislocation of the jaw is a common problem caused by trauma. It may also occur spontaneously in certain individuals by an unusually wide-mouthed yawn or laugh. It is an uncomfortable rather than painful experience.

Serious facial injury requires hospitalization and surgical restoration.

Skin lacerations may have to be sutured and the scars removed by plastic surgery; fractures of the jaw and mouth may require surgical wiring for stabilization and immobilization before healing can take place. In some instances both jaws may be wired together until healing takes place.

Injury to the Rib Cage

Accidents, athletic injuries, and fights account for most injuries to the rib cage. Any blow to the chest can cause rib fractures, which hurt when one coughs or inhales. Hairline and incomplete fractures are less serious than complete fractures, where the fragments are usually sharp and pointed. Such fractured ribs can tear the lungs, causing air to leak into the pleural space, with possibly serious results. The lung can collapse as a result of being punctured. Punctured blood vessels can hemorrhage into the pleural space. The accumulated blood may have to be withdrawn before it reduces the capacity of the lungs to carry out their normal function.

Severe chest injuries—crush injuries with multiple fractures—require hospitalization. The patient must be confined to bed and kept under constant medical observation and treatment. If the lung has collapsed, it has to be reinflated. In simple rib fractures the chest may be strapped to immobilize the fragments and promote rapid healing. Generally, analgesics alone are enough to relieve pain.

Fractures of the sternum are caused by direct blows to the sternal area, as is usually the case with automobile accidents when the steering wheel hits the driver's chest. This injury can be avoided if the driver wears a shoulder-restraining belt, and if his car is equipped with a collapsible steering column.

Chest pains following a blow to the area of the sternum should be medically investigated by means of X-ray diagnosis for possible fracture. The fracture fragments may have to be wired together and remain in place until the injury has healed. For simple fractures, rest may be the only treatment required. The serious complication of a fractured sternum in a steering-wheel accident is contusion of the heart; it should be evaluated by means of an electrocardiogram.

Spinal Injury

Most spinal injuries originate from automobile accidents, industrial mishaps, falls, athletics, or from fights and beatings. Spinal injuries can create fractures that compress or sever the spinal cord, with resultant paralysis. A diving accident or headlong fall may cause a concussion and possible fractures of the cervical spine. Head-on collisions in the sports arena and automobile accidents are the chief causes of cervical spine fractures.

An individual who jumps from a considerable height and lands on his feet, especially on his heels, may easily fracture his spine. Sudden pain in the thoracic spine following a jump should receive immediate medical attention and investigation.

Whiplash

These injuries, the most common form of injury to the spine, occur most often during head-on and rear-end automobile accidents that suddenly jerk the neck and injure the cervical vertebrae. Accident victims thus injured may undergo months of agonizing headaches and pain in the neck. Immobilization of the neck by a surgical collar will reduce some of the pain and aid the healing process.

First Aid for Spinal Injuries

Victims of spinal injuries should be moved as little as possible. While waiting for professional help, the patient should be placed on his back and made as comfortable as possible. If an accident or explosion victim is wedged between debris, attempts should be made to free him, but his body should be kept flat with as little movement as possible. No attempt should be made to have the person sit up or stand before he has been examined by a physician. Unnecessary movement of victims of spinal injury can damage the spinal cord and cause permanent paralysis.

Decompression of Fractures

Anyone with a spinal injury should be taken to the emergency ward of the nearest hospital for X-ray examinations that will reveal possible fractures. If the fracture compresses against the spinal cord, the extremities may be paralyzed. In such cases, a neurosurgeon or an orthopedist may perform a delicate operation, lifting the fracture fragments away from the spinal cord, thereby relieving the pressure and reestablishing control and movement of the paralyzed extremities.

Fractures of the cervical spine can be decompressed by applying traction to the neck. Frequent X-ray rechecks are required to assess the degree of healing and new bone formation. Patients with fractured vertebrae undergo a lengthy rehabilitation with frequent medical rechecks and physical therapy. In some severe cases of spinal fractures that result in paralysis, the individual is never able to walk again.

8

Diseases of the Muscles and Nervous System

We have the capacity to perceive our environment by receiving sensory messages—such as hearing, sight, touch, pain, and awareness of our posture—to associate all the incoming messages, store the information, and then call it back to our consciousness as needed. Another function of the nervous system is the control of the body by sending signals to the muscles to perform movements ranging from the broadest to the most delicate—from wielding a pickax to playing the flute. Further, many aspects of our behavior are not at all mysterious and can be explained in terms of a series of neuroelectrochemical events. In short, our day-to-day existence is a reflection of the state of our nervous system, the normal function of which can be disturbed in many ways.

Diseases of the Nervous System

If any part of the brain has developed abnormally, the usual function of that structure would be expected to be altered. Abnormalities present at birth are called *congenital* defects. If the nervous system does not receive a normal blood supply because of the obstruction of a blood vessel, or if there is a tear in the vessel with subsequent hemorrhage, the cells are deprived of blood and will die. These lesions are *vascular* or *cerebrovascular* accidents. Cerebral injury, or *trauma,* can destroy brain tissue, with consequent loss of normal function; infections of the nervous system may also permanently injure tissue. Finally, brain function can be altered by *metabolic, toxic,* or *degenerative* changes in normal body chemistry. It is not surprising, then, that such a beautifully organized nervous system is vulnerable to the hazards of living.

Diagnostic Tests

A patient who has been referred to a *neurologist,* a physician who specializes in diseases of the nervous system, will be asked to tell the history of the problem in great detail, for that history will describe the nature of the disorder; the neurological examination will help to localize the problem.

After the neurological examination is completed, the physician may order radiographs (X-ray pictures) of the skull and spinal column and an electroencephalogram. The *electroencephalogram* (EEG), or brain wave recording, assists in localizing a brain abnormality or describing the nature of a convulsive disorder. A specific diagnosis is not based upon the EEG alone, but the EEG is used to corroborate the physician's clinical impression of the disease process.

It may also be necessary to perform a *lumbar puncture* (*spinal tap*) in order to obtain a specimen of the *cerebrospinal fluid* (*CSF*), the fluid that bathes the brain and spinal cord. This laboratory test is a benign, relatively painless procedure when performed by a skilled physician and is extremely useful in making a diagnosis. It entails a needle puncture under sterile conditions in the midline of the lower spine as the patient lies on his side or sits upright.

Occasionally, other more specialized diagnostic tests are used to better enable the physician to visualize the structure of the brain and the spinal cord. In a process called *ventriculography,* the cerebrospinal fluid is replaced by air introduced directly into the cavities (*ventricles*) of the brain. In *pneumoencephalography*, the air or other gas is inserted by means of a needle similar to that used in a lumbar puncture. In either case the outlines of the brain structure are photographed by X ray.

Another specialized neuroradiological test is the *angiogram*. A material that is opaque to X rays is injected into the blood vessels that supply the brain. Because the vessels can be plainly seen on the X-ray film, any displacement of those vessels from the normal position is evident.

A more recent diagnostic tool is the *brain scanner* or *CT scanner* (for *computed tomography*). CT scanning may in many cases make angiography, which can be painful and is not without risk, unnecessary. The scanner takes a series of computer-generated X-ray pictures of "slices" of the brain as it rotates about the patient. It can thus provide better pictures of parts of the brain (and of other internal areas of the body) than any older process.

A later version of the CT scanner takes stop-action photos of the beating heart. Called the *cine CT*, the imaging procedure enables cardiologists to measure blood flow through grafted coronary arteries. Only by using a catheter could physicians take such measurements earlier. With the cine CT it is also possible to measure the weights of different parts of the heart with almost 100 percent accuracy and to detect minute holes in the hearts of children suffering from congenital heart defects. Surgeons use these pictures to become familiar with a defective heart before surgery.

More advanced than either the CT scanner or radiography, *nuclear magnetic resonance* (NMR) uses neither X radiation, as does the CT scanner, nor needle-injected contrast fluids. Instead, NMR uses magnetic forces 3,000 to 25,000 times as strong as

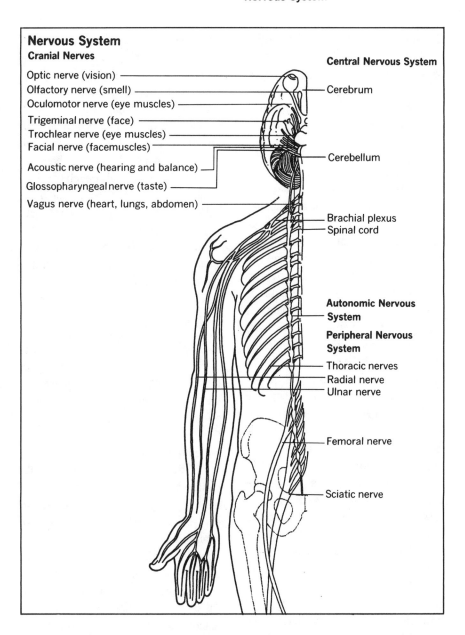

Nervous System
Cranial Nerves

Optic nerve (vision)
Olfactory nerve (smell)
Oculomotor nerve (eye muscles)
Trigeminal nerve (face)
Trochlear nerve (eye muscles)
Facial nerve (facemuscles)
Acoustic nerve (hearing and balance)
Glossopharyngeal nerve (taste)
Vagus nerve (heart, lungs, abdomen)

Central Nervous System

Cerebrum

Cerebellum

Brachial plexus
Spinal cord

Autonomic Nervous System

Peripheral Nervous System

Thoracic nerves
Radial nerve
Ulnar nerve

Femoral nerve

Sciatic nerve

the earth's magnetic field. Taking three-dimensional "pictures" of various parts of the body, NMR "sees" through bones. It can differentiate between the brain's gray and white matter. NMR can also show blood moving through an artery or the reaction of a malignant tumor to therapy.

Another type of contrast study is called a *myelogram*. A radiopaque liquid similar to that used in angiography is introduced through a spinal needle into the sac-enclosed space around the spinal cord. Any obstructive or compressive lesion of the spinal cord is thus seen on the radiograph and

helps to confirm the diagnosis.

Each of these contrast studies helps the physician better understand the structures of the brain or spinal cord and may be essential for him to make a correct diagnosis.

Cerebral Palsy

The term *cerebral palsy* is not a diagnosis but a label for a problem in locomotion exhibited by some children. Definitions of cerebral palsy are many and varied, but in general refer to nonprogressive abnormalities of the brain that have occurred early in life from many causes. The label implies that there is no active disease process but rather a static or nonprogressive lesion that may affect the growth and development of the child.

Symptoms

Included in the category of cerebral palsy are such problems as limpness (flaccidity), *spasticity* of one or all limbs, incoordination, or some other disorder of movement. In some patients, quick jerks affect different parts of the body at different times (*chorea*); in others, slow, writhing, incoordinated movements (*athetosis*) are most pronounced in the hands and arms. Incoordination of movement may also occur in muscles used for speaking and eating, so that speech becomes slurred, interrupted, or jerky; the patient may drool because incoordinated muscle action prevents efficient swallowing of saliva. This does little to improve the physical appearance of the child and, unfortunately, he may look mentally subnormal.

The fact that a patient has an abnormality that is responsible for difficulty in locomotion or speech does not mean that the child is mentally retarded. There is some likelihood that he will be mentally slow, but patients in this group of disease states range from slow to superior in intelligence, a fact that emphasizes that each child must be assessed individually.

A complete examination must be completed, and to determine the patient's functional status complete psychological testing should be performed by a skilled psychologist.

Treatment

Treatment for cerebral palsy is a continuing process involving a careful surveillance of the patient's physical and psychological status. A physical therapist, under the physician's guidance, will help to mobilize and maintain the function of the neuromuscular system. Occasionally, an orthopedic surgeon may surgically lengthen a tendon or in some way make a limb more functional. A speech therapist can provide additional speech training, and a vocational therapist can help the patient to find appropriate work. The key professional is the primary physician, usually the pediatrician, who with care and understanding guides the patient through the years.

Bell's Palsy

Bell's palsy is a paralysis of the facial nerve that was first described by Sir Charles Bell, a Scottish surgeon of the early nineteenth century. It may affect men and women at any age, though it occurs most commonly between the ages of 30 and 50. The onset of the facial paralysis may be abrupt: the patient may awaken one morning unable to move one side of his face. He can't wrinkle one side of his forehead or raise the eyebrow; the eye will not close on the affected side, and when attempting to smile, the face is pulled to the opposite side. Occasionally the patient may experience discomfort about the ear on the involved side. There is no difficulty in swallowing, but because the muscles about the corner of the mouth are weak, drooling is not uncommon, and food may accumulate in the gutter between gum and lip.

Bell's palsy may affect the branch of the facial nerve that supplies taste sensation to the anterior part of the tongue and the branch that supplies a small muscle in the middle ear (the *stapedius*) whose function it is to dampen loud sounds. Depending on the extent to which the facial nerve is affected, the patient may be unable to perceive taste on the side of the paralysis and may be unusually sensitive to sounds, a condition known as *hyperacusis.*

The most probable causes of Bell's palsy are inflammation of the facial nerve as it passes through a bony canal within the skull or inflammation of that bony canal with subsequent swelling and compression of the nerve. It is not uncommon that the patient has a history of exposure to a cold breeze, such as sleeping in a draft or riding in an open car. Any patient who has a facial weakness should be carefully evaluated by a physician, preferably a neurologist, to be quite certain that there is no other neurologic abnormality. When the diagnosis of Bell's palsy is certain, some therapeutic measures can be taken.

Treatment

There is no specific treatment for Bell's palsy, but many physicians recommend massage, application of heat, and exercise of the weak muscles, either passive (by external manipulation) or active (by use). These therapeutic measures do not specifically influence the course of the facial nerve paralysis, but they are thought to be useful in maintaining tone of the facial muscles and preventing permanent deformity. Occasionally a V-shaped adhesive tape splint can be applied to the affected side of the face, from the corner of the mouth to the temple. Some physicians treat the condition with steroids such as cortisone, which may hasten recovery if begun at the onset of the illness.

In treating Bell's palsy, it is important to remember that when the eyelid does not close normally, the conjunctiva and cornea are not fully lubricated, and corneal lesions may develop from excessive dryness or exposure to the air. For this reason, some ophthalmic lubrication may be recommended by the physician.

About 80 percent of the patients with Bell's palsy recover completely in a few days or weeks, and about 10 to 15 percent recover more slowly, over a period of three to six months. The remaining 5 to 10 percent will have some residual facial deformity.

Parkinson's Disease

Patients with *Parkinson's disease,* or *parkinsonism,* are easily recognized because of the characteristic symptoms of tremor, rigidity, and a decrease of movement. This group of symptoms had another name, *shaking palsy,* long before it was scientifically described nearly a century and a half ago by an English physician, James Parkinson. It is associated with degeneration of nerve cells deep within the brain (*basal ganglia*) and the brain surface (*cerebral cortex*). It may follow encephalitis, a brain injury, or exposure to toxic substances, but in most cases, especially when the symptoms appear in a patient who is middle-aged or older, there is no known cause.

The tremor, or shaking, usually involves the fingers and the wrist, but sometimes the arms, legs, or head are involved to the extent that the entire body shakes. Characteristically, the tremor occurs when the patient is at rest. It stops or is much less marked during a voluntary muscle movement, only to start once again when that movement has been stopped. There is no tremor when the patient is asleep.

Early in the disease, the patient is aware that one leg seems a bit stiff; later, the arm does not swing normally at his side when he is walking. He moves about more slowly with stooped-over head and shoulders. Often he has difficulty in starting to walk, but once started he cannot stop unless he grabs at the wall or some

other object. The face appears expressionless, the speech is slurred, and handwriting is small and uneven (*micrographia*) because of the rigidity and the tremor. Mental faculties are usually not impaired but, as might be expected in such a chronic disease in which the patient cannot move or communicate normally, mood disturbances are common.

Treatment

For many years parkinsonism was treated with drugs derived from belladonna. Many other remedies were tried, among them such toxic compounds as strychnine and cigarettes made from jimsonweed. In nearly all cases the results were less than gratifying. Neurosurgical procedures were then devised to produce very small destructive lesions in the brain, with subsequent lessening of the symptoms. The most gratifying improvements following surgery are usually seen in patients under 60 whose symptoms are confined primarily to one side of the body.

Today, three basic categories of drugs are used to relieve the symptoms of parkinsonism: anticholinergics, levodopa-containing compounds, and a single dopamine agonist.

The anticholinergic drugs include trihexyphenidyl hydrochloride (trade name: Artane), benztropine mesylate (trade name: Cogentin), diphenhydramine hydrochloride (trade name: Benadryl), biperiden (trade name: Akineton), and procyclidine hydrochloride (trade name: Kemadrin). All of these drugs reduce tremors and rigidity to a modest degree, but none affects bradykinesia, or slow movement. Patients using the drugs may experience such side effects as gingivitis or inflammation of the gums, constipation, mild dizziness, nausea, nervousness, and slightly blurred vision. More serious side effects could

include urinary retention, confusion, and psychosis.

The levodopa-containing compounds reduce all the main symptoms of parkinsonism. One such compound combines levodopa, also known as L-dopa, with carbidopa (trade name: Sinemet). Levodopa is also sold alone under the trade names Larodopa and Dopar. Because L-dopa's effectiveness may dwindle after several years, physicians sometimes delay treatment until a patient shows more severe symptoms.

Side effects associated with L-dopa include nausea, involuntary movements, some mental changes, cardiac irregularities, and urinary retention. "End-of-dose" akinesia, the return of symptoms a few hours after taking medication, can be relieved in some cases by taking the patient off drugs entirely for three to seven days. The patient is usually hospitalized. During the "drug holiday" some patients take part in physical, occupational, and speech therapy programs.

The one drug in the dopamine agonist class, bromocriptine (trade name: Parlodel), stimulates the brain's dopamine receptors. Used in combination with L-dopa, bromocriptine reduces the end-of-dose response. But clinical studies have not established the drug's safety in long-term use (more than two years). Patients with histories of coronary or peripheral vascular disease should not take bromocriptine. Side effects may include confusion, nasal congestion, liver problems, and swelling of the feet.

One other drug used to treat Parkinson's disease, amantadine hydrochloride (trade name: Symmetrel), has brought rapid improvement when given along with L-dopa. But the drug may also produce such side effects as hypotension, urinary retention, depression, and congestive heart failure.

Epilepsy

Epilepsy is a common disorder of the human nervous system. In the United States, about five persons of every 1,000, or more than one million people, suffer from epilepsy.

Epilepsy affects all kinds of people, regardless of sex, intelligence, or standard of living. Among the more famous epileptics of history were Julius Caesar, Napoleon, Lord Byron, Dostoyevsky, Handel, Mendelssohn, and Mozart. The I.Q. range for epileptics is the same as that of the general population.

Unfortunately, epilepsy has been one of the most misunderstood diseases throughout its long history. Because of the involvement of the brain, epilepsy has commonly been associated with psychiatric disorders. Epilepsy differs strikingly from psychiatric disorders in being manifested in relatively brief episodes that begin and end abruptly.

Causes and Precipitating Factors

A single epileptic seizure usually occurs spontaneously. In some cases, seizures are triggered by visual stimuli, such as a flickering image on a television screen, a sudden change from dark to very bright illumination, or vice versa. Other patients may react to auditory stimuli such as a loud noise, a monotonous sound, or even to certain musical notes. A seizure is accompanied by a discharge of nerve impulses, which can be detected by electroencephalography. The effect is something like that of a telephone switchboard in which a defect in the circuits accidentally causes wrong number calls. The forms that seizures take depend upon the location of the nervous system disturbances within the brain and the spread of the nerve impulses. Physicians have found that certain kinds of epilepsy cases can be traced to specific areas of the brain

where the lesion has occurred.

Epilepsy can develop at any age, although nearly 85 percent of all cases appear before the age of 20 years. Hence, it is commonly seen as an affliction of children. There is no indication that epilepsy itself can be inherited, but some evidence exists that certain individuals inherit a greater tendency to develop the condition from precipitating causes than is true for the general population. According to the Epilepsy Foundation, studies show that if neither parent has epilepsy, the chances are one in 100 that they will have an epileptic child, but the chances rise to one in 40 if one parent is epileptic.

About 70 percent of epilepsy cases are *idiopathic*—that is, they are not attributable to any known cause. In the remaining 30 percent, the recurrent seizures are *symptomatic*—they are symptoms of some definite brain lesion, either congenital or resulting from subsequent injury. Because it can reasonably be assumed that some of the idiopathic cases are a result of lesions that have not been identified, epilepsy is perhaps best regarded not as a specific disease but as a symptom of a brain abnormality due to any of various causes.

Aura Preceding a Seizure

Unusual sensory experiences have been reported to occur before a seizure by about half the victims of epilepsy. The sensation, which is called an *aura,* may appear in the form of an unpleasant odor, a tingling numbness, a sinking or gripping feeling, strangulation, palpitations, or a gastrointestinal sensation. Some patients say the sensation cannot be described. Others report feeling strange or confused for hours or even days before a seizure. Such an early warning is known as a *prodrome.*

The various types of epilepsy can

be broadly grouped under four general categories: grand mal, petit mal, focal, and psychomotor. Only one feature is common to all types of epilepsy—the sudden, disorderly discharge of nerve impulses within the brain.

Grand Mal Seizure

The *grand mal* is a generalized convulsion during which the patient may initially look strange or bewildered, suddenly groan or scream, lose consciousness and become stiff (*tonic phase*), hold the breath, fall to the ground unless supported, and then begin to jerk the arms and legs (*clonic phase*). There may be loss of bowel and bladder control. The tongue may be bitten by coming between clenched jaws. The duration of the entire seizure, both the tonic and clonic phases, is less than two minutes—frequently less than one minute—followed by postconvulsive confusion or deep sleep that may last for minutes or hours.

Following a Seizure

The patient may be able to resume normal activities shortly after the spell has ended. But after recovering from a long postconvulsive sleep, the patient may show a variety of signs or symptoms known as postconvulsive phenomena, which may include headache, mental confusion, and drowsiness.

Variations in the Pattern

The sequence of events in grand mal seizures is not invariable. The tongue-biting and urinary and fecal incontinence do not occur as frequently in children as in adult patients. Children may also demonstrate a type of grand mal seizure in which the patient suddenly becomes limp and falls to the floor unconscious; there is no apparent tonic or clonic phase and the muscles do not become stiff. Other cases may manifest only the tonic phase, with unconsciousness and the muscles remaining in a stiffened, tonic state throughout the seizure. There also is a clonic type of seizure, which begins with rapid jerking movements that continue during the entire attack. In one very serious form of convulsive seizure known as *status epilepticus,* repeated grand mal seizures occur without the victim's becoming conscious between them.

Petit Mal Seizure

Petit mal seizures are characterized by momentary staring spells, as if the patient were suspended in the middle of his activity. He may have a blank stare or undergo rapid blinking, sometimes accompanied by small twitching movements in one part of the body or another—hands, legs, or facial muscles. He does not fall down. These spells, called *absence* or *lapse attacks,* usually begin in childhood before puberty. The attacks are typically very brief, lasting half a minute or less, and occur many times throughout the day. They may go unnoticed for weeks or months because the patient appears to be daydreaming.

Focal Seizure

Focal seizures proceed from neural discharges in one part of the brain, resulting in twitching movements in a corresponding part of the body. Usually, one side of the face, the thumb and fingers of one hand, or one entire side of the body is involved. The patient does not lose consciousness and may in fact remain aware of his surroundings and the circumstances during the entire focal convulsion. Focal

convulsions in adults commonly indicate some focal abnormality, but this is less true in a child who may have a focal seizure without evidence of a related brain lesion.

With their knowledge of the nerve links between brain centers and body muscles, physicians are able to determine quite accurately the site of a brain lesion that is involved with a focal seizure.

Jacksonian Epilepsy

One type of focal seizure has a distinctive pattern and is sometimes called a *Jacksonian seizure,* and the condition itself *Jacksonian epilepsy.* The attack begins with rhythmic twitching of muscles in one hand or one foot or one side of the face. The spasmodic movement or twitching then spreads from the body area first affected to other muscles on the same side of the body. The course of the twitching may, for example, begin on the left side of the face, then spread to the neck, down the arm, then along the trunk to the foot. Or the onset of the attack may begin at the foot and gradually spread upward along the trunk to the facial muscles. There may be a tingling or burning sensation and perspiration, and the hair may stand up on the skin of the areas affected.

Psychomotor Seizures

Psychomotor seizures, or *temporal lobe seizures,* often take the form of movements that appear purposeful but are irrelevant to the situation. Instead of losing control of his thoughts and actions, the patient behaves as if he is in a trancelike state. He may smack his lips and make chewing motions. He may suddenly rise from a chair and walk about while removing his clothes. He may attempt to speak or speak incoherently, repeating certain

words or phrases, or he may go through the motions of some mechanical procedure, like driving a car, for example.

The patient in a psychomotor seizure usually does not respond to questions or commands. If physically restrained during a psychomotor episode, the patient may appear belligerent and obstreperous, or he may resist with great energy and violence. Usually, the entire episode lasts only a few minutes. When the seizure ends, the patient is confused and unable to recall clearly what has happened.

The aura experienced by victims of psychomotor seizures may differ from that of other forms of the disorder. The psychomotor epileptic may have sensations of taste or smell, but more likely will experience a complex illusion or hallucination that may have the quality of a vivid dream. The hallucination may be based on actual experiences or things the patient has seen, or it may deal with objects or experiences that only seem familiar though they are in fact unfamiliar. This distortion of memory, in which a strange experience seems to be a part of one's past life, is known as *déjà vu,* which in French means literally "already seen."

Other visual associations involved in various forms of epilepsy include those in which the patient experiences sensations of color, moving lights, or darkness. Red is the most common color observed in visual seizures, although blue, yellow, and green also are reported. The darkness illusion may occur as a temporary blindness, lasting only a few minutes. Stars or moving lights may appear as if visible to only one eye, indicating that the source of the disturbance is a lesion in the brain area on the opposite side of the head. Visual illusions before an epileptic attack may have a distorted quality, or consist of objects arranged in an unnatural pattern or of an unnatural size.

Auditory illusions, on the other hand, are comparatively rare. Occasionally a patient will report hearing buzzing or roaring noises as part of a seizure, or human voices repeating certain recognizable words.

Treatment of the Epileptic Patient

Usually the physician does not see the patient during a seizure and must rely on the description of others to make a proper diagnosis. Because the patient has no clear recollection of what happens during any of the epileptic convulsions, it is wise to have someone who has seen an attack accompany him to a physician. First, the physician begins the detective work to find the cause of the seizure. He will examine the patient thoroughly, obtain blood tests, an electroencephalogram, and a lumbar puncture, if indicated. Even after all these studies, however, the physician often can find no specific cause that can be eradicated. Efforts are then made to control the symptoms.

The treatment of epilepsy consists primarily of medication for the prevention of seizures. It is usually highly effective. About half of all patients are completely controlled and another quarter have a significant reduction in the frequency and severity of attacks. The medication, usually in tablet or capsule form, must be taken regularly according to the instructions of the physician. It may be necessary to try several drugs over a period of time to determine which drug or combination of drugs best controls the seizures. Phenobarbital and diphenylhydantoin (Dilantin) may be prescribed for the control of grand mal seizures and focal epilepsy, and the physician may find that a combination of these drugs or others offers the best anticonvulsant control. Trimethadione frequently is administered to petit mal patients; primidone or phenobarbital may be prescribed for psychomotor attacks.

Surgery may be recommended when drugs fail to control the seizures. But this approach usually is used only as a last resort and is not always effective.

However, medicine and surgery are not the only treatments for epilepsy patients. Emotional factors are known to influence convulsive disorders. Lessening a patient's anger, anxiety, and fear can help to control the condition. An understanding family and friends are important, as are adequate rest, good nutrition, and proper exercise. The exercise program should not include vigorous contact sports, and some activities such as swimming should not be performed by the patient unless he is accompanied by another person who understands the condition and is capable of helping the epileptic during a seizure.

There is nothing permanent about epilepsy, although some patients may endure the symptoms for much of their lives. It is a disorder that changes appreciably and constantly in form and manifestations. Some experts claim that petit mal and psychomotor cases if untreated may progress to more serious cases of grand mal seizures. On the other hand, epilepsy that is given proper medical attention may eventually subside in frequency and severity of attacks. In many cases, seizures disappear or subside within a short time and treatment can be discontinued gradually.

While some effort has been made by medical scientists to determine if there is an "epileptic personality," evidence indicates there is no typical personality pattern involved. Whatever behavior patterns and emotional reactions are observed are the result of individual personality makeup rather than being directly related to epilepsy. Most epilepsy patients are capable of performing satisfactory work at various jobs; one study showed that only nine percent were partially dependent and four percent were incapable of holding a job. In some areas there may be restrictions on issuing driver's licenses to epileptics or other legal regulations that limit normal activities for epilepsy patients. As a result, some epileptics may conceal their condition or avoid medical treatment that might be reported to government agencies.

Because of ignorance and misinformation, some people regard epilepsy as frightening or mysterious, and patients may suffer unnecessarily and unjustly. In fact, behavioral abnormalities in patients with seizures are commonly the reflection of how they are viewed by others. The patient should be carefully observed by an understanding physician who watches not only for medical but for psychological problems.

When epilepsy has been diagnosed in a child, the parents must be instructed about the condition and the need for continuous careful medical supervision. If the child is old enough to understand, he also should learn more about the nature of the condition. Misbeliefs should be corrected. Both parents and child should understand that seizures are not likely to be fatal and that a brain lesion does not lead to mental deterioration. Parents and child should learn what actions should be taken in the event of a seizure, such as loosening clothing and taking steps to prevent injury. Natural concern should be balanced with an understanding that overprotection may itself become a handicap. The child should be encouraged to participate in social and physical activities at school and in the neighborhood as long as they do not strain his capabilities. Finally, parents should not feel guilty about the child's condition and think that some action of theirs contributed to the child's condition. See "Epileptic Seizures" in Ch. 31, *Medical Emergencies,* for a description of what to do when a seizure occurs.

Further information about epilepsy, including causes, effects, treatment, rehabilitation, and laws regulating employment and driver permits, can be obtained from the Epilepsy Foundation of America, 4351 Garden City Dr., Landover, MD 20785, and from the U.S. Department of Health, Education and Welfare, Public Health Service, National Institutes of Health, Bethesda, MD 20014.

Multiple Sclerosis

Multiple sclerosis is a disease involving the progressive destruction of myelin, the fatty material that covers the nerves of the body. The disease affects mainly the brain and spinal cord. It is termed *multiple* because there are distinct and separate areas of the nervous system involved, seemingly distributed in a random pattern.

Incidence

The incidence of multiple sclerosis is puzzling. It occurs most frequently in the temperate geographic areas of the world; the high-risk regions generally are between 40 and 60 degrees of latitude on either side of the equator, where the incidence is about 40 cases per 100,000 population. Within the high-risk latitudes, however, there are countries in Asia where the disease is relatively rare, and in the Shetland and Orkney Islands to the north of Scotland the incidence of the disease is approximately five times that in the United States, Canada, and Northern Europe. Multiple sclerosis has never been found in certain black populations in Africa, but black persons living in the United States develop the disorder at about the same rate as white persons.

Multiple sclerosis rarely appears before the age of 15 or after 55. A person aged 30 years is statistically at peak risk of developing the disease. The typical patient, statistically speaking, is a woman of 45 who was born and raised in a temperate climate. Women are more susceptible to the disease than men by a ratio of 1.7 to 1, and women are more likely than men to experience the onset of symptoms before the age of 30.

Symptoms and Diagnosis

There are no laboratory tests that are specific for multiple sclerosis, although there are certain tests that may suggest the presence of the disease. Diagnosing the disorder depends to a large extent upon tests that rule out other diseases with similar signs and symptoms. The first symptom may be a transitory blurring of vision or a disturbance in one or more of the limbs, such as numbness, a tingling sensation, clumsiness, or weakness. There may be a partial or total loss of vision in one eye for a period of several days, sometimes with pain in moving the eye, or the patient may experience double vision or dizziness. In some cases, the patient may develop either a lack of sensation over an area of the face or, paradoxically, a severe twitching pain of the face muscles. In more advanced cases, because of involvement of the spinal cord, the patient may have symptoms of bladder or bowel dysfunction and male patients may experience impotence.

When brain tissues become invaded by multiple sclerosis, the patient may suffer loss of memory and show signs of personality changes, displaying euphoria, cheerfulness, irritability, or depression for no apparent reason.

Multiple sclerosis is marked by periods of remission and recurrence of symptoms. Complete recovery can occur. About 20 percent of the patients may have to spend time confined to bed or wheelchair. In severe cases, there can be complications such as infections of the urinary tract and respiratory system.

Treatment

There is no known cure for multiple sclerosis, and treatment techniques generally are aimed at relieving symptoms, shortening the periods of exacerbation, and preventing complications that can be crippling or life-threatening. Most patients experience recurrences of symptoms that last for limited periods of days or weeks followed in cycles by periods of remission that may last for months or years, making it difficult to determine whether the therapy applied is actually effective or if the disease is merely following its natural fluctuating course. Because multiple sclerosis appears to be a disease that affects only humans, medical scientists are unable to use animals in experiments to develop effective remedies.

Among several types of medications now used are anti-inflammatory drugs such as adrenocorticotrophin (ACTH), a hormone that seems to reduce the severity and duration of recurrences. Cortisone and prednisone, two steroid hormones, also can be used and have an advantage over ACTH in that they can be taken by mouth rather than intramuscular injection. But not all patients react favorably to steroid drugs and serious side effects may be experienced. Several immunosuppressive drugs ordinarily used in the treatment of cancer and after organ transplants have been employed but they can be administered only in small doses for limited periods of time without undesirable side effects. Other therapies tested with varying effectiveness include vitamins and special diets.

Physical therapy and antispasmodic medications may be employed for patients suffering weakness or paralysis of the limbs. Bed rest during periods of exacerbation is important; continued activity seems to worsen the severity and duration of symptoms during those periods. Muscle relaxants and tranquilizers may be prescribed in some serious cases and braces could be required for patients who lose some limb functions.

Because of the lower incidence of multiple sclerosis in warmer climates, patients may be led to believe that moving to a "sunshine" state can have curative effects. But experience indicates that once the disease becomes established a change of climate does not change the course of the disorder. Living in a warmer winter climate, however, can lessen the impact of the physical handicaps faced by a multiple sclerosis patient.

Causes

The cause of multiple sclerosis has not been established. Multiple cases of the disease have been reported in only a small percentage of families but they occur often enough to suggest that the risk in brothers and sisters of patients is several times greater than the risk among the population at large. It is possible that patients with multiple sclerosis have inherited a specific susceptibility to the disease, a factor that could explain the vulnerability of members of the same family to acquire the disorder through one of several environmental causes, such as a virus or other infectious organism. Speculation about causes has covered dietary deficiencies, ingestion or inhalation of toxic substances,

and occupation.

A theory that researchers consider promising suggests that a virus similar but not identical to HTLV-I (human T-cell leukemia virus-I) may cause multiple sclerosis. HTLV-I causes an unusual form of leukemia. Some T-cells, a type of white blood cell, have been found to contain genetic material from this virus. These T-cells were taken from the cerebrospinal fluid of multiple sclerosis victims, establishing a possible link between the cells and the virus.

Infections of the Nervous System

Like any other organ system, the brain and its associated structures may be host to infection. These infections are usually serious because of the significantly high death rate and incidence of residual defects. If the brain is involved in the inflammation, it is known as *encephalitis;* inflammation of the brain coverings, or *meninges,* is called *meningitis.*

Encephalitis

Encephalitis is usually caused by a virus, and, because the symptoms are not specific, the diagnosis is usually made by special viral immunologic tests. Both sexes and all age groups can be afflicted. Most patients complain of fever, headache, nausea or vomiting, and a general feeling of malaise. The mental state varies from one of mild irritability to lethargy or coma, and some patients may have convulsions. The physician may suspect encephalitis after completing the history and the physical examination, but the diagnosis is usually established by laboratory tests that include examination of the cerebrospinal fluid (CSF), the EEG, and viral studies of the blood, CSF, and stool. Because there is no specific treatment for viral

encephalitis at the present time, particular attention is paid to general supportive care.

Meningitis

Meningitis can occur in either sex at any time of life. The patient often has a preceding mild respiratory infection and later complains of headache, nausea, and vomiting. Fever and neck stiffness are usually present early in the course of the disease, at which time the patient is commonly brought to the physician for examination. If there is any question of meningitis, a lumbar puncture is performed and the CSF examined. It is not possible to make a specific diagnosis of meningitis without examination of the cerebrospinal fluid.

Meningitis is usually caused by bacteria or a virus. It is important to learn what the infectious agent is in order to begin appropriate therapy. Bacterial infections can be treated by antibiotics, but there is no known specific treatment for viral (*aseptic*) meningitis. Meningitis is a life-threatening disease and, despite modern antibiotic therapy, the mortality rate varies from 10 to 20 percent.

Poliomyelitis

Poliomyelitis is an acute viral illness affecting males and females at any time of life, though most commonly before the age of ten. It is also called *polio, infantile paralysis,* or *Heine-Medin disease.*

Polio is caused by a virus that probably moves from the gastrointestinal tract via nerve trunks to the central nervous system, where it may affect any part of the nervous system. The disease, however, most often involves the larger motor neurons (*anterior horn cells*) in the brain stem and spinal cord, with subsequent loss of nerve supply to the muscle. The neuron may be partially or completely damaged; clinical recovery is, therefore, dependent on whether those partially damaged nerves can regain normal function.

There are two categories of polio victims: asymptomatic and symptomatic. Those persons who have had no observed symptoms of the disease, but in whom antibodies to polio can be demonstrated, belong in the *asymptomatic* group. The *symptomatic* group, on the other hand, comprises patients who have the clinical disease, either with residual paralysis (paralytic polio) or without paralysis (nonparalytic polio).

Symptoms

The symptoms of poliomyelitis are similar to those of other acute infectious processes. The patient may complain of headache, fever, or *coryza* (head cold or runny nose), or he may have loose stools and malaise. One-fourth to one-third of patients improve for several days only to have a recurrence of fever with neck stiffness. Most patients, however, do not improve, but rather have a progression of their symptoms, marked by neck stiffness and aching muscles. They are often irritable and apprehensive, and some are rather lethargic.

Whether or not the patient will have muscle paralysis should be evident in the first few weeks. Some have muscle paralysis with the onset of symptoms; others become aware of loss of muscle function several weeks after the onset. About half of the patients first notice paralysis during the second to the fifth day of the disease. Patients experience a muscle spasm or stiffness, and may complain of muscle pain, particularly if the muscle is stretched.

The extent of the muscle paralysis is variable, ranging from mild localized weakness to inability to move most of the skeletal muscles. Proximal muscles (those close to the trunk, like the shoulder-arm or hip-thigh) are involved more often than distal muscles (of the extremeties), and the legs are affected more often than the arms. When the neurons of the lower brain stem and the spinal cord at the thoracic level and above are affected, the patient may have a paralysis of the muscles used in swallowing and breathing. This circumstance, obviously, is life-threatening, and particular attention must be paid to the patient's ability to handle saliva and to breathe. If independent, spontaneous respiration is not possible, patients must be given respiratory assistance with mechanical respirators.

Treatment

There is no specific treatment for acute poliomyelitis. The patient should be kept at complete bed rest and given general supportive care, assuring adequate nutrition and fluid intake. Muscle spasm has been treated with hot as well as cold compresses, and no one method has been universally beneficial. Careful positioning of the patient with the musculature supported in a position midway between relaxation and contraction is probably of benefit, and skilled physical therapy is of great importance.

Immunization

Since the early 1900s, attempts had been made to produce an effective vaccine against poliomyelitis, with success crowning the efforts of Dr. Jonas Salk in 1953. Today, vaccination is accomplished with either the Salk vaccine (killed virus), which is given intramuscularly, or the Sabin (live attenuated virus), given orally. There is little question that immunization with poliomyelitis vaccine has proven to be highly effective in eradicating the clinical disease within the community, and it is now a part of routine immunization for all children.

Dementia

Dementia is a term for mental deterioration, with particular regard to memory and thought processes. Such deterioration can be brought about in various ways: infection, brain injury, such toxic states as alcoholism, brain tumors, cerebral arteriosclerosis, and so forth.

The presenile dementias (*Alzheimer's disease*) represent a group of degenerative diseases of the brain in which mental deterioration first becomes apparent in middle age. Commonly, the first clue may be demonstrations of unusual unreasonableness and impairment of judgment. The patient can no longer grasp the content of a situation at hand and reacts inappropriately. Memory gradually fades and recent events are no longer remembered, but events that occurred early in life can be recalled. The patient may wander aimlessly or get lost in his own house. There is progressive deterioration of physical appearance and personal hygiene, and, finally, the command of language deteriorates. Unfortunately, there is a relentless progression of the process, and the patient becomes confined to bed and quite helpless.

Whether the mental deterioration seen in some aged patients, senile dementia, is a specific brain degeneration or is secondary to cerebral arteriosclerosis is not yet settled. It does appear, however, that senile dementia is probably secondary to a degenerative process similar to that of Alzheimer's disease but occurring late in life.

Whether or not dementia can be halted depends upon its cause. If, for example, the dementia is secondary to brain infection or exposure to toxic material, eradication of the infectious agent or removal of the toxin may be of distinct benefit in arresting the dementing process. Unfortunately, there is no specific treatment for the brain degenerative processes.

Muscle Diseases

When one hears the words "muscle disease," one may think of only muscular dystrophy and picture a small child confined to a wheelchair. But there are many diseases other than muscular dystrophy in which muscle is either primarily or secondarily involved, and many of these diseases do not have a particularly bad prognosis. Muscle diseases may make their presence known at any time, from early infancy to old age; no age group or sex is exempt.

Any disease of muscle is called a *myopathy*. The hallmark of muscle disease is weakness, or loss of muscle power. This may be recognized in the infant who seems unusually limp or *hypotonic*. Often the first clue to the presence of muscle weakness is a child's failure to achieve the developmental milestones within a normal range of time. He may be unusually clumsy or have difficulty in running, climbing stairs, or even walking. Occasionally a teacher is the first one to be aware that the child cannot keep up with classmates and reports this fact to the parents. The onset of the muscle weakness can be so insidious that it may go unnoticed or be misinterpreted as laziness until there is an obvious and striking loss of muscle power.

This is true in the adult as well who at first may feel tired or worn out and then realize that he cannot keep up

his previous pace. Often his feet and legs are involved in the beginning. He may wear out the toes of his shoes and may then recognize that he must flex his ankles more to avoid tripping or dragging the toes. Or he finds that he must make a conscious effort to raise the legs in climbing stairs; he may even have to climb one step at a time. Getting out of bed in the morning may be a chore, and rising from a seated position in a low chair or from the floor may be difficult or impossible. Those with arm involvement may recognize that the hands are weak; if the shoulder muscles are involved, there is often difficulty in raising the arms over the head. The patient may

take a long time in recognizing the loss of muscle power because the human body can so well compensate or use other muscles to perform the same motor tasks. If the weakness is present for a considerable length of time, there may be a wasting, or a loss of muscle bulk.

Diagnostic Evaluation of Muscle Disease

In evaluating patients with motor weakness, the physician must have a complete history of the present complaints, past history of the patient, and details of the family history. A general physical and neurological examination is required, with particular

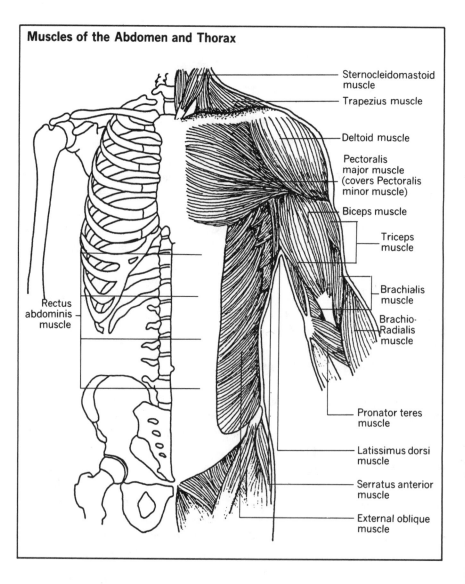

Muscles of the Abdomen and Thorax

Sternocleidomastoid muscle

Trapezius muscle

Deltoid muscle

Pectoralis major muscle (covers Pectoralis minor muscle)

Biceps muscle

Triceps muscle

Brachialis muscle

Brachio-Radialis muscle

Rectus abdominis muscle

Pronator teres muscle

Latissimus dorsi muscle

Serratus anterior muscle

External oblique muscle

reference to the motor, or musculo-skeletal system. In most cases, the physician will be able to make a clinical diagnosis of the disease process, but occasionally the examination does not reveal whether the nerve, the muscle, or both are involved. In order to clarify the diagnosis, some additional examinations may be required, mainly determination of serum enzymes (a good indicator of loss of muscle substance), a muscle biopsy, and an electromyogram.

Serum Enzymes

Enzymes are essential for the maintenance of normal body chemistry.

Because the normal concentration in the blood serum of some enzymes specifically related to muscle chemistry is known, the determination of concentrations of these enzymes can provide additional evidence that muscle chemistry is either normal or abnormal.

Muscle Biopsy

The first step is the surgical removal of a small segment of muscle, which is then prepared for examination under the microscope. The examination enables the physician to see any abnormality in the muscle fibers, supporting tissue, small nerve twigs, and

blood vessels. The muscle biopsy can be of great value in making a correct diagnosis, but occasionally, even in good hands, there is not sufficient visible change from the normal state to identify the disease process.

Electromyograph (EMG)

This is a technique for studying electrical activity of muscle. Fine needles attached to electronic equipment are inserted into the muscle to measure the electrical activity, which is displayed on an *oscilloscope*, a device something like a television screen. It is not a particularly painful process when performed by a skilled physician, and the information gained may be important in establishing a diagnosis.

Muscular Dystrophy

Muscular dystrophy (MD) is defined as an inborn degenerative disease of the muscles. Several varieties of MD have been described and classified according to the muscles involved and the pattern of inheritance. There is no specific treatment for any form of MD, but the patient's life can be made more pleasant and probably prolonged if careful attention is paid to good nutrition, activity without overfatigue, and avoidance of infection. Physical therapists can be helpful in instructing the patient or the parents in an exercise program that relieves joint and muscle stiffness. Sound, prudent psychological support and guidance cannot be overemphasized.

Duchenne's Muscular Dystrophy

In 1886, Dr. Guillaume Duchenne described a muscle disease characterized by weakness and an increase in the size of the muscles and the supporting connective tissue of those

Muscles of the Back

Trapezius muscle

Infraspinatus muscle

Deltoid muscle

Rhomboid muscle

Teres major muscle

Triceps muscle

Latissimus dorsi muscle (covers spinal erector muscle)

External oblique muscle

Internal oblique muscle

Gluteus maximus muscle

muscles. He named the disease *pseudohypertrophic* (false enlargement) *muscular paralysis,* but it is now known as *Duchenne's muscular dystrophy.*

Duchenne's MD is observed almost entirely in males. It is inherited, however, like many other sex-linked anomalies, through the maternal side of the family. The mother can pass the clinical disease to her son; her daughters will not demonstrate the disease but are potential carriers to their sons. More than one-quarter of the cases of Duchenne's MD are sporadic, that is, without any known family history of the disease. There are rare cases of Duchenne's MD in females who have *ovarian dysgenesis,* a condition in which normal female chromosomal makeup is lacking.

The disease process in Duchenne's MD may be apparent during the first few years of life when the child has difficulty in walking or appears clumsy. The muscles of the pelvis and legs are usually affected first, but the shoulders and the arms soon become involved. About 90 percent of the patients have some enlargement of a muscle or group of muscles and appear to be rather muscular and strong; however, as the disease progresses, the muscular enlargement disappears. Most patients progressively deteriorate and at the age of about 10 to 15 are unable to walk. Once the child is confined to a wheelchair or bed, there is a progressive deformity with muscle contracture, with death usually occurring toward the end of the second decade. A small percentage of patients appear to have a remission of the disease process and survive until the fourth or fifth decade. Despite herculean attempts to unravel the riddle of muscular dystrophy, the problem is yet unsolved.

A benign variety of MD, *Becker type,* begins at 5 to 25 years of age and progresses slowly. Most of the reported patients with Becker type are still able to walk 20 to 30 years after the onset of the disease.

Facio-Scapulo-Humoral Muscular Dystrophy

This type of muscular dystrophy affects males and females equally and is thought to be inherited as a dominant trait. The onset may be at any age from childhood to adult life, but is commonly first seen in adolescence. There is not false enlargement of the muscles. The muscles affected, as indicated by the name of the disease, are those of the face and shoulders, usually with abnormal winging of the *scapula* (either of the large, flat bones at the backs of the shoulders). There is also a characteristic appearance of lip prominence, as if the patient were pouting. Occasionally there is an involvement of the anterior leg muscles and weakness in raising the foot. The disease progresses more slowly than Duchenne's type, and some patients can remain active for a normal life span.

Limb-Girdle Muscular Dystrophy

This type of muscular dystrophy is less clearly delineated than the others. Males and females are equally affected and the onset is usually in the second or third decade, but the process may start later. It is probably inherited as a recessive trait, but many cases are sporadic. It may first affect the muscles of the pelvis or the shoulder, but in 10 to 15 years both pelvis and shoulder girdles are usually involved. The disease varies considerably from patient to patient; sometimes the disease process appears to be arrested after involvement of either the pelvis or the shoulder, and the course thereafter may be a benign one. Most, however, have significant difficulty in walking by middle age.

Other Varieties of Muscular Dystrophy

These include ocular, oculopharyngeal, and a distal form (involving the muscles of the hands or feet).

Ocular MD

This type involves the muscles that move the eye as well as the eyelids; occasionally, the small muscles of the face and the shoulder girdle are affected.

Oculopharyngeal MD

This type involves not only the muscles that move the eye and the eyelids but may also affect the throat muscles, so that patients have difficulty in swallowing food (*dysphagia*).

Distal MD

This type is rare in the United States but has been reported in Scandinavia. Both sexes can be affected. Usually after the fifth decade, the patient recognizes weakness of the small muscles of the hands and anterior leg muscles that assist in raising the toes. The disease is relatively benign and progresses slowly.

The Myotonias

This is a group of muscle diseases characterized by *myotonia,* a continuation of muscle contraction after the patient has voluntarily tried to relax that contraction. It is best observed in the patient who holds an object firmly in his hand and then tries to release his grasp suddenly, only to realize that he cannot let go quickly. There are two major members of this group of diseases and several other less common variants.

Treatment

As in the case of muscular dystrophy, there is no specific treatment for myotonia. Some drugs, such as quinine, have limited value in decreasing the abnormally prolonged muscular contractions, but as yet no treatment has been completely effective.

Myotonia Congenita

This condition is usually present at birth, but is recognized later in the first or second decade of life when the child complains of stiffness or when clumsiness is noted. A child with this condition appears very muscular and has been called the "infant Hercules." The unusual muscular development persists throughout life, but the myotonia tends to improve with age.

Myotonic Dystrophy

The other major variety of myotonia, *myotonic dystrophy*, is a disease in which many organ systems in addition to muscle are involved. Both males and females are affected equally, and the onset may occur at any time from birth to the fifth decade. It is not unusual for a patient to recognize some clumsiness, but he may not be aware that he has a muscle disease. The myotonia may range from mild to severe. There is a striking similarity in the physical appearance of patients with myotonic dystrophy, the features of which include frontal baldness in the male, wasting and weakness of the temporal muscles (that control closing the jaws), muscles of the forearm, hands, and anterior leg muscles. Other physical abnormalities include cataracts in about 90 percent of the patients, small testicles, and abnormality of the heart muscle. Thickening and other bony abnormalities have been seen in the skull radiogram and, with time, many patients become demented.

Polymyositis

Polymyositis is a disorder of muscular and connective tissues affecting both sexes, males more commonly than females. It can occur at any age, although usually after the fourth dec-

ade. It is characterized by muscle weakness with associated muscle wasting; about half of the patients complain of muscle pain or tenderness. The disease may begin suddenly, but often follows an earlier mild, febrile illness. Changes in the skin are common, including a faint red-violet discoloration, particularly about the eyelids, and these changes are often associated with mild swelling. There may be a scaly rash. Some patients have ulcerations over the bony prominences. About one-quarter of the patients with polymyositis complain of joint stiffness and tenderness and an unusual phenomenon in which the nail beds become blue (*cyanotic*) after minor exposure to cold.

Treatment

The treatment involves the administration of cortisone preparations, which may be required for many years. General supportive care, including appropriate physical therapy, is recommended.

Myasthenia Gravis

Myasthenia gravis is characterized by muscle weakness and an abnormal muscle fatigability (pathologic fatigue); patients are abnormally weak after exercise or at the end of the day. The disease affects males and females at any period, from infancy to old age, but it is most common during the second to the fourth decades. There is no complete explanation for myasthenia gravis, but it is believed that there is some defect in the transmission of a nerve impulse to the muscle (*myoneural junction defect*). The disease may occur spontaneously, during pregnancy, or following an acute infection, and there appears to be a curious association with diseases in which there is an immunologic abnormality, such as tumors of the thymus gland, increased or decreased activity

of the thyroid gland, and rheumatoid arthritis.

Usually there is an insidious onset of generalized weakness or weakness confined to small groups of muscles. Normal muscle power may be present early in the day, but as the hours pass the patient notices that one or both eyelids droop (*ptosis*) or he may see double images (*diplopia*). If he rests and closes his eyes for a short time, the ptosis and the diplopia clear up, only to return after further muscle activity. The weakness can also be seen in the trunk or the limbs, and some patients have involvement of the muscles used in speaking, chewing, or swallowing (*bulbar* muscles). Some are weak all the time and have an increase in that weakness the longer they use their muscles. The muscles used in breathing may be affected in patients with severe myasthenia, and these patients must be maintained on a respirator for varying periods of time.

Treatment

Myasthenia gravis is treated with drugs that assist in the transmission of the nerve impulse to the muscle. Medication is very effective, but the patient should be carefully observed by the physician to determine that the drug dose and the time of administration are adjusted so that the patient may have the benefit of maximal muscle power. Surgical removal of the thymus gland, *thymectomy*, may prove of benefit to some patients in lessening the symptoms of muscle weakness; however, not all patients have clinical improvement of the disease after thymectomy, and patients must be selected very carefully by the physician. Myasthenia gravis is another chronic disease in which long-term careful observation by the physician is most important in obtaining an optimal medical and psychological outcome.

9

Diseases of the Circulatory System

It's called the river of life, the five or six quarts of blood that stream through the 60,000 tortuous miles of arteries, veins, and capillaries.

Blood contains many elements with specific functions—red cells to transport oxygen from the lungs to body tissues, white cells to fight off disease, and tiny elements called *platelets* to help form clots and repair tears in the blood vessel wall. All float freely in an intricate complex of liquid proteins and metals known as *plasma*.

Because of the blood's extreme importance to life, any injury to it— or to the grand network of channels through which it flows—may have the most serious consequences. The troubles that beset the circulation may be grouped conveniently into two categories: diseases of the blood and diseases of the blood vessels.

Diseases of the Blood

Diseases of the blood include disorders that affect the blood elements directly (as in the case of *hemophilia,* where a deficiency in clotting proteins is at fault) as well as abnormalities in the various organs involved in maintaining proper blood balance (i.e., spleen, liver and bone marrow). The various ills designated and described below are arranged according to the blood component most affected (i.e., clotting proteins, red blood cells, and white blood cells).

Hemorrhagic or Clotting-Deficiency Diseases

The blood has the ability to change from a fluid to a solid and back to a fluid again. The change to a solid is called *clotting*. There are mechanisms not only for sealing off breaks in the circulatory system when serious blood loss is threatened, but also for breaking down the seals, or clots, once the damage has been repaired and the danger of blood loss is eliminated. Both mechanisms are in continuous, dynamic equilibrium, a delicate balance between tissue repair and clot dissolution to keep us from bleeding or literally clogging to death.

Clotting involves a very complex chain of chemical events. The key is the conversion of an inactive blood protein, *fibrinogen,* into a threadlike sealant known as *fibrin*. Stimulus for this conversion is an enzyme called *thrombin,* which normally also circulates in an inactive state as *prothrombin* (formed from vitamin K in the daily diet).

For a clot to form, however, inactive prothrombin must undergo a chemical transformation into thrombin, a step requiring still another chemical—*thromboplastin*. This agent comes into play only when a tissue or vessel has been injured so as to require clot protection. There are two ways for thromboplastin to enter the bloodstream to spark the chain of events. One involves the release by the injured tissue of a substance that reacts with plasma proteins to produce thromboplastin. The other requires the presence of blood platelets (small particles that travel in the blood) and several plasma proteins, including the so-called antihemophilic factor. Platelets tend to clump at the site of vessel injury, where they disintegrate and ultimately release thromboplastin, which, in the presence of blood calcium, triggers the prothrombin-thrombin conversion.

The clot-destroying sequence is very similar to that involved in clot formation, with the key enzyme, *fi-*

brinolysin, existing normally in an inactive state (*profibrinolysin*). There are also other agents (e.g., *heparin*) in the blood ready to retard or prevent the clotting sequence, so that it does not spread to other parts of the body.

Naturally, grave dangers arise should these complex mechanisms fail. For the moment, we shall concern ourselves with hemorrhagic disorders arising from a failure of the blood to clot properly. Disorders stemming from excessive clotting are discussed below under "Diseases of the Blood Vessels" because they are likely to happen as a consequence of preexisting problems in the vessel walls.

Hemophilia

Hemophilia is probably the best known (although relatively rare) of the hemorrhagic disorders, because of its prevalence among the royal families of Europe. In hemophilia the blood does not clot properly and bleeding persists. Those who have this condition are called *hemophiliacs* or bleeders. The disease is inherited, and is transmitted by the mother, but except in very rare cases only the male offspring are affected. Hemophilia stems from a lack of one of the plasma proteins associated with clotting, *antihemophilic factor* (*AHF*).

The presence of hemophilia is generally discovered during early childhood. It is readily recognized by the fact that even small wounds bleed profusely and can trigger an emergency. Laboratory tests for clotting speed are used to confirm the diagnosis. Further investigation may occasionally turn up the condition in other members of the family.

In advanced stages, hemophilia may lead to anemia as a result of excessive and continuous blood loss. Bleeding in the joints causes painful

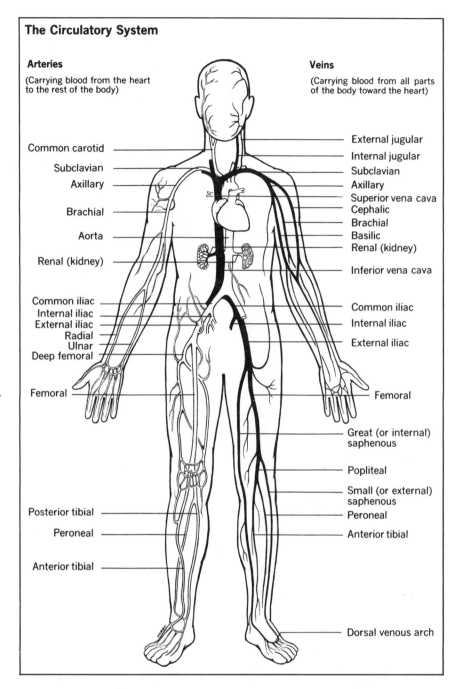

The Circulatory System

Arteries

(Carrying blood from the heart to the rest of the body)

Common carotid
Subclavian
Axillary
Brachial
Aorta
Renal (kidney)
Common iliac
Internal iliac
External iliac
Radial
Ulnar
Deep femoral
Femoral
Posterior tibial
Peroneal
Anterior tibial

Veins

(Carrying blood from all parts of the body toward the heart)

External jugular
Internal jugular
Subclavian
Axillary
Superior vena cava
Cephalic
Brachial
Basilic
Renal (kidney)
Inferior vena cava
Common iliac
Internal iliac
External iliac
Femoral
Great (or internal) saphenous
Popliteal
Small (or external) saphenous
Peroneal
Anterior tibial
Dorsal venous arch

swelling, which over a long period of time can lead to permanent deformity and hemophilic arthritis. Hemophiliacs must be under constant medical care in order to receive quick treatment in case of emergencies.

Treating bleeding episodes may involve the administration of AHF alone so as to speed up the clotting sequence. If too much blood is lost a complete transfusion may be necessary. Thanks to modern blood bank

techniques, large quantities of whole blood can be made readily available. Bed rest and hospitalization may also be required. For bleeding in the joints, an ice pack is usually applied.

Proper dental hygiene is a must for all hemophiliacs. Every effort should be made to prevent tooth decay. Parents of children with the disease should inform the dentist so that all necessary precautions can be taken. Even the most common procedures, such as an extraction, can pose a serious hazard. Only absolutely essential surgery should be performed on hemophiliacs, with the assurance that large amounts of plasma are on hand.

Purpura

Purpura refers to spontaneous hemorrhaging over large areas of the skin and in mucous membranes. It results from a deficiency in blood platelets, elements essential to clotting. Purpura is usually triggered by other conditions: certain anemias, leukemia, sensitivity to drugs, or exposure to ionizing radiation. In newborns it may be linked to the prenatal transfer from the maternal circulation of substances that depress platelet levels. Symptoms of purpura include the presence of blood in the urine, bleeding from the mucous membranes of the mouth, nose, intestines, and uterus. Some forms of the disease cause arthritic changes in joints, abdominal pains, diarrhea and vomiting—and even gangrene of the skin, when certain infectious organisms become involved.

To treat purpura in newborns, physicians may exchange the infant's blood with platelet-packed blood. Sometimes drug therapy with *steroids* (i.e., cortisone) is prescribed. In adults with chronic purpura it may be necessary to remove the spleen, which plays an important role in eliminating worn-out blood components, including platelets, from the circulation. Most physicians prescribe large doses of steroids coupled with blood transfusions. Purpura associated with infection and gangrene also requires appropriate antibiotic therapy.

Red Cell Diseases

Half the blood is plasma; the other half is made up of many tiny blood cells. The biggest group in number is the red blood cells. These cells contain a complicated chemical called *hemoglobin,* which brings oxygen from the lungs to body cells and picks up waste carbon dioxide for expiration. Hemoglobin is rich in iron, which is what imparts the characteristic red color to blood.

Red blood cells are manufactured by bones all over the body—in the sternum, ribs, skull, arms, spine and pelvis. The actual factory is the red bone marrow, located at bone ends. As red cells mature and are ready to enter the bloodstream, they lose their nuclei to become what are called *red corpuscles* or *erythrocytes.* With no nucleus, a red corpuscle is relatively short-lived (120 days). Thus, the red cell supply must be constantly replenished by bone marrow. And a busy factory it is because 20 to 25 trillion red corpuscles normally travel in the circulation. The spleen is responsible for ridding the body of the aged corpuscles, but it is not an indiscriminate sanitizer; it salvages the hemoglobin for reuse by the body.

To measure levels of red cells, physicians make a blood count by taking a smidgen of blood from a patient's fingertip. The average number of red cells in healthy blood is about five million per cubic millimeter for men, and four and one-half million for women.

Anemia

Anemia exists when the red cell count stays persistently below four million. Abnormalities in the size, shape, or hemoglobin content of the erythrocytes may also account for anemic states. Any such irregularity interferes with the red cell's ability to carry its full share of oxygen to body tissues. It also tends to weaken the red cells so that they are more likely to be destroyed under the stresses of the circulation.

Anemia may result from:

- nutritional deficiencies that deprive the body of elements vital to the production of healthy cells

- diseases or injuries to organs associated with either blood cell formation (bone marrow) or blood cell destruction (spleen and liver)

- excessive loss of blood, the consequences of surgery, hemorrhage, or a bleeding ulcer and

- Heredity, as in the case of *sickle cell anemia* (where the red cells are misshapen)

Hemolytic Anemia

There are also several kinds of disorders known as *hemolytic anemias* that are linked to the direct destruction of red cells. Poisons such as snake venom, arsenic, and lead can cause hemolytic anemia. So can toxins produced by certain bacteria as well as by other organisms, such as the parasites that cause malaria, hookworm, and tapeworm. Destruction of red cells may also stem from allergic reactions to certain drugs or transfusions with incompatible blood.

The various anemias range from ailments mild enough to go undetected to disorders that prove inevitably fatal. Many are rare; following are the more common.

Pernicious Anemia

Pernicious anemia, or *Addison's anemia,* is associated with a lack of hydrochloric acid in the gastric juices, a defect which interferes with the body's ability to absorb vitamin B_{12} from the intestine. Because the vitamin acts as an essential stimulus to the production of mature red blood cells by the bone marrow, its lack leads to a reduced output. Moreover, the cells tend to be larger than normal, with only half the lifespan of the normal erythrocyte.

The symptoms are characteristic of most anemias: pale complexion, numbness or a feeling of "pins and needles" in the arms and legs, shortness of breath (from a lack of oxygen), loss of appetite, nausea, and diarrhea (often accompanied by significant weight loss). One specific feature is a sore mouth with a smooth, glazed tongue. Advanced stages of the disease may be marked by an unsteady gait and other nervous disorders, owing to degeneration of the spinal cord. Red cell count may drop to as low as 1,000,000. Several kinds of tests may be necessary to differentiate pernicious anemia from other blood diseases—a test for hydrochloric acid levels, for example.

Pernicious anemia, however, is no longer so pernicious, or deadly, as it once was—not since its cause was identified. Large, injected doses of vitamin B$_{12}$ usually restore normal blood cell production.

Sickle-Cell Anemia

Sickle-cell anemia, an inherited abnormality, occurs almost exclusively among black people. Widespread in tropical Africa and Asia, sickle-cell anemia is also found in this country, affecting perhaps 1 in 500 American blacks. The blood cells are sickle-shaped rather than round, a structural aberration arising from a defect in the manufacture of hemoglobin, the oxygen-carrying component. Such misshapen cells have a tendency to clog very small capillaries and cause the complications discussed below.

A differentiation should be made between sickle-cell anemia, the full-blown disease, and sickle-cell trait. Anemia occurs when the offspring inherits the sickle-cell gene from both

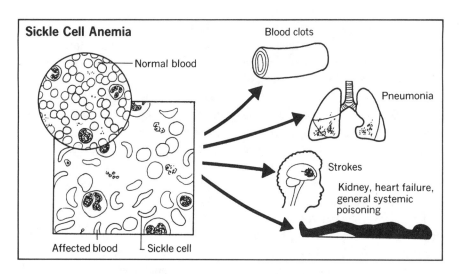

Sickle Cell Anemia — Normal blood — Affected blood — Sickle cell — Blood clots — Pneumonia — Strokes — Kidney, heart failure, general systemic poisoning

parents. For these people life stretches out in endless bouts of fatigue punctuated by a series of crises of excruciating pain lasting days or even weeks. In some cases there is permanent paralysis. The crises often require long-term hospitalization. The misshapen cells increase the patient's susceptibility to blood clots, pneumonia, kidney and heart failure, strokes, general systemic poisoning because of bacterial invasions, and, in the case of pregnant women, spontaneous abortion. Ninety percent of the patients die before age 40, with most dead by age 30. Half are dead by age 20, with a number also suffering from poor physical and mental development.

Those with only one gene for the disease have *sickle-cell trait*. They are not likely to have too much trouble except in circumstances where they are exposed to low oxygen levels (the result, say, of poor oxygenation in a high-altitude plane). Administration of anesthesia or too much physical activity may also bring on some feverish attacks. Those with the trait are also carriers of the disease because they can pass it on to the next generation. Two out of every 25 black Americans are said to be carrying the trait.

Iron-Deficiency Anemia

Iron-deficiency anemia is a common complication of pregnancy, during which time the fetus may rob the maternal blood of much of its iron content. Iron is essential to the formation of hemoglobin. The deficiency can be further aggravated by digestive disturbances (e.g., a lack of hydrochloric acid) that may hinder the absorption of dietary iron from the intestines. Some women may not observe proper dietary habits, thereby aggravating the anemic state. Successful treatment involves increasing iron intake, with iron supplements and an emphasis on iron-rich foods, including eggs, cereals, green vegetables, and meat, especially liver.

Polycythemia

Polycythemia is the opposite of anemia; the blood has too many red corpuscles. The most common form of the disease is *polycythemia vera* (or *erythremia*). In addition to the rise in corpuscle count, there is a corresponding rise—as much as threefold—in blood volume to accommodate the high cell count, and increased blood viscosity. Symptoms include an enlarged spleen, bloodshot eyes, red mouth, and red mucous membranes—all resulting from excess red cells. Other common characteristics are weakness, fatigue, irritability, dizziness, swelling in the ankles, choking sensations, vise-like chest pains (angina pectoris), rapid heartbeat, and sometimes severe headaches. There is also an increased tendency toward both clotting and hemorrhaging.

The disease occurs primarily in the middle and late years and is twice as prevalent in males as in females. The cause is unknown, but polycythemia is characterized by stepped-up bone marrow production activity.

Radioactive phosphorus therapy is one method for controlling this hyperactivity. Low iron diets and several forms of drug therapy have been tried with varying degrees of effectiveness. A one-time panacea, bloodletting—to drain off excess blood—appears to be of considerable value. Many patients survive for years with the disease. Premature death is usually the result of vascular thrombosis (clotting), massive hemorrhage, or leukemia.

The Rh Factor

Rh disease might also be considered a form of anemia—in newborns. The disorder involves destruction of the red blood cells of an as-yet unborn or newborn infant. It is brought about by an incompatibility between the maternal blood and fetal blood of one specific factor—the so-called Rh factor. (Rh stands for rhesus monkey, the species in which it was first identified.) Most of us are Rh positive, which is to say that we have the Rh protein substance on the surface of our red cells. The Rh factor is, in fact, present in 83 percent of the white population and 93 percent of the black. Those lacking it are classified as Rh negative.

A potentially dangerous situation exists when an Rh negative mother is carrying an Rh positive baby in her uterus. Although the mother and unborn baby have separate circulatory systems, some leakage does occur.

When Rh positive cells from the fetus leak across the placenta into the mother's blood, her system recognizes them as foreign and makes antibodies against them. If these antibodies then slip across into the fetal circulation, damage is inevitable.

The first baby, however, is rarely affected because it takes time for the mother's body to become sensitized to the Rh positive cells. But should she become pregnant with another child, the now-sensitized mother's blood produces a large quantity of destructive antibodies that could result in stillbirth, death of the infant shortly after birth or, if the child survives, jaundice and anemia.

Modern medicine has reduced the fatality rate and considerably improved the prognosis. Severely affected newborns are being treated by complete blood transfusion—even while still in the womb—to draw off all the Rh positive cells. After birth and as it grows older, the child will once again produce Rh positive cells in its bone marrow—but by that time the danger from the mother's antibodies is past. Recently an Rh vaccine to prevent the problem from ever occurring was developed. After Rh negative women give birth to their first Rh positive baby, they are immunized with the anti-Rh serum to prevent them from manufacturing these dangerous antibodies.

White Blood Cell Diseases

For every 600 to 700 or more red corpuscles, there is one white blood cell, or *leukocyte*. White cells, unlike red corpuscles, have nuclei; they are also larger and rounder. About 70 percent of the white cell population have irregularly-shaped centers, and these are called *polymorphonuclear leukocytes* or *neutrophils*. The other 30 percent are made up of a variety of cells with round nuclei called *lymphocytes*. A cubic millimeter of blood normally contains anywhere from 5,000 to 9,000 white cells (as compared with the four to five million red cells).

White cells defend against disease, which explains why their number increases in the bloodstream when the body is under infectious assault. There are some diseases of the blood and blood-forming organs themselves that can increase the white count. Disorders of the spleen, for example, can produce white cell abnormalities, because this organ is a major source of lymphocytes (cells responsible for making protective antibodies). Diseases of the bone marrow are likely to affect neutrophil production.

Leukemia

Leukemia, characterized by an abnormal increase in the number of white cells, is one of the most dangerous of blood disorders. The cancerlike disease results from a severe disturbance in the functioning of the bone marrow. Chronic leukemia, which strikes mainly in middle age, produces an enormous increase in neutrophils, which tend to rush into the bloodstream at every stage of their development, whether mature or not. Patients with the chronic disease may survive for several years, with appropriate treatment.

In acute leukemia, more common among children than adults, the marrow produces monster-sized, cancerous-looking white cells. These cells not only crowd out other blood components from the circulation, they also leave little space for the marrow to produce the other elements, especially the red cells and platelets. Acute leukemias run their fatal course in a matter of weeks or months—although there have been dramatic instances of sudden remission. The cause is unknown, but recent evidence strongly suggests that a virus may be responsible for at least some forms of the disease.

Modern treatment—radiation and drugs—is aimed at wiping out all of the malignant cells. A critical stage follows treatment, however. For with the disappearance of these abnormal cells and the temporary disruption of marrow function, the patient is left with his defenses against infection down. He also runs a great risk of hemorrhage. Therefore, he is usually kept in isolation to ward off infections. In addition he may be given white cell and platelet transfusions along with antibiotic therapy. Eventually—and hopefully—the marrow will revert to normal function, freed of leukemic cell production. For additional information on leukemia, see Ch. 18, *Cancer.*

Other White Cell Diseases

Agranulocytosis

Agranulocytosis is a disease brought on by the direct destruction of neutrophils (also called *granulocytes*). Taken over a long period of time, certain types of drugs may bring about large-scale destruction of the neutrophil supply. Symptoms include general debilitation, fatigue, sleeplessness, restlessness, headache, chills, high fever (often up to 105° F.), sore mouth and throat, along with psychologically aberrant behavior and mental confusion. White cell count may fall as low as 500 to 2,000. Sometimes agranulocytosis is confused with leukemia.

Treatment involves antibiotic therapy to ward off bacterial invasion, a likelihood that is increased owing to the lowered body resistance. In advanced cases, hospitalization and transfusions with fresh blood are necessary. Injections of fresh bone marrow may also be prescribed.

Leukopenia

Leukopenia is less severe than agranulocytosis. It too involves a reduction of circulating white cells to counts of less than 5,000. It is usually the result of allergic reactions to some chemical or drug.

Infectious Mononucleosis

Infectious mononucleosis, also known as *glandular fever* or *kissing disease,* is characterized by the presence in the bloodstream of a large number of lymphocytes, many of which are abnormally formed. The disease is mildly contagious—kissing is thought to be one popular source of transmission—and occurs chiefly among children and adolescents. The transmitting agent, however, has yet to be discovered, though some as yet unidentified organism is strongly suspected.

The disease is not always easy to diagnose. It can incubate anywhere from four days to four weeks, at which point the patient may experience fever, headache, sore throat, swollen lymph nodes, loss of appetite, and a general feeling of weakness.

The disease runs its course in a matter of a week or two, although complete recovery may take a while longer. Bed rest and conservative medical management is often enough for complete patient recovery. A few severe cases may require hospitalization because of occasional complications, such as rupture of the spleen, skin lesions, some minor liver malfunctions, and occasionally hemolytic anemia or purpura.

Diseases of the Blood Vessels

Diseases of the blood vessels are the result primarily of adverse changes in the vessel walls, such as hardening of the arteries, stroke, and varicose veins.

A healthy circulation depends to a large extent not only on the condition of the blood-forming organs but on the pipelines through which this life-sustaining fluid flows. The arteries, which carry blood away from the heart, and the veins, which bring it back, are subject to a wide range of maladies. They may become inflamed, as in the case of arteritis, phlebitis, and varicose veins; or they may become clogged—especially the arteries—as a result of atherosclerosis (hardening of the arteries) or blood clots (thrombosis and embolism), which can prevent the blood from reaching a vital organ.

The Inflammatory Disorders

Arteritis

Arteritis, or inflammation of the arterial wall, usually results from infections (e.g., syphilis) or allergic reactions in which the body's protective agents against invading organisms, the antibodies, attack the vessel walls themselves. In these instances, the prime source of inflammation must be treated before the arterial condition can heal.

Phlebitis

Phlebitis is an inflammation of the veins, a condition that may stem from an injury or may be associated with such conditions as varicose veins, malignancies, and infection. The extremities, especially the legs, are vulnerable to the disorder. The symptoms are stiffness and hot and painful swelling of the involved region. Phlebitis brings with it the tendency of blood to form blood clots (*thrombophlebitis*)

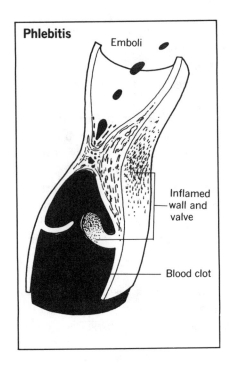

Phlebitis

Emboli

Inflamed wall and valve

Blood clot

at the site of inflammation. The danger is that one of these clots may break away and enter the bloodstream. Such a clot, on the move, called an *embolus,* may catch and become lodged in a smaller vessel serving a vital organ, causing a serious blockage in the blood supply.

Physicians are likely to prescribe various drugs for phlebitis—agents to deal with the suspected cause of the disorder as well as *anticoagulants* (anticlotting compounds) to ward off possible thromboembolic complications.

Varicose Veins

Varicose veins, which are veins that are enlarged and distorted, primarily affect the leg vessels, and are often troublesome to people who are on their feet for hours at a time. Varicose veins develop because either the walls or the valves of veins are weakened. Some people may be born with weakened veins or valves. In others, the damage may develop from injury or disease, such as phlebitis. More women than men seem to have this condition, but it is common among both sexes. In women, the enlarged

veins sometimes occur during pregnancy, but these may well diminish and disappear after delivery. Some elderly people are prone to this condition because the blood vessels lose their elasticity with aging, with the muscles that support the vein growing less sturdy.

In most instances, the surface veins lying just beneath the skin are involved. If there are no other complications, these cases are seldom serious, although they may be disturbing because of unsightliness. Physicians have remedies, including surgery, for making varicose veins less prominent.

When varicose veins become severe, it is usually because the vessels deeper in the leg are weak. Unchecked, this situation can lead to serious complications, including swelling (*edema*) around the ankles and lower legs. The skin in the lower leg may beome thin and fragile and easily irritated. Tiny hemorrhages may discolor the skin. In advanced stages, hard-to-treat leg ulcers and sores may erupt.

Most of the complicating problems can be averted with early care and treatment. Physicians generally prescribe elastic stockings even in the mildest of cases and sometimes elastic bandages to lend support to the veins. They may recommend some newer techniques for injecting certain solutions that close off the affected portion of the vein. On the other hand, surgery may be indicated, especially for the surface veins, in which the varicose section is either tied off or stripped, with the blood being rerouted to the deeper vein channels. See under "Vascular Surgery" in Ch. 20, *Surgery,* for more information about surgical treatment of varicose veins.

While long periods of standing may be hard on varicose veins, so are uninterrupted stretches of sitting, which

may cause blood to collect in the lower leg and further distend the veins. Patients are advised to get up and walk about every half hour or so during any extended period of sitting. A good idea, too, is to sit with the feet raised, whenever possible, to keep blood from collecting in the lower legs.

The Vessel-Clogging Disorders

Atherosclerosis

Atherosclerosis (hardening of the arteries) is the nation's most serious health problem, the underlying cause of a million or more deaths each year from heart attack and stroke. It is the process whereby fats carried in the

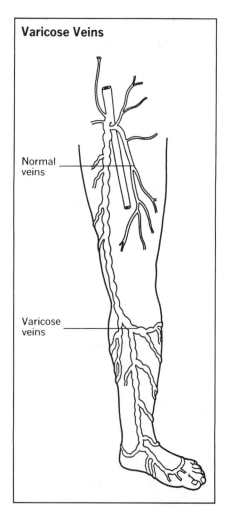

Varicose Veins

Normal veins

Varicose veins

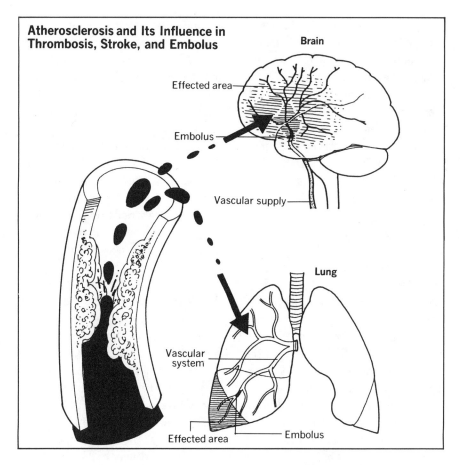

Atherosclerosis and Its Influence in Thrombosis, Stroke, and Embolus

Brain

Effected area

Embolus

Vascular supply

Lung

Vascular system

Effected area

Embolus

roughened wall surfaces, forming clots. If the clot blocks the coronary arteries, it may produce a heart attack—damage to that part of the heart deprived by vessel obstruction. For a detailed account of atherosclerosis and heart attack, see under Ch. 10 *Heart Disease.*

Stroke

Stroke, like heart attack, is a disorder usually resulting from blockage brought on by the atherosclerotic process in vessels supplying the brain. This sets the stage for a *thrombus,* or blood clot fixed within a vessel, which would not be likely to occur in arteries clear of these fatty deposits. A stroke may be a result of an interruption of blood flow through arteries in the brain or in the neck vessels leading to the brain.

Sometimes the shutoff of blood flow, or *embolism,* may be triggered by a wandering blood clot that has become wedged in cerebral vessels. This kind of clot, known as an *embolus,* is a thrombus that has broken free into the circulation.

A stroke may also stem from hemorrhaging, where a diseased artery in the brain bursts. A cerebral hemor-

bloodstream gradually pile up on the walls of arteries, like rust in a pipe. The vessels become brittle and roughened; the channel through which blood flows grows narrower. Eventually the organs and tissues supplied by the diseased arteries may be sufficiently deprived of their normal oxygen delivery so as to interfere with proper function. Such a cutback in the pipeline supply is called *ischemia.* This fat deposit poses its greatest hazard when it occurs in the vessels serving the heart, brain and, sometimes, the lower extremities.

A reduced supply of blood to the lower extremities may cause irreversible damage and ultimately lead to death of the leg tissues unless proper circulation is restored. Bacterial invasion may follow; the area may swell, blacken, and emit the distinctly offensive smell of the deadly infection. Such a condition is known as *gangrene,* a severe disorder that may

require amputation above the site of blockage if other measures, including antibiotic therapy, fail. Diabetics more commonly than others may develop atherosclerotic obstructions in leg arteries. Such persons must take care to avoid leg injuries, because even minimal damage in an already poorly served tissue area can bring on what is termed *diabetic gangrene.*

When the coronary arteries nourishing the heart are involved, even a moderate reduction in blood delivery to the heart muscle may be enough to cause angina pectoris, with its intense, suffocating chest pains.

Thrombosis

Thrombosis, a blood clot that forms within the vessels, is a great ever-present threat that accompanies atherosclerosis. The narrowed arteries seem to make it easier for normal blood substances to adhere to the

Brain Hemorrhage

Displaced brain

Cyst

Blood

rhage is most likely to occur when a patient has atherosclerosis in combination with hypertension (high blood pressure). (For a discussion of hypertension, see "Hypertensive Heart Disease" in Ch. 10, *Heart Disease.*) Hemorrhage is also a danger when an aneurysm forms in a blood vessel. An *aneurysm* is a blood-filled pouch that balloons out from a weak spot in the artery wall. Sometimes, too, pressure from a mass of tissue—a tumor, for example—can produce a stroke by squeezing a nearby brain vessel shut.

When the blood supply is cut off, injury to certain brain cells follows. Cells thus damaged cannot function; neither, then, can the parts of the body controlled by these nerve centers. The damage to the brain cells may produce paralysis of a leg or arm; it may interfere with the ability to speak or with a person's memory. The affected function and the extent of disability depend on which brain region has been struck, how widespread the damage is, how effectively the body can repair its supply system to this damaged area, and how rapidly other areas of brain tissue can take over the work of the out-of-commission nerve cells.

Symptoms

Frequently there are symptoms of impending stroke: headaches, numbness in the limbs, faintness, momentary lapses in memory, slurring of speech, or sudden clumsiness. The presence of these symptoms does not always mean a stroke is brewing; sometimes they are quite harmless. But should they be stroke warning signals, the physician can take some preventive action. He may recommend anticoagulant therapy as well as drugs to bring down elevated blood pressure. In some cases, he might decide to call for surgical replacement of diseased or weakened sections of arteries leading to the brain.

Treatment

Following a stroke, medical personnel may use *single photon emission computed tomography* (SPECT) to assess quickly the effects of a stroke. A refinement of nuclear scanning (See Chapter 26, Physicians and Diagnostic Procedures), SPECT shows the nature and extent of brain damage. The next critical step is intensive rehabilitation. Not everyone needs a rehabilitation regimen; some strokes have little effect. Some persons recover quickly from what appears to be a severe stroke. Others may suffer serious damage, and may take a long time to recover even partially. Treatment can usually help—especially those who are partially paralyzed and those with *aphasia,* the inability to speak properly because of damage to the brain's speech center.

Embolism

An embolus, or thrombus that has broken away into the bloodstream, is, as we have seen, sometimes the direct cause of a stroke. A heart attack may also cause a stroke. Bacterial action may soften a thrombus so that it separates into fragments and breaks free from its wall anchorage. Thrombi are not the only source of emobli; any free-floating mass in the bloodstream, be it an air bubble, clumps of fat, knots of cancer cells, or bacteria, can prove dangerous.

Usually, however, emboli originate as thrombi in the veins, especially the leg veins. Breaking free, the clump of clot material wanders into the bloodstream to be carried towards the right chamber of the heart and then onward into the lungs, unless dissolved before that. Once in the pulmonary arteries there is a growing threat that the moving mass will catch in one of the smaller branches of the lung circulation. This life-threatening blockage is called a *pulmonary embolism.*

This disorder takes at least 50,000 lives a year; most occur during or following prolonged periods of hospitalization and bed rest. The lack of activity slows the blood flow and increases the danger of thrombi—and ultimately emboli. Prevention requires getting the patient out of bed as soon and as often as possible to stimulate leg circulation. The nonambulatory patient, meanwhile, is encouraged to move his legs by raising them, or changing positions so as to step up blood flow.

The detection of a large embolus—symptoms include shortness of breath and chest pains—may require emergency surgery for removal. In most instances, however, treatment means administering anticoagulants to prevent new clots from emerging while allowing the body to rid itself of the embolus.

10

Heart Disease

Heart disease is the commonly used, catch-all phrase for a number of disorders affecting both the heart and blood vessels. A more apt term is cardiovascular disease, which represents America's worst health scourge. More than 68 million Americans of all ages (about 27 percent of the total U.S. population) are afflicted with some kind of cardiovascular disease. When considered together heart and circulatory system diseases, including stroke, account for more than one-half of all deaths each year in the United States, a total of more than one million people. Cardiovascular disease comprises several symptoms and disorders: coronary artery disease (including atherosclerosis, angina pectoris, and heart attack), hypertensive heart disease, rheumatic heart disease, and congenital heart disease.

Coronary Artery Disease

To keep itself going, the heart relies on two pencil-thick main arteries. Branching from the aorta, these vessels deliver freshly oxygenated blood to the right and left sides of the heart. The left artery is usually somewhat larger and divides into two sizable

vessels, the circumflex and anterior branches. The latter is sometimes called the artery of sudden death, since a clot near its mouth is common and leads to a serious and often fatal heart attack. These arteries wind around the heart and send out still smaller branches into the heart muscle to supply the needs of all cells. The network of vessels arches down over the heart like a crown—in Latin *corona*—hence the word *coronary*.

Coronary artery disease is the most frequent cause of death from cardiovascular disease. It is brought on by obstructions (plaque) that de-

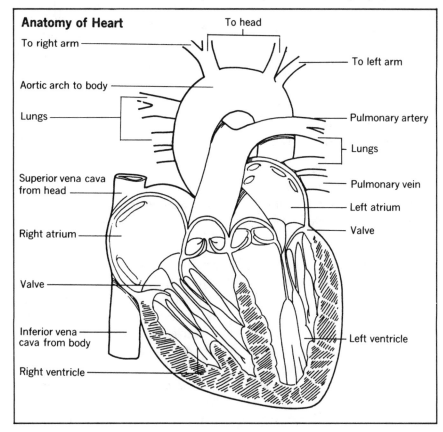

Anatomy of Heart

To head
To right arm
To left arm
Aortic arch to body
Lungs
Pulmonary artery
Lungs
Superior vena cava from head
Pulmonary vein
Left atrium
Valve
Right atrium
Valve
Inferior vena cava from body
Left ventricle
Right ventricle

velop in the coronary vessels nourishing the heart muscle, a condition termed *atherosclerosis*. These fatty blockages impair adequate delivery of oxygen-laden blood to the heart muscle cells. The result may be *angina pectoris:* short episodes of viselike chest pains that strike when the heart fails to get enough blood; or it may be a fullblown attack, where blood-starved heart tissue dies.

Heart attacks strike about 1.6 million annually, killing about 600,000. Overall, more than six million adults either definitely have or are suspected of having some degree of coronary disease; for this reason it has been labeled the "twentieth-century epidemic," or the "black plague of affluence."

Risk Factors of Coronary Artery Disease

1. Sedentary lifestyle
2. High cholesterol
3. High blood pressure
4. Obesity
5. Cigarette Smoking
6. Diabetes

Controlling the Risk Factors of Coronary Artery Disease

- Exercise regularly. Consult your physician for the best program for your age and physical condition.

- Eat less saturated fat and cholesterol. Substitute polyunsaturated vegetable fats or monounsaturated fats. Eat more poultry, fish, and complex carbohydrates.

- Undergo periodic tests of your total cholesterol level. A total cholesterol reading under 200 is desirable; a reading from 200 to 239 ranks as "borderline high" and indicates the need for dietary adjustments; levels above 240 are considered "abnormal" and indicate a need to consult a physician and possibly undergo drug therapy.

- Control high blood pressure. Those whose blood pressure is consistently 140/90 or higher are considered to have high blood pressure. There is some evidence that hypertension in women should be treated differently from that in men.

- Don't smoke. The heart attack death rate is 50 to 200 percent higher, depending on age and number of cigarettes consumed, among men who smoke as compared with nonsmokers. Giving up the habit can decrease the coronary risk to that of the nonsmokers within two years; the danger of smoking is reversible.

- Get down to your proper weight and stay there. Excess weight taxes the heart, making it work harder.

- An aspirin every other day has been shown to lessen the chance of having a heart attack for men at risk. Because aspirin decreases the clotting ability of the blood, it should not be taken by those with high blood pressure, a family history of stroke, bleeding disorders, ulcers, or impaired liver of kidney function. You should consult your physician before taking aspirin regularly.

Atherosclerosis

Coronary artery disease exists when flow of blood is impaired because of narrowed and obstructed coronary arteries. In virtually all cases, this blockade is the result of atherosclerosis, a form of *arteriosclerosis,* the thickening and hardening of the arteries. *Atherosclerosis,* from the Greek for porridge or mush, refers to the process by which fat carried in the bloodstream piles up on the inner wall of the arteries like rust in a pipe. As

more and more fatty substances, including cholesterol, accumulate, the once smooth wall gets thicker, rougher, and harder, and the blood passageway becomes narrower.

This fatty clogging goes on imperceptibly, a process that often begins early in life. To some extent, the body protects itself by developing, over a long period of time, alternative arterial connections, termed *collateral circulation,* through which the blood flow bypasses the diseased arteries. Eventually, however, blood flow may be obstructed sufficiently to cause the heart muscle cells to send out distress signals. The brief, episodic chest pains of angina pectoris announce that these cells are starving and suffering for lack of blood and oxygen. Flow may be so severely diminished or totally plugged up that a region of the heart muscle dies. The heart has been damaged; the person has had a heart attack.

The preventive measures for atherosclerosis are the same as those for a heart attack: exercise regularly, cut down on cholesterol and fat, don't smoke, control high blood pressure, and keep weight down. Avoiding these risk factors greatly decreases the chance of developing serious atherosclerosis.

Angina

Angina pectoris means chest pain (from the Latin *angere* meaning choke and *pectoralis* meaning chest). Angina occurs when the heart is called upon to pump more blood to meet the body's stepped-up needs. To do so means working harder and faster. If one or more of the heart's supply lines is narrowed by disease, the extra blood and oxygen required to fuel the pump cannot get through to a region of the heart muscle. Anginal pain

Angina Pectoralis

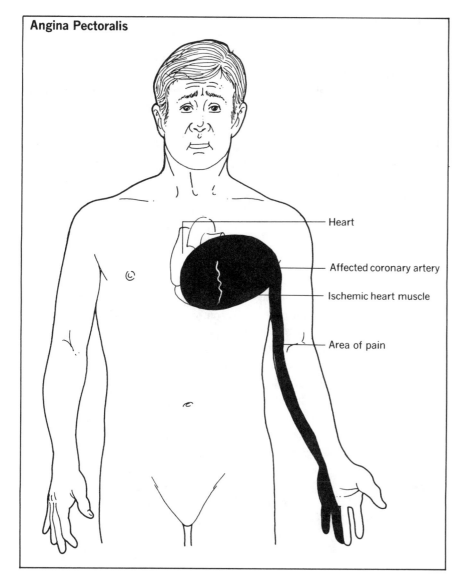

Heart

Affected coronary artery

Ischemic heart muscle

Area of pain

is a signal that muscle cells are being strained by an insufficiency of oxygen; they are, as it were, gasping for air.

The attacks usually are brief, lasting only a matter of minutes. Attacks stop when the person rests. Some people apparently can walk through an attack, as if the heart has gotten a second wind, and the pain subsides.

Symptoms

Angina attacks are likely to appear when sudden strenuous demands are placed on the heart. They may come from physical exertion—walking uphill, running, sexual activity, or the effort involved in eating and digesting a heavy meal. Watching an exciting movie or sporting event can trigger it; so might cold weather. An attack can occur even when the individual is lying still or asleep—perhaps the result of tension or dreams. The most obvious characteristic of an angina attack is pain.

Usually the pain is distinctive and feels like a vest being drawn too tightly across the chest. Sometimes it eludes easy identification. As a rule, however, the discomfort is felt behind the breastbone, occasionally spreading to the arms, shoulders, neck, and jaw. Not all chest pain indicates angina; in most cases it may simply be gas in the stomach.

Treatment

It is important to note that angina is a symptom, not a disorder. In most cases it is the result of atherosclerosis, and thus the program recommended for reducing the risk of atherosclerosis also applies to angina. In addition, treatment may involve merely rearranging activity to avoid overly taxing physical labors or emotional situations likely to induce discomfort. A major medication used for angina is *nitroglycerin*. It dilates small coronary blood vessels, allowing more blood to get through. Nitroglycerine pellets are not swallowed but are placed under the tongue, where they are quickly absorbed by blood vessels there and sped to the heart; discomfort passes in minutes. Nitroglycerin is also available in a sprayable form. Often anginal attacks can be headed off by taking the tablets or spray before activities likely to bring on an attack. Some people experience temporary, mild headaches as a side effect of taking nitroglycerin.

Still other drugs have been found to relieve angina pains. One group, called the beta-blockers, slows down the heart's action and thus its need for oxygen. Widely used to treat high blood pressure as well as heart disease, the beta-blockers may cause shortness of breath. For that reason, physicians usually prescribe other medications for persons with asthma.

The first of the beta-blockers to come into use was *propranolol*. But at least five chemically related drugs may be prescribed: atenolol, timolol, metoprolol, nadolol, and pindalol. Physicians generally try to fit one of these drugs to the problems of the individual patient. There is some evidence that propranolol and nitroglycerin taken together may increase the effectiveness of therapy.

A second group of drugs for angina is known as the calcium slow channel blockers, or simply calcium channel blockers. These drugs prevent coronary spasms, one cause of angina chest pains, by blocking the flow of calcium ions to the heart and thus dilating the arteries and increasing blood flow to the heart. The heart's demand for oxygen is lessened, and blood pressure is lowered. Three chemically different calcium channel blockers in use are verapamil, nifedipine, and diltiazem.

Angina does not mean a heart attack is inevitable. Many angina patients never have one, whether the result of collateral circulation, treatment with medication, or lifestyle changes. Should attacks of angina begin to worsen in spite of these, however, angioplasty or coronary bypass surgery may be necessary.

Heart Attack

Heart attack is the common term for *myocardial infarction,* or death of heart muscle, which is also described as *coronary occlusion* (total closure of the coronary artery) or *coronary thrombosis* (formation of a blood clot, which closes the artery).

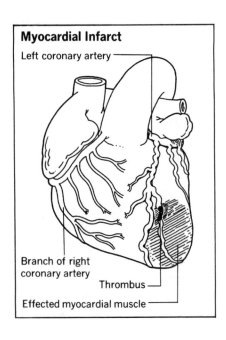

Myocardial Infarct

Left coronary artery

Branch of right coronary artery

Thrombus

Effected myocardial muscle

Although heart attacks can occur at any age, the frequency of heart attacks begins to build rapidly between the ages of 30 and 44 when roughly .05 percent of the total U.S. population experience heart attacks. Of this number only 2 percent are women. Between the ages of 45 and 64 the percentage increases to .2, with 24 percent of that number being women. After age 65 .33 percent of the population experience heart attack, 46 percent of which are women.

Symptoms

Sometimes heart attacks are so vague or indistinct that the victim may not know he has had one. Often a routine electrocardiogram turns up an abnormality indicative of an *infarct,* or injured area, thus the importance of periodic checkups. Special blood tests can also detect an elevation in the number of white blood cells or a rise in the enzyme content, resulting from leakage when heart muscle cells are injured.

Most heart attacks, however, do not sneak by. There are well-recognized symptoms. The most common are:

- A feeling of strangulation, crushing, or compressing

- A prolonged, oppressive pain or unusual discomfort in the center of the chest that may radiate to the left shoulder and down the left arm or up the neck into the jaw

- Abnormal perspiring

- Sudden, intense shortness of breath

- Nausea or vomiting (because of these symptoms, an attack is sometimes taken for indigestion; usually, coronary pains are more severe)

- Occasionally, fainting

Treatment

Knowing these warning signals and taking proper steps may make the difference between life and death. Call a physician or get to a hospital as soon as possible. Time is crucial. Most deaths occur in the initial hours after attack. About 40 percent, for example, die within one hour after onset of a major heart attack.

Often, death is not due to any widespread damage to the heart muscle, but rather to a disruption in the electric spark initiating heart muscle contraction—the same spark measured by the electrocardiogram. These out-of-kilter rhythms, including complete heart stoppage or cardiac arrest, are often reversible with prompt treatment.

For patients whose heart attack is the result of a blood clot (thrombus) the administration of thrombolytic drugs, which dissolve the clot and thus limit the extent of damage to the heart, increase the survival rate by 50 percent. Other drugs used to treat the heart include antiarrhythmics, which restore a regular beat to an irregularly beating heart, and vasopressors or inotropic agents that stimulate the heart and enhance heart function. Among the many cardiostimulants, or inotropic drugs, is a large group called partial beta 1 agonists that accelerate the rehabilitation process and increase exercise tolerance.

Of two other classes of therapeutic drugs, calcium and beta channel blockers are used to slow the heart rate, while angiotensin converting enzyme (ACE) inhibitors increase blood flow to the kidneys. The ACE inhibitors also block an enzyme that raises blood pressure. Among the diuretics are Dyazide and furosemide, marketed as Lasix. Both help to prevent fluid accumulation in the lungs.

Because most heart attacks are the result of reduced blood flow due to clots or buildup of deposits on arterial walls, following a heart attack the problem arteries must be identified. This is done in a procedure called *coronary arteriography* (cardiac catheterization), where blocked arteries are identified by X-ray "movies" taken of an injected opaque dye. Another technique, nuclear magnetic resonance (NMR), uses magnetic forces to scan the interior of the body for abnormalities. In heart disease diagnoses, NMR can identify specific problems in specific areas of the heart and its arteries.

Once clogged arteries are identified, they must be cleared. This is most commonly done by *percutaneous transluminal coronary angioplasty,* or balloon angioplasty. In balloon angioplasty, a catheter is pushed through an artery in the leg or shoulder and maneuvered into a coronary artery that has been narrowed by the build up of cholesterol, minerals, cell debris, and other material (plaque), which cuts off the flow of blood. A balloon attached to the catheter is then inflated, forcing open the affected artery by cracking and crushing the plaque against the arterial walls, compressing it but not removing it. The catheter and balloon are then removed. One problem with angioplasty is re-stenosis, or the return of narrowing deposits, which occurs within six months in 30 percent of coronary arteries. Devices that not only break down but remove plaque are thus being developed.

In cases where the blocked section of the artery is too long, difficult to reach, or located at a tortuous area or branch point of the artery, coronary artery bypass surgery must be performed.

Coronary Care Units

Special hospital centers called coronary care units (CCUs) have been created to provide for heart attack victims. Headed by a cardiologist and staffed by highly trained nurses, the CCU provides around-the-clock electronic devices that keep watch over each patient's vital functions, particularly the heart's electrical activity. The critical period is the first 72 hours, when up to 90 percent of heart attack patients experience some type of electrical disturbance or *arrhythmia* (irregular heartbeat).

Patient rooms in the CCU are designed to ensure privacy and a tranquil, cheerful environment. Rooms may be separated from one another by curtains or partial or full walls. Beds usually stand in a space adequate for movement of heavy equipment such as the portable X-ray apparatus.

Each patient is connected via electrodes attached to the skin to a heart monitor, which records the rhythm and rate of the heartbeat and the blood pressure, enabling nurses to check on a patient's condition without leaving the nurse's station. An alarm system on the monitor notifies the nurse when a major change is taking place in the patient's condition.

Other CCU equipment includes defibrillators for treatment of the condition called ventricular fibrillation (see section on arrhythmias), electroshock equipment, intravenous pacemakers, and a crash cart stocked with such items as the drugs needed for emergency cardiac care (ECC) and endotracheal tubes.

The advent of coronary care has produced striking results. Where in use, these units have reduced heart attack deaths among hospitalized patients up to 30 percent. If all heart victims surviving at least a few hours received such care, more than 50,000 lives could be saved annually.

Emergency Care

Most heart attack victims never reach the hospital. About one-third die before they receive medical care. Evidence suggests that many of these sudden deaths result from ventricular fibrillation or cardiac arrest—reversible disturbances when treated immediately.

These considerations led to the concept of mobile coronary care units—of bringing the advanced techniques of heart resuscitation to the victims. Originated in 1966 in Belfast, Northern Ireland, the practice of having a flying squad of specially equipped ambulances ready to race with on-the-spot aid to heart attack patients has been spreading to more U.S. communities, successfully reducing mortality.

An emergency technique called *cardiopulmonary resuscitation* (CPR), also known as *cardiac massage* or *closed-chest massage,* has also reduced out-of-hospital heart attack mortality figures. Used in conjunction with mouth-to-mouth breathing, cardiac massage is an emergency procedure for treating cardiac arrest. The lower part of the breastbone is compressed rhythmically to keep oxygenated blood flowing to the brain until appropriate medical treatment can be applied to restore normal heart action; often cardiac massage alone is enough to restart the heart. Training for the technique is widely available at hospitals or local branches of the Red Cross. Regular refresher courses are important, however, because improper use of the technique could fracture a rib or rupture a weakened heart muscle if too much pressure is applied.

Coronary Artery Bypass Surgery

Coronary artery bypass surgery involves removing a short length of vein from the leg and using it to reroute blood flow in the heart around severely blocked arteries. One to nine segments of these arteries may receive bypasses, although four to five is the most common.

Instead of a leg vein, it is often preferable to use either of the two (or both) internal mammary arteries for the bypass. (One common problem with using a leg vein is the tendency to develop blockages similar to those in the arteries it was intended to bypass; the mammary arteries are more resistant to the build up of atherosclerosis.

Although coronary artery bypass surgery relieves the debilitating angina or reduces the risk from severely blocked arteries by restoring adequate blood flow to the heart, it does not cure the underlying disease—atherosclerosis. Thus to reduce the risk of further complications or the need for another bypass operation, the patient must take care to follow the recommended dietary and lifestyle changes for reducing atherosclerosis.

Heart Surgery

Direct surgery on the heart is possible because of the development of the heart-lung machine, which takes over the job of oxygenating and pumping blood into circulation, thus giving surgeons time to work directly on a relatively bloodless heart.

Heart surgery is performed to correct congenital defects (see section on congenital heart disease), problems associated with coronary artery disease, hypertension, rheumatic fever, and congestive heart failure (see these sections), and injuries or diseases of the heart. Heart valves and arteries may be repaired or replaced, or the heart itself may be replaced.

The major valves of the heart—mitral, aortic, pulmonary, and tricuspid—may all become either obstructed (thus restricting the blood flow), a condition called *stenosis,* or they may fail to close properly (causing backflow of blood), a condition called *regurgitation.*

Stenosis may be corrected by a valvotomy, which enlarges the constricted valve opening. Some cases of valve regurgitation can be repaired surgically, others require the replacement of the valve.

Heart transplant may be required when such diseases of the heart as *cardiomyopathy* (heart muscle disease), *myocarditis* (inflammation of the myocardium), and *pericarditis* (inflammation of the sac surrounding the heart) do not respond to lifestyle changes or medication.

Heart transplantation has been performed with increasing success for more than 20 years. The best candidates for transplantation are psychologically stable, otherwise healthy individuals under 60. About 80 percent of transplant patients survive for at least a year. Some have lived for more than a decade.

Two problems associated with heart transplantation are the acquisition and storing of donor hearts and overcoming the body's rejection response to transplants. The former means a long waiting list for potential transplant patients. Controlling the latter is becoming increasingly more successful with immunosuppressive drugs. For more information, see "Heart Surgery" in Ch. 20, *Surgery.* See also "Organ Transplants" in Ch. 20, *Surgery.*

Recuperation

Beyond the 72-hour crisis period, the patient will still require hospitalization for three to six weeks to give the heart time to heal. During the first two weeks or so, the patient is made to remain completely at rest. In this period, the dead muscle cells are being cleared away and gradually replaced by scar tissue. Until this happens, the damaged area represents a dangerous weak spot. By the end of the second week, the patient may be allowed to sit in a chair and then to walk about the room. Recently, some physicians have been experimenting with getting patients up and about earlier, sometimes within a few days after their attack. Although most patients are well enough to be discharged after three or four weeks, not everyone mends at the same rate, which is why physicians hesitate to predict exactly when the patient will be released or when he will be well enough to resume normal activity.

About 15 percent of in-hospital heart attack deaths come in the post-acute phase owing to an *aneurysm,* or ballooning-out, of the area where the left ventricle is healing. This is most likely to develop before the scar has toughened enough to withstand blood pressures generated by the heart's contractions. The aneurysm may kill either by rupturing the artery or by so impairing pumping efficiency that the heart fails and the circulation deteriorates.

Most heart attack patients are able to return to their precoronary jobs eventually. Some, left with anginal pain, may have to make adjustments in their jobs and living habits. What kind of activity the patient can ultimately resume is an individual matter to be worked out by the patient with his physician. The prescription usually involves keeping weight down and avoiding undue emotional stress or physical exertion; moderate exercise along with plenty of rest is encouraged.

Before or after a heart attack victim returns to work and more normal life habits, physicians may want to know how he or she will react to stresses, medicines, and other factors and conditions. This is done by using "ambulatory electrocardiographic monitoring"—a portable EKG—which delivers electrocardiographic readings for 6 to 24 hours or longer while the patient goes about his normal activities. Electrodes are attached to the patient's chest over the heart. The electrodes connect with a tape recorder that makes electrocardiograms. Completely portable because of its weight—less than two pounds—the tape recorder/monitor is carried on a strap hung over the patient's shoulder or is attached to the wearer's belt.

The monitor's recordings are especially useful in diagnosing arrhythmias, which may occur at unpredictable times. Patients using the ambulatory monitor are generally asked to supplement the cardiographic record by keeping notes on their activities. These notes show the physician the activities in which the patient was engaged from hour to hour during the day. The notes may be matched up with the EKG to show what stresses accompanied particular activities. Some monitors have a special band on which the patient can record oral reports of his activities. The monitor's tape record and the patient's written or dictated notes help the physician give more specific instructions to the patient regarding his activities to facilitate recovery.

Arrhythmias

A disturbance in the rhythm of the heart is termed *arrhythmia* and can range from a mild "skipped beat" to a life-threatening failure to pump. The latter is called *ventricular fibrillation* and is usually associated with heart disease or occurs soon after a heart attack. The phenomenon of *cardiac arrest* (sudden death) is most often caused by ventricular fibrillation and is the leading cause of death in young and middle-aged men.

In ventricular fibrillation, the lower chambers of the heart contract in an uncoordinated and inefficient manner, causing blood-pumping to cease completely. The patient may experience palpitations, lightheadedness, chest discomfort, shortness of breath, or loss of consciousness. Treated within one minute, the patient has a 90 percent or better chance of surviving. A delay of three minutes means a survival rate of less than 10 percent because of extensive and irreversible brain and heart damage.

Treatment involves the use of an instrument called a *defibrillator*. Through plates applied to the chest, the device sends a massive jolt of electricity into the heart muscle to get the heart back on the right tempo.

More significantly, it is now also possible to head off ventricular fibrillation, so that the already compromised heart will not have to tolerate even brief episodes of the arrhythmia. Ventricular fibrillation is invariably heralded by an earlier, identifiable disturbance in the heartbeat. Most frequently, the warning signal is a skipped or premature ventricular beat. Picked up by the coronary care monitoring equipment, the signal alerts the unit staff to administer heart-calming medicaments that can ward off the danger. One such drug is *lidocaine,* a long-used dental anesthetic found to have the power to restore an irritated heart to electrical tranquility.

Less serious arrhythmias than ventricular fibrillation include *atrial flutter* (where the atria contract too often), *atrial fibrillation* (where they contract in an ineffective and uncoordinated manner), and *paroxysmal atrial tachycardia* (where the heart rate may race at between 140 and 240 beats per minute for minutes or even days).

Most all conditions of arrhythmia are associated with heart disease or heart attacks and can be controlled

with lifestyle changes and medications designed to pace the heart. Others are caused by a malfunctioning mitral valve of the heart or the sinus node (the area of the heart that sends electrical signals to the chambers, controlling the beat; i.e., the heart's pacemaker).

Hypertensive Heart Disease

Hypertension is the most common of the cardiovascular diseases, affecting about 22 million Americans, with more than half having some degree of heart involvement. A little more than 60,000 deaths are directly attributable to hypertension and hypertensive heart disease.

Hypertension, or elevated blood pressure, results from a persistent tightening of the body's very small arterial branches, the *arterioles*. This clenching increases the resistance to blood flow and sends the blood pressure up, just as screwing down the nozzle on a hose builds up pressure in the line. The heart must now work harder to force blood through. Over a period of time, the stepped-up pumping effort may cause the heart muscle to thicken and enlarge. Eventually, the overworked circulatory system may break down, with resultant failure of the heart or kidneys, or the onset of stroke. The constant hammering of blood under high pressure on the walls of the arteries causes them to thicken, making them less flexible (a condition called arteriosclerosis) and also accelerates the development of atherosclerosis and heart attacks.

How Blood Pressure is Measured

Blood pressure is measured in millimeters of mercury with an instrument called a *sphygmomanometer*. The device consists of an inflatable cuff attached to a mercury meter. The physician wraps the cuff around the arm and inflates it with air from a squeeze-bulb. This drives the mercury column up toward the top of the gauge while shutting off blood flow through the brachial artery in the arm. With a stethoscope placed just below the cuff, the physician releases the air and listens for the first thudding sounds that signal the return of blood flow as the blood pressure on the wall of the artery equals the air pressure in the cuff. He records this mercury meter reading. This number represents the *systolic* pressure, the force developed by the heart when it contracts.

By continuing to let air out, the physician reaches a point where he can no longer hear the pulsing sounds of flowing blood. He marks the gauge reading as the *diastolic* pressure, the pressure on the artery when the heart is relaxing between beats. Thus, two numbers are used to record blood pressure the systolic followed by the diastolic.

Recorded when the patient is relaxed, normal systolic pressure for most adults is between 100 and 140, and diastolic between 60 and 90. Many factors, such as age and sex, account for the wide variations in normal readings from individual to individual. Systolic blood pressure, for example, tends to increase with age.

Normally, blood pressure goes up during periods of excitement and physical labor. Hypertension is the diagnosis when repeated measurements show a persistent elevated pressure of 140 or higher for systolic and 90 or more for diastolic.

In addition to the sphygmomanometer reading in the examination for high blood pressure, the physician shines a bright light in the patient's eyes so that he can look at the blood vessels in the retina, the only blood vessels that are readily observable.

Any damage there resulting from hypertension is usually a good index of the severity of the disease and its effects elsewhere in the body.

An electrocardiogram and X ray may be in order to determine if and how much the heart has been damaged. The physician may also perform some tests of kidney function to ascertain whether hypertension, if detected, is of the essential or secondary kind, and if there has been damage to the kidneys as well.

Causes

More than 90 percent of all hypertension cases are classified as essential. This simply means that no single cause can be defined. Rather, pressure is up because of a number of factors—none of which has yet been firmly implicated—operating in some complex interplay.

One theory holds that hypertension arises from excessive activity of the sympathetic nervous system, which helps regulate blood vessel response. This notion could help explain why tense individuals are susceptible to hypertension. Emotional reactions to unpleasant events or other mental stresses prompt the cardiovascular system to react as it might to exercise, including widespread constriction of small blood vessels and increased heart rate.

The theory suggests that repeated episodes of stress may ultimately affect pressure-sensitive cells called *baroreceptors*. Situated in strategic places in the arterial system, these sensing centers are thought to be preset to help maintain normal blood pressure just as a thermostat works to keep a house at a preset temperature. Exposure to regularly recurrent elevated blood pressure episodes may bring about a resetting of the baroreceptors—or *barostats*—to a new, higher normal. Once reset, the

barostats operate to sustain hypertension.

Symptoms

Essential hypertension usually first occurs when a person is in his thirties. In the early stages, one may pass through a transitional or prehypertensive phase lasting a few years in which blood pressure rises above normal only occasionally, and then more and more often until finally it remains at these elevated levels.

Symptoms, if they exist at all, are likely to be something as nonspecific as headaches, dizziness, or nausea. As a result, without a physical examination to reveal its presence, a person may have the disease for years without being aware of it. That can be dangerous, because the longer hypertension is left untreated, the greater the likelihood that the heart will be affected.

About 10 percent of causes fall under the *secondary hypertension* classification because they arise as a consequence of another known disorder. Curing the underlying disorder also cures the hypertension. Usually it is brought on by an obstruction of normal blood flow to the kidney because of atherosclerotic deposits in one or both of its major supply lines, the renal arteries. Adrenal gland problems such as Cushing's Syndrome or a tumor of the adrenal gland can also cause hypertension. Many patients can be cured or substantially improved through surgery.

Treatment

Lifestyle changes are the most important thing an individual can do to reduce his blood pressure. These include reducing intake of salt, alcohol, and caffeine, controlling weight, and increasing physical exercise. Should these changes have no significant effect on the blood pressure after three to six months, a program of medication may be required. The outlook is good for almost all patients with essential hypertension, whether mild or severe, because of the large arsenal of antihypertensive drugs at the physician's disposal. Not all drugs will benefit all patients, but where one fails another or several in combination will almost invariably succeed. Even the usually lethal and hard-to-treat form of essential hypertension described as *malignant* is beginning to respond to new medications. *Malignant hypertension,* which may strike as many as 5 percent of hypertensive victims, does not refer to cancer, but rather describes the rapid, galloping way blood pressure rises.

Mild hypertension often may be readily treated with tranquilizers and mild sedatives, particularly if the patient is tense, or with one of a broad family of agents known as *diuretics*. These drugs flush the body of excess salt decreasing the amount of fluid in blood vessel walls and thus reducing the blood pressure.

Against more severe forms, there are a large number of drugs which work in a variety of ways to offset or curb the activity of the sympathetic nervous system so that it relaxes its hold on the constricted arterioles.

Rheumatic Fever and Rheumatic Heart Disease

Rheumatic heart disease is the possible sequel of rheumatic fever and claims the lives of 13,000 annually. It generally strikes children between the ages of 5 and 15. All told, 1.6 million persons are suffering from rheumatic heart disease, with about 100,000 new cases reported each year. Triggered by streptococcal attacks in childhood and adolescence, rheumatic fever may leave permanent heart scars. The heart structures most often affected are the valves.

Causes

The cause of rheumatic fever is still not entirely understood. It is known that rheumatic fever is always preceded by an invasion of bacteria belonging to the group A beta hemolytic streptococcus family. Sooner or later, everybody has a strep infection, such as a strep throat. Most of us get over it without any complications. But in 1 out of every 100 children the strep infection produces rheumatic fever a few weeks later, even after the strep attack has long since subsided. The figure may rise to 3 per 100 during epidemics in closed communities, such as a children's camp.

The invasion of strep sparks the production of protective agents called antibodies. For some reason, in a kind of biological double cross, the antibodies attack not only the strep but also make war on the body's own tissues—the very tissues they are called upon to protect. Researchers are now suggesting the possible reason, although all the evidence is not yet in. According to a widely held theory, the strep germ possesses constituents (*antigens*) that are similar in structure to components of normal, healthy cartilage and connective tissues—found abundantly in joints, tendons and heart valves—in susceptible individuals. Failing to distinguish between them, the antibodies attack both. The result: rheumatic fever involving joint and valve inflammation and, perhaps, permanent scarring.

Symptoms

Rheumatic fever itself is not always easy to diagnose. The physician must detect at least two of the following major symptoms or one major and two minor symptoms, derived by the American Heart Association.

Major:

- Swelling or tenderness in one or more joints (arthritis); usually, several joints are involved one after the other in migratory fashion

- Carditis or heart inflammation

- An unusual raised skin rash, which often disappears in 24 to 48 hours

- Chorea, or St. Vitus's dance, so-called because of the uncoordinated, jerky and involuntary motions of the arms, legs, or face, which result from rheumatic inflammation of brain tissue; (it may last six to eight weeks and even longer, but when symptoms disappear there is never any permanent damage and the brain and nervous system return to normal)

- Hard lumps, under the skin and over the inflamed joints, usually indicating severe heart inflammation

Minor:

- Joint aches without inflammation

- Fever

- Previous rheumatic fever or evidence of rheumatic heart disease

- Abnormal heartbeat on EKG

- Blood test indicating inflammation

Confirmation of rheumatic fever also requires other clinical and laboratory tests, to determine, for example, the presence of strep antibodies in the patient's blood. Rheumatic fever does not always involve the heart; even when it does, permanent damage is not inevitable. Nor does the severity of the attack have any relationship to the development of rheumatic heart disease.

The real danger arises when heart valve tissue becomes inflamed, affecting the valve's ability to close properly. When the acute attack has passed and the inflammation finally subsides, the valves begin to heal, with scar tissue forming.

Scar tissue may cause portions of the affected valve leaflets to fuse together. (*Leaflets* are the flaps of the heart valves.) This restricts leaflet motion, impeding the full swing action and thereby blood flow through the valve. This condition is called valvular *stenosis*. The leaflets may become shrunken or deformed by healing tissue, causing *regurgitation* or backspill because the valve fails to close completely.

Both stenosis and regurgitation are often present. Most susceptible are the *mitral valve,* which regulates flow from the upper to the lower left chambers of the heart, and the *aortic valve,* the gateway between the left ventricle and the general circulation. Rarely attacked are the two valves in the right chambers.

Treatment

During the acute stages of rheumatic fever, the patient is given heavy doses of antibiotics to rid the body of all strep traces, aspirin to control swelling and fever, and sometimes such hormones as ACTH and cortisone to reduce inflammation.

In the past, rheumatic fever spelled mandatory bed rest for months. Now the routine is to get the patient up and about as soon as the acute episode is over to avert the problem of psychological invalidism. The biggest restriction, especially for young people, is that no participation in competitive sports or other severely taxing exercises is allowed for two to three months while a close watch is kept on cardiac status.

The patient with valve damage can in many cases be treated medically, without the need for surgical intervention. He may, of course, have to desist from certain strenuous activities, but in all other ways he can lead a relatively normal life. Surgical relief or cure is available, however, for patients with severe damage or those who may, with age, develop progressive narrowing or leakage of the valves.

Surgery

Stenotic valves can be scraped clear of excess scar tissues, thereby returning the leaflets to more normal operation. In some cases individually scarred leaflets are replaced with synthetic substitutes. The correction of severe valvular regurgitation requires replacement of the entire valve with an artificial substitute, or, as some surgeons prefer, with a healthy valve taken from a human donor dying of other causes.

Prevention

The development of antibiotics has made rheumatic fever preventable. These drugs can knock out the strep before the germs get a chance to set off the inflammatory defense network sequences, but early detection is necessary. Among the symptoms of strep are a sore throat that comes on suddenly, with redness and swelling; rapidly acquired high fever; nausea and headaches. The only sure way to tell, however, is to have a throat swab taken by passing a sterile piece of cotton over the inflamed area. This culture is then exposed for 24 hours to a laboratory dish containing a substance that enhances strep growth. A positive identification calls for prompt treatment to kill the germs before the complications of rheumatic fever have a chance to set in.

Unfortunately, many strep infections may be mild enough to escape detection. The child may recover so quickly that the parents neglect to take the necessary precautions, but the insidious processes may still be going on in the apparently healthy child. This is a major reason why rheumatic fever is still with us, though in severe decline.

Heart Murmurs and Recurrences of Rheumatic Fever

The prime sign that rheumatic heart disease has developed is a heart murmur—although a heart murmur does not always mean heart disease. The murmur may be only temporary, ceasing once the rheumatic fever attack subsides and the stretched and swollen valves return to normal. To complicate matters more, many heart murmurs are harmless. Such functional murmurs may appear in 30 to 50 percent of normal children at one time or another.

As many as three in five patients with rheumatic fever may develop murmurs characteristic of scarred valves—sounds of blood flowing through ailing valves that fail to open and close normally.

Anyone who has had an attack of rheumatic fever has about a 50–50 chance of having one again unless safeguards are taken. As a result, all patients are placed on a daily or monthly regimen of antibiotics. The preventive dose, although smaller than that given to quell an in-progress infection, is enough to sabotage any attempts on the part of the strep germs to mount an attack.

There is some encouraging evidence that rheumatic fever patients who escape heart damage the first time around will do so again should a repeat attack occur. On the other hand, those with damaged valves will probably sustain more damage with subsequent strep-initiated attacks.

Endocarditis

One of the additional bonuses of antibiotic therapy is that it has all but eliminated an invariably fatal complication to which rheumatic patients were especially vulnerable—an infection of the heart's inner lining, or *endocardium,* called *subacute bacterial endocarditis.* The scar tissue provides an excellent nesting site for bacteria to grow.

The responsible germs are found in most everyone's mouth and usually invade the bloodstream after dental surgery. Fortunately, it is easy to prevent or cure because the germs offer little resistance to antibiotics. As a precaution, dentists are usually advised to give rheumatic fever patients larger doses of penicillin (or other antibiotics to those allergic to penicillin) before, during, and after dental work.

Congenital Heart Disease

Congenital heart disease includes that collection of heart and major blood vessel deformities that exist at birth in 8 out of every 1,000 live births, or 25,000 cases yearly. Nine thousand deaths annually are attributable to these inborn heart abnormalities.

There are some 35 recognized types of congenital heart malformations. Most—including all of the 15 most common types—can be either corrected or alleviated by surgery. The defects result from a failure of the infant's heart to mature normally during development in the womb.

The term *blue baby* refers to the infant born with a heart impairment that prevents blood from getting enough oxygen. Because blood low in oxygen is dark bluish red, it imparts a blue tinge to the skin and lips.

The cause of inborn heart abnormalities is not known in most cases. Some defects can be traced to maternal virus infection, such as German measles (rubella), during the first three months of pregnancy when the fetus' heart is growing rapidly. Certain drugs, vitamin deficiencies or excessive exposure to radiation are among other environmental factors known to be associated with such defects.

Heart abnormalities may come singly or in combination. There may be, for example a hole in the walls separating the right and left heart chambers or a narrowing of a valve or blood vessel which obstructs blood flow, or a mixup in major blood vessel connections—or a combination of all of these.

Diagnosis

A skilled cardiologist often can make a reasonably complete diagnosis on the basis of a conventional physical examination including visual inspection of the infant's general condition, blood pressure reading, X ray, blood tests, and electrocardiogram. For more complex diagnosis, the physician may call for either *angiography* or *cardiac catheterization.* The former, a variation of coronary arteriography, allows direct X-ray visualization of the heart chambers and major blood vessels. In cardiac catheterization, a thin plastic tube or catheter is inserted into an arm or leg vein. While the physician watches with special X-ray equipment, the tube is advanced carefully through the vein until it reaches the heart chambers, there to provide information about the nature of the defect.

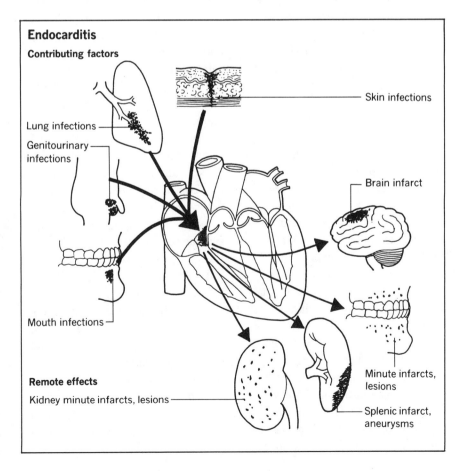

Endocarditis

Contributing factors

Lung infections

Genitourinary infections

Mouth infections

Skin infections

Brain infarct

Minute infarcts, lesions

Splenic infarct, aneurysms

Remote effects

Kidney minute infarcts, lesions

Advanced techniques known as computed tomography (CT), positron emission tomography (PET), and nuclear magnetic resonance (NMR) may also be used. Both the CT and PET scanners require injection of a contrast fluid so that a "picture" can be taken. The CT scanner takes X-ray images of "slices" of the patient's body with the aid of a computer. The PET scanner works on an electronic principle, with detectors located in a circle around the subject. Also computerized, NMR diagnoses by employing magnetic forces to "see" through bones, revealing such details as the differences between healthy and diseased tissues.

Treatment

From these tests, the cardiologist together with a surgeon can decide for or against surgery. Depending on the severity of the disease, some conditions may require an immediate operation, even on days-old infants. In other conditions, the specialists may instead recommend waiting until the infant is older and stronger before surgery is undertaken. In a number of instances, the defect may not require surgery at all.

Open-heart surgery in infants with inborn heart defects carries a higher risk than does the same surgery in older children. Risks must be taken often, however, because about one-third will die in the first month if untreated, and more than half within the first year.

Refinements in surgical techniques and postoperative care have given surgeons the confidence to operate on infants who are merely hours old with remarkable success. Specially adapted miniature heart-lung machines may also chill the blood to produce *hypothermia,* or body cooling. This slows metabolism and reduces tissue oxygen needs so that

the heart and brain can withstand short periods of interrupted blood flow.

A good deal has been learned, too, about the delicate medical management required by infants during the surgical recovery period. All of this accounts for the admirable record of salvage among infants who would have been given up for lost only a few years ago.

Congestive Heart Failure

Heart failure may be found in conjunction with any disease of the heart—coronary artery disease, hypertension, rheumatic heart disease, or congenital defects. It occurs when the heart's ability to pump blood has been weakened by disease. To say the heart has failed, however, does not mean it has stopped beating. The heart muscle continues to contract, but it lacks the strength to keep blood circulating normally throughout the body. Physicians sometimes refer to the condition as cardiac insufficiency or *dropsy,* although the latter term is seldom heard anymore.

When the heart fails to pump efficiently, the flow slows down, causing blood returning to the heart through the veins to back up. Some of the fluid in the blood is forced out through the thin walls of small blood vessels into surrounding tissues. Here the fluid piles up, or congests.

The result may be swelling, or *edema,* which can occur in many parts of the body but is most commonly seen in the legs and ankles. Fluids sometimes collect in the lungs, interfering with breathing and making the person short of breath. Heart failure also affects the ability of the kidneys to rid the body of sodium and water. Fluid retained in this way adds to the edema.

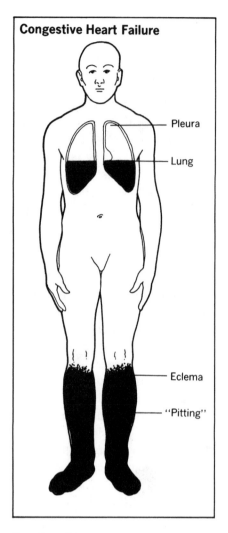

Congestive Heart Failure

- Pleura
- Lung
- Eclema
- "Pitting"

Treatment

Treatment usually includes a combination of rest, drugs, diet, and restricted daily activity. *Digitalis,* in one of its many forms, is usually given to strengthen the action of the heart muscle. It also slows a rapid heartbeat, helps decrease heart enlargement, and promotes secretion of excess fluids. Care must be taken to find the right dose, because this will vary from person to person. When edema is present, diuretics are prescribed to speed up the elimination of excess salt and water. Many improved diuretics are available today. A sodium-restricted diet is generally necessary to reduce or prevent edema. Patients will also probably need bed rest for a while, with gradual return to slower-paced activity.

Most important, however, is the adequate treatment of the underlying disease that led to heart failure in the first place.

Heart Block

Sometimes the scars resulting from rheumatic fever, heart attack, or surgical repair of the heart may damage the electrical network in a way that blocks normal transmission of the signal between the upper and lower chambers. The disruption, called *atrioventricular block*, manifests in three degrees of intensity. First degree heart block is only detectable by an EKG and is merely a short delay in the normal transmission. Second degree heart block shows up as an irregular pulse—some of the beats are blocked. In third degree heart block, none of the beats reach the lower chambers; they begin beating on their own, but at a much slower rate, meaning that blood flow is seriously affected, especially to the brain. Blackouts and convulsions may ensue.

For first degree heart block and many forms of second degree, there are nervous system stimulants to keep the heart from lagging. For third degree heart block and some forms of second degree, however, drugs are not enough. An artificial electronic pacemaker, implanted in the body and connected to the heart by wires, has been successfully applied to many thousands of people throughout the world. This pacemaker fires electrical shocks into the ventricle wall to make it beat at the proper rate. Most devices are powered by tiny lithium batteries that last up to 10 years.

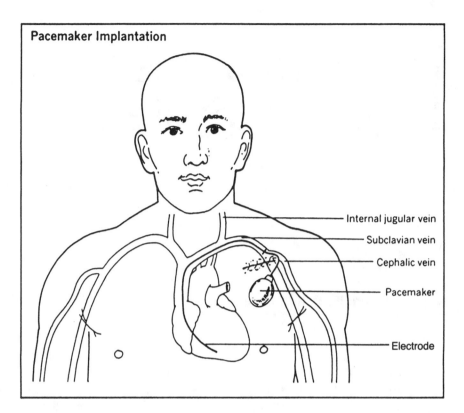

Pacemaker Implantation

Internal jugular vein
Subclavian vein
Cephalic vein
Pacemaker
Electrode

11

Diseases of the Digestive System

Digestive Functions and Organs

The function of the digestive system is to accept food and water through the mouth, to break down the food's chemical structure so that its nutrients can be absorbed into the body, a process called *digestion,* and to expel undigested particles. This process takes place as the food passes through the entire *alimentary tract.* This tract, also called the *gastrointestinal tract,* is a long, hollow passageway that begins at the mouth and continues on through the esophagus, the stomach, the small intestine, the large intestine, the rectum, and the anus. The salivary glands, the stomach glands, the liver, the gallbladder, and the pancreas release substances into the gastrointestinal tract that help the digestion of various food substances.

Digestion

Digestion begins in the mouth where food is shredded by chewing and mixed with saliva, which helps break down starch into sugars and lubricates the food so that it can be swallowed easily. The food then enters the *esophagus,* a muscular tube that for-cibly squeezes the food down toward the stomach, past the *cardiac sphincter,* a ring of muscle at the entrance of the stomach that opens to allow food into the stomach.

The stomach acts as a reservoir for food, churns the food, mixes it with gastric juices, and gradually releases the food into the small intestine. Some water, alcohol, and glucose are absorbed directly through the stomach into the bloodstream. Enzymes secreted by the stomach help break down proteins and fats into simpler substances. Hydrochloric acid secreted by the stomach kills bacteria and prepares some minerals for absorption in the small intestine. Some food may leave the stomach one minute after it enters, while other parts of a meal may remain in the stomach for as long as five hours.

The food passes from the stomach to the first section of the small intestine, the *duodenum,* where it is acted on by pancreatic enzymes that help break down fats, starches, proteins, and other substances. While the food is in the duodenum it is also digested by *bile,* which is produced by the liver and stored in the gallbladder. During a meal, the gallbladder discharges its bile into the duodenum. The bile promotes the absorption of fats and vitamins.

The semidigested food is squeezed down the entire length of the intestines by a wavelike motion of the intestinal muscles called *peristalsis.* Digestion is largely completed as the food passes through 20 feet of small intestine, which absorbs the digested food substances and water and passes them into the bloodstream. The food nutrients are distributed by the bloodstream throughout the body and used by the body cells.

Those parts of the food that are indigestible, such as the skins of fruits, pass into the large intestine, or *colon,* along with bacteria, bile, some minerals, various cells, and mucus. This combination of substances makes up the *feces,* which are stored in the colon until *defecation.* Some water and salts in the feces are absorbed through the walls of the colon into the bloodstream. This conserves the body's fluids and dries the feces. The formation of a semisolid fecal mass helps precipitate defecation.

The Oral Cavity

The Salivary Glands

The smell of food triggers the salivary glands to pour saliva into the mouth; that is what is meant by "mouth-watering" odors. During a meal, saliva is released into the mouth to soften the food as it is chewed.

Stones

Stones will sometimes form in the salivary glands or ducts, blocking the ducts and preventing the free flow of saliva into the mouth. After a meal, the swollen saliva-filled glands and ducts slowly empty. The swelling may sometimes be complicated by infection. Surgical removal of the stones is the usual treatment; sometimes the entire gland is removed.

Tumors

Tumors sometimes invade the salivary gland. An enlarged gland may press on the auditory canal and cause deafness, or it may result in stiffness of the jaw and mild facial palsy. The tumors can grow large enough to be felt by the fingers, and surgery is required to remove them.

Inflammation of the Parotid Glands

Inflammation of the upper (*parotid*) salivary glands may be caused by an infection in the oral cavity, by liver disease, or by malnutrition.

Mumps

One of the commonest inflammations of the salivary glands, called *mumps,* occurs especially in children. It is a highly contagious virus disease characterized by inflammation and swelling of one or both parotid salivary

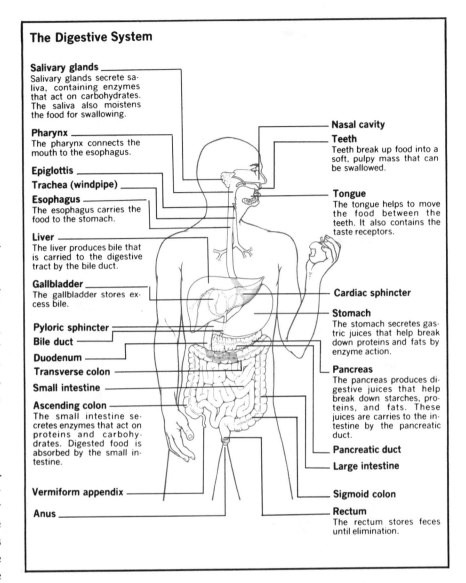

The Digestive System

Salivary glands
Salivary glands secrete saliva, containing enzymes that act on carbohydrates. The saliva also moistens the food for swallowing.

Pharynx
The pharynx connects the mouth to the esophagus.

Epiglottis

Trachea (windpipe)

Esophagus
The esophagus carries the food to the stomach.

Liver
The liver produces bile that is carried to the digestive tract by the bile duct.

Gallbladder
The gallbladder stores excess bile.

Pyloric sphincter

Bile duct

Duodenum

Transverse colon

Small intestine

Ascending colon
The small intestine secretes enzymes that act on proteins and carbohydrates. Digested food is absorbed by the small intestine.

Vermiform appendix

Anus

Nasal cavity

Teeth
Teeth break up food into a soft, pulpy mass that can be swallowed.

Tongue
The tongue helps to move the food between the teeth. It also contains the taste receptors.

Cardiac sphincter

Stomach
The stomach secretes gastric juices that help break down proteins and fats by enzyme action.

Pancreas
The pancreas produces digestive juices that help break down starches, proteins, and fats. These juices are carries to the intestine by the pancreatic duct.

Pancreatic duct

Large intestine

Sigmoid colon

Rectum
The rectum stores feces until elimination.

glands, and can have serious complications in adults. See "Alphabetic Guide to Child Care" in Ch. 2, *The First Dozen Years,* for a fuller discussion of mumps.

Bad Breath (Halitosis)

Poor oral hygiene is the principal cause of offensive mouth odor, or *halitosis.* It can result from oral tumors, abscesses from decaying teeth, and gum disease or infection. The foul smell is primarily a result of cell decay, and the odors are characteristic of the growth of some microorganisms.

When halitosis results from poor oral sanitation, the treatment is obvious—regular daily tooth brushing and the use of an antiseptic mouthwash. If the halitosis is because of disease of the oral cavity, alimentary tract, or respiratory system, the cure will depend on eradicating the primary cause.

Nonmalignant Lesions

The oral cavity is prone to invasion by several types of microorganisms that cause nonmalignant lesions. The most prominent follow.

Canker Sores

These are of unknown origin and

show up as single or multiple small sores near the molar teeth, inside the lips, or in the lining of the mouth. They can be painful but usually heal in a few days.

Fungus Infections

Thrush is the most common oral fungus infection and appears as white round patches inside the cheeks of infants, small children, and sometimes adults. The lesions may involve the entire mouth, tongue, and pharynx. In advanced stages the lesions turn yellow. Malnutrition, especially lack of adequate vitamin B, is the principal cause. Thrush is also one of the opportunistic infections commonly found in persons with AIDS. See also "AIDS" in Ch. 19, *Other Diseases of Major Importance*. Fungus growth may be aided by the use of antibiotic lozenges, which kill normal oral bacteria and permit fungi to flourish.

Tooth Decay and Vitamin Deficiencies

Lack of adequate vitamins in the daily diet is responsible for some types of lesions in the oral cavity. Insufficient vitamin A in children under five may be the cause of malformation in the crown, dentin, and enamel of the teeth. Lack of adequate vitamin C results in bleeding gums. Vitamin D insufficiency may lead to slow tooth development.

An inadequate and improper diet supports tooth decay, which in turn may be complicated by ulcers in the gums and abscesses in the roots of the decaying teeth. A diet with an adequate supply of the deficient vitamins will cause the symptoms to disappear. Infections, abscesses, cysts, or tumors in the mouth require the attention of a physician, dentist, or dental surgeon. See Ch. 22, *The Teeth and Gums*.

Chancres

These are primary syphilis lesions, which commonly develop at the lips and tongue. They appear as small, eroding red ulcers that exude yellow matter. They can invade the mouth, tonsils, and pharynx. Penicillin therapy is usually required.

The Esophagus

Varices

Varices (singular: *varix*) are enlarged and congested veins that appear in the esophagus because of increased blood pressure to the liver in patients with liver cirrhosis. This disease is most common in chronic alcoholics. Esophageal varices can be complicated by erosion of the mucous lining of the esophagus as a result of inflammation or vomiting. This causes hemorrhaging of the thin-walled veins, which can be fatal.

Bleeding esophageal varices may require hospitalization, immediate blood transfusions, and surgery.

Hiatus Hernia

The lower end of the esophagus or part of the stomach can sometimes protrude through the diaphragm. This *hiatus hernia*, sometimes referred to as a *diaphragmatic hernia*, can be a result of congenital malformation; in adults, the principal cause is weakness of the muscles around the opening of the esophagus leading into the stomach.

In individuals who are obese and who have large stomachs, the stomach contents may be forced back into the lower esophagus, causing this area to herniate. Other causes include stooping, bending, or kneeling, which increases pressure in the stomach. Pregnancy may increase abdominal pressure in the same manner as obesity.

Typical symptoms are vomiting when the stomach is full, heartburn with pain spreading to the ears, neck, and arms, swallowing difficulty with the food sometimes sticking in the esophagus, and a swollen abdomen. The vomiting may occur at night, with relief obtained by getting up and walking about for a few minutes. Belching will relieve the distension, and *antacids* (acid neutralizers) may be prescribed to counter gastric hyperacidity.

Conservative treatment involves

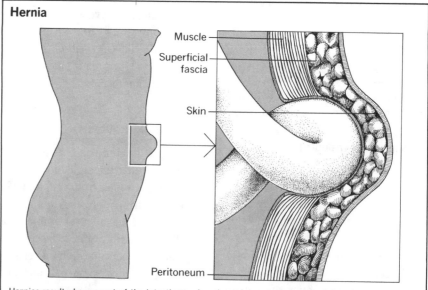

Hernia

Muscle

Superficial fascia

Skin

Peritoneum

Hernias result when a part of the intestine pushes through layers of muscle against the body's layers of skin.

Hiatus Hernia

Esophagus

Herniated stomach

Diaphragm

eating small portions at frequent intervals. Dieting and a reduction in weight cause the symptoms to disappear. When the symptoms are due to pregnancy, they disappear after delivery. When medical management is not successful, surgical repair of the hernia is necessary. See also "Hernias" later in this chapter.

Achalasia

Achalasia is abnormal dilation of the lower esophagus caused by failure of the cardiac sphincter to relax and allow food to enter the stomach. Food collects in the esophagus and does not flow into the stomach. The patient feels as though the food is sticking in the middle of his chest wall. Small amounts of food may eventually pass into the stomach, and the mild pain or discomfort disappears.

If the condition persists, the pain may increase to become a continuous burning sensation at each meal, due to inflammation of the esophagus by accumulated food. If the patient lies down, some of this esophageal content will regurgitate and enter the pharynx. If the vomitus gets into the lungs, the end result may be *aspiration pneumonia*, a form of pneumonia caused by inhaling particles of foreign matter.

The disease is difficult to control,

and the condition tends to return, so that surgery is often used to create a permanent opening between the esophagus and stomach.

Swallowing Difficulty

Difficulty in swallowing is called *dysphagia*, which should not be confused with *dysphasia*, a speech impairment. Dysphagia may be caused by lesions in the mouth and tongue, acute inflammatory conditions in the oral cavity and pharynx (mumps, tonsillitis, laryngitis, pharyngitis), lesions, cancers, or foreign bodies in the esophagus. Strictures in the esophagus—from esophageal ulcers or from swallowing corrosive liquids—will also impair swallowing.

Stomach and Intestines

Indigestion (Dyspepsia)

There are times when the gastrointestinal tract fails to carry out its normal digestive function. The resulting indigestion, or *dyspepsia*, generates a variety of symptoms, such as heartburn, nausea, pain in the upper abdomen, gases in the stomach (*flatulence*), belching, and a feeling of fullness after eating.

Indigestion can be caused by ulcers of the stomach or duodenum and by excessive or too rapid eating or drinking. It may also be caused by emotional disturbance.

Constipation

Constipation is the difficult or infrequent evacuation of feces. The urge to defecate is normally triggered by the pressure of feces on the rectum and by the intake of food into the stomach. On the toilet, the anal sphincter is relaxed voluntarily, and the fecal material is expelled. The

need to defecate should be attended to as soon as possible. Habitual disregard of the desire to empty the bowels reduces intestinal motion and leads to constipation.

Daily or regular bowel movements are not necessary for good health. Normal bowel movements may occur at irregular intervals due to variations in diet, mental stress, and physical activity. For some individuals, normal defecation may take place as infrequently as once every four days.

Simple Constipation

In simple constipation, the patient may have to practice good bowel movement habits, which include a trip to the toilet once daily, preferably after breakfast. Adequate fluid intake and proper diet, including fresh fruits and green vegetables, can help restore regular bowel movement. Laxatives can provide temporary relief, but they inhibit normal bowel function and lead to dependence. When toilet-training young children, parents should encourage but never force them to have regular bowel movements, preferably after breakfast.

Chronic Constipation

Chronic constipation can cause feces to accumulate in the rectum and *sigmoid*, the terminal section of the colon. The colonic fluid is absorbed and a mass of hard fecal material remains. Such impacted feces often prevent further passage of bowel contents. The individual suffers from abdominal pain with distension and sometimes vomiting. A cleansing enema will relieve the fecal impaction and related symptoms.

In the overall treatment of constipation, the principal cause must be identified and corrected so that normal evacuation can return.

Intestinal Obstructions

Obstruction to the free flow of digestive products may exist either in the stomach or in the small and large intestines. The typical symptoms of intestinal obstruction are constipation, painful abdominal distension, and vomiting. Intestinal obstruction can be caused by the bowel's looping or twisting around itself, forming what is known as a *volvulus*. Malignant tumors can either block the intestine or press it closed.

In infants, especially boys, a common form of intestinal obstruction occurs when a segment of the intestine folds into the section below it. This condition is known as *intussusception*, and can significantly reduce the blood supply to the lower bowel segment. The cause may be traced to viral infection, injury to the abdomen, hard food, or a foreign body in the gastrointestinal tract.

The presence of intestinal obstructions is generally determined by consideration of the clinical symptoms, as well as X-ray examinations of the abdomen. Hospitalization is required, since intestinal obstruction has a high fatality rate if proper medical care is not administered. Surgery may be needed to remove the obstruction.

Diarrhea

Diarrhea is the frequent and repeated passage of liquid stools. It is usually accompanied by intestinal inflammation, and sometimes by the passing of mucus or blood.

The principal cause of diarrhea is infection in the intestinal tract by microorganisms. Chemical and food poisoning also brings on spasms of diarrhea. Long-standing episodes of diarrhea have been traced to inflammation of the intestinal mucosa, tumors, ulcers, allergies, vitamin deficiency, and in some cases emotional stress. Diarrhea, in conjunction with

other symptoms, can also indicate infection with human immunodeficiency virus (HIV), the suspected cause of AIDS. See "AIDS" in Ch. 19, *Other Diseases of Major Importance.*

Patients with diarrhea commonly suffer abdominal cramps, lose weight from chronic attacks, or have vomiting spells. A physician must always be consulted for proper diagnosis and treatment; this is especially important if the attacks continue for more than two or three days. Untreated diarrhea can lead to dehydration and malnutrition; it may be fatal, especially in infants.

Dysentery

Dysentery is caused by microorganisms that thrive in the intestines of infected individuals. Most common are *amoebic dysentery,* caused by amoebae, and *bacillary dysentery,* caused by bacteria. The symptoms are diarrhea with blood and pus in the stools, cramps, and fever. The infection is spread from person to person through infected excrement that contaminates food or water. The bacteria and amoebae responsible can also be spread by houseflies which feed on feces as well as on human foods. It is

a common tropical disease and can occur wherever human excrement is not disposed of in a sanitary manner.

Dysentery must be treated early to avoid erosion of the intestinal wall. In bacillary dysentery, bed rest and hospitalization are recommended, especially for infants and the aged. Antibiotic drugs may be administered.

In most cases the disease can be spread by healthy human carriers who must be treated to check further spread.

Typhoid

Enteric fever or *typhoid* is an acute, highly communicable disease caused by the organism *Salmonella typhosa.* It is sometimes regarded as a tropical disease because epidemic outbreaks are common in tropical areas where careless disposal of feces and urine contaminates food, milk, and water supplies. In any location, tropical or temperate, where unsanitary living predominates, there is always the possibility that the disease can occur. Flies can transmit the disease, as can shellfish that live in typhoid-infested waters.

The typhoid bacilli do their damage to the mucosa of the small intestines.

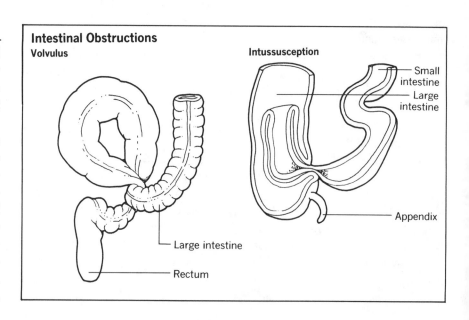

Intestinal Obstructions
Volvulus

Intussusception

—Small intestine
—Large intestine

—Large intestine

—Rectum

—Appendix

They enter via the oral cavity and stomach and finally reach the lymph nodes and blood vessels in the small bowel.

Symptoms

Following an incubation period of about ten days, general bodily discomfort, fever, headache, nausea, and vomiting are experienced. Other clinical manifestations include abdominal pain with tenderness, greenish diarrhea (or constipation), bloody stools, and mental confusion. It is not unusual for red spots to appear on the body.

If untreated, typhoid victims die within 21 days of the onset of the disease. The cause of death may be perforation of the small bowel, abdominal hemorrhage, toxemia, or other complications such as intestinal inflammation and pneumonia.

Treatment and Prevention

A person can best recover from typhoid if he receives diligent medical and nursing care. He should be isolated in a hospital on complete bed rest. Diet should be restricted to highly nutritious liquids or preferably intravenous feeding. Destruction of the bacilli is achieved by antibiotic therapy, usually with Chloromycetin.

The best way to prevent the spread of typhoid is to disinfect all body refuse, clothing, and utensils of the person infected. Isolation techniques practiced in hospitals prevent local spread. Milk and milk products should always be pasteurized; drinking water should be chlorinated.

Human beings can carry the disease and infect others without themselves becoming ill; they are usually not aware that they are carriers. Within recent years, a vaccination effective for a year has been developed.

People traveling to areas where sanitation practices may be conducive to typhoid should receive this vaccination. In such areas, it is usually a good practice to boil drinking water as well.

Foreign Bodies in the Alimentary Tract

Anyone who accidentally swallows a foreign body should seek immediate medical aid, preferably in a hospital. Foreign bodies that enter the gastrointestinal tract may cause obstruction anywhere along the tract, including the esophagus. For emergency procedures, see "Obstruction of the Windpipe" in Ch. 31. *Medical Emergencies.*

Dental plates and large chunks of meat have been known to cause fatal choking. A foreign body in the esophagus may set off a reflex mechanism that causes the trachea to close. The windpipe may have to be opened by means of a *tracheostomy* (incision in the windpipe) to restore breathing. If the object swallowed is long and sharp-pointed, it may perforate the tract.

Foreign bodies in the esophagus are usually the most troublesome. Small fish bones may stick to the walls of the esophagus; large pieces of meat may block the tract. X-ray studies aid the physician in locating the swallowed object and in determining how best to deal with it.

Small objects like coins and paper clips may pass through the digestive tract without causing serious problems. Their progress may be checked by X rays of the abdomen. Examination of stools will indicate whether or not the entire object has been expelled. With larger objects, the problem of blockage must be considered. It is sometimes necessary for a surgeon to open the stomach in a hospital operating room and remove the foreign object.

Ulcers

A *peptic ulcer* is an eroded area of the mucous membrane of the digestive tract. The most common gastrointestinal ulcers are found in the lower end of the esophagus, stomach, or duodenum and are caused by the excessive secretion of gastric acid which erodes the lining membrane in these areas.

The cause of ulcers is obscure, but any factor that increases the gastric acidity may contribute to the condition. Mental stress or conflict, excessive food intake, alcohol, and caffeine all cause the stomach to increase its output of hydrochloric acid.

The disease is sometimes considered to be hereditary, especially among persons with type O blood. Symptoms usually appear in individuals of the 20-to-40 age group, with the highest incidence in persons over age 45. Peptic ulcers of the stomach (*gastric ulcers*) and duodenal ulcers occur more frequently in men than in women. Ulcers are common in patients with arthritis and chronic lung disease.

Symptoms

Early ulcer symptoms are gastric hyperacidity and burning abdominal pain that is relieved by eating, vomiting, or the use of antacids. The pain may occur as a dull ache, especially when one's stomach is empty, or it may be sharp and knifelike.

Other manifestations of a peptic ulcer are the following: nausea, associated with heartburn and regurgitation of gastric juice into the esophagus and mouth; excessive gas; poor appetite with undernourishment and weakness in older victims; and black stools resulting from a bleeding ulcer.

The immediate goal of ulcer therapy is to heal the ulcer; the long-term goal is to prevent its recurrence. An ulcer normally heals through the formation of scar tissue in the ulcer crater. The healing process, under proper medical care, may take several weeks. The disappearance of pain does not necessarily indicate that the ulcer has healed completely, or even partially. The pain and the ulcerative process may recur at regular intervals over periods of weeks or months.

Although treatment can result in complete healing and recovery, some victims of chronic peptic ulcers have a 20-to-30-year history of periodic recurrences. For such patients, ulcer therapy may have to be extended indefinitely to avoid serious complications. If a recurrent ulcer perforates the stomach or intestine, or if it bleeds excessively, it can be quickly fatal. Emergency surgery is always required when perforation and persistent bleeding occur.

Treatment

The basic principles of ulcer therapy are diet, rest, and the suppression of stomach acidity. A patient with an active gastric ulcer is generally hospitalized for three weeks to make certain that he receives the proper diet and to remove him from sources of emotional stress, such as business or family problems. During hospitalization the healing process is monitored by X-ray examination. If there is no evidence of healing within three to four weeks, surgery may be advisable. For patients with duodenal ulcers, a week or two of rest at home with proper diet may be sufficient.

Ulcer diets consist of low-residue bland foods taken in small amounts at frequent intervals, as often as once an hour when pain is severe. The preferred foods are milk, soft eggs, jellies, custards, creams, and cooked cereals. See "Minimal Residue Diet" in Ch. 27, *Nutrition and Weight Control.* Because ulcer diets often lack some essential nutrients, prolonged dietary treatment may have to be augmented with daily vitamin capsules. Antispasmodic medication may be prescribed to reduce contractions of the stomach, decrease the stomach's production of acid, and slow down digestion. Antacids, such as the combination of aluminum hydroxide and magnesium trisilicate, may be required after meals and between feedings. Spicy foods, alcohol, coffee, cola and other caffeine-containing drinks, large meals, and smoking should be strictly avoided.

In addition to common antacids, some new drugs have been introduced to help treat ulcers and other digestive disorders. Tagamet in particular, a brand name for the drug cimetidine, has been found to be effective in treating duodenal ulcers. It has also been used to prevent ulcer-related stomach, esophagus, and duodenal problems. The drug acts primarily to reduce secretions of gastric acid. But side effects have been reported, some of them serious. These include mental confusion, fever, slowed pulse, and others. Metiamide, another drug used to control the production of gastric acids in the digestive system, has been found to attack the leukocytes or white cells of the blood. Other problems have been reported with metiamide.

If the ulcer does not respond to medical therapy, or if pain persists, surgery may be the preferred treatment. Such surgery is elective surgery, a matter of choice, as opposed to the emergency surgery required by large, bleeding, or perforated ulcers. After the removal of the acid-producing section of the stomach, some patients may develop weakness and nausea as their digestive system adjusts to the reduced size of their stomach. A proper diet of special foods and fluids, plus sedatives, can alleviate the condition. The chances for complete recovery are good. For a full description of surgical treatment of peptic ulcers, see "Peptic Ulcers" in Ch. 20, *Surgery.*

Diverticula

A *diverticulum* is an abnormal pouch caused by herniation of the mucous membrane of the digestive tract. The pouch has a narrow neck and a bulging round end. Diverticula are found in the esophagus, stomach, duodenum, colon, and other parts of the digestive tract.

The presence of diverticula in any segment of the digestive tract is referred to as *diverticulosis.* When diverticula become inflamed the condition is known as *diverticulitis.* The latter is a common form of disease of the sigmoid colon and is found in persons past the age of 45.

In mild cases, there may be no symptoms. On the other hand, a diverticulum may sometimes rupture and produce the same symptoms as an acute attack of appendicitis—vomiting and pain with tenderness in the right lower portion of the abdomen. Other symptoms are intermittent constipation and diarrhea, and abdominal pain.

Diverticulosis is treated by bed rest, restriction of solid food and increase of fluid intake, and administration of antibiotics. Surgery is recommended when diverticulosis causes obstruction of the colon or creates an

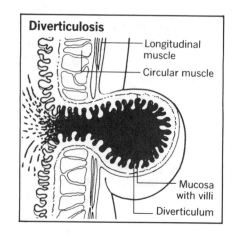

Diverticulosis

Longitudinal muscle

Circular muscle

Mucosa with villi

Diverticulum

opening between the colon and the bladder, or when one or more diverticula rupture and perforate the colon. The outlook for recovery following surgery is good.

Hemorrhoids (Piles)

Hemorrhoids, or *piles,* are round, purplish protuberances at the anus. They are the results of rectal veins that become dilated and rupture. Hemorrhoids are very common and are often caused by straining because of constipation, pregnancy, or diarrhea.

Hemorrhoids may appear on the external side of the anus or on the internal side; they may or may not be painful. Rectal bleeding and tenderness are common. It is important to emphasize, however, that not all rectal bleeding results from hemorrhoids. Small hemorrhoids are best left untreated; large painful ones may be surgically reduced or removed. *Prolapsed* piles—those that have slipped forward—are treated by gentle pressure to return the hemorrhoidal mass into the rectum. The rectal and anal opening must be lubricated to keep the area soft. Other conditions in the large bowel can simulate hemorrhoids and need to be adequately investigated.

Hernias

Hernias in the digestive tract occur

Hemorrhoids

Internal
External

when there is muscular weakness in surrounding body structures. Pressure from the gastrointestinal tract may cause a protrusion or *herniation* of the gut through the weakened wall. Such hernias exist in the diaphragmatic area (*hiatus hernias,* discussed above), in the anterior abdomen (*ventral hernias*), or in the region of the groin (*inguinal hernias*). Apart from hiatus hernias, inguinal hernias are by far the most common.

One of the causes of intestinal obstruction is a *strangulated hernia.* A loop of herniated bowel becomes

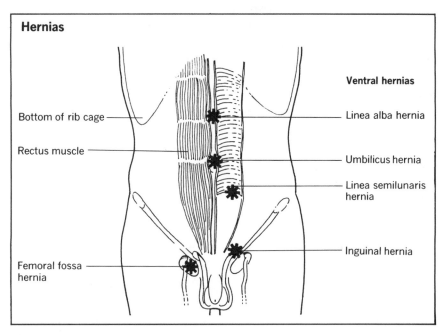

Hernias

Bottom of rib cage

Rectus muscle

Femoral fossa hernia

Ventral hernias

Linea alba hernia

Umbilicus hernia

Linea semilunaris hernia

Inguinal hernia

tightly constricted, blood supply is cut off, and the loop becomes gangrenous. Immediate surgery is required since life is threatened from further complications.

Except for hiatus hernias, diagnosis is usually made simple by the plainly visible herniated part. In men, an enlarged scrotum may be present in untreated inguinal hernias. The herniating bowel can be reduced, that is, manipulated back into position, and a truss worn to support the reduced hernia and provide temporary relief. In all hernias, however, surgical repair is the usual treatment.

Gastritis

Gastritis is inflammation of the mucosa of the stomach. The patient complains of *epigastric* pain—in the middle of the upper abdomen—with distension of the stomach, loss of appetite, nausea, and vomiting.

Attacks of acute gastritis can be traced to bacterial action, food poisoning, peptic ulcer, the presence of alcohol in the stomach, the ingestion of highly spiced foods, or overeating and drinking. Occasional gastritis, though painful, is not serious and may disappear spontaneously. The general treatment for gastritis is similar to the treatment of a gastric ulcer.

Enteritis

Enteritis, sometimes referred to as *regional enteritis,* is a chronic inflammatory condition of unknown origin that affects the small intestine. It is called regional because the disease most often involves the terminal ileum, even though any segment of the digestive tract can be involved. The diseased bowel becomes involved with multiple ulcer craters and ultimately stiffens because of fibrous healing of the ulcers.

Regional enteritis occurs most often in males from adolescence to middle age. The symptoms may exist for a long period before the disease is recognized. Intermittent bloody diarrhea, general weakness, and lassitude are the early manifestations. Later stages of the disease are marked by fever, increased bouts of diarrhea with resultant weight loss, and sharp lower abdominal pain on the right side. This last symptom sometimes causes the disease to be confused with appendicitis, because in both conditions there is nausea and vomiting. Occasionally in women there may be episodes of painful menstruation.

Treatment involves either surgical removal of the diseased bowel or conservative medical management and drug therapy. In acute attacks of enteritis, bed rest and intravenous fluids are two important aspects of treatment. Medical management in less severe occurrences includes a daily diet rich in proteins and vitamins, excluding harder foods such as fresh fruits and vegetables. Antibiotics are prescribed to combat bacterial invasion.

Colitis

Colitis is an inflammatory condition of the colon, of uncertain origin, and often chronic. It may result from a nervous predisposition which leads to bacterial or viral infection. The inflammation can cause spasms that damage the colon, or can lead to bleeding ulcers that may be fatal.

In milder forms, colitis first appears with diarrhea in which red bloody streaks can be observed. The symptoms may come and go for weeks before the effects become very significant. As the disease process advances, the diarrhea episodes become more frequent; more blood and mucus are present in the feces. These are combined with abdominal pain, nausea, and vomiting. Because of the loss of blood, the patient often becomes anemic and thin. If there are ulcer craters in the mucosa, the disease is called *ulcerative colitis.*

Hospitalization is necessary in order to provide proper treatment that will have a long-term effect. Surgery is sometimes necessary if an acute attack has been complicated by perforation of the intestines or if chronic colitis fails to respond to medical management.

Nonoperative treatment includes control of diarrhea and vomiting by drug therapy. Antibiotics are given to control infection and reduce fever, which always accompanies infection. A high protein and vitamin diet is necessary. But if the diarrhea and vomiting persist, intravenous feeding becomes a must. Blood transfusions may be required for individuals who have had severe rectal bleeding. Because there is no absolute cure, the disease may recur.

Appendicitis

The *vermiform appendix* is a narrow tubular attachment to the colon. It can become obstructed by the presence of undigested food such as small seeds from fruits or by hard bits of feces. This irritates the appendix and causes inflammation to set in. If it is obstructed, pressure builds within the appendix because of increasing secretions, a situation that can result in rupture of the appendix. A ruptured appendix can be rapidly fatal if *peritonitis,* inflammation of the peritoneal cavity, sets in.

In most cases the onset of appendicitis is heralded by an acute attack of pain in the center of the abdomen. The pain intensity increases, shifts to the right lower abdomen with nausea, vomiting, and fever as added symptoms. Some individuals, however, suffer from recurrent attacks of dull pain without other signs of gastrointestinal disease, and these may not be significant enough to warrant immediate hospitalization.

Diagnosis of appendicitis is usually dependent on the above symptoms, along with tenderness in the appendix area, increased pulse rate, and decreasing blood pressure. The last two are very significant if the appendix ruptures and peritonitis sets in. Whenever these symptoms are observed, the patient should be rushed to the nearest hospital.

Immediate surgical removal of the diseased appendix by means of a small incision is necessary in all nonperforated acute cases. This type of operation (*appendectomy*) is no longer considered major surgery. If the appendix ruptures and peritonitis is evident, emergency major surgery is necessary to drain the infection and remove the appendix. In the absence of postoperative complications, the patient recovers completely. One of the major problems of appendicitis is early diagnosis to prevent dangerous complications.

Intestinal Parasites

Not all the diseases of man are caused by microscopic organisms. Some are caused by parasitic worms, *helminths,* which invade the digestive tract, most often via food and water. In recent years government health agencies have largely eliminated the prime sources of worm infection: unwholesome meat or untreated sewage that finds its way into drinking water. Nevertheless, helminths still exist. Drugs used to expel worms are called *vermifuges* or *anthelmintics.*

The following are among the major intestinal parasites.

Parasites
Tapeworm

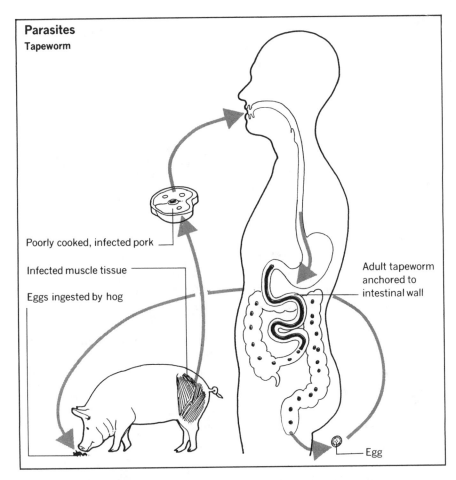

Poorly cooked, infected pork

Infected muscle tissue

Eggs ingested by hog

Adult tapeworm anchored to intestinal wall

Egg

Tapeworms (Cestodes)

These ribbon-shaped flatworms are found primarily in beef, fish, and pork that have not been thoroughly cooked. There are several species ranging from inch-long worms to tapeworms that grow to about 30 feet and live for as long as 16 years.

Tapeworms attach themselves to intestinal mucosa and periodically expel their eggs in excreta. If such feces are carelessly disposed of, the eggs can reach drinking water and be taken in by fish or ingested by grazing cattle. The eggs hatch in the animal's large bowel and find their way into the bloodstream by boring through the intestinal wall. Once in the blood they eventually adhere to muscles and live a dormant life in a capsule.

People who eat raw or partially cooked meat and fish that are infested with tapeworms become infected. The worms enter the bowel, where they feed, grow, and produce eggs. When the egg-filled segments are excreted, the cycle begins anew. Tapeworm infection is usually asymptomatic. It is discovered when egg-laden segments in feces are recognized as such.

Medication must be given on an empty stomach, followed later by a laxative. This will dislodge the worms and enable the body to purge itself of them. A weekly check of stools for segments of the worms may be necessary to confirm that the host is free of the parasites.

Hookworms

There are many species of these tiny, threadlike worms which are usually less than one centimeter long. They are found principally in tropical and subtropical areas of China, North Africa, Europe, Central America, and the West Indies, but they are by no means extinct in the United States.

The eggs are excreted in the feces of infected individuals, and if fecal materials are not well disposed of, the eggs may be found on the ground of unsanitary areas. In warm, moist conditions they hatch into larvae that penetrate the skin, especially the feet of people who walk around barefooted. The larvae can also be swallowed in impure water.

Hookworm-infected individuals, most often children, may experience an inflammatory itch in the area where the larvae entered. The host becomes anemic from blood loss, due to parasitic feeding of the worms, develops a cough, and experiences abdominal pain with diarrhea. Sometimes there is nausea or a distended abdomen. Diagnosis is confirmed by laboratory analysis of feces for the presence of eggs.

Successful treatment requires administration of anthelmintic drugs, preferably before breakfast, to destroy the worms. Weekly laboratory examination of the feces for evidence of hookworm eggs is a necessary precaution in ascertaining that the disease has been eradicated. Untreated hookworm infestation often leads to small bowel obstruction.

Trichinosis

This sometimes fatal disease is caused by a tiny worm, *Trichinella spiralis,* which is spread to man by eating improperly cooked pork containing the tiny worms in a capsulated form. After they are ingested the worms are set free to attach themselves to the mucosa of the small intestines. Here they mature in a few days and mate; the male dies and the female lays eggs that reach the muscles via the vascular system.

Trichinella organisms cause irritation of the intestinal mucosa. The infected individual suffers from abdominal pains with diarrhea, nausea, and vomiting. Later stages of the disease are marked by stiffness, pain, and swelling in the muscles, fever with sweating, respiratory distress, insomnia, and swelling of the face and eyelids. Death may result from complications such as pneumonia, heart damage, or respiratory failure. Despite government inspection of meats, all pork should be well-cooked before eating.

Threadworms (Nematodes)

These worms, also called pinworms, infect children more often than adults. Infection occurs by way of the mouth. The worms live in the bowel and sometimes journey through the anus, where they cause intense itching. The eggs are laid at the anal opening, and can be blown about in the air and spread in that manner. The entire family must be medically treated to kill the egg-laying females, and soothing ointment should be applied at the rectal area to relieve the itching. Good personal hygiene, especially hand washing after toilet use, is an essential part of the treatment.

Roundworms (Ascaris)

These intestinal parasites closely resemble earthworms. The eggs enter the digestive tract and hatch in the small bowel. The young parasites then penetrate the walls of the bowel, enter the bloodstream, and find their way to the liver, heart, and lungs.

Untreated roundworm infestation leads to intestinal obstruction or blockage of pancreatic and bile ducts caused by the masses of roundworms, which usually exist in the hundreds. Ingestion of vermifuge drugs is the required treatment.

Food Poisoning

Acute gastrointestinal illnesses may result from eating food that is itself poisonous, from ingesting chemical poisons, or from bacterial sources. The bacteria can either manufacture *toxins* (poisonous substances) or cause infection. Improperly canned fish, meats, and vegetables may encourage the growth of certain toxin-manufacturing organisms that resist the action of gastric juice when ingested. A person who eats such foods may contract a type of food poisoning known as *botulism*. The symptoms include indigestion and abdominal pain, nausea and vomiting, blurred vision, dryness in the mouth and throat, and poor muscular coordination.

If the toxins become fixed in the central nervous system, they may cause death. Emergency hospitalization is required, where antitoxins are administered intravenously and other measures are taken to combat the effects of botulism.

Salmonella food poisoning is caused by a species of bacteria of that name and is spread by eating contaminated meat, or by eating fish, egg, and milk products that have not been properly cooked or stored or have been inadequately refrigerated. The organisms are also transmitted by individuals who handle well-prepared food with dirty hands. Victims suffer from vomiting, diarrhea, abdominal pain, and fever. This type of food poisoning can be fatal in children and the aged, especially if the latter are ailing. Medical treatment with hospitalization, administration of broad-spectrum antibiotics, and intravenous fluids (to replace water loss due to vomiting) is required.

Some people develop allergic reactions to certain foods and break out in severe rashes after a meal containing any of these foods. Among such foods are fruits, eggs, and milk or milk products. Vomiting or diarrhea

may also occur. The best treatment is to avoid eating such foods and, when necessary, supplement the diet with manufactured protein and vitamins.

Liver Disease

Cirrhosis

Chronic disease of the liver with the destruction of liver cells is known as *cirrhosis*. A common cause is excessive intake of alcoholic beverages along with malnutrition. However, there are other predisposing factors, such as inflammation of the liver (*hepatitis*), syphilis, intestinal worms, jaundice or biliary tract inflammation, and disorders in blood circulation to the liver.

Victims of cirrhosis are usually anemic and have an elevated temperature, around 100° F. Alcoholics very often lose weight, suffer from indigestion, and have distended abdomens.

Accurate diagnosis of cirrhosis depends on complex laboratory tests of liver function, urine, and blood. If liver damage is not too far advanced, treatment of the complications and underlying causes can aid the liver cells in the process of regeneration. In long-standing chronic disease, liver damage may be irreversible. Alcoholics who forgo alcohol may be restored to health, depending on the extent of liver damage, with a proper diet rich in proteins and vitamins.

Successful treatment of liver cirrhosis may require long hospitalization with drug therapy and blood transfusions. During alcoholic withdrawal, the patient may require close medical observation and psychiatric help. If the patient's jaundice improves and his appetite returns, recovery in milder cirrhosis cases is possible.

Jaundice

In diseases of the liver and biliary tract, excessive bile pigment (*bilirubin*) is recirculated into the bloodstream. It enters the mucous membranes and skin, giving them the characteristic yellow pigmentation of the disease.

Gallstones or tumors that obstruct the free flow of bile are one cause of jaundice. Other causes include hepatitis, overproduction of bile pigments with resultant accumulation of bile within the liver, cirrhosis, and congenital closure of the bile ducts, the last a common cause of jaundice in infancy.

Apart from the typical yellow appearance of the skin, jaundice generates such symptoms as body itching, vomiting with bile (indicated by the green appearance and bitter taste), diarrhea with undigested fats present in the stools, and enlargement of the liver with pain and tenderness in the right upper abdomen.

Treatment of jaundice requires continued medical care with hospitalization. Surgery may be necessary to remove stones in the biliary tract or other obstructions. If there is bacterial infection, antibiotic therapy is necessary.

Hepatitis

Inflammation of the liver results in the disease known as *hepatitis*. The most common cause is an infectious process brought on by viruses, jaundice, or high fevers. Other causes of hepatitis include intestinal parasites, circulatory disturbances (such as congestive heart failure), hypersensitivity to drugs, damage to the liver or kidneys, or bacterial infection elsewhere in the body.

One common form of this disease is *infectious hepatitis,* a highly contagious viral infection that often attacks children and young adults, especially those who congregate in large groups. Infectious hepatitis has been known to break out as an epidemic in schools, summer camps, music festivals, and military installations.

The virus is spread by food and water contaminated by feces from infected individuals; good sanitation thus becomes a vital preventive factor. Whole blood used in transfusions can transmit the organisms if the donor is infected. This form of the disease is known as *serum hepatitis* or *hepatitis B.* With the great increase in the use of blood transfusions in recent years in complex surgery, the danger of transmitting hepatitis B by infected blood or infected syringes has become correspondingly greater. Drug addicts are particularly vulnerable to hepatitis B from the use of shared, infected needles.

Symptoms

The incubation period of infectious hepatitis lasts from one to six weeks—that of hepatitis B is longer—followed by fever with headache, loss of appetite (especially for fatty foods), and gastrointestinal distress (nausea, vomiting, diarrhea, or constipation). As the disease progresses, the liver becomes enlarged and the patient jaundiced. There may be some pain in the right upper abdomen.

Treatment

Bed rest, preferably hospital isolation, is a necessary step in the initial treatment stages. Drug therapy with steroids may hasten the recovery process, which may take three to four weeks. When discharged from the hospital, the patient is usually very weak.

Untreated hepatitis causes severe liver damage and may result in coma resulting from liver failure. Sometimes death occurs. Several assaults on the liver reduce the regeneration process and promote cirrhosis. Persons who may have been exposed to the causative virus can receive temporary immunity if they are given an injection of gamma globulin, especially if there is an epidemic. Recent research directed toward the development of a vaccine against serum hepatitis has been very encouraging, and gives rise to the hope that some day wide-scale outbreaks of this disease may become a thing of the past.

Research directed toward the development of a vaccine against hepatitis B, one of three forms of the disease, resulted in the first genetically engineered vaccine. Called Recombivax HB, the vaccine opened a new era in disease prevention. Scientists genetically altered a special type of brewers' yeast to produce a part of the hepatitis B virus. Injected into humans, the vaccine carrying the virus touches off a protective immune system response. Researchers believed similar methods could lead to the development of other vaccines.

An older vaccine for hepatitis B was made from the blood plasma of people infected with the hepatitis B virus. Because the vaccine derived from human blood, there was a small possibility that the vaccine could transmit acquired immune deficiency syndrome (AIDS). The new vaccine eliminates that danger.

Gallbladder Disease

The biliary tract is very often plagued by the presence of stones, either in the gallbladder or in one of the bile ducts. Gallstones are mostly a mixture of calcium carbonate, cholesterol, and bile salts, and can occur either as one large stone, a few smaller ones, or several very small stones.

When fats from the daily diet enter

the small intestines, the concentrated bile from the gallbladder is poured into the duodenum via the bile ducts. Bile is necessary if fats are to be digested and absorbed. If stones are present in the biliary tract, the gallbladder will contract, but little or no bile will reach the fats in the small bowel.

A sharp pain to the right of the stomach is usually the first warning sign of gallstones, especially if the pain is felt soon after a meal of fatty foods—eggs, pork, mayonnaise, or fried foods. The presence of stones very often causes inflammation of the gallbladder and such symptoms as occasional diarrhea and nausea with vomiting and belching. The abdominal area near the gallbladder is usually very tender.

Untreated gallbladder disease leads to several possible complications. The obstructed bile pigments may be recirculated in the bloodstream, causing jaundice. Obstruction of the ducts causes increased pressure and may also result in perforation of the gallbladder or ducts. Acute inflammation of the biliary tract is always a possibility due to the irritation caused by the concentrated bile.

A gallbladder that is full of stones or badly diseased must be surgically removed for the patient's health to improve. In milder cases, other treatment and special diet can prevent attacks.

Treatment and Diagnosis of Gastrointestinal Disorders

Some medications used in treating gastrointestinal disorders, such as antacids and laxatives, can be purchased without prescription. Such medications should be taken only upon a physician's advice.

Treatment of gastrointestinal diseases may require low-residue diets—that is, a diet of foods that pass through the digestive tract very readily without a large amount of solid fecal residue. Included are low-fat meals, liquids, and finely crushed foods. Diagnostic tests may require overnight fasting, fat-free meals, or eating specific foods. Bland meals are vital in the treatment of peptic ulcers and should consist of unspiced soft foods and milk. Raw fruits and vegetables, salads, alcohol, and coffee do not belong in a bland diet. See under Ch. 27, *Nutrition and Weight Control,* for further information on special diets.

X-ray examinations play an important role in diagnosis of gastrointestinal disorders, such as ulcers, diverticula, foreign bodies, malignant lesions, obstruction, achalasia of the esophagus, and varices.

Plain film radiographs are used in initial studies in cases where intestinal obstruction or perforation is suspected. Metallic foreign bodies are easily demonstrated on plain X rays of the digestive tract.

GI Series

By filling the digestive tract with *barium sulfate,* a substance opaque to X rays, a radiologist can locate areas of abnormality. Barium sulfate can be mixed as a thin liquid or paste and be swallowed by the patient during studies of the esophagus, stomach, and small intestines. The type of radiological examination that utilizes such a barium meal is known as a *GI (gastrointestinal) series.* The large bowel is examined with the barium mixture administered through the rectum like a standard enema, known as a *barium enema.* This procedure makes it possible to visualize the inner walls of the colon. For further information on diagnostic procedures, see Ch. 26, *Physicians and Diagnostic Procedures.*

12

Diseases of the Respiratory System

The human body cannot survive for more than a very few minutes in an environment that lacks oxygen. Oxygen is required for the normal functioning of all living body cells. This vital gas reaches the body cells via the bloodstream; each red blood cell transports oxygen molecules to the body tissues. The oxygen comes from the atmosphere one breathes, and it enters the bloodstream through the very thin membrane walls of the lung tissue, a fresh supply of oxygen entering the bloodstream each time a person inhales. As the red blood cells circulating through the walls of the lung tissue pick up their fresh supply of oxygen, they release molecules of carbon dioxide given off by the body cells as a waste product of metabolism. When a person exhales, the lungs are squeezed somewhat like a bellows, and the carbon dioxide is expelled from the lungs.

The automatic action of breathing in and out is caused by the alternate contraction and relaxation of several muscle groups. The main muscle of breathing is the *diaphragm,* a layer of muscle fibers that separates the organs of the chest from the organs of the abdomen. Other muscles of res-

piration are located between the ribs, in the neck, and in the abdomen. As the diaphragm contracts to let the lungs expand, the other muscles increase the capacity of the *thorax,* or chest cavity, when one inhales. The muscles literally squeeze the lungs and chest when an individual exhales.

Any disease of the muscles and bones of the chest wall or of the passages leading from the nose to the lung tissue—containing the small air sacs where the gases are actually exchanged—will interfere to some extent with normal function. As with any organ of the body, there is a great reserve built into the lungs that assures that small to even moderate amounts of diseased tissue can exist without compromising their ability to sustain life. However, when disease of the lungs, air passages, thoracic (rib) cage, or any combination of these parts decreases the capacity of the reserve areas, then the oxygen supply to all the organs and tissues of the body becomes deficient, and they become incapable of performing their vital functions.

Diseases of the thoracic cage are relatively uncommon. Certain forms of arthritis cause fixation of the bony

cage and limit expansion when breathing. Various muscle and nervous system diseases weaken the muscles used to expand the chest for breathing.

Diseases of the *bronchi* or air passages tend to narrow those tubes and thereby limit the amount of air that can pass through to the tiny *alveoli,* or air sacs. Other conditions affect the alveoli themselves, and, if widespread enough, allow no place for the oxygen and carbon dioxide to be exchanged.

The most common forms of lung disease are infections caused by vi-

The Alveoli

Bronchiole

Pulmonary artery

Pulmonary vein

Cross section of alveolus

Capillaries on alveolus

The branches of the pulmonary tree terminate in the alveoli, grapelike clusters of air sacs covered by capillaries, where the gaseous exchange occurs.

Interaction between Heart and Lungs

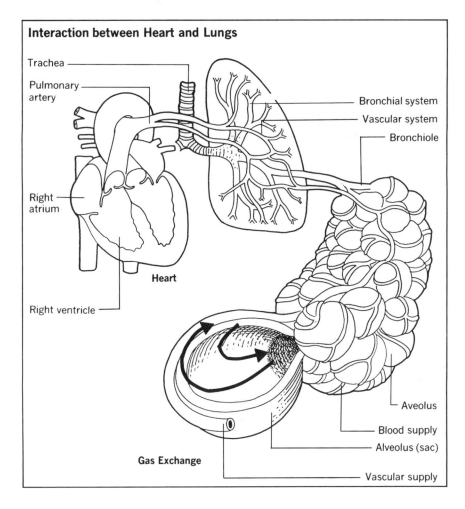

Trachea
Pulmonary artery
Right atrium
Right ventricle
Heart
Bronchial system
Vascular system
Bronchiole
Aveolus
Blood supply
Alveolus (sac)
Vascular supply
Gas Exchange

ruses, bacteria, or fungi. Infection is always a potential threat to the lung because this organ is in constant contact with the outside air and therefore constantly exposed to infectious agents. It is only through elaborate defenses that the body is able to maintain normal functions without interference by these agents.

The major defenses are simply mechanical and consist mainly of the hairs in the nose and a mucous blanket coating the inside of the bronchi. The very small hairs (called *cilia*) in the breathing passage act as a filtering system; mucous membranes of the bronchi help to intercept small particles as they are swept along by the action of the cilia. Whenever these structures are diseased, as in chronic bronchitis, there is a much greater likelihood of acquiring infection.

The Common Cold, Influenza, and Other Viral Infections

The Common Cold

The common cold is the most prevalent illness known to mankind. It accounts for more time lost from work than any other single condition. The infection rate varies from one individual to another.

Surveys indicate that about 25 percent of the population experience four or more infections a year, 50 percent experience two or three a year, and the remaining 25 percent have one or no infections in a year. There is also some variation from year to year for each person, explained often by the amount of exposure to young children, frequent extreme changes in

weather, fatigue, and other factors.

For years it has been felt that chilling plays a role in causing the common cold, and, although difficult to prove, there is almost certainly some truth to the idea. By some as yet unclear process, chilling probably causes certain changes in our respiratory passages that make them susceptible to viruses that otherwise would be harmless.

The common cold affects only the upper respiratory passages: the nose, sinuses, and throat. It sometimes is associated with fever. Several viruses have been implicated as the cause for the common cold. But in the study centers that investigate this illness, isolation of a cold virus is only achieved in about one half of the cases. These viruses are not known to produce any other significant illnesses. Most likely they inhabit the nose and throat, often without producing any illness at all.

Symptoms

The major part of the illness consists of about three days of nasal congestion, possibly a mild sore throat, some sneezing and irritation of the eyes (though not as severe as in hay fever), and a general feeling of ill health often associated with some muscle fatigue and aching. After three days the symptoms abate, but there is usually some degree of nasal congestion for another ten days.

Prevention is difficult, and there is no specific treatment. The natural defenses of the body usually are capable of resolving the infection. Attention should be paid to avoiding further chilling of the body, exhausting activity, and late hours that can further lower the defenses and lead to complications.

Complications

Ear infection may develop because of

blockage of the *Eustachian tube,* which leads from the back of the throat to the inner part of the ear. That complication is heralded by pain in the ear. Bronchitis and pneumonia may be recognized early by the development of cough and production of *sputum* (phlegm). *Sinusitis* develops when the sinus passages are obstructed so that the infected mucus cannot drain into the pharynx (as in postnasal drip). The pain develops near the sinus cavity involved. These complications can and should be treated with specific drugs, and, if they develop, a physician should be consulted.

Influenza

A number of other viruses cause respiratory illness similar to the common cold, but are much more severe in intensity and with frequently serious, and even fatal, complications. The best known member of the group is the *influenza* (flu) virus. It can cause mild symptoms that are indistinguishable from those of the common cold, but in the more easily recognizable form it is ushered in by fever, cough, and what physicians refer to as *malaise*—chills, muscle ache, and fatigue.

The symptoms of influenza appear quickly; they develop within hours and generally last in severe form from four to seven days. The disease gradually recedes over the following week. The severity of the local respiratory and generalized symptoms usually forces the influenza patient to stay in bed.

Not only is the individual case often severe, but an outbreak of influenza can easily spread to epidemic proportions in whole population groups, closing factories, schools, and hospitals in its wake. There have been 31 very severe *pandemics* (epidemics that sweep many countries) that have occurred since 1510. The most devastating of these pandemics occurred in 1918; it led to the death of 20 million people around the world. Rarely is death directly attributable to the influenza virus itself, but rather to complicating bacterial pneumonia or to the failure of vital organs previously weakened by chronic disease.

Flu Shots

Inoculation is fairly effective in preventing influenza, but is not long-lasting and has to be renewed each year. Unfortunately, there are several different types of influenza virus, and a slightly different vaccine is needed to provide immunity to each type of infection. Each recent epidemic in the United States has been the result of a different strain, and although there have been several months' warning before the epidemics started, it has been difficult to mass-produce a vaccine in time to use it before the epidemic developed.

Treatment

Once acquired, there is no cure for influenza, but the body defenses are usually capable of destroying the virus if given the necessary time and if the defenses are not depressed by other illness. Fluids, aspirin, and bed rest help relieve the symptoms. Special attention should be paid to sudden worsening of fever after seeming recovery, or the onset of sputum production. In elderly people more intensive medical care is often necessary, including hospitalization for some.

Pneumonia

Pneumonia might be defined as any inflammation of the lung tissue itself, but the term is generally applied only to infections of an acute or rapidly developing nature caused by certain bacteria or viruses. The term is generally not used for tuberculous or fungal infections. The most common severe pneumonia is that caused by the *pneumococcus bacterium.*

Pneumonia develops from inhaling infected mucus into the lower respiratory passages. The pneumococcus is often present in the nasal or throat secretions of healthy people, and it tends to be present even more often in the same secretions of an individual with a cold. Under certain conditions these secretions may be *aspirated,* or inhaled, into the lung. There the bacteria rapidly multiply and spread within hours to infect a sizable area. As with the common cold, chilling and fatigue often play a role in making this sequence possible. Any chronic debilitating illness also makes one very susceptible to pneumonia.

Symptoms

Pneumonia develops very suddenly with the onset of high fever, shaking chills, chest pain, and a very definite feeling of total sickness or malaise. Within hours enough pus is produced within the lung for the patient to start coughing up thick yellow or greenish sputum that often may be tinged or streaked with blood. The patient has no problem in recognizing that he has suddenly become extremely ill.

Prior to penicillin the illness tended to last about seven days, at which time it would often suddenly resolve almost as quickly as it started, leaving a healthy but exhausted patient. But it also could frequently lead to death or to serious complications, such as abscess formation within the chest wall, meningitis, or abscess of the brain. Because penicillin is so very effective in curing this illness today, physicians rarely see those complications.

Treatment

The response of pneumococcal pneumonia to penicillin is at times one of the most dramatic therapeutic events in medicine. After only several hours of illness the patient presents himself to the hospital with a fever of 104° F, feeling so miserable that he does not want to eat, talk, or do anything but lie still in bed. Within four to six hours after being given penicillin he may have lost his fever and be sitting up in bed eating a meal. Not everyone responds this dramatically, but when someone does, it is striking.

Prevention

There is no guaranteed way to prevent pneumonia. The advice to avoid chilling temperatures, overexertion, and fatigue when one has a cold is directed principally toward avoiding pneumonia. Anybody exposed to the elements, especially when fatigued and wearing damp clothing, is particularly susceptible to pneumonia; this explains its frequent occurrence among army recruits and combat troops. The elderly and debilitated become more susceptible when exposed to extremes of temperature and dampness.

Pneumonia is not really a contagious illness except in very special circumstances, so that isolation of patients is not necessary. In fact, all of us carry the pneumococcus in our noses and throats, but we rarely have the constellation of circumstances that lead to infection. It is the added physical insults that allow pneumonia to take hold.

Other Kinds of Pneumonia

All bacteria are capable of causing pneumonia and they do so in the same manner, via the inhalation of infected upper airway secretions. Some diseases, such as alcoholism, tend to predispose to certain bacterial pneumonias. Usually these are not as dramatic as those caused by the pneumococcus, but they may be much more difficult to treat and thereby can often be more serious.

Far less severe are the pneumonias caused by certain viruses or a recently discovered organism that seems to be intermediate between a virus and a bacterium. The term *walking pneumonia* is often applied to this type, because the patient is often so little incapacitated that he is walking about and not in bed. These pneumonias apparently occur in the same way as the bacterial pneumonias, but the difference is that the infecting agent is not capable of producing such severe destruction. These pneumonias are usually associated with only mild temperature elevation, scant amount of sputum production, and fewer general body symptoms. They should be suspected when coughing dominates the symptoms of a cold, especially if it turns from a dry or nonproductive cough to one that produces sputum. Antibiotic therapy tends to hasten recovery and prevent the complication of bacterial pneumonia.

Pleurisy

No discussion of pneumonia is complete without mention of *pleurisy*. This term refers to any inflammation of the lining between the chest wall and the lung. Infection is only one of the causes, but probably the most common, of inflammation of the *pleura*. Pleurisy is almost always painful, the pain being felt on inhaling and exhaling but not when the breath is quietly held for a brief period. It is a symptom that always deserves the attention of a physician and investigation of its cause. The same type of pain on breathing can often be mimicked by a strain of the chest wall muscles, but the difference can usually be determined by a physician's examination. If not, a chest X ray will help to reveal the cause of the pain.

Tuberculosis

At the turn of the century *tuberculosis* was the leading cause of death in the world; now it is eighteenth. The change in status is due both to the discovery of antibiotics and to modern preventive measures. In this century most other infectious diseases have likewise decreased in incidence and severity for similar reasons. The general decline leaves tuberculosis still at the top of the list as the leading cause of death among infectious diseases. And tuberculosis remains a very serious health problem, accounting for 40,000 new illnesses every year in the United States. In contrast to a disease like influenza, physicians already have the tools with which to eliminate tuberculosis. But many factors, primarily social, make that a very distant possibility.

Tuberculosis is caused by one specific type of bacterium. Certain ethnic groups seem particularly susceptible to the disease, but the reasons are unclear. The American Indian and the Eskimo are two susceptible groups. However, there is no recognized hereditary factor. The disease is different from many commonly known infections in several ways. Unlike pneumonia, tuberculosis is a chronic and painless infection, measured more in months than in days. Because of this pattern, it not only takes a long time to develop serious disease, but it also takes a long time to effect a cure.

Another very important difference between tuberculosis and many other infections is its ability to infect individuals without causing symptoms of illness, but then to lie dormant as a potential threat to that person for the rest of his life. The early stages of the disease do not produce any symptoms. Consequently a patient develops large areas of diseased tissue before he begins to feel sick. Screening procedures, therefore, are very important in detecting early disease in patients who feel perfectly healthy. Another is the skin testing of schoolchildren, which is carried out routinely in many communities today.

How Tuberculosis Spreads

Tuberculosis is contracted by inhaling into the lungs bacteria that have been coughed into the air by a person with advanced disease. It is, therefore, contagious, but not as contagious as measles, mumps, or chicken pox. Unlike those illnesses, it usually requires fairly close and prolonged contact with a tuberculous patient before the infection is passed on. Once the bacteria are inhaled, the body defenses are usually capable of isolating them into small areas within the tissues, thereby preventing any significant destruction or disease. However, though defenses are able to isolate the bacteria, they are not able to destroy all of them. Some bacteria persist in a state in which they are unable to break out and destroy tissue, but they always maintain the potential to do so at a time when the body defenses are impaired.

In about 20 percent of individuals the body defenses are not initially capable of isolating the tubercle bacilli. These individuals, mostly children, develop progressive tuberculosis directly following their initial contact. Others are successful in preventing actual disease at the time of initial contact, but they join a large group with the potential for active disease at some time in the future. Most of the new cases of active tuberculosis come

from this second group; their defenses break down years after the initial contact and resultant infection.

Weight loss, malnutrition, alcoholism, diabetes, and certain other chronic illnesses are particularly likely to lead to deterioration of the defense mechanisms holding the tuberculosis organisms in check. Still other individuals develop active disease with no recognizable condition to account for the loss of defenses. In fact, the most likely age group to develop active disease as a result of breakdown of past infection is the 20- to 30-year-old group.

Once active disease has appeared it usually involves the chest, although it can develop anywhere in the body. There is gradual spread of inflammation within lung tissue until large areas are involved. Holes, or cavities, are formed as a result of tissue destruction. These contain large numbers of tuberculosis organisms and continue to enlarge as new tissue is destroyed at the edges. At any stage of this development organisms may find their way into the bloodstream and new foci of disease can spring up throughout the body. The sputum becomes loaded with organisms that are coughed into the air and go on to infect other individuals. The infected sputum from one area of the lung may gain access to other areas and cause development of diseased tissue there as well.

Treatment

Before the modern era of drug treatment all these events followed an inexorable course to death in 85 percent of people with active tuberculosis. Only a lucky few were able to survive as cured, usually because their disease was found at an early stage. That survival was often at the expense of years confined to a sanatorium. Because of its almost uniform

outcome and the required separation from family and home, tuberculosis was formerly looked upon with quite as much dread as cancer is today.

The sanatorium rest cure of tuberculosis was first developed in the midnineteenth century at a time when the cause of the disease was unknown. In 1882, Robert Koch first demonstrated the tuberculosis organism, thereby proving the disease was an infection. As the twentieth century progressed, general public health measures helped limit the number of new cases, and new surgical procedures were developed to treat the disease. These measures were effective enough to arrest tuberculosis in another 25 percent of cases, brightening somewhat the dismal outlook of the past century.

But the discovery of specific antibiotics in the 1940s made the real difference in tuberculosis. Because of drug treatment, surgery is rarely resorted to today, although it still may be helpful in certain patients. Now patients with tuberculosis can face a relatively bright future without having to be hospitalized for prolonged periods or enduring periods of endless disability.

Tuberculosis Control

People still contract tuberculosis, and people still die from it. Two of the principal causes of death are delayed therapy and interruptions in therapy, the latter leading to the development of tuberculosis organisms that are unaffected by drugs. Both of these causes are often under the control of the patient. The first can be avoided by seeing a physician whenever one develops a cough that lasts more than two weeks, especially when it is not associated with the typical symptoms of a cold at the outset. The other symptoms of developing tuberculosis are also seen in other illnesses, and should always lead one to recognize that he is sick and needs to consult his physician. These symptoms are weight loss, loss of appetite, fever, and night sweats. When tuberculosis is diagnosed, the patient must follow carefully the directions regarding medication, which is always continued for a long time after the patient has regained his feeling of well-being.

There are other ways, however, to attack tuberculosis, even before one becomes sick. Once a person has had contact with tuberculosis, even though he usually does not develop active disease, he produces antibodies against the bacteria. A person with such antibodies can be recognized by injecting under the skin specially prepared material from dead tuberculosis bacteria, which gives rise to a reaction within the skin after two days. This material is called *tuberculin* and the test is known as the *tuberculin test.*

There are now many mass screening programs of tuberculin testing for schoolchildren, hospital personnel, and industrial groups. Those with positive skin test reactions are screened further for the presence of active disease. If they are found to be active cases, they are treated during what is usually an early and not very severe stage of the disease. The other people with positive tuberculin tests, without any evidence of active disease, are candidates for *prophylactic* (preventive) *therapy.* This therapy employs *isoniazid* (*INH*), the most effective of many drugs for the treatment of tuberculosis and one that has virtually no side effects. Treatment for one year has been shown to reduce greatly the chance of future progress from the merely infected state to the state of active disease.

The goal of prophylactic therapy is chiefly to prevent the far more serious development of active disease. But in addition, by preventing disease

before it develops, physicians can prevent the infection of others, since the typical patient with tuberculosis has already infected some of those living with him before he becomes ill and seeks medical attention. The surface has just been scratched in this regard, however, as there are estimated to be 25 million people in the United States who would demonstrate reactions to tuberculin tests. Many of these people have never been tested and are not aware of the potential threat within them.

In most foreign countries the tuberculosis problem is much more serious. An estimated 80 percent of the populations of the countries of Asia, Africa, and South America would show positive tuberculin skin tests, with the number of active cases and deaths being proportionately high.

Sarcoidosis

Sarcoidosis (or *Boeck's sarcoid*), a disease that affects black people more often than whites, has symptoms closely resembling those of tuberculosis and other diseases. The most obvious symptom is the formation of skin nodules, often of the face, but the nodules, called *granulomas* (small tumors composed chiefly of granulation tissue), commonly occur in many other places as well, especially in the lungs and lymph nodes. They can occur also in the liver, bones, eyes, and other tissues.

Although sarcoidosis occurs all over the world, it is more common in temperate regions, and in the United States occurs more frequently in the southeastern states than elsewhere. Men and women are about equally affected. The onset of the disease occurs usually in the third or fourth decade of life.

Diagnosis and Treatment

The disease is diagnosed by an ex-

amination of chest X rays, which will show the proliferation of nodules in the lungs. Surgical biopsy and microscopic examination of skin tissue or tissue from a lymph node is usually necessary to confirm the presence of the disease.

There is no specific treatment for sarcoidosis, and in spite of its similarities in some respects to tuberculosis, no connection between the two disorders has been established. Steroids are sometimes used to treat the skin lesions, but in many cases the skin nodules clear up eventually without any treatment. About half of the patients, however, do not recover completely, and the disease becomes chronic—though of varying severity. Ultimately the granulomas can change into fibrous scars that may pose serious threats to the patient, depending upon where the scarring occurs. Respiratory distress, heart failure, and glaucoma, for example, can result from tissue changes in the lungs, heart, and eyes, respectively.

Respiratory Diseases Caused by Fungi

Two fungal diseases affecting respiration are of great importance in particular regions of the United States. They are both caused by types of fungi capable of growing within mammalian tissue, thereby infecting and destroying it. Both cause chronic diseases very similar to tuberculosis and may lead to death, though that is a far less common outcome—even when untreated—than in tuberculosis.

The spores of the fungi are inhaled from the air, and the response of the body is similar to that in tuberculosis in that most people become merely infected (the spores being contained by body defenses) while a few develop progressive disease. The body also produces anitbodies, and consequently skin tests similar to the tuberculin test can identify infected individuals.

Histoplasmosis (named for a fungus called *histoplasma*) organisms are prevalent in the Midwest, generally in the areas of the Ohio, Mississippi, and Missouri rivers. Largely unknown prior to World War II, histoplasmosis has been studied extensively since. Local epidemics have brought it to public attention on several occasions. The fungus grows readily in soil containing large amounts of bird (chickens, pigeons, starlings) or bat excrement. One of the better ways to assure exposure is to clean out an old chicken coop. The concentration of organisms may reach such high levels in bat caves that entry by spelunkers may prove fatal. In contrast to tuberculosis, the amount of exposure seems to play a very important role in determining the extent of the disease. There also seem to be few cases of late breakdown (the rule in tuberculosis). Most people develop the active disease, if at all, at the time of their initial exposure.

Coccidioidomycosis (for *Coccidioides* fungus) also generates in the soil, in this case in California, the southwest United States, and Mexico. It grows best in hot, dry soil. The common names for this disease are *desert rheumatism* or *valley fever.* Infection and disease occur in a similar pattern to that of histoplasmosis. Skin testing of large population groups for both these fungi in the appropriate geographical areas indicates that the majority of exposed individuals quite adequately contain the initial infection and never develop any illness or active disease.

Because Americans travel into infected regions, these diseases are being seen more frequently in people who do not live where the fungi are found. Both conditions, fortunately, are often self-limited, even when active disease develops. For more se-

vere cases there is a drug, *amphotericin-B,* which is quite effective; however, because it is also quite toxic to the patient, it must be given in progressive doses starting with a small initial dose, to permit the body's tolerance to build up. It is hoped that less toxic agents will be found in the future that will be just as effective against the fungus.

Allergic Respiratory Diseases

Hay fever (*allergic rhinitis*) and *asthma* are two very common allergic diseases of the respiratory tract. The two have much in common as to age at onset, seasonal manifestations, and causation. Hay fever involves the *mucosa,* or lining, of the upper respiratory tract only, whereas asthma is confined to the bronchial tubes of the lower respiratory tract. Physicians usually distinguish two main types of asthma, allergic and infectious. The infectious type of asthma resembles bronchitis, with cough and much wheezing as well. The discussion here will be confined to the allergic form of asthma.

In hay fever and asthma the allergenic substance causing the reaction is usually airborne, though it can be a food. In most cases the offender is pollen from a plant. The pollen is inhaled into the nostrils and alights upon the lining of the respiratory passages. In the allergic individual, antibodies react with the proteins in the pollen and cause various substances to be released from the tissue and blood cells in the immediate area. These substances, in turn, produce vessel enlargement in the area and an outpouring of mucus, plus certain irritating symptoms that result in a stuffy or runny nose and itchy eyes. The same reactions occur in the bronchial lining in asthma, but the substances released there also cause constriction of the bronchial muscle and conse-

quent narrowing of the passages. This muscular effect and the narrowing caused by greatly increased amounts of mucus in the passages are both responsible for the wheezing in asthma.

Hay Fever

Hay fever is never a threat to life, but in severe cases it can upset one's life patterns immensely. For unknown reasons it is more common in childhood, where it is often seen in conjunction with eczema or asthma. The tendency to develop hay fever, eczema, and asthma is hereditary. The transmission of the hereditary factors is complex, so that within a family group any number of individuals or none at all may exhibit the trait.

Most people with hay fever have their only or greatest difficulty in the summer months because of the airborne pollens from trees, grasses, flowers, and molds that are prevalent then. The most notorious of all pollens is the ragweed pollen. This weed pollinates around August 15 and continues to fill the air until late September. In many cities an official pollen count is issued every day, and those with severe difficulty can avoid some trouble by staying outside as little as possible on high-count days. *Antihistamine* drugs are used to counteract the nasal engorgement in hay fever. These drugs counteract the effect of *histamine,* which is one of the major substances released by the allergic reaction.

Allergic Asthma

Allergic asthma is the result of the allergic reaction taking place in the bronchial mucosal lining rather than in the nasal lining. A person may suffer from both asthma and hay fever. The common inciting factors are pollens, hair from pets (especially cats), house dust, molds, and certain foods (especially shellfish). When foods are responsible, the reaction initially occurs within the bloodstream, but the major effect is felt within the lung, which is spoken of as the target organ.

Most allergic asthma is seen in children. For unclear reasons it usually disappears spontaneously at puberty. In those who continue to have difficulty after puberty, the role of infection as a cause for the asthma usually becomes more prominent. Allergic asthma attacks start abruptly and can usually be aborted rather easily with medication.

People with asthma are symptom-free much of the time. When exposed to high concentrations of pollen they begin wheezing and producing sputum. Wheezing refers to the high-pitched squeaking sound that is made by people exhaling through narrowed bronchi. Associated with the wheezing and sputum is a distinct sensation of shortness of breath that varies in severity according to the nature of the attack. Milder attacks of asthma often subside spontaneously, merely with relaxation. This is especially true when the wheezing is induced by nonspecific factors, such as a cloud of dust, cold air, or exercise. Asthmatic individuals have more sensitive air passages and they are more easily bothered by these nonspecific irritants.

Treatment

For more severe attacks of asthma there are several types of treatment.

There are oral medications that dilate the bronchi and offset the effects of the allergic reaction. (Antihistamines, however, exert no effect on asthma and may even worsen the condition.) Also available are injectable medications, such as adrenaline, and sprays that contain substances similar to adrenaline and that can be inhaled. Any or all of these methods may be employed by the physician. During times of high exposure it is often helpful to take one of the oral medications on a regular basis, thereby avoiding minor episodes of wheezing.

A recently discovered remedy for asthma is particularly useful to persons—primarily infants and small children, who cannot swallow tablets. The remedy comes in capsules containing tiny pellets of the drug theophylline. Once the capsule is twisted open, the pellets can be sprinkled on soft foods, including strained baby food, applesauce, pudding, or hot or cold cereal. The pellets give relief for about 12 hours, long enough to protect children during sleep.

The best therapy for asthma and hay fever is avoidance of the allergen responsible for attacks. Obviously, cats and certain foods can be avoided more readily than pollens and other airborne substances. The first requisite, however, is to identify the offender. The most important method of identification is the patient's medical history. Sometimes the problem is easy, as when the patient states that he only has trouble during the ragweed season. At other times a great

amount of detective work may be required. Skin testing is used to complement the history. The skin test merely involves the introduction under the skin (usually within a tiny scratch) of various materials suspected of being allergens. If the individual has antibodies to these substances he will form a hive at the site of introduction. That he reacts does not necessarily mean that his asthma is due to that test substance, because many people have reactions but no hay fever or asthma. The skin test results need to be interpreted in the light of the history of exposure.

If the substance so identified cannot be avoided, then hyposensitization may prove useful. This form of treatment is based on the useful fact that the human body varies its ability to react depending upon the degree and the frequency of exposure. In a hyposensitizing program small amounts of pollen or other extract are injected frequently. Gradually the dose of extract is increased. By this technique many allergic individuals become able to tolerate moderate exposure to their offending material with few or no symptoms. Hyposensitization does not succeed in everyone, but it is usually worth attempting if other approaches are unsuccessful. For more information see Ch. 21, *Allergies and Hypersensitivities.*

13

Lung Disease

Two present-day problems of major proportions are not diseases in themselves, but both are detrimental to health. These are smoking and air pollution. The former is a habit that, in some users, can produce as serious results as narcotics or alcohol addiction. Knowledge of air pollution has grown with the increased public awareness of our environment. It is quite clear that there are many serious consequences produced by the products with which we foul our air. Both tobacco and air pollution are controllable: one by individual will, the other by public effort.

Smoking

Eighty-five million Americans smoke, and the vast majority of these people smoke cigarettes. This discussion will therefore center on cigarettes. The number of new smokers is increasing, which offsets the number of quitters, thereby producing a new gain in smokers each year. There was a temporary absolute decline in 1964 when the first U.S. Surgeon General's report on smoking outlined the many hazards, but that trend quickly reversed itself. The tobacco industry spends $280 million per year to promote smoking. The U.S. Public Health Service and several volunteer agencies spend $8 million in a contrary campaign to discourage smoking.

Dangers of Smoking

Scientists know much about the ways in which smoking produces health dangers. As they burn, cigarettes release more than 4,000 different substances into the atmosphere. Carried in the cigarette smoke, these substances enter the smoker's lungs or simply dissipate in the air. Three of the substances, carbon monoxide, "tar," and nicotine, are the primary threats to health.

Smoking has "mainstream" effects on the smoker who inhales. But there are "sidestream" effects as well. For example, persons who habitually breathe the smoke from others' cigarettes may be inhaling higher concentrations of possibly harmful chemicals than the smokers themselves. These nonsmokers may experience such unpleasant symptoms as watery eyes and headaches. If they have lung or heart diseases, suffer from asthma or some allergies, or wear contact lenses, the nonsmokers may find that their symptoms are worsening.

Some of the direct effects of breathing tobacco smoke suggest its capacity for producing disease in the smoker. Smoking lowers skin temperature, often by several degrees, principally through the constricting effect of nicotine on blood vessels. Carbon monoxide levels rise in the blood when a person is smoking. Even a single cigarette may impair somewhat the smoker's ability to expel air from the lungs. Adverse changes in the activity of several important chemicals in the body can be demonstrated after smoking.

Smoking has been strongly implicated in bronchitis and emphysema, lung and other cancers, heart disease, and peripheral vascular disease. Cigarette smoking causes more "preventable" deaths in the United States than any other single factor. Of the five leading causes of American deaths, smoking is related to four. According to verified statistics, a smoker faces a 70 percent greater risk of dying prematurely than a nonsmoker of comparable age. Smoking-related diseases take six times as many American lives annually as automobile accidents.

Lungs

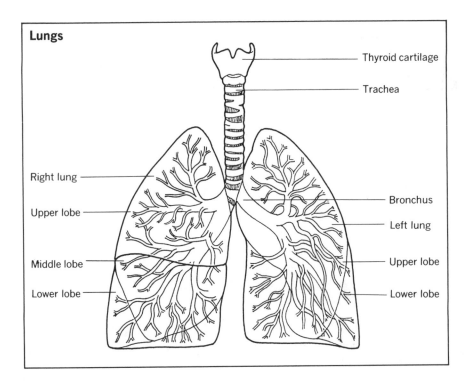

Thyroid cartilage

Trachea

Right lung

Upper lobe

Middle lobe

Lower lobe

Bronchus

Left lung

Upper lobe

Lower lobe

A Cause of Cancer

Lung cancer takes more American lives annually than any other type of cancer. Some 80 percent of all lung cancer deaths, over 90,000 in a typical year, may be attributed to cigarette smoking. On average, 7 in 10 lung cancer patients die within a year of diagnosis.

The cigarette smoker's risks are not confined to lung cancer. Such serious and sometimes fatal diseases as cancers of the mouth, pharynx, larynx, and esophagus may also be smoking-related. Of all cancer deaths, 30 percent are related to smoking. Smoking leads to 10 times as many cancer deaths as all other reliably identified cancer causes combined.

Heart Disease

Heart disease caused by smoking cigarettes takes more American lives than does cancer. But smoking is implicated in about 30 percent of all deaths resulting from coronary heart disease, the most common cause of American deaths. In 1982, about 170,000 U.S. citizens died of heart disease resulting from smoking.

In the mid-1980s, statistics showed that one living American in every 10 would die prematurely as a result of smoking-related heart disease. The smoker who refused to give up smoking after a heart attack was inviting a second attack to a significant degree. But the person who quit smoking would after some 10 years face a heart-disease risk about equal to that of a nonsmoker.

Women and Smoking

Where women accounted for one lung cancer death in six in 1968, one-fourth of all such deaths occurred among women in 1979. Those figures suggest what later statistics have borne out: that lung cancer would soon replace breast cancer as the leading cause of cancer death among women.

Women were once thought to be less susceptible to smoking-related diseases than men. But later epidemiological studies have proved the opposite. When the earlier studies were conducted, women had simply not been smoking as long as men, or in such numbers. As the picture has changed, the statistics have changed. Like men, women smokers who experience other heart disease risk factors, including hypertension and high serum cholesterol levels, face a greatly increased risk of coronary heart disease.

The Dose-Response Relationship

The number of cigarettes an individual smokes is one of the determinants of eventual damage even though individual susceptibility is also important. Thus a definite dose-response relationship exists between smoking and disease. If a person smokes one pack a day for one year he has smoked one pack-year; if he smokes one pack a day for two years or two packs a day for one year, he has smoked two pack-years, and so on. Calculating by pack-years, it appears that 40 pack-years is a crucial time period above which the incidence of cancer of the lung, emphysema, and other serious consequences rises rapidly. Smoking three packs a day, it takes only about 13 years to reach this critical level.

Breaking the Smoking Habit

Obviously, the best way not to smoke is never to start. Unfortunately, young people are continuing to join the smoking ranks at a rapid rate. The teenager often is one of the hardest persons to convince of the hazards of smoking. He is healthy, suffers less from fatigue, headaches, breathlessness, and other immediate effects of smoking, and he often feels the need to smoke to keep up with his peers. Once he starts, it is not long before he becomes addicted. The addiction to cigarettes is very real. It is more psychological dependency than the physical addiction associated with narcotics, but there are definite physical addiction aspects to smoking that are mostly noted when one stops.

For most people it is quite a challenge to stop smoking. There are many avenues to travel and many sources now available to aid one on the way. They include smoking clinics that offer group support and medical guidance to those anxious to quit. The clinics vary in their format but basically depend on the support given the smoker by finding other individuals with the same problems and overcoming the problems as a group. The medical guidance helps people recognize and deal with withdrawal symptoms as well as helping them with weight control.

Withdrawal Symptoms

Withdrawal symptoms vary from person to person and include many symptoms other than just a craving for a cigarette. Many people who stop smoking become jittery and sleepless, start coughing more than usual, and often develop an increased appetite. This last withdrawal effect is especially disturbing to women, and the need to prevent weight gain is all too often used as a simple excuse to avoid stopping the cigarette habit or to start smoking again. The weight gained is usually not too great, and one generally stops gaining after a few weeks. Once the cigarette smoking problem is controlled, then efforts can be turned to weight reduction. Being overweight is also a threat to health, but ten extra pounds, even if maintained, do not represent nearly the threat that confirmed smoking does.

Despite all efforts, many individuals who would like to stop smoking fail in their attempts. The best advice

for them is to keep trying. Continued effort will at least tend to decrease the amount of smoking and often leads to eventual abstinence, even after years of trying. If a three-pack-per-day smoker can decrease to one pack a day or less, he has helped himself even though he is still doing some damage. For prospective quitters it is important to remember that cigarette smoking is an acquired habit, and that the learning process can be reversed. The problem most people have is too little knowledge of the dangers and too much willingness to believe that disease and disability cannot strike them, just the other fellow.

Air Pollution

While 85 million Americans pollute the air they breathe individually with cigarettes, all 210 million of us collectively pollute the atmosphere we all breathe. Some people are obviously more responsible than others, but air, water, and land pollution is a disease of society and can only be solved through a concerted effort by the whole society. Pollution has always been a problem to man. As we have become more urbanized the problem has grown. It has now reached what many consider to be crisis proportions in our large cities and even in some of our smaller ones.

We have had ample warning. In 1948 a killer smog engulfed Donora, Pennsylvania, killing 20 persons and producing serious illness in 6,000 more. In 1952 a lingering smog over London was blamed for 4,000 deaths in a few weeks. New York City has had several serious encounters with critical smog conditions that have accounted for many illnesses and deaths. The exteriors of many buildings in our cities are showing signs of vastly increased rates of decay due to the noxious substances in the air. It

is estimated that air pollution costs the United States $11 billion a year in damage, illness, and in other ways. Even if all this loss of life and property were not a result it would clearly be more pleasant to live in a clean atmosphere than in a foul one.

Emphysema and Bronchitis

Emphysema and chronic bronchitis are diseases that involve the whole lung. They can be of varying severity, and both are characterized by the gradual progression of breathlessness.

Because chronic bronchitis is almost invariably associated with pulmonary emphysema, the combined disorder frequently is called *obstructive-airway disease*. The disease involves damage to the lung tissue, with a loss of normal elasticity of the air sacs (*emphysema*), as well as damage to the *bronchi*, the main air passages to the lungs. In addition, chronic bronchitis is marked by a thickening of the walls of the bronchi with increased mucus production and difficulty in expelling these secretions. This results in coughing and sputum production.

The condition known as *acute bronchitis* is an acute process generally caused by a sudden infection, such as a cold, with an exaggeration of bronchitis symptoms. If a spasm of the bronchi occurs, accompanied by wheezing, the ailment is called infectious or nonallergic asthma.

Obstructive-airway disease is very insidious, and characteristically people do not, or will not, notice that they are sick until they suddenly are very sick. This is partly because of chronic denial of the morning cough and breathlessness, but also because we are fashioned in such a way as to have great reserve strength in our organs. As the disease progresses one starts using up his reserve for exertion. Be-

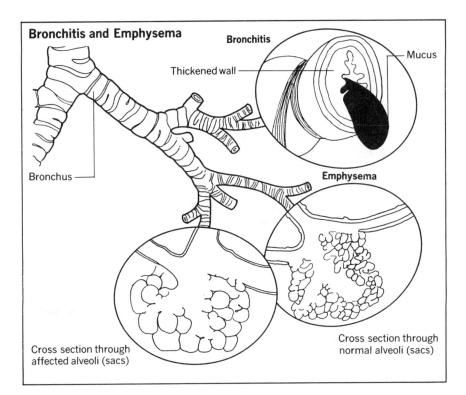

Bronchitis and Emphysema

Bronchitis

Thickened wall

Mucus

Bronchus

Emphysema

Cross section through affected alveoli (sacs)

Cross section through normal alveoli (sacs)

cause most people's life styles allow them to avoid exertion easily, the victim of this disease may have only rare chances to notice his breathlessness. Then, suddenly, within a period of a few months he becomes breathless with ordinary activity because he has used up and surpassed all his reserve. He goes to a physician thinking he has just become sick. Usually this event occurs when the patient is in his fifties or sixties and little can be done to correct the damage. The time for prevention was in the previous 30 years when elimination of smoking could have prevented much or all of the illness.

Chronic cough and breathlessness are the two earliest signs of chronic bronchitis and emphysema. A smoker's cough is not an insignificant symptom. It indicates that very definite irritation of the bronchi has developed and it should be respected early. Along with the cough there is often production of phlegm or sputum, especially in the morning, because of less effective emptying of the bronchial tree during the relatively

motionless period of sleep. Another early manifestation of disease is the tendency to develop chest infections along with what would otherwise be simple head colds. With these chest infections there is often a tightness or dull pain in the middle chest region, production of sputum and sometimes wheezing.

Treatment

Once emphysema or bronchitis are diagnosed there are many forms of therapy that can help. Stopping smoking is the most important measure, and will in itself often produce dramatic effects. The more bronchitis the patient has, the more noticeable the effect, as the bronchial irritation and mucous production decrease, cough lessens, and a greater sense of well-being ensues. The emphysema component does not change, as the damage to the air sacs is irreversible, but the progression may be greatly slowed. When chest infections develop they can be treated with antibiotics.

For more severe disease a program of breathing exercises and graded exertion may be beneficial. When these people develop heart trouble as a result of the strain on the heart, a treatment to strengthen the heart is rewarding. For those with the most advanced stage of the disease new methods of treatment have been devised in recent years. One of the most encouraging is the use of controlled oxygen administration, treatment that can sometimes allow a patient to return to an active working life from an otherwise helpless bed-and-chair existence. But it must be remembered that all these measures produce little effect if the patient continues to smoke.

Vaporizers, Nebulizers, IPPB

Mechanical methods have been developed to help control emphysema, bronchitis, acute and chronic asthma, and other respiratory disorders. These methods include the use of vaporizers, nebulizers, and intermittent positive pressure breathing (IPPB).

The vaporizer is a device that increases the moisture content of a home or room. In doing so, the vaporizer relieves the chronic condition that makes breathing difficult: the increased humidity loosens mucus and reduces nasal or bronchial congestion. One simple type of vaporizer or humidifier is the "croup kettle" or hot-steam type that releases steam into the air when heated on the stove or electrical unit. A more formal type of vaporizer is the electric humidifier that converts water into a spray. In dispersing the spray into the atmosphere, the vaporizer raises the humidity level without increasing the temperature.

The nebulizer also converts liquid into fine spray. But the nebulizer dispenses medications, such as isoproterenol hydrochloride, directly into the throat through a mouthpiece and pressure-injector apparatus like an atomizer. Used in limited doses according to a physician's instructions, nebulization can relieve the labored or difficult breathing symptoms common to various respiratory diseases, among them asthma and bronchitis. The patient controls the dosage while using the nebulizer simply by employing finger pressure and obeying instructions.

In IPPB, a mask and ventilator are used to force air into the lungs and enable the patient to breathe more deeply. The ventilator supplies intermittent positive air pressure. The IPPB method of treatment has been used to help persons suffering from chronic pulmonary disease that makes breathing difficult. But IPPB may also be used with patients who cannot cough effectively; these patients include those who have recently undergone surgery. Newer IPPB units are highly portable; but they must be cleaned carefully with an antibacterial solution before use, and should always be used carefully to avoid producing breathing difficulties or aggravating heart problems.

Smoking and Obstructive Diseases

The problems encountered by patients with obstructive disease do not encompass merely that disease alone. Because of their smoking history these patients are also prone to develop lung cancer. All too often a person with a potentially curable form of lung cancer is unable to undergo surgery because his lungs will not tolerate the added strain of surgery. Patients with obstructive disease are also more prone to pneumonia and other infectious pulmonary conditions. When these develop in the already compromised lung, it may be impossible for the patient to maintain adequate oxygen supply to his vital

tissues. If oxygen insufficiency is severe and prolonged enough, the patient dies from pulmonary failure.

Despite the emphasis placed on smoking as the predominant factor for the development of obstructive disease, there are people with the disease who have never smoked. For many of these individuals there is no known cause for their disease. However, a group of younger people with obstructive disease has been found to be deficient in a particular enzyme. (Enzymes are agents that are necessary for certain chemical reactions.) Individuals with this deficiency develop a particularly severe form of emphysema, become symptomatic in their third or fourth decade, and die at a young age. They may not smoke, but if they do, the disease is much more severe. Just how the enzyme deficiency leads to emphysema is not clear, but a great amount of research is being conducted on this new link to try to learn more about the causes of emphysema.

The Pneumoconioses

Pneumoconiosis is a chronic reaction of the lung to any of several types of inhaled dust particles. The reaction varies somewhat but generally consists of initial inflammation about the inhaled particle followed by the development of scar tissue. The pneumoconioses develop predominantly from various occupational exposures to high concentrations of certain inorganic compounds that cannot be broken down by the cells of the body. The severity of the disease is proportional to the amount of dust retained in the lung.

Silica is the most notorious of these substances. People who work in mining, steel production, and any occupation involved with chipping stone, such as manufacturing monuments, are exposed to silica dust. Many of the practices associated with these occupations have been altered over the years because of the recognition of the hazard to workers. Other important pneumoconioses involve talc and asbestos particles, cotton fibers, and coal dust. Coal dust has gained wide attention in recent years with the heightened awareness of *black lung,* a condition seen in varying degrees in coal miners. The attention has resulted in a federal black lung disease law under which more than 135,000 miners have filed for compensation.

Although there are individual dif-

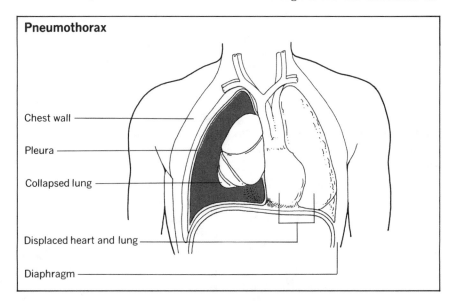

Pneumothorax

Chest wall

Pleura

Collapsed lung

Displaced heart and lung

Diaphragm

ferences in reaction to the varied forms of pneumoconiosis, the ultimate hazard is the loss of functioning lung tissue. When enough tissue becomes scarred, there is interference with oxygenation. Those people with pneumoconiosis who smoke are in great danger of compounding their problem by adding obstructive disease as well.

Prevention

Once the scarring has taken place there is no way to reverse the process. Therefore, the answer to the pneumoconioses is to prevent the exposure. Attention to occupational diseases in the United States has lagged about 30 years behind Europe, so that we are just now beginning to show concern about certain industrial practices condemned as hazardous in many European countries in the 1940s. New lung diseases caused by inhaled substances are discovered every year, and more will undoubtedly be found in the future. People in industries in which there is exposure to industrial dust should be aware of the potential danger and should be prepared to promote the maintenance of protective practices and the investigation of new ideas and devices. Where masks have been supplied, the workers should wear them, a practice too often neglected.

Pulmonary Embolism

Pulmonary embolism is a condition in which a part of a blood clot in a vein breaks away and travels through the heart and into the pulmonary circulatory system. Here the vessels leading from the heart branch like a tree, gradually becoming smaller until finally they form *capillaries,* the smallest blood vessels. Depending on its size, the clot will at some point reach a vessel through which it cannot pass, and there will lodge itself. The clot disrupts the blood supply to the area supplied by that vessel. The larger the clot, the greater is the area of lung that loses its blood supply, and the more drastic the results to the patient.

This condition develops most commonly in association with inflammation of the veins of the legs (*thrombophlebitis*). People with varicose veins are particularly susceptible to thrombophlebitis. Because of constrictions produced by garters or rolled stockings, or just sitting with crossed legs for a long time, the sluggish blood flow already present is aggravated, and a clot may form in a vessel. Some people without varicose veins can also develop clots under the same conditions. The body often responds to the clot with the reaction of inflammation, which is painful. However, when there is no inflammatory response, there is no warning to tell that a clot has formed. In either situation there is always a chance that a piece may break off the main clot and travel to the lung. Of recent concern in this regard are studies that appear to link oral contraceptives with the incidence of clotting, thereby leading to pulmonary embolism. The number of women affected in this way by the use of oral contraceptives is small, but enough to be of concern.

The symptoms of pulmonary embolism are varied and may be minor or major. Most common are pleurisy—marked by chest pain during breathing—shortness of breath, and cough with the production of blood. Once the pulmonary embolism is diagnosed the treatment is simple in the less severe cases, which are the majority. But in cases of large clots and great areas of lung deprived of blood supply there may be catastrophic effects on the heart and general circulation.

Prevention

Certain preventive measures are worthwhile for all people. Stockings should not be rolled, because that produces a constricting band about the leg that impairs blood flow and predisposes to clot formation. Especially when taking long automobile or airplane rides one should be sure to stretch the legs periodically. Individuals with varicose veins or a history of thrombophlebitis should take these precautions more seriously. People who stand still for long periods during the day should wear elastic support stockings regularly and elevate their feet part of the day and at night.

When considering the use of oral contraceptives the physician must weigh the risks of developing clots from the drug against the psychological, social, and physical risks of pregnancy. The risk from oral contraceptives is lessened if the woman does not have high blood pressure. Any persistent pain in the leg, especially in the calf or behind the knee, deserves the attention of a physician. Anyone with varicose veins or anyone taking oral contraceptives should be especially attentive to these symptoms.

Pneumothorax

Another less common lung condition is spontaneous *pneumothorax* or collapse of a lung. This most commonly occurs in the second and third decade of life and presents itself with the sudden development of pain in the chest and breathlessness. The collapse occurs because of a sudden leak of air from the lung into the chest cavity.

The lung is ordinarily maintained in an expanded state by the rigid bony thorax, but if air leaks out into the space between the thorax and the lung, the lung collapses. This condition is rarely very serious but the patient needs to be observed to be sure that the air leak does not become greater with further lung collapse.

Treatment

Often a tube has to be placed in the chest, attached to a suction pump, and the air pumped out from the space where it has collected. When the air is removed the lung expands to fill the thoracic cage again. Some individuals tend to have several recurrences. Because the reason for the collapse is poorly understood, there is no satisfactory method of preventing these recurrences except by surgery. This is rarely required. In a person with a proven propensity for recurrence it is usually advisable to open the chest and produce scarring of the lung surface so that it becomes fixed to the thoracic cage. Although it is usually successful, even this procedure does not always solve this bothersome problem.

14

Diseases of the Endocrine Glands

Glands are organs that produce and secrete substances essential for normal body functioning. There are two main types of glands: the *endocrine* and the *exocrine*. The endocrines, or *ductless*, glands send their secretions directly into the bloodstream. These secretions, which are biochemically related to each other, are called *hormones*. The exocrines, such as the sebaceous or sweat glands, the mammary (or milk) glands, and the lachrymal (or tear) glands, have ducts that carry their secretions to specific locations for specific purposes.

The exocrine glands are individually discussed elsewhere in connection with the various parts of the body where they are found. This section is devoted to diseases of the ductless glands, which include:

- The *pituitary*, which controls growth and the activity of the adrenal, thyroid, and sex glands

- The *thyroid*, which controls the rate of the body's chemical activity or metabolism

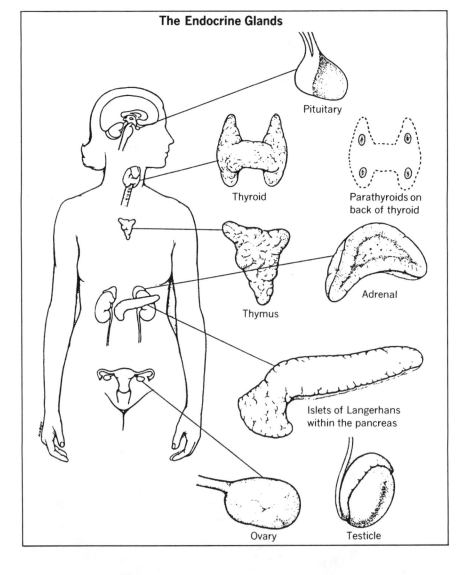

The Endocrine Glands

Pituitary

Thyroid

Parathyroids on back of thyroid

Thymus

Adrenal

Islets of Langerhans within the pancreas

Ovary

Testicle

- The *adrenals,* which affect metabolism and sex characteristics

- The *male gonads* or testicles and the *female gonads* or ovaries

- The *parathyroids,* which regulate bone metabolism

Unlike the exocrine glands, which can function independently of one another, the endocrines form an interrelated system. Thus a disorder in one of them is likely to affect the way the others behave. Glandular disorder can sometimes be anatomical, but it is usually functional. Functional disease can result in the production and release of too little or too much of a particular secretion.

When too much of a hormone is being secreted, the prefix *hyper-* is used for the condition, as in *hyperthyroidism.* When too little is being secreted, the prefix *hypo-* is used, as in the word *hypofunction,* to indicate that a gland operates below normal.

Abnormalities of the endocrine glands that cause changes in their functioning are responsible for a wide variety of illnesses. These illnesses are almost always accompanied by symptoms that can be recognized as distinctly abnormal. Prompt and accurate diagnosis can usually prevent the occurrence of irreversible damage. For many people with glandular disorders, treatment may have to be lifelong. They can feel well and function almost normally, but they must follow a program of regulated medication taken under a physician's supervision.

Anterior Pituitary Gland

The anterior pituitary gland, also called the *hypophysis,* is located in the center of the brain. It produces two types of secretions: a growth hor-

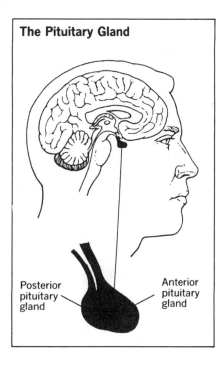

The Pituitary Gland

Posterior pituitary gland

Anterior pituitary gland

mone and hormones that stimulate certain other glands.

The anterior pituitary gland is subject to neurochemical stimulation by

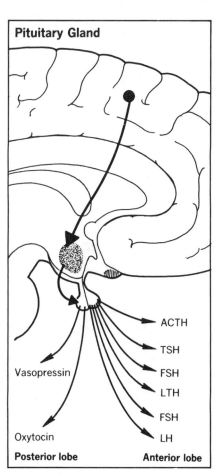

Pituitary Gland

Vasopressin

Oxytocin

ACTH
TSH
FSH
LTH
FSH
LH

Posterior lobe   **Anterior lobe**

the *hypothalamus,* a nearby part of the brain. This stimulation results in the production of the hormones that promote testicular and ovarian functioning, and does not occur normally until around 12 years of age in girls and 14 in boys. The beginning of this glandular activity is known as the onset of *puberty.*

Puberty is sometimes delayed for no apparent reason until age 16 or 17. Because the hypothalamus is affected by emotional factors, all of the endocrine glands governed by the anterior pituitary can also be affected by feelings. Psychological factors can therefore upset the relationships in the glandular system and produce the physical symptoms of endocrine disorders.

It is extremely rare for the anterior pituitary to produce too much or too little of its hormones, but sometimes hypofunction may follow pregnancy because of thrombosis or changes in the blood vessels.

A truly hypofunctioning anterior pituitary gland can cause many serious disturbances: extreme thinness, growth failure, sexual aberration, and intolerance for normal variations in temperature. When appropriate diagnostic tests determine the deficiency, the patient is given the missing hormones in pill form.

Absence of the growth hormone alone is unknown. Most cases of *dwarfism* result from other causes. However, excess production of the growth hormone alone does occur, but only rarely. If it begins before puberty when the long bones are still growing, the child with the disorder will grow into a well-proportioned giant. When it begins after puberty, the head, hands, feet, and most body organs except the brain slowly enlarge. This condition is called *acromegaly.* The cause of both disorders is usually a tumor, and radiation is the usual treatment.

The thyroid, adrenal cortex, testicles, ovaries, and pancreatic glands are target glands for the anterior pituitary's stimulating hormones, which are specific for the functioning of each of these glands. Therefore, a disorder of any of the target organs could be caused either by an excess or a deficiency of a stimulating hormone, creating a so-called *secondary disease*. There are various tests that can be given to differentiate primary from secondary disorders.

The Thyroid Gland

The thyroid gland is located in the front of the neck just above its base. Normal amounts of *thyroxin,* the hormone secreted by the thyroid, are necessary for the proper functioning of almost all bodily activities. When this hormone is deficient in infancy, growth and mental development are impaired and *cretinism* results.

Hypothyroidism

In adulthood, a deficiency of thyroxin hormone is caused primarily by a lack of sufficient iodine in the diet. In *hypothyroidism,* the disorder resulting from such a deficiency, the metabolic rate is slower than normal, the patient has no energy, his expression is dull, his skin is thick, and he has an intolerance to cold weather.

Treatment consists of increasing the amount of iodine in the diet if it is deficient or giving thyroid hormone medication. Normal metabolic functioning usually follows, especially if treatment is begun soon after the symptoms appear.

Hyperthyroidism

An excess amount of thyroid hormone secretion is called *hyperthyroidism* and may relate to emotional stress. It causes physical fatigue but mental alertness, a staring quality in the eyes, tremor of the hands, weight loss with increased appetite, rapid pulse, sweating, and intolerance to hot weather.

Long-term treatment is aimed at decreasing hormone production with the use of a special medicine that inhibits it. In some cases, part of the gland may be removed by surgery; in others, radiation treatment with radioactive iodine is effective.

Hyperthyroidism may recur long after successful treatment. Both hypothyroidism and hyperthyroidism are common disorders, especially in women.

Other Thyroid Disorders

Enlargement of part or all of the thyroid gland occurs fairly often. It may be a simple enlargement of the gland itself caused by the lack of iodine, as in *goiter,* or it may be caused by a tumor or a nonspecific inflammation. Goiter is often treated with thyroxin, but it is easily prevented altogether by the regular use of iodized table and cooking salt. Treatment of other problems varies, but surgery is usually recommended for a tumor, especially if the surrounding organs are being obstructed.

The Adrenal Glands

The adrenals are paired glands located just above each kidney. Their outer part is called the *cortex.* The inner part is called the *medulla* and is not governed by the anterior pituitary. The cortex produces several hormones that affect the metabolism of salt, water, carbohydrate, fat, and protein, as well as secondary sex characteristics, skin pigmentation, and resistance to infection.

An insufficiency of these hormones

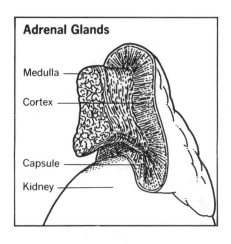

Adrenal Glands

Medulla
Cortex
Capsule
Kidney

can be caused by bacterial infection of the cortex, especially by *meningococcus;* by a hemorrhage into it; by an obstruction of blood flow into it; by its destruction because of tuberculosis; or by one of several unusual diseases.

In one type of sudden or acute underfunctioning of the cortex, the patient has a high fever, mental confusion, and circulatory collapse. Unless treated promptly, the disorder is likely to be fatal. When it persists after treatment, or when it develops gradually, it is called *Addison's disease* and is usually chronic. The patient suffers from weakness, loss of body hair, and increased skin pigmentation. Hormone-replacement treatment is essential, along with added salt for as long as hypofunction persists.

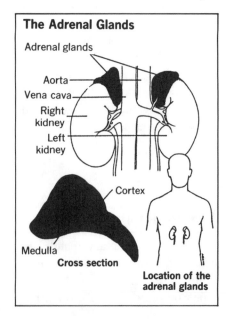

The Adrenal Glands

Adrenal glands
Aorta
Vena cava
Right kidney
Left kidney
Cortex
Medulla
Cross section
Location of the adrenal glands

The formation of an excess of certain cortical hormones (i.e., hormones produced in the adrenal cortex)—a disorder known as *Cushing's syndrome*—may be caused by a tumor of the anterior pituitary gland, which produces too much specific stimulating hormone, or by a tumor of one or both of the adrenal glands. It is a rare disease, more common in women, especially following pregnancy. Symptoms include weakness, loss of muscle tissue, the appearance of purple streaks in the skin, and an oval or "moon" face.

Treatment involves eliminating the overproducing tissue either by surgery or irradiation and then replacing any hormonal deficiencies with proper medication.

An excess of certain other cortical hormones because of an increase in cortical tissue or a tumor can result in the early onset of puberty in boys, or in an increase in the sexuality of females of any age. Surgical removal of the overproducing tissue is the only treatment.

The Adrenal Medulla

The medulla of the adrenal glands secretes two hormones: *epinephrine* (or *adrenaline*) and *norepinephrine*. Although they contribute to the proper functioning of the heart and blood vessels, neither one is absolutely indispensable. Disease caused by hypofunction of the medulla is unknown. Hyperfunction is a rare cause of sustained high blood pressure. Even more rarely, it causes episodic or paroxysmal high blood pressure accompanied by such symptoms as throbbing headache, profuse perspiration, and severe anxiety. The disorder is caused by a tumor effectively treated by surgical removal. Cancer of the adrenal medulla is extremely rare and virtually incurable.

Changes in hormone production can be caused by many intangible factors and are often temporary disorders. However, persistent or recurrent symptoms should be brought to a physician's attention. The accurate diagnosis of an endocrine disease depends on careful professional evaluation of specific laboratory tests, individual medical history, and thorough examination. No one should take hormones or medicines that affect hormone production without this type of evaluation, since their misuse can cause major problems.

Male Sex Glands

The male sex glands, or *gonads,* are the two testicles normally located in the *scrotum.* In addition to producing sperm, the testicles also manufacture the male hormone called *testosterone.* This hormone is responsible for the development and maintenance of secondary sex characteristics as well as for the male *libido,* or sexual impulse. Only one normal testicle is needed for full function.

Testicular Hypofunction

Hypofunction of one or both of the testicles can result from an abnormality in prenatal development, from infections such as mumps or tuberculosis, from injury, or from the increased temperature to which undescended testicles are exposed.

When hypofunction occurs before puberty, there is failure in the development of secondary sex characteristics. The sex organs do not enlarge; facial, pubic, and armpit hair fails to appear; and the normal voice change does not occur. Fertility and libido also fail to develop. A person with this combination of abnormalities is called a *eunuch.*

If the disorder is secondary to anterior pituitary disease, it is called *Froehlich's syndrome.* When it occurs after puberty, the body changes are less striking, but there may be a loss of fertility and libido. The primary disease is usually treated by surgery, and testosterone may be given. If the disorder is secondary to anterior pituitary disease, the gonad-stimulating hormone should be administered.

Testicular hypofunction is rare because it results only when both testicles are damaged in some way. Although mumps may involve the testicles, it is rarely the cause of sterility, even though this is greatly

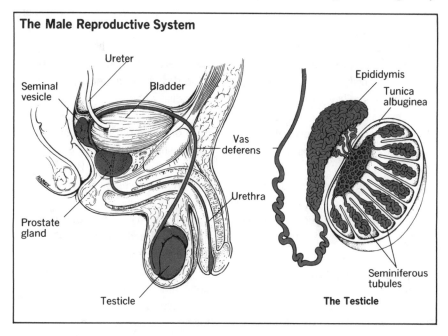

The Male Reproductive System

Ureter

Seminal vesicle

Bladder

Vas deferens

Urethra

Prostate gland

Testicle

Epididymis

Tunica albuginea

Seminiferous tubules

The Testicle

feared. Even so, everyone should be immunized against mumps in infancy.

It is advisable to wear an appropriate athletic supporter to protect the testicles when engaged in strenuous athletics or when there is a possibility that they might be injured. However, nothing that restricts scrotal movement should be worn regularly, since movement is essential for the maintenance of constant testicular temperature.

A sudden decrease in sexual drive or performance may be caused by disease, trauma, or emotional factors. In certain cases administering male hormones may relieve the condition. However, a decrease in sexual drive is one of the natural consequences of aging. It is not a disease and should not be treated with testosterone.

Testicular Hyperfunction

Testicular hyperfunction is extremely rare and is usually caused by a tumor. Before puberty, the condition results in the precocious development of secondary sex characteristics; after puberty, in the accentuation of these characteristics. Such a tumor must be removed surgically or destroyed by irradiation.

Cancer can develop in a testicle without causing any functional change. It is relatively uncommon. When it appears, it shows up first as a painless enlargement. The cancer cells then usually spread quickly to other organs and have a fatal result. Prompt treatment by surgery and irradiation can sometimes arrest the condition.

Because an undescended testicle may become cancerous, it should be repositioned into the scrotum by surgery or removed.

Female Sex Glands

The female gonads are the *ovaries,* situated on each side of and close to

Female Reproductive Organs

Ovary
Fallopian tube
Bladder
Uterus
Rectum
Cervix
Urethra
Vagina

the uterus or womb. In addition to producing an *ovum* or egg each month, they manufacture the female hormones *estrogen* and *progesterone,* each making its special contribution to the menstrual cycle and to the many changes that go on during pregnancy. Estrogen regulates the secondary sex characteristics such as breast development and the appearance of pubic and axillary hair.

The periodicity of the menstrual cycle depends on a very complicated relationship between the ovaries and the anterior pituitary. Birth control pills, most of which contain estrogen and progesterone, interrupt this relationship in such a way that no ovum is produced and pregnancy therefore should not occur.

Changes in normal ovarian hormone function create problems similar to changes in normal testicular hormone function, except of course

for the female–male differences. In general, the diseases responsible for these changes are the same in males and females. However, changes in female hormone function are very often caused by emotional stress or by other unspecific circumstances.

Ovarian Hypofunction

Hypofunction of the ovaries may cause failure to menstruate at all or with reasonable regularity. A disruption of the menstrual cycle is an obvious indication to the woman past puberty that something is wrong. Less obvious is the reduction or complete loss of fertility that may accompany the disorder.

Both menstrual and infertility problems should be evaluated by a trained specialist, preferably a gynecologist, to find out their cause. If it should be hormonal deficiency, treatment may consist of replacement hormone therapy. In many cases, however, effective treatment consists of eliminating the emotional stress that has affected the stimulation relationship between the anterior pituitary and the ovaries, thereby inhibiting hormone production. Occasionally, hormone treatment for infertility causes several ova to be produced in the same month, increasing the possibility of a multiple pregnancy.

Menopause

All women eventually develop spontaneous ovarian hypofunction. This usually happens between the ages of 45 and 50 and is called the *climacteric* or *menopause*. When it happens before the age of 35, it is called premature menopause.

Normal menopause results from the gradual burning out of the ovaries so that estrogen is deficient or absent altogether. Most women experience very few changes or symptoms at this time other than the cessation of menstruation, usually preceded by progressive irregularity and reduction of flow.

A few women become excessively irritable, have hot flashes, perspire a great deal, gain weight, and develop facial hair. Such women, as well as those who have premature menopause, are likely to benefit greatly from estrogen replacement therapy for a few years. However, because recent statistical studies have implicated sustained use of estrogen therapy as increasing the risk of uterine cancer in postmenopausal women, the American Cancer Society has cautioned physicians to supervise such women closely. At the present time, most physicians feel that the treatment should be given temporarily and only when menopause symptoms are causing special discomfort.

Ovarian Hyperfunction

Hyperfunction of the ovaries after puberty is one cause of increased menstrual flow during or at the end of each cycle. This is called functional bleeding and is caused by excess estrogen. The disorder is treated with progesterone, which slows down estrogen production. In cases where this treatment fails, it is sometimes necessary to remove the uterus by an operation called a *hysterectomy*.

Some diseases of the ovaries, such as infections, cysts, and tumors, do not necessarily cause functional changes, but they may call attention to themselves by being painful, or a physician may discover them during a pelvic examination. Treatment may be medical, surgical, or by irradiation, depending on the nature of the disorder. See Ch. 25, *Women's Health,* for fuller treatment of ovarian and other disorders affecting women.

A rather common cause of short-lived ovarian pain is connected with *ovulation,* which occurs about 14 days before the next expected menstrual period. This discomfort is called *mittelschmerz,* which is German for "middle pain," and can be treated with aspirin or any other simple analgesic.

The Pancreas

The pancreas, a combined duct and endocrine gland, is to some extent regulated by the anterior pituitary. See Ch. 15, *Diabetes Mellitus,* for a discussion of the pancreas and diabetes.

Posterior Pituitary Gland

The posterior lobe of the pituitary gland, the parathyroid glands, and the adrenal medulla are not governed by the anterior pituitary gland. The posterior pituitary produces a secretion called *antidiuretic hormone* which acts on the kidneys to control the amount

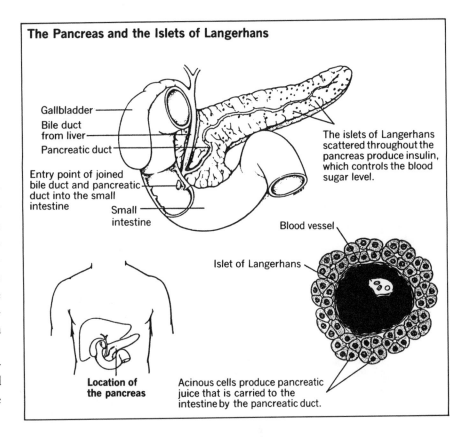

The Pancreas and the Islets of Langerhans

Gallbladder

Bile duct from liver

Pancreatic duct

Entry point of joined bile duct and pancreatic duct into the small intestine

Small intestine

The islets of Langerhans scattered throughout the pancreas produce insulin, which controls the blood sugar level.

Blood vessel

Islet of Langerhans

Location of the pancreas

Acinous cells produce pancreatic juice that is carried to the intestine by the pancreatic duct.

The Pancreas and the Islets of Langerhans

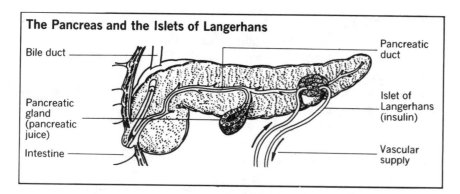

Bile duct

Pancreatic gland (pancreatic juice)

Intestine

Pancreatic duct

Islet of Langerhans (insulin)

Vascular supply

of urine produced. A deficiency of this hormone causes *diabetes insipidus,* which results in the production of an excessive amount of urine, sometimes as much as 25 quarts a day. (A normal amount is about one quart.) The natural consequence of this disorder is an unquenchable thirst. It is an extremely rare disease, the cause of which is often unknown, although it may result from a brain injury or tumor. Treatment involves curing the cause if it is known. If not, the patient is given an antidiuretic hormone.

The Parathyroid Glands

The parathyroid glands are located in or near the thyroid, usually two on each side. They are important in the regulation of blood calcium and phosphorus levels and therefore of bone metabolism. Hypofunction of these glands almost never occurs except when they have been removed surgically, usually inadvertently during a thyroid operation. In underfunctioning of the parathyroids, blood calcium levels fall and muscle spasm results. The patient is usually given calcium and replacement therapy with parathyroid hormone to correct the disorder.

Hyperfunction is rare and is slightly more common in women. A benign tumor, or *adenoma,* is the usual cause. The amount of calcium in the blood rises as calcium is removed from the bones, which then weaken and may break easily. The excess calcium is excreted in the urine and may coalesce into kidney stones, causing severe pain. Treatment for hyperfunction of the parathyroids consists of surgical removal of the affected glands.

15

Diabetes Mellitus

A lot of people have diabetes and they live a long time with it. In the United States there are around four million diabetics, or people who have diabetes. About a third of them at any one time are undiagnosed. This figure constitutes about two percent of the population, and ranges from one one-hundredth percent of people under 24 years of age to seven percent of those over 64.

Diabetes can develop at any age. Susceptibility gradually increases up to age 40, and then rapidly increases. After age 30 it more commonly affects women than men.

History of Diabetes

Diabetes has been known for several thousand years. Because people with this disease, when untreated, may urinate frequently and copiously, the Greeks named it diabetes, meaning "siphon." In the late seventeenth century the name *mellitus*, meaning "sweet", was added. In early days, diagnosis was made by tasting the urine. The sweetness is caused by the presence of sugar (*glucose*) in the urine; its presence distinguishes diabetes mellitus from the much rarer

diabetes insipidus, an entirely different problem. See under Ch. 14, *Diseases of the Endocrine Glands,* for a discussion of diabetes insipidus.

Discovery of Insulin

Late in the nineteenth century, when diabetes was well recognized as an abnormality in carbohydrate metabolism, several scientists discovered that the experimental removal of certain cells, the *islets of Langerhans,* from the pancreas, produced diabetes in dogs. This observation led to the 1921 discovery and isolation of insulin by two Canadian doctors, Frederick Banting and Charles Best. Insulin is a hormone produced by these islets. Injection of insulin proved to be the first and remains the most effective means of treating diabetes. And so began a real revolution in improving the outcome of this disease. Previously death occurred in a few years for almost every diabetic. Often death was much quicker, especially for people who were under 30 years of age when they developed diabetes—because this age group tends to have a more severe form of the disease. Since 1921 new knowledge and techniques have made it possible to do more and

more for diabetics.

An early pioneer in the treatment of diabetes with insulin was Dr. Elliott Joslin of Boston. Dr. Joslin realized that the diabetic patient needed to have a full understanding of his disease so that he could take care of himself. He knew that the diabetic, with the chronic abnormality of a delicate and dynamic metabolic process, could not be cared for successfully solely by knowledgeable physicians. The patient and his family had to be informed about the disease and had to make day-to-day decisions about managing it.

In many ways this marked the beginning of what have become ever-increasing efforts to educate patients about all their diseases, especially chronic ones. The results have been rather remarkable.

Characteristics of Diabetes

The fundamental problem in diabetes is the body's inability to metabolize glucose, a common form of sugar, fully and continually. This is a vital process in creating body cell energy. Glucose is a chemical derivative of the carbohydrate in foods after they have been ingested. Carbohydrates are mostly of plant origin and may be called starch, saccharide, sucrose, or simply sugar. Glucose is stored under normal conditions in the form of *glycogen,* or animal starch, in the liver and muscles for later use, at which time it is reconverted to glucose.

Need for Insulin

Insulin is necessary for both the storage and reconversion of glucose. The metabolic failure may come about because of an insufficiency of insulin, an inability of the body to respond normally to it for a number of complex chemical reasons, or a combination of both factors. In any event, the failure to metabolize glucose results in an abnormal accumulation of sugar in the bloodstream.

This failure is somewhat similar to starvation. A starved person eats no food, whereas the diabetic eats food but cannot use the carbohydrate in it and cannot get sufficient energy from the protein and fat content of food. After the starving person has used his previously stored glycogen, which the diabetic without insulin cannot do, the body has to metabolize its stored fat for energy. This results in a loss of weight and is often an early indication of diabetes.

A by-product of fat metabolism is the formation of *ketone bodies* (chemical compounds) which, when excessive, cause a condition known as diabetic *acidosis*. This can cause coma and death if not treated with insulin and the right kind of intravenous fluids. Before insulin was discovered, this was the way most diabetics died.

Excess Urine Production

As glucose accumulates above normal levels in the diabetic's bloodstream it is filtered by his kidneys and remains in the urine. Additional amounts of u-

rine are produced to contain the excess glucose. This situation results in copious and frequent urination that in turn causes dehydration and an often insatiable thirst. These are classically the first signs of the presence of diabetes.

This is diabetes described largely in terms of changes in carbohydrate metabolism. But protein and fat metabolism are also involved, as are almost invariably some changes in the nerves, muscles, eyes, kidneys, and blood vessels.

No one knows why diabetes develops. In some ways diabetes resembles premature aging, and the causes of diabetes, if known, might shed some light on the causes of aging.

The body's need to obtain energy from glucose and to convert glucose to glycogen and vice versa is continuous but always changing quantitatively. Meeting these needs requires constantly fluctuating amounts of effective insulin. Nondiabetics produce these amounts no matter what they eat or do, thus maintaining a steady state of metabolism. Diabetics, however, cannot achieve this steady state simply by taking insulin; they must also control their diets and their activities. They may have to change the amounts of their medications from time to time.

Diabetes is not an all-or-nothing phenomenon. It can be mild, moderate, or severe, and can fluctuate in degree in any one individual over a long period of time, or even from day to day. Very little is known about the reasons for these differences and changes. It is known, however, that diabetes generally gets worse in the presence of illness, particularly infections (even colds). It is also affected adversely by hyperfunctioning diseases of the anterior pituitary, thyroid, and adrenal glands, by emotional and physical stress, and during pregnancy.

Diabetes Diagnosis

The diagnosis of diabetes is not ordinarily a difficult one. Especially in children, the symptoms of rapid weight loss, extreme hunger, generalized weakness, frequent and copious urination, and insatiable thirst make it easy to recognize. Finding glucose in the urine along with increased levels of glucose in the blood generally confirms the diagnosis. However, glucose in the urine does not always indicate the presence of diabetes. A few people with unusual kidney function have glucose in their urine with normal blood levels, a condition known as *renal glycosuria.*

Moreover, an adult with diabetes may not have such a definite set of symptoms for months or years after he has actually developed the disease. Instead he may have vague fatigue or persistent skin infections. A woman may have a persistent genital itch that a physician might suspect is due to diabetes. Proof is provided by urine and blood tests. Glucose in the urine at the time of a routine physical examination might provide the first clue. Once diagnosed, treatment should be begun.

Treatment of Diabetes

Diet

The diet of a diabetic, although a major part of his treatment, is similar to what a normal person of the same age should eat. However, some radical dietary changes may be ordered if the previous diet has not been a proper one. This is particularly true in regard to reducing the calories in food eaten by overweight diabetics.

Diet is the only treatment needed by many adult diabetics, particularly those who are obese when they develop the disease, provided they can lose and not regain their excess weight. Because obese people are more likely to develop diabetes, they should have urine or blood sugar tests yearly after the age of 40. But it is more important for them to make every effort to lose weight before they become diabetics.

Individualized Diets

Each diabetic's diet has to be individualized to a certain extent. This is done originally by the physician when the diagnosis is made and periodically thereafter. The physician must learn the eating habits, customs, and preferences of his diabetic patient. Because eating is so much a part of the patient's personality and has such great psychological importance, its pattern should be changed radically only when necessary.

Certain principles that may not involve major changes should be kept in mind. For example, the diet should conform to the patient's customary cultural and ethnic pattern. It should not make him feel weak and without energy. If it does, he needs more food and more insulin.

Some nonobese diabetics, especially elderly ones, need only to eliminate sugar, soft drinks, and pastry from their diets. A mild diabetic often needs only to reduce the amount of carbohydrate in his diet and replace it with fats and proteins. Alcohol can be a part of a diabetic's diet under certain circumstances, which he should discuss with his physician. Sugar-free foods and beverages enable a diabetic to enjoy some of life's minor luxuries.

Children should, if possible, have diets that are similar to those of their friends, although they must be helped to understand that they should avoid eating foods containing concentrated sugars, like soda pop, candy, jams, and jellies.

Diet Guides

Most physicians have available printed diet guides to help their patients adjust their diets as needed. These indicate the number of calories and amount of protein, carbohydrate, and fat per household measure in all foods. See also Ch. 27, *Nutrition and Weight Control,* for additional reading on this subject.

When to eat is another matter, and this often necessitates some changes in eating habit patterns, especially for people taking insulin. Most important is regularity in relation to the patient's rest-activity time patterns. In general, almost half of the day's carbohydrates should be eaten at lunch because this is usually when activity and energy expenditure are greatest. The remainder should be divided between breakfast and dinner.

Insulin

Until recent years, insulin was prepared commercially in the United States from beef or pork pancreas. More recently, researchers have developed an insulin drug that is manufactured with a synthetic duplicate of human genes. Until this drug, called Humulin, appeared diabetics who were allergic to insulin products made from animal cells had to resort to more complex drugs such as steroids. Unlike animal insulins, Humulin, the first consumer health product made with DNA (*deoxyribonucleic acid*), can be produced in unlimited quantities.

Insulin has to be given by injection, usually *subcutaneous injection,* just beneath the skin, because it is destroyed by gastric secretions when taken orally.

The method of preparation also determines the timing of its action, and it is classified into three basic types:

TYPE OF INSULIN	TIME (HOURS) OF ACTION AFTER INJECTION		
	Onset	Peak	Duration
Rapid	½–1	2–8	4–14
Intermediate	2–4	6–12	10–26
Prolonged	4–8	12–24	24–36

There are two or three different insulin preparations for each type—rapid, intermediate, and prolonged.

Ideally, insulin injected once a day should more or less mimic the normal insulin action of a nondiabetic. That is the purpose of the intermediate and long-acting insulins, with which a rapid insulin is sometimes combined. Many diabetics are able to take insulin only once a day, particularly when their diet and activity pattern is sufficiently constant. Others, however, require two or more injections. The usual time to take insulin is before breakfast. This should be the same time every day. Second injections are often taken at suppertime.

A diabetic's basic insulin dose has to be established initially according to the severity of his disease. The dose is determined largely by his blood and urine glucose levels, the physician's judgment, and trial and error. Once established, the dosage has to be assessed daily and adjusted as necessary on the basis of the amount of sugar in the urine, diet, activity, and other factors.

Many diabetics take the same dose daily for years; others need to readjust theirs constantly. The number of units taken per day varies greatly from person to person, but probably most diabetics take between 10 and 40 units a day. The cost generally is less than one cent a unit. Insulin comes in 10-cc vials that must be refrigerated until first used. Thereafter they can be kept at room temperature.

Self-medication

Most diabetics self-inject their insulin. One can learn the technique of self-injection by practicing injecting an orange before trying it on oneself. The needle should always be sharp. It is important to change the exact site of the injection from day to day. Too frequent use of the same site may impair insulin absorption. The specially calibrated syringe and the needle can be either presterilized and discarded after one use, or they can be reused after resterilization by boiling for five minutes.

Insulin Shock

When injected insulin is active in the body system it must be matched by a sufficient amount of blood sugar. If not matched because of too much insulin, too much exercise, or too little ingested carbohydrate, the blood sugar level falls, a condition known as *hypoglycemia,* and the brain is deprived of an essential source of energy. This is most apt to occur at the time of the insulin's peak activity.

The first sign of an insulin reaction or *insulin shock* is usually mild hunger. Then come, and rather quickly, sweating, dizziness, palpitation, shallow breathing, trembling, mental confusion, strange behavior, and finally loss of consciousness. Prompt treatment is important. A lump of sugar or a piece of candy taken when symptoms first begin to appear will usually provide enough glucose to abort the reaction.

It is sometimes necessary to give intravenous glucose to counter insulin shock. This terminates the reaction almost immediately. Diabetics who use insulin should always have a lump or two of sugar or some candy with them and learn to recognize an oncoming insulin reaction. In general they should eat a small snack of glu-

Injection of Insulin Dose

1. Wipe site of injection with cotton swab dipped in alcohol.
2. With one hand, pinch up skin at injection site. Place syringe perpendicularly to the skin and quickly insert needle for its entire length in order to insure injection of sufficient depth *(see illustration).*The more rapidly the needle is inserted, the less the pain will be. Stainless steel needles are preferred.
3. Inject insulin dose.

Sites of Insulin Injections

It is important to change the site of injection daily for best absorption of insulin.

cose of some sort about the time their insulin activity reaches its peak.

Insulin reaction or shock can happen to any diabetic taking insulin. It is one of the liabilities of insulin therapy. Repeated and prolonged episodes of insulin reaction can be damaging to the brain. All diabetics, and especially those taking insulin, should have an identification bracelet or necklace indicating they have diabetes so that anyone examining them in an unconscious state can quickly realize the probable cause of their uncon-

sciousness. This can be supplemented by a card in the wallet or purse with additional details. These are available from the Medic Alert Foundation, Turlock, CA 95380, at a very modest cost. It is also vital that at least a few persons with whom the diabetic regularly associates know about his disease so that they can take prompt action if they see problems developing.

The Insulin Pump

Development of a pump for infusion of insulin into the body may offer a better method of treating diabetics with keto-acidosis, or ketosis. The pump method of continuous intravenous (IV) infusion has been used with moderate success in such cases.

Some advantages have been noted. A reduced amount of hypoglycemia has been reported, for example. Because the insulin is injected directly into the bloodstream, a smaller amount is required for control. Shots, or injections, under the skin have not been necessary while the patient has been receiving infusion treatment. Some physicians believe, however, that the older method of administering insulin by injection will remain useful. These physicians point out that better control of the treatment results when shots are given and the amount of urine glucose is monitored closely. Also, patients can observe how the insulin is given when the needle is used.

The insulin pump system generally includes a reservoir for the insulin; a peristaltic pump, one that impels the fluid by contracting and expanding; and a "power pack" containing batteries that activate the pump. The entire assembly, with associated tubings, typically weighs about 1.5 pounds (525 grams). The system is rugged enough to withstand rough treatment under difficult weather and environmental conditions.

If widely accepted and used, the insulin pump system may answer a basic need for improved ways to introduce drugs into the body. Earlier methods, including the subcutaneous, or needle, technique, have been described as faulty because they are "nonphysiologic"—they do not deliver the drugs where they can be used immediately by the body.

Oral Drugs

Oral *hypoglycemic drugs* have been available since the late 1950s. They are mainly helpful in controlling mild diabetes that develops in people 45 and over. However, younger people can occasionally be maintained on these drugs rather than on insulin. They stimulate the release of *endogenous* (self-produced) *insulin* from the pancreas or foster insulin activity in other ways. Chemically composed of *sulfonylurea,* they are remotely related to sulfa drugs but are not true sulfas. An entirely different oral hypoglycemic agent is *DBI* (*phenformin*). Some physicians urge that such drugs be prescribed only in cases that cannot be controlled effectively by other techniques.

For these drugs to work, some of the islet cells must be producing insulin or be capable of producing it. They either work well or not at all. The dose varies from one to eight tablets taken before meals and throughout the day. They cost a few cents a tablet. Insulin reactions do not occur although some diabetics take insulin also and are thereby vulnerable to insulin reactions. The decision about treating a given diabetic with these pills, insulin, or both has to be left to the patient's physician.

Diabetic Coma

Prolonged *hyperglycemia,* or excess sugar in the blood, from insufficient insulin activity can cause *diabetic coma.* This condition involves the increasing buildup of ketone bodies, the by-product of fat metabolism, which creates an *acidotic* condition (chemical imbalance in the blood, marked by an excess of acid). When this has been present for several days, perhaps a week or longer, symptoms begin to develop that are similar to those associated with the onset of diabetes. They include excessive urination and thirst, dry and hot skin, drowsiness, and finally, coma. The earliest stage of the problem is called *diabetic ketosis;* a slightly later stage is known as *diabetic acidosis.* From the beginning there are increasing amounts of glucose as well as ketone bodies in the urine. The unconscious patient will have deep, labored breathing, and a fruity odor to his breath.

Diabetic acidosis resembles an insulin reaction, although they can be distinguished from each other. If you find a diabetic in coma and you do not know the cause, assume the cause is an insulin reaction and treat him initially with sugar. This will give immediate relief to an insulin reaction but will not affect diabetic acidosis.

Diabetic acidosis occurs for many reasons. The patient does not take his insulin or oral hypoglycemic drugs for several days. He may take too little insulin because he is confused about the dosage. He may overeat or underexercise for a number of days, perhaps because he feels ill or has a cold.

Treatment

In its early stages ketosis generally can be treated by the patient himself with directions from his physician, usually by telephone. The fundamentals of this treatment involve taking rapid-acting insulin—every diabetic should keep a bottle of this on hand—every three or four hours until the urine has less glucose and no longer contains ketone bodies. Ketone bodies can be tested in the urine along with glucose. If there is a treatable underlying cause for the acidosis, such as an infection, it should be treated as well. In the later stages, hospital treatment with larger amounts of insulin, often given intravenously, and specific intravenous fluid therapy is essential.

Diabetes Control

An occasional insulin reaction is almost unavoidable, but diabetic acidosis occurs mainly because the diabetes was not well controlled. Good control means feeling well with only small amounts of sugar, or none, in the urine. This is possible for most but not all diabetics. A few diabetics can never achieve good control for a variety of reasons relating largely to the vagaries of this disease.

Personal Glucose Tests

The amount of glucose in the urine provides a kind of barometer of diabetic control. The amount in the blood at a given point in time provides a better barometer but is more difficult to check for obvious reasons. Therefore all diabetics should test their urine daily and sometimes more often, particularly in the beginning or when they are having control problems.

The ordinary urine specimen contains urine collected in the bladder over a period of several hours or overnight. The glucose in it is an average indication of what the blood sugar has been during a previous period. To get an idea of the blood sugar level at the time of the urine test, the urine that has accumulated in the bladder must first be discarded. Then a second specimen of urine should be passed about a half hour later and that specimen tested for glucose.

Several types of tests are available for this purpose. Some utilize chemically treated paper which, when dipped in urine, turns different colors to indicate varying amounts of glucose in the urine. Others use tablets that change to different colors when dropped into small amounts of urine. Adjustments in diet, activity, and insulin or oral hypoglycemic agents can be made on the basis of these test results. It costs a few cents to do each test.

Making Lifelong Adjustments

Once a diabetic has learned the fundamentals of his diet, his insulin or oral hypoglycemic agent medication, and has stabilized sufficiently his daily physical activities, he is well on his way to leading a normal life. There are, however, still a few psychological roadblocks.

First is the hard business of adjusting to the disease and coming to accept the fact that it can be lived with even though there is no cure. Initial depression is understandable and common. It does not persist. Then comes the often difficult task of regularizing one's life in terms of eating schedules, taking insulin, testing the urine, and exercising regularly.

Not many diabetics can maintain good control if they go to a Saturday night party, postpone their dinner time by four or five hours, and sleep until noon on Sunday. Maintaining one's usual schedule while traveling is another obstacle. The diabetic may feel that people treat him differently from the way they used to treat him or from the way they treat others. He will have to get used to seeing his physician frequently and regularly and having blood drawn to determine his blood sugar. He will have to spend a certain amount of money for insulin or oral hypoglycemic drugs, syringes and needles, urine-testing materials,

special sugar-free foods, and medical care.

Self-pity and then rebellion against these factors are not unusual, especially in children. And with rebellion comes an increased likelihood of insulin reactions or diabetic ketosis. Some diabetics use their disease as a way to manipulate others and thus create trying interpersonal relationships. The sensitive physician is aware of all of this and will give his patient the opportunity to verbalize his feelings.

Those with whom the diabetic lives—parents, siblings, spouse, and children—are also affected in various ways. The family's food style may be changed to some extent. Parents may have a sense of guilt about what they erroneously presume to be their part in the child's development of diabetes. They may have difficulty differentiating normal adolescent moods from those associated with the diabetic's fluctuating carbohydrate metabolism. They may become controlling and coddling or rejecting and resentful. Either reaction pattern will affect the child adversely. Parents should be helped to understand the disease as well as its effect on their child.

Juvenile Insulin Dependent Diabetes (JIDD)

Boys and girls develop diabetes in approximately equal numbers. For both sexes, the average age of onset is about eight years. For both sexes, too, diabetes may be discovered in the first hours or days of life. More frequently, diabetes appears at the age of puberty.

In severe cases, the youthful victim of diabetes suffers from a critical shortage of insulin. Acidosis may occur. The child in this situation usually has what is known as juvenile insulin dependent diabetes (JIDD). Insulin therapy may be required throughout the young person's life.

Therapy need not adversely affect the child's activities, growth rate, or psychological or intellectual development. The young person on continuous insulin therapy can usually be allowed to eat as much as he or she wants; but if abnormally large quantities of food are consumed, or if hunger continues even after meals, a physician should be consulted.

What kind of diet is best for the child with juvenile insulin dependent diabetes? High-carbohydrate diets appear to meet this child's need best. But animal fats should be restricted; ice cream in particular should be avoided. Ice milk may serve as a substitute. The rule restricting the intake of animal fats also means that commercially baked cookies, candy containing fat, including chocolate mixtures, and similar foods are unsuitable.

Some kinds of candy, fruit juices, meat, and eggs may be included in the young JIDD child's diet. "Permissible" candy may contain honey, or it may be made from sorbitol. Some health-food shops stock sesame crunch that the diabetic child can enjoy. Because they contain protein and vegetable oil, nuts make good snack foods.

Fruit juices, meat, and eggs supply a number of nutrients that the diabetic child needs. Orange and grapefruit juices, for example, contain potassium, fructose, and vitamins C and A. Meat provides protein, and should be included in the diet. Eggs supply lecithin, which keeps cholesterol from building up in blood vessels, and amino acids, essential to body-building. Eggs should be soft- or hard-boiled or poached, not fried in butter or other kinds of fat.

Fresh fish, chicken, and turkey belong properly in the diabetic child's diet, as do peanut butter and jelly sandwiches. Peanut butter made from fresh-ground nuts is preferred, but cannot be obtained in all stores. For essential whole grains, the child should eat whole wheat bread, millet, oatmeal, and other cereals—but dried cereals should be ruled out. Fresh vegetables may be served if the child does not like cooked vegetables.

Adequate amounts of sugar and starches will usually prevent hypoglycemic reactions in the JIDD child. But where such a reaction does set in, the child should drink fruit juice or some kind of rapidly digestible carbohydrate. The prepared child always carries hard candy or a box of raisins. Both help terminate hypoglycemic attacks.

Pregnancy and Diabetes

Pregnancy is a very special time in any woman's life, but it is particularly special for a diabetic and her unborn child. Diabetes is not a factor of any magnitude as far as conception is concerned, but pregnancy affects the diabetic's carbohydrate metabolism dramatically. In general there is an increase in blood glucose levels and an ever-increasing need for insulin. However, there can be periodic and unpredictable reductions in insulin need. Therefore, urine glucose and blood glucose need to be tested more frequently than under ordinary circumstances.

The urine should be tested three or four times a day and the blood glucose at every visit to the obstetrician. With good management during a diabetic's pregnancy, her baby has an excellent chance of being as normal and healthy as that of the nondiabetic mother.

Diabetes in Later Life

The association between aging and diabetes relates largely to a gradual loss of elasticity in the cells of the blood vessels, kidneys, eyegrounds (the inner sides of the backs of the eyeballs), and nerve tissues. These cellular changes may not become apparent for many years after the development of diabetes. However, occasionally they are present before or appear several years after the diabetes is recognized. This is particularly apt to be true in older people who develop diabetes.

The nerve-tissue changes can cause a diminished sensation to touch and pain and sometimes a loss of motor function of the extremities as well as sexual impotence. The eyeground changes damage the retina in various ways and can cause varying degrees of loss of vision. In about eight percent of cases this progresses to blindness.

The changes in the kidneys affect their filtration functions, causing *albuminuria,* a loss of protein from the blood serum into the urine and the development of high blood pressure in roughly 23 percent of diabetics. The vascular changes, which are rather diffuse, contribute to the specific organ changes noted above, and frequently cause a reduction in blood supply to the legs and heart muscle. This ultimately causes heart damage in perhaps 20 percent of diabetics. Medicine can do much to reduce the effects of these many changes but cannot cure them.

Some degree of prevention is possible, and good diabetic control generally is thought to contribute to a reduction and delay in the development of these complications. Because the nerve and vascular changes make the feet particularly vulnerable to infections that can be serious and even lead to amputation—gangrene occurs in about three percent of diabetics— proper and daily care of the feet is essential to prevent the development of infections. The older diabetic should be careful to keep his feet clean and dry and cut his toenails frequently and evenly. Some physicians recommend that diabetics have their toenails cut only by a podiatrist.

Early Detection

Anyone who does not have diabetes might very well wonder whether he or she is at all likely to get it, and, if so, what can be done to prevent it. One answer is clear. If you are obese, whatever your age, try to lose weight. This is especially important if you have grandparents, parents, brothers, sisters, or children who developed diabetes in middle age or earlier. It is important also if you are a mother who has had babies weighing nine or more pounds at birth.

A fairly simple laboratory test, called a *glucose tolerance test* (GTT), has been developed to identify a person who is prediabetic. The subject either swallows a drink containing 100 grams of glucose or is given the same amount intravenously. Thereafter his blood sugar is determined at set intervals over a three-to-six-hour period. If his blood sugar level remains abnormally high for too long, he is said to be a prediabetic or to have *chemical diabetes.*

All adults should have their urine tested at least once a year for the presence of sugar. Some adults and younger persons should have more frequent urine tests and perhaps periodic glucose tolerance tests.

Genetically, diabetes has many characteristics of a Mendelian recessive inherited disease. Theoretically the chances are one in four of a child developing diabetes if one parent has the disease; it is almost inevitable if both have it. These are obviously important factors for diabetics to consider before they have children, particularly when both prospective parents have diabetes.

16

Diseases of the Eye and Ear

Most people never experience any impairment of the senses of smell, taste, and touch. But it is indeed lucky and unusual to reach old age without having some problems connected with sight or with hearing or both.

The Eyes

All sensations must be processed in the brain by a normally functioning central nervous system for their proper perception. In addition, each sensation is perceived through a specific sense organ. Thus, sight is dependent on at least one functioning eye.

The eye is an optical system that can be compared to a camera, because the human lens perceives and the retina receives an image in the same way that a camera and its film does. Defects in this optical system are called errors in refraction and are the most common type of sight problem.

Myopia

Nearsightedness or *myopia* is a refractive error that causes faraway objects to be seen as blurred and indistinct. The degree of nearsightedness can be measured by testing each eye with a Snellen Test Chart. Normal vision is called 20/20. This means that at 20 feet the eye sees an image clearly and accurately.

Eyesight of less-than-normal acuity is designated as 20/50 or 20/100 and so on. This means that what the deficient eye can see accurately at a distance of 20 feet or less, the normal eye can see accurately at 50 or 100 feet.

Myopia is the most common of all the refractive errors and usually results from an elongation of the eyeball. The cause of this abnormality is unknown, but it prevents the image from being focused on the retina. Those who are affected by myopia usually develop it between the ages of 6 and 15. They are likely to become aware of the condition when they can no longer see as well as they used to in school or at the movies or as well as their friends can. Individually prescribed eyeglasses or contact lenses can correct the refractive error and produce normal vision.

Farsightedness and Astigmatism

The opposite of myopia is *hyperopia*, or farsightedness, which results from a shortening of the eyeball. The two conditions may be combined with *astigmatism,* in which vertical and horizontal images do not focus on the same point, mainly because of some abnormality of the front surface of the cornea. Properly fitted glasses can correct all of these deficiencies.

Presbyopia

A fourth refractive error combines with the other three to make up about 80 percent of all visual defects. It is known as *presbyopia,* or old-sight, and results from an inability of the lens to focus on near objects. Almost everyone is affected by presbyopia some time after the age of 40, because of the aging of the lens itself or the muscles which expand and contract it. The condition is usually noticed when it becomes necessary to hold a book or newspaper farther and farther away from the eyes in order to be able to read it. Although presbyopia is a nuisance, it can be easily corrected with glasses.

All these conditions represent variations in the sight of one or both eyes from what is considered the norm.

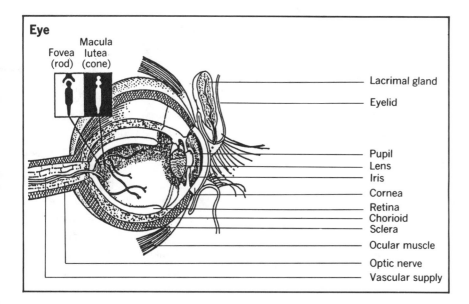

Eye

Fovea (rod)
Macula lutea (cone)

Lacrimal gland
Eyelid
Pupil
Lens
Iris
Cornea
Retina
Chorioid
Sclera
Ocular muscle
Optic nerve
Vascular supply

Because seating distance from a school blackboard, the size of print, and the distance at which signs must be read are all based on what is considered to be normal vision, eye defects are handicaps, some mild and some severe.

Many people can function normally without glasses if the defects are minor. But because uncorrected refractive errors can cause headaches and general fatigue as well as eye aches and eye fatigue, they should receive prompt medical attention.

Color Blindness

Color blindness is a visual defect that occurs in about eight percent of men but is extremely rare in women. It is hereditary, and usually involves an inability to differentiate clearly between red, green, and blue. It is a handicap for which there is no known cure at the present time.

Glaucoma

Glaucoma is a serious problem that affects about two percent of those people who are over 40. It is caused not only by the aging process, but also and more importantly by anatomical changes inside the eye that pre-

vent the normal drainage of fluid. The pressure inside the eye is therefore increased, and this pressure causes further anatomical change that can lead to blindness.

Glaucoma may begin with occasional eye pain or blurred vision, or it may be very insidious, cause no symptoms for years, and be discov-

ered only at an eye examination. Glaucoma is the number one cause of blindness, and an annual check for its onset by a specialist is particularly recommended for everyone over 40. The test is quick, easy, and painless, and should symptoms appear, early treatment, either medical or surgical or both, can reduce the likelihood of partial or complete loss of sight.

Cataracts

Another serious eye problem is the development of *cataracts*. These are areas in the lens that are no longer transparent. The so-called *senile cataract* is common among elderly people because of degenerative changes in the lens. The condition causes varying degrees of loss of vision which are readily noticed by the patient. If the vision is reduced a great deal, the entire lens can be removed surgically and appropriate glasses or contact lenses can be provided.

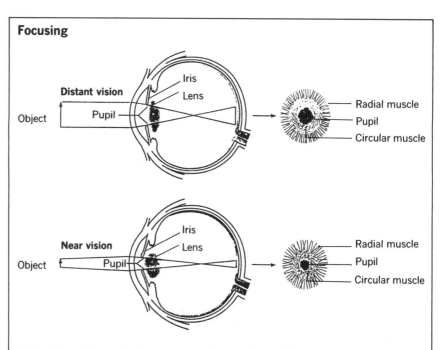

Focusing

Distant vision
Object
Iris
Lens
Pupil
Radial muscle
Pupil
Circular muscle

Near vision
Object
Iris
Lens
Pupil
Radial muscle
Pupil
Circular muscle

When viewing a distant object (more than 20 feet away), the lens flattens and the pupil dilates, allowing more light to enter the eye. The pupil is dilated by the action of the outer radial muscles of the iris, which contract and thus stretch the previously contracted circular muscles. When viewing a near object, the lens becomes more oval and the pupil contracts as more light enters the eye. This prevents overstimulation of the retina. The pupil is reduced in size by the contraction of the inner circular muscles, which serve to stretch the previously contracted radial muscles.

Eye Surgery

Eye muscle
Catarct
Cornea transplant

Lens

Cornea

Cataract

Corneal transplant

Cornea
Iris

Retinal vessels

Laser

Retina

Retinal detachment

Vitreous humor

Canal

Aqueous humor

Glaucoma

Detached Retina

Among the most serious eye disorders is the condition known as *separated* or *detached retina*. It occurs when fluid from inside the eye gets under the retina (the inner membrane at the back of the eye, on which the image is focused) and separates it from its bed, thus breaking the connections that are essential for normal vision. The most common cause of the detachment is the formation of a hole or tear in the retina. However, the condition may also develop following a blow to the head or to the eye, or because of a tumor, nephritis, or high blood pressure.

The symptoms of the onset of retinal separation are showers of drifting black spots and frequent flashes of light shaped like pinwheels that interfere with vision. These disturbances are usually followed by a dark shadow in the area of sight closest to the nose.

A retinal detachment is treated by surgical techniques in which the accumulated fluid is drained off and the hole in the tissue is sealed. About 60 percent of all cases are cured or considerably improved after surgery. The earlier the diagnosis, the more favorable is the outcome. Proper postoperative care usually involves several weeks of immobilization of the head so that the retinal tissue can heal without disturbance.

Trauma

Like any other part of the body, the eye can be injured by a major accident or *trauma,* although it is somewhat protected by the bones surrounding it. Trauma can cause most of the problems previously described. In addition, small objects can get into the eye easily, and particles of soot and other wind-borne dirt can cause great discomfort. The tearing that results

from the irritation usually floats foreign substances away, but occasionally they have to be removed by an instrument.

When a particle in the eye or under the eyelid is not easily dislodged and begins to cause redness, it should be removed by someone qualified to do so. The eye should never be poked at or into by untrained hands.

Leaving contact lenses in the eye for too long can cause discomfort that lasts for quite a while even after they have been taken out. Bacterial or viral infections of the outer surface of the eye such as *conjunctivitis* or *pinkeye,* or of the eyelids, are quite common and should be treated by a physician if they are extensive or chronic.

Contact Lenses

Contact lenses, which are fitted directly over the iris and pupil of the eye in contact with the cornea (the tissue covering the outer, visible surface of the eye), are preferred by some people for the correction of vision defects. In some cases of severe astigmatism or nearsightedness, or following cataract surgery, contact lenses can be more effective and comfortable than eyeglasses. But the chief reason for their popularity has been cosmetic. They are practically invisible.

Hard contact lenses adhere to the eye by suction; a partial vacuum is created between the inner surface of the lens and the outer surface of the eyeball.

Soft plastic contact lenses are *hydrophilic* (literally, water-loving) and adapt their shape to the shape of the moist cornea, to which they adhere. Thus they are relatively easily fitted, and patients seldom experience discomfort in adjusting to them. It is virtually impossible for dust particles to get under them. Many ophthalmologists, however, advise that the soft lens be sterilized daily.

The soft lens has proved valuable in the treatment of some eye disorders. But it often leads to problems among wearers. It may scratch or tear, for example, and generally it has

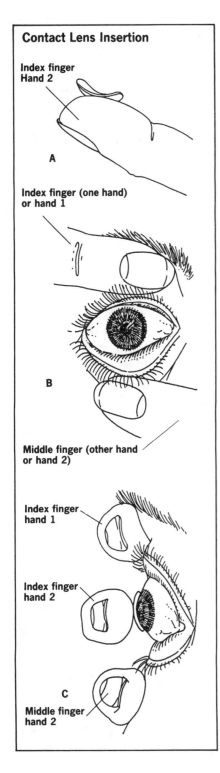

Contact Lens Insertion

Index finger
Hand 2

A

Index finger (one hand)
or hand 1

B

Middle finger (other hand
or hand 2)

Index finger
hand 1

Index finger
hand 2

C

Middle finger
hand 2

been limited to the correction of certain kinds of nearsightedness and farsightedness.

Extended wear lenses (EWLs) were introduced in the 1970s. Made of soft plastic like the older lenses, but thinner and more porous, they could be worn as long as 30 days. But wearing EWLs too long was found to cause such problems as scarring of the cornea; neurovascularization, the growth of tiny blood vessels that can cloud the vision and in extreme cases threaten the wearer's sight; the development of microcysts during sleep; and bacterial infections of the eye or eyelid, such as *Acanthamoeba keratitis.*

Disposable lenses and cosmetic contacts appeared in the late 1980s. Worn for a week and then discarded, disposable lenses reduce the danger of keratitis and other infections. But they cost about 50 percent more than the regular EWLs. Cosmetic contacts simply change the color of the eyes. Disposables should not be worn longer than prescribed, and cosmetic lenses should not be shared to prevent the spread of eye diseases and other infections. Clean the lenses according to instructions and seek medical help quickly if problems arise.

Diseases That Affect Vision

In addition to the various disorders involving only the eye, there are a number of generalized diseases that affect vision. Among these are arteriosclerosis, diabetes mellitus, and hypertension or high blood pressure, which often cause abnormalities in the blood vessels of various parts of the eye. These abnormalities can lead to tissue changes that cause the patient to see spots or to notice that his vision is defective.

Diseases of the brain, such as mul-

tiple sclerosis, tumors, and abscesses, although rare, can result in double vision or loss of lateral or central vision. Any sudden or gradual changes in vision should be brought to a physician's attention promptly, since early diagnosis and treatment is usually effective and can prevent serious deterioration.

The Ears

The ear, like the eye, is a complicated structure. Its major parts consist of the auditory canal, middle ear, and inner ear. Hearing results from the perception of sound waves whose loudness can be measured in decibels and whose highness or lowness of pitch can be measured by their frequency in cycles per second.

Sound waves usually travel through the auditory canal to the eardrum or *tympanic membrane,* vibrating it in such a way as to carry the vibrations to and along the three interlocking small bones in the middle ear to the inner ear. Here the vibrations are carried to the auditory nerve through a fluid-filled labyrinth called the communicating channel.

An abnormality at any of these points can produce a hearing deficiency. Normal hearing means the ability to hear the spoken voice in a relatively quiet room at a distance of about 18 feet. How well a person hears can be tested by an audiometer, which measures decibels and frequency of sound.

Wax Accumulation

A very common cause of hearing deficiency is the excessive accumulation of wax in the auditory canal, where it is continually being secreted. When the excess that blocks the passage of sound waves is removed—sometimes by professional instrumenta-

Ear

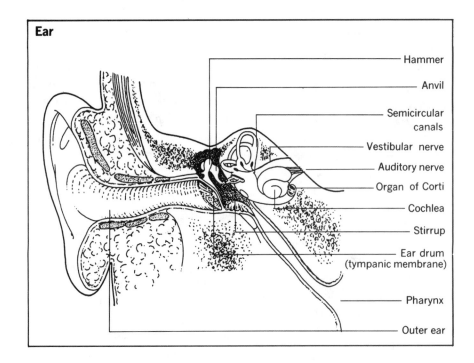

- Hammer
- Anvil
- Semicircular canals
- Vestibular nerve
- Auditory nerve
- Organ of Corti
- Cochlea
- Stirrup
- Ear drum (tympanic membrane)
- Pharynx
- Outer ear

tion—hearing returns to normal. Anyone whose hearing is temporarily impaired in this way should avoid the use of rigid or pointed objects for cleaning out the accumulated wax.

Infection

Infections or other diseases of the skin that lines the auditory canal can sometimes cause a kind of local swelling that blocks the canal and interferes with hearing. Although such a condition can be painful, proper treatment, usually with antibiotics, generally results in a complete cure.

A major cause of hearing deficiency acquired after birth is recurrent bacterial infection of the middle ear. The infecting organisms commonly get to the middle ear through the *Eustachian tube,* which connects the middle ear to the upper throat, or through the eardrum if it has been perforated by injury or by previous infection.

The infection can cause hearing loss, either because it becomes chronic or because the tissues become scarred. Such infections are usually painful, but ever since treatment with antibiotics has become pos-

sible, they rarely spread to the mastoid bone as they used to in the past.

Disorders Caused by Pressure

The Eustachian tube usually permits the air pressure on either side of the eardrum to equalize. When the pressure inside the drum is less than that outside—as occurs during descent in an airplane or elevator, or when riding through an underwater tunnel, or during skin diving—the eardrum is pushed inward. This causes a noticeable hearing loss or a stuffy feeling in the ear that subsides as soon as the pressure equalizes again. Yawning or swallowing usually speeds up the return to normal.

When the unequal pressure continues for several days because the Eustachian tube is blocked, fluid begins to collect in the middle ear. This is called *serous* (or *nonsuppurative*) *otitis media* and can cause permanent hearing damage.

Eustachian tube blockage is more commonly the result of swelling around its *nasopharyngeal* end because of a throat infection, a cold, or an allergy. Nose drops help to open

up the tube, but sometimes it may be necessary to drain the ear through the eardrum or treat the disorder with other surgical procedures.

Otosclerosis

A very common cause of hearing loss that affects about 1 in 200 adults—usually women—is *otosclerosis.* This disorder is the result of a sort of freezing of the bones in the middle ear caused by an overgrowth of tissue. The onset of the disorder usually occurs before age 30 among about 70 percent of the people who will be affected. Only one ear may be involved, but the condition does get progressively worse. Although heredity is an important factor, the specific cause of otosclerosis is unknown. In some cases, surgery can be helpful.

Injury

A blow to the head, or a loud noise close to the ear such as the sound of a gunshot or a jet engine, especially when repeated often, can cause temporary and sometimes permanent hearing defects. Anyone who expects to be exposed to damaging noise should wear protective earmuffs. Injury to the auditory nerve by chemicals or by medicines such as streptomycin can also cause loss of hearing.

Ringing in the Ears

Sometimes people complain of hearing noises unrelated to the reception of sound waves from an outside source. This phenomenon is called *tinnitus* and occurs in the form of a buzzing, ringing, or hissing sound.

It may be caused by some of the conditions described above and may be relieved by proper treatment. In many cases, however, the cause is unknown and the patient simply has to learn to live with the sounds and ignore them.

Impairment of Balance

The *labyrinths* of the inner ear are involved not only in hearing but also in controlling postural balance. When the labyrinths are diseased, the result can be a feeling of *vertigo* or true dizziness. This sensation of being unable to maintain balance is quite different from feeling lightheaded or giddy.

Vertigo can be an incapacitating disorder. Sometimes it is caused by diseases of the central nervous system such as epilepsy or brain hemorrhage, but more often by inflammation sometimes caused by infection of the labyrinth. It can be sudden and recurrent as in *Ménière's disease,* or somewhat gradual and nonrecurrent. It may or may not be accompanied by vomiting or hearing loss. Treatment for the condition varies depending on the cause.

Deafness

Deafness at birth or in a very young baby is an especially difficult problem because hearing is necessary for the development of speech. Although the deafness itself may be impossible to correct, its early recognition and management can usually prevent muteness from developing.

Many communities now have special schools for deaf children, and new techniques and machines are constantly being devised for helping them to learn how to speak, even if imperfectly. Any doubt about an infant's ability to hear should therefore be brought to a physician's attention immediately.

Deafness at birth can be caused by a maternal infection such as rubella (German measles) during pregnancy. Because children are often the ones who spread this disease, youngsters should be immunized against it.

Hearing Aids

Hearing loss that cannot be treated medically or surgically can often be compensated for by an accurately fitted hearing aid. This device, which now comes in many sizes, shapes, and types, converts sound waves into electrical impulses, amplifies them, and reconverts them into sound waves. A hearing aid can be placed in the auditory canal for air conduction of sound waves, or it can be worn behind the ear for bone conduction. See under "Hearing Loss" in Ch. 6, *The Later Years,* for further information about hearing aids.

17

Diseases of the Urinogenital System

The parts of the urinogenital tract that produce and get rid of urine are the same for men and women: the kidneys, ureters, bladder, and urethra. To understand some of the problems that can arise from diseases of the urinary tract, it is necessary to know a few facts about the anatomy and function of these parts.

The two kidneys are located on either side of the spinal column in the back portion of the abdomen between the last rib and the third lumbar vertebra of the spine. They are shaped like the beans named after them but are considerably larger.

Their function is to filter and cleanse the blood of waste substances produced in the course of normal living and, together with some other organs, to maintain a proper balance of body fluids. The kidneys do this job by filtering the fluid portion of the blood as it passes through them, returning the necessary solids and water to the bloodstream, and removing waste products and excess water, called *urine*. These products then flow into the *ureters,* the ducts that connect the kidneys and bladder.

The *bladder* holds the urine until voiding occurs. The duct from the bladder to the urinary opening is called the *urethra*. In the male, it passes through the penis; in the female, in front of the anterior wall of the vagina.

Symptoms of Kidney Disorders

Normal kidney function can be disrupted by bacterial or viral infection, by tumors, by external injury, or by congenital defects. Some of the common symptoms that may result under these circumstances are:

- *Anuria:* inability to produce or void urine

- *Dysuria:* pain, often of a burning quality, during urination

- Frequency: abnormally frequent urination, often of unusually small amounts

- Hesitancy: difficulty in starting urination

- Urgency: a very strong urge to urinate, often strong enough to cause loss of urine

- *Oliguria:* reduced production of urine

- *Polyuria:* voiding larger than normal amounts of urine

- *Nocturia:* frequent voiding at night

- *Hematuria:* voiding blood in the urine

Because any of these symptoms may indicate a disease of the urinary tract, their appearance should be brought to the attention of a physician without delay.

Kidney Failure

Kidney failure can occur gradually—either from kidney disease or as a secondary condition resulting from another disease—or suddenly, as from an infection.

Acute Kidney Failure

The sudden loss of kidney function over a period of minutes to several days is known as acute kidney failure. It may be caused by impairment of blood supply to the kidneys, by severe infection, by nephritis (discussed below), by poisons, and by various other conditions that injure both kidneys.

Urogenital Systems

The body can function adequately throughout a normal lifespan with only one healthy kidney, but if both are impaired sufficiently over a short period of time, there will be symptoms of acute kidney failure: production of a decreased amount of urine (*oliguria*) sometimes with blood in it; fluid retention in body tissues, a condition known as *edema;* increasing fatigue and weakness; nausea and loss of appetite.

If damage to the kidneys has not been too severe, the patient begins to have a *diuresis,* or greater than normal urine output. When this happens—usually after one or two weeks of reduced urine output—he is kept on a restricted diet and reduced fluid intake after recovery until normal kidney function returns.

Causes

Heredity is rarely a factor in acute kidney failure, although people born with one kidney or with congenital defects of the urinary tract may lack the normal reserve capacity to prevent it. It is also unusual for external injury to result in a loss of function in both kidneys. However, severe internal shock accompanied by a reduction of blood flow to the kidneys can cause acute kidney failure.

Prevention and Treatment

Acute kidney failure can occur at any age. Prevention hinges on the proper control of its many causes. About 50 percent of patients with this disease may succumb to it; in cases of severe kidney failure involving widespread destruction of tissue, mortality may be almost 100 percent.

When acute kidney failure occurs as a complication of another serious illness, its prevention and treatment are usually managed by physicians in a hospital. If the patient is not already under a physician's supervision when he has the characteristic symptoms, he should immediately be brought to a medical facility for diagnosis and treatment.

Chronic Kidney Failure and Uremia

Many progressive kidney diseases can eventually lead to a group of symptoms called *uremia.* Other diseases, such as severe high blood pressure, diabetes, and those leading to widespread damage of kidney tissue, can also cause uremia.

In this condition, as in acute kidney failure, waste products and excess fluid accumulate in the body and cause the symptoms of chronic kidney failure. Certain congenital defects in the urinogenital system such as *polycystic kidney disease,* in which cysts in the kidneys enlarge slowly and destroy normal kidney tissue, may lead to uremia. Hereditary diseases such as hereditary nephritis may cause chronic kidney failure, but this is uncommon. Injury is also rarely the cause of uremia.

Although kidney failure is more likely to occur in older people because of the decreased capacity of the body to respond to stress, uremia can occur in any age group if kidney damage is severe enough. The onset of uremia may be so gradual that it goes unnoticed until the patient is weak and seems chronically ill. Voiding unusually large amounts of urine and voiding during the night are early symptoms.

Sleepiness and increasing fatigue set in as the kidney failure progresses, and there is a loss of appetite accompanied sometimes by nausea and hiccups. As the disease gets more serious, increasing weakness, anemia, muscle twitching, and sometimes internal bleeding may occur. High blood pressure is another characteristic symptom. Because of fluid retention, there will often be marked signs of facial puffiness and swelling of the legs.

Kidney damage that leads to chronic kidney failure is irreversible and the outlook for the victim of uremia is poor. The technique of dialysis (discussed below) has, however, prolonged many lives and continues to be a life-saving procedure for many.

Dialysis

An effective method of treatment of kidney failure developed in the 1960s is based on an artificial kidney that cleanses the patient's blood if his own kidneys are not functioning properly. The procedure, known as *dialysis* (or *hemodialysis*), removes dangerous waste products and excess fluids from the patient's bloodstream. It is the accumulation of waste products and fluids that probably causes the symptoms of acute kidney failure and that can be fatal if not reversed in one way or another.

Dialysis for Chronic Kidney Failure

For patients suffering chronic kidney failure or uremia, dialysis is a life-preserving but unfortunately expensive

Dialysis

Intermediate mechanical support system

Circulating blood

Outflow

Inflow

Vein

Artery

Supporting mesh

Flat tubing

Washing solution

To drain pump

procedure. The patient must be dialyzed with the artificial kidney unit two or three times a week, usually for six to eight hours at a time. Although the technique does not cure uremia, it can keep the patient comfortable provided that his diet is carefully restricted and supervised.

Dialysis in the Home

One approach that promises to be helpful in reducing the excessive cost is the development of home dialysis programs prepared with the cooperation of hospitals having departments specializing in kidney disease. Home dialysis is not suitable for everyone; the patient must be mature and stable enough to be relied on to undertake the procedure on schedule and in the prescribed manner. The overall costs of home dialysis, however, are about one-third those of in-hospital dialysis.

Medicare Coverage

Medicare coverage is now available for a part of the costs for dialysis maintenance for those suffering from permanent kidney failure, even if they are under 65 years of age. Coverage includes training in self-dialysis and the cost of dialysis equipment and applies to dialysis done in the home as well as in hospitals or other approved facilities. For details of this coverage, see your local social security office or write for the free booklet, *Medicare Coverage for Kidney Dialysis and Kidney Transplant Services,* published by the Social Security Administration.

Kidney Transplant Surgery

Some people suffering from kidney disease may benefit greatly from the surgical transplant of a donor's kidney. The donor kidney may be taken from a live relative or from someone recently deceased. The organ is removed from the donor's abdomen, usually flushed with a salt solution, and then reattached to a large artery and vein in the recipient's abdomen and to his ureter.

The successfully transplanted kidney functions just as the patient's own did when he was healthy, removing wastes and excess fluids from his bloodstream and excreting the resulting urine through the bladder. The recipient of a kidney transplant must take special medication to prevent the rejection of the newly installed organ by his own body tissues. With proper medical care, recipients have lived for many years with their transplanted organs.

Medicare Coverage

Medicare coverage is now available for a part of the costs of kidney transplant surgery for those under 65 as well as those over 65. This coverage includes hospital charges for costs incurred by the donor. For details of this coverage, see your local social security office or write for the free booklet, *Medicare Coverage of Kidney Dialysis and Kidney Transplant Services,* published by the Social Security Administration.

Nephritis

Nephritis is a disorder characterized by inflammation of the *glomeruli* of the kidneys. The glomeruli are tiny coiled blood vessels through which the liquid portion of the blood is filtered as it enters the outer structure of the kidneys. There are about one million of these tiny blood vessels in each kidney. The fluid from the blood passes from them into many little ducts called *tubules*. Water and various substances are secreted into and

absorbed from the liquid in the tubules. The final product of this passage of filtered fluid from the glomeruli through the tubules to the ureters and then to the bladder is urine. It contains the excess fluid and waste products produced by the body during normal functioning.

When the glomeruli become inflamed, the resulting disease is called *glomerulonephritis.* There are several forms of this disease. One type is thought to be caused by the body's allergic reaction to infection by certain streptococcal bacteria. Another type sometimes accompanies infection of the valves of the heart. The relationship between glomerulonephritis and strep infections is not fully understood at present, and the same may be said for nephritis, which is associated with allergic reaction to certain drugs and to heart valve infections.

Glomerulonephritis may occur ten days to two weeks after a severe strep throat infection. For this reason, any severe sore throat accompanied by a high fever should be seen and diagnosed by a physician. Prompt treatment with antibiotics may decrease the possibility of kidney involvement.

Nephritis Symptoms

The inflammation and swelling of the glomeruli cause a decrease in the amount of blood that the kidney is able to filter. As a result of the slowing down of this kidney function, the waste products of metabolism as well as excess fluid accumulate in the body instead of being eliminated at the normal rate.

In a typical case, a person will develop a severe sore throat with fever and a general feeling of sickness. These symptoms will disappear, but after one or two weeks, there will be a return of weakness and loss of appetite. The eyes and the face may be-

come puffy, the legs may swell, and there may be shortness of breath— all because of the retention of excess fluid in the body. The amount of urine is small and the color is dark brown, somewhat like coffee. Abdominal pain, nausea, and vomiting may occur, always accompanied by fatigue. In most cases, the blood pressure increases, leading to headaches.

Although there is a hereditary type of nephritis, the more common types of the disease have other causes. When the disease is suspected, the physician examines a specimen of urine under a microscope and looks for red blood cells. These cells, which usually do not pass through the walls of the normal glomerulus in large numbers, do pass through the damaged walls of the inflamed blood vessels characteristic of nephritis. Evidence of decreased kidney function is also found by special blood tests.

Nephritis occurs in all age groups. Children under ten have an excellent chance of recovery, about 98 percent. In adults, from 20 to 50 percent of the cases may be fatal or may progress to chronic nephritis, which often leads to uremia and death.

Treatment

It is absolutely essential for anyone with a streptococcal infection, which may lead to acute glomerulonephritis, to receive prompt and proper treatment. Penicillin is considered the most effective antibiotic at present.

Once acute nephritis is present, the treatment consists of bed rest, some fluid restriction, and protein restriction if kidney failure occurs. If there is a total loss of kidney function, a specially restricted diet is prescribed. Complete lack of urine output—*anuria*— may last as long as ten days, but the patient can still make a full recovery if the treatment is right. Usually a gradual return of kidney function occurs over a period of several months.

Nephrosis

The *nephrotic syndrome,* commonly referred to as *nephrosis,* is a disease in which abnormal amounts of protein in the form of *albumin* are lost in the urine. Albumin consists of microscopic particles of protein present in the blood. These particles are important in maintaining the proper volume of fluids in the body, and they have other complicated functions as well. The loss of albumin in the urine affects the amount that remains in the blood, and it is this imbalance, together with other body changes, that results in the retention of excess fluid in the tissues, thus causing facial puffiness and swelling of the legs.

The disease is caused by damage to the glomeruli, but at the present time the exact nature of the damage is uncertain. It may be caused by an allergic reaction, by inflammation, or it may be a complication of diabetes. The nephrotic syndrome may also appear because of blood clots in the veins that drain the kidneys.

Although the disease is more common among children than among adults, it may affect a person of any age. The main symptom is painless swelling of the face, legs, and sometimes of the entire body. There is also loss of appetite, a tired, rundown feeling, and sometimes abdominal pain, vomiting, and diarrhea.

Recovery from nephrosis varies with age. More than 50 percent of child patients are completely free of kidney ailments after the first attack. Adults are more likely to develop some impairment of kidney function, or the disease may become chronic, with accompanying high blood pressure. In some people, protein loss may continue over the years, al-though the kidneys function in an apparently normal manner without any visible symptoms.

Treatment

Treatment of the nephrotic syndrome has been greatly helped by the use of the adrenal hormones known as *steroids.* The treatment is effective for about two-thirds of child patients and for about one-fourth to one-third of adults. Some patients may relapse after therapy is completed, sometimes years after such therapy has been discontinued. For this reason, steroids are sometimes continued after initial treatment but in reduced dosage, to avoid some of the unpleasant side effects such as acne and facial swelling.

Unlike the dietary treatment for uremia, a high protein diet is used with nephrotic patients so that the protein loss can be replaced. Salt intake is usually restricted because salt contributes to fluid retention and may cause high blood pressure or heart failure. If fluid retention doesn't respond to steroid treatment, other medicines called *diuretics,* which increase urinary output, are used.

Anyone with unusual swelling of the face, limbs, or abdomen should see a physician promptly. Even though the swelling is painless, it may be the first sign of the onset of a serious kidney problem.

Infection in the Urinary Tract

Infection in the urinary tract is a common disorder that can be serious if the kidneys themselves are involved.

Cystitis

Infection of the bladder is called *cystitis.* The symptoms include a burning sensation when urine is passed, the frequent need to urinate, occasionally blood in the urine, and sometimes difficulty in starting to urinate. Cystitis is rarely accompanied by high fever.

The problem may be recurrent and is more usual with women than men, probably because the female urethra is shorter and closer to the rectum, permitting bacteria to enter the bladder more easily. These bacteria multiply in the urine contained in the bladder, causing irritation to the bladder walls and producing the symptoms described above.

Cystitis should be treated promptly because the infection in the bladder can easily spread to the kidneys, with serious consequences. Treatment usually consists of antibiotics after urine analysis and culture have determined the type of bacteria causing the infection. Cystitis and other kidney infections are especially common during pregnancy because of the body changes that occur at this time. At no time is cystitis itself a serious disease, but it must be diagnosed and treated promptly to avoid complications.

Other Causes of Infection

Infection of the bladder and kidneys may occur because of poor hygiene in the area of the urethra, especially in women. It is also caused by some congenital defects in the urinary tract or by the insertion of instruments used to diagnose a urinary problem.

Sometimes bacteria in the bloodstream can settle in and infect the kidneys. Patients with diabetes seem to be more prone to urinary infections—indeed to infections generally—than other people. Any obstruction to the flow of urine in the urinary tract, such as a kidney stone, increases the possibility of infection in the area behind the obstruction. Damage to the nerves controlling the bladder is another condition that increases the chances of infection in that area.

Pyelonephritis

Infection in the kidneys is called *pyelonephritis*. Although it sometimes occurs without any symptoms, a first attack usually causes an aching pain in the lower back, probably due to the swelling of the kidneys, as well as nausea, vomiting, diarrhea, and sometimes severe pain in the front of the abdomen on one or both sides, depending on whether one or both kidneys are involved. Fever may be quite high, ranging from 103° F to 105° F, often accompanied by chills.

Although the symptoms of pyelonephritis may disappear in a few days without treatment, bacterial destruction of the kidney tissue may be going on. This silent type of infection may eventually disrupt normal kidney function and result in a chronic form of the disease, which in turn can lead to uremia. If the disease is not halted before this, it can be fatal.

Anyone with symptoms of acute pyelonephritis must have prompt medical attention. To diagnose the disease properly, the urine is analyzed and the number and type of bacteria in the urine are determined. The disease is brought under control by the right antibiotics and by administering large amounts of fluids to flush out the kidneys and urinary tract, thus decreasing the number of bacteria in the urine. In its chronic form the disease is much more difficult to cure because bacteria that are lodged deep in the kidney tissue do not seem to be susceptible to antibiotics and are therefore almost impossible to get rid of.

Kidney Stones

Another cause of infection in the bladder and kidneys is obstruction in the urinary tract by *kidney stones*. These stones, crystallizations of salts that form in the kidney tissue, may be quite small, but they can grow large enough to occupy a considerable part of one or both of the kidneys. The smaller ones often pass from the kidney through the ureters to the bladder, from which they are voided through the urethra. However, obstruction of the flow of urine behind a kidney stone anywhere in the urinary tract usually leads to infection in the urine. This type of infection may lead to attacks of acute pyelonephritis.

Removal of Stones

Kidney stones must be removed unless they cause no symptoms of infection. Removal may be accomplished by flushing out the urinary tract with large fluid intake, by surgical methods, or by lithotripsy, a method of dissolving the stones with electrical shock waves so that the fragments can be flushed out of the body. Any accompanying infection may be treated with antibiotics. A drug, *potassium citrate,* may also be used to keep kidney stones from forming. See "Urinary Stones" in Ch. 20, *Surgery.*

Why kidney stones form in some people and not in others is not clearly understood. Because of metabolic disorders, certain substances may build up in the body. The increased excretion of these substances in the urine as well as excessive amounts of calcium in the blood may encourage kidney stone formation. People who have gout are also likely to develop them.

Renal Colic

Sometimes the formation and passage of stones cause no symptoms. However, when symptoms do occur with the passage of a kidney stone, they can be uncomfortably severe. The pain that results from the passage of a stone through the ureter, referred

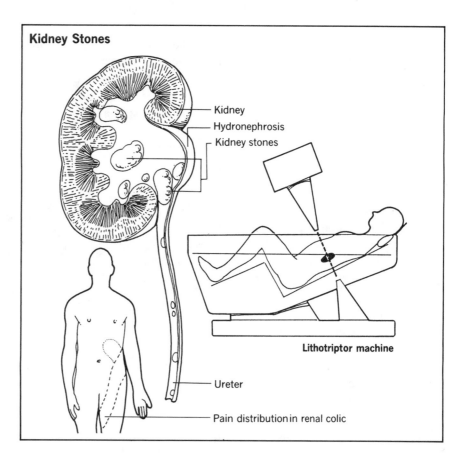

Kidney Stones

Kidney
Hydronephrosis
Kidney stones

Lithotriptor machine

Ureter

Pain distribution in renal colic

to as *renal colic,* is usually like an intense cramp. It begins in the side or back and moves toward the lower abdomen, the genital region, and the inner thigh on the affected side. The attack may last for a few minutes or for several hours. Sometimes bloody urine may be passed accompanied by a burning sensation.

Kidney stones are more likely to form in middle-aged and older people than in young ones. A history of stones is sometimes found in several generations of a family, since the metabolic disorders encouraging their formation have a hereditary basis.

Treatment for an acute attack of renal colic usually relieves the pain several hours after the patient has taken medication and fluids. If they are not promptly treated, kidney stones may lead to serious infection and eventual impairment of function.

Tumors of the Urinary Tract

Benign and malignant tumors of the kidney are not common problems. However, anyone with pain in the midback, blood in the urine, or a mass in the abdomen should have the symptoms diagnosed. If a malignant tumor is discovered early enough, it can be removed with the affected kidney, and normal function can be maintained by the healthy kidney that remains.

Malignant kidney tumors are most often found in children or adults over 40, and more often in men than in women. A tumor of any type can usually be diagnosed by X-ray studies. Where this technique is inadequate, an operation is necessary to search for the suspected growth. About one-fourth of all patients with a malignant kidney tumor live for more than ten years after surgery.

A malignant tumor of the bladder is a serious problem because it obstructs kidney drainage and may cause death from uremia. The main symptom is the painless appearance of blood in the urine, although sometimes a burning sensation and a frequent need to urinate are also present. Treatment usually includes surgical removal of the bladder followed by radiation treatment of the affected area to destroy any malignant cells that remain after the operation.

Some malignant bladder tumors grow very slowly and do not invade the bladder wall extensively. Surgical treatment for this type, called *papillary tumors,* is likely to be more successful than for tumors of the more invasive kind.

The Prostate Gland

The *prostate gland,* which contributes to the production of semen, encircles the base of the male urethra where it joins the bladder. When it begins to enlarge, it compresses the urethra and causes difficulty in voiding. Urination may be difficult to start, and when the urine stream appears it may be thinner than normal.

Because urine may remain in the bladder, there is the possibility of local infection that may spread to the kidneys. If the kidneys become enlarged because of this type of obstruction, a condition of *hydronephrosis* is said to exist. This disease can cause impaired kidney function and lead to uremia.

Benign Prostatic Enlargement

Enlargement of the prostate gland occurs in about half the male population over 50, and the incidence increases with increasing age. The condition is called *benign prostatic enlargement* and must be treated surgically if sufficient obstruction is present. For temporary relief, a catheter can be inserted into the bladder through the urethra, allowing the urine to drain through the catheter and out of the body. If surgery is necessary, the entire prostate may be removed or only that part of it that surrounds the urethra.

Symptoms of benign prostatic enlargement are quite distinctive: increased difficulty in voiding; an urge to continue to urinate after voiding has been completed; burning and frequent urination, caused in part by infection from urine retained in the bladder.

The cause of benign prostatic en-

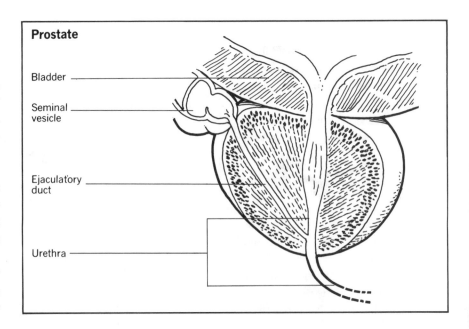

Prostate

Bladder

Seminal vesicle

Ejaculatory duct

Urethra

largement is thought to be a change during the aging process in the hormones that affect prostate tissue, but the exact nature of the change and its effect is not clear. It is likely that hormone-containing medicines will eventually be developed that will prevent or reverse prostate tissue growth.

Acute Prostatitis

Acute prostatitis occurs typically in young men. Symptoms include pain on urinating, sometimes a discharge of pus from the penis, pain in the lower back or abdomen indicating a tender and enlarged prostate, and fever. It is caused by a bacterial infection and usually responds promptly to antibiotics.

Cancer of the Prostate

Cancer of the prostate is a common type of malignancy in older men. It accounts for about 10 percent of male deaths from cancer in the United States. The disease may be present without any symptoms or interference with normal function and is therefore difficult to diagnose. A very high proportion of men over 80—probably more than 50 percent—has been found to have had cancer of the prostate at autopsy.

When symptoms are present, they are likely to be the same as those of benign prostatic enlargement. The disease can be diagnosed only by a biopsy examination of a tissue sample taken from the prostate during surgery. If malignancy is found, the gland is surgically removed when feasible to do so; the testes are removed too so that the level of male hormones in the body is lowered.

Male hormones increase the growth of malignant prostate tissue, but because female hormones slow it down, they may be administered after a diagnosis of prostate malignancy. If the tumor has spread to bone tissue,

radiation treatment of the affected areas may slow down cancerous growth and relieve pain.

Men over 40 should have a rectal examination once a year, since tumors of the prostate and benign prostatic enlargement can often be diagnosed early in this way.

Bedwetting

Enuresis, the medical term for bedwetting, is the unintentional loss of urine, usually during sleep at night. Infants do not have sufficiently developed nervous systems to control urination voluntarily until they are about two-and-a-half or three years old. Controlling urination through the night may not occur until after the age of three. A child who wets his bed recurrently after he has learned to control urination has the problem of enuresis.

There are many causes of enuresis. It may occur because of a delay in normal development or as a result of emotional stress. About 15 percent of boys and 10 percent of girls are bedwetters at the age of 5. By 9, about 5 percent of all children still have the problem, but most children outgrow it by the time they reach puberty.

Children who are bedwetters should be examined to rule out any physical abnormality in the urinary tract. Obstruction at the neck of the bladder where it joins the urethra or obstruction at the end of the urethra may cause uncontrollable dribbling of urine, but this usually occurs during the day as well as at night.

Disease of the nerves controlling the bladder, sometimes hereditary, can cause loss of urine. It can also occur in children who are mentally retarded or mentally ill, or because of an acute or chronic illness. In the latter cases, the problem disappears when the child regains his health.

Emotional Problems

If all physical abnormalities for bedwetting have been explored and eliminated as possible causes, the emotional problems of the child and his family should be examined. An understanding attitude rather than a hostile or punitive one on the part of the parents is extremely important in helping a child who is a bedwetter. He may be anxious about school or angry at a favored younger child, or he may feel insecure about parental acceptance. In such cases, an effort to bring the child's hidden feelings into the open and to deal with them sympathetically usually causes the problem to disappear.

Sexually Transmitted Diseases

The name of Venus, the Roman goddess of love, is preserved in the term *venereal disease* because they are transmitted by sexual contact. But today the broader phrase *sexually transmitted disease* (STD) is more commonly used to refer to both venereal and other diseases that may be passed from one person to another during sexual activity. STDs include some diseases, among them *acquired immunodeficiency syndrome,* or AIDS (see "AIDS" in Ch. 19, *Other Diseases of Major Importance*), that had not been identified as separate disorders until the 1970s or 1980s.

Sexually transmitted diseases were spreading at epidemic rates by the middle 1980s. Because all are contagious by definition, and can often cause serious complications, the symptoms should be treated without delay. At least two of the STDs, AIDS and genital herpes, or herpes simplex type II, are incurable. Some drugs and medications can, however, ameliorate specific symptoms of both diseases.

Except for pelvic inflammatory disease (PID), a serious complication among women, STDs afflict both men and women. Of the 11 most common STDs, chlamydia is the most prevalent. Public health officials believe the disease has spread because it has no obvious symptoms and victims can live for years without realizing they have it.

AIDS

While neither a disease of the urinogenital system nor an STD, strictly speaking, acquired immunodeficiency syndrome (AIDS) ranks as one of the most feared diseases today. Because the disease may be transmitted by intravenous needles that are shared by drug abusers as well as through sexual contact and contaminated blood it cannot strictly be called an STD. The disease strips the body of its acquired immunity against infection and leaves its victims susceptible to a variety of opportunistic infections. These include a rare form of pneumonia and Karposi's sarcoma, a rare type of cancer. AIDS is uniformly fatal.

A virus called the *human immunodeficiency virus* (HIV) is thought to be the cause of AIDS. Researchers speculate, however, that more than one virus may be the causative agent in AIDS. Exposure to the disease does not mean inevitably that a person will contract AIDS. Perhaps no more than 10 to 20 percent of the individuals who have been exposed to HIV will develop full-blown cases of AIDS. Many will develop what has been termed ARC, AIDS-related complex, which is less often fatal and not considered by authorities to be AIDS per se.

Diagnosis

No simple means of diagnosing AIDS exists. Physicians can test for certain opportunistic infections. They also study symptoms as reported by individuals. Damage to white blood cells (specifically the T-cells), revealed by tests, may indicate the presence of the disease. The only test available now, commonly called the "AIDS test," can only test for the presence of antibodies. These antibodies are indicative of exposure to HIV and do not indicate the presence of the virus itself. Because the test was developed for blood donor screening its use by individuals concerned about possible exposure to HIV is not advocated by most health professionals. A positive test showing AIDS antibodies does not necessarily mean that the person will contract the disease, nor does a negative test mean the person has not become infected. The present blood screening test has a relatively high degree of unreliability and so should therefore not be relied upon as the sole indicator of exposure to AIDS.

The symptoms of AIDS range across a broad grouping of complaints that are common to various illnesses. Because these complaints are so common, diagnosis becomes even more difficult. The symptoms include night sweats, diarrhea, fatigue, weight loss of 10 or more pounds over a short period, swollen lymph nodes, fever, and loss of appetite. The symptoms may appear from six months to five years or more after infection.

Treatment

There is no treatment for AIDS as yet; therefore, physicians can only treat the specific symptoms that occur from the various opportunistic diseases that attack AIDS patients. Also, an antiserum has been found to keep the AIDS virus from invading human cells in laboratory tests. The antiserum, a blood substance, reacts with a thymus gland hormone called thymosin alpha 1. Researchers hope the antiserum will eventually lead to development of an AIDS vaccine. The development of such a vaccine, however, is thought to be some years away.

Chlamydia

Chlamydia is a bacterial infection that can cause sterility in men and women and has been called "the disease of the '80s." Most women with the disease have no obvious symptoms. For that reason, physicians suggest that sexually active women undergo tests for chlamydia at least once a year. The disease is spreading more rapidly than any other STD.

Persons at highest risk of contracting chlamydia are under 35 years of age. A bacterium, *Chlamydia trachomatis,* causes the disease, which is spread to adults during sexual contact and to babies of infected mothers during birth. Complications affect both sexes: both men and women may become infertile, and women may have pregnancy problems that could kill a fetus. In some cases the disease may be fatal for the mother. Babies infected during birth may develop infections of the eyes, ears, or lungs.

Diagnosis

A new diagnostic technique has led to hope that chlamydia can be brought under control. The technique, *antigen detection testing,* is a relatively simple and painless laboratory procedure.

Symptoms that indicate the possibility of chlamydia may or may not appear. Men may experience a discharge from the penis or a burning sensation while urinating. Women may have vaginal itching, bleeding between menstrual periods, and chronic abdominal pain. The symptoms may appear two to four weeks after infection.

Treatment

Even though chlamydia is spreading more rapidly than other STDs, it ranks among the lesser STD threats. Treatments involve drug therapies with tetracycline or doxycycline. Erythromycin has also been used successfully. The drugs usually take effect in about seven days. The partner of a person who is undergoing treatment for chlamydia should also be treated.

Gonorrhea

The second most common STD, *gonorrhea,* has afflicted mankind for centuries. Gonorrhea, caused by the bacteria gonococcus, lives in the mucous membranes of the body, including the vagina, rectum, throat, or hollow of the cheek. Cervical, penile, or rectal gonorrhea are contracted through intercourse; oral sex may lead to throat gonorrhea. Women may acquire gonorrhea in a single contact with an infected male; but men face only about a 20 to 40 percent risk of contracting the disease from a female.

Untreated, gonorrhea can lead to various complications. Women can suffer from pelvic inflammatory disease. In relatively unusual cases gonococci can enter the bloodstream and cause blood poisoning. The babies of infected mothers may be born blind. Gonococci settling in joints may cause arthritis. Very rarely the disease leads to *endocarditis,* an inflammation of the lining of the heart, or to *meningitis,* an inflammation that destroys the membrane surrounding the brain and spinal cord.

Except for PID, men experience most of the basic symptoms of untreated gonorrhea. Thus male problems can range from back pains to sterility.

Diagnosis

Anyone suspecting the presence of gonorrhea should arrange for a medical examination as quickly as possible. A test "just in case" may be advisable if, for example, a sex partner indicates that he or she has contracted the disease. Women are cautioned against douching before a visit to a physician or public health clinic; nor should self-treatment with antibiotics be attempted. In either case diagnosis may become more difficult.

Gonorrhea is more difficult to detect in women than in men. As many as four out of five women infected with cervical gonorrhea may not realize for days or weeks that they have the disease. When symptoms do appear, they include vaginal discharges and discomfort when urinating. These symptoms, appearing three to eleven days after exposure, may become steadily worse. Urinating may become extremely painful. With rectal gonorrhea, burning sensations, bleeding or mucous discharges may accompany defecation. Approximately nine of ten males know within a week to ten days that they have been infected. Male symptoms are, commonly, a puslike discharge from the penis and a burning sensation while urinating.

Treatment

Penicillin is the most effective treatment for gonorrhea. For persons allergic to penicillin, physicians usually prescribe tetracycline or erythromycin in oral doses. All three drugs are effective in most cases.

Researchers believe the possibility that they will find a vaccine for gonorrhea is strong. Experimental vaccines have been successfully tested on laboratory animals.

Genital Herpes

Genital herpes, or herpes simplex type II, is transmitted by physical—usually sexual—contact. The virus is one of the herpesviruses that also cause shingles, mononucleosis, or chicken pox. The disease is transmitted through skin-to-skin contact with herpes sores or the secretions of an infected person. The virus enters the body through the mucous membranes of the genitals, mouth, or anus.

The first attack of genital herpes usually occurs one to two weeks after exposure. Sores may appear; the afflicted person may have difficulty urinating or defecating. The symptoms usually disappear in ten days to three weeks, but for most herpes victims a recurrence can be expected within six months. Later attacks may be milder, but the disease is incurable and can be transmitted even when no symptoms are visible.

Stress and depression, authorities say, can trigger herpes attacks. Women suffering from the disease face increased risks of cervical cancer. They may also pass the virus to babies during delivery. So exposed, the babies may die within a few weeks; some newborns are deformed, blind, or mentally handicapped. Because of the danger that the herpesvirus poses to newborns, women with genital herpes should alert their obstetricians so that delivery can be by cesarian section. By avoiding vaginal mucous membranes, the infant will not be exposed to the virus.

Diagnosis

Physicians can usually diagnose herpes by visual examination while the characteristic sores are evident. A physician may also take a herpes culture from the base of the lesion.

Treatment

While no cure for genital herpes exists, the drug acyclovir has been found to reduce the severity of the flareups. Acyclovir is applied as a topical ointment, usually for initial outbreaks. In an oral form the drug alleviates subsequent attacks. The oral preparation has been reported to be effective in about seven cases out of ten.

Whether treated or not, later outbreaks of herpes are generally shorter and less severe than the first. Physicians agree that acyclovir effects improvement in the majority of cases, but some reserve judgment concerning the drug's long-term effects.

Trichomoniasis

A type of leukorrhea, *trichomoniasis* is caused by the *Trichomonas vaginalis,* an organism that causes an irritating itching condition in women. Men usually have no symptoms. The organism, a parasite, favors warm, moist areas, such as genital tissues; but some experts believe it can sometimes survive in damp cloths, douching syringes, towels, around toilet seats, on beaches, and around swimming pools. Thus the disease can, it is believed, be spread without sexual contact.

Complications can follow trichomoniasis. Women victims experience discomfort and pain. Chronic infection, according to some researchers, may make a woman more susceptible to cervical cancer. Constant irritation of the cervix is said to produce such susceptibility.

Diagnosis

The trichomoniasis leukorrhea consists of a yellow to green frothy discharge. The itching that accompanies the infection tends to begin or worsen immediately after a menstrual period. Some women report a burning sensation when they urinate. In diagnosis the physician uses a test similar to a Pap smear (see "Pap Smear" in Ch.

25, *Women's Health*), made with a specimen taken from the vagina. Under a microscope the trichomonas organisms are easy to identify because they are pear-shaped and have three to five whiplike tails.

Treatment

Several drugs are available for treating trichomoniasis. They include tablets taken orally and suppositories inserted in the vagina. Most commonly prescribed is metronidazole. Cures may be effected quickly. One dose of two grams (eight 250 mg tablets) may be adequate for both the victim and his or her partner. The oral medication may, however, be continued for weeks or months if the infection resists the drug.

Trichomoniasis victims have reported such side effects as nausea, depression, and hives. Because many persons are allergic to metronidazole, physicians may suggest the use of vaginal douches made up of vinegar and water, or of vaginal suppositories. The latter relieve trichomoniasis symptoms, but do not cure the disease.

Venereal Warts

Venereal warts, also called *genital warts,* may be painless but they can be serious and thus require medical attention. If left untreated, researchers say, venereal warts can increase the risk of penile cancer in men and cervical cancer in women. A pregnant woman with these growths may transmit the virus to her infant during delivery. Warts may then develop in the newborn's windpipe, causing later breathing problems.

The *human papilloma viruses* cause venereal warts, which may appear in a variety of places in the pubic area. The growths are usually small pink bumps, but they can grow to-

gether to resemble tiny cauliflowers. In most cases, the growths itch and produce a foul-smelling discharge.

Diagnosis

A physician can usually diagnose venereal warts from their external appearance. To make certain that the warts are not syphilis growths, however, the physician may take a biopsy. A tiny part of the wart is removed for study under a microscope. The papilloma virus can then be identified.

Women with external venereal warts may also have the growths on the cervix. A Pap test is required for detection of these internal warts.

Treatment

The drug podophyllin can be used in solution to remove venereal warts. The solution is painted on the growths, left for six hours, then washed off. The warts usually disappear within a few days. The treatment may have to be repeated several times. If any wart cells remain, the problem will most likely recur.

Podophyllin is not effective in all cases. Where it cannot achieve a cure, other methods, including surgery, may have to be attempted. Among these other methods, which are not always successful, are freezing and burning of the growths. Some studies have indicated that the hormone interferon can prevent recurrences of the disease. Interferon therapy may, however, produce such flulike side effects as fatigue and fever.

Syphilis

Historically, syphilis has ranked among mankind's chief health scourges. Modern medicine has brought it largely under control, but it can still be life-threatening.

Syphilis strikes men about three times as often as women. Approximately half of the male victims are homosexuals. A spiral-shaped bacterium called *Treponema pallidum* causes the disease. Transmittal takes place during sex with a person in the infectious stage in which open sores or rashes are typical symptoms. The *Treponema* bacteria fill the sores and in infecting another person invade the mucous membranes of the genitals, mouth, or rectum. The *spirochete,* or spiral bacterium, succumbs to heat, dryness, ordinary antiseptics, or even soap and water. But it can tolerate cold and survive freezing.

Stages

Unless it is treated early, syphilis progresses from a primary to secondary and sometimes tertiary stages. In the primary stage, the victim may have a painless chancre, or ulcer, that may be small, single, or multiple and that may look like any common skin ulcer. The reddish-brown ulcers generally appear between ten days and three months after exposure to the disease, with a typical incubation time of three weeks.

The secondary and latent stages of syphilis can lead to serious complications unless treatment is undertaken. A month to six weeks after the first ulcers appear, secondary lesions may develop, taking the form of a rash or almost any other kind of skin eruption. The lesions may appear on the trunk of the body, on the face, the arms and legs, or the palms of the hands and soles of the feet. The lesions may or may not itch, and they may not appear at all. The victim may, however, experience fevers and flu symptoms as well as hair loss. A latent stage of many years' duration follows untreated secondary syphilis. In this stage only a blood test can reveal

the presence of the bacteria in the body.

If still untreated, late or tertiary-stage syphilis follows the secondary and latent stages in about one case in four. Tertiary syphilis involves the gradual destruction of the central nervous system, the heart, the bones, the liver, the stomach, or other organs. The bacteria can cause paralysis, convulsions, heart failure, insanity, and even death. Attacking the circulatory system, syphilis can cause an *aneurysm,* dilated section, of the aorta just above the heart. The blood flow to the heart is reduced; a ruptured aneurysm can produce a fatal hemorrhage. While gummas, rubbery syphilitic tumors inside organs, may respond to antibiotics in the late stage of syphilis, damage to the heart valves and arteries may be irreversible.

General Paresis

Permanent tissue damage to the brain and nerves can result from syphilitic invasion of the central nervous system; this the chronic, progressive form of syphilis known as *general paresis.* The damage occurs gradually, and early symptoms may include headaches, a tendency to forget things, or difficulty in concentrating. Mental effects may progress from memory loss to psychotic symptoms of delusions of grandeur.

Tabes Dorsalis

Late syphilis involving deterioration of the sheaths of spinal nerves (demyelination) and other destructive changes in the spinal cord is known as *tabes dorsalis.* The patient may become uncoordinated in movement. Tremors of the hands and fingers may be noticed, as well as tremors of the lips and tongue. Vision may be affected, and sensory effects can range

from sharp sudden pains to a loss of feeling. The patient may lose control of bladder function or the ability to walk.

Congenital Syphilis

The latent syphilitic condition is not uncommon, and it is a period of great danger to the fetus if an infected woman, especially a recently infected woman, becomes pregnant at this time. The fetus can acquire syphilis through the placenta and be born with congenital syphilis. Or it can be still-born or die shortly after birth. Some of the signs of syphilis in an infant born with the congenital form of the disease are similar to those of secondary syphilis. Others are very different, more closely resembling tertiary syphilis. Because of the hazards to the child, most physicians test the mother's blood for the presence of the spirochete during the first three months of pregnancy and during the last three months; syphilis acquired during pregnancy is especially likely to affect the fetus. Treatment of the mother has the added benefit of treating the fetus. Treatment begun before the eighteenth week of pregnancy will prevent syphilis from developing; treatment begun after the eighteenth week will cure the fetus of syphilis.

Diagnosis

Because the symptoms of syphilis may appear sporadically or not at all, and because they so closely resemble the symptoms of other diseases, diagnosis usually calls for a blood test. If a chancre has developed, the physician may take a scraping from the lesion and order a special microscopic examination.

Treatment

Long-lasting penicillin, given by intravenous injection, usually cures syphilis. But the disease can, as noted, cause irreversible damage if allowed to spread unchecked. For persons who are allergic to penicillin, physicians may prescribe tetracycline or erythromycin. Both are effective as treatments.

Pelvic Inflammatory Disease

Pelvic inflammatory disease (PID) is a serious complication of STDs. It affects women as a result of infection from a number of diseases including chlamydia and gonorrhea. To produce PID, a disease has to progress to the point where it leads to inflammation and abscesses of a victim's Fallopian tubes, ovaries, and pelvis.

One woman in about seven who contract PID becomes infertile. On the average, three of four women experiencing attacks of the disease will be unable to conceive.

Diagnosis and Treatment

Physicians can diagnose PID by conducting abdominal and pelvic examinations as well as various laboratory tests.

Antibiotics are prescribed in some cases. In more severe cases, surgery may be necessary. The surgery usually results in infertility.

Lymphogranuloma Venereum

This disease, also known as LGV and *lymphogranuloma inguinale,* is a venereal disease that produces a primary lesion like a small blister, which ruptures to form a small ulcer. It is caused by a virus that is spread by sexual intercourse, although sexual contact is not necessary for transmission of the disease. It can be acquired by contact with the fluid excreted by a lesion.

The primary lesion usually appears in the genital area within one to three weeks after contact with an infected person. It may appear only briefly or be so small as to go unnoticed. But the disease spreads to neighboring lymph nodes, where the next sign of the disorder appears 10 days to a month later. The swelling of the lymph nodes (forming *buboes*) is often the first symptom to be noted by the patient; the lymph nodes become matted together and hard, forming channels (or *fistulas*) through which pus drains to the surface of the skin. Enlargement of the lymph nodes may produce painful swelling of the external genitalia. The lymph-node involvement may spread to the anal region, leading to rectal constriction and painful bowel movements.

Diagnosis and Treatment

Because the lesions of lymphogranuloma venereum may resemble those of syphilis, chancroid, or certain nonvenereal diseases, physicians usually make a number of tests to determine whether or not the condition is, in fact, LGV. Therapy includes administration of antibiotics and sulfa drugs for a period of about a week to a month, depending on the severity of the infection.

Chancroid

Chancroid, or *soft chancre,* is a venereal disease transmitted by a bacterium that causes a tender, painful ulcer. The ulcer, which may erode deeply into the tissues, follows the formation of a primary pustule at the site of infection. The pustule appears within five days after contact with an infected person. While essentially a venereal disease, like other venereal diseases it is transmissible without sexual intercourse. Physicians, for

example, have been known to develop a soft chancre on a finger after examining an infected patient.

Diagnosis and Treatment

Physicians usually do tests to make sure that the lesion is not a syphilitic chancre. Although the disease can spread from the genital region to other parts of the body, the soft chancre generally is self-limiting. Therapy consists of administration of sulfa drugs or tetracycline.

Granuloma Inguinale

Granuloma inguinale, also called *granuloma venereum,* is not the same, in spite of the similarity in name, as lymphogranuloma venereum. The former is an insidious, chronic venereal disease that produces lesions on the skin or mucous membrane of the genital or anal regions. The first sign of the infection may be a painless papule or nodule that leaves an ulcer with a reddish granular base. If untreated, the lesions tend to spread to the lower abdomen and thighs. In time, the sores produce a sour, pungent odor.

Treatment

Antibiotics such as streptomycin and tetracycline are prescribed. Relapses may occur and cure may be slow, especially in cases of long standing.

External Venereal Maladies

The two conditions described below, one related to viruses and one a parasitic infestation, may generally be considered sources of discomfort and disfigurement rather than threats to general health. Both of these STDs are transmissible by other means besides sexual contact.

Molluscum Contagiosum

A viral disease transmitted during sexual intercourse is known by the medical term *molluscum contagiosum*. The disease can also be transmitted by ordinary person-to-person contact, as between members of a family or children in a classroom. The virus causes raised lesions containing a waxy white material. The lesions, which may be very small or as large as an inch in diameter, occur on the skin or mucous membranes, commonly in the anal or genital area but sometimes on the face or torso. The lesions may last for several months or several years, then disappear spontaneously, or they may be removed by medications or surgery.

Pubic Lice

Infestations of pubic lice constitute a unique kind of venereal disease. Pubic lice, known popularly as crabs, are a species somewhat larger than body and head lice but still almost invisible to the naked eye. These whitish, oval parasites usually remain in the hair of the anal and genital regions, but they may sometimes be found attached to the skin at the base of any body hair, including eyelashes and scalp. A very few pubic lice in the anal and genital areas can cause intense irritation and itching. The itching results in scratching which, in turn, produces abrasions of the skin. The lice may also produce patches of bluish spots on the skin of the inner thighs and lower abdomen. Another sign of their presence is the appearance of tiny brown specks deposited by the lice on the inside of undergarments.

Pubic lice are commonly spread by sexual contact, but they can be acquired from toilet seats, clothing, towels, bedclothes, combs, or any article of intimate use. Creams or ointments containing various parasiticides are available for disinfestation. They are applied every night for several nights, but overuse should be avoided because of the danger of injury to the tender tissues of the genital and anal region. Some physicians recommend soaking the infested part of the body several times daily in a mild solution of potassium permanganate. Lice on the eyebrows and eyelashes may have to be removed individually with a pair of tweezers. Treatment must be repeated after one week to kill the nits (eggs) that have hatched since the first treatment. Clothing and other contaminated materials must be cleaned to prevent reinfestation.

Complications of an infestation of pubic lice include intense itching (known medically as *pruritus*) and secondary infections from scratching. These may require special medical care and administration of antibiotics, corticosteroid creams, or other appropriate remedies.

18
Cancer

Cancer has always figured uniquely in the diseases of mankind. For centuries people spoke of it only in whispers, or not at all, as if the disease were not only dreadful but somehow shameful as well. Today, the picture is changing and rapidly. This decade may see the time—undreamt of only scant years ago—when half of those stricken by cancer will survive its ravages. And much of the mystery that cloaked the disease in an awful shroud has been dissipated, although the last veils remain to be stripped away.

Of course, cancer remains a formidable enemy. More than a million Americans are under medical care for cancer; an estimated 500,000 will die of it each year. Of all Americans now alive, one in three will be stricken. Cancer is the greatest cause of lost working years among women and ranks third after heart disease and accidents in denying men working years.

But in context, the picture is not as bleak as it might seem. At the beginning of the twentieth century, survival from cancer was relatively rare. At the end of the 1930s, the five-year survival rate (alive after five years) was one in five or fewer. Ten years

later it had shot up to one in four, and in the mid-fifties to one in three. This figure has remained relatively stable because the survival rate for some of the more widespread cancers has leveled off despite the best efforts of physicians to devise better forms of treatment. For such cancers, which include those of the breast, colon, and rectum, improvements will come through earlier detection and even prevention. Dr. Richard S. Doll, Professor of Medicine at Oxford University, has said that we could prevent 40 percent of men's cancer deaths and 10 percent of women's simply by applying what we already know. For example, according to the American Cancer Society, the risk of death from lung cancer is 15 to 20 times greater among men who smoke cigarettes than among men who have never smoked. The relative risk of lung cancer among women smokers is five times that of women who have never smoked.

Considerable progress is being made on many fronts in the war against cancer. It ranges from advances in early detection to breakthroughs in treatment. The past 25 years have seen a 50 percent dip in the death rate from cervical cancer,

mostly because of increasing acceptance of the Pap test, which can detect the disease at a very early stage. At the same time, children with acute lymphocytic leukemia, which used to be invariably fatal in weeks or months, have benefited from new therapies, with at least half now surviving three years, some more than five years, and a few on the verge of being pronounced cured. Similar advances in the treatment of a cancer of the lymph system called *Hodgkin's disease* have improved the five-year survival rate from 25 percent at the end of World War II to about 55 percent today.

What Is Cancer?

Cancer would surely be easier to detect and treat if it were a single entity with a single simple cause. But it is not. Experts agree that there are actually some 100 different diseases that can be called cancers. They have different causes, originate in different tissues, develop for different reasons and in different ways, and demand vastly different kinds of treatment. All have one fatal element in common,

Normal cells

1. Cell surface bonding is strong.
2. Cells remain in place.
3. Electrical voltage level is high.
4. Cells divide at a low rate.

Malignant cells

1. Cell surface bonding is very weak.
2. Cells spread and invade normal tissue.
3. Electrical voltage level is low.
4. Cells divide at a rapid pace.

however; in every case, normal cells have gone wild and lost their growth and development controls.

Initial Stages

The cancer may start with just one or a few cells somewhere in the body that undergo a change and become malignant, or cancerous. The cells divide and reproduce themselves, and the cancer grows.

Most cancers arise on the surface of a tissue, such as the skin, the lining of the uterus, mouth, stomach, bowel, bladder, or bronchial tube in the lung, or inside a duct in the breast, prostate gland, or other site. Eventually, they grow from a microscopic clump to a visible mass, then begin to invade underlying tissues. As long as the cells remain in one mass, however, the cancer is localized.

Later Stages

At some later phase, in a process called *metastasis,* some of the cancer cells split off and are swept into the lymph channels or bloodstream to other parts of the body. They may be captured for a while in a nearby lymph node (a stage called *regional involvement*), but unless the disease is arrested, it will rapidly invade the rest of the body, with death the almost

certain result. Some cancers grow with a malevolent rapidity; some are dormant by comparison. Some respond to various therapies, such as radiation therapy; others do not. About half of the known types of cancer are incurable at any stage. Of the remaining half, it is obviously imperative to diagnose and treat them as early as possible.

How Cancers Are Classified

The cancers described above, arising in *epithelial* (covering or lining) tissue, are called *carcinomas* as a group. Another class of malignant tumors, similar in most basic respects, is the *sarcomas,* which originate in connective tissue, such as bones and muscles. A third group of cancers—*leukemia* and the *lymphomas*—includes diseases of the blood-forming organs and the lymphatic system, respectively, and does not produce tumors. They arise and spread in a basically different way.

What Causes Cancer?

In its battle with cancer, medical science devotes constant attention to a search for those factors in our environment that can produce cancer in human beings. They include a large number of chemical agents such as

those in tobacco smoke, and including asbestos fibers and other occupational chemical hazards; ionizing radiation such as that from X rays, nuclear bombs, and sunlight; injury or repeated irritation; metal or plastic implants; flaws in the body's immune reaction; genetic mistakes; parasites; and—many scientists believe— viruses.

It is this last factor that is generating perhaps the most interest among medical scientists today. It has been shown that viruses cause a variety of cancers in animals; yet they have never been proved responsible in human cancer, although they have been linked to at least six different ones. Recently, researchers discovered an enzyme in a virus believed to cause cancer and also in the tissues of leukemia patients. This enzyme may be the key to the mechanism by which a virus induces a malignant change in normal cells.

Scientists have also discovered that certain substances in the environment which by themselves may not stimulate the growth of a cancer can be dangerously activated to become carcinogenic by the presence of one or more other substances. Each of these potential cancer-causing agents is called a *cocarcinogen.* It is possible that some cocarcinogens are present in ordinary fruits and vegetables, in certain food additives, and in such other substances as the synthetic estrogen diethylstilbestrol (DES). For more information on DES, see Ch. 25, *Women's Health.*

Major Forms of Cancer

The following material includes discussions of the major forms of cancer with the exception of those cancers that affect women only. For additional information on many kinds of tumors for which surgery may be indicated, see also Ch. 20, *Surgery*.

Breast Cancer

See under *Women's Health,* Ch. 25.

Lung Cancer

Lung cancer kills more Americans than any other cancer. The average annual death toll for recent years is more than 90,000 men and more than 45,000 women. It represents 36 percent of all cancers in men, 20 percent of all cancers in women. There has been a dramatic increase in the incidence of lung cancer in women over the past 35 years to where it has surpassed breast cancer as the leading cause of cancer death among women. The five-year survival rate for this disease is between 10 and 20 percent.

Symptoms

Although some early lung cancers do not show up on an X-ray film, they are the ones that usually produce coughing as an early symptom. For this reason, any cough that lasts more than two or three weeks—even if it seems to accompany a cold or bronchitis—should be regarded as suspicious and investigated in that light. Blood in the sputum is another early warning sign that must be investigated immediately; so should wheezing when breathing. Later symptoms include shortness of breath, pain in the chest, fever, and night sweats.

Detection

If many lives could be saved by preventing lung cancer in the first place, others could be saved by early detection. By the time most lung cancers are diagnosed, it is too late even for the most radical approach to cure—removal of the afflicted lung. Experts estimate that up to five times the present cure rate could be achieved if very early lung cancers could be spotted. They therefore recommend a routine chest X ray every six months for everyone over 45.

Causes

Lung cancer is one of the most preventable of all malignancies. Most cases, the majority of medical experts agree, are caused by smoking cigarettes. The U.S. Public Health Service has indicted smoking as "the main cause of lung cancer in men." Even when other agents are known to produce lung cancers—uranium ore dust or asbestos fibers, for example—cigarette smoking enormously boosts the risk among uranium miners and asbestos workers. Smoking accounts for 90 percent of all lung cancer deaths.

It is known that the lungs of some cigarette smokers show tissue changes before cancer appears, changes apparently caused by irritation of the lining of the *bronchi*—the large air tubes in the lung. Physicians believe these changes can be reversed before the onset of cancer if the source of irritation—smoking—is removed. This is why a heavy smoker who has been puffing away for many years but then stops smoking has a better chance of avoiding lung cancer than one who continues smoking.

Until recently, the evidence linking cigarette smoking and lung cancer was purely statistical, although overwhelming. No one had succeeded in producing lung cancer in laboratory animals by having them ingest smoke. However, lung cancer has been induced in dogs specially trained to in-

hale cigarette smoke, as reported by the American Cancer Society.

Cigarette smoking has also been implicated in other kinds of lung disease, including the often-fatal emphysema, and in cardiovascular diseases. To any sensible person, then, the options would seem clear: If you don't smoke, don't start. If you do smoke, stop. If you can't stop, cut down, and switch to a brand low in tars and nicotine—suspected but not proved to be the principal harmful agents in cigarette smoke.

Colon-Rectum Cancer

Cancer of the colon (large intestine) and rectum is the second leading cause of cancer death in the United States. Each year it claims an estimated 55,000 lives, and produces about 150,000 new cases—more than any other kind of cancer except skin cancer. It afflicts men and women about equally. The five-year survival rate from this form of cancer, usually after surgery, is 60 to 70 percent where the cancer was localized and 30 to 40 percent where there was regional involvement. However, authorities now believe that this rate could be upped substantially through early diagnosis and prompt treatment.

Symptoms

It is important, then, to be alert to the early symptoms of these cancers. Cancers of the colon often produce changes in bowel habits that persist longer than normal. The change may be constipation or diarrhea, or even both alternating. Cancers of the colon also often produce large quantities of gas, which cause abdominal discomfort ranging from a feeling of overfullness to pain, intermittent at first and then coming as regular cramps.

Both colon cancer and rectal cancer may also cause bleeding. Sometimes such bleeding is evidenced in the stool or on the tissue (the most frequent first sign of rectal cancer); but if the bleeding is slight and occurs high enough up the colon, it may not be visible at all. After a period of weeks, however, the persistent bleeding causes anemia in the patient.

All such symptoms should be investigated promptly. Unfortunately, many persons tend to ignore them. Chronic constipation, for example, or gas, is easy to dismiss for the nuisance that it usually is. Even rectal bleeding, which demands immediate medical consultation, is often ignored by hemorrhoid sufferers, who fail to realize that hemorrhoids and cancer, though unrelated, can and sometimes do exist in the same persons at the same time.

Detection

For these reasons, the key to successful and early diagnosis of colon and rectum cancer lies in making a *proctoscopy* part of the regular annual health checkup. In this procedure, performed in a physician's office, a lighted tube called a *proctoscope* is passed into the rectum. Through it, the physician can examine the walls visually for signs of tumor. If the physician thinks it advisable to check the sigmoid colon also, the procedure is called a *proctosigmoidoscopy,* and a similar instrument called a *sigmoidoscope* is used. The American Cancer Society now recommends that everyone over age 40 have a proctoscopy or proctosigmoidoscopy in routine annual checkups.

Therapy

The indicated treatment for colon-rectum cancer is surgical removal of the affected part of the bowel. Adjacent portions and related lymph nodes may also be removed, and if the surgeon sees that the cancer is widespread, he may have to perform extensive surgery. This may require that he create a *colostomy*—a temporary or permanent opening in the abdominal wall through which solid wastes may pass. Although this method of voiding the bowels is somewhat inconvenient at first, most colostomy patients adjust to it very easily and lead perfectly normal, active, and healthy lives. The wall of prudish silence that used to surround the disease and the colostomy is fortunately crumbling. An organization for colostomy patients called the United Ostomy Association keeps up with current information on diet, colostomy equipment, and other problems the members have in common.

Radiotherapy is sometimes used before the operation (occasionally to make surgery possible) and sometimes afterward to treat recurrence of the cancer. Various chemical agents have been found useful in treating colon-rectum cancer that has spread to the lymph nodes or more widely.

Skin Cancer

With as many as 500,000 new cases occurring annually, skin cancer is the largest single source of malignancy in the United States. An estimated 6,000 persons die of this disease each year. Since 1980, the number of cases of malignant melanoma, the most deadly form of skin cancer, has risen by more than 90 percent.

Experts believe that many cases of skin cancer could be prevented if more people avoided exposure to the sun. Radiation in sunlight not only burns and dries the skin; it also is thought to suppress the human immune system and thus contribute indirectly to skin problems. Long and continued exposure to the sun has been associated with cataracts as well as with skin aging and wrinkling.

Symptoms

Persons with skin problems should report promptly to their physicians any sores that refuse to heal, or changes in warts or moles. Pimples that itch and recur may also be symptoms of skin cancer.

Therapy

Most skin cancers remain localized. They can usually be removed by excisional surgery, with an electric needle, or by cryosurgery (freezing). X-ray irradiation and chemotherapy may also be used.

Causes

Most skin cancers appear after the age of 40. Scientists point to the ultraviolet radiation in sunlight as the primary cause, with ultraviolet-B (UV-B), the shorter wavelength band, as the more dangerous. But dermatologists recommend that ultraviolet-A (UV-A), used often in high-intensity sunlamps and tanning beds, be avoided as well. While UV-A is spread more evenly throughout the day, UV-B is largely concentrated around midday.

Fair-skinned individuals who burn readily, rather than tanning, are more vulnerable to radiation-caused cancer than darker-skinned persons. Geographic location is also important. Skin cancer occurs more frequently in the southern belt of states, particularly in the sunny Southwest.

Chemicals, too, can cause skin cancer. Before the relationship was discovered, skin cancer was an occupational hazard for many thousands of unprotected workers who dealt with arsenic and various derivatives of coal and petroleum.

Kinds

Of the three primary kinds of skin cancer, two are both common and relatively curable. These are basal-cell and squamous-cell *carcinoma.* Early detection almost ensures that a cure can be effected.

A *melanoma,* or so-called *black cancer,* is a malignant tumor that arises from a mole. The moles may begin as flat, soft, brown, and hairless protrusions, but they can change suddenly into darker, larger growths that itch and bleed. They can also metastasize, spreading cancer cells to other parts of the body through the bloodstream and the lymphatic system.

Unlike other types of skin cancer, melanomas may grow in skin areas not usually exposed to the sun, such as the feet, in the genital area, or under the belt or collar. Chronic irritation from tight clothing is one suspected cause. Melanomas rarely occur before middle age; nearly three-fourths of the victims are women.

Oral Cancer

Cancers of the mouth and lips strike an estimated 24,000 persons in the United States each year and kill a shocking 8,500. Shocking because anyone with the aid of a mirror and a good light can see into his mouth and therefore spot even very small cancers early in their development.

Symptoms

Any sore, lump, or lesion of the mouth or lips should be regarded as suspicious if it persists more than two weeks without healing, and a physi-

cian or dentist should then be consulted without delay. The five-year survival rate for localized mouth cancers—when they are usually no larger than the little fingernail—is 67 percent—about two out of three. But if regional involvement occurs, the rate falls to 30 percent—fewer than one out of three.

Detection

Just as the Pap test screens for cervical cancer by scraping up sloughed-off cells that are then examined under a microscope, so one day your dentist may routinely scrape mouth cells to detect oral cancer. When more than 40,000 patients were screened over a five-and-one-half-year period at the Western Tennessee Cancer Clinic, about 230 cases of oral cancer were diagnosed, of which 35 percent would have been missed otherwise.

Right now, a weekly or monthly personal inspection of your mouth is the best detective method available. The American Cancer Society has materials explaining the best way to conduct such an examination.

Therapy

Oral cancers are treated by surgical removal or by irradiation.

Causes

No one can pinpoint the causes of oral cancer definitely, but there are a number of leading suspects. They are smoking, in all its forms; exposure to wind and sun (for lip cancer); poor mouth hygiene; sharp or rough-edged teeth or improperly fitted, irritating dentures; dietary inadequacies, and constant consumption of alcohol or very hot foods and liquids.

Ovarian and Uterine Cancer

See under *Women's Health,* Ch. 25.

Stomach Cancer

Before World War II, cancer of the stomach was the most common type of cancer among men and women in the United States. The death rate from stomach cancer in the 1930s was about 30 per 100,000 population. In recent years, stomach cancer has declined in proportion to other forms of the disease, such as lung, breast, and uterine cancer. However, stomach cancer is still one of the more frequently diagnosed types of cancer and the death rate is relatively high, at nearly 10 per 100,000 population.

Today, men are twice as likely to be victims of stomach cancer as women. The disease is seldom found in persons under 40 years of age, but after that age the incidence increases steadily, reaching a peak before the age of 60. One of the disease's mysterious incidental factors is its peculiar geographical distribution, the highest rates of occurrence being in Japan, Chile, Iceland, northern Russia, and the Scandinavian countries.

Symptoms

Stomach cancer seems to develop slowly and insidiously, with initial symptoms that may be disregarded by the patient because they mimic ordinary gastric distress. The victim may experience a distaste for foods, particularly meats, and display a slow but progressive loss of weight. There may be sensations of fullness, bloating, or pain after meals. The same symptoms may be noted between meals and be aggravated by eating. The pain may vary from intermittent stomachaches to intense pain that seems to extend into the patient's back. The patient also experiences fatigue or weakness and anemia, and, as the cancerous condition progresses, may have periods of vomiting. The vomitus is dark, much like the color of coffee grounds, and there may be other signs of bleeding in the patient's stools.

Cancer's Seven Warning Signals*

1. Change in bowel or bladder habits
2. A sore that does not heal
3. Unusual bleeding or discharge
4. Thickening or lump in breast or elsewhere
5. Indigestion or difficulty in swallowing
6. Obvious change in wart or mole
7. Nagging cough or hoarseness

If you have a warning signal, see your doctor without delay.

*from the American Cancer Society

Detection

X rays of the stomach and examination of the stomach interior by gastroscopy usually locate and define the cancerous area; they may also reveal another cause of the symptoms, such as a peptic ulcer. During the physical examination, the physician may find a tissue mass and tenderness in the stomach area. The laboratory report usually will show signs of anemia from blood loss, the presence of blood in a stool sample, and the level of hydrochloric acid in the stomach; a lack of hydrochloric acid is found in more than half the stomach cancer patients. A biopsy study of the suspected tissue usually completes the diagnosis.

Therapy

Unfortunately, because of the insidious nature of stomach cancer, the disease becomes easier to diagnose as it progresses. By the time cancer has been confirmed, the most expedient form of treatment is surgery to remove the affected area of the stomach. If the cancer is small and has not spread by metastasis to lymph nodes in the region, the chances are relatively good that the patient will survive five years or more; the odds against surviving five years without surgery are, by comparison, about 50 to 1 at best. Chemotherapy treatments may be used in cases where surgery is not feasible, but the use of medicines instead of surgery for stomach cancer is not a routine procedure and generally is not recommended.

Occasionally, a stomach tumor is found to be noncancerous. The tumor may be a polyp, a *leiomyoma* (a growth consisting of smooth muscle tissue), or a *pseudotumor* (false tumor), such as an inflammatory fibroid growth. Such benign tumors produce symptoms ranging from gastric upset to internal bleeding and should be removed by surgery.

Causes

Many possible factors have been suggested as causes of stomach cancer. Dietary factors include hot food and beverages, as well as fish and smoked foods. Food additives have been implicated despite the fact that the incidence of stomach cancer has been declining during the period in which the use of additives has been increasing. Cured meats and cheeses, preserved with nitrites to retard spoilage, reportedly foster the development of carcinogenic chemical compounds in the digestive tract.

On the other hand, the widespread use of refrigeration has been offered as an explanation for the declining incidence of stomach cancer, since refrigeration reduces the need for chemical food preservatives.

Beyond the influence of diet, medical epidemiologists have found that genetic factors may play a role in the development of stomach cancer. Statistical analysis of large population studies of stomach cancer shows a tendency for the disease to occur in persons with blood type A, or with below-normal levels of hydrochloric acid in the stomach, or with inherited variations in the stomach lining. There also seems to be a good possibility that stomach cancers evolve from noncancerous changes in the stomach lining, as from polyps or peptic ulcers.

Bladder Cancer

As with stomach cancer, the incidence of cancer of the bladder rises progressively with age and occurs much more frequently in men than in women. Extensive occurrence of bladder cancer is commonly associated with industrial growth, but internationally its incidence ranges from a high rate in England to a low one in Japan; in the United States, the highest incidence of bladder cancer is in southern New Jersey. A study by the Roswell Park Memorial Institute, a cancer research center in Buffalo, New York, found that persons of Italian-American parentage were more likely to have bladder cancer than those of different parentage, and that women living in urban areas were more likely to develop the disease than their country cousins. American blacks have less bladder cancer than American whites.

Bladder cancer appears at an annual rate of about 40,000 new cases each year in the United States and causes more than 15,000 deaths annually.

Symptoms

A change in bladder habits is among the first signs of bladder cancer. The change might be the presence of pain while urinating, a noticeable difficulty in urinating, or a difference in the frequency of urination.

Another symptom of the disease is the appearance of blood in the urine. The degree of blood coloration is not necessarily related to the severity of the cancer; any sign of blood in the urine should be investigated. Nor should the absence of pain be allowed to minimize the seriousness of urinary bleeding as a symptom of a diseased bladder. Even without pain, the presence of blood can indicate a problem such as an obstruction to the urinary flow that can lead to uremia, a toxic condition caused by retention of urinary waste products in the system.

Detection

Cancer of the bladder is frequently diagnosed from common signs and symptoms, particularly the appearance of blood in the urine. A laboratory examination of the patient's urine may also reveal the presence of cancer cells that have been washed out of the bladder. The disease can be detected by a *pyelogram*—a kind of X-ray picture made by filling the urinary system with a fluid that makes tissue details appear in sharp contrast—and by examination of the membrane lining the bladder. The bladder lining may be examined by surgical biopsy or by *cystoscopy*, the viewing of the interior of the bladder by means of a device inserted in the urethra—or both.

Examination of the bladder lining is needed to determine the type of tumor that may be the cause of the symptoms. One type, called a *papillary tumor*, or *papilloma*, is relatively harmless and usually does not invade the wall of the bladder as does the more dangerous type, sometimes described as a solid lesion. The degree of invasion of the bladder tissues by

the infiltrating mass determines the type of treatment recommended. However, any tumor found in the lining of the bladder must be removed, because the papillary type can progress into a solid lesion if not treated.

Therapy

The cure of a bladder tumor can be approached in several ways, the choice of treatments depending upon the size and type of growth, the location of the tumor, and so on. Chemotherapy, using drugs such as thiotepa, has been successful in treating papillary bladder tumors; the chemical is applied directly to the bladder lining. A kind of electric cautery known as *fulguration* also may be used to destroy the tissue growth; it may be employed by cystoscopy or as part of a surgical approach. Radiation therapy also may be used by implanting radium needles in the affected bladder tissue. Surgical excision of the cancerous area, with or without radiation, chemotherapy, or cautery, may be the procedure chosen. In advanced cases of bladder cancer, the bladder may be removed and its function performed by the construction of a substitute organ from other tissues or by the relocation of the upper ends of the ureters at other urine-collecting points.

Causes

Cancer of the bladder may be caused by irritation from bladder stones or by toxic chemicals excreted from the kidneys. A high incidence of bladder cancer has been found among persons who are heavy cigarette smokers; a possible explanation is that certain carcinogenic tobacco-burning by-products are absorbed into the blood and excreted through the kidneys. The evidence includes studies show-

ing that when such patients quit smoking, the carcinogens no longer appear in their urine.

Occupational factors have been associated with cancer of the bladder since 1895, when it was discovered that persons who worked with aniline chemical dyes were among those most likely to develop the disease. The incidence of the disease among chemical workers was found to be 30 times greater than that of the general population. The aniline dye workers developed bladder cancer at an average age 15 years younger than among the general population. The effect of the chemical dyes was verified by the development of cancer in the bladders of laboratory animals exposed to the dyes. In recent years, it has been found that many other chemicals can cause bladder cancer.

Besides the influence of industrial environmental factors, bladder cancer is associated with *schistosomiasis,* a disease occurring in Africa, Asia, South America, and other regions. Schistosomiasis develops after bathing or wading in water infested by a blood fluke. The organisms penetrate the skin and migrate to the intestines or urinary bladder, producing an inflammation that eventually leads to cancer. See Ch. 19, *Other Diseases of Major Importance,* for a fuller description of the disease.

Cancer of the Prostate

Cancer of the prostate is one of the most common cancers among men and is second only to lung cancer as a lethal type of tumor for men. About 30,000 people die of prostate cancer each year. The incidence increases with advancing age from the fifth decade of life, when prostatic cancer cells are found in nearly 20 percent of all men examined, to those in their 70s, an age when 60 percent of the men have been found to have cancer cells in their prostate glands. Fortunately, only 15 percent of the men with evidence of latent carcinoma of the prostate ever develop clinical symptoms of cancer before death. But after the age of 75, there are almost as many deaths, due to prostatic cancer as to lung cancer.

Symptoms

Cancer of the prostate is a disease noted for its secondary symptoms. It usually is detected because a physician begins analyzing symptoms that could suggest other disorders. There may, for example, be blood in the urine, indicating a serious problem that could be located anywhere along the urinary tract. Because the prostate encircles the urethra, which is the outlet from the bladder, any prostatic problem can cause disturbances in the normal passage of urine, including increased frequency of urination or discomfort in urinating. However, these also could be the symptoms of ailments other than cancer of the prostate.

Detection

Diagnosis of prostatic cancer usually begins with an examination of the prostate through the wall of the rectum. This technique is a regular part of a physical examination for men over the age of 40. If during the examination of the prostate the physician feels a lump or hardened area, further tests are ordered. The presence of a lump in the prostate need not be evidence of cancer; about half of the lumps and nodules are caused by fibrosis, calcium deposits, or other noncancerous bodies. Transrectal ultrasound is a newer detection method used in conjunction with the traditional digital rectal examination.

Additional tests may include examination by a cystoscope, which is inserted through the urethra to provide a view of the tissues of the area, plus a laboratory examination of tissue samples and prostatic fluid samples. A microscopic study of the samples may reveal the presence of cancer cells. The examination of prostatic cells for signs of cancer is similar to the technique used in the Pap test for cancer of the cervix in women.

In the search for evidence of cancer of the prostate, diagnostic clues may be found in blood chemistry tests and by the examination of a urinary pyelogram that could indicate obstructions from the prostate walls. Additional information may be forthcoming from an evaluation of the patient's medical history; low back pain complaints, for example, may result from prostate disorders.

Therapy

Surgery is the usual treatment for cancer of the prostate when the tumor is confined to the prostate gland. The surgical removal of the prostate may be supplemented by the administration of estrogens, or hormone therapy. If the cancer has spread to other areas, a frequent complication of prostatic cancer, an additional form of therapy could be the administration of radioactive drugs or some other form of radiation. An additional measure may be *orchiectomy,* the surgical removal of the testicles, performed because of the close physiological relationship between the testicles and the prostate. Impotence is a major result of prostate cancer, and if female hormones are administered, water retention, painful breast enlargement, and cardiovascular complications can result. An alternative to orchiectomy or hormone therapy is the monthly injection of luteinizing hormone-

releasing hormone agonists, which disrupts the normal production of testosterone.

Causes

Cancer of the prostate seems to be associated with activity of the sex hormones in men. It has been reported that all patients with prostatic cancer previously had a normal history of sex-hormone activity. The cancer symptoms begin to appear at a period of life when male sex-hormone activity is waning. Laboratory studies of the urine of patients show a decrease in levels of male sex hormones after the age of 40. As in female breast cancer, which also is related to sex-hormone activity, there are certain tissues of the body that appear to be more sensitive to influences of hormones. Changes in hormonal activity lead to increasing numbers of cells in those tissues and abnormal tissue growth.

Cancer of the Kidney

Cancer of the kidneys is most likely to occur in young children or in adults over the age of 40. The most common form of kidney cancer in children is known as *Wilms' tumor.* In adults, kidney cancer is usually in the form of a growth called *Grawitz's tumor,* or *hypernephroma,* a malignant growth that occurs chiefly among men.

Wilms' Tumor

Wilms' tumor, also called *nephroblastoma,* accounts for perhaps 25 percent of all cancers in children. About 90 percent of the cases develop before the age of seven; it has been diagnosed in infants less than five months old.

Symptoms

The symptoms can include fever, abdominal pain, weight loss, lack of appetite, blood in the urine, and an abdominal mass that may grow quickly to enormous size. The growth may be accompanied by symptoms of hypertension.

Detection

Examination of the patient may show the tumor to be on either the left or the right kidney. In a small percentage of the cases both kidneys are affected. A biopsy usually is performed in order to verify the presence of cancer cells in the growth.

Therapy

Treatment is most effective when the disease is diagnosed before the age of two. Surgery, radiation, and chemotherapy may be employed. The choice of chemotherapeutic agents may be varied as follow-up examinations reveal side effects or tumor resistance to one of the previously administered medications.

The five-year survival rate for victims of Wilms' tumor is about 65 percent when surgery and other measures are employed at an early stage. If not controlled, the cancer cells from Wilms' tumor tend to spread by metastasis to the lungs, liver, and other organs.

Causes

Wilms' tumor is believed to be congenital in nature. Studies of the tumor cells indicate that it may develop from embryonic kidney tissue that fails to evolve as a normal part of that organ.

Grawitz's Tumor

In about half of the cases of Grawitz's tumor, the common adult kidney cancer, the disease manifests itself through a combination of three symptoms: abdominal mass, pain in the area of the kidneys, and blood in the urine. In the other half of the cases, the cancer has metastasized and is found in the brain, lung, liver, or bone.

Detection

The physician may get important information about the seriousness of the tumor through laboratory studies of blood and urine samples; these can indicate the presence of substances that appear in body fluids when cancer cells are active.

Information can also be obtained by angiogram studies. An angiogram is an X-ray picture of an organ that has been injected with a dye to make the blood vessels, which carry the dye, markedly visible. A kidney angiogram shows different dye patterns for a normal organ, a kidney with a cyst, or a kidney with a tumor. The diagnosis usually is confirmed by biopsy or surgical exploration.

Therapy

Surgery and radiation treatment are the usual forms of therapy for adult kidney tumors, and the chances of ten-year survival, even after removal of a cancerous kidney, are fairly good.

Causes

Causes of adult kidney tumors remain largely unknown, but they have been thought to be associated with other disorders, such as infections or the presence of kidney stones.

Cancer of the Pancreas

Pancreatic cancer affects men about twice as frequently as women and accounts for about five percent of the cancer deaths. It is most likely to develop after the age of 40, and persons who are diabetic seem to be particularly susceptible to the disease.

Symptoms

The pancreatic cancer patient complains of apparent digestive disorders, such as abdominal pain, nausea, loss of appetite, and perhaps constipation. The abdominal distress may improve or worsen after eating and the pain may increase when the patient lies on his back. He will suffer weight loss and there will be jaundice. Many victims of pancreatic cancer also complain of itching sensations. Abdominal pain is usually persistent.

Detection

Along with signs of jaundice and scratching, the examining physician will evaluate laboratory reports of urine, blood, and stool analyses. Glucose tolerance tests and bilirubin levels are helpful in defining the source of the disorder. Negative findings of X-ray studies of the gastrointestinal tract, kidney-bladder area, and gallbladder can suggest a pancreatic disorder; by their normal condition, the physician can conclude that the disease is elsewhere in the abdominal region.

Therapy

Surgery is the usual treatment recommended for cancer of the pancreas; the precise location of the tumor within the pancreas may determine the exact surgical procedure to be undertaken. Removal of the tumor surgically has a more hopeful outcome if it is located at the head of the pancreas; cancers in the body or tail of the pancreas usually are not detected until the disease has spread to other parts of the body. Radiation and chemotherapy are not as effective in the treatment of pancreatic cancer as in other organs.

Cancer of the Liver

Cancer of the liver is commonly found to be the result of metastasis from other parts of the body. Cancers that originate in the liver account for less than 2 percent of the cancers reported in the United States and occur more frequently in men than in women, most frequently after the age of 40. Cancer of the liver is usually fatal.

Symptoms

Weakness, weight loss, and pain in the upper abdomen or right side of the chest are among the symptoms of liver cancer. A fever apparently unrelated to any infection also may mark the onset of liver cancer.

Detection

An enlarged liver with masses of abnormal tissue may be detected by an examining physician. Laboratory tests usually reveal alterations in metabolism that are associated with changes in the liver cells caused by the cancer growth. A biopsy test of the abnormal liver tissue may confirm the presence of cancer. A more direct approach is to perform exploratory surgery for examination of the liver.

Therapy

If the tumor is located during exploratory surgery and the area can be ex-

cised, part of the liver is removed. Chemotherapy may also be used.

A nonsurgical therapy for liver cancer involves the use of so-called "radiolabeled antibodies." To these molecules of antibodies, the defensive compounds of the body, radioactive substances are attached. The antibodies then seek out the cancer cells, and the radioactivity helps them destroy the cancer. The procedure has been used experimentally on patients whose tumors were too large for surgical instruments.

Causes

While the exact cause of primary liver cancer is unknown, a large proportion of cases is associated with cirrhosis of the liver. In recent years, some types of liver cancer have been traced to exposure of industrial workers to chemicals known to be carcinogenic. The high incidence of primary liver cancer in Asia and Africa is related to *aflatoxins* (molds) in grains and legumes, such as peanuts.

Secondary cancers of the liver are the result of primary cancers in other body areas; the liver is vulnerable to metastasis from cancers in every organ except the brain because of the pattern of blood circulation that carries cancer cells through the body.

Cancer of the Brain

Cancers in the brain tissue frequently are the result of metastasis from other body organs. They travel through the bloodstream, primarily from cancers of the lung, kidney, gastrointestinal tract, and breast. They become implanted in both the cerebrum and cerebellum, and, although there is wide distribution of the cancer cells, they are clustered mainly near the surfaces of the brain tissues. Primary brain tumors are more com-

mon among children than among adults; in children, other cancer sites are not likely to have had time to develop to the stage of metastasis required for the transmission of malignant cells to the brain.

A cancer that seems to originate in the brain tissues is known as *glioblastoma multiforme,* a malignant growth that may strike at any age but is more likely to occur during middle age. The glioblastoma may develop in nearly any part of the brain structure, including the brain stem, and spread extensively into a large tumorous mass.

Symptoms

Symptoms of brain cancer may include headache, dizziness, nervousness, depression, mental confusion, vomiting, and paralysis. The symptoms sometimes are interpreted as those of a psychiatric disorder, and treatment of the organic disease may be postponed until too late.

Detection

Diagnosis may be difficult, and the physician must evaluate the symptoms in terms of other findings from laboratory tests, X rays, and other techniques. In some cases, cancer cells may be detected in samples of spinal fluid.

Therapy

Treatment of brain cancers usually requires surgery or radiation or both, depending upon the type of tumor, its location, and other factors. Whether or not the brain tumor is a true cancer is not as important as early treatment; any abnormal tissue growth in the brain causes destructive pressure against vital tissues.

Cancer of the Larynx

Cancer of the larynx is chiefly a disease of men, afflicting about eight times as many men as women, usually around the age of 60. It is not one of the major types of cancer, with about 9,000 new cases appearing each year in the United States; but more than 35 percent of these cases are fatal. About 70 percent involve tumors on the vocal cords and are classed as *intrinsic* cancers of the larynx. The remainder of the cases involve tissues originating outside the vocal cords and are designated as *extrinsic*.

Symptoms

One of the first symptoms of intrinsic cancer of the larynx is hoarseness. Later the patient loses his ability to speak and has difficulty breathing. The same series of symptoms occurs in cases of extrinsic cancer except that there is an initial period of pain or discomfort in the throat before hoarseness begins. *Adenopathy,* or swelling of the lymph nodes in the area, also may be an early symptom of extrinsic cancer of the larynx.

Detection

Diagnosis of cancer of the larynx is relatively simple because the throat's interior can be examined by a physician and tissue samples can be removed for biopsy study. Detection of extrinsic cancer may be complicated by the fact that it is more likely to metastasize than intrinsic forms.

Therapy

In early cases of intrinsic cancer, or for small lesions that appear in the middle of the vocal cords, radiation may be the therapy of choice.

Surgery may be required for more serious cases, with radiation treatments before or after surgery, or both. The surgery, called a *laryngectomy,* may involve partial or total removal of the larynx. If a partial laryngectomy is performed, an effort is made to save as much of the vocal cords as possible. The voice will be changed after surgery, but it will be functional. The respiratory tract will be preserved. When total laryngectomy is required, the entire larynx is removed and the neck is dissected to determine if cancer cells have migrated to the lymph nodes in the neck. A new trachea is constructed by plastic surgery to permit normal or nearly normal respiration.

Thyroid Cancer

Cancer of the thyroid gland is relatively uncommon, with fewer than three new cases per 100,000 population per year. The death rate is even less, about one thyroid-cancer death per year per 200,000 persons. One reason for the low death rate is that many of the cancers are detected during examination or surgery for goiter or other throat symptoms.

Symptoms

These include rapid growth of the thyroid gland, hoarseness, paralysis of nerves in the larynx, and enlarged lymph nodes in the neck and surrounding area. Diagnosis is aided by the rate at which suspected areas of cancer in the thyroid gland absorb radioactive iodine; the pattern of radioactive uptake helps pinpoint tissue abnormalities.

Therapy

Treatment may include surgery to remove the cancer and part of the surrounding tissue, plus removal of lymph nodes that may contain cancer cells that have metastasized from the thyroid tumor. In addition, other lymph nodes that are in the path of drainage from the thyroid gland may be removed. Surgery usually is more successful in young patients than in older persons. Radiation sometimes is used, either from an external source or by injection of large doses of radioactive chemicals.

Causes

Among causes of cancer of the thyroid gland is exposure of children and young adults to radiation therapy of the head and neck region; many such patients later develop thyroid cancer.

Hodgkin's Disease

Hodgkin's disease is one of the *lymphomas*—cancers of the lymphatic system. It occurs most commonly among young adults, although it can appear at any age. Men are more likely to be victims than are women.

Symptoms

One of the first symptoms of Hodgkin's disease is a painless enlargement of a lymph node, usually in the area of the neck. The enlarged lymph nodes usually are firm and rubbery at first. The patient may experience a severe and persistent itching for several weeks or months before the first enlarged lymph node appears.

Other symptoms may include shortness of breath, fever, weight loss, anemia, and some pressure or pain as the disease progresses and nerve tissue becomes involved. Gradually, the lymph nodes that originally were separate and movable become matted and fixed, and sometimes inflamed. Over a period of months to years, the disease spreads through other parts of the body.

Therapy

Hodgkin's disease is ordinarily confirmed by removal of an affected lymph node for biopsy study. If the disease is limited to one or two localized areas the usual therapy is radiation treatments. Surgical excision of the nodes may be employed in special cases, as when a mass of nodes threatens a vital organ. But intense radiation exposure is generally more effective than surgery. Radiation treatments when properly applied may have a cure rate of as high as 95 percent. In cases where the disease has spread over a large area of the body, the treatment of choice may be chemotherapy utilizing nitrogen mustard, steroid drugs, and other substances.

Causes

The cause of Hodgkin's disease is unknown. Because of the fever and other symptoms associated with the disorder, and because it appears to occur more frequently among members of the same family or community than in the population as a whole, it has been suggested that Hodgkin's disease is a viral disease that has a malignant effect on the human lymphatic system.

Leukemia

Because leukemia involves blood cells circulating through the body rather than a fixed mass of tissue, leukemia is sometimes not considered a true cancer. However, leukemia cells, when studied under the microscope and in cell cultures, behave like cancer cells found in tumors.

There are at least ten different kinds of blood cells that have been identified with various forms of the disease. In addition, there are both acute and chronic forms of leukemia, such as *acute granulocytic leukemia* and *chronic lymphocytic leukemia,* named after the particular kind of white blood cells that are most affected.

Leukemia affects the blood-forming tissues, such as the bone marrow, resulting in an overproduction of white blood cells. The disease is particularly lethal to children under the age of 15; more than 10 percent of the leukemia deaths each year are among children. The incidence by age group varies according to the specific type of leukemia, however; one variety of acute granulocytic leukemia can occur at any age, but chronic lymphocytic leukemia usually does not appear before the age of 40. Men are more likely than women to be the victims of one of the various forms of leukemia.

Symptoms

Common symptoms to all leukemias include fever, weight loss, fatigue, bone pain, anemia as expressed in paleness, and an enlarged spleen or masses under the skin caused by an accumulation of leukemic cells. There may be skin lesions and a tendency to bleed. Infections may become more common and less responsive to treatment because of a loss of the normal blood cells needed to resist disease.

Detection

Diagnosis of leukemia from early symptoms may be difficult because they resemble those of mononucleosis and other infections. Biopsies of bone marrow and careful blood studies usually identify the disease.

Therapy

Treatment usually is directed toward reducing the size of the spleen and the number of white cells in the blood, and increasing the level of blood hemoglobin to counteract the effects of anemia. Antibiotics may be included to help control infections when natural resistance to disease has been lowered. X-ray treatments, radioactive phosphorus, anticancer drugs, and steroid hormone medications are administered according to the needs of the individual patient and the type of leukemia being treated.

Acute leukemia may be fatal within a few weeks of the onset of symptoms. But chronic cases receiving proper treatment have been known to survive more than 25 years. Remission rates are improving, partly because of new drugs and methods of treatment. The new chemotherapeutic approaches include the following:

- For acute leukemia in children, *methotrexate* has been used with increasing success. One of the antimetabolites, the family of drugs that interfere with development of essential cell components, methotrexate reduces the production in the blood of folic acid. In that way the drug competes with the cancer cells for the vital enzyme folic reductase—and inhibits the cancer's growth.

- In adults, chronic and acute forms of leukemia may be treated with *chlorambucil* or *cyclophosphamide.* Both drugs are types of nitrogen mustard. Both may produce such side effects as suppression of bone marrow, loss of hair, nausea, dizziness, and vomiting.

- In cases of acute leukemia in childhood, the vinca alkaloid drugs have proved valuable. These drugs, such as *vincristine sulfate,* are extremely powerful. They attack active cancer cells more directly than they attack normal cells. They may lead to such side effects as headaches, convulsions, and loss of some muscular control.

Other drugs in the alkaloid and other drug families have been used to treat leukemia. The others include *cytosine arabinoside,* which works to prevent cell synthesis—including cancer-cell synthesis; 6-Mercotopurine, which inhibits some metabolic processes; and *busulfan* and similar drugs, which work against multiplication of the cancer cells. Antitumor antibiotics that prevent growth of cancer cells include daunoribicin, doxorubicin, and bleomycin.

Causes

There is no general theory about the cause of leukemia. Animals are known to be susceptible to a form of leukemia transmitted by virus, but there is no solid evidence that human leukemias are caused by viral infections. Survivors of nuclear explosions as well as persons exposed to large doses of X rays have developed leukemia at a higher-than-normal rate than other people. There is evidence that at least one type of acute leukemia may be a result of an inherited genetic defect.

Other Cancers

Lymphosarcoma

Another of the cancers that involve the lymphatic system is called *lymphosarcoma*—a malignant lymphoma that tends to metastasize in lymphatic tissue. The most common first symptom is a swelling of the lymph nodes, and the diagnosis and treatment are similar to those of Hodgkin's disease. Lymphosarcoma can occur at any time and in any part of the body where there is lymphatic tissue, including the gastrointestinal tract, the tonsils, the tongue, or the nasopharynx area.

Reticulum-Cell Sarcoma

The lymphomas also include *reticulum-cell sarcoma.* (A sarcoma is a malignant tumor in the connective tissue. Reticulum cells are a particular kind of connective tissue.) The disease is marked by the invasion of normal tissue by increased numbers of reticulum cells or fibers. As in the treatment of leukemia, it is important to know which of the various types of cancer has affected the lymphatic system, because each of the lymphomas responds to a different therapeutic routine.

Myeloma and Multiple Myeloma

Myelomas, once considered rare but now reported in increasing numbers, are cancerous growths that seem to originate in the bone marrow. The average age at onset is about 65. Men are twice as likely as women to be victims of myelomas.

The disease is marked by bone destruction, mainly in the pelvis, ribs, and spine. The bones break easily, sometimes causing collapse of the spinal column and pressure on the spinal cord. There also may be anemia, kidney damage, and changes in the blood chemistry. When the myelomas occur at numerous sites in the bone marrow throughout the body, the disease is known as *multiple myeloma.*

Treatment

Various methods of treating lymphomas have evolved despite serious difficulties. Lymphomas appear in many different forms, and can change form in the process of spreading to another part of the body. Different types may be found in a single lymph gland.

Despite these difficulties, many chemotherapeutic agents have been found useful in treatment of lymphomas. To an extent, the preferred drugs fall in the same categories as those used in treating leukemia. The principal drugs, thus, include:

- alkalyting agents, such as nitrogen mustard, cyclophosphamide, and chlorambucil;

- vinca alkaloids, among them vincristine and vinblastine;

- procarbazine, which works like the alkalyting agents;

- antibiotics, which work to reduce or eliminate tumors, including Adriamycin and actinomycin D; and

- the corticosteroids, combinations of agents including hormones, acids, and other body elements.

These and other drugs have been used in various combinations in the treatment of lymphomas. One of the more successful has been named for the four drugs that are included in the protocol, or treatment series. The four are nitrogen mustard, vincristine (Oncovin), Procarbazine, and Prednisone; the combination treatment is known as MOPP. The treatment is used at certain stages of lymphoma, and has encouraged medical specialists to consider lymphoma as potentially curable.

In addition to drug therapy, methods of treating lymphomas include irradiation therapy, or radiotherapy, and a combination of drugs and radiotherapy.

19

Other Diseases of Major Importance

This chapter discusses a number of diseases of major importance that are not dealt with elsewhere: acquired immune deficiency syndrome (AIDS), a disease characterized by a defect in the body's natural immune system; plague, of great historical importance but fortunately now uncommon in the United States; two infectious diseases—tularemia and Rocky Mountain Spotted Fever; and seven tropical diseases that afflict millions of people in the warmer regions of the world and that occasionally occur elsewhere—malaria and yellow fever, leishmaniasis, trypanosomiasis, filariasis, schistosomiasis, and leprosy.

AIDS

First reported widely in 1981, AIDS has become a priority of the U.S. Public Health Service. Researchers have isolated a virus, the *human immunodeficiency virus* (*HIV*), that they believe causes AIDS. This virus was initially called the *human T-cell leukemia virus III* (*HTLV-III*). Persons with AIDS (PWAs) are susceptible to a variety of unusual or rare illnesses called *opportunistic diseases*. These include *Pneumocystis carinii* pneu-

monia (PCP); Kaposi's sarcoma; thrush, or *Candida albicans*; dementia (AIDS dementia complex or ADC); herpes simplex; and meningitis.

Groups at highest risk of contracting AIDS include homo- and bisexual men and intravenous drug users in large cities; hemophiliacs; female prostitutes; heterosexuals with multiple partners in areas where AIDS is common; and recipients of multiple blood transfusions from areas where the disease was common between 1983 and 1985. Evidence suggests that the HIV virus may also be affecting more and more young people, particularly runaways. In "passive transmission," a mother can pass AIDS to her child before or during birth.

Increasingly, medical authorities view AIDS as a disease with which victims may live for years. But AIDS is incurable. No treatment has successfully restored the immune system of an AIDS patient to normal functioning. Making the task of researching AIDS more difficult, the virus can lie inactive in the human body for as long as 10 years without causing any symptoms. Where this occurs, a "carrier" of AIDS can infect others with the disease.

Symptoms

Once infection with AIDS occurs, the human body may take from six weeks to a year or more to produce antibodies. These appear in response to the virus's invasion of the blood stream. The symptoms that can follow may resemble those of flu or even the common cold. Symptoms may include swollen glands, or enlarged lymph nodes, in the neck, armpits, or groin; night sweats; fever; unexplained rapid weight loss; chronic, unexplained diarrhea; fatigue; loss of appetite, and bruising and bleeding that do not heal.

Prevention

To prevent the spread of AIDS, the U.S. Public Health Service has recommended that persons at risk of contracting the disease should:

- Not donate blood or plasma, sperm, body organs, or other tissues

- Limit sexual contacts and be assertive with sexual partners about engaging only in safe sexual practices

- Not engage in sexual acts in which

exchange of body fluids, including semen, takes place

- Refrain from sharing toothbrushes, razors, or other implements that could be contaminated with blood

- If a drug user, limit drug use, do not let others use needles you have used, and do not leave needles or other drug paraphernalia where others might find and use them

- If a woman who has had a positive antibody test (see below), or who is the sexual partner of a man with a positive antibody test, avoid or postpone pregnancy

The Public Health Service has reported that no evidence indicates that the AIDS virus can be transmitted through casual kissing or other casual social contacts. But persons who have had positive antibody tests should let their physicians and dentists know about the test results. The physician and dentist can then cooperate in preventing the spread of the virus if the patient has become infected. There has been no risk of contracting AIDS through blood donations or transfusions since the introduction of blood-screening procedures in 1985.

Treatment

Although there is no known cure, a blood test called the *ELISA* (enzyme-linked immunosorbent assay) test has been developed to detect the presence of antibodies to the AIDS virus in human blood. The test has helped to eliminate nearly all questionable blood and plasma from the nation's blood supply—not to diagnose individuals. Laboratories have also used the Western Blot test to verify positive results from ELISA. In 1989, the FDA approved marketing of the HIVAG-1 test, the first designed to help physicians detect the AIDS virus

and to monitor its development in the human body. Already in use, a rapid screening test, the Recombigen HIV-1 Latex Agglutination test, can detect AIDS virus antibodies in five minutes.

More than 50 pharmaceutical companies have begun to develop vaccines, antiviral drugs, and other diagnostic tests for AIDS patients. The drugs in use include zidovudine, or AZT, the only compound proven effective against AIDS; alpha interferon, used to treat AIDS-generated cancer; and aerosolized pentamidine, approved in 1989 for broadened use with patients afflicted at least once with Pneumocystis pneumonia. AZT offered hope to some 600,000 Americans infected with AIDS after it was discovered that the drug can delay the onset of active symptoms.

At least 25 potential anti-HIV compounds were in various stages of testing in the late 1980s. The drugs worked in different ways. Researchers believed some of the agents might be most effective when used in combination. For example, alpha interferon has been combined in tests with AZT to reduce AZT's toxic effects, including anemia and liver problems. Various experimental drugs are designed to prevent the AIDS virus from binding to body cells, from entering into cells, or from developing into "virus factories" once inside human cells. Still others are designed to combat groups of AIDS symptoms, known as AIDS-Related Complex (ARC). Among the test drugs were several natural human products that bolster the immune system or antiviral defenses, including Imreg-2, interleukin-2, and virus-fighting interferons.

The FDA has taken steps to reduce the time elapsing between testing of drugs for treating life-threatening diseases and introduction of those compounds into the marketplace. The goal is to make possible

decisions on the approvability of various drugs much sooner than would once have been possible. In line with this program, the FDA approved expanded studies of the drugs foscarnet and ganciclovir, both of them potential compounds for the prevention of AIDS-related blindness.

Plague

Bubonic plague, one of the many diseases transmitted to humans through direct or indirect contact with animals, usually is listed among the scourges of past centuries. At least three great epidemics of bubonic plague have been recorded, including the Black Death of the 14th century, when the disease claimed at least 50 million lives. The most recent worldwide epidemic of the plague occurred in the 1800s. While recent cases of the plague in North America have been relatively rare, the disease organism is still carried by rodents, including squirrels, rats, and rabbits; and cases of the plague still occur in the western United States. Increased activity in western areas by hunters, campers, and other outdoor enthusiasts has resulted in a higher incidence of the disease among humans in recent years. The disease also is fairly common in Asia, Africa, and South America.

Symptoms

The infection is transmitted from animals to man through the bite of a flea carrying the disease organism. Symptoms usually develop in several days but may take as long as two weeks after the flea bite. The victim experiences chills and fever, with the temperature rising above 102° F. He may experience headaches, a rapid heart beat, and difficulty walking. Vomiting and delirium also are among the symptoms of plague. There may be pain and tenderness of the lymph nodes, which become inflamed and swollen; the enlarged lymph nodes are known as *buboes,* a term that gives its name to the type of plague involved. The buboes occur most frequently in the legs and groin because these are the most frequent sites for flea bites.

The site of the flea bite may or may not be found after the symptoms develop. If present, it may be marked by a swollen, pus-filled area of the skin.

Diagnosis of plague can be confirmed by laboratory tests that might include examination of the bacteria taken in samples from buboes or other diseased areas of the body, inoculation of laboratory animals with suspected disease organisms, and studies of the white blood cells of the patient.

Complications can include pneumonia and hemorrhages, with bleeding from the nose or mouth or through the gastrointestinal or urinary tracts, and abscesses and ulcerations. The pneumonic form of plague can be transmitted from one person to another like colds or other infectious diseases; in other words, plague organisms are spread by being exhaled by one person and inhaled by another.

Treatment and Prevention

As in other infectious diseases, early treatment is most effective. Antibiotics are administered every day for a period of one to two weeks, and buboes are treated with hot, moist applications. The buboes may be drained if necessary after the patient has responded to antibiotic medications. Antibiotics have reduced the fatality rate from plague infections from a high of 90 percent to a maximum of about 10 percent. Vaccines are available but are of limited and temporary

value. Prevention requires eradication of rats and other possibly infected rodents (some 200 species are known to carry the disease), use of insecticides to control fleas, and avoidance of contact with wild animals in areas where plague is known to exist. Domestic animals also should be protected from contact with possibly infected wild animals.

Tularemia

An infectious disease known as *tularemia,* sometimes called *rabbit fever,* is transmitted from animals to humans who come in contact with the animal tissues. It also can be transmitted through the bites of ticks or flies or by drinking contaminated water. Like the plague-disease organism, tularemia can be transmitted by inhalation of infected particles from the lungs of a diseased person, although such occurrences are rare.

Symptoms

Within a couple of days to perhaps two weeks after exposure to the tularemia germ, the patient develops chills and a fever with temperatures rising to 103° F. or higher. Other symptoms include headache, nausea and vomiting, extreme weakness, and drenching sweats. Lymph nodes become enlarged and a pus-filled lesion develops at the site of the infection. Usually only one pustular papule develops on a finger or other skin area, marking the point of the insect bite or contact with infected animal tissues; but there may be several such sores in the membranes of the mouth if that is the point of infection. It is not uncommon for the eyes or lungs to become involved.

Laboratory tests, along with a record of contact with wild animals or game birds, eating improperly cooked

meats, being bitten by deer flies or ticks, or drinking water from ponds or streams, usually helps verify the cause of the symptoms as tularemia. In some cases the contact with the disease organism can be made through bites or scratches of infected dogs or cats, but most frequently the disease of humans originates through handling of the meat or fur of wild animals or by camping or hiking in areas where the disease is endemic.

Treatment

Treatment includes bed rest and administration of antibiotics. Adequate fluid intake is important and oxygen may be required. Aspirin usually is given also, to relieve headache and muscle aches. Hot compresses are applied to the enlarged lymph node areas; it may be necessary to drain the swollen, infected nodes. If the disease is complicated by pneumonic tularemia or infection of the eye, the patient usually is hospitalized. Success of the therapy depends upon early and adequate treatment. The disease is rarely fatal when properly treated with antibiotics, but it can be lethal if the symptoms are ignored. Anyone who develops the symptoms of tularemia after handling wild animals or being exposed to biting insects or contaminated water in rural or rugged country should seek immediate medical help.

Hunters, campers, hikers, and others venturing into the great outdoors should protect their bodies against invasion by ticks by wearing long-sleeved shirts and long trousers with cuffs securely fastened. Regular checks should be made of the scalp, groin, and armpits for ticks. Any ticks found should be detached quickly and the bite area cleansed with soap and water, followed by an alcohol cleansing. If the head of the tick breaks off, it can be removed by the same techniques used to remove a splinter from the skin. Raw water from ponds and streams should be boiled or disinfected with chemicals before using. Rubber gloves should be worn while dressing the meat of wild game or birds, and the meat should be thoroughly cooked. On the positive side, once the disease occurs, the recovered patient develops immunity to tularemia.

Rocky Mountain Spotted Fever

The name of an increasingly common tick-borne disease, *Rocky Mountain spotted fever,* is misleading, because humans are most likely to become infected in regions far from the Rocky Mountains. The disease, also known as *tick fever,* has become most prevalent in rural and suburban areas of the southern and eastern United States. It is caused by a rickettsial organism transmitted by a tick bite. Wild rodents are a reservoir of the infected ticks that carry the disease.

Symptoms

Rocky Mountain spotted fever may be relatively mild or dangerously severe. The symptoms of headache, chills, and fever may begin suddenly and persist for a period of two or three weeks. Fever temperatures may reach 104° F and may be accompanied by nausea and occasional vomiting. Headaches have been described in some cases as excruciating, with the pain most intense along the forehead. Muscles of the legs, back, and abdomen may ache and feel tender. The most serious cases seem to develop within a few days after a tick bite; milder cases usually are slower to develop. A rash usually develops a few days after the onset of other symptoms and is most likely to be concentrated on the forearm, ankles, feet,

wrists, and hands. If untreated, Rocky Mountain spotted fever symptoms may abate in two weeks, but the infection can be fatal, particularly in persons over the age of 40.

Treatment

Treatment includes administration of antibiotics and, in some cases, steroid hormones. Careful nursing care and adequate intake of protein foods and liquids also are needed.

Preventive measures are similar to those recommended to guard against tularemia. Wear adequate protective clothing that forms a barrier against tick invasion of the skin surfaces, check the scalp and other hairy body areas regularly for ticks, and remove and destroy any ticks found. In addition, ground areas known to be inhabited by wood ticks should be sprayed with an effective insecticide safe for humans; insect repellents also should be applied to clothing and exposed skin surfaces when venturing into wooded or brushy areas. Ticks may become attached to dogs and other animals and care should be used in removing them from the pets, because the disease organism can enter the body through minor cuts and scratches on the skin. A vaccine is available for protection of persons who are likely to use possibly infested tick areas for work or recreation. Immunity usually is established by two inoculations, about a month apart, and booster shots as needed.

Tropical Diseases

Most people living in the temperate climates of North America and Europe are spared the ravages of

some of the most lethal and debilitating diseases known to mankind. They include malaria, which probably has killed more people than any other disease in history, yellow fever, leishmaniasis, trypanosomiasis, filariasis, schistosomiasis, and leprosy.

While many persons probably have never heard of some of these diseases and at least a few doctors might have trouble in diagnosing the symptoms, they affect hundreds of millions of people each year and could pose a threat to persons living in any part of the world. They are generally classed as tropical diseases, but so-called tropical or exotic diseases have been prevented from spreading into temperate regions partly because of alert medical care and preventive measures by public health experts. Malaria, for example, has been found as far north as the Arctic Circle, as far south as the tip of South America, and at one time was a disease of epidemic proportions in such northern cities as Philadelphia and London. These diseases have altered the course of history, ending the life of Alexander the Great as he tried to conquer the world, nipping in the bud Napoleon's plans to retake Canada from the English, defeating French efforts to build the Panama Canal, and contributing to the black-slave trade between Africa and the Americas.

The major tropical diseases are caused by a variety of organisms, including viruses, protozoa, and worms. Some are transmitted by insect bites, some by contact with contaminated water, and others, like leprosy, are spread by means that remain a mystery despite centuries of medical experience with millions of cases of the disease. Space does not permit detailed discussion of all tropical diseases; only those regarded by medical authorities as among the most significant to world health are described in this chapter.

Malaria

Malaria, one of the most common diseases in the world, gets its name from an Italian word for "bad air" because of an ancient belief that a mysterious substance in the air was the cause of the ailment. It is now known that the disease is caused by any of at least four parasites carried by Anopheles mosquitoes. According to the World Health Organization (WHO), some 200 million persons are affected by the disease, including one-fourth of the adult population on the continent of Africa. WHO estimates that at least one million children die each year of malaria. The disease was relatively rare in the United States until the 1960s, when hundreds of cases began to appear among military personnel who apparently contracted the disease in southeast Asia but did not develop symptoms until they returned to the United States; the disease later occurred in soldiers who had never left the United States, apparently transmitted by domestic Anopheles mosquitoes that had become infested with the malaria parasites.

Symptoms

The symptoms of malaria differ somewhat among various patients because the four known kinds of plasmodia, or protozoa, that cause the infection do not produce the same specific effects. However, the general symptoms common to all forms of malaria are fever, chills, headache, muscle pains, and, in some cases, skin disorders such as cold sores, hives, or a rash. A malaria attack may begin with a severe chill that lasts from twenty minutes to an hour, followed by a fever lasting from three to eight hours with temperature rising to more than 104° F. The fever usually is accompanied by profuse sweating, and the afflicted person is left exhausted by the cycle of chills and fever. The attacks be-

come more or less successively milder, less frequent, and more irregular, and finally cease, although there may be relapses.

One kind of malarial organism seems to cause attacks that occur every other day, while another type produces attacks that appear quite regularly on every third day; still another type of malaria plasmodium seems to cause a fever that is continuous. While the liver seems to be a favored target organ, other body systems can be involved, with related complications. If the organism reaches the brain, the patient may suffer convulsions, delirium, partial paralysis, or coma. If the organism invades the lungs, there may be coughing symptoms and blood-stained sputum. In some cases, there may be gastrointestinal symptoms with abdominal pain, vomiting, or diarrhea.

Medical examination of malaria patients frequently reveals signs of anemia, an enlarged spleen, liver abnormalities, and edema, or swelling because of fluid accumulation. Blood studies may show the malaria parasites in the blood, damaged red blood cells, and an abnormal white blood cell count. The four species of malaria organism are distinctive enough to be identified in laboratory tests.

Treatment

Treatment includes administration of antimalarial drugs such as quinine, chloroquine, or primaquine. Newer antimalarial drugs are sometimes used in combinations because of the development of drug-resistant strains of the organism in South America and Asia. There is no vaccine that protects against malaria.

Causes

The protozoa that cause malaria are carried by the Anopheles mosquito,

How Malaria Is Transmitted

Infected mosquito → Protozoa multiply in human bloodstream → Mosquito is infected and will transmit disease to next victim

A mosquito infected with malaria protozoa bites a human. The protozoa produce daughter cells within the human bloodstream. These cells are transmitted to another mosquito that bites the infected human. This mosquito will infect the next human it bites, thus perpetuating the malaria cycle.

but humans are the intermediate host. This means that both infected humans and infected mosquitoes are needed to continue the life cycle of the organism. The disease therefore can be controlled if Anopheles mosquito populations are eradicated and humans are not carrying the protozoa in their blood. When these organisms get into human blood, they invade the red blood cells and multiply until the blood cells rupture to release offspring called *daughter cells*. When the mosquito bites a human for a blood meal, the daughter cells enter the mosquito stomach, where they complete their life cycle and migrate to the mosquito's salivary gland to be injected into the next human, and so on. It takes from ten days to six weeks following a mosquito bite for the first malaria symptoms to develop, the time differences varying with the species of protozoa involved. The malaria mosquito in recent years has developed resistance to insecticides, and areas of infestation have spread in some countries where irrigation for farming has been expanded.

Yellow Fever

Yellow fever, which sometimes produces symptoms similar to those of malaria, also is transmitted by a mosquito. But yellow fever is a virus disease carried by the Aedes mosquito.

Yellow fever also can be harbored by other animals, while the malaria organism that affects humans is not transmitted between humans and lower animals. Like malaria, yellow fever has in past years spread deeply into North America with cases reported along the Gulf Coast, the Mississippi River Valley, and as far north as Boston. A vaccine is available for protection against yellow fever.

Leishmaniasis

Leishmaniasis is similar to malaria in that the disease organisms are protozoa transmitted to humans by an insect bite, but the insect in this case is the sandfly. There are several forms that leishmaniasis can take. The kind considered most lethal, with a mortality rate of up to 95 percent of untreated adults, is known as *kala-azar,* a term derived from the Hindi language meaning "black disease". Kala-azar also is known as *black fever, dumdum fever,* and *visceral leishmaniasis.* It occurs from China through Russia and India to North Africa, the Mediterranean countries of Europe, and in parts of Central and South America. Kala-azar has appeared in the United States in cases contracted overseas.

Symptoms

The symptoms may not appear for a period of from ten days to more than three months after the bite of a sandfly, although the disease organism may be found in blood tests before the first symptoms occur. Symptoms include a fever that reaches a peak twice a day for a period of perhaps several weeks, then recurs at irregular intervals while the patient experiences progressive weakness, loss of weight, loss of skin color, and a rapid heartbeat. In some cases, de-

pending upon the type of infection, there may be gastrointestinal complaints and bleeding of the mucous membranes, particularly around the teeth. There also can be edema, an accumulation of fluid in the tissues that conceals the actual loss of body tissue. Physical examination shows an enlarged spleen and liver plus abnormal findings in blood and urine tests.

American Cutaneous Leishmaniasis

The American cutaneous form of leishmaniasis usually begins with one or more skin ulcers resulting from sandfly bites, with the skin of the ear the target site of the insect in many cases. The skin lesion may enlarge, with or without secondary infection by other disease organisms, and spread into the lymphatic system of the body. From the lymph system, the infecting protozoa may invade the mouth and nose, producing painful and mutilating skin ulcers and other destructive changes in the tissues. Bacterial infections and respiratory problems can lead to the death of the patient. In some areas of Central and South America, more than 10 percent of the population suffer from the disfiguring effects of leishmaniasis. Diagnosis usually is confirmed by medical tests that identify the leishmaniasis organism in the patient's tissues.

Old World Cutaneous Leishmaniasis

A milder form, sometimes known as Old World cutaneous leishmaniasis, occurs from India westward to the Mediterranean countries and North Africa. An ulcer appears at the site of a sandfly bite, usually several weeks after the bite, but it heals during a period of from three months to a year. A large pitted scar frequently remains to mark the site of the ulceration, but the invading organism does not

spread deeply into the body tissues as in the severe types of leishmaniasis.

Treatment

Therapy for leishmaniasis cases includes administration of various medications containing antimony, along with antibiotics for the control of secondary infections. Bed rest, proper diet, and, in severe cases, blood transfusions also are advised.

Causes

The leishmaniasis organisms injected into the human body by the sandfly bite multiply through parasitic invasion of the tissue cells, particularly blood cells that usually resist infection. They may invade the lymph nodes, spleen, liver, and bone marrow, causing anemia and other symptoms. In populated areas, sandflies can be eradicated by insecticides. Unfortunately, rodents and other wild and domestic animals serve as a reservoir for the leishmaniasis protozoa and tend to perpetuate the disease in rural and jungle areas of warm climates.

Trypanosomiasis

Trypanosomiasis is a group of diseases caused by similar kinds of parasitic protozoa. The diseases, which include two kinds of African *sleeping sickness* and *Chagas' disease* of Central and South America, affect about 10 million people. The sleeping-sickness forms of trypanosomiasis are transmitted by species of the tsetse fly, while Chagas' disease is carried by insects known as *assassin bugs* or *kissing bugs.* Besides affecting humans, the trypanosomiasis organisms infect other animals, including cattle, horses, dogs, and donkeys, and have made an area of nearly four million square miles of Africa uninhabitable. According to the World Health Organization, the African land devastated by trypanosomiasis contains large fertile areas capable of supporting 125 million cattle, but domestic animals cannot survive the infestation of tsetse flies.

Sleeping Sickness

The two kinds of African sleeping sickness, Gambian and Rhodesian, are similar. Gambian, or mid-African, sleeping sickness is transmitted by a tsetse fly that lives near water; Rhodesian, or East African, sleeping sickness is carried by a woodland species of tsetse fly that uses antelopes as a reservoir of the infectious organism. The most likely victims of tsetse fly bites are young men, probably because they are more likely to be exposed to the insects.

Symptoms

The symptoms of trypanosomiasis infections from tsetse fly bites can vary considerably according to various factors, such as the general health of the victim. A small area of inflammation, called a *chancre,* appears at the site of the tsetse fly bite about two days after the incident; some patients complain of pain and irritation in the area around the bite for several weeks, but others have no symptoms. Then, for a period of perhaps several months, episodes of fever occur, with temperatures rising to 106° F. The bouts of fever may be accompanied by skin rashes, severe headaches, and heart palpitations. Loss of appetite and weight follow, with insomnia, an inability to concentrate, tremors, and difficulty in speaking and walking. There also may be signs of anemia and delayed reaction to a painful stim-

ulus. Eventually, the protozoa can invade the central nervous system, producing convulsions, coma, and death.

Sleeping sickness, which may progress gradually, gets its name from the appearance of the patient, who develops a vacant expression and drooping eyelids, along with blurred speech, general lethargy, and occasional periods of paralysis.

Gambian and Rhodesian Varieties

A major difference between the Gambian and Rhodesian forms of African sleeping sickness is that the Rhodesian variety, which has similar symptoms, is more acute and progresses more rapidly than the Gambian. The fevers are higher, weight losses greater, the disease more resistant to treatment, and the span of time from first symptoms to death much shorter. Even with intensive treatment, Rhodesian sleeping sickness patients have only a 50–50 chance of survival, while 90 to 95 percent of the Gambian sleeping sickness patients recover when properly treated for the disease.

Treatment

Several chemotherapeutic agents are available for treatment of Gambian and Rhodesian sleeping sickness; they include suramin, pentamidine, and tryparsamide given by injection. Good nutrition, good nursing care, and treatment of secondary infections are additional therapeutic measures.

Chagas' Disease

Chagas' disease, or American trypanosomiasis, is a primary cause of heart disease from Mexico through much of South America. The protozoan infection is rare in the United

States, but cases have been reported. The first symptoms may be edema of the face. The accumulation of fluid occuring in the area of the eyelids, conjunctivitis, hard reddish nodules on the skin, along with the fever and involvement of the heart, brain, and liver tissues. The assassin or kissing bugs by which the disease is spread tend to bite the face, especially around the lips or eyelids, accounting for the swelling of those facial areas. The bite may be painful, or if the victim is sleeping at the time, it may not be noticed at all.

Symptoms

The protozoa multiply rapidly at the site of the bug bite, frequently producing symptoms resembling those of leishmaniasis—intermittent fever, swollen spleen, and enlarged liver, after signs of an insect bite. After several days, the trypanosomiasis organisms spread from the site of infection into other tissues, especially the heart and brain, where they cause tissue destruction, inflammation, and often death.

Treatment

There is no specific treatment for Chagas' disease, and, except for experimental drugs, most therapeutic measures are intended to treat the symptoms.

Like the African sleeping sickness forms of trypanosomiasis, the American type can involve reservoirs of wild and domestic animals; the disease has been found in cats and dogs as well as in opossums and armadillos. Persons traveling in endemic areas should use preventive measures that are appropriate, such as insect sprays and repellents. Efforts to eradicate large areas of insects carrying the trypanosomiasis organisms have been futile; in some instances it has been found to be more effective to move villages away from the insects than to try to remove the insects from the villages.

Filariasis

The species of mosquitoes that transmit malaria and yellow fever, diseases caused by protozoa and viruses, also transmit *filariasis,* caused by a parasitic worm—a nematode or roundworm. Filariasis affects 300 million people living in tropical and subtropical areas of the world. The worm invades the subcutaneous tissues and lymph system of the human body, blocking the flow of lymph and producing symptoms of inflammation, edema, abscesses, and, in one form of the disease, blindness. Filariasis is not unknown to Americans; some 15,000 soldiers contracted the disease during World War II fighting in the Pacific Theater, and cases have been reported along the Carolina coast area. But most of the victims of filariasis live in a region extending from Africa through Asia to the islands of New Guinea and Borneo.

Symptoms

Symptoms of filariasis can develop insidiously during an incubation period that may last from three months to a year after infection. There can be brief attacks of a low-grade fever, with chills and sweating, headache, nausea, and muscle pain. The patient also may feel sensitive to bright lights. Signs and symptoms more specifically related to filariasis are the appearance of red, swollen skin areas with tender spots that indicate the spread of the threadlike worms through the lymphatic system. Most likely sites for the first signs of filariasis are the lymph vessels of the legs, with later involvement of the groin and abdomen, producing the swollen lower frontal effect known as *elephantiasis.* Diagnosis of the disease is confirmed by finding the tiny worms in the lymph; the infecting organism also may be found in blood tests, but only at certain times. The worms of one form of the disease are only 35 to 90 millimeters long in the adult stage, and those of a second type of the disease are only half that size. Larvae, or embryos, of the worms may be only 200 microns (one-fifth of a millimeter) in size.

Treatment

An oral medication, diethylcarbamazine, is available to kill the larvae in the system; the drug has only limited value in destroying the adult worms. The drug is taken orally for three weeks, but courses may have to be repeated over a period of two years because relapses can occur. Other therapeutic measures include bed rest during periods of fever and inflammation, antibiotics to control secondary infections, and, occasionally, surgery to remove damaged tissues that may interfere with normal working activities following recovery.

Onchocerciasis

The type of filariasis that causes blindness is transmitted by a species of blackfly that introduces or picks up the worm larvae while biting. As in mosquito-transmitted filariasis, the worms work their way through the skin to the lymphatic system but tend to migrate to eye structures. Blackfly filariasis, also called *onchocerciasis,* occurs most frequently in Africa and from southern Mexico to northern South America. More than one million cases of onchocerciasis have been found in the upper basin of the Volta River of Africa, with thousands of patients already blinded by the infection.

Loiasis

A third variation of filariasis is called *loiasis.* It is carried from man to monkey or from monkey to man by a biting fly. The larvae develop into adult worms that migrate under the skin and sometimes through the eye. Migration of a worm through the skin causes swelling, irritation, and redness. The disease is treated with drugs to kill the larvae, as well as by antihistamines and, occasionally, surgery to remove the adult worms.

Control of filariasis requires eradication of the flies and mosquitoes that transmit the parasitic worms and perhaps the wild animals that can serve as reservoirs. As in the examples of other tropical diseases, it frequently is easier to separate the humans from the areas infested by the insects than to eradicate the insects.

Schistosomiasis

A worm of a different sort—the trematode, a flatworm of the class *Trematoda,* which includes the flukes—is responsible for *schistosomiasis.* This disease occurs in various forms in Africa, Asia, South America, and the Caribbean, including Puerto Rico. About 200 million people are infected with schistosomiasis, also called *bilharziasis.*

Life Cycle of the Fluke Parasite

The process of infection by one kind of fluke involves free-swimming larvae that penetrate the skin of a human who has entered waters containing the organism. The larvae follow the human bloodstream to the liver, where they develop into adult worms. The adult worms then move into the blood vessels of the host and lay eggs. Some of the eggs find their way into the intestine or urinary bladder and are excreted with the urine or feces of the host. If they find their way to fresh water, the eggs hatch and the released organisms find their way to the body of a snail. Inside the snail they multiply into thousands of new larvae over a period of one or two months, after which they return to the water and invade the skin of another human. In this manner the fluke worm continues its life cycle, infecting more humans who venture into the contaminated waters.

Symptoms

Skin rashes and itching, loss of appetite, abdominal discomfort, and diarrhea are among early symptoms of schistosomiasis infections. There also may be fever and generalized aches and pains. During a period of from one to two or more months after the initial infection, more severe symptoms may occur as a result of a growing number of adult worms and eggs in the body, which produce allergic reactions. Those symptoms may include diarrhea, abdominal pain, coughing spells, and high fever and chills. Medical examination may reveal a tender and enlarged liver plus signs of bleeding in the intestinal tract. Complications may result from obstruction by masses of worms and eggs or by rupturing of the walls of body organs during migration of the organisms. Diagnosis usually can be confirmed by examination of the victim's stools or of the lining of the rectum for the presence of eggs of the fluke worms.

Treatment

Therapy may consist of administration of antimony-based drugs, tartar emetic, measures to relieve the symptoms, and, when deemed necessary, surgery. In some cases, a medication may be administered to flush the eggs of the fluke worm

through a specific part of the circulatory system during a surgical procedure in which a filter is inserted in a vein to trap the eggs; thousands of fluke worms can be removed by this technique. Some of the medications used in treating schistosomiasis can have serious side effects and are used cautiously. However, the alternative may be prolonged emaciation of the victim, with a bloated abdomen and early death by cancer or other causes related to the infection. The female fluke worm has been known to continue depositing eggs during a life span of 30 years, causing frequent recurrence of acute symptoms.

Other Forms of Schistosomiasis

There are several other forms of schistosomiasis that cause variations in symptoms. One kind involves the liver and central nervous system, resulting in death of the victims within as little as two years after infection. Another form seems to involve the urinary bladder, causing frequent, painful, and blood-tinged urination with bacterial infection as a complication.

Swimmer's Itch

A mild form of schistosomiasis is known by the popular name *swimmer's itch*. It can occur anywhere from Asia to South America and as far north as Canada and western Europe, affecting bathers in both fresh water and sea water. As in the severe forms of schistosomiasis, snails are the intermediate hosts, and wild animals and birds provide a reservoir of the organism. The effects are treated as a skin allergy, and shallow local waters used for swimming are treated with chemicals to eradicate the snails. Careful drying and examination of the skin after swimming in possibly infected waters can control to some de-

gree the invasion of the skin by fluke larvae. A chemical skin cream that tends to repel fluke larvae also is available as a protective measure.

Leprosy

More than 10 million people are victims of *leprosy,* an infectious disorder also known as *Hansen's disease.* Although leprosy is more common in tropical regions, where up to 10 percent of some population groups may be affected, the disease also occurs in several northern countries, including the United States, where the disease is found in coastal states from California through Texas and Louisiana, and from Florida to New York. Ancient medical writings indicate that leprosy was known in China and India about 3,000 years ago but did not spread to the eastern Mediterranean until A.D. 500 or 600. Thus, the disease described in the Bible as leprosy probably was not the same disease known today by that name.

Symptoms

The manifestations of leprosy resemble those of several other diseases, including syphilis, sarcoidosis, and vitiligo, a skin disease marked by patches where pigmentation has been lost. The lesions of leprosy, which may begin as pale or reddish areas of from one-half inch to three or four inches in diameter, appear on body surfaces where the temperature is cooler than other body areas. These cooler surfaces include the skin, nose and throat, eyes, and testicles. The early cosmetic symptoms are followed gradually by a loss of feeling in the affected areas because of involvement of the nerve endings in those tissues. At first the patient may notice a loss of ability to distinguish hot and cold sensations in the diseased area.

Then there may be a loss of tactile sensation. Finally, there is a loss of pain sensation in the affected tissues.

A case of leprosy may progress into one of two major forms, *tuberculoid leprosy* or *lepromatous leprosy,* or a combination of the two forms. The advanced symptoms can include more severe nerve damage and muscular atrophy with foot drop and contracted hands, plus damage to body areas from burns and injuries that are not felt but that can become infected. Damage to nose tissues can lead to breathing difficulties and speech problems. Crippling and blinding are not uncommon in untreated causes of leprosy, and death may occur as a result of secondary infections.

Treatment

A number of different sulfone drugs have been found effective against the mycobacterium that apparently causes leprosy, but the drugs also produce such side effects as fever and anemia. When intolerance to sulfones occurs, other medications are offered, including thiourea, mercaptan, and streptomycin. Steroid hormones are used to help control adverse reactions.

Causes

The disease organism, *Mycobacterium leprae,* or *Hansen's bacillus,* is believed to enter the skin or the respiratory system of the victim, probably during childhood. It rarely infects adults except under unusual circumstances, as through skin tattooing. Some medical scientists believe the infection may be transmitted through an insect bite, since the disease organism has been found in insects. However, the true process of leprosy infection remains unknown, and efforts to cultivate the mycobacterium in laboratory tissue cultures have been futile, although the disease can be induced in the footpads of experimental animals. Doctors have not found it necessary to isolate patients with the disease except during the period when treatments begin. Regular and thorough skin examinations of persons who have been in contact with leprosy patients and early detection and treatment of the disease by specialists are the recommended means of control.

20
Surgery

What You Should Know Before Undergoing Surgery

Almost everyone can expect to be wheeled into an operating room at some point in his lifetime. The range of surgical procedures performed every year is vast—correction of broken bones, organ transplants, facial uplifts, hernia repairs, hysterectomies, caesarian sections, vasectomies, appendectomies, and so on. It is obviously impossible for a work of this sort to describe more than a fraction of the thousands of surgical procedures and their variations that are widely performed. For a representative sampling of some specific surgical procedures, see "Common Surgical Procedures" later in this chapter.

The seriousness of surgical procedures within the same category can vary widely. For example, one case of inguinal hernia may be repaired quickly and simply in a young man physically able to leave the hospital on the same day he arrived. Another inguinal hernia case could be a real emergency if a portion of the small intestine were to become trapped in the hernia sac protruding into the abdominal wall, resulting in the death of

the bowel-tissue cells. Easy generalizations about the seriousness of a given procedure are simply not warranted.

Types of Surgery

Surgery is sometimes categorized according to whether it is vital to life, necessary for continued health, or desirable for medical or personal reasons. Although there are many ways in which surgical procedures are classified, the following breakdown is one that is widely accepted among surgeons.

Emergency Surgery

Most disorders requiring surgery do not improve by delaying the trip to the hospital. Some can be planned and scheduled so as to coincide with periods in which a few days in the hospital will be unlikely to interfere with job or family responsibilities. But, unfortunately, there are also unpredictable events that precipitate an immediate need for surgery. An

automobile accident, a fire, a violent crime, or even a sudden change in a chronic medical problem, like a perforated ulcer or a strangulated hernia, can create situations in which the life of the patient depends upon the time it takes to get the victim into the hands of a trained surgeon. Emergency surgery cases typically involve the treatment of gunshot and stab wounds, fractures of the skull and other major bones, severe eye injuries, or life-threatening situations, such as obstruction of the windpipe caused by choking on a piece of food.

Emergency surgery may be one of the most common routes for patients entering the operating room. Accident patients, according to one estimate, require four times as many hospital beds as cancer patients and more hospital beds than all heart patients. They account for more than a half-million deaths and disabilities in America each year. They present tremendous challenges to surgeons, because emergency room patients frequently have multiple injuries involving several organ systems.

Such victims are often unconscious or otherwise unable to communicate coherently about their injuries, and there may be little or no time to obtain medical histories or information about their blood types, allergies to medicines, etc.

When possible, vital information about the patient and the circumstances surrounding the injury or sudden need for surgery is obtained by medical personnel who question anybody who might provide one or more clues. Efforts to maintain life are begun even while blood samples are taken for laboratory analysis and X-ray photographs made of the chest, abdomen, and other body areas that may be involved. Many *heroic* measures—extreme measures taken when life is in immediate peril—may be used in critical cases; for example, resuscitation, induction of anesthesia, and surgery might proceed simultaneously as soon as a diagnosis is made. When several teams are working on the patient at the same time, a general surgeon may be called upon to coordinate the multiple operating room procedures.

Urgent Surgery

Next in priority for the surgeon are cases in which an operation is vital but can be postponed for a few days. A person injured in an automobile accident but conscious and suffering a minor bone fracture may be classed as an urgent rather than emergency surgery case, and the delay would give surgeons and other medical personnel time to study X rays carefully, evaluate blood tests and other diagnostic data, and otherwise plan corrective therapy while under less pressure. A penetrating ulcer of the stomach likely would be classed as urgent surgery, but the ulcer case would become emergency surgery if it were to rupture through the stomach wall. An acute, inflamed gall bladder, kidney stones, or cancer of a vital organ would be examples of urgent surgery cases.

Elective Surgery

Elective surgery is usually subdivided into three categories: required, selective, and optional.

Required Surgery

Physical ailments that are serious enough to need corrective surgery but that can be scheduled a matter of weeks or months in advance generally are designated as required surgery cases. Conditions such as a chronically inflamed gall bladder, cataracts, bone deformities, or diseased tonsils and adenoids would be examples of conditions that require surgery. Also in this classification might be cases of uncomplicated inguinal hernia, hiatal hernia, and surgery of the reproductive organs which do not need immediate attention.

Selective Surgery

Selective surgery covers a broad range of conditions that are of no real threat to the health of the patient but nevertheless should be corrected by surgery in order to improve his comfort and well-being. Certain congenital defects such as cleft lip (harelip) and cleft palate would be included in this classification, as well as removal of certain cysts and nonmalignant fatty or fibrous tumors. Selective surgery also might include operations to correct crossed eyes in children so that normal binocular vision can develop properly.

Optional Surgery

Of the lowest priority are operations that are primarily of cosmetic benefit, such as removal of warts and other nonmalignant growths on the skin, blemishes of the skin, and certain cases of varicose veins. Optional surgery also includes various kinds of plastic surgery undertaken for cosmetic effect. Among popular types of plastic surgery are operations to change the shape of female breasts; this would include the correction of unusually large or pendulous breasts as well as the enlargement of unusually small breasts. Other common plastic surgery procedures are *rhinoplasty,* or nose shaping; *otoplasty,* the correction of protruding ears; *blepharoplasty,* the removal of bags under the eyes; and *rhytidoplasty,* known popularly as a facelift. Rhytidoplasty is relatively simple, virtually painless, and effective; because the benefits usually are temporary, it is an operation that many patients volunteer to undergo more than once. For fuller information on these procedures, see "Plastic and Cosmetic Surgery" later in this chapter.

Since the end of World War II, there has been a proliferation of surgical specialties. The general surgeon of past eras who handled all kinds of operations is gradually being replaced by a battery of highly specialized experts who may work only on the nervous system, the eye, the ear, the bones and muscles, and so on. When warranted, a patient's case may be handled by several different surgical specialists. The result has been safer, more effective surgical treatment for the average patient.

Laser Surgery

Advancing technology has made laser surgery an accepted method of treating a growing number of physical disorders (see sections in this chapter titled "Cataract"; "Glaucoma"; "Retinal Detachment or Disease"; and

"Brain Tumor"). Surgeons have found that laser beams provide a noninvasive operating technique, or a less invasive one than the traditional method. The laser promotes coagulation of vessels, including blood vessels, while also keeping the operating area sterile. The laser can reach otherwise inaccessible body parts. Because of this flexibility, repair of many organs is possible without removing them.

An acronym for **L**ight **A**mplification by **S**timulated **E**mission of **R**adiation, the laser is a precisely controlled light beam that is narrowly focused and that can be aimed at a minute target. In each laser, the light is all one frequency, or wavelength, and contains only one color. The color determines how the beam will interact with particular kinds of tissue, and may be different for different kinds of surgery. Lasers may function continuously or in pulsed bursts. The type of laser determines the number of pulses per second and the duration of the pulses.

Three kinds of lasers have been found to be of special value as surgical tools:

The *argon laser,* functioning in the blue-green frequencies, utilizes a very high electric current passed through argon gas. Because it readily coagulates the blood in the operating area, the argon laser has been especially useful in the fields of ophthalmology, plastic surgery, and dermatology.

The *carbon dioxide laser,* with a wavelength in the far infrared spectrum, penetrates tissue to a depth of only one millimeter. Utilizing a gas mixture of CO_2, nitrogen, and helium, the carbon dioxide laser can cut tissue to a precisely controlled depth. It has thus been used widely as a surgical scalpel to treat some types of cancer, gynecological disorders, and brain tumors.

The *neodymium YAG laser* (YAG representing "yttrium-aluminum garnet") has a wavelength in the near infrared spectrum. Applications of the YAG laser include the treatment of bleeding in the esophagus and digestive tract, treatment of some cancers and glaucoma, burn therapy, and some types of neurosurgery.

Preoperative Procedures

Preparation of a patient for surgery involves a variety of procedures determined by the urgency of the operation, the anatomical area involved, the nature of the disease or injury requiring surgery, the general condition of the patient, and other factors. Emergency surgery of an accident victim in critical condition obviously requires a greatly accelerated pace of preparing the patient for the operating room; medical personnel may cut away the clothing of the victim in order to save precious minutes. An operation on the intestine, on the other hand, may require a full week of preparation, including the five or so days needed to sterilize the bowel with drugs and evaluate laboratory tests. However, most *preop* procedures, as they are commonly called, generally follow a similar pattern designed to insure a safe and sound operation. Even in a case of emergency surgery, certain information must be compiled to help guide the surgeon and other hospital staff personnel in making the right decisions affecting proper care of the patient during and after the operation.

Medical History

This pattern begins with a medical history of the patient. The medical history should reveal the general health of the patient and any factors that might increase the risk of surgery. Perhaps one of his parents or another close relative suffered from heart disease or diabetes; such facts might suggest a predisposition of the patient to problems associated with those disorders. The data should also show whether the patient has a tendency to bleed easily and whether he has been following a special diet, such as a sodium-restricted diet.

It is important that the patient reveal quite frankly to his own physician, the surgeon, and the anesthetist the names of any drugs or other medications used. It also is vital that the medical personnel have a complete record of any patient experiences, including allergic reactions to certain drugs, that might help predict drug sensitivities that could complicate the surgery. The simple fact that a patient suffers from asthma or hay fever might indicate that he may be more sensitive than other individuals to drugs that might be administered.

Allergic Reactions

Some patients are allergic to penicillin or other antibiotics. Others may be sensitive to aspirin or serums. Still others could be allergic to iodine, Merthiolate, or even adhesive tape. All of these factors if they are known and if they apply to the patient about to undergo surgery, should be brought to the attention of the medical staff.

Medications Currently Being Used

Among medications routinely used by the patient that should be brought to the attention of the surgeon and anesthetist are insulin for diabetes, digitalis drugs for heart diseases, and cortisone for arthritis. Depending upon various factors relating to the individual case, the patient may be directed to continue using the medication as usual, change the size of the dose before or after surgery, or discontinue the drug entirely for a while.

A patient who has been taking certain sedatives or drinking alcoholic beverages regularly for a prolonged period before surgery may have developed a tolerance for the anesthetic used, which means that he would require a larger than usual dose to get the desired effect. A patient who has been using epinephrine-type eye drops for glaucoma may be asked to increase the dosage before surgery as an adjustment to one of the drugs used in conjunction with a general anesthetic.

Diuretics, tranquilizers, and anticoagulant drugs are among other medications commonly used by patients that could affect the manner in which a surgical procedure is carried out. When possible, the patient should take a sample of the medication, a copy of the prescription, or the pharmacist's label from a container of the medication to the hospital so the medical staff can verify the type of drug used.

Psychological Evaluation

Of increasing importance in recent years has been a psychological evaluation of the patient. Individuals with a past history of mental disease or patients whose complaints may be based on psychoneurotic factors may react differently to surgery than persons who could be described as psychologically well balanced. The preoperative interviews also may seek to obtain information about the patient's use of drugs of abuse or alcohol; a patient who has developed a physical dependence upon alcohol could develop withdrawal symptoms after suddenly being separated from alcoholic beverages during his hospital stay.

Physical Examination

In addition to the medical history evaluation, the surgeon will need vital information about the physical condition of the patient. This requires a complete physical examination, including a chest X ray, an electrocardiogram of the heart activity, a neurological examination, and a check of the condition of the blood vessels in various areas of the body. Other body areas may be checked as warranted by complaints of the patient or by the type of surgery to be performed. An examination of the rectum and colon may be suggested, for example, if the medical history includes problems related to the digestive tract. Adult women patients usually receive a Pap test and possibly a pelvic examination. Samples of blood and urine are taken for laboratory analysis, including blood typing in the event a transfusion is needed. The laboratory tests for older patients frequently are more detailed and may include an examination of a stool sample.

Many hospitals and surgeons will accept information obtained from a preop examination conducted several days or more before admission to the hospital for surgery, especially for elective surgery. By completing the blood and urine tests, physical examination, X rays, electrocardiograms, and medical history interview in advance of the trip to the hospital, the patient can reduce the length of the hospital stay. In some instances, the patient may be able to report to the hospital the night before the surgery is scheduled or even a few hours ahead of actual surgery. However, additional blood and urine samples may be taken immediately after admission to recheck the body chemistry, and a brief physical examination may be made to make sure the patient does not have any open wounds or infections that might complicate the chances of recovery or introduce a dangerous strain of bacteria into the sterile environment of the operating room.

Preparation for Anesthesia

After the patient is settled in his assigned bed, he is visited by the anesthetist who will be working with the surgeon. The anesthetist usually has an advance copy of all the information obtained by the surgeon and other physicians who have examined the patient, along with laboratory reports of blood chemistry, etc. He may want to review the information with the patient and examine him briefly to learn more about his particular problem. If the patient uses a medication that might interfere with the intended effects of the anesthetic to be used, the anesthetist will make a decision regarding the best way to avoid a possible chemical conflict during surgery.

Other Preparations

In a typical case of elective surgery, the patient can expect to experience the actual preoperative preparations on the afternoon or evening before surgery is scheduled. If blood transfusions may be required, there will be a final check by the hospital staff to make sure enough units of the correct cross-matched type are available.

If the surgery involves the lower digestive tract, or is an abdominal operation that may result in a disturbance of normal bowel function, the patient can expect to be given an enema. However, enemas are not administered routinely to surgery patients who are being prepared for other kinds of operations. An exception to the rule would be patients who complain of constipation.

Legal Authorization

Before the preoperative preparations are completed, chances are good that a member of the hospital staff will make sure that the patient has signed a permit authorizing the operation. The permit is a legal form describing the operation to be performed, or a special diagnostic or therapeutic procedure other than surgery if that is the purpose of the hospitalization. The statement may be signed by a close relative or legal guardian if for some reason the patient is unable to take responsibility for this action. For example, a parent will be asked to sign a permit authorizing an operation on his or her child.

Exceptions may be made in cases of emergency surgery where the patient is unable to sign a permit and a relative or guardian cannot be located in time. But there are in-house procedures of consultation among staff members who accept the responsibility. Laws regarding permission to perform surgery may vary locally; and in some communities, for example, a married patient cannot authorize surgery that may affect his or her reproductive organs without consent of the spouse. Abortion, likewise, may be illegal in some areas without the husband's consent.

Preop Meals

A light but adequate evening meal is served if the surgery is scheduled for the following morning, but no solid food is permitted for 12 hours before surgery. No fluids are allowed during the eight hours before surgery. Children and patients with certain diseases, such as diabetes, may be given special orders regarding nutrients. An infant, for example, may be allowed sweetened orange juice up to four hours before surgery in order to prevent the child from developing restless anxiety because of hunger.

Preparation of the Skin Area

The area of the skin around the surgery site is carefully prepared beginning the evening before the operation. A member of the hospital staff may assist or direct the cleaning of the area with soap and warm water. The cleansing may be done in a shower or tub, or simply with a pan of water and soap brought to the patient's bedside. The cleaned skin area is usually scrubbed again in the operating room as further protection against possible infection.

Shaving

Whether or not the skin area is to be shaved depends upon the amount of hair present. If there is no hair, the tiny nicks or cuts made by a razor would constitute an unnecessary hazard of infection. Where hair is present, however, shaving is essential in order to make available a very clean skin surface. Also, it is important that no hair or hair fragments be close enough to the surgical incision to fall beneath the skin; the bit of hair beneath the skin could cause a serious infection after surgery. Thus, to clean an area for an inguinal hernia, the patient's abdomen may be shaved and scrubbed from a point above the navel down to the mid-thigh level.

Sedation

After all these preop steps have been completed, the patient usually is given a bedtime sedative or other medication and additional sedatives plus special medications in the morning, about 30 minutes to an hour before surgery is scheduled to begin.

The Surgical Team

Most surgical operations are performed not by the surgeon alone but by a surgical team. Depending upon the complexity of the surgical procedure involved, the surgeon may have one or more assistants working with him. The assistants may be interns or hospital residents who participate in the operation as a part of their advanced training in surgical techniques, or they may be other surgeons who are specialists in a particular field. An abdominal surgeon or orthopedic surgeon, for example, may be assisted by a neurosurgeon if the operation is likely to require a special knowledge of the nervous system as it affects another organ system.

The Anesthetist

The anesthetist, who is also likely to be a physician, specializes in maintaining the proper degree of anesthesia in the patient, while also helping to maintain the body's life systems. The job of the anesthetist is more complicated than one might suppose, because in addition to making the patient unaware of pain during the operation—sometimes by making him unconscious, sometimes without affecting consciousness—the muscles and nervous reflexes must be kept in proper state for the type of surgery to be performed. Each of the various functions—muscle relaxation, reflex paralysis, etc.—requires a different anesthetic drug. Their performance must be perfectly coordinated to prevent complications during the operation. In some cases, it may be necessary for the patient to remain awake during the procedure so that he can follow instructions of the surgeon in moving certain muscle groups. At the same time, the patient must have an anesthetic that eliminates pain. Obviously, the anesthetist must prepare a different combination of drugs for a child, an elderly person, a pregnant woman in labor, or a man with a heart disease.

Other Members of the Surgical Team

As noted earlier, there are occasions when several surgeons are working more or less simultaneously on an accident victim with injuries to multiple organ systems. In such cases of emergency surgery, a general surgeon may supervise and coordinate the work of the other surgeons. The nursing staff in the operating room also may be headed by a Chief Operating Room Nurse, whose responsibility is to supervise and coordinate the activities of the scrub nurses who assist the surgeon in the actual operation, and the supply and circulating nurses who aid the rest of the surgical team by making available as needed the various towels, drapes, sponges, sutures, instruments, and other equipment.

One or more of the nurses wear gowns and gloves that have been sterilized so they can work directly with the surgeon and hand him equipment or supplies that he requests. Such a nurse is called a *scrub nurse* because she scrubs her hands and arms for ten minutes before the operation—just as the surgeon does. Other nurses in the operating room, who do not wear sterilized gowns and gloves, are not permitted to handle equipment directly but may be permitted to pick up sterilized materials with an instrument that has been sterilized. One or more orderlies, who are responsbile for lifting the patient and keeping the operating room in tidy condition, complete a typical surgical team.

Operating Room Equipment

When the operating room is in use by the surgical team, an impressive array of equipment is mobilized. The center of activity, of course, is the operating table, a massive metal device equipped with numerous levers and gears to permit the surface of the table to be raised, lowered, tilted to various angles, or to raise or lower the head, feet, or other parts of the

patient's body. The table is equipped with straps to hold the patient firmly in place during the surgical procedure.

Above the operating table is a very large and powerful lamp with lenses designed to focus a bright, shadowless light on the area in which the surgical team is working. Additional lights also are available to provide illumination at various sides or angles not adequately lighted by the overhead lamp.

Near the head of the operating table is a cart containing tanks of gases used as general anesthetics, plus oxygen tanks and equipment for administering anesthetics and monitoring the life processes of the patient.

Also in the operating room are a variety of other wheeled carts, small tables, and stands containing myriad instruments, and suction machines to clear mucus from the patient's throat and blood and other fluids from the incision area. Several stands in the area hold basins that, during an operation, can be filled with sterile solutions for rinsing hands, cleaning instruments, or moistening towels and sponges used by the surgeon and his assistants. One tall metal stand near the operating table is designed to hold bottles of intravenous fluids or containers of blood for transfusions. Another special stand is used to collect sponges used in the operation. One cart contains jars or bottles of alcohol and other solutions, soap, and gauze pads, all of which are available for careful cleansing and sterilizing of the skin around the area of the incision just before the surgeon begins the actual operation.

A large clock on the wall of the operating room is intended for timing various functions and procedures involved in an operation, such as the number of minutes that have elapsed since sterilization of certain instruments was started. For many patients

the clock is the last thing they see in the operating room before they begin the deep sleep of anesthesia; patients who remain conscious under a local anesthetic like to keep one eye on the clock face so they can tell how much time the operation requires.

Anesthetics and How They Are Used

Anesthesia is a word derived from ancient Greek, meaning "without perception," or a loss of sensation. During a major or minor operation, as in having a tooth extracted by a dentist, it is helpful to both the patient and the physician if there is a lack of sensation during the procedure. But eliminating pain isn't the only consideration in the choice of anesthetic and other drugs used in conjunction with it. The age of the patient, chronic ailments, the site of the operation, and the emotional status of the patient are among factors considered. If a patient has undergone surgery previously and had an adverse effect from a particular kind of anesthesia, this information would have an important influence on the choice of an alternative type of anesthetic.

For many types of surgery, the kind of anesthetic chosen may be the result of an agreement among the surgeon, the patient, and the anesthetist. Some patients, given a choice, would prefer to remain conscious during an appendectomy or hernia repair; others would rather not. The surgeon frequently recommends the use of a general anesthetic because the procedure may require more time than the patient can be comfortable with in an operating room situation. Therefore, patients should realize that when a surgeon recommends a general anesthetic for an operation in which a local or spinal anesthetic might be adequate, it is for their own welfare.

General Anesthetics

General anesthetics are those that produce "sleep," or unconsciousness, along with *analgesia,* or absence of pain. They also cause a kind of amnesia in that the patient remembers nothing that occurs during the period in which the anesthetic is effective. At the same time, general anesthetics produce a certain loss of muscle tone and reflex action. A general anesthetic, however, should not interfere significantly with such normal bodily functions as respiration and circulation, nor should it produce permanent damage to body tissues.

How They Work

General anesthetics cause the patient to fall into a kind of sleep state by depressing the central nervous system, an effect that is reversible and lasts only until the drug has been eliminated by the body tissues. The general anesthetic reaches the central nervous system rather quickly because it is introduced directly or indirectly into the bloodstream. The use of a gas to produce anesthesia is an indirect method of producing unconsciousness.

A gas-type anesthetic, such as nitrous oxide or cyclopropane, can be delivered under compression from tanks or cylinders, or it may be stored in the operating room as a liquid that is converted to a vapor, like ether or halothane. The compressed-gas anesthetics are administered with the help of an anesthetic machine. The liquid forms of gases may be dripped through a mask over the patient's face; or the liquid may be vaporized and directed to the patient by anesthetic equipment. Whether the source of the anesthetic is compressed gas or a volatile liquid, the purpose is the same: to get the anesthetic into the patient's lungs.

There the gas enters the bloodstream through the walls of the blood vessels of the tiny sacs that make up the lungs.

Kinds of General Anesthetics

Nearly a dozen different kinds of gases are available as general anesthetics. Each has certain advantages and disadvantages and interacts differently with other drugs used by the patient. The effects of each on chronic diseases of the patient must be weighed. Some gases induce anesthesia more rapidly than others; some are tolerated better by patients. These are among the many factors that can determine which gas or mixture of gases might be selected by the anesthetist for a particular surgical procedure.

Intravenous Anesthetics

Not all general anesthetics come in the form of compressed gases or volatile liquids. Several commonly used general anesthetics are administered intravenously, by injection into the bloodstream. The group includes barbiturates, such as thiopental, and narcotics, such as morphine. Ketamine is a general anesthetic drug that can be injected into the muscles as well as into the bloodstream. The intravenous anesthetics may be used instead of the gaseous general anesthetics or in combination with them. Thiopental is often administered to a patient first, to bring on sleep quickly, after which an inhaled general anesthetic is applied. Like the gaseous general anesthetics, each of the injected general anesthetics has its own peculiarities and may have different effects on different individuals. The rate of recovery from thiopental anesthesia varies according to the ability of a patient's body tissue to eliminate the drug; narcotics can affect the patient's respiration; ketamine may produce hallucinations in some patients.

Regional Anesthetics

Regional anesthetics include *local anesthetics* and *spinal anesthetics.* They are more likely to be used than general anesthetics when the patient is ambulatory and the surgery involves removal of moles or cysts, plastic surgery, certain eye, ear, nose, and throat procedures, and certain operations such as hernia repair that generally are uncomplicated. Regional anesthetics also may be recommended by the surgeon for operations to correct disorders in the arms or legs.

The surgical procedure may require that the patient remain conscious so he can follow instructions of the surgeon in manipulating muscles or bones to test the function of a body part being repaired. In such cases, a regional anesthetic would be preferred; a regional also would be advised for a patient with severe heart or lung disease that might be complicated by the effects of a general anesthetic. A restless child, on the other hand, might be given a general anesthetic for a relatively minor operation, because the youngster would not be likely to remain motionless for the duration of the operation.

Topical Anesthetics

Regional anesthetics generally are administered by infiltration of a drug into the tissues involved or into the nerve trunks leading into the area of incision. A simple kind of regional anesthesia is the topical application of a substance to a sensitive membrane of a body organ. For example, the eye drops applied by an ophthalmologist may anesthetize a patient's eyes to make it easier for him to examine them. Topical anesthetics are not very effective when applied to the skin, which forms a tough barrier against most invasive substances, but they can effectively anesthetize the inner surfaces of the mouth, nose, throat, and other inner body surfaces. The anesthetic might be administered by sprays, gargles, or by direct application. Topical anesthetics commonly are used to prepare the throat and upper lung passages for examination with medical instruments.

Local Anesthetics

Local anesthetics, which are similar to those used by the dentist, are usually injected via a hypodermic needle into the tissues surrounding the area to be operated on. The injection of an anesthetic into the tissue area sometimes is referred to as a *field block.* A variation of this technique is the *nerve* or *plexus block,* in which a hypodermic needle is used to inject the drug into the region of one or more key nerve trunks leading to the site of the incision. Local anesthetics are not recommended by most surgeons if there is an inflammation or infection of the tissues around the surgery site. The drugs used for local anesthetics can lower the patient's resistance to the infection while at the same time the inflammation may reduce the effectiveness of the drug as a pain-killer.

Intravenous Administration

Sometimes a regional anesthetic is administered intravenously by injecting it into a vein that runs through the site of the surgery. The drug is confined to the area, such as an arm or leg, by applying a tourniquet about the limb. Because of the possible dangers in suddenly releasing a potent anesthetic drug into the general bloodstream after the operation is ended, the tourniquet is intermit-

tently tightened and released to slow the flow to a mere trickle. A sudden release also would quickly end the pain-killing effect in the area of the incision.

Spinal Anesthetics

Spinal anesthesia is similar to a nerve or plexus block method of eliminating pain sensation in a region of the body, except that the nerves receive the drug at the point where they leave the spinal cord. The drugs may be the same as those used as local anesthetics. They are injected either by hypodermic needle or by catheter into tissues surrounding the spinal cord. Although there are several variations of spinal anesthesia—each involving the precise layer of tissue or space around the spinal cord which is the immediate target area of the injection—for all practical purposes the objective is the same. They are all intended to produce a lack of sensation in the spinal nerves along with a loss of motor function so there will be no movement of the body area to be operated on during surgery.

The spinal anesthetic may affect not only the targeted nerve system but neighboring spinal nerves as well, generally all the spinal nerves below the point of drug injection. For its purposes, spinal anesthesia can be a highly effective alternative to a general anesthetic. However, side effects are not uncommon. Severe headache is one of the most frequent complaints of patients. Temporary adverse effects can occur after use of other regional anesthetics as well and may be owing in part to individual allergic reactions to the drug used.

Care after Surgery

The last thing you may remember as a patient, before receiving a general anesthetic, is being wheeled into the

operating room and lifted by hospital orderlies onto the operating table. You may not see the surgeon, who could be scrubbing for the operation or reviewing the information compiled on your case. The anesthetist and a few nurses may be in the operating room. You are feeling relaxed and drowsy because of the preanesthetic medications. A tube may be attached to your arm to drip an intravenous solution into a vein. The anesthetist may administer a dose of a drug such as sodium pentothal, a not unpleasant medication that brings on a deep sleep within a matter of seconds.

The Recovery Room

You will probably remember nothing after that point until you gradually become aware of the strange sounds and sights of a recovery room. The recovery room may contain a number of patients who have undergone surgery at about the same time, especially in a large hospital. Each is reclining in bed equipped with high railings to prevent a groggy, confused patient just recovering from a general anesthetic from falling onto the floor.

Nurses move briskly about the room, checking the conditions of the various patients. As each patient gains some awareness of the situation, a nurse puts an oxygen mask over his face and explains the purpose: to help restore the tiny air sacs of the lungs to their normal condition. During administration of the anesthetic, the air sacs can become dry and partially collapsed. The humidified oxygen mixture helps restore moisture to the inner surfaces of the lungs; by breathing deeply of the oxygen, the patient expands the air sacs to their normal capacity. Before the use of oxygen masks in the recovery room and deep-breathing techniques for patients recovering from the effects of an anesthetic gas, there was a much greater danger of pneumonia developing as a postoperative complication.

Nurses assigned to the recovery room are given a report on each patient arriving from the operating room and instructions about such matters as the position of the patient in the bed. One patient may have to lie flat on his back, another on his side, a third in a sitting position, and still another with the head lower than the feet. If the patient has received a general anesthetic, the nurses may be instructed to turn him from one side to the other at regular intervals until he is able to turn himself.

The patient's blood pressure, pulse, and respiration are checked at regular intervals by the recovery room nurses, who also watch for any signs of bleeding or drainage from the area of incision. The surgeon is notified immediately of any signs of complications. Because the recovery room usually is located next to the operating room, the surgeon can quickly identify complications and attend the problem without delay. Most surgical patients will remain in the recovery room for a few hours at the most, and when they appear to be able to manage somewhat on their own they are returned to their beds in the regular nursing area of the hospital.

The Intensive Care Unit

Critically ill patients or those with heart, lung, kidney, or other serious disorders usually are assigned to an intensive care unit where each bed may be isolated from the others in a glass booth designed to provide privacy and quiet during the recovery period. Patients can still be clearly observed from the central nursing station.

Patients in an intensive care unit are given continuous care by nurses.

Electronic equipment is used to monitor pulse, blood pressure, heartbeat, and, when needed, brain function and body temperature. Other devices are available for making bedside measurements of bodily function and to obtain laboratory data such as blood chemistry without moving the patient from his bed.

Pain

Most surgical patients will be concerned about how much pain they will feel after leaving the operating room. It is not unusual to expect greater pain than is actually experienced; the incision may cause no more discomfort than the problem that required surgical therapy. Obviously, a minor operation will result in less painful discomfort than a major operation. Generally, the pain or discomfort associated with a surgical incision may last for one or two days, then subside over a period of perhaps three or four days. After that an occasional twinge may be felt in the area of the incision when shifting the body puts extra stress on the muscles or other tissues involved in the operation. During the hospital stay, medications will be available to help relieve any serious pain resulting from the operation.

Signs of Recovery or Complication

While the patient may be concerned about pain following surgery, the physicians and nurses are more likely to direct their attention toward other signs and symptoms that will help them to gauge the rate of recovery, such as the patient's body temperature, skin coloring, urine output, and his ability to cough. The health professionals are well aware that surgery, and drugs or anesthetics administered in conjunction with surgery, can be disruptive to normal bodily ac-

tivities. A major operation is more likely to cause changes in the patient's physiology than a minor operation.

Vital Signs

Nurses can be expected to make regular checks of temperature, pulse, and respiration because these common measures of the body functions (sometimes called *vital signs*) can provide early-warning signals of possible post operative complications. A patient may have a temperature of 100° F. even after a major operation, but because of increased metabolic activity of the body following surgery, a slightly elevated thermometer reading is considered normal. The pulse and respiration also may be slightly above the patient's rate before surgery, but the mild change again is caused by the normal stress reaction of the body. However, a temperature rising above 100° F. and/or a significantly faster pulse or respiration rate suggests that a complication may have developed.

If a nurse seems interested in the patient's ability to cough, it is because the cough reflex helps the patient get rid of mucus accumulation in his lungs, especially after the use of a general anesthetic. If coughing is difficult, a plastic tube may be inserted into the patient's throat to help clear the breathing passages. Normal breathing can also be restored by steam inhalation, aerosol sprays of water or special medications, or positive pressure breathing equipment that forces air into the lungs. Failure to expand the air passages of the lungs leads to serious respiratory complications.

Urine output is also checked. This is just one more way of watching the rate of recovery of a patient and alerting the staff to any signs of complications. If for some reason the patient is unable to pass urine, a *catheter*, or plastic tube, is inserted into the bladder to drain it. The volume of urine drained is collected and measured.

The Incision Area

Some blood may accumulate under the skin in the area of the incision or in nearby tissues, causing a discoloration of the skin. But this effect is seldom a serious matter, and the discoloration gradually vanishes. In some cases of excess blood accumulation, the surgeon may simply remove one or two sutures and drain away the blood. Any continued bleeding about the incision would, of course, be a complication.

A more common complication is infection of the incision area by bacteria that enter the wound. An infection may develop any time from one day to one week after an operation. However, most postoperative infections of incision wounds are easily controlled by antibiotics, drainage, or natural defenses against disease. The surgeon or other physicians will make regular inspections of the incision during the first few days after surgery to make sure it is healing properly.

Postoperative Nourishment

A light meal may be offered the patient a few hours after surgery. The patient may or may not feel like eating, especially if he still feels a bit nauseated from the effects of a general anesthetic. At this stage fluid intake is probably more important, especially if the patient has not been allowed to have even a sip of water since the previous evening. If the surgery was not performed on the stomach or intestinal tract, a small amount of water or tea may be permitted within a few hours after the operation. It is unlikely in any case that the patient will feel a great desire for fluid, because intravenous solutions

may have been dripping slowly into a vein since he entered the operating room. Intravenous solutions can satisfy hunger as well as thirst because they may contain proteins, carbohydrates, and essential vitamins and minerals dissolved in a finely formulated broth. Perhaps unnoticed by the patient, the amount of fluid intake will be routinely measured by members of the hospital staff.

Ambulation

Ambulation—getting the patient out of bed and moving about—is an important part of postoperative care. Experience has shown that recovery from surgery is more effective if the patient spends increasing amounts of time each day in simple physical activity. The degree of ambulation depends upon the magnitude of the surgery and the general physical health of the patient. But in a typical case of hernia surgery or an appendectomy, the patient may be asked, on the first or second day after the operation, to sit on the edge of his bed and dangle his legs for a while. On the second or third day, he may be allowed to walk about the room, and may in fact prefer to walk to the bathroom rather than use a bedpan or urinal. On the following day, he may walk up and down the halls with the help of a nurse or other hospital staff member.

Each patient is encouraged to handle the ambulation phase of recovery at his own pace, and there are few hard and fast rules. Of two persons entering the operating room on the same day for the same kind of elective surgery, one may feel like walking to the bathroom a few hours after surgery while the second may prefer to remain in bed and use a bedpan a week after surgery. The surgeon and attending physicians may encourage and in some cases even insist upon early ambulation, however, because it reduces the rate of complications.

Back at Home

Dressings used to cover the incision are changed regularly, as the incision is inspected once each day, more frequently if warranted. If the patient is anxious to be discharged from the hospital as early as possible, the surgeon may give him instructions for changing his own dressings. The surgeon will also outline a plan for recovery procedures to be followed after he leaves the hospital. The plan will include a schedule of visits to the surgeon's office for removal of stitches that may remain and a final inspection of the incision. The surgeon will also offer his advice on how the patient should plan a return to normal activities, including a return to his job and resumption of sports or recreational programs.

Special Diets

Proper foods are as important as proper medicines in helping a patient recover from surgery. Despite the common complaints about hospital meals, the nutrients that are provided in certain special diets for surgical patients are as carefully prescribed and prepared as are some medications that are served in pill or capsule form.

Surgical nutrition has become increasingly important in recent years because of an awareness by physicians that an operation, minor or major, is not unlike an organic disease that creates physiological stresses and a nutritional imbalance in the patient's body. To help compensate for alterations in the patient's physiology as it recovers from the effects of surgery, special diets may be ordered.

Bland Soft Diet

A bland soft diet frequently is ordered for patients who are unable to handle a regular diet but whose condition is not serious enough to require a liquid diet. The foods are selected because they are low in cellulose and connective tissue; they are bland, smooth, and easily digested. The choice of food, nevertheless, represents as great a variety as one might be served in a restaurant or at home, except for an absence of spices and other substances that would be stimulating to the gastrointestinal tract. Included in the surgical soft diet might be lean meat, fish, poultry, eggs, milk, mild cheese, cooked tender or pureed fruits and vegetables, refined cereals and breads with butter or margarine, plus gelatin desserts, puddings, custards, and ice cream.

Liquid Diet

Liquid diets for surgical patients may be prepared with or without milk. They are usually ordered for patients with impaired function of the gastrointestinal tract. A liquid diet without milk may include a cereal gruel made with water, clear bouillon or broth, gelatin, strained fruit juce, and coffee or tea. Liquid diets with milk are similar but may also include creamed soups, sherbets, ice cream, cereal gruel made with milk instead of water, cocoa and beverages of milk or cream. Beverage options permitted are tomato juice and some carbonated beverages such as ginger ale.

Diets Following Particular Kinds of Surgery

Peptic Ulcers

A special diet for peptic ulcer patients may include a half-and-half mixture of milk and cream, plus mashed potatoes, eggs, toast and butter, pureed vegetables, cottage cheese, rice, plain puddings and gelatin desserts. But meat soups, tea, coffee, raw vegetables, and fried foods are prohibited.

Rectal Surgery

Following rectal surgery, and other procedures in which it is necessary to prevent bowel movements for a period of several days, a low residue diet is ordered. A low residue diet (or *minimal residue diet,* as it is also called) might offer eggs, poached or boiled, rice, soda crackers, cereals made with water, butter, bouillon or clear broths, carbonated beverages, tea, coffee, and certain meats, including oysters, sweetbreads, and tender bits of beef or veal. An alternative low residue diet is the bland soft diet with all milk-containing items eliminated.

Gallbladder Surgery

Gallbladder surgical patients may expect a modified fat diet that eliminates as much as possible fats and gas-producing food items. It includes foods that provide protein and carbohydrate sources of energy to replace fats and includes primarily fish, poultry, lean cuts of beef, cottage cheese, cereal products and bread, and certain fruits and vegetables. However, foods prohibited are mainly pork products and fatty cuts of other meats, cream, chocolate, melons, apples, fried foods of any kind, onions, cabbage, turnips, cucumbers, radishes, green peppers, and dried beans and peas.

Restricted Salt Intake

Chronic heart failure patients and those with liver ailments or edema are placed on a low-sodium diet before and after surgery. The low-sodium diet is fairly simple in that it is prepared mainly with foods from which sodium or salt either is naturally absent or has been removed. Many salt-free or low-sodium foods are available commercially from manufacturers that also supply special dietetic foods for persons suffering from diabetes.

Fractures or Burns

Special consideration is given the diets of patients who are recovering from accidents that result in fractures or burns. Because of complex body responses to such injuries, there may be an abnormal loss of nitrogen from the tissues and a breakdown of muscle tissue, which is a rich source of nitrogen, an important component of protein. As a result, adequate amounts of protein need to be provided to surgical patients with burn injuries and broken bones.

Potassium Loss

Normal body stores of potassium also may be diminished during and immediately after surgery, but potassium can be replaced in the tissues by including in the meals adequate amounts of meats, fish, poultry, bananas, raisins, figs, dates, and prunes, as well as dried peaches and dried apricots. Prune, tomato, orange, and pineapple juices also are a rich source of potassium for postoperative patients.

Replacement of Water Losses

While water is not always thought of as a food, it is an important part of the gastronomic intake of the surgical patient; adequate amounts of water need to be provided the person recovering from an operation. The postoperative patient usually requires larger than normal amounts of water even though he may not feel inclined to help himself to as much fluid intake as he would at home or on the job. In addition to normal water losses through perspiration, urine, and breathing, there may be additional water losses through vomiting. Water replacement may be provided through sufficient amounts of fruit juices and other beverages offered during meals and between meals.

Apprehensions about Surgery

Most people feel anxious when faced with the need for surgery. This is to be expected. After all, a certain amount of anxiety normally accompanies any prolonged or incapacitating illness or infirmity. When surgery is the recommended therapy, it's natural for the patient to feel some anxiety about the surgery even if he's optimistic about a favorable result.

Factors That Reduce the Risk of Modern Surgery

Much of the risk of surgery these days is eliminated through the careful preoperative screening examinations reviewed earlier. A patient with a chronic disease who might have been a surgical risk a generation ago may have one or more options not available in past years, such as regional anesthetics that allow surgeons alternatives to general anesthetics that would be less than satisfactory. Antibiotics and other backup medications are available to control possible complications after surgery. Recovery room techniques and intensive care units with electronic monitoring of vital life systems provide added insurance of safe recovery. And, of course, surgeons today have the added experience of many millions of successful operations involving a range of procedures such as kidney and heart transplants, open heart surgery, and replacement of important organ parts with plastic substitutes. These and other procedures, including the implanting of electronic heart pacemakers, were beyond the dreams of surgeons of past years.

Surgery for the Older Patient

With the rapid increase in the proportion of older people in the population, the surgical patient is more likely to be an older person with problems as-sociated with aging. An older man who underwent surgery to remove his prostate gland before World War II had a life expectancy of a few years after the operation. Today, such procedures in older men are considered routine cases with little or no effect on longevity. It is not unusual nowadays to find men and women in their 70s and 80s who have undergone five or six major operations since reaching the traditional retirement age and without any significant restrictions on their physical activities.

Part of the reason for the greatly improved outlook for surgery on older patients may be that older persons today are simply in better health because of the improved medical care available. Thus they are better surgical risks than their parents would have been at the same age. Advanced preoperative and postoperative care has also improved the outlook for the older patient. He may be admitted to the hospital a few days earlier than the younger patient for more intensive examinations, and he may remain a few days longer for postoperative care. Convalescence for the older patient may take longer, and in some instances the recovery may not be as complete as that of a younger person. But in general, modern surgical techniques are likely to offer a safe and effective therapy for people of advanced age with complaints that can be corrected by an operation.

In addition to the physical benefits, surgery may improve the mental capacity, personality, and sensitivity of older persons who had been depressed about a disorder before surgery. The patient who complained that he is no longer the person he used to be physically may have assumed that his medical problem was simply a result of growing old and overlooked the possibility that the complaint was due to a disease that might respond to treatment.

Surgery for the Child

A child, on the other hand, may have his own reasons to be apprehensive about the trip to a hospital for surgery. Most children seem to worry that the operation will hurt or that other procedures, such as taking a blood sample for testing, will be painful.

Telling the Truth

Many surgeons recommend that the child be told as realistically as possible, in terms he can understand, what can be expected. The youngster should not be given a sugar-coated story about the operation which might give the impression that he is embarking upon a happy adventure. At the same time, the child should not be frightened by suggestions that he may be given drugs to make him unconscious while he is strapped to a table so that strangely masked and gowned strangers can cut him open with sharp knives.

Children are more likely to appreciate surgery if they are told that a friendly person will help them go to sleep; that the operation will hurt a little but the pain will go away after a while; and that the operation will make them feel better or help correct a problem so they can be more active like other children. A small child should always understand that he may have to remain overnight at the hospital without his parents, but that he will have other adults to take care of him and there probably will be other children at the hospital to keep him company.

Common Surgical Procedures

In this section some of the more

common surgical procedures are described. The operations discussed are organized by the system or region of the body with which they are concerned. The following areas are covered in this order:

- Male Reproductive System (for surgical procedures involving the female reproductive system, see Ch. 25, *Women's Health*);

- Urinary Tract;

- Abdominal Region;

- Oral Cavity and Throat;

- Ear Surgery;

- Eye Surgery;

- Chest Region;

- Vascular Surgery;

- Orthopedic Surgery; and

- Neurosurgery.

Many of the conditions treated in this chapter from a surgical point of view are also treated elsewhere, in the chapter devoted to diseases of the appropriate body system or organ; the reader is invited to turn to those chapters for additional information. For example, although heart surgery is discussed in this chapter, heart disease is treated in greater detail in Ch. 10, *Heart Disease*.

Male Reproductive System

Surgical procedures of the prostate, testis, scrotum, and penis are considered in this section. Undescended testicles and vasectomy are also among the subjects discussed.

Prostate Surgery

The prostate gland is a small cone-shaped object that surrounds the male urethra, the tube that carries urine from the urinary bladder to the penis.

It is normally about one-half inch long and weighs less than an ounce. Ejaculatory ducts empty through the prostate into the urethra, and other ducts drain glandular secretions of the prostate into the urethra. Because of the intimate association of the prostate gland and the urinary tract, a disorder in one system can easily affect the other. A urinary infection can spread to the prostate and an abnormality of the prostate can interfere with the normal excretion of urine.

Enlargement of the Prostate

A relatively common problem is the tendency of the prostate to grow larger in middle-aged men. The gradual enlargement continues from the 40s on, but the symptoms usually go unnoticed until the man is in his 60s. At that point in life, the prostate may have become so enlarged that it presses on the urethra and obstructs the flow of urine from the neighboring bladder. The older man may experience various difficulties in emptying his bladder. He may have to urinate more frequently, and suddenly find himself getting out of bed at night to go to the bathroom. He may not be able to develop a urine stream of the size and force he had in earlier years. He may have trouble getting the stream of urine started and it may end in a dribble.

In addition to the somewhat embarrassing inconveniences caused by prostate enlargement, the urinary bladder may not drain properly and can eventually lose its own muscle tone needed for emptying. Residual urine in the bladder can become a source of infection, and backflow into the ureters can gradually affect those tissues and the kidneys. It has been estimated that 20 percent of all older men may need treatment of some kind, including surgery, for correcting this problem of the prostate gland.

Factors Indicating the Need for Surgery

Factors that may decide in favor of surgical removal of the prostate include residual urine in the patient's bladder; blood in the urine, with evidence that the blood comes from the prostate; the severity of the inconveniences associated with irregular urination; and complications such as the presence or threat of failure of the wall of the urinary bladder, the formation of stones, and symptoms and signs of infection.

Surgical Methods

There are several methods of performing a *prostatectomy* (excision of all or part of the prostate) for relief of the symptoms of an enlarged prostate, a condition that may appear on the patient's medical records as *benign prostate hyperplasia*. All of the methods are relatively safe and in none of the techniques is the entire prostate removed. One method, called *transurethral resection*, requires insertion of an instrument into the urethra through the penis. The instrument, a *resectoscope,* uses a high-frequency electric current to cut away the tissue inside the gland. This technique avoids open surgery and requires a postoperative hospital stay of only a few days.

Open Surgery

The other techniques involve *open surgery,* that is, surgery in which an incision is made in the pelvic or rectal area to make the prostate gland accessible so that its inner tissues can be removed. The differences in the various open surgery techniques depend upon such factors as where the incision should be made and the risks associated with the approaches. The incision is made either in the *perineum,* the region between the rectum

Prostate

Bladder

Seminal vesicle

Ejaculatory duct

Urethra

and the testicles, or through the abdomen. Only a small percentage of patients experience complications or regrowth of the prostate tissues to produce a second enlargement problem. Impotence is usually not an aftereffect of the surgery, and libido is normal.

Infections of the Prostate

Infections of the prostate gland can involve obstruction of the urethra, but the problem usually can be resolved by the use of medications and techniques other than surgery. An abscess, however, may require an incision to drain the prostate. Surgery also may be recommended for the treatment of stones, or calculi, that develop in the prostate and cause obstruction or contribute to infections.

Cancer of the Prostate

Cancer of the prostate also may occur in older men, causing obstruction or the urinary flow or contributing to infection of the urinary tract. If examination including biopsy studies confirms the presence of cancer, the surgeon may recommend radical prostatectomy. In this procedure an

incision is made either through the lower abdomen or through the perineum to remove the entire prostate gland and surrounding tissues, such as the seminal vesicles. Hormonal therapy, chemotherapy, and radiation treatments also may be administered.

Tumors of the Testis

Tumors of the testis occur most frequently in men between the ages of 18 and 35. Such a tumor appears as a firm and enlarged testis and usually without pain unless bleeding is involved as a symptom. Testicular tumors generally are malignant and spread rapidly to other parts of the body, including the lungs. The onset of the disorder can be so insidious that the patient may seek medical advice for a more obvious secondary problem, such as the apparent development of mammary glands on his chest, the result of disruption of his normal male hormonal balance.

Special laboratory tests and other examination techniques usually are required to determine which of several possible kinds of testicular tumors may be involved and the extent of the metastasis of the cancer cells to other body areas. If cancer of a

testicle is confirmed, it is removed by an incision through the groin area, and neighboring lymph nodes also will be taken out. The surgical procedure usually is supplemented with chemotherapy and radiation. The prognosis, or chances for recovery, following surgical removal of a testicular tumor depends upon the particular kind of cancer involved and how far the disease had progressed before medical treatment was begun.

Tumors of the Scrotum and Penis

Tumors of the scrotum and penis are relatively uncommon but do occur. Cancer of the scrotum is usually associated with exposure to cancer-causing chemicals. Boys who worked as chimney sweeps a century ago tended to develop cancer of the scrotum from body contact with soot in coal-burning fireplaces. Cancer of the penis occurs usually in men who have not been circumcised. In either type of cancer, the treatment usually requires removal of the affected tissues. This can mean castration in the case of scrotal cancer or amputation of a part or all of the penis, depending upon the extent of the cancerous growth. Surgery that requires removal of a part of the reproductive system can have a devastating psychological effect on a man, but the alternative is likely to be early death from the spread of cancer.

Undescended Testicles

About 10 percent of cases of tumors of the testis occur in men with an undescended testicle. Because the chances of a tumor developing in an undescended testicle are as much as 50 times greater than the incidence for the normal male population, the existence of an undescended testicle can warrant corrective surgery.

Ordinarily, the testicles descend

from their fetal location in the abdomen into the scrotum about two months before birth. But in one case in 200 male births, a child is found with a failure of one or, less commonly, both testicles to descend properly into the scrotum. In addition to the risk of cancer, undescended testicles are associated with lack of fertility and other problems, such as hernias.

Cryptorchidism

In male babies and young boys, an undescended testicle sometimes can be encouraged to enter the scrotum by manipulation or administration of hormones. Many surgeons recommend that the developmental problem of undescended testicles, or *cryptorchidism*, be corrected before a child enters school, although the surgical procedure for correcting the situation can be postponed until adolescence or adulthood. The operation for correcting an undescended testicle is called *orchidopexy* and involves an incision in the groin to release the testicle and its attached cord from fibrous tissue holding it in the abdomen. The testicle may be brought directly down into the scrotum, where it may be anchored temporarily with a suture, or it may be brought down in stages in a series of operations to permit the growth and extension of blood supply to the testis. The original location of the undescended testicle determines which procedure is used.

Vasectomy

Vasectomy is a birth control technique that is intended to make a man permanently sterile. It does not involve the removal of any of the male reproductive system and does not result in a loss of potency or libido. A vasectomy is a relatively simple operation that can be performed in a physician's office in less than 30 minutes and requires only a local anesthetic. The operation is similar to but much less complicated than the procedure in which a woman may be sterilized by cutting or tying her Fallopian tubes. A vasectomy requires no hospitalization, and the man is able to return to work or other normal activities after a day or two.

How the Procedure Is Done

The vasectomy procedure requires a small incision, about one-half inch in length, on either side of the scrotum. The surgeon removes through the incision a short length of the *vas deferens*, the tube that carries spermatozoa from the testicles, and ties a piece of surgical thread at two points about an inch apart. Then a small piece of the vas deferens between the tied-off points is snipped out of the tube. The procedure is done on each side. With the ducts of the vas deferens cut and tied, sperm from the testicles can no longer move through their normal paths to the prostate, where they would become mixed with semen from the prostate and seminal vesicles and be ejaculated during sexual intercourse.

Sterility Is Usually Permanent

A vasectomy does not immediately render a man sterile. Sperm already stored in the seminal "pipeline" can still be active for a period of a month to six weeks, and a woman who has intercourse with a vasectomized man during that period can become pregnant. On the other hand, a man who undergoes a vasectomy should not expect that the severed ducts can be connected again should he want to become a father in the future. Sperm banks have been offered as a possible alternative for the man who might want to store some of his spermatozoa for future use, but there is little

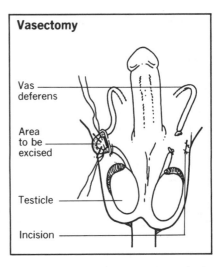

Vasectomy

Vas deferens

Area to be excised

Testicle

Incision

evidence that the sperm will remain fertile in a sperm bank for more than a year or 18 months. In rare cases, men who have undergone vasectomies have unintentionally become fertile again because of *canalization*, or creation of a new channel connecting the severed ends of the vas deferens; in one case the canalization occurred 8 years after the vasectomy was performed.

The vasectomy is regarded as an extremely safe operation, and complications are infrequent. Some swelling and discomfort are reported by a small percentage of men undergoing the operation. Steroid hormone drugs are sometimes administered to control these aftereffects.

Urinary Tract

Surgical procedures involving urinary stones and tumors of the bladder, ureter, urethra, and kidney are considered in this section. Also discussed are kidney cysts and conditions affecting the adrenal glands which might require surgery.

Urinary Stones

Most stones that occur in the urinary tract are formed in the kidneys, but kidney stones can travel to other areas, such as the ureters, and cause problems there. Various types of stones can develop in the kidneys from several different causes. A common cause is a metabolic disorder involving calcium, proteins, or uric acid. Other causes are infections or obstructions of the urinary tract, the use of certain drugs, such as diuretics, or vitamin deficiency.

Symptoms

Kidney stones seldom cause problems while they are forming, but movement of the stones irritates the urinary tract and can cause severe pain; the irritation of the tissues may cause bleeding that will ultimately show up in the urine. Other symptoms may indicate obstruction of the flow of urine, and infection. In some cases obstruction of a ureter can lead to failure of the kidney. X-ray techniques can usually verify the cause of the patient's symptoms and locate the urinary stone. Most stones cast a shadow on X-ray film, and by injecting special dyes into the urinary system, the degree of obstruction by a stone can be determined.

Ureter Stones

Most stones released by the kidney are small enough to pass through a ureter to the bladder and be excreted while urinating. But if a stone is large enough it can become lodged in a ureter, causing excruciating pain that may be felt both in the back and in the abdomen along the path of the ureter. Ureter stones often can be removed by manipulation, using catheter tubes that are inserted through the bladder. If the stuck stone cannot be manipulated from the ureter, an operation in a hospital is required. However, the surgical procedure is relatively simple and direct. An incision is made over the site of the stuck stone, and the ureter is exposed and opened just far

enough to permit removal of the stone. The operation is safe and requires perhaps a week in the hospital.

Kidney Stones

If the urinary stone is lodged in the kidney, the surgical procedure also is a relatively safe one although more complicated and requiring a longer hospital stay. The surgeon must work through skin and muscle layers to reach the kidney, then cut into the kidney if necessary to remove the stone. If the obstruction has been serious enough to impair normal kidney function or if infection has damaged the kidney tissue, the surgeon may elect to remove the affected kidney. Fortunately, the human body can get along fairly well with one good functioning kidney, so a *nephrectomy*, as the procedure is called, may not be as drastic a maneuver as the patient might imagine. If, on the other hand, the affected kidney has not been seriously damaged, the stone or stones can be removed with instruments or by the surgeon's fingers and the incision in the kidney sewed up so that it can resume its normal functions.

More modern techniques for removing kidney stones include two that hold promise of eliminating nearly all surgical methods. One involves the use of the lithotriptor, a machine that shatters the stones with an electrical shock wave. The wave is focused on the stones with the aid of a reflector and two sophisticated X-ray machines that "aim" the target beam. No surgery is required, and the patient is usually back at work within a week. A second means of attacking kidney stones is a drug, *potassium citrate*, which keeps the stones from forming. The drug actually corrects the metabolic disorders that cause the formation of kidney stones.

Vesical Stones

Occasionally, urinary stones are found in the neck of the bladder or in the bladder itself. They are called *vesical stones* and, depending upon their size and other factors, may be removed by several techniques, including use of a cystoscope inserted through the urethra. In some cases the stone can be broken into smaller pieces for removal. If it appears unlikely that the stone can be removed directly or by crushing it, the surgeon can make an incision directly to the bladder in a manner similar to the approach used in removing a stone from the ureter.

Bladder Tumors

About three-fourths of the tumors of the bladder occur in men past the age of 45. Although the specific cause of bladder tumors is unknown, physicians suspect that a cancer-producing chemical is involved. Several studies have found an association between the disease and cigarette smoking or occupations that require contact with organic chemicals used in making dyes. Tumors that appear in the female bladder are less likely to be cancerous than those that occur in the male bladder.

Symptoms and Diagnosis

The first symptom of bladder tumor is blood in the urine. The tumor itself may cause no pain, but an early complication could be an infection producing inflammation and discomfort in the region of the bladder. If the tumor blocks the normal flow of urine, the patient may feel pain or discomfort in the area of the kidneys; this condition is most likely to happen if the tumor is located at the opening of a ureter leading from a kidney to the bladder. An early examination of the bladder may fail to locate a small tumor, although X rays might show the growth as a bit of shadow on the film, and obstruction of a ureter could be seen. Nonetheless, examination of the interior of the bladder by a cystoscope is necessary to confirm the presence of the tumor. A biopsy can be made by removing a few tissue cells from the area in a manner quite like the procedure for making a Pap-smear test for possible cancer of the cervix in a female patient.

Treatment

Most early and simple cases of bladder tumor can be corrected by a procedure called *saucerization* by an instrument that removes the abnormal tissue, leaving a shallow wound that normally will grow over with healthy tissue cells. But a tumor that invades deeply into the wall of the bladder requires more radical therapy, such as surgery to cut away the part of the bladder that is affected by the growth. Radiation also may be employed to control the spread of tumor cells, particularly if laboratory tests indicate that the type of tumor cells involved are sensitive to radiation.

Surgical Procedure

If it is necessary to cut away a part of the bladder, the surgeon simply shapes a new but smaller organ from the remaining tissues. If a total *cystectomy* is required to save the life of the patient, the entire bladder is removed, along with the prostate if the patient is a man. When the bladder is removed, a new path for the flow of urine is devised by the surgeons, usually to divert the urine into the lower end of the intestinal tract.

Tumors of the Ureter or Urethra

Tumors of the ureter, above the bladder, or of the urethra, below the bladder, may begin with symptoms resembling those of a bladder tumor, although X rays might show the growth as a bit of shadow on the normal flow of urine. Treatment also usually requires removal of the affected tissues with reconstructive surgery as needed to provide for a normal flow of urine from the kidneys.

Kidney Tumors

Wilms' Tumor

Tumors of the kidney generally occur either in children before the age of eight or in adults over the age of 25. The type of tumor that affects children usually is the Wilms' tumor, one of the most common kinds of cancer that can afflict a youngster. The tumor grows rapidly and may be painful even though there may be no obvious signs of urinary tract disorder in the child's urine. The tumor frequently becomes so large that it appears as an abdominal swelling. A Wilms' tumor usually occurs only on one side of the body, but in a small percentage of the cases the disorder can develop in both right and left kidneys. Kidney function may continue normally during growth of the tumor, but cancerous cells from the tumor may be carried by the bloodstream to other parts of the body, by metastasis, causing the problem to spread to the lungs and other vital organs.

Treatment usually requires surgical removal of the affected kidney and radiation therapy; the tumor cells responsible for the growth are sensitive to radiation. The younger the child and the earlier treatment is started, the better are the child's chances for recovery from a Wilms' tumor.

Adult Kidney Tumor

The adult type of kidney tumor, which is more likely to affect men than women, may also appear as an enlarged abdominal mass. But, unlike the Wilms' tumor, the adult kidney tumor presents as an early symptom blood in the urine. Bleeding from the kidney may be painless. X-ray studies may show an enlarged and sometimes distorted kidney. The patient may have symptoms indicating metastasis of the tumor cells to the lungs, bones, or other body systems. Adult kidney tumors are almost always malignant.

Treatment usually requires nephrectomy, or surgical removal of the diseased kidney. Radiation therapy may be provided in addition to the surgery, although the kind of tumor cells involved in the adult type of kidney tumor usually are resistant to radiation. Chemotherapy also may be offered. The chances for complete recovery from a kidney tumor depend upon several factors, such as the location of the tumor in the kidney and the extent of metastasis of the cancerous cells to other organ systems.

Kidney Cysts

A cyst is a small pouch enclosed by a membrane; technically, the urinary bladder and gall bladder are cysts. But the cysts of medical disorders are small pouches or sacs filled with a fluid or viscous substance; they may appear on the skin, in the lungs, or in other body systems, such as the kidneys.

Symptoms

Kidney cysts produce symptoms that resemble the symptoms of cancer of the kidney; in a few cases kidney cysts are associated with tumors that cause bleeding into the cysts. In addition to the troublesome symptoms of flank pain and blood in the urine, untreated cysts can grow until they damage normal kidney tissue and impair the function of the organ's functions. Simple or solitary kidney cysts usually do not occur before the age of 40.

Diagnosis

X-ray techniques are made to determine the exact nature of kidney cyst symptoms, but in some cases exploratory surgery is recommended to differentiate a cyst from a tumor. The cyst is excised, frequently by cutting away the exposed wall of the growth. The chances of the cyst reforming are very slight.

Polycystic Kidney Disease

A different kind of kidney cyst disease, consisting of many small cysts, may be found in younger persons, including small children. The symptoms again may be flank pain and blood in the urine; examination may show some enlargement of the kidney. This form of the disease, sometimes called *polycystic kidney disease,* can be complicated by uremia and hypertension as the patient grows older. Treatment usually is medical unless the cysts interfere with urine flow by obstructing the upper end of the ureter. If the outlook for recovery through conservative treatment is poor, the surgeon may consider a kidney transplant operation.

Adrenal Glands

The adrenal glands are small hormone-producing organs that are located just above the kidneys. Although the combined weight of the two glands may be only one-fourth of an ounce, the adrenals affect a number of important body functions, including carbohydrate and protein metabolism and fluid balance. Surgery of the adrenal glands may be needed for

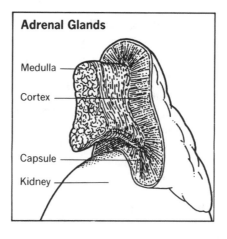

Adrenal Glands

Medulla

Cortex

Capsule

Kidney

the correction of various bodily disorders associated with oversecretion of the adrenal hormones; it may also be indicated to help control of cancer of the breast in women and cancer of the prostate in men.

Tumors of the Adrenal Glands

Tumors of the adrenal glands produce a disorder known as *primary hyperaldosteronism,* which is marked by symptoms of muscle weakness, hypertension, abnormally large outputs of urine, and excessive thirst. Another kind of tumor invasion of the adrenal glands can produce symptoms of hypertension with headaches, visual blurring, and severe sweating. Still another adrenal-related disorder, called *Cushing's syndrome,* tends to affect women under the age of 40. The symptoms may range from hypertension and obesity to acne, easy bruising, and *amenorrhea* (cessation of menstruation). Adrenal tumors may also alter secondary sex characteristics of men and women; they may result in body hair and baldness in women and increased sex drive in men.

Despite the tiny size of the adrenal glands, they are complex organs, and the varied disorders caused by tumors of the glands may depend upon the precise kind of tumor cells involved and the precise area of the glands affected by the tumor, as well

as the interactions of the adrenal hormones with hormones from other glands, such as the pituitary, or master gland of the body, located at the base of the brain.

Preoperative Tests

Before adrenal surgery for correction of a disorder is begun, the surgeon may ask for detailed laboratory tests and other diagnostic information. A radioactive scan to help locate and identify the kind of tumor more precisely may be ordered. Women patients who have been using oral contraceptives usually have to discontinue use of "the pill" for two months or more, because the medication can interfere with laboratory studies of hormones in the bloodstream.

Long-Range Effects

Physicians handling the case also must evaluate the long-range effects of an adrenal gland operation because normal metabolism is likely to be disrupted by removal of the glands, if that should be necessary. Hormone medications usually are needed in such cases to replace the hormones normally secreted. An *adrenalectomy* (removal of an adrenal gland) sometimes is explained as the substitution of a controllable disease for a life-threatening disease that cannot be controlled by medical therapy. If only one of the adrenal glands must be removed, however, the patient may be able to recover and resume a normal life without the need for hormone medications.

Surgical Procedure

The surgical approach to the adrenal glands is similar to that used in kidney operations. The incision may be made through the abdomen or through the flank. The surgery may be primarily exploratory, or the surgeon may excise a part of a gland, an entire gland, or both glands, depending upon the extent of the disease, or upon other factors, such as the need to control cancers in other parts of the body.

Abdominal Region

This section discusses the following procedures or conditions: appendicitis, peptic ulcers, hiatus hernia, adhesions, cancer of the stomach and of the intestines, gallbladder surgery, inguinal hernia, and hemorrhoids.

Appendicitis

Inflammation of the appendix is one of the most common causes of abdominal surgery today, particularly among children. But appendicitis was not recognized as a disease until 1886, leading some doctors to believe that this digestive tract infection may be related to a change in eating habits that occurred within the past century. The vermiform appendix, the site of the inflammation, is a short, wormlike (or *vermiform*) appendage at the junction of the small and large intestines. Its function in humans is unknown; plant-eating animals have an appendix, but carnivorous animals, like cats, do not. Humans live quite well without an appendix, so it seems reasonable to have a diseased appendix removed.

Symptoms

The appendix can cause trouble if it becomes obstructed by a foreign body, a tumor, an infection, or other cause of inflammation. Pain is a common symptom; there may be two kinds of pain at the same time: one, localized on the lower right side of the abdomen, near the site of the appendix; the other, more generalized and

colicky, of the kind sometimes associated with gas in the intestine. Some patients experience diarrhea or a constant urge to defecate, an effect attributed to irritation of the bowel by the abnormal activity of the appendix. Frequently there is loss of appetite, nausea and vomiting, and a fever.

The symptoms of appendicitis may begin suddenly, but frequently take from 6 to 18 hours to develop into a pattern typical of the disease, so most cases permit ample time for a doctor to examine the patient and make a diagnosis before the problem becomes critical. During the period that any symptoms suggest a possibility of appendicitis, the patient should avoid the use of any laxatives.

Ruptured Appendix

A potentially serious complication of untreated appendicitis is rupture of the appendix, which can produce a slightly different set of symptoms because of the onset of *peritonitis,* a dangerous inflammation of tissues outside the intestinal tract. The contents of the ruptured appendix leak into the body cavity, spreading the bacterial infection and irritating the lining (peritoneum) of the abdominal cavity. Diarrhea and a fever of more than 101° F. are frequently associated with a perforated or ruptured appendix. The colicky pain may disappear suddenly, because the internal pressure ends with perforation of the wall of the appendix, but it is quickly replaced by the pain of peritonitis. The severe pain of peritonitis usually is made worse by any body movement, including the abdominal muscle movement required for coughing or sneezing.

Appendicitis with perforation is much more common in older persons, perhaps because the early symptoms of colicky pain that younger people notice are not felt by older people, so

the disease is not detected until it has reached an advanced stage. Appendicitis also requires special attention in pregnant women, because the enlarged uterus crowds and repositions segments of the intestinal tract and the potential threat grows more serious during the last trimester of pregnancy.

Surgical Procedure

Laboratory tests usually are checked before surgery proceeds if there is no evidence of perforation. The usual symptoms of appendicitis can be produced by a number of other ailments, and the symptoms may diminish with bed rest, time, and medications. However, appendicitis must be considered in any case of acute abdominal complaints, and many surgeons and physicians follow the rule of "When in doubt, operate." Surgery for appendicitis is fairly simple and safe if the appendix has not perforated. An incision is made in the lower right side of the abdomen, the connection between the end of the large intestine and appendix tied off with surgical thread, and the appendix cut away from the stump. The actual operation, if uncomplicated by peritonitis or other factors, may require only a few minutes. A hospital stay of a few days is usually required during which the diet is readjusted from nothing by mouth at first, to a liquid diet, then a soft diet, etc. Normal work activities usually can be resumed within two or three weeks following surgery. Complications other than those related to peritonitis are rare. In untreated cases involving peritonitis, however, the risk is very high.

Peptic Ulcers

The cause of peptic ulcers is still unknown, although the disease affects about 10 percent of the population at some time in life. Men are four times as likely as women to develop ulcers; the incidence is highest in young and middle-aged men. Peptic ulcers may occur in the stomach, where they are called *gastric ulcers,* or in the duodenum, where they are called *duodenal ulcers.* Ninety percent of the ulcer cases that reach the physician's office for treatment are in the duodenum, a short length of the small intestine just beyond the stomach. Autopsy studies indicate that gastric ulcers may be as common as duodenal ulcers, but are frequently not detected during the life of the individual.

Causes

The development of ulcers is associated with the possible action of gastric acid on the lining of the stomach and duodenum in people who may have inherited a sensitivity to the substances. Ulcers are also related to the use of certain drugs and exposure to severe burns, injury, emotional stress, and disease.

Symptoms

A common symptom is a gnawing pain in the area of the stomach from 30 minutes to several hours after eating; the pain is relieved by food or antacid medications. The pain sometimes is likened to heartburn and may be described as radiating from the abdomen to the back. Some patients report the discomfort is more like a feeling of hunger or cramps; they may be awakened from sleep by the feeling that is relieved by a midnight snack of milk or other foods. Attacks of ulcers may be seasonal, occurring in certain patients only in the spring and autumn. In severe cases there may be bleeding without any sensation of abdominal pain; bleeding occurs from erosion of the lining of the stomach or duo-

denum and penetration of blood vessels in those membranes.

Complications other than bleeding can include perforation of the wall of the stomach or duodenum by continued erosion, or inflammatory swelling and scarring by an ulcer at a narrow part of the digestive tract, causing an obstruction. A duodenal ulcer can erode into the head of the pancreas, which secretes its digestive juices into the small intestine in that area. The pain may then become more or less continuous regardless of efforts to palliate it with food or antacids.

Symptoms vary only slightly between duodenal and gastric ulcers. Gastric ulcer pain usually begins earlier after a meal, attacks generally last longer, and symptoms, including vomiting and loss of appetite, may be more severe than in duodenal ulcer. But because of the similarities, physicians usually rely on laboratory tests and X-ray studies to determine the precise location in the digestive tract of the peptic ulcer.

Duodenal Ulcers

Duodenal ulcers nearly always occur within an inch of the pyloric valve separating the stomach from the small intestine. The pain or discomfort follows a cycle. The patient may experience no pain until after breakfast. The pain is relieved by the noon meal but returns in the afternoon and occurs again in the evening. Milk or other bland food or medications relieve the pain that may appear at various times in the cycle. The symptoms of duodenal ulcers also go through periods of remission and recurrence over months or years. Most duodenal ulcers are treated with diet, drugs, and measures that encourage rest and relaxation.

Surgical Procedures

Surgery for either duodenal or gastric

ulcer is designed to reduce gastric acid secretion rather than simply to excise the ulcer from the normal digestive tract tissue. One surgical approach, called *subtotal gastrectomy,* involves cutting away a portion of the stomach in the area where it joins the duodenum. There are several variations of this technique, including one in which the remaining portion of the stomach is attached to the jejunum, a segment of the small intestine. The ulcerated portion of the duodenum may be removed during the reconstructive surgery of the digestive tract, or it may be left in the duodenal segment that is closed during the gastrectomy procedure. An interesting effect is that a duodenal ulcer usually heals, when left in place, after the gastric juices are routed into the intestine through the jejunum. The reconstructed stomach and stomach-to-intestine connection cause no serious problems in eating after the patient has recovered.

A second surgical approach, called a *vagotomy,* involves cutting a part of the vagus nerve trunk that controls the secretion of stomach acid. There are several variations of vagotomy, each technique affecting a different portion of the vagus nerve distribution to the stomach.

Gastric Ulcers

Stomach or gastric ulcers tend to develop in older persons more often than duodenal ulcers, and the problem seems to be less importantly related to the overproduction of gastric acid. The real hazard of stomach ulcers is that a significant percentage are found to be a kind of cancer and do not respond to the usual therapies for controlling peptic ulcer symptoms. If it is determined that a stomach ulcer is a malignant growth, a partial gastrectomy is performed in the same manner as an operation of the type for duodenal ulcers. The vagotomy approach is not used for treatment of a stomach ulcer unless the ulcer is excised at the same time.

Hiatus Hernia

The term *hiatus hernia* actually describes a diaphragmatic hernia or weakness in the diaphragm, the horizontal muscular wall separating the organs of the chest from the organs of the abdomen. A *hernia* is an abnormal protrusion of an organ or tissue through an opening. A *hiatus,* or opening, occurs naturally to permit the esophagus to carry food from the mouth to the stomach. Blood vessels and nerves also pass through the diaphragm. The diaphragm is an important group of muscles for contracting and expanding the lungs, forcing air in and out of the lung tissues.

Hiatus hernias are rare in children, but as people grow older, there may be a weakening of the diaphragm muscles and associated tissues. Aided by a tendency toward obesity and the use of girdles and other tight garments, a portion of the stomach may be pushed through the opening designed by nature for use of the esophagus. Aside from the discomfort of having a part of the stomach in the chest, there are potential dangers of incarceration of the stomach, with obstruction, strangulation, and hemorrhage with erosion of the stomach lining. In severe complications, the entire stomach along with intestines and other abdominal organs may be forced through the hiatus hernia into the chest area.

The most common kind of hiatus hernia is sometimes called *sliding hiatus hernia* from the tendency of the stomach to slide in and out of the thorax, or chest cavity, when the patient changes body positions or as a result of the pressure of a big meal in the gastrointestinal tract. Sometimes

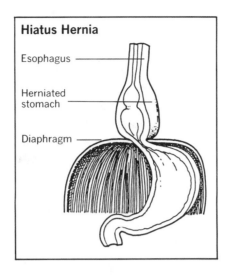

Hiatus Hernia

Esophagus

Herniated stomach

Diaphragm

the herniated stomach does not move at all but remains fixed, with a significant portion of the stomach above the diaphragm. Hiatus hernia causes heartburn symptoms, including regurgitation of digested food and gastric acid from the stomach, when one is lying down or straining or stooping. The effect also may be noticeable in a woman during pregnancy.

Nonsurgical Treatment

Many cases of hiatal hernia can be treated without surgery through a change of eating habits and the use of antacid medications. The patient may be advised to eat small amounts more frequently during the day with dietary emphasis on high-protein, low-fat foods. Some physicians recommend that patients use liquid antacid medications rather than antacid tablets or lozenges.

Surgical Treatment

When surgery is recommended to correct hiatus hernia, the repair may be performed either through the abdominal wall or through the chest. About three-fourths of the procedures are handled through abdominal incisions, because surgeons often find other abdominal problems that need to be corrected at the same time,

such as peptic ulcers or gall bladder disease. The opening through the diaphragm is firmly closed with sutures to prevent upward movement of the stomach. The stomach and lower end of the esophagus may be anchored in place in the abdomen. The chances of recurrence are about one in ten, although some patients may continue to have a few of the symptoms of the disorder for a while after the hernia repair.

Adhesions

Adhesions may develop between various abdominal organs and the peritoneum, the membrane lining the abdominal cavity. The bowel may acquire adhesions that result in obstruction of the intestinal tract. Adhesions may form between the liver and the peritoneum or between the liver and the diaphragm. The symptoms may be pain or cramps in the area where tissues are literally stuck together; in more serious cases that involve bowel obstruction, symptoms may include constipation, vomiting, and distension of the abdomen. Adhesions do not show on X-ray film and can be difficult to diagnose unless the patient's medical history suggests a cause for the bands or filaments of tissues responsible for the adhesions.

Causes

The causes may be peritonitis, injury, infection, internal bleeding, or foreign objects. Adhesions occur after an operation, perhaps because of a bit of blood resulting from surgery or as a result of a speck of talc from the surgeon's glove or a fiber from a surgical drape which produces a foreign-body reaction, much like an allergic reaction, when it comes in contact with abdominal tissues. Disease organisms may enter the female abdominal cavity through the Fallopian tubes to produce adhesions, especially in the case of gonorrhea, which can escape early detection in women because of the lack of obvious symptoms.

Complications

Adhesions can cause complications, such as changing the position of the intestinal tract through twisting or otherwise distorting its path so that bowel movements are obstructed. If the involved portion of the intestine becomes so seriously damaged that it no longer functions properly, the surgeon may have to remove that section. Generally, when the surgeon is correcting the problem of adhesions, a relatively simple procedure of cutting away the tissue bands or filaments holding organs in abnormal ways, he inspects the organs to determine if they appear to be in good working order. That part of the operation may add 15 or 20 minutes to the time spent on an operating table, but it helps insure that the patient will not have to be returned soon for further surgery.

Cancer of the Stomach

There are several possible types of stomach tumors, but one kind, called *adenocarcinoma,* is one of the greatest killers of men over the age of 45. Although the incidence of stomach cancer in the United States has declined considerably since the end of World War II, the death rate from this problem in the United States alone is about 15,000 per year. In central and eastern Europe the incidence of stomach cancer is about four times, and in Japan seven times, that of the United States. Almost two-thirds of the stomach cancers develop near the pylorus, the opening from the stomach into the small intestine; only five percent involve the entire stomach area.

Symptoms

Symptoms include a feeling of heaviness rather than pain following a meal. The patient in many cases mysteriously loses his appetite for meat and begins to lose weight. There may be vague symptoms of an upset stomach, with some vomiting, especially if the tumor begins to obstruct the pylorus such that stomach contents cannot be emptied into the intestine. The vomitus usually is the color of coffee grounds, suggesting a loss of blood from the stomach lining because of the tumor, and the patient's stools also may be dark in coloration because of internal bleeding. The physician frequently can confirm his suspicions about the cause of the symptoms by laboratory analysis of a specimen of cells from the stomach, by X-ray studies of the stomach, or by an examination with a gastroscope that permits a direct view of the interior of the stomach. In some cases the physician will be able to feel an abnormal mass in the stomach by palpating the stomach area of the abdomen with his hands.

Treatment

Treatment is by cutting away the tumor and surrounding tissues that may be involved, including parts of neighboring organs. The lymph nodes in the region of the stomach are also removed. The remaining part of the stomach is used to build a new digestive organ, as in a case of partial gastrectomy for correcting a peptic ulcer problem. However, before beginning reconstructive surgery, the physician usually orders biopsy tests of the remaining tissues to make sure the new stomach will not be made of tissues in which tumor cells have spread. If the edges of the remaining stomach wall are found to contain tumor cells, the surgeon simply extends the area

to be removed. As in subtotal gastrectomy for peptic ulcers, the remaining portion of the stomach may be connected directly to the upper portion of the small intestine, at the duodenum or the jejunum.

Meals are provided in the form of intravenous feedings for the first few days following surgery. Sips of water may be permitted on the second or third day after the operation with the amounts gradually increased to one or two ounces of water per hour as the new digestive system adjusts to fluid intake. Then soft or bland foods can gradually be taken orally in a half-dozen small feedings each day. It may take three or four months for the new stomach to distend and adjust to normal eating habits of the patient.

Postoperative Effects

Some patients may experience a variety of symptoms ranging from nausea to cramps and diarrhea while recovering from stomach surgery. The symptoms form what is known as the *dumping syndrome,* which occurs within a half hour after a meal, presumably by rapid distension of the upper portion of the small intestine as fluid rushes, or is dumped, into that part of the digestive tract from the new stomach. The effects can be controlled by a change of diet to eliminate starches and sugars, by delaying the intake of fluids until after the meal, by medications, and by training the patient to lie in a recumbent or semi-recumbent position to lessen discomfort following a meal. The symptoms occur in only a small proportion of stomach surgery patients, and they usually diminish gradually during the period of recovery.

Cancer of the Intestines

Small Intestine

Tumors of the small intestine are not

common, but they also are not rare. It has been estimated that less than five percent of all tumors of the gastrointestinal tract occur in the small intestine. Of tumors that do develop in this portion of the gastrointestinal tract, about 90 percent are benign, or noncancerous, growths. The symptoms of small intestine tumors may include bleeding, obstruction, and perforation of the intestinal wall. However, most tumors of the small intestine produce no symptoms at all. When tumors are found in the small intestine they usually are found at the same time in other parts of the body, and usually in a patient over 40 years of age, although the more malignant growths can occur in younger persons. Treatment of a cancer of the small bowel is by removing the affected section and administration of radiation therapy for certain kinds of cancerous tumors.

Large Intestine

Tumors of the large intestine, unlike those of the small bowel, account for a large proportion of cancers of the human body and for most of the malignant growths of the entire gastrointestinal tract. More than 40,000 deaths each year in the United States are a result of cancers of the colon and rectum portions of the large bowel. And about three-fourths of all large-intestine tumors develop near the rectal portion of the bowel, where, ironically, they should be easily available for detection during physical examination.

Tumors of the large intestine can be found in persons of any age, but they occur most frequently in patients who are of middle age or older, reaching a peak of incidence around the age of 65. Men are more likely to develop cancer of the rectum, but women are more frequently affected by cancer of the colon. While cancer of the large intestine tends to occur among members of the same families at a rate that is two or three times the normal incidence, it is believed that family environment factors, such as life style and diet, are the causative influences, rather than hereditary factors. People who develop cancer of the large intestine usually eat foods that are low in cellulose and high in animal fats and refined carbohydrates.

Bowel cancers appear to grow in size at a very slow rate, doubling about once every 20 months, so a number of years may elapse between the start of a bowel tumor and the appearance of signs or symptoms of cancer.

Symptoms

The location of the growth can influence the types of symptoms experienced. Cancer in the right colon may be found as an abnormal mass during a physical examination by a physician after complaints of fatigue and weakness and signs of anemia. The tumor can develop to a rather large size without producing signs of blood in the stools. Cancer in the left colon, by contrast, may be found after complaints of alternate periods of constipation and frequent urge to defecate, pain in the abdomen, and stools marked by dark and bright red blood. When the cancer is in the rectum, the patient may find blood mixed with the bowel movements but experience no pain in the early stages. Other symptoms of cancer of the large intestine may mimic those of appendicitis, hemorrhoids, peptic ulcer, or gall bladder disease.

As noted above, most cancers of the large bowel are close enough to the end of the intestinal tract to be observed directly by palpation or the use of fiberoptic instruments, such as a sigmoidoscope or colonoscope, which can be inserted into the rectum or colon. Biopsy samples can be removed for study and X-ray pictures taken after administration of a barium enema, which coats the bowel membrane in such a way that abnormal surfaces are clearly visible.

Surgical Procedures

Surgical procedures for treatment of cancer of the large intestine vary somewhat according to the location of the growth, but the objective is the same: to remove the affected portion and reconstruct the bowel so that normal digestive functions can resume. Radiation therapy and chemotherapy may be used in the treatment of certain advanced cases. When surgical treatment is begun soon after the first symptoms are diagnosed, the chances of curing cancer of the large bowel are very good.

If there are complications, such as obstruction of the portion of the large intestine, the surgery may be conducted in a series of stages over a period of several weeks. The several stages involve a colostomy procedure in which an opening is made in the wall of the abdomen to permit a portion of the intestinal tract to be brought to the surface of the body. After the complicating problem is treated and resection of the cancerous segment is completed, the colostomy is closed by sewing the open end of the bowel to the remaining portion and closing the opening in the abdomen.

Preoperative Steps

Some special preoperative measures are ordered for patients awaiting surgery for treatment of bowel cancer. They consist primarily of several days of liquid diets, laxatives, and enemas to make the interior of the intestinal tract as clean as possible. Other measures will be directed toward correction of anemia and compensation for possible loss of blood resulting from the cancer's invasion of bowel tissues.

Gallbladder Surgery

Gallbladder disease is one of the most common medical disorders in the United States. It has been estimated that more than 15 million Americans are affected by the disease and about 6,000 deaths a year are associated with it. The incidence increases at middle age; 1 of every 5 women over the age of 50 and 1 of every 20 men can expect to be treated for gallbladder symptoms. Approximately 1,000 people in the United States enter operating rooms each day for removal of gallstones, a primary cause of the symptoms of the disorder.

Gallstones

Gallstones generally are formed from crystals of cholesterol that gradually increase in size in the gallbladder; some, however, are formed from other substances, such as bile salts and breakdown products of red blood cells. Because they are very small in size, the stones may produce no symptoms at first. But as they grow in size they become more threatening and eventually can block the normal flow of bile from one of the bile ducts emptying into the intestine. Bile contains substances needed by the body to digest fats in the diet.

Symptoms

A common symptom of *chronic cholecystitis,* or gallstone disease, is a pain that appears suddenly in the upper abdomen and subsides slowly over a period of several minutes to several hours. The pain may occur after a meal or with no apparent relationship to meals. There can be tenderness in the upper right side of the body, with pain extending to the shoulder. The pain also can appear on the left side or near the center of the upper abdomen, producing misleading

symptoms suggesting a heart attack. Nausea, heartburn, gas, indigestion, and intolerance to fatty foods are among other possible symptoms. The gallbladder attacks may occur frequently or there may be remissions (periods without symptoms) lasting for several months or years.

A careful and extensive physical examination, including X-ray studies of the gallbladder area, may be needed to confirm the presence of gallstones. Until recently, the most commonly used test was the oral cholecystogram (OCG), in which the patient swallowed an iodine-based "dye," or contrast agent. X rays taken about 12 hours after administration of the dye might or might not provide useful "pictures" of the gallstones. As a result, ultrasound has largely replaced X rays as a primary test for suspected gallstones.

Acute Cholecystitis

About three-fourths of the cases of acute cholecystitis are patients who have had previous attacks of gallstone disease. In the acute phase there is persistent pain and abdominal tenderness, along with nausea and vomiting in many cases and a mild fever. Complications may include perforation, or rupture, of the gallbladder, leading to peritonitis, or development of adhesions to neighboring organs such as the stomach or intestine.

Treatment

Surgical treatment of chronic or acute cholecystitis is basically an elective procedure that can be scheduled at a time convenient to the patient. But acute cases with complications may require emergency operations. The patient can usually be maintained, after surgery, on intravenous fluids and pain-killing medications.

A number of alternatives to surgery have been developed. A gastroenterologist may use an endoscope on older patients or those in poor health. The endoscope, a tube inserted through the chest wall, enables the physician to view the gallbladder's duct area and to widen its opening so that small gallstones can slip through the small intestine. Using a small basket on the endoscope, the physician can sometimes catch and withdraw or crush the stones.

In gallstone surgery, the abdomen is opened so that the surgeon can examine the gall bladder and the ducts leading from it for stones. The gallbladder may be freed of stones and a temporary drainage tube inserted, with an opening to the outside of the upper abdomen. But usually the surgeon removes the entire gallbladder in an operation called a *cholecystectomy.* The bile duct, which remains as a link between the liver and the small intestine, gradually replaces the gallbladder in function. Most patients require no more than ten days to two weeks of hospitalization, and can resume normal work activities in a month to six weeks.

Other nonsurgical treatments include chemical preparations. Chenodeoxycholic acid, or chenodiol, has been given orally to dissolve smaller, floating cholesterol stones. But the drug has little effect against pigment stones or stones with a high calcium content, and can cause diarrhea as a side effect. Researchers have worked experimentally with ursodeoxycholic acid and other drugs that have been found to dissolve gallstones in both animals and humans.

Among the most advanced techniques is *choledocholithotripsy,* a nonsurgical method using shock waves to destroy gallstones. Already in use as a method of shattering kidney stones, lithotripsy requires only a local anesthetic and the recovery period lasts only a few days. The physician uses a hollow tool—the lithotriptor—that is inserted through the patient's chest until it approaches the stones. With a foot switch, the physician then triggers a jolt of high-voltage, low-current electricity that shatters the stones.

In another advance, drugs have been utilized to dissolve gallstones. A drug called *methyl tertbutyl ether* (MTHE) has been found to break down gallstones as large as golf balls. Still partly experimental, the compound could replace most surgical operations for gallstones.

Inguinal Hernia

An inguinal hernia (hernia of the groin) can develop in either men or women at almost any age from infancy to late adult years. But the incidence of inguinal hernia is much more common in males. An inguinal hernia is one in which the intestinal tract protrudes through the opening of one of the inguinal rings on either side of the groin. In males, the inguinal rings are temporary openings through which the testicles descend into the scrotum before birth; in females, the openings permit the passage of a ligament supporting the ovary.

Causes

Normally, the inguinal rings are closed after the birth of the child. However, they may fail to close completely or the muscles and connective tissues may become stretched or weakened in later years to permit a portion of the abdominal contents, usually part of the intestine, to protrude. A number of factors can contribute to the development of a hernia, including physical strain from exercise or lifting, straining over a bowel movement, coughing spells, pregnancy, pressure of abdominal organs, or obesity.

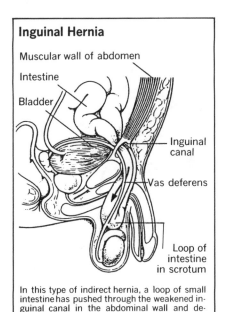

Inguinal Hernia

Muscular wall of abdomen
Intestine
Bladder
Inguinal canal
Vas deferens
Loop of intestine in scrotum

In this type of indirect hernia, a loop of small intestine has pushed through the weakened inguinal canal in the abdominal wall and descended into the scrotal sac.

Reducible and Irreducible Hernias

The hernia may be *reducible,* that is, the bulge in the abdominal wall may disappear when the body position is changed, as in lying down, only to reappear upon standing. An *irreducible* hernia does not allow the hernia sac contents to return to the abdominal cavity; an irreducible hernia also may be called *incarcerated,* a term aptly describing the hernia as being trapped. A serious complication is strangulation of the hernia contents, which usually involves obstruction of normal blood flow and resulting damage or destruction of the incarcerated intestines. A strangulated hernia may be life-threatening because of the possibility of gangrene in body tissues damaged by incarceration.

Surgical Procedure

Some hernias are called *direct,* some *indirect,* for purposes of medical records. These terms indicate to the surgeon specific layers of muscle and connective tissue that have been breached and are of no real significance to the patient, because the sur-

gical repair procedures are essentially the same for either type. In the absence of complications, the operation is fairly simple and usually can be performed with either a general or a local anesthetic. An incision is made in the lower abdomen in the area of the hernia, the protruding organ is returned to its normal position, and the weakened or ruptured layers of muscle and connective tissue are repaired and reinforced to provide a strong internal wall that will hold the abdominal contents in place. In some cases the surgeon will use available tissues from the patient's own body in building a new wall against future hernias. The surgeon also may use a variety of materials, including silk, catgut, stainless steel, tantalum mesh gauze, or mesh screens made of plastics, in building a new barrier.

Recovery

The hospital stay for hernia repair is relatively brief, usually from three days to a week; some healthy children undergo surgery early in the morning and return home in the evening of the same day. The patient usually is instructed to avoid exercise or exertion for a couple of weeks and can return to work in a month to six weeks, depending upon the work load expected. Hernias tend to recur in only a small percentage of cases among adults and very rarely in children.

Femoral Hernia

About five percent of all hernias of the groin area are femoral hernias, with the hernia bulge appearing along the thigh. Femoral hernias occur about four times as frequently among women and usually appear in middle age. While a femoral hernia is not necessarily limited to obese patients, it is more likely to be associated with being overweight, and the movement

Femoral Hernia

Inguinal ligament

Femoral vessels

Bowel hernia

Bladder hernia

of a bowel segment or the urinary bladder into the hernia frequently is preceded by a fat pad—a mass of fatty tissue. Femoral hernias are more prone to incarceration and strangulation than inguinal hernias. The surgical treatment of femoral hernias is similar to that used in the repair of inguinal hernias, although the incision may be made through the thigh in a few cases.

Hemorrhoids

Hemorrhoid, a term derived from Greek words meaning "blood flowing," refers to a system of arteries and veins that serve the rectal area. The medical problem known as *hemorrhoids,* or *piles,* is a tortuous enlargement of the hemorrhoidal veins, a problem similar to the varicose veins of the legs. Causes of the varicosities of the hemorrhoidal veins include the human peculiarity of standing and walking in an erect posture—animals that walk on all fours do not get hemorrhoids.

Women during pregnancies are particularly subject to hemorrhoidal problems because of the pressure on the veins of the lower body area. Other causes are constipation and straining at stool; diseases of the digestive tract resulting in anal infec-

tion; and cirrhosis of the liver, which obstructs blood flow and puts increased pressure on the hemorrhoidal veins.

Symptoms

Symptoms usually include bleeding, which may stain the patient's clothing; irritation and discomfort, including itching, in the anal region; and occasionally pain with inflammation. Because rectal bleeding also can be a sign of a number of other diseases, the physician usually makes a thorough examination to rule out other possible causes, such as cancer or ulcerative colitis.

Treatment

If the hemorrhoids do not warrant surgery, medical treatments may be

Hemorrhoids

Internal

External

prescribed. *Prolapsed hemorrhoids* (veins that protrude from the anus) can be reduced by gentle pressure. Bed rest, warm baths, and medications are also a part of medical treatments. A type of injection chemotherapy sometimes is used to control bleeding and eliminate the varicosed veins.

Surgery can be used to excise all the affected tissues, and the disorder also can be treated by cryosurgery in which the hemorrhoids are destroyed by a probe containing supercold liquid nitrogen or carbon dioxide. The patient usually is able to recover and return to work within one or two weeks after surgical removal of the hemorrhoidal tissues.

Oral Cavity and Throat

This section discusses oral cancers, tonsils and adenoids, and surgery of the thyroid. For a discussion of cosmetic surgery of the face area, see "Plastic and Cosmetic Surgery" later in this chapter.

Oral Cancers

There are many potential problems of the mouth, or oral cavity, besides an occasional toothache. Surgical treatment frequently is needed to correct a disorder or to prevent a life-threatening situation from developing. Cancers of the lips, tongue, hard and soft palate, and other areas of the mouth, for example, affect about 25,000 people in the United States each year. Elsewhere in the world, the incidence varies considerably according to sex and location; the rate in Hong Kong for men is three times the figure for women, and the incidence of oral cancer for women in Hong Kong is nearly 10 times as high as that of women in Japan. Environmental factors such as tobacco and contact with chemical and physical agents have been suggested as causes, although one form of oral cancer, known as *Burkitt's lymphoma,* is believed to be transmitted by a mosquito-borne virus.

Cancer of the Lip

Oral cancers tend to occur after the age of 45. Some types of oral cancer, particularly when the lips are affected, are found most frequently in persons exposed to a great deal of sunlight. Farmers, sailors, and other outdoor workers develop such tumors around the age of 60, with the lesion appearing on the lower lip. Like other cancers, cancer of the lip may begin as a tiny growth, but, if untreated, can spread through neighboring tissues and eventually destroy part of the chin. Treatment may include both radiation therapy and surgical excision of the growth; if surgery is performed when the tumor is small, the scar is likewise small. Obviously, the larger the tumor is allowed to grow, the more difficult the treatment.

Cancer of the Cheek

Similarly, cancers that develop on the inner surface of the cheek usually can be excised and the wound closed with simple surgery if treatment is started early. If the cancer is allowed to grow before treatment, the surgery becomes more complicated with removal of tissues extending to the outer skin layers and repair of the wound with skin grafts. Radiation therapy also may be used to augment the surgical repair.

Cancer of the Mouth

Cancer of the floor of the mouth may be second only to lip cancer in rate of occurrence of oral cavity tumors; together they may account for half of the oral cavity cancers in the United States. A tumor of the floor of the mouth may involve the under surface of the tongue, the lower jawbone, and other tissues of the area. A small lesion detected early can be controlled in most cases by excision of the growth and radiation therapy.

Cancer of the Tongue

The tongue may be the site of cancerous growths beginning in the 30s of the patient's life, particularly if the individual is a heavy user of tobacco and alcohol and has been neglectful of proper oral hygiene, such as brushing the teeth regularly. If the growth is at the tip of the tongue rather than underneath or along the sides, the operation is easier and there is less chance that the normal function of the tongue will be impaired by removing the growth and surrounding tissue cells. Radiation therapy for cancer of the tongue sometimes involves the implantation of needles containing radium into the tongue. The procedure is done while the patient is under a general anesthetic. Tumors at the base of the tongue, as well as some growths on the floor of the mouth, sometimes are approached through an incision in the neck.

Other Surgery

Apart from cancers, surgery of the oral cavity may be needed to treat genetic defects, such as cleft lip and cleft palate, damage to tissues from injuries, and noncancerous tumors of the soft tissues, such as cysts.

Tonsils and Adenoids

Tonsils and adenoids are glands of lymphoid tissue lying along the walls near the top of the throat. The tonsils are located on the sides of the pharynx, or throat, near the base of the tongue. Unless an adult's tonsils are inflamed, they may not be easily visible to a physician or other person looking into the throat, but when inflamed and swollen they can be seen without difficulty. The adenoids are located higher in the pharynx and cannot be seen by looking into the back of the mouth without special instruments, because the palate, or roof of the mouth, blocks the view.

Tonsillitis

The function of the tonsils and adenoids apparently is that of trapping infectious organisms that enter the body through the nose and mouth. But sometimes the glands do such a good job of collecting infections that they lose their effectiveness, becoming enlarged and inflamed, a condition known as *tonsillitis.* The patient develops fever and sore throat and the breathing passages become obstructed. The infections can spread through the nearby Eustachian tubes to the ears, causing *otitis media* (inflammation of the middle ear), resulting in deafness. Disease organisms also can spread from the tonsils and adenoids to the kidneys, joints, heart, eyes, and other body areas. Many youngsters survive occasional bouts of tonsillitis, and the infections can be treated with antibiotics and medications to relieve pain and fever symptoms. But many surgeons recommend that the tonsils and adenoids be removed if tonsillitis occurs repeatedly.

Tonsillectomy

A *tonsillectomy* (removal of the tonsils) is not a complicated operation, but it usually is performed under a general anesthetic if the patient is a child. A local anesthetic may be used for an adult. The adenoids usually are removed at the same time; they consist of the same type of lymphoid tissue in the same general area, and adenoids develop similar problems from the same kinds of infectious agents. An overnight stay in the hospital may be required or it may be possible for the patient to have the tonsils and adenoids removed in the morning and be released from the hospital in the evening of the same day, after a few hours of postoperative rest under medical observation.

Preoperative and Postoperative Care

The patient may receive antibiotic medications two or three days prior to surgery and is instructed to avoid eating foods or drinking fluids for at least 12 hours before the operation. If the patient has a cold or other viral infection, the surgery may be delayed or postponed. Some surgeons also prefer to avoid tonsillectomy operations during the hay-fever season. If there is any evidence of bleeding after the patient is released, such as spitting blood, he is returned to the hospital and the surgeon is notified; the bleeding usually can be controlled without difficulty. The patient also returns for checkups a couple of weeks after the operation and again about six months later.

Adenoidectomy

In some cases, a surgeon may recommend an *adenoidectomy* (removal of the adenoids) without a tonsillectomy. This is particularly true when the patient suffers from recurrent ear infections and hearing loss. An adenoidectomy is a relatively simple operation performed under a local anesthetic when the patient is an adult or older teenager; a general anesthetic is preferred for younger patients.

The surgeon can reach the adenoid mass through the open mouth of the patient. The tissue grows on a palate ledge near the point where the nasal passage enters the back of the mouth cavity. Using a special instrument, the surgeon cuts away the adenoid tissue within a few minutes. A medicated pack is inserted into the postnasal area to help control bleeding and the patient is moved to a recovery room. The only aftereffects in most cases are a soreness in the postnasal area for a few days and, occasionally, a temporary voice change that is marked by a nasal tone while the wound heals.

Thyroid Surgery

The thyroid gland lies along the trachea, or windpipe, at a point just below the Adam's apple. Secretions of the thyroid gland are vital for metabolic activities of the body, and the gland's functions are closely orchestrated with those of other endocrine glands of the body. When the thyroid is less active than normal, mental and physical functions are slow and the patient gains weight. When the gland is overly active, body functions operate at an abnormally fast pace, with symptoms of weight loss, irritability, heart palpitations, and bulging eyes. Occasionally, lumps develop on the thyroid, requiring medical or surgical treatment. A lump on the thyroid gland may be a nodular, or nontoxic, goiter. Or it could be a tumor. A nodular goiter poses several threats: it can make the thyroid gland become overactive, it can press on the windpipe and cause hoarseness, or it can develop into a cancer. Some growths of the thyroid gland can be treated effectively with medications, radiation, or a combination such as radioactive iodine. However, when conservative forms of therapy no longer appear to control the condition, or when it is suspected that a thyroid growth may be a malignant cancer,

The Thyroid Gland

surgical removal of the affected area is advised promptly.

Surgical Procedure

The operation itself is fairly simple. An incision is made through the skin folds of the neck, neck muscles beneath the skin are separated, and the affected portion of the gland is cut away. The neck and throat area may be sore and painful for a few days after the operation; within a few weeks the patient can resume normal activities. A thin scar remains at the line of incision, but it is usually partly concealed by skin folds of the neck.

Ear Surgery

Surgical treatment of the ear usually is directed toward restoring the function of normal hearing which may have been lost or impaired by disease or injury. The eardrum, or tympanic membrane, can be perforated or ruptured by direct injury, by the shock waves of an explosion, or by an infection of the middle ear. Infection or injury also can disrupt hearing function by damaging the ossicles, a chain of tiny bones that transmit sound waves from the eardrum to the inner ear. Disease, aging effects, and exposure to loud noises can cause hearing loss or impairment.

Surgery of the ear usually involves working with the middle ear, the compartment between the eardrum and the inner ear, which contains the nerve endings that carry impulses to the auditory centers of the brain. The middle ear contains three ossicles, known by their common names of *hammer, anvil,* and *stirrup*—terms that suggest their functions in translating movements of air molecules into the vibrations the brain understands as sounds.

Otitis Media

One common disease of the middle ear is otitis media, which can occur by infection from a number of different kinds of organisms. Otitis media also can develop from secretions or fluids such as milk being forced into the ear through the Eustachian tube, particularly in infants who are fed while they are in a reclining position. The symptoms of otitis media are pain in the ear, fever, and loss of hearing; a small child may indicate the symptoms by crying and tugging at the ear.

Surgical Procedure

Many cases of otitis media respond to medical treatment, such as the use of antibiotics, but for patients who suffer severe pain or who have middle ears filled with pus, a surgical procedure called *myringotomy* is performed. "Myringotomy" means simply perforating the eardrum. But the operation usually is peformed in a hospital, under a local anesthetic, and with great care to avoid disturbing the ossicles or other ear structures beyond the eardrum. The middle ear is drained and the eardrum either heals spontaneously or can be subsequently repaired with a graft from the patient's own tissues.

Surgery to Correct Hearing Loss

Occasionally surgery is required to correct a conductive hearing loss in-

volving the structures of the middle ear. Such problems happen more frequently among older persons because of abnormal tissue growths that in effect "freeze" the ossicles, so that they no longer work with normal flexibility. Ossicular disorders also can occur in younger persons, including children, because of congenital defects, injury, or repeated infections, as of otitis media. The exact procedure for restoration of hearing depends upon the type of disorder. If one of the ossicles has slipped out of position or has become rigidly attached to another structure, like the tympanic membrane, the tiny bones can be repositioned or freed from the tissues that may have immobilized them. It is not unusual for the surgeon, working in a space about the size of a pea and viewing his progress through a microscope, to literally take the middle ear structures apart, rebuild the organ with bits of plastic or metal shaped like the ossicles, and reconstruct the eardrum with tissue grafts. This kind of surgery is called *microsurgery.*

Inner Ear Disturbances

Disorders of the inner ear usually are treated with medications. Surgery in that area is seldom performed unless there is a great risk to the life of the patient. Little can be done to restore hearing loss caused by nerve deafness except with hearing aids; these are designed to pick up sounds on the affected side of the head and route the sounds by electronic circuitry to an area where they can be picked up by remaining functional auditory nerves.

Eye Surgery

Among common types of eye surgery are procedures for correcting eye muscles, glaucoma, cataracts, cornea

and retina disorders. Operations on the eye muscles are intended to correct crossed eyes or similar problems in which the two eyes fail to work together.

Crossed Eyes

The condition technically known as *strabismus,* in which one eye drifts so that its position is not parallel with the other, is caused by a congenitally weak muscle. Infants often appear to have crossed eyes, but in most cases the drifting corrects itself by the time the baby is six months old. If the condition persists beyond that time, a physician should be consulted. He may recommend the use of an eye patch over the stronger eye so that the weaker one will be exercised. If this does not achieve the desired result, he may prescribe special glasses and eye exercises as the child gets older, so that there is no impairment of vision.

Corrective Surgery

If corrective surgery proves necessary after these measures, it is usually done before the child enters school. The operation is a simple one involving the muscle and not the inside of the eye itself. Each eye has six *extraocular* muscles—muscles originating outside the eyeball—to move the eye up, down, left, right, etc.; the surgeon lengthens or shortens these muscles, as may be required, to coordinate the eye movements. The operation is safe and requires only a brief hospital stay.

Amblyopia

If the lack of eye coordination is not corrected, a kind of blindness called *amblyopia* can result in one of the eyes. This condition occurs particularly in young children who depend upon the vision of one good eye; the function of the other eye is allowed to deteriorate. It has been estimated that about two million Americans have lost a part of their vision in this manner. Crossed eyes should receive professional attention early enough to prevent a permanent visual handicap.

Cataract

Cataract is a condition in which there is a loss of transparency of the lenses of the eyes. Each lens is made up of layers of cells naturally formed to focus a visual image on the retina at the rear of the eyeball. As a result of aging, or because of an injury to the eye, the lens may develop cloudy or opaque areas, or *cataracts,* that result in a blurring of vision. About five percent of the population of the United States have cataracts. Some physicians claim that anyone who lives long enough can expect to have cataracts, although age is not the only determining factor.

Surgical Correction

The condition can be corrected rather easily by several different kinds of surgical procedures. Among these, a relatively simple, advanced technique involves a microsurgery procedure called *extracapsular extraction* followed by implantation of a new lens. Using this method, the surgeon first makes a tiny incision in the cornea. Reaching through that incision, the surgeon then makes a circle of tiny cuts in the lens. The lens and its cataract are then drawn through the opening in the cornea. The back part of the lens remains in place to support the implant lens.

Extracapsular extraction has begun to replace older techniques.

These include dissolving the tissues holding the lens in place with a liquid enzyme, freezing the lens with a supercold probe, and grinding the lens tissue with a high-speed instrument. Extracapsular extraction requires only a local anesthetic injected into the facial muscles. Because the sutures are tiny, healing time can be as short as a few weeks.

Laser surgery has also been used effectively following cataract lens replacements. The neodymium yttrium-aluminum garnet (Nd:YAG) laser has helped to clear the capsular membrane that sometimes clouds the eye after such surgery.

The timing of cataract surgery presents the patient with a difficult decision. To help you make up your mind, the physician may use a potential acuity meter (PAM) to show what kind of vision you should have after a cataract is removed. The PAM projects a light beam that flashes a standard eye chart through tiny clear areas in the cataract. Because the beam hits your retina directly, you can read the chart without interference.

Lens implants normally effect greatly improved vision. But for optimum results most patients need to wear eyeglasses or contact lenses after the operation. Because implanted lenses cannot focus as your eye's natural lens does, you will probably need reading glasses. The artificial lenses may require some adjustments to compensate for visual illusions as to distances and shapes, but the blurring of progressive blindness will have been eliminated.

Sometimes after cataract operations, patients notice that the rear part of the lens left in to support the implant has begun to cloud. In such a case a surgeon may use a laser beam to punch a tiny hole in the clouded area. The hole lets light rays reach the retina unimpeded.

Cornea Transplant

The cornea of the eye is a clear window of several cells in thickness at the very front of the eye. While it is protected by the constant sweeping of the corneal surface by the eyelid and the washing of the surface by the tears, it is vulnerable to injury and infection, allergies, and metabolic disorders. The simple habit of rubbing the eyes can distort the shape of the cornea, changing the normal round shape to a cone shape. Eventually, a cornea may degenerate from wear and tear and become so clouded that the patient can no longer see clearly, if at all. It is possible, however—and has been since the 1930s—to replace a clouded cornea with an undamaged cornea from a deceased person. Corneas are contributed by donors and stored in eye banks.

Surgical Procedures

When only a portion of the cornea needs to be replaced, as is often the case, a disk encompassing the damaged cornea is carefully cut out and a piece of new cornea of precisely the same size and shape is sewn into the remaining tissue of the old cornea. The reconstructed cornea is treated with antibiotics and bandaged for several weeks. More than three-fourths of the cornea transplants are successful; the chances of success depend upon many factors, including the health of the remaining tissues of the original cornea.

Glaucoma

Glaucoma, a leading cause of blindness, is a disease caused by a failure of the fluid produced inside the eye to drain properly. The fluid, or *aqueous humor,* is produced in the anterior chamber of the eye, between the cornea and the lens. In a normal eye it drains through a duct at the base of the cornea at the same rate at which it is produced. But if the drainage system is obstructed, fluid buildup creates pressure backward through the eye. If untreated, such pressure can cause gradual blindness by crushing the nerves at the back of the eye.

Treatment

Some cases of glaucoma can be treated with medications that control the rates of fluid production and drainage. But when medications are no longer effective or when an acute attack occurs, with symptoms of severe eye pain sometimes accompanied by abdominal pain, nausea, and vomiting, surgery within a matter of hours is recommended. Several surgical procedures for the treatment of glaucoma are available; all are designed to release the fluid pressure in the eye. One common procedure involves cutting a small opening in the iris. Another technique is to insert a fine wire into the duct that normally drains the fluid and literally ream it open.

Other surgical and nonsurgical treatments for glaucoma have been developed. For example, laser surgery has proved effective for treating both open-angle and closed-angle glaucoma. In the former, the eye's internal drain system does not work properly, causing pressure to build up in the eye. In closed-angle glaucoma, fluid cannot pass properly from the front to the back of the eye, again producing dangerous pressure. The neodymium yttrium-aluminum garnet (Nd:YAG) laser is usually used in treatment to "drill" a tiny hole and destroy swollen blood vessels that block normal fluid drainage. Because marihuana has also been found to reduce pressure in the eye, manufacture of the chemical known as THC (delta-9-tetrahydrocannabinol), the key marihuana ingredient, was authorized by the Food and Drug Administration in 1985 and begun in 1986. THC has also been used to relieve the nausea accompanying cancer chemotherapy and to slow multiple sclerosis.

An estimated 10 million people in the world are afflicted by glaucoma, and the chances of developing increase with age. Women are twice as likely to develop the disease as men, and there is some evidence that the risk is hereditary. However, it also is easily preventable and controllable, since glaucoma usually develops slowly and can be detected during routine eye examinations in its early stages.

Retinal Detachment or Disease

Retinal detachment can occur from bleeding in the retinal area, an injury, a change in the shape of the eyeball, or other causes. The surgical treatment to correct the problem usually is related to the specific cause. For example, if fluid or blood has accumulated behind the retina, it is drained away. Alternatively, pressure may be directed within the eyeball to push the retina back into its proper position. For some cases, such as those associated with *diabetic retinopathy,* a kind of retinal bleeding in diabetes patients, a laser beam is used to seal the blood vessels responsible for the tiny hemorrhages in the eye.

Chest Region

This section deals with surgery of the lungs and heart. For a discussion of cosmetic surgery of the chest area, as of the breast, see "Plastic and Cosmetic Surgery" later in this chapter.

The Lungs

Before the era of modern drugs such as antibiotics, lung disorders were the leading cause of death in the United States. Lung diseases are still common enough. With every breath taken in, the lungs are vulnerable to damage from disease organisms, chemicals, and air pollutants, many of which did not exist 50 years ago when pneumonia and tuberculosis were among the greatest threats to human life. Because the lungs are not as sensitive to pain as some other organs, a respiratory disorder may develop insidiously with few or no symptoms. When pain is felt in the chest area, the source of the pain may be the chest wall, the esophagus, or the bronchial tubes that branch from the trachea into smaller units that distribute air through the lung tissues. Other symptoms of respiratory disease may be coughing, shortness of breath, or sputum that contains blood.

Tuberculosis

Any of the above signs or symptoms could be associated with tuberculosis, which also can cause loss of appetite, weight loss, lethargy, and heavy perspiration, especially during the night. Tuberculosis is still one of the most common causes of death in the world, and new cases are found in the United States each year at a rate of 18 per 100,000 population. In addition, an estimated 35 million Americans are tuberculin-positive, indicating they have been in contact with the infectious organism but have developed an immune response to it. For an explanation of how tuberculosis is spread and of tests devised to check its spread, see "Tuberculosis" in Ch. 12, *Diseases of the Respiratory System.*

Surgical Treatment of Tuberculosis

A dozen different drugs are available for medical treatment of tuberculosis and several types may be taken in combination by a patient. Intensive treatment may require a hospital stay of several months and use of the drugs for at least 18 months. However, because of the adverse side effects of drugs, resistance of the bacterium to the drugs, and other reasons, surgery may be required. If one of the five lobes of lung tissue—the right lung has three lobes, the left lung two—has been severely damaged by tuberculosis, it may be removed by surgeons. In some instances, physicians may recommend that surgery be undertaken to allow one of the lungs to rest while it recovers from the infection. This is accomplished by crushing the phrenic nerve, under a local anesthetic, creating a partial paralysis of the diaphragm. Partial lung collapse also can be accomplished by removing parts of the ribs over the affected lung.

Lung Cancer

Cancer of the lung may appear with early symptoms of coughing, wheezing, or the appearance of blood in sputum; in about 10 percent of cases there is chest pain or shortness of breath. However, it is not unusual for the lung cancer patient to have no complaints of illness. Chest X rays during a routine physical examination may reveal the disease. In many cases, the cancer develops from metastases of cancers that have spread from other body systems. Medical therapy for lung cancer patients, including the use of radiation, is primarily for the purpose of relieving pain or other symptoms. The only effective cure is surgical excision of the affected lung tissue along with the nearby lymph nodes. Surgical treatment is most effective in young adults when the tumor has not invaded neighboring tissues, although the five-year survival rate for lung cancer is still poor.

Heart Surgery

Heart surgery procedures that are routine in many hospitals today were unheard of a generation ago. Since World War II, techniques have been devised to permit attachment of a heart-lung machine to the human body so that the patient's blood can be circulated and refreshed with oxygen while the heart itself is stopped temporarily for surgery.

Heart Valve Repair

While the blood flow is shunted away from the heart, surgeons can replace a diseased heart valve that may have become calcified with deposits that keep it from closing normally. An artificial valve made of metal and plastic may be used to replace the patient's diseased mitral valve that no longer effectively controls the flow of blood from the left atrium to the left ventricle of the heart. Artificial valves also can be installed between the right chambers of the heart. In some cases, a diseased valve leaf may be repaired with a graft of tissue from the patient's body.

Installation of artificial heart valves has had a remarkably good record of success; some surgeons recommend the procedure over other techniques for treatment of heart valve diseases and report the operation has been well tolerated by patients over 70. While some activites may be restricted, life expectancy is increased for most patients, and they are able to have comfortable and more normal lives after such operations.

Septal Defect

Another kind of heart surgery is used to correct a septal defect. The right and left atria of the heart are separated by a septum, a wall of muscular tissue. A similar but much thicker septum separates the left and right ventricles. Occasionally, usually because of a birth defect, the septum does not close completely and blood flows from one side to the other through the opening in the heart wall. The problem is solved by putting the patient on a heart-lung machine while the heart is opened and the septum closed either by sewing the opening or by stitching into the septum a patch of plastic material.

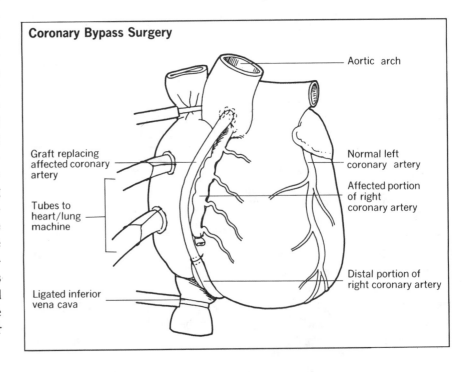

Coronary Bypass Surgery

Aortic arch

Graft replacing affected coronary artery

Tubes to heart/lung machine

Ligated inferior vena cava

Normal left coronary artery

Affected portion of right coronary artery

Distal portion of right coronary artery

Coarctation of the Aorta

An equally dramatic bit of heart surgery is used to correct a defect called *coarctation,* or narrowing, of the aorta, the main artery leading from the heart. This short, pinched section interferes with normal blood flow. If untreated, the patient may die of a ruptured aorta or heart failure. Treatment requires an operation in which the narrowed section of the aorta is cut away and the two normal-sized ends sewed together. In some cases, a piece of plastic material is sewed into the reconstructed aorta to replace the coarctated section.

Aortal-Pulmonary Artery Shunt

A comparatively simple bit of heart surgery is employed to correct a defect that occurs in some newborn children. Before birth, when the lungs are not needed because fresh blood is supplied from the placenta via the umbilical cord, the aorta is connected by a shunt to the pulmonary artery. After birth the shunt closes in most cases so the pulmonary artery can carry the blood from the heart to the lungs for oxygenation. In some children this shunt fails to close. To correct the defect and prevent heart failure, the surgeon opens the child's chest, ties off the open shunt, and cuts the ligated connection.

Vascular Surgery

This section consists of discussions of aneurysms, varicose veins, phlebitis, and intermittent claudication.

Aneurysm

When a blood vessel develops a balloonlike malformation the defect is called an *aneurysm.* A common complication of the aneurysm is that it may rupture if not treated. A ruptured

Aortal-Pulmonary Artery

Aorta
Superior vena cava
Right atrium
Heart
Pulmonary artery

aneurysm of a large blood vessel, or of a small blood vessel in a critical area such as the brain, can be fatal or severely disabling.

Surgical Procedures

If the aneurysm develops at a vital site such as the aorta, heroic surgical measures may be required to correct the problem. Before the important artery can be clamped off, the patient may have to be attached to a heart-lung machine and the body temperature lowered so as to reduce normal body functions to a minimum. After the aneurysm is removed, that section of the aorta may have to be replaced with a piece of plastic artery. Not all aneurysms require such complicated methods of repair; if the ballooning section of artery develops as a saclike appendage, it frequently can be tied off and removed while the relatively small opening between the blood vessel and the sac is sewed closed.

Surgical removal of an aneurysm is the only available treatment for the disorder. The surgery is much less complicated if the abnormal section of the blood vessel is replaced before it ruptures than after. When the patient has recovered from correction of the aneurysm, he can resume a rather active, normal life style.

Varicose Veins

Varicose veins can develop in many parts of the body. But they are most obvious and commonly a problem when they appear in the legs, especially in the *saphenous veins,* large veins that lie close to the surface of the skin.

Causes

The cause of varicose veins is a failure of tiny valves in the blood vessels to function properly, so that venous blood destined for the heart flows backward and forms pools that can make the veins distended, tortuous, and painful. Varicose veins are related to the erect posture of humans; the heart pumps blood through arteries to the extremities, but the return flow must fight the pull of gravity. Ordinarily, venous blood gets a boost up the legs by a pumping action of leg-muscle contractions. Valves in the legs are designed to let the blood move upward but are supposed to block any backward flow. People whose jobs require them to stand all day are among those likely to suffer from a breakdown of the normal functioning of the valves. Women who have had multiple pregnancies and obese individuals are also apt to develop varicose veins.

Ulceration

Varicose veins can cause ulcers in the lower leg near the ankle that bleed through the skin after an injury to the area.

Treatment

One kind of surgical treatment of the varicosed vein is *ligation,* which means "tying" or "binding". An incision is made in the leg, usually in the area of the groin. The diseased saphenous vein is severed from its connection with the larger, femoral vein and is tied off. The function of a ligated vein is taken over by other veins in the leg. An alternate kind of surgery for varicose veins, sometimes called *stripping,* requires either a series of small incisions along the path of the vein, from the groin to the ankle, or an internal stripping by use of a special, long, threadlike instrument. The diseased vein is then removed and any connections with other veins ligated.

Varicose vein surgery is used for treatment of the *superficial* veins—those that are close to the skin. The operation is simple and can be performed under a local anesthetic in many cases. When multiple varicose veins are on both legs, all of the problem veins can be stripped and ligated at the same time. A hospital stay of several days may be required, and dressings are needed on the treated legs for two or three weeks after the operation.

Phlebitis

A problem related to varicose veins is *phlebitis,* a disease that usually involves the larger, deep veins of the legs with inflammation, pain, and swelling. Phlebitis is much more serious than varicose veins because a large vein is involved and a clot usually forms, obstructing return blood flow of the limb. The danger is that the clot will break loose—that is, become an *embolus*—and travel to the lungs, where it can obstruct a vital blood vessel, with serious or even fatal results. The obstructing clot is called an *embolism.*

Causes and Treatment

Causes of phlebitis can be injury, infection, poor circulation, or simply sitting for long periods of time. Medical therapy may include wet dressings and medications, especially anticoagulant drugs to thin the blood and reduce the chances of clot formations. Supportive bandages, leg exercises, and elevation of the legs may also be recommended.

Surgical Procedure

Surgery is reserved usually for cases in which medical therapy fails to control the risk of emboli forming. The surgical procedure is directed toward treatment of the deep vein that is the source of the phlebitis symptoms. The surgeon may open the vein to remove the clot, or a device can be inserted in the vein to strain out any clots that may form in the vein and travel toward the lungs. In some cases the surgeon may block the upward flow of blood from the affected vein, allowing other veins in the leg to assume that function. However, if other veins already have been stripped or ligated in the treatment of varicose veins, it is unlikely that a surgeon would occlude or block the flow of blood in a deep leg vein.

Intermittent Claudication

Intermittent claudication is a disorder of blood circulation of the legs involving the arteries. It is primarily a disease of aging, with gradual, progressive narrowing of the lumen (interior space) of the arteries by atherosclerosis. Atherosclerosis of the arteries occurs in other parts of the body, including the arms. Intermittent claudication is marked by muscle fatigue and pain when the leg muscles are used, as in walking. The symptoms are relieved by rest. The condition can be relieved by drugs, particularly medications that help dilate the arteries, but in severe cases surgery to reconstruct the leg arteries is the solution.

Surgical Procedure

The surgeon may build a bypass artery by grafting a length of plastic tubing into the affected blood vessel and around the area blocked by atherosclerotic narrowing. Sometimes surgeons will use a piece of a vein from the patient's body to make a bypass artery; for example, a vein from the arm may be transformed into an artery for the leg. Another procedure involves simply removing the portion of the artery blocking the normal flow of blood.

Orthopedic Surgery

Orthopedics originally was the name given the subject of treating deformities in children; the original Greek term could be translated as "normal child." But the medical world now uses the word to describe treatment of the bones, muscles, joints, and associated tissues of the body's locomotion apparatus. Orthopedic surgery, therefore, might involve repair of a broken big toe, as well as treatment of a whiplash injury to the neck.

This section discusses disorders of the spine, including herniated (or "slipped") disk, fractures, and torn ligaments.

Slipped Disk

The spinal column of 33 stacked vertebrae is a common source of painful problems that require orthopedic treatment. In addition to helping support the weight of the body above the hips, the vertebrae are subjected to a variety of twists, turns, and strains during a typical day. Much of the nearly continuous shock exerted on the spinal column is absorbed by the gel-like disks between the vertebrae.

Symptoms

Eventually, one of the disks may *her-*

niate, or slip out of place, causing pressure on a spinal nerve. The result can be severe pain that radiates along the pathway of the nerve as far as the lower leg. The pain may be accompanied by muscular weakness and loss of reflexes, even perhaps by a loss of feeling in part of the leg affected by a pinched or squeezed nerve. This condition, known popularly as a *slipped disk,* has symptoms of low back pain or leg pain that are similar to those of other disorders, such as intermittent claudication, arthritis, strained muscles, and prostatitis. Also, a herniated disk can occur near the top of the spinal column with symptoms of head and neck-area pains. But more than 90 percent of herniated disk cases involve the lumbar region of the spinal column, in the lower back.

Diagnosis

Physicians usually can confirm a herniated disk problem by a technique called *myelography,* in which a dye is injected into the spinal canal and X-ray pictures taken. Another procedure, called *electromyography,* can help determine which nerve root is involved.

Treatment

Conservative measures generally are used at first to reduce the pain and other symptoms. They include bed rest on a hard mattress, medications, and sometimes the use of traction and back braces. If conservative therapy fails to correct the problem and the diagnosis has been well established by a myelogram, surgery may be advised to remove the herniated disk.

Spinal Fusion

The surgeon may recommend a procedure called *spinal fusion,* in which

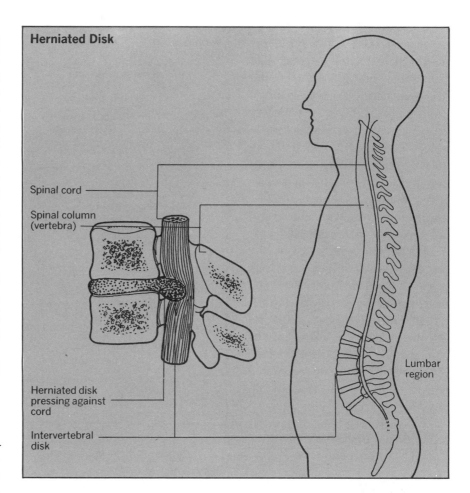

Herniated Disk

Spinal cord

Spinal column (vertebra)

Herniated disk pressing against cord

Intervertebral disk

Lumbar region

Spinal Fusion

Scrapped vertebra

Pelvis

Pelvic bone chips

Sacrum

the edges of several of the vertebrae are roughened and a piece of bone from the pelvis grafted onto the roughened edges. The bone graft will fuse with the vertebrae and in effect make the several vertebrae a single bone. However, the fused vertebrae will not interfere noticeably with body movements after the fusion is completed, which takes about six months. The operation requires a hospital stay of from one to two weeks and the patient must wear a body cast for the first few weeks and then use a back brace for a period of possibly several months. The patient usually can return to work and resume some normal activities within a couple of months after the operation. Strenuous activity, however, is usually restricted after an operation on the spinal column.

Other Spinal Disorders

Spondylolisthesis

Spinal fusion surgery also may be used to correct two other kinds of spinal disorders. One disorder is known as *spondylolisthesis*, a condition in which one of the vertebrae slips out of alignment. Spondylolisthesis usually occurs at the bottom of the group of lumbar vertebrae, where that section of the spinal column rests on the sacrum.

Scoliosis

The other disorder is *scoliosis*, or abnormal curvature of the spinal column. If the case of scoliosis is mild and causes no severe symptoms, it may be treated with conservative measures such as braces and special exercises. Surgical treatment of scoliosis may involve not only spinal fusion but reinforcement of the spinal column with metal rods attached to

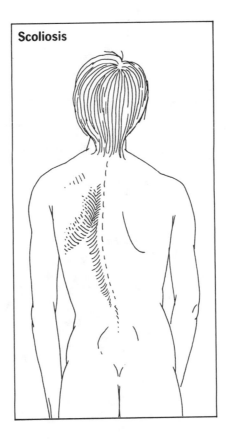

Scoliosis

the vertebrae to hold them in proper alignment.

Disorders of the cervical portion of the spinal column, in the area of the neck, may cause symptoms similar to those of a herniated disk in the lower back. But there is pain in the neck and shoulders and weakness in the arms. Surgical treatment also is similar, with removal of a herniated disk portion or fusion of cervical vertebrae when conservative therapy, with bed rest, neck braces, and medications, does not prove helpful.

Fractures

Many fractures of the spinal column also are treated by fusion operations, use of casts, braces, bed rest, or traction, in addition to therapy directed toward the specific problem. Spinal fractures frequently are compression fractures of vertebrae caused by falling in a sitting or standing position or mishaps in which a bony process of a vertebra is broken.

Spinal fractures that result in permanent damage to the spinal cord, with resulting paralysis, are relatively uncommon.

Reduction of Fractures

Fractures of the long bones of the arms and legs are treated by a method called *reduction,* the technique of aligning the broken ends of the bones properly so the healing process will not result in a deformity. Reduction also requires that the muscles and surrounding tissues be aligned and held in place by immobilizing them as the break heals.

If the break is simple enough, the limb can be immobilized by putting a plaster cast around the part of the involved limb after the fractured ends of the bone and associated tissues have been realigned. In complicated cases with a number of bone fragments resulting from the fracture and surrounding tissues in some disarray, the patient usually is given a general anesthetic while the surgeon recognizes the shattered limb like a player assembling pieces of a jigsaw puzzle. If some of the needed pieces are missing, the surgeon may fill the gaps with bone from a bone bank, although bank materials usually are not as effective in the healing process as pieces of the patient's own bones.

Use of Internal Appliances

A common technique of modern fracture surgery is the application of wires, screws, pins, metal plates, and other devices to provide internal fixation of a broken long bone during the healing process. Nails and pins may be used to fasten the fractured neck of a femur, the long bone of the upper leg, to the shaft of that bone. A steel rod may be driven through the shaft of a long bone to align the broken sections. Screws may be used to hold together bone ends of a fracture in which the break runs diagonally across the shaft. Screws also may be employed to hold a metal plate or strip of bone from the patient's own body across the break. The screws, nails, and other devices generally are well tolerated by the body and may be left in the bones indefinitely if they do not cause adverse reactions after the healing process is completed.

Traction

Traction frequently is employed to hold a limb in alignment while a fracture is healing. A clamp sometimes is placed at one end of the fractured limb and a weight attached by wires over a pulley is connected to the clamp. Depending upon the kind of fracture and type of traction prescribed, a system of several weights and pulleys may be rigged around the bed of a patient to fix the bone and related tissues in correct positions.

Torn Cartilage

Joints of the body can be vulnerable to damage from sudden twisting and turning actions, particularly when the force of the individual's body weight is added to the pressure on the joint. The effect of such forces on the knee joint can result in tearing of the half-moon-shaped cartilages that cushion friction of the upper and lower leg bones where they are joined. Sports fans are particularly aware of the vulnerability of the knee joint because of the high incidence of knee injuries to athletes, especially in football and basketball. Obese individuals are also particularly liable to develop cartilage problems in the knee.

Symptoms

When a cartilage of the knee joint is torn, the patient may feel pain and weakness in the area of the injury. Swelling usually occurs, and in more than half the cases the knee cannot be straightened, because it has become "locked" by the cartilage. There may be a remission of symptoms, but surgery frequently is required sooner or later.

Surgical Procedure

The surgeon makes an incision in the area of the kneecap and cuts away the torn cartilage. Full recovery takes several weeks after the first few postoperative days, during which the patient remains in bed with the affected leg elevated. Special exercises are required to overcome muscle weakness in the leg and to help the patient learn to use the leg with part of the cartilage cushion missing.

Neurosurgery

Neurosurgery may be employed to treat a wide assortment of disorders involving the nervous system, from the brain to nerve endings in the fingers and toes. Neurosurgery may involve treatment of epilepsy, Parkinson's disease, and psychiatric disorders, as well as herniated disks of the spinal column and aneurysms that affect the nervous system. Causes of neurosurgical problems can be injury, tumors, infectious diseases, or congenital disorders.

This section includes discussions of trigeminal neuralgia, brain tumors, and head injuries.

Trigeminal Neuralgia

Trigeminal neuralgia is one of many types of pain that sometimes can be treated by surgery. The disorder, also known as *tic douloureux* or *facial neuralgia,* tends to develop in persons between 40 and 60 years of age, causing attacks of acute pain and muscular twitching in the area of the face containing branches of the trigeminal nerve. The painful attacks occur with no apparent reason but seem to be associated with certain stimuli, such as touch or temperature changes, at points around the face and mouth. During periods of attacks, the patient may avoid eating, shaving, or any other activity that might trigger a spasm of severe pain. But the pain attacks also may cease, with or without treatment, for three or four months, only to resume for weeks or months.

Treatment

Alcohol injections and medications may offer relief of symptoms, but when symptoms continue, surgery frequently is recommended. The operation consists of an incision to reach the root of the nerve and cut the divisions that appear to be involved with the painful symptoms. However, cutting the nerve can result in loss of feeling for the entire side of the face, including the cornea of the eye, so that the patient must wear special glasses to protect the cornea. An alternative procedure that is not always effective involves exposing the nerve root and rubbing it, a technique that seems to produce a temporary loss of sensation in the nerve fibers.

Brain Tumor

Brain tumors are popularly associated with neurosurgery skills. And while brain surgery requires great skill and knowledge of brain anatomy, which in itself is quite complicated, most brain tumor operations are conducted safely and successfully. Diagnosing, locating, and identifying a brain tumor are challenges faced by the physician before surgery begins. There are a

Brain Tumors
Frequent locations of common lesions

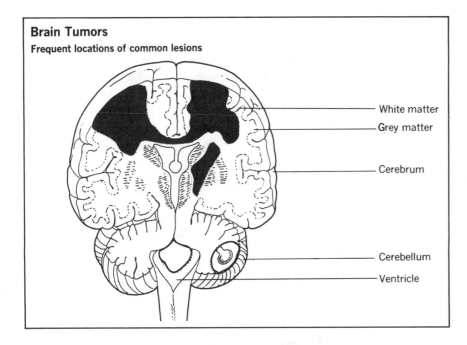

White matter

Grey matter

Cerebrum

Cerebellum

Ventricle

dozen major types of brain tumors plus some minor types. The types of tumors tend to vary according to the age of the patient; the patient's age and the type of tumor may suggest where it develops.

Symptoms

Because brain tumors can cause organic mental changes in the patient, the symptoms of changed behavior can be mistaken for neurotic or psychotic disorders, with the result that a patient may spend valuable time receiving psychiatric treatment rather than surgical treatment; autopsies of a significant number of patients who die in mental hospitals reveal the presence of brain tumors. In addition to mental changes, the person suffering from a brain tumor may complain of headaches, experience convulsions, or display signs of neurological function loss, such as abnormal vision.

Diagnosis

The specific signs and symptoms, along with X-ray studies, electroen-cephalograms, and other tests, help the physicians determine the site and extent of growth of a brain tumor. A recently developed technique called *CT scanning* (for *computed tomography*) aids the neurosurgeon by producing a series of X-ray pictures of the interior of the skull as if they were "slices" of the brain taken in thicknesses of about two-thirds of an inch. The detailed anatomical portrait of the patient's brain helps pinpoint the disorder and indicate whether it is a tumor or another kind of abnormality.

Surgical Procedure

The usual method of removing a brain tumor after it has been diagnosed and located is a procedure called a *craniotomy*. The entire head is shaved and cleaned to eliminate the possibility that a stray bit of hair might fall into the incision that is made in the scalp. After the scalp has been opened, a series of holes are drilled in a pattern outlining the working area for the surgeon; a wire saw is used to cut the skull between the drilled holes.

Removing the tumor is a delicate operation, not only because of the need to avoid damage to healthy brain tissue but because accidental severing of a blood vessel in the brain could produce a critical hemorrhage. The surgeon tries to remove the entire tumor, or as much of the tumor as appears possible without damaging vital brain tissues or blood vessels. All the various types of brain tumors are considered dangerous, whether malignant or benign, because within the rigid confines of the skull there is no opportunity for outward release of pressure. Therefore any growth may compress or destroy vital brain tissues if left untreated.

After the tumor is removed, the piece of skull removed at the start of the operation is replaced and the scalp flap is sewed in place. Radiation therapy may be administered for a month to six weeks after surgery to destroy any tumor tissue left behind or tumor cells that may have drifted into the spinal canal. Some tumors near the base of the brain may be treated effectively with radiation alone if the tumor cells are radiosensitive. Tumors of the pineal gland and the pituitary gland also may be treated with radiation.

Laser Surgery

In an alternative procedure, *laser neurosurgery*, a brain surgeon may use a laser beam to vaporize the tumor. The hair is removed from all or part of the skull; a section of the skull is removed with a power or hand saw after being marked out with tiny holes; and the surgeon then uses the laser to destroy the tumor. Typically, the surgeon may actually control two laser beams: a helium-neon type that guides the surgical work, and a carbon dioxide (CO_2) laser that does the vaporizing.

Because the "no-touch" CO_2 laser works slowly, an operation may require 10 or more hours. The laser beam can focus on and destroy one tumor cell at a time, targeting areas of tissue 1/50th the thickness of a human hair, or it can attack a number of cells in a group. The surgeon controls the electrical power that activates the beam with a foot pedal. In effect, the laser causes the tumor cells to heat up beyond the boiling point and then to explode into vapor. At the same time, the beam coagulates the tiny blood vessels that it passes through, preventing bleeding.

Head Injuries

Brain Hemorrhage

Head injuries, such as a blow to the head, can produce massive hemorrhages within the skull. As in the case of brain tumors, the expanding pool of blood within the skull gradually compresses the brain tissue and can result in death unless the problem is corrected. The damage of a brain hemorrhage can be insidious, with no immediate signs or symptoms of the problem until irreversible changes have occurred in the brain tissue. The patient may receive what may appear to be a minor head injury, for exam-

Brain Hemorrhage

Displaced brain

Cyst

Blood

ple, and not lose consciousness. Or he may be unconscious for a brief period, then recover and seem very alert. But gradually, over a period of hours or even days, neurological signs of disintegrating brain function appear.

Treatment

The treatment requires a procedure similar to that used for removing brain tumors. An opening is made in the skull to remove the blood or blood clot and relieve pressure upon the brain tissues. The chances for full recovery depend somewhat upon the extent of brain damage caused by the hemorrhage before treatment.

Skull Fracture

Surgical treatment for a skull fracture may combine techniques of various other methods for fractures and brain injuries. The scalp is shaved and cleaned carefully so the surgeon can determine the extent of the injury and its location with respect to vital tissues under the skull. With the help of X rays and signs of neurological damage, the surgeon frequently can tell how severe the fracture may be and whether there is bleeding beneath the skull.

Treatment

If the skull appears to be intact but there are signs of a brain hemorrhage, the skull is opened to remove the blood or blood clot and relieve pressure on the brain. If the skull fracture is compound and depressed, or with skull fragments in the brain tissue, efforts also must be made to elevate the depressed bone section so it does not press on vital brain areas and to remove bits of bone or other foreign materials that may have en-

tered the brain.

Surgeons frequently can rebuild a fractured skull by replacing missing bits of bone or adding appropriate synthetic materials such as a piece of metal plate. Full recovery depends upon such factors as the age of the patient and the severity of damage before treatment was started. Younger patients generally respond better to the repair procedures, but full recovery from a severe skull fracture may take as long as a year.

Aneurysm in the Brain

Aneurysms can develop in blood vessels of the brain, and like aneurysms in other parts of the body they can be corrected surgically. A ruptured aneurysm produces a brain hemorrhage. The condition is most likely to develop in people over the age of 30; in patients over 40, women are more likely than men to be victims of the disorder. The approach to repair of an intracranial aneurysm depends upon the condition of the patient and the location and size of the aneurysm, which frequently can be identified by X-ray pictures after an opaque dye has been injected into the bloodstream. The diseased blood vessel may be ligated, reinforced, or repaired, depending upon the conditions found by the surgeon after the aneurysm has been exposed and examined.

Plastic and Cosmetic Surgery

The use of surgical techniques for the correction of physical deformities is by no means a modern development. The practice goes back to ancient India, where as early as the sixth century B.C. Hindu specialists were reconstructing noses, reshaping ears, and grafting skin for reducing scar tissue.

Through the centuries, improvements in procedure and new types of operations became part of the common fund of information. During World War I, great technical advances were made when the Medical Corps of the United States Army created a special division of *plastic surgery* to treat the deformities caused by battle injuries. Today's plastic surgery is based on many of the procedures perfected then and during World War II.

In recent years, attention has been focused not only on birth and injury deformities but on lesser irregularities as well. Surgeons in the field of *cosmetic surgery* perform such procedures as nose reconstruction, face lifting, reshaping of breasts, removal of fatty tissue from upper arms and legs, and the transplanting of hair to correct baldness.

There is no longer any reason for someone to suffer from the emotional and professional problems caused by abnormalities in appearance. No child should be expected to live with the disability of a cleft lip or crossed eyes. A young woman tormented by what she considers to be a grotesque nose can have it recontoured to her liking. An older woman who finds wrinkles a social liability can have them removed. Anyone interested in undergoing any form of cosmetic surgery should stay away from so-called beauty experts, and deal only with a reputable surgeon or physician.

Some surgical specialists, called *plastic surgeons,* perform cosmetic or plastic surgery exclusively. Other surgeons and physicians, including general surgeons, dermatologists, ophthalmologists, and others, are qualified to do some kinds of plastic surgery, usually the techniques related to their particular specialties. The kind of surgery desired should first be discussed with the family doctor, who can then evaluate the problem and recommend a qualified surgeon to deal with it.

Before undergoing any kind of plastic surgery, the prospective patient should realize that it is neither inexpensive nor totally painless. Most cosmetic surgery is performed in hospitals, which means that in addition to the surgeon's fees there can be a bill for the anesthetist, use of the operating and recovery rooms, and the hospital stay itself. Also, because cosmetic surgery is often optional surgery, surgery not needed to ensure the patient's physical health, it may not be covered by a health-insurance policy.

Reshaping the Nose

Known technically as a *rhinoplasty,* the operation for the reconstruction of the nose is not only one of the oldest but also one of the most common forms of cosmetic surgery. Depending upon the demands of facial symmetry and individual taste, the nose can be shortened, straightened, narrowed, or even lengthened. If a nose deformity has caused breathing problems, the surgeon will take the correction of this into account in planning the reconstruction.

Barring accidents, most children's noses are perfectly adequate until they enter their teens, when the facial bones begin to take on the contours determined by inheritance. Teenagers are especially sensitive about their looks. If nose surgery seems advisable, therefore, it is usually undertaken when the child is between 14 and 16 years of age, though the operation is also performed on adults.

Cosmetic Breast Surgery

Breast Lifting

Breasts that sag even though they are not too large can be lifted to a more attractive contour by an operation that consolidates the tissue. The surgical procedure consists of removing strips of skin from the base of the breasts and bringing the rest of the skin together under tension so that it is tight enough to support the tissue in an upward position.

Breast Reduction

In spite of all the publicity given to breast augmentation, most cosmetic surgery involving the breasts is concerned with reducing rather than enlarging them. Breast reduction is frequently undertaken not only to improve appearance but also for purposes of health and comfort.

The operation, called a *mastoplasty,* is performed under general anesthesia and consists in cutting out fatty tissue and skin. Although the incision may be large, the resulting scars are not thicker than a hairline and are hidden in the fold below the breasts.

The most remarkable thing about this type of surgery—and the reason for its being considerably more complicated than breast enlargement—is the repositioning of the nipples so that they are properly placed relative to the newly proportioned breast contours.

Breast Enlargement

The techniques used in this operation, called a *mammoplasty,* have changed over the years. Early operations to augment the size of the breasts involved the injection of paraffin, but this was soon abandoned as unsatisfactory. Considerable experimentation with the use of various synthetics, as well as with the use of fatty tissue taken from the buttocks, didn't provide good results either.

Silicone—a form of man-made plastic material of great versatility—

was first used in this connection in the form of sponges, and later was injected in liquid form directly into the tissue. However, the federal Food and Drug Administration has ruled that the use of liquid silicone is unsafe and illegal because its presence would mask signs of malignancy. Another problem with liquid silicone is that it has a tendency to drift to other parts of the body.

In the latest techniques of breast augmentation, a silicone gel or saline solution is placed in a flexible silicone bag shaped to resemble the breast. The bags are inserted through incisions under the breast tissue, and to date appear to be the safest and most satisfactory solution to the problem of breast enlargement.

Face Lift

Face lifting, or *rhytidoplasty,* is a form of cosmetic surgery designed to eliminate as far as possible signs of aging, such as wrinkles, pouches under the chin and eyes, and sagging tissue generally. About 7,000 such operations are performed each year with satisfactory results.

In deciding on the advisability of a face lift, a reputable surgeon will take into account the person's age, emotional stability, and physical condition. The main procedure involves tightening the skin after the surplus has been removed. The resulting scars are usually hidden in the hair and behind the ears. Those directly in front of the ears are visible only under very close scrutiny. Even after a face lift, however, the same wrinkles will eventually reappear, owing to the characteristic use of the individual's facial muscles.

Eyelids

The shape and size of the eyelids can

Face Lift — Incision line behind hairline — Separating skin from the face — Tying loose subcutaneous tissue — Excess skin to be cut off

be changed by an operation called a *blepharoplasty.* In this procedure, an incision is made in the fold of the upper eyelid, and excess skin and fat are removed. The technique can be used to correct congenital deformities, such as hanging upper eyelids that do not fully open. When a comparable incision is made below the lash line on the lower lid, the surgeon can remove the fat that causes bags under the eyes.

Ears

Surgery to correct protruding or overlarge ears is called *otoplasty.* Though it can be performed on adults, it is usually performed on children before they enter school, to prevent the psychological problems that often re-

sult from teasing. In the procedure, an incision is made behind the ear, cartilage is cut, and the ear is repositioned closer to the skull. Otoplasty can also build up or replace an ear missing because of a birth defect or accident.

Scar Reduction

Unsightly scars that are the result of a birth defect or an injury can usually be reduced by plastic surgery to thin hairlines. The procedure is effective only if there has been no extensive damage to surrounding areas of underlying tissue, as sometimes occurs in severe burns. The operation involves the removal of the old scar tissue, undermining the surrounding skin, and pulling it together with very fine stitches.

Uncommon Surgical Procedures

Organic Transplants

The notion of man's ability to rebuild human bodies from the parts of other humans or from artificial organs probably is as old as the dreams that men might someday fly like birds or travel to the moon. Some of the oldest documents, thousands of years old, tell of medical efforts to transplant organs, limbs, and other tissues to save lives or enable disabled persons to pursue normal activities. In recent decades, medical scientists have discovered how to overcome some of the obstacles to organ transplanting, just as other scientists have learned to fly higher and faster than birds and travel beyond the moon.

Tissue Compatibility

A major obstacle to organ transplants has been one of *histoincompatibility* (*histo* means "tissue"): the tissues of the person receiving the transplant tend to reject the tissues of the transplanted organs. The problem is quite similar to that of allergies or the body's reaction to foreign bodies, including infectious organisms. Each individual has a set of antigens that are peculiar to that person, because of genetic variations among different persons. The histoincompatible antigens are on the surfaces of the tissue cells. But in most cases the antigens on the cells of the transplanted organ do not match those of the person receiving the transplant, so the recipient's body in effect refuses to accept the transplant.

The major exception to this rule is found in identical twins, who are born with the same sets of antigens. The organs of one twin can be transplanted to the body of the other twin with a minimum risk of rejection. Antigens on the tissue cells of brothers and sisters and of the parents will be similar, because of the biological relationship, but they will not be as compatible as those of identical twins. Even less compatible are antigens of people who are not related.

Types of Grafts

There is virtually no problem in transferring tissues from one area to another of the same patient. Skin grafts, bone grafts, and blood-vessel transplants are commonly made with a patient's own tissues, which have the same antigens, as in spinal fusions, repair of diseased leg arteries, and so on. Tissue transplants within an individual's body are called *autografts*. Transplants of tissues or organs from one human to another are called *homografts*. *Heterografts* are tissues from one species that are transplanted to another; they offer the greatest risk of histoincompatibility and are used mainly as a temporary measure, such as covering a severely burned area of a person with specially treated pieces of pigskin. The heterograft will be rejected, but it will provide some protection during the recovery period.

Much of the experience of surgeons in handling tissue transplants between humans came from early experiments in skin grafting. It was found that histoincompatibility in transplants of skin appeared to sensitize the recipient tissues in the same way that allergy sensitivity rises. Thus, when a second skin graft from the same donor is attempted, the graft is rejected more rapidly than the first graft because of the buildup of antibodies from the first rejection. The same sort of rejection reaction can occur in transplants of kidneys, hearts, and other organs unless the problem of histoincompatibility is overcome.

Immunosuppressive Chemicals

In order to make the host body more receptive to an organ transplant, *immunosuppressive* chemicals are injected into the recipient's tissues to suppress their natural tendency to reject the foreign tissue. However, the technique of suppressing the immune response of the host tissues is not without hazards. By suppressing the natural rejection phenomenon, the transplant recipient is made vulnerable to other diseases. It has been found, for example, that persons who receive the immune response suppression chemicals as part of transplant surgery develop cancers at a rate that is 15 times that of the general population. Transplant patients also can become extremely vulnerable to infections, such as pneumonia.

Antigen Matching

The breakthrough in human organ transplantation was helped by the development of a system of matching antigens related to lymphocytes—a type of white blood cell—of the donor and recipient. At least a dozen lymphocyte antigens have been identified, and it is possible to match them by a process similar to matching blood factors of patients before making a blood transfusion. If all or most of the antigens of the donor tissue and the recipient match, the chances for a successful transplanting procedure are greatly enhanced.

Antigen matching is less important in some kinds of homografts, such as replacing the cornea of the eye. The cornea is a unique kind of tissue with no blood vessels, and therefore is unlikely to be invaded by antibodies of the recipient. Pieces of human bone also may be used in homografts with a minimum risk of rejection, although surgeons usually prefer to use bone from the patient's own body in repairing fractures and in other orthopedic procedures.

Types of Transplants

Cornea Transplant

Cornea transplants helped to pioneer the art of homografts. The first successful cornea transplants were made during the 1930s. In addition to the absence of rejection problems because of incompatible antigens, cornea transplants probably succeeded in the early days of homografts because only small pieces of the tissue were used.

Kidney Transplant

Kidney transplants began in the 1950s. Antigen typing was unknown at that time, but physicians had learned of the genetic factors of blood groups and found from experience that although kidney transplants from siblings and parents could eventually be rejected, the rejection phenomenon was delayed. The first truly successful kidney transplant operation was performed in Boston in 1954 between twin brothers; doctors had tested the tissue compatibility of the twins first by making a small skin transplant to see if it would be rejected. Knowledge acquired later of immunosuppressive drugs enabled surgeons to make kidney transplants between persons who were not twins.

More than 5,000 kidney transplant operations have been performed with an 82 percent survival rate of two years or more when the donor was related to the recipient. When a ca-

daver kidney was transplanted, the two-year survival rate was 65 percent. It has been estimated that as many as 10,000 kidney disease patients each year could benefit from a transplanted organ, but a lack of available kidneys in satisfactory condition restricts the number of transplants. An alternative for some kidney patients awaiting an organ transplant is hemodialysis, a process that performs as an artificial kidney.

Heart Transplant

The first successful human heart transplant was performed by Dr. Christiaan Barnard in Cape Town, South Africa, in 1968. The patient survived more than 18 months and led a relatively active life until the second heart failed because of a rejection reaction. Many heart transplant operations have been performed since 1968, with varying success, sometimes leading to complete recovery and sometimes to recovery for long periods of time. Heart transplants were found to be more difficult than some other organ transplants, such as of the kidney, because the heart must be taken from the donor at virtually the moment of death and immediately placed in the body of the recipient. Because of concern about determining the moment of death, the medical profession has offered guidelines for answering this complex ethical and legal question.

Success of a heart transplant operation may depend on the health of other organ systems in the patient's body; persons in need of heart transplants usually have medical problems involving the lungs and kidneys as a result of the diseased heart. And heart transplant patients frequently seem less able to tolerate the use of immunosuppressive drugs that must be administered after surgery. The introduction of cyclosporine as an im-

munosuppressant changed the picture substantially, however. Medical evidence indicated that cyclosporine would lead to a five-year survival rate among heart transplant patients of 50 percent or more. Because cyclosporine speeds rehabilitation after an operation, average hospital stays for patients receiving the immunosuppressant have been reduced from 72 to 42 days.

Conducted before cyclosporine came into common use, one study of a group of transplant patients showed that fewer than 40 percent survived beyond the first year. Several lived more than two years after the operation.

Bone-Marrow Transplant

Limited success has been reported in efforts to perform bone-marrow transplants. Bone-marrow transplants are performed to supply patients with active leukocytes to fight cancer and other diseases. The successful early cases have involved transplants between sisters and brothers who had been typed for tissue compatibility.

Other Kinds of Transplants

Surgeons also have experimented with varying success with human transplants of livers, lungs, and pancreas tissue. Lung transplant efforts have been hampered by infection, rejection, and hemorrhage. Because the lungs are exposed to pathogenic organisms in the environment they are especially vulnerable to infections when the host tissues have been treated with immunosuppressive chemicals. Liver transplants are difficult to perform because of a lack of satisfactory donor organs and the complex circuitry of arteries, veins, and bile duct that must be connected to the recipient before the liver can begin to function.

Most major organ transplants are considered only in terms of a "last ditch" effort to prolong the life of a patient who is critically ill. While homografts are not always a perfect success and may lengthen a patient's life by only a few years, remarkable strides in these surgical techniques have been made over a relatively short period of time. Surgeons who specialize in organ transplants state that even greater progress could be made if a greater supply of donor organs were available.

Reattachment of Severed Members

Because an individual's tissues present no histocompatibility problem with other parts of his own body, severed fingers and other members can be rejoined to the rest of the body if vital parts are not damaged beyond repair. Children sometimes suffer amputation of a part of a finger during play or in accidents at home. For example, a finger tip can be severed when caught in a closed door of an automobile. If the severed part of the finger is saved and the patient is given immediate medical care, the finger usually can be rejoined and sutured in place with a very good chance of survival of the graft.

Rejoining a Severed Limb

One of the most dramatic cases of a rejoined limb in American medical annals involved a 12-year-old whose right arm was severed at the shoulder when he was crushed between a train and a tunnel wall in 1962. Railroad workers called an ambulance, and the boy, his severed arm still encased in his sleeve, was rushed to a hospital. The boy was given plasma by physicians who packed the severed arm in ice and flushed out the blood vessels of the arm with anticoagulant drugs and antibiotics. During three hours of surgery, the major veins and artery of the arm were carefully stitched to the vessels at the shoulder. For the next five hours, surgeons joined the bones, located the main nerve trunks and connected them to the nerve ends in the shoulder, and repaired the muscles. The boy was released from the hospital three weeks after the accident but returned for additional operations to connect various nerve fibers. That operation was a success, but similar attempts to rejoin severed arms of middle-aged men have failed despite heroic attempts by surgeons to restore the limbs as functioning parts of the body.

A Chinese factory worker suffered accidental amputation of his right hand when it was caught in a metal-punching machine, and was rushed to a hospital in Shanghai. Chinese medical reports of the case indicate that a procedure similar to the one used on the American boy was followed. Blood vessels were rejoined first to permit the flow of blood to tissues. This was followed by surgery to connect the tendons and main nerve trunks. The bones of the forearm, where the amputation occurred, were joined and held in place with metal plates and screws. Physicians reported that the graft was successful, and the patient, a 27-year-old man, was able to move his fingers again within three weeks after the accident.

Medical records indicate that major reattachments of severed limbs are still rare, although rejoined finger tips, ears, and other parts not involving main arteries, veins, or nerve trunks are not as uncommon.

21

Skin and Hair

Not many people have perfectly proportioned faces and bodies, but practically anyone, at any age, can present an attractive appearance if skin is healthy-looking and glowing and hair is clean and shining. Healthy skin and hair can be achieved through good health habits, cleanliness, and personal grooming. Expensive skin-and-hair products may boost self-confidence, but they are a poor substitute for proper diet, exercise, enough sleep, and soap and water or cleansing creams.

The condition of skin and hair reflects a person's physical and emotional health. Of course, general appearance is determined not only by what is going on inside the body but also by outward circumstances, such as extremes of temperature or the use of harsh soaps. Appearance can also be altered temporarily by cosmetics and permanently by surgery.

The Skin

The skin is one of the most important organs of the body. It serves as protection against infection by germs and shields delicate underlying tissue against injury. Approximately one-third of the bloodstream flows through the skin, and as the blood vessels contract or relax in response to heat and cold, the skin acts as a thermostat that helps control body temperature. The two million sweat glands in the skin also regulate body temperature through the evaporation of perspiration. The many delicate nerve endings in the skin make it a sense organ responsive not only to heat and cold but also to pleasure, pain, and pressure.

Certain cells in the skin produce a protective pigmentation that determines its color and guards against overexposure to the ultraviolet rays of the sun. By absorption and elimination, the skin helps regulate the body's chemical and fluid balance. One of the miracles of the skin is that it constantly renews itself.

Structure of the Skin

The skin is made up of two layers. The outer later, or *epidermis,* has a surface of horny, nonliving cells that form the body's protective envelope. These cells are constantly being shed and replaced by new ones, which are made in the lower or inner layer of the epidermis.

Underneath the epidermis is the *dermis,* the thicker part of the skin. It contains blood vessels, nerves, and connective tissue. The sweat glands are located in the dermis, and they collect fluid containing water, salt, and waste products from the blood. This fluid is sent through tiny canals that end in pores on the skin's surface.

The oil, or *sebaceous,* glands that secrete the oil that lubricates the surface of the skin and hair are also located in the dermis. They are most often associated with hair *follicles.* Hair follicles and oil glands are found over most of the body, with the exception of the palms of the hands and the soles of the feet.

The layer of fatty tissue below the dermis, called *subcutaneous* tissue, acts as an insulator against heat and cold and as a shock absorber against injury.

Skin Color

The basic skin color of each person is determined at birth, and is a part of his heritage that cannot be changed.

Anatomy of the Skin

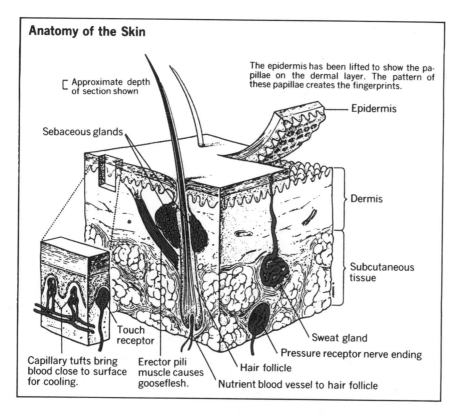

Approximate depth of section shown

The epidermis has been lifted to show the papillae on the dermal layer. The pattern of these papillae creates the fingerprints.

Sebaceous glands

Epidermis

Dermis

Subcutaneous tissue

Touch receptor

Sweat gland

Pressure receptor nerve ending

Capillary tufts bring blood close to surface for cooling.

Erector pili muscle causes gooseflesh.

Hair follicle

Nutrient blood vessel to hair follicle

Melanin

There are four pigments in the normal skin that affect its color: melanin, oxygenated hemoglobin, reduced hemoglobin, and various carotenes. Of these, *melanin* is the most powerful. The cells that produce it are the same in all races, but there is wide variation in the amount produced, and wide variation in its color, which ranges from black to light tan. Every adult has about 60,000 melanin-producing cells in each square inch of skin.

Melanin cells also affect eye color. When the cells are deep in the eye, the color produced is blue or green. When they are close to the surface, the eye is brown. An *albino*, a person with no melanin, has eyes that appear pink, because the stronger pigment that ordinarily masks the blood vessels is lacking.

Hemoglobin

The pigment that gives blood its color, called *hemoglobin,* has the next greatest effect on skin color. When it is combined with oxygen, a bright red is the result, and this in turn produces the rosy complexion associated with good health in light-skinned people. When such people suffer from reduced hemoglobin because of anemia, they appear to be excessively pale. A concentration of reduced hemoglobin gives the skin a bluish appearance. Because hemoglobin has a weaker coloring effect than the melanin that determines basic skin color, these variations are more visible in lighter-skinned individuals.

Carotenes

The weakest pigments in the skin are the *carotenes*. These produce a yellowish tone that is increased by eating excessive amounts of carrots and oranges. In people with black or brown skin, excess carotene is usually masked by the melanin pigment.

Aging Skin

Skin appearance is affected by both internal and external factors. A baby's skin has a silken quality because it has not yet begun to show the effects of continued exposure to sun and wind. The skin problems associated with adolescence reflect the many glandular changes that occur during the transition to adulthood. As the years pass, the skin becomes the most obvious indicator of aging.

Heredity, general health, and exposure to the elements are some of the factors that contribute to aging skin. Because people with darker skin have built-in protection against the ravages of the sun, their skin usually has a younger appearance than that of lighter-skinned people of comparable age.

In general, the skin of an older person is characterized by wrinkles and shininess. It feels thinner when pinched because it has lost its elasticity and part of the underlying fat that gives firmness to a younger skin.

Constant exposure to sunlight is now thought to play a more important role in the visible aging of skin than the aging process itself. Such exposure also appears to be directly related to the greater frequency of skin cancer among farmers, sailors, and others who spend most of their working hours out of doors.

Care of the Skin

Healthy, normal skin should be washed regularly with mild soap and warm water to remove grease, perspiration, and accumulated dirt. For those with a limited water supply or inadequate bath and shower facilities, sponge baths are a good substitute if the sponge or washcloth is thoroughly rinsed as various parts of the body are washed. Many people feel that a shower is a much more efficient way of getting clean than a bath, since the bath water becomes the receptacle for the dirt washed from the body, instead of its being rinsed away.

No matter what method is used, all soap should be thoroughly rinsed off the skin after washing. Unless specifically prescribed by a physician, medicated or germicidal soaps should not be used, since they may be an irritant. Skin should be dried with a fluffy towel, and bath towels should never be shared. Hands should be washed several times a day, and fingernails kept clean.

Facial skin requires special care because of its constant exposure. The face should be cleaned in the morning and before bedtime. Some women may prefer to use a cleansing cream rather than soap and water. Everyone should avoid massaging soap into the skin, because this may cause drying.

Dry and Oily Skin

Both heredity and environment account for the wide variation in the amount of oil and perspiration secreted by the glands of different people. Also, the same person's skin may be oily in one part of the body and dry in another.

Dry Skin

This condition is the result of loss of water from the outer surface of the epidermis and its insufficient replacement from the tissues below. Some causes of the moisture loss are too frequent use of soap and detergents, and constant exposure to dry air. Anyone spending a great deal of time in air-conditioned surroundings in which the humidity has been greatly lowered is likely to suffer from dry skin.

To correct the condition, the use of soap and water should be kept to a minimum for those parts of the body where the skin is dry. Cleansing creams or lotions containing lanolin should be used on the face, hands, elbows, and wherever else necessary. If tub baths are taken, a bath oil can be used in the water or applied to the skin after drying. Baby oil is just as effective and much cheaper than glamorously packaged and overadvertised products. Baby oil or a protective lotion should also be used on any parts of the body exposed to direct sunlight for any extended length of time. Applying oil to the skin will not, however, prevent wrinkles.

Oily Skin

The amount of oil that comes to the surface of the skin through the sebaceous glands is the result not only of heredity but also of temperature and emotional state. In warm weather, when the skin perspires more freely, the oil spreads like a film on the surface moisture. Nonoily foundation lotions can be helpful in keeping the oil spread to a minimum, and so can frequent washing with soap and water. When washing is inconvenient during the day, cleansing pads packaged to fit in pocket or purse are a quick and efficient solution for both men and women.

Too much friction from complexion brushes, rough washcloths, or harsh soaps may irritate rather than improve an oily skin condition.

Deodorants and Antiperspirants

Sweat glands are present almost everywhere in the skin except for the lips and a few other areas. Most of them give off the extremely dilute salt water known as sweat, or perspiration. Their purpose is to cool the body by evaporation of water. Body odors are not produced by perspiration itself but by the bacterial activity that takes place in the perspiration. The activity is most intense in warm, moist parts of the body from which perspiration cannot evaporate quickly, such as the underarm area.

Deodorants

The basic means of keeping this type of bacterial growth under control is through personal cleanliness of both skin and clothing. Deodorant soaps containing antiseptic chemicals are now available. Though they do not kill bacteria, they do reduce the speed with which they multiply.

Underarm deodorants also help to eliminate the odor. They are not meant to stop the flow of perspiration but rather to slow down bacterial growth and mask body odors with their own scent. Such deodorants should be applied immediately after bathing. They are usually more effective if the underarm area is shaved, since the hair in this unexposed area collects perspiration and encourages bacterial growth.

Antiperspirants

Antiperspirants differ from deodorants in that they not only affect the rate of bacterial growth but also reduce the amount of perspiration that reaches the skin surface. Because the action of the chemical salts they contain is cumulative, they seem to be more effective with repeated use. Antiperspirants come under the category of drugs, and their contents must be printed on the container. Deodorants are considered cosmetics, and may or may not name their contents on the package.

No matter what the nature of the advertising claim, neither type of product completely stops the flow of perspiration, nor would it be desirable to do so. Effectiveness of the various brands differs from one person to another. Some may produce a mild allergic reaction; others might be too weak to do a good job. It is practical to experiment with a few different brands, using them under similar conditions, to find the type that works best for you.

Creams and Cosmetics

The bewildering number of creams and cosmetics on the market and the exaggerated claims of some of their advertising can be reduced to a few simple facts. Beauty preparations should be judged by the user on their merits rather than on their claims.

Cold Creams and Cleansing Creams

These two products are essentially the same. They are designed to remove accumulated skin secretions, dirt, and grime, and should be promptly removed from the skin with a soft towel or tissue.

Lubricating Creams and Lotions

Also called night creams, moisturizing creams, and conditioning creams, these products are supposed to prevent the loss of moisture from the skin and promote its smoothness. They are usually left on overnight or for an extended length of time. Anyone with dry skin will find it helpful to apply a moisturizer under foundation cream. This will help keep the skin from drying out even further, and protect it against the effects of air-conditioning.

Vanishing Creams and Foundation Creams

These products also serve the purpose of providing the skin with moisture, but are meant to be applied immediately before putting on makeup.

Rejuvenating Creams

There is no scientific proof that any of the "royal jelly," "secret formula," or "hormone" creams produce a marked improvement on aging skin. They cannot eliminate wrinkles, nor can they regenerate skin tissue.

Medicated Creams and Lotions

These products should not be used except on the advice of a physician, since they may cause or aggravate skin disorders of various kinds.

Lipsticks

Lipsticks contain lanolin, a mixture of oil and wax, a coloring dye, and pigment, as well as perfume. Any of these substances can cause an allergic reaction in individual cases, but such reactions are uncommon. Sometimes the reaction is caused by the staining dye, in which case a "nonpermanent" lipstick should be used.

Cosmetics and the Sensitive Skin

Anyone with a cosmetic problem resulting from sensitive skin should consult a *dermatologist,* a physician specializing in the skin and its diseases. Cosmetic companies will inform a physician of the ingredients in their products, and he or she can then recommend a brand that will agree with the patient's specific skin problems. The physician may also recommend a special nonallergenic preparation.

Eye Makeup

Eye-liner and mascara brushes and pencils—and lipsticks, for that matter—can carry infection and should never be borrowed or lent.

Hypoallergenic makeup, which is specially made for those who get allergic reactions to regular eye makeup, is available and should be used by anyone so affected.

Suntanning Creams and Lotions

Growing awareness that exposure to the sun may cause skin cancer (see "Skin Cancer" in Ch. 18, *Cancer*) has led to a demand for a variety of skin creams and lotions. The preparations protect the skin or speed the tanning process. Many of the "sunblocks" and "sunscreens" keep the ultraviolet radiation in sunlight from reaching the skin. They are adapted to six basic skin types, ranging from type 1, which burns easily and never tans, to types 5 and 6, which never burn and usually tan well.

Skin lotions and creams are rated according to a "sun protection factor" (SPF). Among the basic ratings are SPF 4, providing "moderate protection;" SPF 8, a "maximal" sunscreen; and SPF 15, with "ultra" protection. Other ratings range up to SPF 50. Some medical authorities question the need for sunscreens rated higher than 15 or 20. Food and Drug Administration ratings go only to SPF 15. Many newer sunscreens are greaseless, hypoallergenic, waterproof, or PABA-free. PABA, or para-aminobenzoic acid, is a sunscreen chemical that can irritate skin and stain clothing.

Sunscreen ratings indicate, in theory, how long the user can stay in the sun without burning. A lotion or cream with a rating of SPF 2 should allow users to remain exposed twice as long as they could with no protection at all. The Skin Cancer Foundation believes that persons who burn in the sun should uniformly wear an SPF 15 protective preparation.

Persons who want suntans have many products from which to choose. "Tanning accelerators" in lotion form speed up the tanning process. A pocket-sized "sun exposure meter" operated electronically alerts the user when overexposure may be taking place. The meter is programmed with the individual's skin type and SPF.

Tanning Pills

Case-studies have proven that tanning pills can cause serious medical problems, possibly resulting in death. Ailments include aplastic anemia (a decrease in the production of red blood cells), orange skin, headaches, weight loss, easy bruising, and increased fatigue. Treatment involves blood transfusion therapy. Physicians believe that the ingredient canthaxanthin is responsible for the disorders.

This drug is not approved as a prescription or an over-the-counter preparation by the Federal Drug Administration. Ultimately, this product serves no purpose, and it is best to avoid using it.

Hair

Hair originates in tiny sacs or follicles deep in the dermis layer of skin tissue. The part of the hair below the skin surface is the root; the part above is the shaft. Hair follicles are closely connected to the sebaceous glands, which secrete oil to the scalp and give hair its natural sheen. Hair grows from the root outward, pushing the shaft farther from the scalp.

Texture

Each individual hair is made up of nonliving cells that contain a tough protein called *keratin*. Hair texture differs from one part of the body to another. In some areas, it may be soft and downy; in others, tough and bristly. Hair texture also differs between the sexes, among individuals, and among the different races.

If an individual hair is oval in cross-section, it is curly along its length. If the cross-section is round, the hair is straight. Thick, wiry hair is usually triangular or kidney-shaped. The fineness or coarseness of hair texture is related to its natural color.

Curling

Anyone using a home permanent preparation should read and follow instructions with great care. If a new brand is tried, the instructions should be read all over again, since they may be quite different from the accustomed ones.

Electric curling irons are not safe, because they may cause pinpoint burns in the scalp that are hardly noticeable at the time but may lead to permanent small areas of baldness. The danger can be minimized, however, if instructions for use are followed exactly. It is especially important that the iron not be hot enough to singe the hair. Setting lotions used with rollers or clips have a tendency to dull the hair unless they are completely brushed out.

Straightening

The least harmful as well as the least effective way of straightening the hair temporarily is the use of pomades. They are usually considered unsatisfactory by women because they are too greasy, but are often used by men with short, unruly hair. Heat-pressing the hair with a metal comb is longer-lasting but can cause substantial damage by burning the scalp. The practice of ironing the hair should be discouraged, since it causes dryness and brittleness, with resultant breakage.

Chemical straighteners should be used with great care, since they may cause serious burns. Special efforts must be made to protect the eyes from contact with these products.

Hair Color

In the same way that melanin colors the skin, it also determines hair color. The less melanin, the lighter the hair. As each hair loses its melanin pigment, it gradually turns gray, then white. It is assumed that the age at which hair begins to gray is an inherited characteristic and therefore can't be postponed or prevented by eating special foods, by taking vitamins, or by the external application of creams. The only way to recolor gray hair is by the use of a chemical dye.

Dyes and Tints

Anyone wishing to make a radical change in hair color should consult a trained and reliable hairdresser. Trying to turn black hair bright red or dark red hair to blond with a home preparation can sometimes end up with unwanted purplish or greenish results. When tints or dyes are used at home to lighten or darken the hair color by one or two shades, instructions accompanying the product must be followed carefully. Anyone with a tendency to contract contact dermatitis should make a patch test on the skin to check on possible allergic reactions. Hair should be tinted or dyed no more often than once a month.

Dye Stripping

The only safe way to get rid of an unwanted dye color that has been used on the hair is to let it grow out. The technique known as stripping takes all color from the hair and reduces it to a dangerously weak mass. It is then redyed its natural color. Such a procedure should never be undertaken by anyone except a trained beautician, if at all.

Bleaching

Hydrogen peroxide is mixed with a hair lightener to prebleach hair before applying blond tints. Bleaching with peroxide alone can cause more damage to the hair than dyeing or tinting it with a reliable commercial preparation, because it causes dryness, brittleness, and breakage.

General Hair Care

Properly cared for hair usually looks clean, shiny, and alive. Unfortunately, too many people mask the natural good looks of their hair with unnecessary sprays and "beauty" preparations.

Washing the Hair

Hair should be washed about once a week—more often if it tends to be oily. The claims made by shampoo manufacturers need not always be taken too seriously, since most shampoos contain nothing more than soap or detergent and a perfuming agent. No shampoo can restore the natural oils to the hair at the same time that it washes it. A castile shampoo is good for dry hair, and one containing tincture of green soap is good for oily hair.

Thorough rinsing is essential to eliminate any soap deposit. If the local water is hard, a detergent shampoo can be rinsed off more easily than one containing soap.

Drying the Hair

Drying the hair in sunlight or under a heat-controlled dryer is more satisfactory than trying to rub it dry with a towel. Gentle brushing during drying reactivates the natural oils that give hair its shine. Brushing in general is excellent for the appearance of the hair. Be sure to wash both brush and comb as often as the hair is washed.

Hair pomades should be avoided or used sparingly, since they are sometimes so heavy that they clog the pores of the scalp. A little bit of olive oil or baby oil can be rubbed into dry hair after shampooing. This is also good for babies' hair.

There is no scientific evidence that creme rinses, protein rinses, or beer rinses accomplish anything for the hair other than making it somewhat more manageable if it is naturally fine and flyaway.

Dandruff

Simple dandruff is a condition in which the scalp begins to itch and flake a few days after the hair has been washed. There is no evidence that the problem is related to germ infection.

Oiliness and persistent dandruff may appear not only on the scalp but also on the sides of the nose or the chest. In such cases, a dermatologist should be consulted. Both light and serious cases often respond well to prescription medicines containing tars. These preparations control the dandruff, but there is no known cure for it.

Nits

Head lice sometimes infect adults as well as children. These tiny parasites usually live on the part of the scalp near the nape of the neck, and when they bite, they cause itching. They attach their eggs, which are called *nits,* to the shaft of the hair, and when they are plentiful, they can be seen by a trained eye as tiny, silvery-white ovals. This condition is highly contagious and can be passed from one head to another by way of combs, brushes, hats, head scarfs, and towels. A physician can be consulted for information on effective ways of eliminating nits—usually by the application of chemicals and the use of a fine-tooth comb.

Baldness

Under the normal circumstances of combing, brushing, and shampooing, a person loses anywhere from 25 to 100 hairs a day. Because new hairs start growing each day, the loss and replacement usually balance each other. When the loss rate is greater than the replacement rate, thinning and baldness are the result.

Alopecia

The medical name for baldness is *alopecia,* the most common form of which is *male pattern baldness.* Dr. Eugene Van Scott, Professor of Dermatology of Temple University's Health Sciences Center, sums up the opinion of medical authorities on the three factors responsible for this type of baldness: sex, age, and heredity. Unfortunately, these are three factors over which medical science has no control.

Other Causes of Baldness

Other forms of baldness may be the result of bacterial or fungal infections, allergic reactions to particular medicines, radiation, or continual friction. It has also been suggested that constant stress from hair curlers or tightly pulled ponytails can cause loss

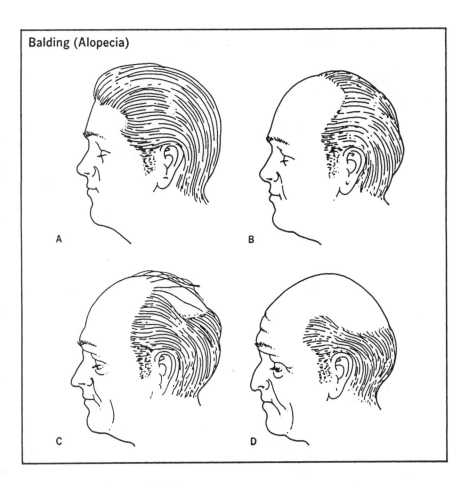

Balding (Alopecia)

A   B   C   D

of hair. These forms of baldness usually disappear when the cause is eliminated.

Although diet has very little to do with baldness, poor nutrition can result in hair that is dry, dull, and brittle enough to break easily. Any serious illness can lead to hair loss as well. It is thought that vitamin A taken in grossly excessive amounts can contribute to hair loss.

Women ordinarily lose some of their hair at the end of pregnancy, after delivery, and during the menopause, but regrowth can be expected in a few months.

It is now possible for anyone suffering from temporary baldness or from male pattern baldness to choose from a wide variety of attractively styled wigs and hairpieces.

A surgical procedure for treating male pattern baldness and baldness in women is called hair transplantation; it is discussed in Ch. 20, *Surgery*.

Hair Removal

Over the centuries and around the world, fashions in whiskers and beards come and go, but the average American male still subjects at least part of his face to daily shaving. Although feminine shaving practices are a more recent phenomenon, most American women now consider it part of good grooming to remove underarm and leg hair with a razor as often as twice a week. Shaving removes not only the dead skin cells that make up the protective layer of the body's surface but also some of the living skin underneath. Instead of being harmful, this appears to stimulate rather than damage new skin growth.

Male Shaving

The average beard grows about two-tenths of an inch a day. However, the density of male face hair varies a great deal depending on skin and hair color. In all races, the concentration is usually greatest on the chin and in the area between the nose and upper lip.

There is no proof that an electric razor is safer or better for all types of skin than a safety razor. Both types result in nicks and cuts of the living skin tissue, depending on the closeness of the shave.

Twice as many men prefer wet shaving to dry because the use of soap and hot water softens the hair stubble and makes it easier to remove. Shaving authorities point out that thorough soaking is one of the essentials of easy and safe shaving. Leaving the shaving lather on the face for at least two minutes will also soften whiskers a good deal.

The razor should be moistened with hot water throughout the process, and the chin and upper lip left for last so that the heavier hair concentration in these areas has the longest contact with moisture and lather.

Oily Skin

Men with oily skin should use an aerosol shaving preparation or a lather type applied with a brush. These are really soaps and are more effective in eliminating the oils that coat the face hair, thus making it easier to shave.

Dry Skin

A brushless cream is advisable for dry skin, since it lubricates the skin rather than further deprives it of oil.

Ingrown Hairs

One of the chief problems connected with shaving is that it often causes ingrown hairs, which can lead to pore-clogging and infection. Hair is more likely to turn back into the skin if it is shaved against the grain, or if the cutting edge of the blade is dull and rough rather than smooth. Men with coarse, wiry, curly, rather than fine, hair may find that whisker ends are more likely to become ingrown than men with fine hair. The problem is best handled by shaving with the grain, using a sharp blade, and avoiding too close a shave, particularly in the area around the neck.

Shaving and Skin Problems

For men with acne or a tendency to skin problems, the following advice is offered by Dr. Howard T. Behrman, Director of Dermatological Research, New York Medical College:

- Shave as seldom as possible, perhaps only once or twice a week, and always with the grain.

- If wet shaving is preferred, use a new blade each time, and shave as lightly as possible to avoid nicking pimples.

- Wash face carefully with plenty of hot water to make the beard easy to manage, and after shaving, rinse with hot water followed by cold.

- Use an antiseptic astringent face lotion.

- Instead of plucking out ingrown hairs, loosen them gently so that the ends do not grow back into the skin.

- Although some people with skin problems find an electric shaver less irritating, in most cases, a wet shave seems best.

Female Shaving

Millions of American women regularly shave underarm and leg hair, and most of them do so with a blade razor.

In recent years, various types of shavers have been designed with blade exposure more suited to women's needs than the standard type used by men. To make shaving easier and safer, the following procedures are recommended.

- Since wet hair is much easier to cut, the most effective time to shave is during or immediately following a bath or shower.

- Shaving cream or soap lather keeps the water from evaporating, and is preferred to dry shaving.

- Underarm shaving is easier with a contoured razor designed for this purpose. If a deodorant or antiperspirant causes stinging or irritation after shaving, allow a short time to elapse before applying it.

- Light bleeding from nicks or scrapes can be stopped by applying pressure to a sterile pad placed on the injured area.

Unwanted Hair

The technical word for excess or unwanted hair on the face, chest, arms, and legs is *hirsutism*. The condition varies greatly among different ethnic strains, and so does the attitude toward it. Women of southern European ancestry are generally hairier than those with Nordic or Anglo-Saxon ancestors. Caucasoid peoples are hairier than Negroid peoples. The sparsest amount of body hair is found among the Mongolian races and American Indians. Although heredity is the chief factor of hirsutism, hormones also influence hair growth. If there is a sudden appearance of coarse hair on the body of a young boy or girl or a woman with no such former tendency, a glandular disturbance should be suspected and investigated by a physician.

A normal amount of unwanted hair on the legs and under the arms is usually removed by shaving. When the problem involves the arms, face, chest, and abdomen, other methods of removal are available.

Temporary Methods of Hair Removal

Bleaching

Unwanted dark fuzz on the upper lip and arms can be lightened almost to invisibility with a commercially prepared bleach or with a homemade paste consisting of baking soda, hydrogen peroxide (bleaching strength), and a few drops of ammonia. Soap chips can be used instead of baking soda. The paste should be left on the skin for a few minutes and then washed off. It is harmless to the skin, and if applied repeatedly, the hair will tend to break off as a result of constant bleaching.

Chemical Depilatories

These products contain alkaline agents that cause the hair to detach easily at the skin surface. They can be used on and under the arms, and on the legs and chest. However, they should not be used on the face unless the label says it is safe to do so. Timing instructions should be followed carefully. If skin irritation results, this type of depilatory should be discontinued in favor of some other method.

Abrasives

Devices that remove hair from the skin surface by rubbing are cheap but time-consuming. However, if an abrasive such as pumice is used regularly, the offending hairs will be shorter with each application. A cream or lotion should be applied to the skin after using an abrasive.

Waxing

The technique of applying melted wax to the skin for removal of excess facial hair is best handled by an experienced cosmetician. The process involves pouring hot wax onto the skin and allowing it to cool. The hairs become embedded in the wax, and are plucked out from below the skin surface when the wax is stripped off. Because this method is painful and often causes irritation, it is not very popular, although the results are comparatively long-lasting.

Plucking

The use of tweezers for removing scattered hairs from the eyebrows, face, and chest is slightly painful but otherwise harmless. It is not a practical method for getting rid of dense hair growth, however, because it takes too much time.

Permanent Hair Removal by Electrolysis

The only permanent and safe method of removing unwanted hair is by *electrolysis*. This technique destroys each individual hair root by transmitting electric current through fine wire needles into the opening of the hair follicle. The hair thus loosened is then plucked out with a tweezer. The older type of electrolysis machine uses galvanic current. The newer type, sometimes called an *electrocoagulation machine,* uses modified high-frequency current. In either case, the efficiency and safety of the technique depends less on the machine than on the care and skill of the operator.

Because the process of treating each hair root is expensive, time-consuming, and uncomfortable, it is not recommended for areas of dense hair growth, such as the arms or legs. Before undertaking electrolysis either at a beauty salon or at home, it would be wise to consult a dermatologist about individual skin reaction.

Nails

Fingernails and toenails are an extension of the epidermis, or outer layer of the skin. They are made of elastic tissue formed from keratin, the substance that gives hair its strength and flexibility.

Some of the problems associated with fingernails are the result of too much manicuring. White spots, for example, are often caused by too much pressure at the base of the nail when trying to expose the "moon"— the white portion that contains tissue not yet as tough as the rest of the nail.

To ensure the health of toenails, feet should be bathed once a day and the nails cleaned with a brush dipped in soapy water. Shoes should fit properly so that the toenails are not subjected to pressure and distortion. To avoid ingrown toenails, trimming should be done straight across rather than by rounding or tapering the corners.

Splitting

Infection or injury of the tissue at the base of a fingernail may cause its surface to be rigid or split. Inflammation of the finger joints connected with arthritis will also cause nail deformity. For ordinary problems of splitting and peeling, the nails should be kept short enough so that they don't catch and tear easily. For practical purposes, the top of the nail should not be visible when the palm is held about six inches from the eye. As the nails grow stronger, they can be grown longer without splitting.

Brittleness

This condition seems to be caused by such external factors as the chemicals in polish removers, soaps, and detergents. It is also a natural consequence of aging. Commercial nail-hardening preparations that contain formaldehyde are not recommended, because they are known to cause discoloration, loosening, or even loss of nails in some cases.

Nail damage can be reduced by wearing rubber gloves while doing household chores. Hand cream mas-

Nail Anatomy

Dead cells

Germinal layer

Bone

Nail root

Cuticle

saged into the skin around the nails will counteract dryness and lessen the possibility of hangnails. Although nail polish provides a shield against damage, it should not be worn all the time, particularly if the nail is polished right down to the base; this prevents live tissue from "breathing."

Disorders of the Skin

The skin is subject to a large number of disorders, most of which are not serious even though they may be temporarily uncomfortable. A disorder may be caused by one or another type of allergy; by excessive heat or cold; or by infection from fungi, bacteria, viruses, or parasites. Many skin ailments are caused or aggravated by emotional disturbances.

The symptoms and treatment of the more common disorders are discussed in the following pages. Any persistent change in skin condition should be brought to the attention of a physician.

Allergies and Itching

Itching and inflammation of the skin may be caused by an allergic reaction, by exposure to poisonous plants, or by a generalized infection.

Dermatitis

Dermatitis is the term used for an inflammation of the skin. The term for allergic reactions of the skin resulting from surface contact with outside agents is *contact dermatitis*. This condition is characterized by a rash and may be brought out by sensitivity to cosmetics, plants, cleaning materials, metal, wool, and so on. Other forms of dermatitis can be caused by excesses of heat or cold, by friction, or by sensitivity to various medicines. Dermatitis is usually accompanied by itching at the site of the rash.

Poison Ivy

This common plant, unknown in Europe but widespread everywhere in the United States except in California and Nevada, produces an allergic reaction on the skin accompanied by a painful rash and blisters. Some people are so sensitive to it that they are affected by contact not only with the plant itself but with animal fur or clothing that might have picked up the sap weeks before.

A mild attack of poison ivy produces a rash and small, watery blisters that get progressively larger. The affected area of the skin becomes crusty and dry, and after a few weeks, all symptoms vanish. If the exposed area is thoroughly washed with laundry soap immediately after contact, the poison may not penetrate the skin.

If the symptoms do develop, they can be relieved with Burow's solution—one part solution to fifteen parts of cool water—or with the application of calamine lotion. If the symptoms are severe, and especially if the area around the eyes is involved, a physician should be consulted. He may prescribe an application or an injection of cortisone.

The best way to avoid the unpleasantness of a poison ivy attack is to learn to recognize the plant and stay away from it. Children especially should be warned against putting the leaves and berries in their mouths.

Poison oak and poison sumac produce somewhat the same symptoms and should also be avoided.

Under no circumstances should these plants be burned to eliminate them, because the inhaling of the contaminated smoke even from a distance can cause a serious case of poi-soning. The application of special sprays, if the instructions are followed carefully, will get rid of the plants without affecting people or the neighborhood greenery.

Hives

These are large, irregularly shaped swellings on the skin that burn and itch. The cause is unknown, but allergic reactions to certain foods and medicine or to insect bites have been suggested as possible causes. The swellings of hives usually disappear within a day or so, but they can be very uncomfortable while they last. The itching and burning can often be relieved by applying cold water and a calamine solution. However, some people are sensitive to cold and develop wheals when subjected to intense cold. Commercial preparations containing surface anesthetics are seldom effective and may cause allergic reactions.

If the outbreak of hives can be traced to a specific food, such as shellfish or strawberries, the food should be eliminated from the diet. If a medicine such as penicillin or a sulfa drug is the cause, a physician should be told about the reaction.

Eczema

This condition is an allergic reaction that produces itching, swelling, blistering, oozing, and scaling of the skin. It is more common among children than among adults and may sometimes cover the entire body, although the rash is usually limited to the face, neck, and folds of the knees and elbows. Unlike contact dermatitis, it is likely to be caused by an allergy to a food or a pollen or dust. Advertised cures for eczema cannot control the cause and sometimes make the condition worse. A physician should be consulted if the symptoms are severe, particularly if the patient is an infant or very young child.

Itching

The technical name for the localized or general sensation on the skin that can be relieved by scratching is *pruritus*. Itching may be caused by many skin disorders, by infections, by serious diseases such as nephritis or leukemia, by medicines, or by psychological factors such as tension. A physician should always be consulted to find the cause of persistent itching, because it may be the symptom of a basic disorder. Repeated scratching may provide some relief, but it can also lead to infection.

Anal Pruritus

If itching in the anal area is so severe that only painful scratching will relieve it, the condition is probably *anal pruritus*. It is often accompanied by excessive rectal mucus that keeps the skin irritated and moist. This disorder is most commonly associated with hemorrhoids, but many other conditions, such as reactions to drugs, can cause it. Anxiety or tension can also contribute to it. Sitz baths with warm water are usually recommended. Every effort should be made to reduce scratching and to keep the anal skin clean and dry. Cortisone cream may be prescribed in persistent cases.

Skin Irritations and Weather

Extremes of weather produce local inflammations and other skin problems for many people.

Chapping

In cold weather, the sebaceous glands slow down the secretions that lubricate the skin, causing it to become dry. When dry skin is exposed to wintry weather, it becomes irritated and is likely to crack, particularly around the lips. Chapped skin is especially sensitive to harsh soaps. During such periods of exposure, the skin can be protected with a mild cream or lotion. A lubricating ointment should be used on the lips to prevent them from cracking. Children who lick their lips continually no matter what the weather can benefit from this extra protection. Chapped hands caused by daily use of strong soaps and detergents can be helped by the use of a lubricating cream and rubber gloves during housework.

Frostbite

Exposure to extreme cold for a prolonged period may cause freezing of the nose, fingers, toes, or ears, thus cutting off the circulation to the affected areas. Frostbitten areas are of a paler color than normal and are numb. They should not be rubbed with snow or exposed to intense heat. Areas should be thawed gradually, and a physician should be consulted for aftercare in extreme cases.

Chilblain

A localized inflammation of the skin called *chilblain* is common among people who are particularly sensitive to cold because of poor circulation. Chilblain may occur in the ears, hands, feet, and face, causing itching, swelling, and discoloration of the skin. Anyone prone to chilblain should dress protectively during the cold weather and use an electric pad or blanket at night. Affected parts should not be rubbed or massaged, nor should ice or extreme heat be applied directly, since these measures may cause additional damage. Persistent or extreme attacks of chilblain should be discussed with a physician.

Chafing

This condition is an inflammation of two opposing skin surfaces caused by the warmth, moisture, and friction of their rubbing together. Diabetics, overweight people, and those who perspire heavily are particularly prone to chafing. Chafing is accompanied by itching and burning, and sometimes infection can set in if the superficial skin is broken. Parts of the body subject to chafing are the inner surfaces of the thighs, the anal region, the area under the breasts, and the inner surfaces between fingers and toes.

To reduce the possibility of chafing, lightweight clothing should be worn and strenuous exercise avoided during hot weather. Vaseline or a vitamin A and D ointment may be applied to reduce friction. In general, the treatment is the same as that for diaper rash in infants. If the condition becomes acute, a physician can prescribe more effective remedies.

Prickly Heat

This skin rash is usually accompanied by itching and burning. It is caused by an obstruction of the sweat ducts such that perspiration does not reach the surface of the skin but backs up and causes pimples the size of a pinhead. If the obstruction is superficial, the pimples are white; if it is deeper, they are red. The condition can be brought on by other minor skin irritations, by continued exposure to moist heat, such as a compress, or by exercise in humid weather. Infants and people who are overweight are especially prone to prickly heat.

The discomfort can be eased by wearing lightweight, loose-fitting clothing, especially at night, and keeping room temperature low. Alcoholic beverages, which tend to dehydrate the body, should be avoided. Tepid baths and the application of cornstarch to the affected skin areas will usually relieve itching. If the rash remains for several days, a physician should be consulted to make sure it does not arise from some other cause.

Calluses and Corns

As a result of continued friction or pressure in a particular area, the skin forms a tough, hard, self-protecting layer known as a *callus*. Calluses are common on the soles of the feet, the palms of the hands, and, among guitarists and string players, on the tips of the fingers. A heavy callus that presses against a bone in the foot because of poorly fitted shoes can be very painful. The hard surface can be reduced somewhat by the use of pumice, or by gently paring it with a razor blade that has been washed in alcohol.

Corns are a form of callus that appear on or between the toes. They usually have a hard inner core that causes pain when pressed against underlying tissue by badly fitted shoes. A hard corn that appears on the surface of the little toe can be removed by soaking for about ten minutes and applying a few drops of ten percent salicylic acid in collodion. The surface should be covered with a corn pad to reduce pressure, and the corn lifted off when it is loose enough to be released from the skin. Anyone suffering from a circulatory disease and particularly from diabetes should avoid home treatment of foot disturbances. Those with a tendency to callus and corn formations should be especially careful about the proper fit of shoes and hose. A *chiropodist* or *podiatrist* is a trained specialist in foot care who can be visited on a regular basis to provide greater foot comfort.

Fungus Infections

Fungi are plantlike parasitic growths found in the air, in water, and in the soil. They comprise a large family that includes mushrooms, and are responsible for mildew and mold. Only a small number cause disease.

Ringworm

This condition is caused not by a worm but by a group of fungi that live on the body's dead skin cells in those areas that are warm and damp because of accumulated perspiration. One form of ringworm attacks the scalp, arms, and legs, especially of children, and is often spread by similarly affected pets. It appears as reddish patches that scale and blister and frequently feel sore and itchy. Ringworm is highly contagious and can be passed from person to person by contaminated objects such as combs and towels. It should therefore be treated promptly by a physician. Ringworm can best be prevented by strict attention to personal cleanliness.

Athlete's Foot

Another form of ringworm, *athlete's foot,* usually attacks the skin between the toes and under the toenails. If not treated promptly, it can cause an itching rash on other parts of the body. Athlete's foot causes the skin to itch, blister, and crack, and as a result, leaves it vulnerable to more serious infection from other organisms. The disorder can be treated at home by gently removing the damaged skin, and, after soaking the feet, thoroughly drying and dusting between the toes with a medicated foot powder. Some of the powder should be sprinkled into shoes. If the condition continues, a fungicidal ointment can be applied in the morning and at night. Persistent cases require the attention of a physician.

Scabies

An insectlike parasite causes the skin irritation called *scabies,* otherwise known as "the itch." The female itch mite burrows a hole in the skin, usually in the groin or between the fingers or toes, and stays hidden long enough to build a tunnel in which to deposit her eggs. The newly hatched mites then work their way to the skin surface and begin the cycle all over again. There is little discomfort in the early period of infestation, but in about a week, a rash appears, accompanied by extreme itching, which is usually most severe at night. Constant scratching during sleep can lead to skin lesions that invite bacterial infection.

Scabies is very contagious and can spread rapidly through a family or through a community, such as a summer camp or army barracks. It can also be communicated by sexual contact.

Treatment by a physician involves the identification of the characteristic tunnels from which sample mites can be removed for examination. Hot baths and thorough scrubbing will expose the burrows, and medical applications as directed by the physician usually clear up the condition in about a week.

Bacterial Infections

The skin is susceptible to infection from a variety of bacteria. Poor diet and careless hygiene can lower the body's resistance to these infectious agents.

Boils

These abscesses of the skin are caused by bacterial infection of a hair follicle or a sebaceous gland. The pus that accumulates in a boil is the result of the encounter between the bacteria and the white blood cells that fight them. Sometimes a boil subsides by itself and disappears. Sometimes the pressure of pus against the skin surface may bring the boil to a head; it will then break, drain, and heal if washed with an antiseptic and covered with a sterile pad. Warm-water compresses can be applied for ten minutes every hour to relieve the pain and to encourage the boil to break and drain. A fresh, dry pad should be applied after each period of soaking.

Anyone with a serious or chronic illness who develops a boil should consult a physician. Since the bacteria can enter the bloodstream and cause a general infection with fever, a physician should also be consulted for a boil on the nose, scalp, upper lip, or in the ear, groin, or armpit.

Carbuncles

This infection is a group of connected boils and is likely to be more painful and less responsive to home treatment. Carbuncles may occur as the result of poor skin care. They tend to occur in the back of the neck where the skin is thick, and the abscess tends to burrow into deeper tissues. A physician usually lances and drains a deep-seated carbuncle, or he may prescribe an antibiotic remedy.

Impetigo

This skin infection is caused by staphylococcal or streptococcal bacteria, and is characterized by blisters that break and form yellow crusted areas. It is spread from one person to another and from one part of the body to another by the discharge from the sores. Impetigo occurs most frequently on the scalp, face, and arms and legs. The infection often is picked up in barber shops, swimming pools, or from body contact with infected people or household pets.

Special care must be taken, especially with children, to control the spread of the infection by keeping the fingers away from infected parts. Bed linens should be changed daily, and disposable paper towels, as well as paper plates and cups, should be used during treatment. A physician should be consulted for proper medication and procedures to deal with the infection.

Barber's Itch

Sycosis, commonly called *barber's itch,* is a bacterial infection of the hair follicles of the beard, accompanied by inflammation, itching, and the formation of pus-filled pimples. People with stiff, curly hair are prone to this type of chronic infection, because their hair is more likely to curve back and reenter the skin. The infection should be treated promptly to prevent scarring and the destruction of the hair root. In some cases, physicians recommend antibiotics. If these are not effective, it may be necessary to drain the abscesses and remove the hairs from the inflamed follicles. During treatment, it is best to avoid shaving, if possible. If one must shave, the sterilization of all shaving equipment and the use of a brushless shaving cream are recommended.

Erysipelas

An acute streptococcal infection of the skin, *erysipelas* can be fatal, particularly to the very young or very old, if not treated promptly. One of its symptoms is the bright redness of the affected areas of the skin. These red patches enlarge and spread, making the skin tender and painful. Blisters may appear nearby. The patient usually has a headache, fever, chills, and nausea. Erysipelas responds well to promptly administered antibiotics, particularly penicillin. The patient is

usually advised to drink large amounts of fluid and to eat a nourishing, easily digested diet.

Viral Infections

The most common skin conditions caused by viruses are cold sores, shingles, and warts, discussed below.

Cold Sores

Also called fever blisters, *cold sores* are technically known as *herpes simplex.* They are small blisters that appear most frequently in the corners of the mouth, and sometimes around the eyes and on the genitals. The presumed cause is a virus that lies dormant in the skin until it is activated by infection or by excessive exposure to sun or wind. There is no specific cure for cold sores, but the irritation can be eased by applying drying or cooling agents such as camphor ice or cold-water compresses. Recurrent cold sores, especially in infants, should be called to a physician's attention.

Recent studies have shown that a variety of the herpes simplex virus called HSV-II (for herpes simplex virus-Type II) can be a serious danger to the fetus of a pregnant woman. For a discussion of this condition, see Ch. 25, *Women's Health.* The variety that causes cold sores is called Type I.

Shingles

The virus infection of a sensory nerve, accompanied by small, painful blisters that appear on the skin along the path of the nerve—usually on one side of the chest or abdomen—is called *shingles.* The medical name for the disorder, which is caused by the chicken pox virus, is *herpes zoster,* Latin for "girdle of blisters." When a cranial nerve is involved, the blisters appear on the face near the eye. The preliminary symptom is neuritis with severe pain and, sometimes, fever. The blisters may take from two to four weeks to dry up and disappear. Although there is no specific cure, the pain can be alleviated by aspirin. In severe cases, or if the area near the eye is involved, a physician should be seen.

Warts

These growths are caused by a virus infection of the epidermis. They never become cancerous, but can be painful when found on the soles of the feet. In this location, they are known as *plantar warts*, and they cause discomfort because constant pressure makes them grow inward. Plantar warts are most likely to be picked up by children because they are barefooted so much of the time, and by adults when their feet are moist and they are walking around in showers, near swimming pools, and in locker rooms. Warts can be spread by scratching, by shaving, and by brushing the hair. They are often transmitted from one member of the family to another. Because warts can spread to painful areas, such as the area around or under the fingernails, and because they may become disfiguring, it is best to consult a physician whenever they appear.

In many ways, warts behave rather mysteriously. About half of them go away without any treatment at all. Sometimes, when warts on one part of the body are being treated, those in another area will disappear. The folklore about "witching" and "charming" warts away has its foundation in fact, because apparently having faith in the cure, no matter how ridiculous it sounds, sometimes brings success. This form of suggestion therapy is especially successful with children.

There are several more conventional ways of treating warts. De-pending on their size and the area involved, electric current, dry ice, or various chemicals may be employed. A physician should be consulted promptly when warts develop in the area of the beard or on the scalp, because they spread quickly in these parts of the body and thus become more difficult to eliminate.

Sebaceous Cysts

When a sebaceous gland duct is blocked, the oil that the gland secretes cannot get to the surface of the skin. Instead, it accumulates into a hard, round, movable mass contained in a sac. This mass is known as a *sebaceous cyst*. Such cysts may appear on the face, back, ears, or in the genital area. A sebaceous cyst that forms on the scalp is called a *wen*, and may become as large as a billiard ball. The skin in this area will become bald, because the cyst interferes with the blood supply to the hair roots.

Some sebaceous cysts just disappear without treatment. However, those that do not are a likely focus for secondary infection by bacteria, and they may become abscessed and inflamed. It is therefore advisable to have cysts examined by a physician for possible removal. If such a cyst is superficial, it can be punctured and drained. One that is deeper is usually removed by simple surgical procedure in the physician's office.

Acne

About 80 percent of all teenagers suffer from the skin disturbance called *acne*. It is also fairly common among women in their twenties. Acne is a condition in which the skin of the face, and often of the neck, shoulders, chest, and back, is covered to a greater or lesser extent with pimples, blackheads, whiteheads, and boils.

The typical onset of acne in adolescence is related to the increased activity of the glands, including the sebaceous glands. Most of the oil that they secrete gets to the surface of the skin through ducts that lead into the pores. When the surface pores are clogged with sebaceous gland secretions and keratin, or when so much extra oil is being secreted that it backs up into the ducts, the result is the formation of the skin blemishes characteristic of acne. Dirt or makeup does not cause acne.

The blackheads are dark not because they are dirty but because the fatty material in the clogged pore is oxidized and discolored by the air that reaches it. When this substance is infected by bacteria, it turns into a pimple. Under no circumstances should such pimples be picked at or squeezed, because the pressure can rupture the surrounding membrane and spread the infection further.

Although a mild case of acne usually clears up by itself, it is often helpful to get the advice of a physician so that it does not get any worse.

Cleanliness

Although surface dirt does not cause acne, it can contribute to its spread. Therefore, the affected areas should be cleansed with a medicated soap and hot water twice a day. Hair should be shampooed frequently and brushed away from the face. Boys who are shaving should soften the beard with soap and hot water. The blade should be sharp and should skim the skin as lightly as possible to avoid nicking pimples.

Creams and Cosmetics

Nonprescription medicated creams and lotions may be effective in reducing some blemishes, but if used too often, they make the skin dry. They should be applied according to the manufacturer's instructions and should be discontinued if they cause additional irritation. If makeup is used, it should have a nonoily base and be completely removed before going to bed.

Forbidden Foods

Although acne is not caused by any particular food, it can be made worse by a diet overloaded with candy, rich pastries, and fats. Chocolate and cola drinks must be eliminated entirely in some cases.

Professional Treatment

A serious case of acne, or even a mild one that is causing serious emotional problems, should receive the attention of a physician. He or she may prescribe antibiotics, usually considered the most effective treatment, or recommend sunlamp treatments. A physician can also be helpful in dealing with the psychological aspects of acne that are so disturbing to teenagers.

Psoriasis

Psoriasis is a noncontagious chronic condition in which the skin on various parts of the body is marked by bright red patches covered with silvery scales. The areas most often affected are the knees, elbows, scalp, and trunk, and less frequently, the areas under the arms and around the genitals.

The specific cause of psoriasis has not yet been discovered, but it is thought to be an inherited abnormality in which the formation of new skin cells is too rapid and disorderly. In its mild form, psoriasis responds well to a variety of long-term treatments.

When it is acute, the entire skin surface may be painfully red, and large sections of it may scale off. In such cases, prompt hospitalization and intensive care are recommended.

Conditions That Can Bring On an Outbreak

The onset or aggravation of psoriasis can be triggered by some of the following factors:

- bruises, burns, scratches, and overexposure to the sun

- sudden drops in temperature—a mild, stable climate is most beneficial

- sudden illness from another source, or unusual physical or emotional stress

- infections of the upper respiratory tract, especially bacterial throat infections and the medicines used to cure them

Treatment

Although there is no specific cure for psoriasis, these are some of the recommended treatments:

- controlled exposure to sunlight or an ultraviolet lamp

- creams or lotions of crude coal tar or tar distillates, used alone or in combination with ultraviolet light

- psoralen and ultraviolet light (PUVA), a combined systemic-external therapy in which a psoralen drug is taken orally before exposure to ultraviolet light

- systemic drugs, such as methotrexate, which can be taken orally

- steroid hormone medications applied to the skin surface under dressings

Pigment Disorders and Birthmarks

The mechanism that controls skin coloration is described above under "Skin Color." Abnormalities in the creation and distribution of melanin result in the following disorders, some of which are negligible.

Freckles

These are small spots of brown pigment that frequently occur when fair-skinned people are exposed to the sun or to ultraviolet light. For those whose skin gets red rather than tan during such exposure, freckles are a protective device. In most cases, they recede in cold weather. A heavy freckle formation that is permanent can be covered somewhat by cosmetic preparations. No attempt should be made to remove freckles with commercial creams or solutions unless supervised by a physician.

Liver Spots

Flat, smooth, irregularly placed markings on the skin, called *liver spots,* often appear among older people, and result from an increase in pigmentation. They have nothing to do with the liver and are completely harmless. Brownish markings of similar appearance sometimes show up during pregnancy or as a result of irritation or infection. They usually disappear when the underlying cause is eliminated.

Liver spots are permanent, and the principal cause is not aging but the accumulated years of exposure to sun and wind. They can be disguised and treated in the same way as freckles. A liver spot that becomes hard and thick should be called to a physician's attention.

Moles

Clusters of melanin cells, called *moles,* may appear singly or in groups at any place on the body. They range in color from light tan to dark brown; they may be raised and hairy or flat and smooth. Many moles are present at birth, and most make their appearance before the age of 20. They rarely turn into malignancies, and require medical attention only if they become painful, if they itch, or if they suddenly change in size, shape, or color.

There are several ways of removing moles if they are annoying or particularly unattractive. They can be destroyed by the application of an electric needle, by cauterizing, and by surgery. A mole that has been removed is not likely to reappear. The hairs sometimes found in moles can be clipped close to the surface of the skin, or they can be permanently removed. Hair removal often causes the mole to get smaller.

Vitiligo

The condition called *vitiligo* stems from a loss of pigment in sharply defined areas of the skin. There is no known cause for this abnormality of melanin distribution. It may affect any part of the body and may appear any time up to middle age. It is particularly conspicuous when it occurs among blacks, or when a lighter skinned person becomes tanned except around the paler patches. There is no cure for vitiligo, but cosmetic treatment with pastes and lotions can diminish the contrast between affected areas and the rest of the skin.

Birthmarks

About one-third of all infants are born with the type of birthmark called a *hemangioma,* also known as a vascular birthmark. These are caused by a clustering of small blood vessels near the surface of the skin. The mark, which is flat, irregularly shaped, and either pink, red, or purplish, is usually referred to as "port wine stain." There is no known way to remove it, but with cosmetic covering creams, it can usually be successfully masked.

The type of hemangioma that is raised and bright red—called a strawberry mark—spontaneously disappears with no treatment in most cases during early childhood. If a strawberry mark begins to grow rather than fade, or if it begins to ulcerate, a physician should be promptly consulted.

See Ch. 18, *Cancer,* for a discussion of skin cancer; see Ch. 3, *The Teens,* for a discussion of adolescent skin problems; see Ch. 23, *Aches, Pains, Nuisances, Worries,* for further discussion of minor skin problems.

22

The Teeth and Gums

Although a human baby is born without teeth, a complete set of 20 *deciduous,* or baby, teeth (also called *primary teeth*) already has formed within the gums of the offspring while it still is within the mother's womb. The buds of the permanent or secondary teeth are developing even before the first baby tooth appears at around the age of six months. The baby teeth obviously are formed from foods eaten by the mother. Generally, if the mother follows a good diet during pregnancy, no special food items are required to ensure an adequate set of deciduous teeth in the baby.

It takes about two years for the full set of deciduous teeth to appear in the baby's mouth. The first, usually a central incisor at the front of the lower jaw, may erupt any time between the ages of three and nine months. The last probably will be a second molar at the back of the upper jaw. As with walking, talking, and other characteristics of infants, there is no set timetable for the eruption of baby teeth. One child may get his first tooth at three months while another must wait until nine months, but both would be considered within a normal range of tooth development.

The permanent teeth are never far behind the deciduous set. The first permanent tooth usually appears around the age of six years, about four years after the last of the baby teeth has erupted. But the last of the permanent molars, the third molars or *wisdom teeth,* may not break through the gum line until the offspring is an adult.

Types of Teeth

The permanent teeth number 32. In advancing from deciduous to permanent teeth, the human gains six teeth in the lower jaw, or *mandible,* and six in the upper jaw, or *maxilla,* of the mouth. The primary set of teeth includes the following:

UPPER JAW	LOWER JAW
2 central incisors	2 central incisors
2 lateral incisors	2 lateral incisors
2 cuspids	2 cuspids
2 first molars	2 first molars
2 second molars	2 second molars

The permanent set of teeth has an equivalent combination of incisors, cuspids, and first and second molars. But it also includes:

2 first bicuspids	2 first bicuspids
2 second bicuspids	2 second bicuspids
2 third molars	2 third molars

An *incisor* is designed to cut off particles of food, which is then pushed by muscles of the tongue and cheeks to teeth farther back in the mouth for grinding. The front teeth, one on each side, upper and lower, are central incisors. Next to each central incisor is a lateral incisor.

A *cuspid* is so named because it has a spear-shaped crown, or *cusp.* It is designed for tearing as well as cutting. Cuspids sometimes are called *canine teeth* or *eyeteeth; canine teeth* owe their name to the use of these teeth by carnivorous animals, such as dogs, for tearing pieces of meat. There are four cuspids in the mouth, one on the outer side of each lateral incisor in the upper and lower jaws.

Bicuspids sometimes are identified

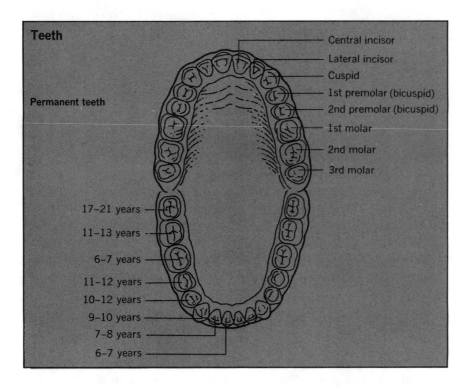

Teeth

Permanent teeth

Central incisor
Lateral incisor
Cuspid
1st premolar (bicuspid)
2nd premolar (bicuspid)
1st molar
2nd molar
3rd molar

17–21 years
11–13 years
6–7 years
11–12 years
10–12 years
9–10 years
7–8 years
6–7 years

Dentin

Beneath the enamel surface of a tooth is a layer of hard material—though not as hard as enamel—called *dentin*, which forms the bulk of a tooth. The dentin forms at the same time that enamel is laid down on the surface of a developing tooth, and the portion beneath the crown of the tooth probably is completed at the same time as the enamel. However, the dentin, which is composed of calcified material, is not as dense as the enamel; it is formed as myriad tubules that extend downward into the pulp at the center of the tooth. There is some evidence that dentin formation may continue slowly during the life of the tooth.

Cementum

The *cementum* is a bonelike substance that covers the root of the tooth. Though harder than regular bone, it is softer than dentin. It contains attachments for fibers of a periodontal ligament that holds the tooth in its socket. The periodontal ligament serves as a kind of hammock of fibers that surround and support the tooth at the cementum surface, radiating outward to the jawbone. This arrangement allows the tooth to move a little while still attached to the jaw. For example, when the teeth of the upper and lower jaws are brought together in chewing, the periodontal ligament allows the teeth to sink into their sockets. When the teeth of the two jaws are separated, the hammocklike ligament permits the teeth to float outward again.

Pulp

The cavity within the dentin contains the *pulp*. There is a wide pulp chamber under the crown of the tooth and a pulp canal that extends from the chamber down through the root or

as *premolars*. The term "bicuspid" suggests two cusps, but a bicuspid may in fact have three cusps. The function of the bicuspids is to crush food passed back from the incisors and cuspids. The permanent set of teeth includes a total of eight bicuspids.

The *molars*, which also number eight and are the last teeth at the back of the mouth, are the largest and strongest teeth, with the job of grinding food. The third molars, or wisdom teeth, are smaller, weaker, and less functional than the first and second molars.

Structure of the Tooth

The variety of shapes of teeth make them specialized for the various functions in preparing food for digestion—biting, chewing, and grinding. All varieties, however, have the same basic structure.

Enamel

The outer covering of the part of the tooth that is exposed above the gum line is *enamel*, the hardest substance in the human body. Enamel is about 97 percent mineral and is as tough as some gemstones. It varies in thickness, with the greatest thickness on the surfaces that are likely to get the most wear and tear.

Enamel begins to form on the first tooth buds of an embryo at the age of about 15 weeks, depending upon substances in the food eaten by the mother for proper development. Once the tooth has formed and erupted through the gum line, there is nothing further that can be done by natural means to improve the condition of the enamel. The enamel has no blood supply, and any changes in the tooth surface will be the result of wearing, decay, or injury.

While the health and diet of the mother can affect the development of tooth enamel in the deciduous teeth, certain health factors in the early life of a child can result in defective enamel formation of teeth that have not yet erupted. Some infectious or metabolic disorders, for example, may result in enamel pitting.

roots. Some teeth, such as the molars, may contain as many as three roots, and each of the roots contains a pulp canal.

The pulp of a tooth contains the blood vessels supplying the tooth and the lymphatic system. Although the blood supply arrangement is not the same for every tooth, a typical pattern includes a dental artery entering through each passageway, or *foramen,* leading into the root of a tooth. The artery branches into numerous capillaries within the root canal. A similar system of veins drains the blood from the tooth through each foramen. A lymphatic network and nerve system also enter the tooth through a foramen and spread through the pulp, as branches from a central distribution link within the jawbone. The nerve fibers have free endings in the tooth, making them sensitive to pain stimuli.

Supporting Structures

The soft, pink gum tissue that surrounds the tooth is called the *gingiva,* and the bone of the jaw that forms the tooth socket is known as *alveolar bone.* The gingiva, alveolar bone, and periodontal ligaments sometimes are grouped into a structural category identified as the *periodontium.* Thus, when a dentist speaks of periodontal

disease, he is referring to a disorder of these supporting tissues of the teeth. The ailment known as *gingivitis* is an inflammation of the gingiva, or gum tissue around the teeth.

Care of the Teeth and Gums

Years ago, loss of teeth really was unavoidable. Today, thanks to modern practices of preventive dentistry, it is possible for nearly everyone to enjoy the benefits of natural teeth for a lifetime. But natural teeth can be preserved only by daily oral-hygiene habits and regular dental checkups.

The Dental Examination

During the teen years, careful supervision by the dentist and cooperation from the teenager are especially necessary. The poor eating habits of many youngsters are reflected in high cavity rates, which may be greater during adolescence than in later life. Neglect of proper dental care also occurs in the middle years when an often used excuse is that eventual loss of teeth is inevitable. After the permanent teeth are established, the dentist should be visited every six months, or at whatever intervals he recommends for an individual patient who may need more or less care than the typical patient.

The dentist, like the family physician, usually maintains a general health history of each patient, in addition to a dental health history. He examines each tooth, the gums and other oral tissues, and the *occlusion,* or bite. A complete set of X-ray pictures may be taken on the first visit and again at intervals of perhaps five to seven years. During routine visits, the dentist may take only a couple of X-ray pictures of teeth on either side of the mouth; a complete set of X rays may result in a file of 18 or 20 pictures covering every tooth in the mouth.

X rays constitute a vital part of the dental examination. Without them the dentist cannot examine the surfaces between the teeth or the portion of the tooth beneath the gum, a part that represents about 60 percent of the total length of the tooth. The X rays will reveal the condition of the enamel, dentin, and pulp, as well as any impacted wisdom teeth and the alveolar bone, or tooth sockets. Caps, fillings, abscessed roots, and bone loss resulting from gum disease also are clearly visible on a set of X rays.

Other diagnostic tests may be made, such as a test of nerve response. Sometimes the dentist will make an impression of the teeth, an accurate and detailed reverse reproduction, in plaster of paris, plastic impression compound, or other material. Models made from these impressions are used to study the way the teeth meet. Such knowledge is often crucial in deciding the selection of treatment and materials.

After the examination, the dentist will present and explain any proposed treatment. After oral restoration is completed, he will ask the patient to return at regular intervals for a checkup and *prophylaxis,* which includes cleaning and polishing the teeth. Regular checkups and prophylaxis help prevent periodontal diseases affecting the gum tissue and un-

Structure of Tooth

Lymphatic system
Gingiva
Alveolar bone of jaw
Periodontal ligament

Enamel
Dentin
Nerve supply
Vascular supply
Pulp
Cement

derlying bone. Professional cleaning removes hard deposits that trap bacteria, especially at the gum line, and polishing removes stains and soft deposits.

Dental Care in Middle Age

Although periodontal (gum) disease and cavities—called *dental caries* by dentists—continue to threaten oral health, two other problems may assume prominence for people of middle age: replacing worn-out restorations, or fillings, and replacing missing teeth. No filling material will last forever. The whitish restorations in front teeth eventually wear away. Silver restorations tend to crack and chip with age because they contract and expand slightly when cold or hot food and drinks come in contact with them. Even gold restorations, the most permanent kind, are subject to decay around the edges, and the decay may spread underneath.

If a needed restoration is not made or a worn-out restoration is not replaced, a deep cavity may result. When the decay reaches the inner layer of the tooth—the dentin—temporary warning twinges of pain may occur. If the tooth still is not restored, the decay will spread into the pulp that fills the inner chamber of the tooth. A toothache can result from inflammation of the pulp, and although the pain may eventually subside, the pulp tissue dies and an abscess can form at the root of the tooth.

Dental Care during Pregnancy

It may be advisable for a pregnant woman to arrange for extra dental checkups. Many changes take place during pregnancy, among them increased hormone production. Some pregnant women develop gingivitis (inflammation of the gums) as an indirect consequence of hormonal changes. A checkup by the dentist during the first three months of pregnancy is needed to assess the oral effects of such changes, and to make sure all dental problems are examined and corrected. Pregnant women should take special care to brush and floss their teeth to minimize these problems.

Infection

To avoid the problem of toxic substances or poisons circulating in the mother's bloodstream, all sources of infection must be removed. Some of these sources can be in the mouth. An abscessed tooth, for example, may not be severe enough to signal its presence with pain, but because it is directly connected to the bloodstream it can send toxic substances and bacteria through the mother's body with possible harmful effects to the embryo.

It is during pregnancy that tooth buds for both the deciduous and permanent teeth begin to form in the unborn child. If the mother neglects her diet or general health care during this period, the effects may be seen in the teeth of her child.

Maintaining Good Oral Hygiene

Fluoridation

Among general rules to follow between dental checkups are using fluorides, maintaining a proper diet, and removing debris from the teeth by brushing and by the use of dental floss. Fluorides are particularly important for strengthening the enamel of teeth in persons under the age of 15. Many communities add fluorides to the water supply, but if the substance is not available in the drinking water, the dentist can advise the patient about other ways of adding fluoride to water or other fluids consumed each day. Studies show that children who drink fluoridated water from birth have up to 65 percent fewer cavities than those who do not drink fluoridated water. However, using excessive amounts of fluoride in the drinking water can result in mottled enamel.

Diet

Although a good diet for total health should provide all of the elements needed for dental health, several precautions on sugars and starches should be added. Hard or sticky sweets should be avoided. Such highly refined sweets as soft drinks, candies, cakes, cookies, pies, syrups, jams, jellies, and pastries should be limited, especially between meals. One's intake of starchy foods, such as bread, potatoes, and pastas, should also be controlled. Natural sugars contained in fresh fruits can provide sweet flavors with less risk of contributing to decay if the teeth are brushed regularly after eating such foods. Regular chewing gum may help remove food particles after eating, but it deposits sugar; if you chew gum, use sugarless gum.

Because decay is promoted each time sugars and other refined carbohydrates are eaten, between-meals snacks of sweets should be curtailed to lessen the chances of new or additional caries. Snack foods can be raw vegetables, such as carrots or celery, apples, cheese, peanuts, or other items that are not likely to introduce refined carbohydrates into the mouth between meals.

Brushing

Brushing the teeth is an essential of personal oral hygiene. Such brushing rids the mouth of most of the food

Brushing

Begin by brushing the tops of the upper and lower molars, using a scrubbing motion without much pressure. A soft toothbrush with a straight handle is most recommended.

Next, keeping the brush parallel to the teeth, angle the bristles against the lower gums and brush back and forth with short strokes against both sides of every tooth. Use the same technique for the upper teeth.

Apply the tip of the brush to the backs of upper and lower front teeth. Scrub in an up-and-down motion holding the brush handle directly out in front.

for claims about whether toothbrushes should have bristles with square corners or rounded shapes, a dentist may point out that there are both curved and straight surfaces in the mouth, so what one design offers in advantages may be offset by equivalent disadvantages. There also are special brushes for reaching surfaces of crooked teeth or cleaning missing-tooth areas of the mouth.

Although several different methods may be used effectively, the following is the technique most often recommended. Brush the biting surfaces, or tops, of the back upper and lower teeth. The lines and grooves on these surfaces make them prone to decay. They should be brushed first, before moisture has softened the brush. The cheek and tongue surfaces of the lower teeth are brushed next. Hold the brush parallel to the teeth with the bristle edges angled against and touching the gums. Using short strokes, move the brush back and forth several times before proceeding to the next one or two teeth. Use the same technique on all the inner surfaces of your teeth as well. For the hard-to-brush inner surfaces of the front teeth, hold the handle of the brush out in front of the mouth and apply the tip in an up-and-down motion. For all brushing, a scrubbing motion—but without too much pressure—should be used.

Some people prefer electric toothbrushes, which require less effort to use than ordinary toothbrushes. These are available with two basic motions—up and down and back and forth. Your dentist may advise which kind best serves an individual's needs and proper use of equipment. Some dentists point out that back-and-forth brushing applied with too much pressure can have an abrasive effect on tooth enamel because it works against the grain of the mineral deposits. The American Dental Association also

evaluates electric toothbrushes and issues reports on the safety and effectiveness of various types.

Removing Debris with Dental Floss

Brushing often does not clean debris from between the teeth. But plaque and food particles that stick between the teeth usually can be removed with dental floss. A generous length of floss, about 18 inches, is needed to do an effective job. The ends can be wrapped several times around the

Flossing

(1) Wrap floss several times around middle fingers and pull center section taut between thumbs or index fingers. (2) Insert floss between teeth and gently slide back and forth against every tooth. Work floss into the space between tooth and gumline. (3) To remove, pull floss gently downward along the angle of the tooth. Snapping it in and out may cause gum irritation.

debris that encourages bacterial growth, which is most intense 20 minutes after eating. Therefore, the teeth should be cleaned as soon as possible after a meal.

There is no one kind of toothbrush that is best for every person. Most dentists, however, recommend a soft toothbrush with a straight handle and flat brushing surface that can clean the gums without irritating them. As first joint of the middle finger of each hand. Using the thumbs or index fingers, the floss is inserted between the teeth with a gentle, sawing, back-and-forth motion. Then it is slid gently around part of a tooth in the space at the gum line and gently pulled out; snapping the floss in and out may irritate the gums. After brushing and flossing, the mouth should be rinsed with water. A mouthwash is unnecessary, but it may be used for the good taste it leaves in the mouth.

The dentist may recommend the use of an oral irrigating device as part of dental home care. These units produce a pulsating stream of water that flushes food debris from between teeth. They are particularly useful for patients wearing orthodontic braces or for those who have had recession of the gums, creating larger spaces between the teeth.

The person who wants to see the areas of plaque on his teeth can chew a *disclosing tablet*, available at most pharmacies, which leaves a harmless temporary stain on plaque surfaces. Some dentists recommend the use of disclosing tablets about once a week so that patients can check on the effectiveness of their tooth-cleaning techniques.

Tooth Decay

In addition to wear, tear, and injury, the major threat to the health of a tooth is bacteria. Bacteria can cause tooth decay, and the human mouth is a tremendous reservoir of bacteria because the mouth is warm, dark, moist, and usually contains tiny particles of food that help nourish the organisms. The bacteria found in the mouth are of two kinds, *aerobic* and *anaerobic*. Aerobic bacteria need oxygen to survive; anaerobic bacteria do not. Anaerobic bacteria can find their way through cracks and crevices into areas of the mouth or teeth where there is little or no oxygen and continue their *cariogenic,* or decay, activity.

Saliva

Saliva offers some protection against the decay germs, for reasons not well understood, but there are crevices and deep pockets around the teeth and gums where saliva does not penetrate. Paradoxically, saliva itself contains millions of different bacterial organisms. Dental scientists have calculated that one ounce of saliva may contain as many as 22 billion bacteria. Even a presumably healthy mouth may contain more than ten varieties of bacteria, plus protozoa and yeast cells. The yeast cells and at least three of the different kinds of bacteria are capable of producing acids that erode the tough enamel surface of a tooth.

Bacterial Acids and Plaque

The acids produced by decay bacteria actually are waste products of the organisms' digestive processes; bacteria, like other living creatures, eventually excrete waste products after a meal. As unpleasant as the thought may be, tooth decay can be the result of feeding a colony of germs in the mouth. Bacterial growth—hence the production of harmful acids—is encouraged by the consumption of too many foods composed of refined sugars. The sugars of candies, cakes, soft drinks, and the like are easier for the bacteria to eat and digest than those of fruits, vegetables, and other less thoroughly processed foods. Even a tiny bit of food remaining in the mouth after a meal may be enough
to support many millions of bacteria for 24 hours or more.

An additional contributing factor to tooth decay is *plaque* formation. Plaque is a sticky, transparent substance that forms a film over the surface of the teeth. Plaque forms every day, which is the reason that the teeth must be brushed every day. Plaque frequently begins with deposits of soft food debris along the gum line after a meal; it consists mainly of bacteria and its products. When mixed with mucus, molds, tissue cells from the membranes lining the mouth, and mineral salts, it takes the form of a white, cheesy substance called *materia alba.* If not removed regularly by brushing and the use of dental floss, this substance becomes a thick, sticky mass that has been compared to epoxy cement. Then it becomes a rough-surfaced hard substance with the texture of stone, otherwise known as *dental calculus,* or *tartar.*

Other Causes of Decay

Bacterial acid is not the only way in which the tooth enamel may be damaged to permit the entry of decay bacteria. Certain high-acid foods and improper dental care can erode the molecules of enamel. Temperature extremes also can produce cracks and other damage to the enamel; some dental scientists have suggested that repeated exposure to rapid temperature fluctuations of 50° F., as in eating alternately hot and cold foods or beverages, can cause the enamel to develop cracks.

Complications of Tooth Decay

Once decay activity breaks through the hard enamel surface, the bacteria can attack the dentin. Because the dentin is about 30 percent organic material, compared to 5 percent in the enamel layer, the decay process can advance more rapidly there. If the tooth decay is not stopped at the dentin layer, the disease organisms can enter the pulp chamber, where they will multiply quickly, producing an acute inflammation and, if unchecked, spread through the blood vessels to other parts of the body. Osteomyelitis, an infection of the membrane covering the skeletal bones, and endocarditis, an extremely dangerous heart ailment, are among diseases in other parts of the body that can begin with untreated tooth decay.

Periodontal disease, described below, is another possible complication of tooth decay.

Treatment of Tooth Decay

The portion of a tooth invaded by decay is called a *cavity;* it may be compared to an ulcer that develops because of disease in soft tissues. In treating the decay process, the dentist tries to prevent further destruction of the tooth tissue. The dentist also tries to restore as much as possible the original shape and function of the diseased tooth. The procedure used depends on many factors, including the surfaces affected (enamel, dentin, etc.) and the tooth face and angle involved, as well as whether the cavity is on a smooth area or in a pit or fissure of the tooth surface.

The decayed portions of the tooth are removed with various kinds of carbide burrs and other drill tips, as well as with hand instruments. The dentist may also use a caries removal system that reduces or eliminates drilling. In this system two solutions are combined in one liquid and squirted in a pulsating stream onto the decayed area. The stream does not harm gums or healthy teeth; rather, it softens the caries so that it can easily be scraped away. Used, generally, in conjunction with rotary or hand instruments, the "squirt" sys-

Tooth Restoration

The portion of the tooth affected by decay is known as a *cavity.* After removal of this diseased area (2), using drill, hand instrument, or other method, the dentist fills the cleaned cavity with a base or liner material (3). Finally, the tooth is filled with a restorative substance such as an amalgam, inlay, or ceramic material.

tem may make anesthesia unnecessary.

In other cases an anesthetic may be injected for the comfort of the patient. The dentist usually asks whether the patient prefers to have an anesthetic before work commences. In the cleaning process, an effort is made to remove all traces of diseased enamel or dentin, but no more of the tooth material than is necessary.

The cleaned cavity is generally filled in a layering procedure. The layers of liners and bases used before insertion of the filling are determined by the depth of the cavity and other factors. If pulp is exposed, special materials may be applied to help the pulp recover from the irritation of the procedure and to form a firm base for the amalgam, inlay, or other restorative substance that becomes the filling.

In the 1980s, new ceramic materials came into use for fillings. Many dentists believed that ceramics could provide more natural-looking restorations. With ceramics, also, teeth would be less sensitive to changes of temperature—a problem with some more traditional materials.

Tooth Extraction

When it becomes necessary to re-

move a diseased, damaged, or malpositioned tooth, the procedure is handled as a form of minor surgery, usually with administration of a local anesthetic to the nerves supplying the tooth area. However, there is no standard routine for extraction of a tooth, because of the numerous individual variations associated with each case. The dentist usually has a medical history of the patient available, showing such information as allergies to drugs, and medications used by the patient that might react with those employed in oral surgery. Because the mouth contains many millions of bacteria, all possible precautions are taken to prevent entry of the germs into the tooth socket.

The condition of the patient is checked during and immediately after tooth extraction, in the event that some complication develops. The patient is provided with analgesic (painkilling) and other needed medications, along with instructions regarding control of any postoperative pain or bleeding. The dentist also may offer special diet information with suggested meals for the recovery period, which usually is quite brief.

Dry Socket

Severe pain may develop several days after a tooth has been extracted if a blood clot that forms in the socket becomes dislodged. The condition, commonly called *dry socket*, can involve infection of the alveolar bone that normally surrounds the roots of the tooth; loss of the clot can expose the bone tissue to the environment and organisms that produce *osteitis*, or inflammation of the bone tissue. Dry socket may be treated by irrigating the socket with warm salt water and packing it with strips of medicated gauze. The patient also is given analgesics, sedatives, and other medications as needed to control the pain and infection.

General anesthetics are sometimes necessary for complicated oral surgery. In such cases, there are available dental offices or clinics that are as well equipped and staffed as hospital operating rooms.

Endodontic Therapy

Tooth extraction because of caries is less common today than in previous years, although an estimated 25 million Americans have had all of their teeth removed. Modern preventive dentistry techniques of *endodontics* now make it possible to save many teeth that would have been extracted in past decades after the spread of decay into the pulp canal. The procedures include *root canal therapy, pulp capping,* and *pulpotomy.*

Root Canal Therapy

Once the tooth has fully developed in the jaw, the nerve is not needed, so if the pulp is infected the nerve as well as the pulp can be removed. Only minor effects are noticeable in the tooth structure after the pulp is removed, and the dentist compensates for these in filling the tooth after root canal therapy.

Briefly, the procedure of root canal

Root Canal Therapy

(1) The first step of root canal, or removal of the nerve of a tooth, begins with examining the infected pulp to determine its vitality. (2) The depth of the root is measured by X ray and, after administering local anesthetic, the dentist extracts the pulp with drill or hand instrument marked to indicate when the end of the root has been reached. (3) When the entire pulp and nerve have been removed the canal is sterilized to prevent infection. (4) After filling the tooth with silver or a tough plastic substance known as *gutta‑percha,* or sometimes a combination of both, the dentist then caps the tooth.

work begins by examination and testing of the pulp viability. The pulp may be tested by heat, cold, or an electrical device called a *vitalometer,* which measure the degree of sensation the patient feels in a tooth. If the pulp is dead, the patient will feel no sensation, even at the highest output of current.

After the degree of vitality in the pulp has been determined, a local anesthetic is injected and the dentist begins removing the pulp, using rotary drills and hand instruments. By means of X-ray pictures, the dentist measures the length of the root, which may be about one and a half times the length of the crown. Stops or other markers are placed on the root excavation tools to show the dentist when the instrument has reached the end of the root. The canal is then sterilized and filled with gutta-percha—a tough plastic substance—silver, or a combination of the two, and a cap is added.

Pulp Capping

Pulp capping consists of building a cap over the exposed pulp with layers of calcium hydroxide paste, which is covered by zinc oxide and topped with a firm cement.

Pulpotomy

A pulpotomy procedure involves removal of the pulp in the pulp chamber within the crown of the tooth, while leaving the root canal pulp in place. The amputated pulp ends are treated and a pulp-capping procedure is used to restore the crown of the tooth.

Periodontal Disease

It is important in the middle years of life and later to continue good oral-hygiene habits and the practice of having regular dental checkups. Studies have found that after the age of 50 more than half the people in America have periodontal disease. At the age of 65, nearly everybody has this disease.

The Course of the Disease

The combination of bacterial action described above and the roughness of the resulting calculus injures the surrounding gum tissue and makes it susceptible to infection and recession. The irritation causes swelling, inflammation, and bleeding into the crevices between the teeth and gums, which is one of the early signs of impaired tissue health.

The inflammation of the gums, known as *gingivitis,* can spread to the roots of the teeth if not treated. The gums separate from the teeth, forming pockets that fill up with more food particles and colonies of bacteria. As the disease progresses, the bone support for the teeth is weakened and the affected teeth begin to loosen and drift from their normal position. Finally, unless the disease is treated in time, the teeth may be lost.

Periodontal disease is sometimes called *pyorrhea,* a Greek word meaning a discharge of pus. But "pyorrhea" is a somewhat misleading term, because it identifies only one manifestation of the disease, an abscess that usually forms along the side of an affected tooth. In some cases, a membrane forms around the abscess, creating a pus-filled cyst in the tooth socket.

Other Signs and Complications

Another manifestation of periodontal disease is periodontal atrophy, or recession of the gingiva, or gum tissue, and the underlying bone away from the outer layer of the tooth that joins it to its socket. Recession tends to expose the dentin below the gum line, which is not protected by a layer of enamel. The exposed dentin may be hypersensitive to hot or cold foods or beverages, air, and sweet or sour food flavors.

Inflammation of the gingival tissue in periodontal disease may be increased in intensity by toxic chemicals from tobacco smoke, bacterial infections, vitamin deficiencies, and defective dental restorations. The normal pink color of the gingival tissue may be altered by periodontal disease to a bright red or a darker coloration ranging to bluish purple.

The inflamed gingival tissue may lead to a complication called *periodontitis* in which the bone under the gum tissue is gradually destroyed, widening the crevice between the tooth and surrounding tissues. Pregnant women seem particularly vulnerable to periodontitis and gingivitis if they have been experiencing periodontal disorders, because the temporary hormonal imbalance of the pregnancy tends to exaggerate the effects of this condition.

One kind of gingivitis that involves projections of gum tissue between the teeth is sometimes referred to as *trench mouth,* because it was not an uncommon form of periodontal disease affecting soldiers during World War I. The infection is associated with poor oral hygiene, along with nutritional deficiencies and general depressed condition of health.

Causes

At one time it was assumed that periodontal diseases were associated with the life styles of persons living in more technologically advanced societies, where soft, rich foods are eaten regularly, providing materials toward the formation of plaque and support of bacteria in the plaque. But recent investigations show that people living in the less developed nations, who are relatively free of tooth decay, eventually develop periodontal disease. However, this does not alter the fact that the accumulation of plaque and harmful bacteria are the chief causes of periodontal disease, as well as of tooth decay.

Although periodontal disease generally becomes troublesome in middle age, there is some evidence that early symptoms of gingival disorders occur during childhood or adolescence. Also, because more people live longer today, periodontal disease has become more common than in the past.

Bruxism

Bruxism—the nervous habit, often unconsciously done, of clenching and grinding the teeth—can contribute to the development of periodontal disease. Bruxism frequently occurs during sleep.

Malocclusion

Another contributing cause to periodontal disease is repeated shock or undue pressure on a tooth because of

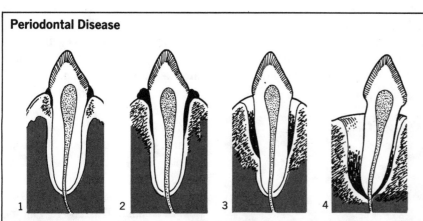

Periodontal Disease

(1) If allowed to build up at the gumline, deposits of plaque and calculus result in damage to the gum tissues (periodontal disease). (2) As gums become increasingly irritated and inflamed, they may bleed easily and begin to recede from the tooth itself. (3) Untreated, the inflammation spreads to the roots of the teeth. Bacteria and particles of food lodge in the pockets between tooth and gums, aggravating the condition. (4) A tooth held by the diseased gum loses most of its bony support structure, causing it to loosen and move out of position. Eventually, such teeth may need to be extracted.

malocclusion, or an improper bite. This effect accelerates damage to the tooth and gum structure during such simple activities as biting and chewing.

Treatment

Periodontal treatment may include a variety of techniques ranging from plaque removal to oral surgery to form new contours on the alveolar bone surrounding the tooth. If treatment is not begun until periodontal disease is well advanced, it may be difficult to fit replacement teeth, or *dentures,* as substitutes for lost teeth. Dentures fit over the ridges of the jaws, and if the top edge of the ridge has been destroyed by periodontal disease, the procedure for holding the denture firmly in place will be complicated.

Dentures

If it becomes necessary to have some teeth removed, they should be replaced as soon as possible with a *bridge*—a mounting for false teeth anchored to natural teeth on either side—or a partial or full denture.

Why Missing Teeth Must Be Replaced

Chewing ability and clarity of speech may be impaired if missing teeth are not replaced. Also, each tooth functions to hold the teeth on either side and opposite it in place. If a tooth is lost, the tooth opposite may erupt further and the teeth on either side shift in their positions because there is no counterforce to keep them in place. Food particles lodge in the spaces created by the shifting teeth, plaque

forms, and periodontal disease develops, causing the loss of additional teeth. This loss may take years if the movement of intact teeth is slow, but if they tilt and shift rapidly into the empty spaces, the remaining teeth may be lost in a much shorter time.

The loss of a few teeth can also alter a person's appearance. The cheeks may become puckered and the lips drawn together, making the individual look older.

Fitting of Dentures

Modern techniques and materials of construction and the skill of modern dentists should assure well-fitting, natural-looking dentures. The dentist selects the tooth shade and shape that are best for an individual's face size, contours, and coloring. No one, however, has perfectly arranged, perfectly white natural teeth. Tooth coloring depends upon genetic factors and changes as one grows older. These factors must be considered in designing dentures.

Bridges and Partial Dentures

Several different types of dental appliances may be constructed to fill empty spaces. Some, such as dental bridges, may be attached to the remaining natural teeth by cementing them. Others, such as complete sets of dentures, are removable.

A bridge may be made entirely of gold, a combination of gold and por-

Partial Denture

Anchoring teeth

Denture

Upper palate

celain, or combinations of gold and porcelain and other materials. If there is a sound natural tooth on either side of the space, a *pontic,* or suitable substitute for the missing tooth, may be fused to the metal bridge. The crown retainer on either side of the pontic may then be cemented to the crowns of the neighboring natural teeth.

If there are no natural teeth near the space created by an extracted tooth, a partial denture may be constructed to replace the missing teeth. This appliance usually fastens by a clasp onto the last tooth on each side of the space. A bar on the inside of the front teeth provides stability for the partial denture.

A "Maryland bridge," a fixed partial denture developed by the University of Maryland's Baltimore College of Dental Surgery, eliminates the need for crowns to anchor false teeth. With the Maryland bridge, hidden metal "wings" are used to anchor the partial denture. The wings are bonded to the backs of neighboring teeth. Because it eliminates the need for drilling, the Maryland bridge saves healthy teeth, makes anesthesia unnecessary, and reduces costs considerably.

New materials have brought bonding into more common use as an alternative to crowning and for cosmetically restoring chipped, malformed, stained, or widely spaced teeth. In the bonding process the dentist isolates a tooth with a rubber dam, cleans and dries the tooth, and applies a phosphoric acid solution that produces microscopic pores in the enamel. The etched area is then filled in with a liquid plastic. To that base the dentist applies thin layers of tooth-colored plastics known as composite resins. The layers can be sculpted, hardened with a beam of light or by some other method, contoured, and polished.

A removable partial denture should

be taken out and cleaned whenever the natural teeth are brushed. A special brush, usually cone-shaped to fit into the clasp, is available as a cleaning tool. The pontic, or tooth substitute of a bridge, remains in place permanently and is brushed like a natural tooth.

A bridge or partial denture helps prevent further deterioration of the mouth if it is kept clean and in good condition. But a dentist should check bridges and partial dentures periodically to make sure they have not become loosened. A loose clasp of a partial denture can rock the teeth to which the device is attached, causing damage and possible loss.

Complete Dentures

Before a full set of removable dentures is constructed, the dentist will take X rays to determine whether there are any abnormalities in the gum ridges, such as cysts or tooth root tips that may have to be removed. If the gums are in poor condition, treatments may be needed to improve the surfaces of the ridges on which the dentures will be fitted. The dentist may also have to reconstruct the bone underlying the gums—the alveolar ridge. Human bone "harvested" from another part of the patient's body has for decades been used in such reconstruction, but is today giving way to ceramic materials.

Two ceramic materials used in such surgery are hydroxylapatite and beta tricalcium phosphate. Oral surgeons have reported good results with both. The new materials are said to be safer and simpler to use and less expensive than human bone. They also eliminate the need for preliminary surgery to obtain transplants of the patient's bone.

With preliminary work done, the dentist makes an impression of the patient's mouth. Tooth and shade choices are discussed. Several other appointments may be arranged before the new dentures are delivered to the patient. Appointments may be needed for "try-ins" of dentures as they are being constructed and for adjustments after completion of the set.

Although dentures do not change with age, the mouth does. Therefore, it is necessary for the denture-wearer to have occasional dental checkups. At denture checkup appointments, the dentist examines oral tissues for irritation and determines how the dentures fit with respect to possible changing conditions of the mouth. If the dentures no longer fit properly, a replacement may be recommended. The dentist also seeks to correct any irritations of the oral tissues of the mouth and polishes the dentures, making them smooth and easier to keep clean between checkups. If any of the teeth in the dentures has become damaged, the dentist can repair or replace the denture tooth.

Care of Dentures

Dentures should be cleaned daily with a denture brush and toothpaste; once a week they should be soaked for seven or eight hours in a denture cleaner. To avoid breaking them during the brushing process, fill a wash basin with water and place it under the dentures while they are being cleaned; if they are dropped, the dentures will be cushioned by the water. A harsh abrasive that could scratch the denture surface should not be used. Scratches allow stains to penetrate the surface of the dentures, creating permanent discoloration.

The use of adhesives and powders is only a temporary solution to ill-fitting dentures. In time, the dentist may rebuild the gum side of the denture to conform with the shape of the patient's gum ridge. The patient should never try to make his own changes in the fit of dentures. Rebuilding the gum side of the dentures, or *relining,* as it is called, usually begins with a soft temporary material if the patient's gums are in poor condition, and requires several appointments over a period of two or three weeks while the gum tissues are being restored to good health.

Most patients show some concern over the replacement of natural teeth with dentures, even when a set of complete dentures is needed to replace an earlier set. Some people associate the loss of teeth with old age in the same way that others resist the advice that they should wear eyeglasses or a hearing aid. The fact is that many millions of persons of all ages have found they can improve their eating, speaking, and physical appearance by obtaining attractive and well-fitted dentures.

Orthodontics

*O**rthodontics** is a term derived from the Greek words for straight, or normal, teeth. Straight teeth are easier to keep clean and they make chewing food more efficient. There also is a cosmetic benefit in being able to display a smile with a set of straight teeth, although many dentists consider the cosmetic aspect of orthodontics as secondary to achieving proper occlusion, or bite.

Causes of Improper Bite

Orthodontic problems can be caused by hereditary factors, by an infectious or other kind of disease, by the premature loss of primary teeth, by the medications used in treatment, or by individual factors such as injury or loss of permanent teeth. A person may have congenitally missing teeth resulting in spaces that permit drifting

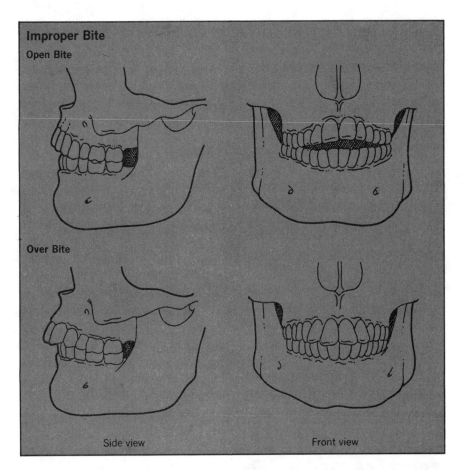

Improper Bite
Open Bite

Over Bite

Side view   Front view

of neighboring teeth or collapse of the dental arch. Or he may develop extra (supernumerary) teeth resulting from an inherited factor. The supernumerary teeth may develop during the early years of life while the deciduous teeth are in use. A supernumerary tooth may force permanent teeth into unnatural positions.

Nutritional disorders can also affect the development of jaws and teeth, while certain medications can cause abnormal growth of gingival, or gum, tissues, resulting in increased spaces between the teeth.

Teeth that erupt too early or too late, primary teeth that are too late in falling out when permanent teeth have developed, and habits such as grinding of the teeth, thumb-sucking, or pushing the tongue against the teeth are among other factors that can result in *malocclusion,* or improper bite, and the need for orthodontic treatment.

Diagnosis of Orthodontic Problems

Each child should visit a dentist before the eruption of his permanent teeth for an examination that may determine the need for orthodontic treatment. Because there are many genetic and other influences that help shape the facial contours and occlusion of each individual, there are no standard orthodontic procedures that apply to any or all children. The dentist may recommend what treatment, if any, would be needed to produce normal occlusion and when it should begin; some dentists advise only that necessary procedures for correcting malocclusion be started before the permanent set of teeth (excluding wisdom teeth) has become established, or around the age of 12 or 13. However, there are few age limits for orthodontic care, and an increasing number of adults are receiving treatment today for malocclusion problems that were neglected during childhood.

In the normal or ideal occlusion positions of the teeth, the first and second permanent upper molars fit just slightly behind the same molars of the lower jaw; all of the teeth of the upper jaw are in contact with their counterparts of the lower jaw. In this pattern of occlusion, all of the biting surfaces are aligned for optimum use of their intended functions of cutting, tearing, or grinding.

There are numerous variations of malocclusion, but generally, in simple deformities, the teeth of the upper jaw are in contact with lower jaw teeth once removed from normal positions. Other variations include an *open bite,* in which the upper and lower incisors do not contact each other, or *closed bite,* in which there is an abnormal degree of overlapping (*overbite*) of the front teeth.

Diagnosis is made with the help of X-ray pictures, photographs of the face and mouth, medical histories, and plaster models of the patient's teeth and jaws. The plaster models are particularly important because the dentist can use them to make experimental reconstructions without touching an actual tooth of a patient. For example, the dentist can remove one or more teeth from the plaster model and reorganize neighboring teeth in the jawbones to get an accurate representation of the effects of extracting teeth or forcing teeth into different developmental situations.

Orthodontic Appliances

Once a plan of orthodontic treatment has been determined by the dentist, he may choose from a dozen or more types of bands, braces, or other orthodontic appliances, some removable and some nonremovable, for shaping the teeth and jaws of the patient. A typical orthodontic appliance may include small curved strips or loops of metal cemented to the surfaces of the

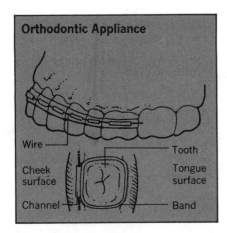

Orthodontic Appliance

Wire

Cheek surface

Channel

Tooth

Tongue surface

Band

teeth as anchors for arch wires that pass around the dental arch. Springs and specially designed rubber bands, called elastics, are sometimes used to bring about alignment of the two jaws, or to align teeth within a dental arch.

In addition to the appliances that are attached to and between the upper and lower dental arches, the dentist may prescribe the use of an elastic tape device with a strap that fits around the back of the patient's neck and is attached also to the arch wire inside the mouth, thus providing a force from outside the mouth to bring teeth into alignment.

Orthodontic appliances are custom-designed and built for the individual patient. This requires several rather long sessions or one all-day session in the dental chair while the appliance is being organized and properly anchored. Thereafter, the patient must return at regular intervals spaced a few weeks to a month apart so the dentist can make adjustments in the appliance, determine if any of the bands have pulled away from tooth surfaces, and prevent plaque from building up in places that the braces may make impervious to brushing.

The patient, meanwhile, must follow a diet that prohibits sticky foods or items that may damage the appliance or any of its parts. A conscientious program of oral hygiene, including regular cleaning by the dentist or hygienist, also is necessary because, as indicated above, it is more difficult to do a thorough job of cleaning the teeth when orthodontic appliances are in the mouth.

Orthodontics for Adults

Although orthodontic treatment originally was applied only to children, the technique has been requested with increasing frequency for the correction of a variety of facial and dental disorders. Receding chins, buck teeth, sunken cheeks, sunken mouths, and other abnormalities have been treated successfully in adults beyond the age of 40. Orthodontists have observed that adult patients usually are more patient and cooperative during the long periods of treatment than youngsters.

The upper age limit for orthodontic work has not really been established, but doctors at the National Institute of Dental Research believe it is possible to treat adult patients with protrusion of the upper jaw and related disfigurements until the age of 70. This is possible because the upper jaw does not completely unite with the frontal bone of the skull, according to the experts, until after the age of 70 in most people.

Orthodontic treatments can be relatively expensive and involve many visits to a dentist's office over a long period of time. Any parent of a prospective patient or a responsible older patient seeking orthodontic work for himself should have a frank discussion with the dentist regarding the time and money to be invested in the corrective procedures before making an agreement to begin the work. In nearly every case some arrangement can be made for covering the costs of dental work that is vital to the health and welfare of a patient.

23

Aches, Pains, Nuisances, Worries

And Other Things You Can Live With But Could Get Along Very Well Without

None of the variety of discomforts discussed in this chapter is a laughing matter. The best thing about most of them is that they will pass, given your commonsense attention, or will disappear if you follow your physician's advice. This includes taking the medications prescribed by your physician exactly as directed. In a few cases, such as allergies or gout, long-term drug therapy may be necessary on a self-supervised basis, once treatment has been established by a physician. Of course, when symptoms of any kind persist or get worse, you should waste no time in seeking a professional diagnosis.

There may be somebody, somewhere, who has never felt rotten a day in his life. But most of us are not so fortunate. Among the most common nuisance ailments are:

- upper respiratory infections

- allergies

- occasional headaches

- backaches

- weight problems

- weather discomforts

- disturbances of normal sleep patterns

- aching feet

- indigestion

The unpleasant feeling associated with any of these common disorders can almost always be banished with a modicum of care and thought. For example, allergic reactions to particular foods can be curtailed by identifying the offending food and avoiding it. Self-diagnosis and self-discipline can often enable one to cope with weight problems. A backache may be cured by attention to posture, or adjusting your office chair. A sensible approach to clothing and exposure can often do away with weather discomforts.

For many minor disorders and discomforts, particularly those caused by stress, massage may be the an-

swer. Massage is a process that is at least 3,000 years old and has been used to help relieve tension, increase muscle tone, improve blood and oxygen circulation, and aid major body functions. Massage has also helped alleviate aches and pains resulting from exercise, improve posture, and increase joint flexibility. Among the disorders for which massage should not be used are osteoporosis, varicose veins, inflamed joints, herniated discs, tumors, and some cardiovascular problems.

Massage invariably involves kneading, manipulation, and methodical pressure on various body parts. The process should never be painful. The three kinds of massage in most common use are Swedish, a pleasant, muscle-kneading procedure; Shiatsu, or "acupressure," which depends on finger and hand pressure on so-called energy meridians in the body; and reflexology, a system that calls for pressure on various points of the foot.

When symptoms do not respond to

self-help—as when sporadic difficulty in sleeping burgeons into a string of near-sleepless nights, or when abdominal pain you interpret as indigestion is intense or frequent in spite of avoiding rich or heavy foods, it's time to see a physician.

The Common Cold and Upper Respiratory Infections

Common cold is the label attached to a group of symptoms that can be caused by one or more of some 20 different viruses. Colds are considered highly contagious, but some physicians think that people don't entirely catch others' colds—in a sense they catch their own. While the viruses that carry the infection are airborne and practically omnipresent, somebody in good health is usually less susceptible to a cold than someone who is run down. Both environmental factors (such as air pollution) and emotional ones (such as anxiety or depression) seem to increase susceptibility.

Symptoms

Symptoms differ from person to person and from cold to cold with the same person. Generally, a cold starts with sneezes, a running nose, teary eyes, and a stuffed head. Sometimes the nasal membranes become so swollen that a person can breathe only through the mouth; sometimes the senses of smell and taste simply disappear. The throat may be sore; a postnasal drip may cause a constant cough when the person is lying down at night.

When these symptoms are acute and are accompanied by fever and aching joints, the illness is usually referred to as influenza or "the flu." There are many different viruses that cause influenza, and new ones are always turning up. Unfortunately, there is as yet no medicine that can cure either a cold or a flu attack, although many people do get relief from symptoms by taking various cold remedies. Antibiotics are sometimes prescribed by doctors to prevent more serious bacterial diseases, such as pneumonia, from developing, but antibiotics are not effective against the cold viruses.

Treatment

Some people can get away with treating a cold with contempt and an occasional aspirin, and go about their business. Others are laid low for a few days. If you are the type who is really hit hard by a cold, it isn't coddling yourself to stay home for a couple of days. In any event, a simple cold usually runs its course, lasting anywhere from a few days to two weeks.

Discomfort can be minimized and recovery speeded by a few simple steps: extra rest and sleep, drinking more liquids than usual, and taking one or two aspirin tablets every four hours. Antihistamine preparations or nose drops should be avoided unless specifically prescribed by a physician.

A painful sore throat accompanied by fever, earache, a dry, hacking cough, or pains in the chest are symptoms that should be brought to the attention of a physician.

Prevention

Although taking massive doses of vitamin C at the first sign of a cold is said by some authorities to prevent the infection from developing, there is not yet general agreement on the effectiveness of this treatment.

Actually, there are several commonsense ways of reducing the risk of infection, particularly for those people who are especially susceptible to catching a cold. For most people, getting a proper amount of sleep, eating sensibly, avoiding exposure to sudden chill, trying to stay out of crowds, and trying to keep emotional tensions under control can increase resistance to colds and other minor respiratory infections.

Inoculation against particular types of viruses is recommended by many physicians in special cases: for pregnant women, for the elderly, and for those people who have certain chronic heart and lung diseases. Flu shots are effective against a particular virus or viruses for a limited period.

Allergies

Discomforts of various kinds are considered allergies when they are brought on by substances or conditions that ordinarily are harmless. Not too long ago, perturbed allergy sufferers would say things like:

"I can't use that soap because it gives me hives."

"Smelling roses makes me sneeze."

"Eating almonds gives me diarrhea."

Nowadays, such complaints are commonly recognized as indications of allergies.

Symptoms

Allergic symptoms can range from itching eyes, running nose, coughing, difficulty in breathing, welts on the skin, nausea, cramps, and even going into a state of shock, depending upon the severity of the allergic individual's response. Almost any part or system of the body may be affected, and almost anything can pose an allergic threat to somebody.

Allergens

Substances that trigger an allergic reaction are called *allergens*. The system of an allergic individual reacts to such substances as if they were germs, producing *antibodies* whose job it is to neutralize the allergens. But the body's defense mechanism overreacts: in the process of fighting off the effects of the allergens, various chemicals, particularly *histamines,* are dumped indiscriminately into the bloodstream. It is the overabundance of these "good" chemicals that causes the discomforts associated with allergies.

Allergens are usually placed in the following categories:

- Those that affect the respiratory tract, or *inhalants,* such as pollens, dust, smoke, perfumes, and various airborne, malodorous chemicals. These bring on sneezing, coughing, and breathing impairment.

- Food substances that affect the digestive system, typically eggs, seafood, nuts, berries, chocolate, and pork. These may cause not only nausea and diarrhea but also hives and other skin rashes.

- Medicines and drugs, such as penicillin, or a particular serum used in inoculations.

- Agents that act on the skin and mucous membranes, such as insecticides, poison oak, and poison ivy, particular chemical dyes, cosmetics, soaps, metals, leathers, and furs.

- Environmental agents, such as sunlight or excessive cold.

- Microbes, such as particular bacteria, viruses, and parasites.

Treatment

In general, approaches to treatment for allergies fall into three categories: removing or avoiding as many allergens from the environment as possible; using creams, inhalers, pills, and other medications to control the symptoms; and undergoing immunotherapy (allergy shots) to reduce the allergic response. The type of treatment selected often depends on test findings that indicate what is causing the allergic reaction; the tests may produce such identification quickly or they may have to be continued for weeks or months before the allergen is finally tracked down.

As soon as the source of the allergen is identified, the obvious course is to avoid it, if possible. Avoidance may not, however, be possible. Few persons can avoid breathing pollen in the spring and fall. Giving up a house pet may be almost as difficult, but may be necessary as a health or comfort measure.

New medications that control the symptoms of allergies have been marketed in recent years. Newer antihistamines, for example, relieve allergic reactions but do not cause the drowsiness associated with earlier medications. Other medicines that have been used to treat allergies include adrenaline, ephedrine, and cortisone. Aerosol drugs may be used to attack specific symptoms. Some, for example, may be inhaled to treat the linings of the nose and throat.

In addition to histamines, other body chemicals are released during an allergy "attack." Researchers have found that these chemicals include leukotrienes. Consequently, antileukotrienes have tested as medications.

Direct or specific immunotherapy constitutes the third approach to treatment of allergy. The shots are effective in reducing allergic responses. A person with a substance allergy receives increasing amounts of the substance over a period of years. For example, a person who is allergic to insect stings receives injections of the particular insect's venom.

A life-threatening allergic reaction calls for emergency treatment, usually with adrenalin. Physicians suggest that persons with very intense food allergies or who are allergic to insect stings should carry special kits that include an adrenalin-filled syringe. The allergy victims administer the medication to themselves in case of *anaphylaxis*— an acute, life-threatening response (see "Allergic Shock" in Ch. 31, *Medical Emergencies*).

Persons subject to severe, disabling allergy attacks by a known allergen should also carry a card describing both the allergen and the allergic reactions. Detailed information on the latest developments in allergy treatment is available from the Asthma and Allergy Foundation of America, 1302 18th St., NW, Suite 800, Washington, DC 20036. See also Ch. 24, *Allergies and Hypersensitivities*.

Headaches

The common headache is probably as ancient as primitive man. The headache, a pain or ache across the forehead or within the head, may be severe or mild in character, and can last anywhere from under half an hour to three or four days. It may be accompanied by dizziness, nausea, nasal stuffiness, or difficulty in seeing or hearing. It is not a disease or illness but a symptom.

Causes

Headaches in today's modern world can arise from any of a number of underlying causes. These include excessive drinking or smoking, lack of sleep, hunger, drug abuse, and eyestrain. Eyestrain commonly results from overuse of the eyes, particularly under glaring light, or from failure to correct defective vision.

Headaches can also be caused by exposure to toxic gases, such as carbon monoxide and sulfur dioxide, which are common components in polluted air. Some headaches are symptoms of illness or disease, including pneumonia, constipation, allergy, high blood pressure, and brain tumor. Finally, emotional strain or tension can cause headache by muscle constriction in the head and neck. Many of these causes give rise to the common physiological cause of headache—dilation of the blood vessels in the head.

Headaches may be suffered on an occasional basis, or they may be chronic. Chronic headaches are usually *tension* or *migraine headaches.*

Migraine

Migraine, also called *sick headache,* is a particularly severe, intense kind of headache. An attack may last several days and necessitate bed rest. Dizziness, sensitivity to light, and chills may accompany a migraine headache.

The exact cause of migraine is unknown, but researchers suspect a hereditary link, since the majority of migraine patients have one or more close relatives with migraine.

Migraine headaches can be precipitated by changes in body hormone balance (as from oral contraceptives), sudden changes in temperature, exposure to bright light or noise, shifts in barometric pressure, or by the intake of alcoholic beverages or the abuse of drugs. An attack can also be triggered by allergic responses to certain foods or beverages, such as chocolate or milk, and by emotional stress. Women, who outnumber men by a 2 to 1 ratio in the incidence of migraine, may have an attack brought on by premenstrual tension. Many migraine sufferers have been found to

conform to a personality type characterized as compulsive; their standards of achievement are exacting, their manner of work meticulous, and they tend to avoid expression of their anxieties.

Anyone suffering from very severe or chronic headaches should see a physician and get a complete physical checkup.

Tension Headaches

Tension headaches can be avoided by getting adequate amounts of sleep and exercise and by learning to cope with frustrations and anxieties. Find time to relax each day, and resist the temptation to be a perfectionist or overachiever in all things. Tension headaches can be helped by neck massage, use of a heating pad, or a long, hot bath.

Headache Relief

Aspirin is often effective against headaches, but should be taken according to directions. A double dose is dangerous, and is not doubly effective. A cup of coffee or other caffeine beverage may prove helpful, because caffeine helps constrict blood vessels. In some cases headaches can be helped by nothing more than a few deep breaths of fresh air. Excess use of alcohol and tobacco should be avoided. If you must skip a meal, have a candy bar, piece of fruit, or some soup to prevent or relieve a hunger headache.

Take care of your eyes. Do not read in dim or glaring light. Have your eyes checked regularly, and if you have glasses, wear them when you need them.

Backaches

"Oh, my aching back" is probably the most common complaint among peo-

ple past the age of 40. Most of the time, the discomfort—wherever it occurs, up or down the backbone—can be traced to some simple cause. However, there are continuous backaches that have their origin in some internal disorder that needs the attention of a physician. Among the more serious causes are kidney or pancreas disease, spinal arthritis, and peptic ulcer.

Some Common Causes

Generally a backache is the result of strain on the muscles, nerves, or ligaments of the spine. It can occur because of poor posture, carelessness in lifting or carrying heavy packages, sitting in one position for a long time in the wrong kind of chair, or sleeping on a mattress that is too soft. Backache often accompanies menstruation, and is common in the later stages of pregnancy. Emotional tension can also bring on back pain.

Prevention

In general, maintaining good posture during the waking hours and sleeping on a hard mattress at night—if necessary, inserting a bed board between the mattress and bedsprings—are the first line of defense against backaches. Anyone habitually carrying heavy loads of books or groceries, or even an overloaded attaché case, should make a habit of shifting the weight from arm to arm so that the spine doesn't always get pulled in one direction. Workers who are sedentary for most of the day at a desk or factory table should be sure that the chair they sit in provides firm support for back muscles and is the right height for the working surface.

Treatment

Most cases of simple backache respond to rest, aspirin, and the application of heat, applied by a hot water bottle or heating pad. In cases where the pain persists or becomes more acute, a physician should be consulted. He may find that the trouble is caused by the malfunctioning of an internal organ, or by pressure on the sciatic nerve (*sciatica*). With X rays he may also locate a slipped disk or other abnormality in the alignment of the vertebrae of the spine. See "Back Pain and Its Causes" in Ch. 7, *Diseases of the Skeletal System.*

Weight Problems

A few people can maintain the weight that is right for their body build without ever having to think about it. However, most experts believe that just about half the people in the United States may be risking shorter lives because they are too heavy. By one estimate, approximately one out of five American men and one out of four American women are 10 percent or more overweight, a group that may be called the borderline obese.

There is no longer any reasonable doubt that, if you are overweight, you have statistically a greater chance of high blood pressure, diabetes, and *atherosclerosis* (lumpy deposits in the arteries). And because atherosclerotic heart disease alone accounts for 20 percent of deaths among adults in the United States, it is understandable why physicians consider weight truly a national problem.

Causes

In practically all cases, weighing too much is the result of eating too much and exercising too little. In many cases, the food eaten is of the wrong kind and leisure time is used for riding around in a car rather than walking, or for watching television rather than playing tennis.

Many people like to think that they weigh too much only because they happen to like good food; but the real explanations may be considerably more complicated. In some cases, overeating has been found to have emotional sources: feelings of inadequacy; the need to compensate for a lack of affection or approval, or an unconscious desire to ward off the attention of the opposite sex. Psychological weight problems of this kind can be helped by consulting a psychiatrist or psychologist.

Treatment

There are many overweight people who merely need the support and encouragement that come from participating in a group effort, and for them, joining one of the various weight-control organizations can be extremely beneficial in taking off extra pounds and keeping them off.

Permanent results are rarely achieved by crash diets, faddish food combinations, or reducing pills. Not only are such solutions usually temporary; they may actually be harmful. See "Weight" in Ch. 27, *Nutrition and Weight Control,* for further information about weight problems.

Weather Discomforts

Using good sense about clothing, exercise, and proper diet is probably our best protection against the discomforts caused by extremes of temperature. Sometimes circumstances make this exercise of good sense impossible, with unpleasant but rarely serious results, if treatment is promptly administered. Following are some of the more common disorders resulting from prolonged exposure to excessive heat or cold, and what you can do to alleviate them.

Heat Cramps

In a very hot environment, a person may drink great quantities of water while "sweating buckets" of salty perspiration. Thus, the body's water is replaced, but its salt is not. This salt–water imbalance results in a feeling of faintness and dizziness accompanied by acute stomach cramps and muscle pains in the legs. When the symptoms are comparatively mild, they can be relieved by taking coated salt tablets in five-to-ten-grain doses with a full glass of tepid or cool—not iced—water. Salt tablets along with plenty of fluids should be taken regularly as a preventive measure by people who sweat a great deal during hot weather.

Sunburn

If you have not yet been exposed to much sun, as at the beginning of summer, limit your exposure at first to a period of 15 to 20 minutes, and avoid the sun at the hours around midday even if the sky is overcast. Remember, too, that the reflection of the sun's rays from water and beach sand intensifies their effect. Some suntan lotions give effective protection against burning, and some creams even prevent tanning; but remember to cover all areas of exposed skin and to reapply the lotion when it's been washed away after a swim.

Treatment

A sunburn is treated like any other burn, depending upon its severity. See "Burns" in Ch. 31, *Medical Emergencies.* If there is blistering, take care to avoid infection. Extensive blistering requires a physician's attention.

Heat Exhaustion

This condition is different from heatstroke or sunstroke, discussed below. Heat exhaustion sets in when large quantities of blood accumulate in the skin as the body's way of increasing its cooling mechanism during exposure to high temperatures. This in turn lowers the amount of blood circulating through the heart and decreases the blood supply to the brain. If severe enough, fainting may result. Other symptoms of heat exhaustion include unusual pallor and profuse cold perspiration. The pulse may be weak, and breathing shallow.

Treatment

A person suspected of having heat exhaustion should be placed in a reclining position, his clothing loosened or removed, and his body cooled with moist cloths applied to his forehead and wrists. If he doesn't recover promptly from a fainting spell, smelling salts can be held under his nose to revive him. As soon as he is conscious, he can be given salt tablets and a cool sugary drink—either tea or coffee—to act as a stimulant. Don't give the patient any alcoholic beverages.

Sunstroke or Heatstroke

Sunstroke is much more of an emergency than heat exhaustion and requires immediate attention. The characteristic symptom is extremely high body temperature brought on by cessation of perspiration. If hot, dry, flushed skin turns ashen gray, a physician must be called immediately. Too much physical activity during periods of high temperature and high humidity is a direct contributing cause.

Treatment

See "Heatstroke" in Ch. 31, *Medical Emergencies,* for a description of the emergency treatment recommended for this condition.

Chapped Skin

One of the most widespread discomforts of cold weather is *chapped skin.* In low temperatures, the skin's sebaceous glands produce fewer oils that lubricate and protect the skin, causing it to become dry. Continued exposure results in reddening and cracking. In this condition, the skin is especially sensitive to strong soaps.

Treatment

During cold, dry weather, less soap should be used when washing, a bath oil should be used when bathing, and a mild lotion or creme should be applied to protect the skin from the damaging effects of wind and cold. A night cream or lotion containing lanolin is also helpful, and the use of cleansing cream or oil instead of soap can reduce additional discomfort when cleansing chapped areas. The use of a colorless lip pomade is especially recommended for children when they play out of doors in cold, dry weather for any length of time.

Chilblain

A *chilblain* is a local inflammation of the skin brought on by exposure to cold. The condition commonly affects people overly sensitive to cold because of poor circulation. When the hands, feet, face, and ears are affected, the skin in these areas itches and burns, and may swell and turn reddish blue.

Treatment

The best way to avoid chilblains is to wear appropriate clothing during cold weather, especially warm socks, gloves, and ear coverings. The use of bed socks and a heating pad at night is also advisable. Once indoors, cold, wet feet should be dried promptly, gently, and thoroughly. Rubbing or massaging should be avoided, because these can cause further irritation. People who suffer from repeated attacks of chilblains should consult a physician for diagnosis of circulatory problems.

Frostbite

Frostbite is a considerably more serious condition than chilblains, because it means that a part or parts of the body have actually been frozen. The fingers or toes, the nose, and the ears are most vulnerable. If frostbitten, these areas turn numb and pale and feel cold when touched. The dangerous thing about frostbite is that pain may not be a warning. If the condition is not treated promptly, the temperature inside the tissues keeps going down and eventually cuts off blood circulation to the overexposed parts of the body. In such extreme cases, there is a possible danger of gangrene.

Treatment

In mild cases, prompt treatment can slowly restore blood circulation. The frozen parts should be rewarmed *slowly* by covering them with warm clothing or by soaking them in lukewarm water. Nothing hot should be applied—neither hot water nor a heating pad. Nor should the patient be placed too close to a fireplace or radiator. Because the affected tissues can be easily bruised, they should not be massaged or rubbed. If you are in doubt about restoring circulation, a physician should be called promptly or the patient taken to a hospital for emergency treatment.

Sleep and the Lack of It

Until rather recently, it was assumed that sleep was the time when the body rested and recovered from the activities of wakefulness. Although there is still a great deal to learn about why we sleep and what happens when we are sleeping, medical researchers have now identified several different phases of sleep, all of them necessary over the long run, but some more crucial than others.

How much sleep a person needs varies a great deal from individual to individual; and the same individual may need more or less at different times. Children need long periods of unbroken sleep; the elderly seem to get along on very little. No matter what a person's age, too little sleep over too long a time leads to irritability, exhaustion, and giddiness.

Insomnia

Almost everybody has gone through periods when it is difficult or impossible to fall asleep. Excitement before bedtime, temporary worries about a pressing problem, spending a night in an unfamiliar place, changing to a different bed, illness, physical discomfort because of extremes of temperature—any of these circumstances can interfere with normal sleep patterns.

But this is quite different from *chronic insomnia,* when a person consistently has trouble falling asleep for no apparent reason. If despite all your commonsense approaches insomnia persists, a physician should be consulted about the advisability of taking a tranquilizer or a sleeping pill. Barbiturates should not be taken unless prescribed by a physician.

The Vulnerable Extremities

Aches and pains in the legs and feet occur for a wide variety of reasons, some trivial and easily corrected, others serious enough to require medical attention. Those that originate in such conditions as arthritis and rheumatism can often be alleviated by aspirin or some of the newer prescription medications.

Gout

Gout, which is usually a metabolic disorder, is a condition that especially affects the joint of the big toe, and sometimes the ankle joint, causing the area to become swollen, hot, and acutely painful. Although the specific cause of gout is not yet clearly understood, the symptoms can be alleviated by special medication prescribed by a physician. An attack of gout can be triggered by a wide variety of causes: wearing the wrong shoes, eating a diet too rich in fats, getting a bad chill, surgery in some other part of the body, or chronic emotional anxiety, as well as the use of certain medicines, such as diuretics ("waterpills"). See also "Gout" in Ch. 7, *Diseases of the Skeletal System.*

Fallen Arches

Fallen arches can cause considerable discomfort because the body's weight is carried on the ligaments of the inside of the foot rather than on the sole. When the abnormality is corrected by orthopedic shoes with built-in arches for proper support, the pressure on the ligaments is relieved. A physician rather than a shoe salesman should be consulted for a reliable diagnosis. In some cases, the physician may also recommend special exercises to strengthen the arch.

Flat Feet

Flat feet can usually be revealed by a simple test—making a footprint on level earth or hard-packed sand. If the print is solid rather than indented by a curve along the big-toe side of the foot, the foot is flat. Aching ligaments in the area of the instep are often a result, but can be relieved by proper arch supports inside the shoes. Corrective arch supports are particularly important for young children, for anyone who is overweight, and for anyone who has to stand a great deal of the time.

Blisters

Although blisters are sometimes a sign of allergy, fungus infection, or sunburn, they most commonly appear on the feet because of the friction of a shoe or of hosiery that does not fit properly. A *water blister* is a collection of lymph that forms inside the upper level of the skin; a *blood blister* goes down deeper and contains some blood released from broken capillaries. A normal amount of walking in shoes and hosiery that fit comfortably—neither too loose nor too tight—rarely results in blisters. When blisters do appear, it is best to protect them from further friction by the use of a sterile bandage strip.

Treatment

A blister that causes acute pain when one is walking can be treated as follows: after cleaning the area with soap and water, pat it dry and swab it with rubbing alcohol. Sterilize the tip of a needle in a flame, let it cool a little, and then puncture the edge of the blister, absorbing the liquid with a sterile gauze. The loose skin can be removed with manicure scissors that have been sterilized by boiling for ten minutes. The surface of raw skin should then be covered with an adhesive bandage. This procedure is best done before bedtime so that healing can begin before shoes are worn again.

If redness appears around the area of any blister and inflammation appears to be spreading, a physician should be consulted promptly.

Bunions

A *bunion* is a deformation in the part of the foot that is joined by the big toe. The swelling and pain at the joint is caused by inflammation of the *bursa* (a fluid-filled sac) that lubricates the joint. Although bunions often develop because of wearing shoes that don't fit correctly, they most frequently accompany flat feet. Pain that is not too severe can be relieved by the application of heat; the condition may eventually be cured by doing foot exercises recommended by a physician, who will also help in the choice of correct footwear. A bunion that causes acute pain and difficulty in walking can be treated by a simple surgical procedure.

Calluses

A *callus* is an area of the skin that has become hard and thick as a result of constant friction or pressure against it. Pain results when the callus is pressed against a nerve by poorly fitting shoes. A painful callus can be partially removed by rubbing it—very cautiously—with a sandpaper file or a pumice stone sold for that purpose. The offending shoes should then be discarded for correctly fitted ones. Foot care by a podiatrist is recommended for anyone with recurring calluses and corns (see below), and especially for those people who have diabetes or any disorder of the arteries.

Corns

A *corn* is a form of callus that occurs on or between the toes. When the thickening occurs on the outside of the toe, it is called a *hard corn;* when it is located between the toes, it is called a *soft corn*. The pain in the affected area is caused by pressure of the hard inside core of the corn against the tissue beneath it. The most effective treatment for corns is to wear shoes that are the right size and fit. Corns can be removed by a podiatrist, but unless footwear fits properly, they are likely to return.

Treatment

To remove a corn at home, the toes should be soaked in warm water for about ten minutes and dried. The corn can be rubbed away with an emery file, or it can be treated with a few drops of 10 percent salicylic acid in collodion, available from any druggist. Care should be exercised in applying the solution so that it doesn't reach surrounding tissue, because it is highly irritating to normal skin. The area can then be covered with a corn pad to relieve pressure. This treatment may have to be repeated several times before the corn becomes soft enough to lift out. Diabetics or those suffering from any circulatory disorder should never treat their own corns.

Housemaid's Knee

Housemaid's knee is actually a form of *bursitis,* in which the fluid-filled bursa in front of the kneecap becomes inflamed by injury or excessive pressure, as because of constant kneeling. When the inflammation is mild, it can usually be corrected by rest. In the acute stage, the knee becomes swollen and painful, particularly when bent. It is especially prone to infection if scratched, bruised, or cut. Acute housemaid's knee is usually treated by anti-inflammatory-type drugs, injections of cortisone, or surgery under local anesthesia in a physician's office. Anyone whose daily activities involve a great deal of kneeling should make a habit of using a thick rubber mat.

Tennis Elbow

This disorder can affect not only tennis players but also people who have injured their elbow joint or subjected it to various stresses and strains. It may be a form of bursitis similar in nature to housemaid's knee, but it is more correctly called *tendinitis,* that is, an inflammation of the tendons that can affect any joint in the arms and legs. Rest and the application of heat usually relieve the painful symptoms. If the pain becomes acute, a physician should be consulted.

Tenosynovitis

Tenosynovitis is an inflammation of a tendon sheath. One of the commoner sites of trouble is that of the wrist muscles. It can be caused by injury, infection, or constant use of the wrist muscles in piano playing, typing, or some form of labor involving the wrist. The condition is usually treated by splinting the wrist and resting it for a while. Pain can be relieved with aspirin.

Writer's Cramp

Writer's cramp is a muscular pain caused by constant use of a set of muscles for a particular activity. The same set of muscles will function with no difficulty when the activity is changed. The best way to treat the discomfort is to give the muscles a rest from the habitual activity and to relieve the pain with heat and aspirin.

Other Muscle Cramps

A sharp cramp or pain in the leg muscles, and sometimes in the arm, can occur because blood circulation has been impaired, either by hardening of the arteries or because of undue pressure, such as habitually sitting with one leg tucked under the upper thigh. The cramp is usually relieved either by changing the activity involved or by shifting the position of the affected limb. Constant or acute muscle cramps should be brought to the attention of a physician.

The Exposed Integument

Common skin and scalp annoyances such as rashes, itches, dandruff, excessive perspiration, and infections of various kinds (such as athlete's foot and ringworm), as well as acne, wrinkles, and baldness, are discussed in Ch. 21, *Skin and Hair.*

Splinters

If lodged superficially in the hand, a splinter will usually work its own way out, but a splinter of no matter what size in the sole of the foot must be removed promptly to avoid its becoming further embedded by pressure and causing infection. The simplest method of removal is to pass a needle through a flame; let the needle cool; then, after the skin surface has been washed with soap and water or swabbed with alcohol, press the point of the needle against the skin, scraping slightly until the tail of the splinter is visible and loosened. It can then be pulled out with tweezers that have been sterilized in boiling water or alcohol.

Hangnails

Hangnails are pieces of partly living skin torn from the base or side of the fingernail, thus opening a portion of the underskin to infection. A hangnail can cause considerable discomfort. It should not be pulled or bitten off; but the major part of it can be cut away with manicuring scissors. The painful and exposed area should then be washed with soap and water and covered with a sterile adhesive bandage. Hangnails are likely to occur when the skin is dry. They can therefore be prevented by the regular use of a hand cream or lotion containing lanolin.

"Normal" Disorders of the Blood and Circulation

Almost everybody is bothered occasionally by minor disturbances of the circulatory system. Most of the time these disturbances are temporary, and in many cases where they are chronic they may be so mild as not to interfere with good health. Among the more common disturbances of this type are the following.

Anemia

Anemia is a condition in which there is a decrease in the number of red blood cells or in the hemoglobin content of the red blood cells. *Hemoglobin* is the compound that carries oxygen to the body tissues from the lungs. Anemia in itself is not a disease but rather a symptom of some other disorder, such as a deficiency of iron in the diet; excessive loss of blood resulting from an injury or heavy menstrual flow; infection by industrial poisons; or kidney or bone marrow disease. A person may also develop anemia as a result of hypersensitivity (allergy) to various medicines.

In the simple form of anemia, caused by a deficiency of iron in the diet, the symptoms are rarely severe. There may be feelings of fatigue, a loss of energy, and a general lack of vitality. Deficiency anemia is especially common among children and pregnant women, and can be corrected by adding foods high in iron to the diet, such as liver, lean meat, leafy green vegetables, whole wheat bread, and dried peas and beans.

If the symptoms persist, a physician should be consulted for diagnosis and treatment. For more information on anemia, see "Diseases of the Blood" in Ch. 9, *Diseases of the Circulatory System.*

Varicose Veins

Varicose veins are veins that have become ropy and swollen, and are therefore visible in the leg, sometimes bulging on the surface of the skin. They are the result of a sluggish blood flow (poor circulation), often combined with weakened walls of the veins themselves. The condition is common in pregnancy and occurs frequently among people who find it necessary to sit or stand in the same position for extended periods of time. A tendency to develop varicose veins may be inherited.

Even before the veins begin to be visible, there may be such warning symptoms as leg cramps, feelings of fatigue, or a general achiness. Unless the symptoms are treated promptly, the condition may worsen, and if the blood flow becomes increasingly impeded, ulcers may develop on the lower area of the leg.

Treatment

Mild cases of varicose veins can be kept under control, or even corrected, by giving some help to circulation, as follows:

- Several times during the day, lie flat on your back for a few minutes, with the legs slightly raised.

- Soak the legs in warm water.

- Exercise regularly.

- Wear lightly reinforced stockings or elastic stockings to support veins in the legs.

If varicose veins have become severe, a physician should be consulted. He or she may advise injection treatment or surgery. See also "The Inflammatory Disorders" in Ch. 9, *Diseases of the Circulatory System.*

Chronic Hypertension

Hypertension, commonly known as *high blood pressure,* is a condition that may be a warning of some other disease. In many cases, it is not in itself a serious problem and has no one underlying specific cause: this is called *functional, essential,* or *chronic hypertension.* The symptoms of breathing difficulty, headache, weakness, or dizziness that accompany high blood pressure can often be controlled by medicines that bring the pressure down, by sedatives or tranquilizers, and in cases where overweight is a contributing factor, by a change in diet, or by a combination of these.

More serious types of high blood pressure can be the result of kidney disease, glandular disturbances, or diseases of the circulatory system. Acute symptoms include chronic dizziness or blurred vision. Any symptoms of high blood pressure call for professional advice and treatment. See "Hypertensive Heart Disease" in Ch. 10, *Heart Disease.*

Tachycardia

Tachycardia is the medical name for a condition that most of us have felt at one time or another—abnormally rapid heartbeat, or a feeling that the heart is fluttering, or pounding too quickly. The condition can be brought on by strong feelings of fear, excitement, or anxiety, or by overtaxing the heart with sudden exertion or too much exercise. It may also be a sign

of heart disease, but in such cases, it is usually accompanied by other symptoms.

The most typical form of occasional rapid heartbeat is called *paroxysmal tachycardia,* during which the beat suddenly becomes twice or three times as fast as it is normally, and then just as suddenly returns to its usual tempo. When the paroxysms are frequent enough to be disturbing and can be traced to no specific source, they can be prevented by medicines prescribed by a physician.

Nosebleed

Nosebleeds are usually the result of a ruptured blood vessel. They are especially common among children, and among adults with high blood pressure. If the nosebleed doesn't taper off by itself, the following measures should be taken: the patient should be seated—but not lying down—clothing loosened, and a cold compress placed on the back of the neck and the nose. The soft portion of the nostril may be pressed gently against the bony cartilage of the nose for at least six minutes, or rolled wads of absorbent cotton may be placed inside each nostril, with part of the cotton sticking out to make its removal easier. The inserted cotton should be left in place for several hours and then gently withdrawn.

Fainting

Fainting is a sudden loss of consciousness, usually caused by an insufficient supply of blood and oxygen to the brain. Among the most common causes of fainting are fear, acute hunger, the sight of blood, and prolonged standing in a room with too little fresh air. Fainting should not be confused with a loss of consciousness resulting from excessive alcohol intake or insulin shock. A person about to faint

usually feels dizzy, turns pale, and feels weak in the knees.

Treatment

If possible, the person should be made to lie down, or to sit with his head between his knees for several minutes. Should he lose consciousness, place him so that his legs are slightly higher than his head, loosen his clothing, and see that he gets plenty of fresh air. If smelling salts or aromatic spirits of ammonia are available, they can be held under his nose. With these procedures, he should revive in a few minutes. If he doesn't, a physician should be called.

Troubles Along the Digestive Tract

From childhood on, most people are occasionally bothered by minor and temporary disturbances connected with digestion. Most of the disturbances listed below can be treated successfully with common sense and, if need be, a change in habits.

The Mouth

The digestive processes begin in the mouth, where the saliva begins chemically to break down some foods into simpler components, and the teeth and the tongue start the mechanical breakdown. Disorders of the teeth such as a malocclusion or poorly fitted dentures that interfere with proper chewing, should promptly be brought to the attention of a dentist.

Inflammation of the Gums

Also known as *gingivitis,* inflammation of the gums is caused by the bacteria that breed in food trapped in the spaces between the gums and the teeth. The gums become increasingly swollen, may bleed easily, and be sore enough to interfere with proper chewing. The condition can be prevented by cleaning the teeth thoroughly and frequently, which includes the use of dental floss or the rubber tip on the toothbrush to remove any food particles lodged in the teeth after eating. Because gingivitis can develop into the more serious condition of *pyorrhea,* persistent gum bleeding or soreness should receive prompt professional treatment. See Ch. 22, *The Teeth and Gums.*

Canker Sores

Canker sores are small ulcers inside the lips, mouth, and cheeks. Their specific cause is unknown, but they seem to accompany or follow a virus infection, vitamin deficiency, or emotional stress. They may be additionally irritated by citrus fruit, chocolate, or nuts. A canker sore usually clears up in about a week without special treatment. A bland mouth rinse will relieve pain and, in some cases, speed the healing process.

Coated Tongue

Although a coated tongue is commonly supposed to be a sure sign of illness, this is not the case. The condition may occur because of a temporary lack of saliva.

Glossitis

Glossitis, an inflammation of the tongue causing the tongue's surface to become bright red or, in some cases, glazed in appearance, may be a symptom of an infection elsewhere in the body. It may also be a symptom of anemia or a nutritional deficiency, or it may be an adverse reaction to certain forms of medication. If the in-flammation persists and is accompanied by acute soreness, it should be called to a physician's attention.

Halitosis or Bad Breath

Contrary to the millions of commercial messages on television and in print, bad breath cannot be cured by any mouthwash, lozenge, spray, or antiseptic gargle now on the market. These products can do no more than mask the odor until the basic cause is diagnosed and cured. Among the many conditions that may result in bad breath (leaving out such fleeting causes as garlic and onions) are the following: an infection of the throat, nose, or mouth; a stomach or kidney disorder; pyorrhea; respiratory infection; tooth decay; improper mouth hygiene; and excessive drinking and smoking. Anyone who has been made self-conscious about the problem of bad breath should ask his physician or dentist whether his breath is truly offensive and if it is, what to do about it.

Gastritis

Gastritis, one of the most common disorders of the digestive system, is an inflammation of the lining of the stomach that may occur in acute, chronic, or toxic form. Among the causes of *acute gastritis* are various bacterial or viral infections; overeating, especially heavy or rich foods; excessive drinking of alcoholic beverages; or food poisoning. An attack of acute gastritis may be severely painful, but the discomfort usually subsides with proper treatment. The first symptom is typically sharp stomach cramps, followed by a bloated feeling, loss of appetite, headache, and nausea. When vomiting occurs, it rids the stomach of the substance causing the attack but usually leaves the patient temporarily weak. If painful cramps persist and are accompanied by fever, a physician should be consulted about the possibility of medication for bacterial infection. For a few days after an attack of acute gastritis, the patient should stay on a bland diet of easily digested foods, taken in small quantities.

Toxic Gastritis

Toxic gastritis is usually the result of swallowing a poisonous substance, causing vomiting and possible collapse. It is an emergency condition requiring prompt first aid treatment and the attention of a physician. See "Poisoning" in Ch. 31, *Medical Emergencies.*

Chronic Gastritis

Chronic gastritis is a recurrent or persisting inflammation of the stomach lining over a lengthy period. The condition has the symptoms associated with indigestion, especially pain after eating. It can be caused by excessive drinking of alcoholic beverages, constant tension or anxiety, or deficiencies in the diet. The most effective treatment for chronic gastritis is a bland diet from which caffeine and alcohol have been eliminated. Heavy meals should be avoided in favor of eating small amounts at frequent intervals. A tranquilizer or a mild sedative prescribed by a physician may reduce the tensions that contribute to the condition. If the discomfort continues, a physician should be consulted about the possibility of ulcers. See Ch. 11, *Diseases of the Digestive System.*

Gastroenteritis

Gastroenteritis is an inflammation of the lining of both the stomach and the intestines. Like gastritis, it can occur in acute or toxic forms as a result of food poisoning, excessive alcohol intake, viral or bacterial infections, or food allergies. Vomiting, diarrhea, and fever may be more pronounced and of longer duration. As long as nausea and vomiting persist, no food or fluid should be taken; when these symptoms cease, a bland, mainly fluid diet consisting of strained broth, thin cereals, boiled eggs, and tea is best. If fever continues and diarrhea doesn't taper off, a physician should be called.

Diarrhea

Diarrhea is a condition in which bowel movements are abnormally frequent and liquid. It may be accompanied by cramps, vomiting, thirst, and a feeling of tenderness in the abdominal region. Diarrhea is always a symptom of some irritant in the intestinal tract; among possible causes are allergy, infection by virus or bacteria, accidentally swallowed poisonous substances, or excessive alcohol. Brief attacks are sometimes caused by emotions, such as overexcitement or anxiety.

Diarrhea that lasts for more than two days should be diagnosed by a physician to rule out a more serious infection, a glandular disturbance, or a tumor. Mild attacks can be treated at home by giving the patient a light, bland diet, plenty of fluids, and the prescribed dosage of a kaolin-pectin compound available at any drugstore.

Constipation

Many people have the mistaken notion that if they don't have a bowel movement every day, they must be constipated. This is not necessarily so. From a physician's viewpoint, constipation is determined not by an arbitrary schedule of when the bowel should be evacuated but by the indi-

vidual's discomfort and other unpleasant symptoms. In too many instances, overconcern and anxiety about bowel movements may be the chief cause of constipation.

The watery waste that results from the digestion of food in the stomach and small intestine passes into the large intestine, or colon, where water is absorbed from the waste. If the waste stays in the large intestine for too long a time, so much water is removed that it becomes too solid and compressed to evacuate easily. The efficient removal of waste material from the large intestine depends on wavelike muscular contractions. When these waves are too weak to do their job properly, as often happens in the elderly or the excessively sedentary, a physician may recommend a mild laxative or mineral oil.

Treatment

Constipation is rarely the result of an organic disorder. In most cases, it is caused by poor health habits; when these are corrected, the disorder corrects itself. Often, faulty diet is a major factor. Make sure that meals contain plenty of roughage in the form of whole-grain cereals, fruit, and leafy green vegetables. Figs, prunes, and dates should be included from time to time. Plenty of liquid intake is important, whether in the form of juices, soups, or large quantities of water. Scheduling a certain amount of exercise each day strengthens the abdominal muscles and stimulates muscle activity in the large intestine. Confronting the sources of worries and anxieties, if necessary with a trained therapist, may also be helpful.

An enema or a laxative should be considered only once in a while rather than as regular treatment. The colon should be given a chance to function properly without relying on artificial stimulation. If constipation resists

these commonsense approaches, the problem should be talked over with a physician.

Hemorrhoids

Hemorrhoids, commonly called *piles,* are swollen veins in the mucous membrane inside or just outside the rectum. When the enlargement is slight, the only discomfort may be an itching sensation in the area. Acute cases are accompanied by pain and bleeding. Hemorrhoids are a very common complaint and occur in people of all ages. They are usually the result of straining to eliminate hard, dry stools. The extra pressure causes a fold of the membranous rectal lining to slip down, thus pinching the veins and irritating them.

Because hemorrhoids may be a symptom of a disorder other than constipation, they should be treated by a physician. If neglected, they may bleed frequently and profusely enough to cause anemia. Should a blood clot develop in an irritated vein, surgery may be necessary.

Treatment

Advertised cures should be avoided because they are not only ineffective but can cause additional irritation. Laxatives and cathartics, which may temporarily solve the problem of constipation, are likely to aggravate hemorrhoids.

If pain or bleeding becomes acute, a physician should be consulted promptly. Treatment can be begun at home. Sitting for several minutes in a hot bath in the morning and again in the evening (more frequently if necessary) will provide temporary relief. Preventing constipation is of the utmost importance.

Anal Fissure

This is a condition in which a crack or

split or ulcerated place develops in the area of the two anal sphincters, or muscle rings, that control the release of feces. Such breaks in the skin are generally caused by something sharp in the stool, or by the passage of an unusually hard and large stool. Although discomfort often accompanies a bowel movement when there is a fissure, the acute pain typically comes afterward. Healing is difficult because the injured tissue is constantly open to irritation. If the condition persists, it usually has to be treated by a minor surgical procedure. Intense itching in this area is called *anal pruritis*.

Minor Ailments in the Air Pipes

In addition to all the respiratory discomforts that go along with the common cold, there are various other ailments that affect breathing and normal voice production.

Bronchitis

Usually referred to as a chest cold, *bronchitis* is an inflammation of the bronchial tubes that connect the windpipe and the lungs. If bronchitis progresses down into the lungs, it can develop into pneumonia. Old people and children are especially susceptible to acute bronchitis. The symptoms include pain in the chest, a feeling of fatigue, and a nagging cough. If the infection is bacterial, it will respond to antibiotics. If it is viral, there are no specific medicines. The attack usually lasts for about ten days, although recovery may be speeded up with bed rest and large fluid intake.

Chronic Bronchitis

Chronic bronchitis is a condition that may recur each winter, or may be present throughout the year in the form of a constant cough. The condition is aggravated by smoking and by irritants such as airborne dust and smog. The swollen tissues and abnormally heavy discharge of mucus interfere with the flow of air from the lungs and cause shortness of breath. Medicines are available that lessen the bronchial phlegm and make breathing easier. People with chronic bronchitis often sleep better if they use more than one pillow and have a vaporizer going at night.

Coughing

Coughing is usually a reflex reaction to an obstruction or irritation in the trachea (windpipe), pharynx (back of mouth and throat), or bronchial tubes. It can also be the symptom of a disease or a nervous habit. For a simple cough brought on by smoking too much or breathing bad air, medicines can be taken that act as sedatives to inhibit the reflex reaction. Inhaling steam can loosen the congestion (a combination of swollen membranes and thickened mucus) that causes some types of coughs, and hot drinks such as tea or lemonade help to soothe and relax the irritated area. Constant coughing, especially when accompanied by chest pains, should be brought to a physician's attention. For a discussion of whooping cough and croup, see the respective articles under the "Alphabetic Guide to Child Care" in Ch. 2, *The First Dozen Years*.

Laryngitis

Laryngitis is an inflammation of the mucous membrane of the larynx (voice box) that interferes with breathing and causes the voice to become hoarse or disappear altogether. This condition may accompany a sore throat, measles, or whooping cough, or it may result from an allergy. Pro-

longed overuse of the voice, a common occupational hazard of singers and teachers, is also a cause. The best treatment for laryngitis is to go to bed, keep the room cool, and put moisture into the air from a vaporizer, humidifier, or boiling kettle. Don't attempt to talk, even in a whisper. Keep a writing pad within arm's reach and use it to spare your voice. Drinking warm liquids may help to relieve some of the discomfort. If you must go out, keep the throat warmly protected.

Chronic laryngitis may result from too many acute laryngitis attacks, which can cause the mucous membrane to become so thick and tough that the voice remains permanently hoarse. The sudden onset of hoarseness that lasts for more than two weeks calls for a physician's diagnosis.

Hiccups

Hiccups (also spelled *hiccoughs*) are contractions of the diaphragm, the great muscle responsible for forcing air in and out of our lungs. They may be brought on by an irritation of the diaphragm itself, of the respiratory or digestive system, or by eating or drinking too rapidly. Common remedies for hiccups include sipping water slowly, holding the breath, and putting something cold on the back of the neck. Breathing into a paper bag is usually effective because after a few breaths, the high carbon dioxide content in the bag will serve to make the diaphragm contractions more regular, rather than spasmodic. If none of these measures helps, it may be necessary to have a physician prescribe a sedative or tranquilizer.

The Sensitive Eyes and Ears

Air pollution affects not only the lungs but the eyes as well. In addition to all the other hazards to which the eyes are exposed, airborne smoke, chemicals, and dust cause the eyes to burn, itch, and shed tears. Other common eye troubles are discussed below.

Sty

This pimplelike inflammation of the eyelid is caused by infection, which may be linked to the blocking of an eyelash root or an oil gland, or to general poor health. A sty can be treated at home by applying clean compresses of hot water to the area for about 15 minutes at a time every two hours. This procedure should cause the sty to open, drain, and heal. If sties are recurrent, a health checkup may be indicated.

Pinkeye

Pinkeye, an acute form of *conjunctivitis,* is an inflammation of the membrane that lines the eyelid and covers the eyeball, causing the eyes to become red and the lids to swell and stick together while one is sleeping. The condition may result from bacterial or viral infection—in which case it is extremely contagious—or from allergy or chemical irritation. A physician should be consulted.

Conjunctivitis can be treated by washing the eyes with warm water, drying them with a disposable tissue to prevent the spread of infection, and applying a medicated yellow oxide of mercury ophthalmic ointment (as recommended by your physician) on the inner edges of the lids. This should be done upon rising in the morning and upon retiring at night. The eyes should then be closed until the ointment has spread. Apply compresses of hot water three or four times a day for five-minute periods.

Eyestrain

Eyestrain—with symptoms of fatigue, tearing, redness, and a scratchy feeling in the eyelids—can be caused by a need for corrective glasses, by a disorder of the eye, or by overuse of the eyes. One of the most common causes of eyestrain, however, is improper lighting. Anyone engaged in close work, such as sewing or miniature model building, and at all times when reading, should have light come from behind and from the side so that no shadow falls on the book or object being scrutinized. The light should be strong enough for comfort—not dazzling. Efforts should be made to avoid a shiny or highly polished work surface that produces a glare. To avoid eyestrain when watching television, be sure the picture is in sharp focus; the viewer should sit at least six feet from the screen; and see that the room is not in total darkness.

Ear Infections

Ear infections related to colds, sore throats, or tonsillitis can now be kept from spreading and entering the mastoid bone by the use of sulfa drugs and antibiotics. Any acute earache should therefore be called to a physician's attention promptly. Aspirin can be taken for temporary relief from pain; holding a heating pad or a hot-water bottle to the affected side of the face may also be helpful until proper medication can be prescribed.

Earwax

An excessive accumulation of earwax can sometimes cause pain as well as interfere with hearing. When the ear canal is blocked in this way, gently rotating a small wad of cotton may clean it. The ears should never be cleaned with sharp objects such as hairpins or matchsticks. If earwax has hardened too much to be removed with cotton, it can be softened by a few drops of hydrogen peroxide. When the wax is so deeply and firmly imbedded that it can't be removed at home, a physician may have to flush it out with a syringe.

Ear Blockage

A stopped-up feeling in the ear can be caused by a cold, and also by the change in air pressure experienced when a plane makes a rapid descent. The obstruction of the Eustachian tube can usually be opened by swallowing hard or yawning.

Ringing in the Ear

The general word for a large variety of noises in the ear is *tinnitus.* People who experience such noises describe the sounds in many ways: hissing, ringing, buzzing, roaring, whistling. When they are heard only occasionally for brief periods, without any other symptoms, they can be ignored. However, when they are constant, they should be considered a symptom of some disorder, such as an infection, high blood pressure, allergy, or an improper bite (malocclusion). Sounds in the ears may also be caused be excessive smoking or drinking, or by large doses of aspirin or other medicines. In cases where the source of the ear disturbance can't be diagnosed and the noises become an unsettling nuisance, the physician may recommend a sedative or tranquilizer.

The Path from the Kidneys

Cystitis

Cystitis is the general term for inflammation of the bladder caused by various types of infection. It is more common in women than in men. Infecting microbes may come from outside the body by way of the urethra, or from some other infected organ, such as the kidney. When the bladder becomes inflamed, frequent and painful urination results.

Cystitis may also occur as a consequence of other disorders, such as enlargement of the prostate gland, a structural defect of the male urethra, or stones or a tumor in the bladder. Although there is no completely reliable way to prevent cystitis, some types of infection can be prevented by cleansing the genital region regularly so that the entrance of the urethra is protected against bacterial invasion. Cystitis is usually cured by medicines prescribed by a physician. For a detailed discussion of cystitis and related conditions affecting women, see "Disorders of the Urinary System" in Ch. 25, *Women's Health*.

Prostatitis

Prostatitis is an inflammation of the prostate gland (present in males only), caused by an infection of the urinary tract or some other part of the body. It may occur as a result of venereal infection. The symptoms of painful and excessive urination generally respond favorably to antibiotics. *Acute prostatitis* is less common: the patient is likely to have a high fever, as well as a discharge of pus from the penis. These symptoms should be brought to a physician's attention without delay.

Excessive Urination

A need to empty the bladder with excessive frequency can be merely a nuisance caused by overexcitement or tension, or it can be the sign of a disorder of the urinogenital system. A physician should be consulted if the problem persists.

The All-Important Feet

The *podiatrist* is the specialist who treats foot problems. Causes of foot ailments range from lack of cleanliness to ill-fitting shoes and overindulgence in athletic activities (see "Care of the Feet" in Ch. 5, *The Middle Years*, "The Vulnerable Extremities" in Ch. 23, *Aches, Pains, Nuisances, Worries*).

An ache, pain, or other disorder of the foot can be particularly annoying because it usually hampers mobility. A severe problem can keep a person bedridden, sometimes in the hospital, for substantial periods of time. As humans, we move about on our feet. They deserve the best of care from us, as their owners, and from the podiatrist in case a serious problem arises.

Podiatry, the science of foot care, has become more and more important as Americans have taken to athletics and exercises of various kinds. Most of these activities require the use of the feet. Increasing numbers of persons in the adult years are also taking up walking, jogging, or running as diversions or exercises.

Podiatrists believe that some persons "walk old"—they give the appearance, by the way they walk, of greater age than their chronological years. Others "walk young," or walk normally. Those who walk old may be inviting foot problems, and a fact of podiatric science is that every foot problem has its reflection in another part, or other parts, of the body.

By contrast, good foot and body posture often suggests that the owner of the feet enjoys good health in other parts of the body. Foot care may in effect help other body parts to function better. Because many problems with parts of the body remote from the feet make good foot posture and normal walking difficult or impossible, individuals with diverse problems, such as back pains, sometimes go to

a podiatrist for treatment. The back pain may disappear when the feet have been brought into good working order.

Diabetes and the Feet

"Care" for the feet of diabetics means prevention. The diabetic tries to keep his feet so healthy that he avoids major problems. He knows that diabetes affects blood circulation, and that the leg and foot are extremely vulnerable to circulatory problems. Where blood cannot reach a limb or member, gangrene becomes a possibility.

Foot Care

What kind of care serves the diabetic best? Effective care means that the diabetic takes steps quickly to treat such problems as abrasions or ulcers that refuse to heal. Other conditions that warn of possible future problems are dry skin, numbness, and dry or brittle nails. Ulcers that appear in the skin of the foot and that appear to have roots in deeper layers of tissue serve as danger signals. Such ulcers may appear on the site of an injury, cut, or scratch. A physician will usually prescribe medication, dietary adjustments, or other measures.

Ulcers may result from neglect of a corn or callus. But such neglect itself indicates the risks that diabetics incur: they may neglect to have a foot problem such as a corn treated because their disease has, over time, reduced the sensitivity of their feet. They may lose much of their ability to feel pain, heat or cold, or stress in the foot. Because of such problems, diabetics generally follow certain rules of foot care, including the following:

- Give the feet a daily examination for cuts, bruises, or other abnormalities

- Use only prescribed medications in caring for the feet—and avoid over-the-counter preparations

- Visit a podiatrist regularly, as often as once a month, and avoid medical "treatment" of one's own feet or even cutting one's own toenails

- Wash the feet daily in warm, not hot, water and dry them carefully, including the area between the toes

- Use a gentle lubricant on the feet after washing and drying—and never go barefoot

- Avoid the use of items of clothing that may interfere with circulation, including wraparound garters and support hosiery

- Avoid "holey" socks, darned socks, or anything else that may irritate the soles of the feet and

- Avoid constrictive boots or shoes

Jogging and Running

The podiatrist usually tries to learn about a patient's work, his hobbies and sports, and other facts before undertaking treatment. In particular, the podiatrist asks whether the patient runs or jogs or takes part in other strenuous exercises. With such background information, he or she can suggest appropriate treatment.

A podiatrist will advise runners or joggers on the kind of footwear that would be best—especially if problems have been encountered or may be expected. Shoe inserts may be custom-designed if needed. The podiatrist may also advise runners and joggers to run on softer surfaces rather than cement. Jogging or running "in place," without forward movement, is to be avoided if possible; even when jogging inside the home or apartment, the jogger should move from room to room.

Podiatrists point out that even the more serious knee and ankle problems incurred in running and jogging can be treated. "Jogger's ankle," pain resulting from too much jogging and the attendant strain, can be controlled if the jogger will use moderation. Beginning joggers in particular should start slowly and gradually increase their level of participation. Runners' knee problems may be cured in many cases by treatment that enables the feet to carry the weight of the body properly. In part, the treatment requires practice in throwing the body weight onto the balls of the feet, not on the inner sides of the feet. The remainder of the body, including the knees, can be kept in proper alignment with the feet if the weight falls where it should.

Podiatrists also advise runners, joggers, and others taking part in sports to make certain *all* their clothing and equipment are appropriate. That applies especially in skiing, ice-skating, and other sports requiring extensive foot use. Proper equipment helps runners and joggers avoid colds and similar respiratory problems.

With proper equipment, including good shoes, and a moderate approach, runners and joggers can avoid many other potentially troublesome physical difficulties that could require podiatric care. These others include fallen arches; corns, calluses, and bunions; and "aging feet" that grow weaker from lack of proper foot attention.

24

Allergies and Hypersensitivities

*A*llergy is a broad term used to describe an unusual reaction of the body's tissues to a substance that has no noticeable effect on other persons. About 17 out of every 100 persons in America are allergic, or hypersensitive, to one or more substances that are known to precipitate an unusual reaction. Such substances, known as *allergens*, include a variety of irritants, among them mold spores, pollens, animal dander, insect venoms, and house dust. Some individuals are allergic to substances in soap, which produce a skin irritation. Others react to the smell of a rose by sneezing. Still others react with an outbreak of hives, diarrhea, or other symptoms to allergens in foods.

How Allergens Affect the Body

Allergic symptoms can range from itching eyes, running nose, coughing, difficulty in breathing, and welts on the skin to nausea, cramps, and even going into a state of shock, depending upon the severity of the particular individual's sensitivity and response. Almost any part or system of the body can be affected, and almost anything can pose an allergic threat to somebody.

The Role of Antibodies

The system of an allergic individual reacts to such substances in the way it would react to an invading disease organism: by producing *antibodies* whose job it is to neutralize the allergen. In the process of fighting off the effects of the allergen, the body's defense mechanism may overreact by dumping a chemical mediator, *histamine*, indiscriminately into the individual's bloodstream. It is the overabundance of this protective chemical that causes the discomforts associated with allergies.

At the same time, the antibodies can sensitize the individual to the allergen. Then, with each new exposure to the allergen, more antibodies are produced. Eventually the symptoms of allergy are produced whenever the allergen is encountered. Most allergic reactions, including hay fever, asthma, gastrointestinal upsets, and skin rashes, are of the type just described; their effect is more or less immediate. A second type,

known as the delayed type, seems to function without the production of antibodies; contact dermatitis is an example of the delayed type.

Eosinophils

Some individuals seem to be sensitive to only one known allergen, but others are sensitive to a variety of substances. Persons who suffer acute allergic reactions have abnormally high levels of a type of white blood cell called *eosinophil*. The eosinophil contains an enzyme that may have some control over the allergic reaction, and varying degrees of the enzyme's efficiency appear to account for individual differences in the severity of allergic reactions.

Allergic Symptoms in Children

Many of the common allergies appear during the early years of life. It has been estimated that nearly 80 percent of the major allergic problems begin to appear between the ages of 4 and 9. Allergic youngsters may have nasal speech habits, breathe through the mouth, have coughing and wheezing spells, or rub their eyes, nose, and ears because of itching. A not uncommon sign of allergic reaction in a child may be dark circles under the eyes caused by swelling of the mucous membranes to such an extent that blood does not drain properly from the veins under the lower eyelids. Nose twitching and mouth wrinkling also are signs that a youngster has allergic symptoms.

Common Allergens

The allergens responsible for so many unpleasant and uncomfortable symptoms take a variety of forms too numerous and sometimes too obscure for any book to enumerate. Discussed below are some of the more common types of allergens.

Foods

Foods are among the most common causes of allergic reactions. While nearly any food substance is a potential allergen to certain sensitive individuals, those most frequently implicated are cow's milk, orange juice, and eggs, all considered essential in a child's diet. However, substitute foods are almost always available. Many natural foods contain vitamin C, or ascorbic acid, found in orange juice. Ascorbic acid also is available in vitamin tablets. All of the essential amino acids and other nutrients in cow's milk and eggs also can be obtained from other food sources, although perhaps not as conveniently packaged for immediate use. Other common food offenders are chocolate, pork, seafoods, nuts, and berries. An individual may be allergic to the gluten in wheat, rye, and oats, and products made from those grains.

Inhaled Allergens

Allergens also may affect the respiratory tract, bringing on sneezing, coughing, and breathing impairment. The substances involved can be pollens, dust, smoke, perfumes, and various airborne chemicals.

Mold Spores

A person also can become allergic to a certain mold by inhaling the spores, or reproductive particles, of fungus. In the nose, the mold spores trigger a reaction in cells of the tissues beneath the mucous membranes that line the nasal passages. This in turn leads to the symptoms of allergy. Because they are small, mold spores can evade the natural protective mechanisms of the nose and upper respiratory tract to reach the lungs and bring on an allergic reaction in that site. Usually, this leads to the buildup of mucus, wheezing, and difficulty in breathing associated with asthma.

Less frequently, inhaling mold spores can result in skin lesions similar to those of eczema or chronic hives. In all but the very warmest areas of the United States, molds are seasonal allergens, occurring from spring into late fall. But unlike pollens, molds do not disappear with the killing frosts of autumn. Actually, frost may help increase the activity of molds, which thrive on dying vegetation produced by cold temperatures.

Dust and Animal Hair

House dust and animal hair (especially cat and dog hair) are also responsible for respiratory allergies in many people. Asthma attacks are often triggered by contact with these substances. Symptoms of dust allergy are usually most severe in the spring and fall, and tend to subside in the summer.

Man-Made Allergens

An example of respiratory allergy caused by man-made allergens is the complaint known as "meat wrappers' asthma," which results from fumes of the price-label adhesive on the polyvinyl chloride film used to package foods. The fumes are produced when the price label is cut on a hot wire. When the fumes are inhaled, the result is burning eyes, sore throat, wheezing and shortness of breath, upset stomach, and other complaints. Studies show that exposure to the fumes from the heat-activated label adhesive for as little as five minutes could produce airway obstruction in food packagers.

Another source of respiratory allergy is the photochemical smog produced by motor vehicle exhaust in large city areas. The smog is composed of hydrocarbons, oxides of nitrogen, and other chemicals activated by the energy of sunlight. When inhaled in the amounts present along the nation's expressways, the smog has been found to impair the normal function of membranes in the lungs.

Drugs

Medicines and drugs, such as penicillin, or serums used in inoculations, can cause allergic reactions. Estimates of the incidence of allergy among those receiving penicillin range from one to ten percent. The National Institutes of Health has calculated that just three common drugs—penicillin, sulfonamides, and aspirin—account for as much as 90 percent of all allergic drug reactions. The allergic reactions include asthmatic symptoms, skin rash, shock, and other symptoms similar to tissue reactions to other allergens. Medical scientists theorize that chemicals in certain drugs probably combine with protein molecules in the patient's body to form a new substance that is the true allergen. However, it also has been noted that some persons show allergic reactions to placebo drugs, which may contain sugar or inert substances rather than real drugs.

Insect Venom

Insect stings cause serious allergic reactions in about four of every 1,000 persons stung by bees, fire ants, yellow jackets, wasps, or hornets. A single sting to a sensitive person may lead to a serious drop in blood pressure, shock, and possibly death. There are more than 50 reported fatalities a year, and experts suspect that other deaths occur as a result of insect stings but are listed as heart attacks, stroke, or convulsions.

Sensitivity tests of persons who might be acutely allergic to insect stings have been difficult to develop, because allergic individuals reacted in the same way as nonallergic persons to skin tests performed with extracts from insect bodies. More recently, physicians have found that using pure insect venom produces a reaction that determines whether a person is allergic to the sting. Medical scientists also have isolated the major allergen in an insect venom for use in diagnosing and treating patients who are particularly sensitive to stings.

Skin Allergies

Allergies affecting the skin take many forms, the most common being eczema, urticaria (hives), angioedema (swelling of the subcutaneous tissues), and contact dermatitis. Among the most common causes are foods, cosmetics, fabrics, metals, plants and flowers, plastics, insecticides, furs and leather, jewelry, and many industrial chemicals. Studies of patients who seem to be especially sensitive to skin allergies show that they have higher than average amounts of a

body protein called *immunoglobulin E* in their systems.

In certain instances, a person who is sensitive to an allergen in a plant food also may be allergic to the pollen of the plant. The fava bean, for example, produces severe reactions when eaten by individuals who are allergic to the food; inhaling the pollen of the growing plant can cause similar reactions.

Poisonous Plants

Poison ivy, poison oak, and poison sumac contain an extremely irritating oily resin that sensitizes the body; repeated contact seems to increase the severity of the allergic reactions. About 50 percent of the population who come in contact with the resin will experience a severe form of dermatitis, and up to 10 percent will be temporarily disabled by the effects. Exposure to the resin may come from direct contact with the plant, from contact with other objects or animals that have touched the plant, or from inhaling smoke from the burning plant.

Cosmetics and Jewelry

A wide variety of cosmetics and jewelry can cause allergic reactions through skin contact. Even jewelry that is presumably pure gold can contain a certain amount of nickel that will produce a mild reaction that causes a skin discoloration, sometimes aided by chemical activity resulting from perspiration in the area of jewelry contact. Among cosmetics that may be involved in allergic reactions are certain permanent-wave lotions, eyelash dyes, face powders, permanent hair dyes, hair-spray lacquers, and skin-tanning agents. Of course, not all persons are equally sensitive to the ingredients known to be allergens, and in most cases a similar product

with different ingredients can be substituted for the cosmetic causing allergic reactions. For more information on skin allergies, see "Disorders of the Skin" in Ch. 21, *Skin and Hair.*

Environmental Allergies

Environmental agents such as sunlight, excessive cold, and pressure are known to produce allergic reactions in certain individuals. Cold allergy, for example, can result in hives and may even lead to a drop in blood pressure, fainting, severe shock, and sometimes death. Research into the causes of cold allergy has shown that cold urticaria, or hives, results from a histamine released from body tissues as they begin to warm up after a cold stimulus. Extremely high histamine levels coincide with episodes of very low blood pressure, the cause of fainting.

Although reaction of the body tissues to the invasion of microbes, such as bacteria, viruses, and other microorganisms, generally is not thought of as an allergic situation, the manner in which the body musters its defenses against the foreign materials is essentially the same as the way the antibodies are mobilized to neutralize other allergens. Thus, there is a similarity between infectious diseases and allergies.

Temporary Allergies

Occasionally, a change in the body's hormonal balance may trigger a hypersensitivity to a substance that previously had no effect on the individual. Pregnant women are especially susceptible to these temporary allergies, which almost always disappear after childbirth. Some women during pregnancy, on the other hand, experience complete relief from allergies that have plagued them since childhood.

People who suffer from seasonal allergies, such as hay fever, often have heightened allergic reactions to dust, animal dander, and even certain foods, such as chocolate and pineapple, during the season when ragweed pollen or other airborne allergens are plentiful.

Diagnosis of Allergies

Some allergic reactions are outgrown; some don't develop until adulthood; some become increasingly severe over the years because each repeated exposure makes the body more sensitive to the allergen. In many instances, the irritating substance is easily identified, after which it can be avoided. In other cases, it may take a long series of tests before the offending allergen is tracked down.

Medical History

If a person suspects he may have an allergy, the first thing he should do is consult a physician to see if the help of an allergy specialist should be sought. The physician or allergist will first take a complete medical history and check the patient's general health. Not infrequently the source of an allergy can be found by general questioning about the patient's life style. For example, the reaction may occur only on or immediately after the patient eats seafood. Or a patient may have an apparently chronic allergy but be unaware that it may be related to daily meals that include milk and eggs. A patient who keeps several cats or sleeps every night with a dog in the bedroom may not realize that an asthmatic condition actually is an allergic reaction to dander from the fur of a pet animal.

The history taken by the physician will include questions about other known allergies, allergies suffered by other members of the family, variations in symptoms according to the weather, time of day, and season of the year. The symptoms may be related to a change in working conditions or the fact that the symptoms, if perhaps a result of house dust, diminish during periods of outdoor exercise. A person sensitive to cold may unwittingly exacerbate the symptoms with cold drinks, while another person who is sensitive to heat may not realize that symptoms can be triggered by hot drinks but relieved by cold drinks, and so on.

Skin Testing

If the patient is referred to an allergy specialist, the allergist will continue the detective story by conducting skin tests.

Scratch Test

Based on information in the medical history of the patient and the allergist's knowledge of molds, pollens, and other airborne allergens in the geographical area, "the allergist" will conduct what is called a *scratch test*.

A diluted amount of a suspected allergen is applied to a small scratch on the patient's arm or back. If the results of the scratch test are inconclusive, a more sensitive test may be tried.

Intracutaneous Test

In the *intracutaneous* test, a solution of the suspected allergen is injected into the underlayer of skin called the *dermis*. The intracutaneous test also may be used to verify the results of a positive scratch test. With either test, a positive reaction usually consists of a raised reddish welt, or *wheal*. The welt should develop within 15 or 20 minutes if that particular allergen is the cause of the symptoms.

Culture Plates

If the allergen has been identified, or if the allergist still suspects a substance in the environment of the patient despite negative or inconclusive tests, the patient may be given a set of culture plates to place around his home and office or work area. If the allergen has been identified, the culture plates can help the physician and patient learn where his exposure to the substance takes place. If the allergen is not known, the cultures may pick up samples of less common allergens that the specialist can test.

Mucosal Test

Another kind of approach sometimes is used by allergists when skin tests fail to show positive results despite good evidence that a particular allergen is the cause of symptoms. It is called the *mucosal test*. The allergist using the mucosal test applies a diluted solution of the suspected allergen directly to the mucous membranes of the patient, usually on the inner surface of a nostril or by aerosol spray into the bronchial passages. In some cases, the allergic reaction occurs immediately and medication is administered quickly to counter the effects. Because of the possibility of a severe reaction in a hypersensitive patient, the mucosal test is not employed if other techniques seem to be effective.

Relief from Allergies

Other Tests

Allergists have other ways to test for allergies. They can, for example, use the *prick test,* a kind of skin test in which a physician or nurse pricks the skin as many as 30 or 40 times. On each pricked spot a drop of a watery solution is dropped; the solution contains a small amount of one allergen. A red welt appears on the spot within 15 to 30 minutes if the patient is allergic. Using another approach, an *elimination diet,* an allergist may specify a diet that omits certain foods for stated periods. Improvement in the patient's condition while avoiding certain foods usually indicates that the individual has an allergy to that food.

A variation of the prick test involves injection of small amounts of food in solution under the skin or application of the solution under the tongue. If the injection or drops provoke reactions, an allergy is indicated.

Avoidance

For a patient sensitive to a particular type of allergen, such as molds, complete avoidance of the substance can be difficult, but some steps can be taken to avoid undue exposure. For example, the mold allergy sufferer should avoid areas of his home, business, or recreational areas that are likely spots for mold spores to be produced. These would include areas of deep shade or heavy vegetation, basements, refrigerator drip trays, garbage pails, air conditioners, bathrooms, humidifiers, dead leaves or wood logs, barns or silos, breweries, dairies, any place where food is stored, and old foam, rubber pillows and mattresses.

Medication

To supplement avoidance measures, the allergist may prescribe medications that will significantly reduce or relieve the irritating symptoms of the allergic reaction. Antihistamines, corticosteroids, and a drug called cromolyn sodium are among medications that may be prescribed, depending upon the nature and severity of the patient's reactions to the allergen.

Immunotherapy

If avoidance measures and medications do not control the symptoms effectively, the allergist may suggest *immunotherapy.* Immunotherapy consists of injections of a diluted amount of the allergen, a technique similar to that used in the skin tests. A small amount of a very weak extract is injected once or twice a week at first. The strength of the extract is gradually increased, and the injections are given less frequently as relief from the symptoms is realized. The injections are continued until the patient has experienced complete relief of the symptoms for a period of two or three years. However, some people may have to continue the injections for longer time spans. Even though the treatments may relieve the symptoms, they may not cure the allergy.

Identification Cards

Any person subject to severe disabling allergy attacks by a known allergen should carry a card describing both the allergic reaction and the allergen. Detailed information can be obtained from the Asthma and Allergy Foundation of America, 1302 18th St., NW, Washington, DC 20036. See also "Allergic Respiratory Diseases" in Ch. 12, *Diseases of the Respiratory System,* and "Asthma Attack" in Ch. 31, *Medical Emergencies.*

25

Women's Health

The special health matters that are related to a woman's reproductive system belong to the branch of medicine known as *gynecology. Obstetrics* is a closely related specialty associated with pregnancy and childbirth. The distinction is something of a technicality for most patients, since obstetricians usually are quite capable of handling gynecological cases and vice versa. The practice of obstetrics and gynecology is commonly combined in a medical service identified by the contraction *Ob-Gyn.* However, there are medical matters that are specifically concerned with female reproductive organs and related tissues but have little to do with obstetrics. For a discussion of obstetrics, see "Infertility, Pregnancy, and Childbirth" in Ch. 4, *The Beginning of a Family.*

The Gynecological Examination

What should a woman expect on her first visit to a gynecologist? First, the gynecologist will interview her, asking about her family, her medical history, and any fears or apprehensions she may have about her personal health. The woman's answers and comments are written into her medical records for future reference. The information can contain important clues that may help in diagnosing any present or future disorders.

A sample of urine and a sample of blood are usually obtained for laboratory tests. During the ensuing physical examination, the woman lies on a special examination table with her feet in metal stirrups and her knees apart. A nurse will be present to assist the doctor. While she is in the *lithotomy position,* the woman's abdomen will be palpated for lumps or other abnormalities. The breasts also will be palpated for possible lumps. Then an external inspection of the vulva and surrounding areas is made by the physician, followed by internal inspection, in which a speculum is used to spread apart the sides of the vagina so that the cervix is exposed. A digital examination (using the fingers) is made of the walls of the vagina and rectum and the neighboring tissue areas, in a search for possible growths or other abnormal conditions. And a sample of cells and secretions from the cervix is taken for a Pap-smear test.

In addition to the examination of the breasts and reproductive system, the gynecologist usually conducts a general physical examination, recording information about height, weight, blood pressure, heart and lung condition, and so on. The routine physical examination, like the medical history, provides additional clues that, when added to the results of the examination of the breasts and reproductive system, will give a complete picture of the patient's gynecological health.

Following the examination, the gynecologist discusses his appraisal of the woman's condition and answers questions. He will discuss whatever treatment she needs. Medications can be explained at this time, including reasons why certain drugs can or should not be taken. If any surgery or further testing is recommended, those aspects of the health picture also should be discussed in some detail.

Results of some laboratory tests and the Pap smear are not usually available for several days. But the physician or nurse will contact the patient when the results are available and advise if she should return in the near future for follow-up testing. The American Cancer Society and the American College of Physicians and Gynecologists agree (1) that all

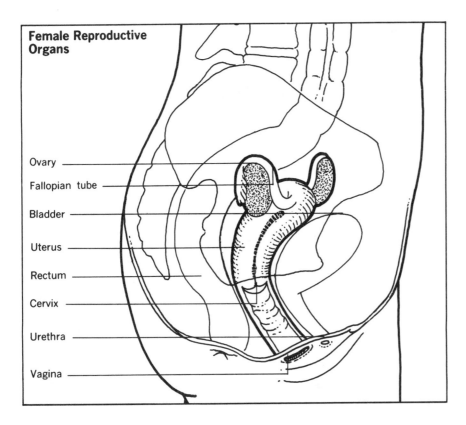

Female Reproductive Organs

Ovary

Fallopian tube

Bladder

Uterus

Rectum

Cervix

Urethra

Vagina

women should have their first Pap smear when they become sexually active or at age 18, whichever occurs first; (2) that every woman should have a yearly Pap smear for the following two years; and (3) that later tests should be administered at the physician's discretion if the first three Pap smears are negative. The woman also should discuss arrangements for future checkups or Pap smear tests rather than wait until signs or symptoms of a serious disorder warrant an immediate visit.

Menstrual Disorders

Among the health concerns of women that specifically belong to gynecology are menstrual disorders. Normally, the first menstrual period (menarche) occurs about age 12 or 13, or sometimes earlier or later. Periods are generally irregular for the first year or two, and then they tend to recur at intervals of 24 to 32 days. Each period begins about two weeks after ovulation, or the release of an egg cell (ovum) from the ovary—unless, of course, the ovum happens to be fertilized in the interval and pregnancy interrupts the whole process.

The menstrual flow, which lasts from three to seven days, is composed mainly of serum, mucus, and dead cells shed from the lining (endometrium) of the uterus. The loss of blood is minimal, usually from two to four ounces. The volume of flow, as well as the time schedule, tends to be fairly regular for most women. When one's menstrual pattern varies noticeably from the expected pattern, and in the absence of pregnancy, it may be a sign of a physical or emotional disorder.

Amenorrhea

Failure to menstruate is called *amenorrhea*. Amenorrhea is a natural effect of pregnancy and of nursing a baby. In an older woman, it may be a sign of menopause. But if a nonpregnant or nonnursing woman after menarche and before menopause (say between the ages of 17 or 18 and 52) fails to menstruate for two or more periods, she should bring it to the attention of a doctor—unless, of course, she has undergone a hysterectomy or other surgical or medical treatment that eliminates menstruation.

Primary Amenorrhea

When menarche has not occurred by the age of 16 or 17, the absence of menstruation is called *primary amenorrhea*. In such a case, a physical examination may show that an imperforate hymen or a closed cervix is obstructing the flow of menses, or a congenital defect may be interfering with menstruation. In almost all cases, menarche can be started with a bit of minor surgery, by treatment of any existing systemic disease, or by the injection of sex hormones; or it will start spontaneously later.

Secondary Amenorrhea

When menstrual periods cease after menarche, the condition is known as *secondary,* or *acquired, amenorrhea*. Secondary amenorrhea may involve missing a single menstrual period or many periods in consecutive months. Among possible causes of interrupted menstruation are certain medications, drugs of abuse, emotional stress, normal fluctuations in ovarian activity in the first few years after menarche, and a number of organic diseases. Medicines that can disrupt normal menstrual activity include tranquilizers and other psychotropic (mind-affecting) drugs that apparently influence hormonal activity in the brain centers, amphetamines, and oral contraceptives. When a particular medication is found to be the cause of amenorrhea, the medical treatment may be judged to be more important than maintaining normal menstrual cycles. When the use of oral contraceptives is followed by amenorrhea for six or more months, normal menstrual activity may resume eventually, but it can often be started sooner by a prescribed medication. Among drugs of abuse known to cause amenorrhea are alcohol and opium-based drugs.

Just as the mind-altering effects of psychotropic drugs involve the hypothalamus and pituitary glands in the brain, which control the hormones that regulate menstrual functions, emotional stress seems to have a parallel influence on the incidence of amenorrhea. *Anorexia nervosa,* a disorder associated with emaciation resulting from an emotional disturbance, also can result in an interruption of menstruation.

Other factors contributing to secondary amenorrhea are measles, mumps, and other infections; cysts and tumors of the ovaries; changes in the tissues lining the vagina or uterus; premature aging of the ovaries; diabetes; obesity; anemia; leukemia; and Hodgkin's disease. In many cases, normal or near-normal menstrual function can be restored by medical treatment, such as administration of hormones, or by surgery, or both. In one type of amenorrhea, marked by adhesion of the walls of the uterus, curettage (scraping of the uterus) is followed by insertion of an intrauterine contraceptive device (IUD) to help hold the uterine walls apart.

Menorrhagia

Almost the opposite of amenorrhea is *menorrhagia,* an excessive menstrual flow. The causes of menorrhagia are as varied as those associated with amenorrhea. They include influenza and other infectious diseases, emotional stress, polyps of the cervical or uterine tissues, hypertension, congestive heart failure, leukemia, and blood coagulation disorders. Menorrhagia may occur during the early stages of a young woman's reproductive life soon after reaching puberty, and medical treatment may be necessary to control the excessive loss of blood. In some cases, dilation and curettage is recommended in addition to the administration of hormones and other medications, such as iron tablets to correct anemia resulting from the loss of red blood cells.

Dilation and Curettage

Dilation and curettage, generally referred to as *D and C,* is a procedure in which the cervix is dilated and the cavity of the uterus is cleaned out by a scooplike instrument, a curette. The same procedure is sometimes used to abort an embryo or to remove a tumor or a polyp.

Although it takes only a few minutes to perform a D and C, the procedure is done in a hospital while the patient is anesthetized. There is no afterpain, only a dull discomfort in the lower pelvic region similar to menstrual awareness.

A physical examination is usually made to determine if there are tumors anywhere in the reproductive organs. Except where tumors are found to be a causative factor, most women will resume normal menstrual cycles after treatment of menorrhagia with medications and D and C. For women beyond the age of 40, the physician may recommend a hysterectomy to prevent recurrence of excessive menstrual blood loss.

Polymenorrhea and Metrorrhagia

These medical terms refer to two other ways in which menstrual periods may depart from typical patterns. *Polymenorrhea* is abnormally frequent menstruation, so that menstrual periods occur at intervals of less than 21 days. This short interval may be the natural established pattern for some women. If it is not, the cause may be physical or emotional stress. *Metrorrhagia* is marked by menstrual bleeding that occurs erratically at unpredictable times. It may be the result of a cyst in the lining of the uterus, a tumor in the reproductive tract, polyps, or some hormonal imbalance, including a disorder of the thyroid gland.

Dysmenorrhea

Abdominal or pelvic pain occurring just before or along with the onset of menstruation is known as *dysmenorrhea.* The symptoms include severe colicky abdominal cramps, backache, headache, and, in some cases, nausea and vomiting. As with amenorrhea, there are two general types of dysmenorrhea, primary and secondary.

Primary Dysmenorrhea

This type includes all cases in which no organic disorder is associated with the symptoms, which are presumed to be a result of uterine contractions and emotional factors. More than 75 percent of all cases are of this type. Primary dysmenorrhea generally begins before age 25, but it may appear at any time from menarche to menopause. It frequently ends with the birth of the first child.

Since primary dysmenorrhea by definition occurs in the absence of organic disease, the diagnosis can be made only after a careful medical history is compiled and a special study of the reproductive organs is made to ensure that no disorder has been overlooked. In some cases, oral contraceptives may be prescribed because of the effect such drugs have in suppressing ovulation; the contraceptives prevent the natural production of the hormone progesterone, which is responsible for certain tissue changes associated with the discomfort of dysmenorrhea. Analgesic drugs to relieve pain and medications that help to relax muscles may be prescribed. Medication is often less beneficial, however, than emotional support—including the easing of any stress at home, school, or work, and reassurance about the worries sometimes associated with menstruation.

Secondary Dysmenorrhea

This condition comprises all menstrual pain that is a result of or associated with an organic disease of the reproductive organs, such as endometriosis, to cite just one example. Secondary dysmenorrhea can occur at any age.

Premenstrual Syndrome

Premenstrual syndrome (PMS) has emerged in recent years as a major challenge to the medical profession. PMS clinics have begun to offer specialized counseling, physical examinations, and treatment for women unable to cope with the disorder. Treatment regimens or therapies range from aspirin to large doses of sex hormones, diet programs, and exercise.

A group of related symptoms, PMS involves both psychological and physical changes. Among the psychological are lethargy, tension, irritability, depression, and feelings of aggression. The physical signs may include headache, bloating, asthma,

and more exotic problems, such as recurrent herpes or hives. In all, more than 300 different symptoms have been attributed to PMS.

The symptoms, gynecologists warn, should become "disturbing" before they are labeled PMS. Restlessness, minor cramps, and other premenstrual problems may indicate that menstruation is about to start but do not necessarily point to PMS. Such minor problems are called *menstrual molimina*. Cramping and other painful conditions occurring during menstruation are referred to as *dysmenorrhea* (see above).

Of the many treatments for PMS, none has proved uniformly effective. This is because the cause or causes of PMS are not totally understood. Most commonly, physicians believe the disorder represents some basic imbalance in the major female hormones, estrogen and progesterone. Thus one treatment calls for administration of "natural" progesterone to correct the supposed imbalance.

Another common treatment suggested for PMS is vitamin B_6, although the treatment remains partly experimental. Some researchers and physicians, however, have reported

disturbing neurological side-effects.

Other theories and treatments exist. Some physicians who have studied PMS and its symptoms believe *prolactin*, a pituitary hormone that stimulates milk secretion, and PMS are associated. A diet and nutrition theory has evolved out of findings that some women report improvement after going on a hypoglycemic diet.

Treated over a substantial period, PMS victims often find that diagnostic tests combined with diet and exercise regimens and vitamin therapy bring good results. If such initial attempts fail, the physician may prescribe medications. In all cases of PMS, according to researchers, psychological support for the sufferer may be important to treatment effectiveness.

Minor Menstrual Problems

Blood Clots

There is not usually any cause for alarm if blood clots are expelled during menstruation. Ordinarily, the menstrual flow is completely liquefied, but a few clots tend to appear

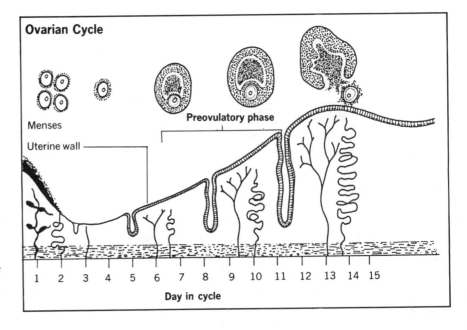

Ovarian Cycle

Menses

Uterine wall

Preovulatory phase

Day in cycle

when the flow is profuse. However, if many clots appear and the flow seems excessive, medical advice is recommended, since these conditions may be a sign of fibroid tumors in the uterus.

Oral Contraceptives

Women on combination birth-control pills can expect to see a changed menstrual pattern. The flow becomes slighter than before and very regular. For a discussion of oral contraceptives, see "Family Planning" in Ch. 4, *The Beginning of a Family.*

Odor

The menstrual flow of a healthy woman generally has a mild odor that develops when it is exposed to the air or to the vulva. Some women are concerned about this odor, although it usually is not offensive. When it is, it tends to be associated with inadequate bathing. Detergents are added to some commercial tampons and pad products, and special deodorants have been developed to mask the odor. However, such materials produce allergic reactions in some women, and they can have the unfortunate effect of masking an odor that may be the sign of an abnormal condition.

Onset of Menopause

Menstrual irregularities almost always precede the natural cessation of menstrual function. For a full discussion of menopause, see Ch. 5, *The Middle Years.*

Postmenopausal Bleeding

Bleeding that occurs after the final cessation of menstrual activity should be seen as an urgent signal to seek medical advice. The bleeding may be painless or painful and may range from occasional spotting that is brownish or bright red to rather profuse bleeding that continues for several days or more. The various signs and symptoms should be noted carefully because they can help suggest to a physician the possible cause of bleeding. Bleeding after the menopause is often a sign of cancer of the cervix or the lining of the uterus, but there is a wide variety of other possible causes, including polyps, ulcers, hypertensive heart disease, an ovarian tumor, or infection. In many cases, the problem can be treated by dilation and curettage or withdrawal of any hormone medications, such as estrogens prescribed for menopausal symptoms, or both. In these cases, if D and C and treatment and discontinuance of hormone therapy fail, the physician may advise a hysterectomy.

Infections of the Reproductive Tract

Vaginal and other reproductive tract infections are among the most common gynecological problems, and among the most stubborn to treat successfully.

Leukorrhea

A whitish, somewhat viscid discharge from the vagina, which is known medically as *leukorrhea,* may be quite normal, especially if it is not continual but occurs only intermittently—prior to menstruation, for example, or associated with sexual excitation. It may also be increased when oral contraceptives are used.

Constant leukorrhea, on the other hand, often is a symptom of an abnormality. Leukorrhea resulting from disease can occur at any age. It is generally associated with an infection of the lower reproductive tract. The discharge may occur without any discomfort, but in some cases there is itching, irritation, and *dyspareunia*—or painful intercourse.

Laboratory tests of vaginal secretions may be needed to help identify the precise cause of the discharge. Leukorrhea can result from vaginal ulcers; a tumor of the vagina, uterus, or

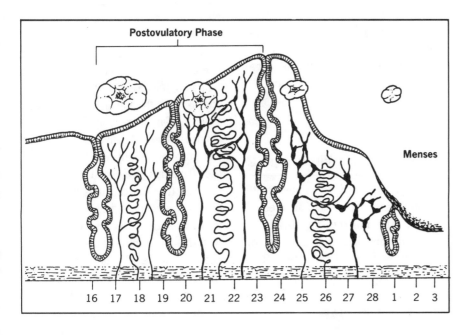

Postovulatory Phase

Menses

16 17 18 19 20 21 22 23 24 25 26 27 28 1 2 3

fallopian tubes; gonorrhea; or infection by any of various disease organisms of the vulva, vagina, cervix, uterus, or tubes. It may also result from an abnormality of menstrual function, or even emotional stress.

Treatment, of course, depends on the cause. If the discharge is because of an infection, care must be taken to avoid being reinfected or transmitting the disease organism through sexual contact or possibly contaminated underclothing, etc.

Moniliasis

Moniliasis, also known as *candidiasis,* is an infection by a yeastlike fungus that invades mucous membrane and sometimes skin in various parts of the body. Inside the mouth, the organism causes thrush, most commonly in babies. When the organism invades the vaginal area, it causes a scant white discharge of a thick consistency resembling that of cottage cheese. There is itching, burning, and swelling of the labial and vulvar areas. The symptoms tend to worsen just before the menstrual period. The occurrence of the disease is thought by some researchers to be fostered by oral contraceptives. Antibiotic therapy, may increase the moniliasis organism, because it destroys many of the benign organisms that regularly share the same environment.

Moniliasis is treated with suppositories, creams, and other medications. The woman's partner should be treated at the same time to prevent a cycle of reinfection because the fungus will otherwise spread to the genital tissues of the man.

Trichomoniasis

A type of leukorrhea that consists of a copious yellow to green frothy and fetid discharge is caused by infection by the *Trichomonas* organism. The organism causes an irritating itching condition that tends to set in or worsen just after a menstrual period. The condition is diagnosed by a test similar to a Pap smear, made with a specimen taken from the vagina. Trichomonas organisms, if present, are easy to identify under a microscope; they are pear-shaped protozoa with three to five whiplike tails.

The organism favors warm, moist areas, such as genital tissues, but it can also survive in damp towels and washcloths, around toilet seats, and on beaches and the perimeters of swimming pools. Thus it can spread from one member of a family to other members and from one woman to other women. *Trichomoniasis* is not technically a venereal disease, but it can be transmitted by sexual contact. When one partner is infected with trichomoniasis, both must be treated at the same time and a condom must be worn during intercourse.

Several drugs are available for treating trichomoniasis, including tablets taken orally and suppositories inserted in the vagina. The tablets are taken for ten days, then an examination is made to determine if any *Trichomonas* organisms are still present. Medication may be continued for several months if the infection resists the drug—studies show that the organism appears to survive in about 10 percent of treated cases.

Herpes Simplex Virus Type 2

Herpes is acquired by contact with the mucous membranes of an infected person. The mucous membrane of the mouth and lips, the genitals, or the rectum may be affected. The causative agent is known as *herpes simplex virus Type II,* or *HSV-II*. It is similar to but not the same as the virus that causes fever blisters, or cold sores, which is Type *I* (HSV-I). The virus is associated with some spontaneous abortions. If the mother has blisters at the time of delivery, the virus can be transmitted to the baby as he or she passes through the vagina. The central nervous system, including the brain, may be damaged by the virus if the baby becomes infected. To avoid exposure to the virus, a caesarian delivery is recommended.

Symptoms

Patients with their first HSV-II infection usually complain of intense itching, painful blisterlike eruptions, and ulcerated patches with a discharge. Other symptoms may include genital pain and vaginal bleeding. Fever, swelling, difficult urination, and a general feeling of ill health and lack of appetite may accompany the infection.

Symptoms may subside after a few weeks, but recurrences are common, though they are less painful and of shorter duration. There is no known cure for the viral infection.

Treatment

No drug has been found to attack the viruses while they are "hibernating" in cells at the base of the spine. But one antiviral drug, *acyclovir,* has been found to reduce recurrent outbreaks and to block flareups for up to several months. Taken orally in pill form, acyclovir is ingested daily. Some patients can stop treatment and have no further flare-ups. Researchers have discovered that the capsules kill or neutralize the herpes viruses only when they are active. Because of evidence that the virus may be related to the subsequent development of cervical cancer, women sufferers should have Pap-smear tests at intervals of six months instead of the usual twelve.

Pelvic Inflammatory Disease

Pelvic inflammatory disease, or PID, is on the increase in the female population. Commonly caused by bacteria from other diseases such as chlamydia or gonorrhea, PID may go for years without detection. Frequently symptomless, PID infects and destroys the interior of the reproductive system. It attacks the fallopian tubes and uterine lining, leaving permanent scarring. The increase in the number of ectopic pregnancies (fallopian tube pregnancies) is believed to stem from the increase in women who have scarring from PID. The increase in sterility in the population is also linked directly to PID scarring.

One is seven women in the United States has been infected with PID. Treatment for both partners involves antibiotics to kill the bacteria, and treatment of any original disease that may have caused it. Douching should be avoided if PID is suspected. Symptoms include abdominal tenderness or pain, vaginal discharge, or dull ache or twitching in the uterine cavity.

Blood tests and cultures for chlamydia or other diseases should be done. Two-thirds of PID cases are from sexual transmission. If left untreated, PID can cause sterility, miscarriage, ectopic pregnancy, blood infection, and eventually death.

Disorders of the Urinary System

Both men and women are subject to disorders of the urinary system, but there are a few disorders that affect women chiefly or women only, for reasons related to anatomical structure. See also Ch. 17, *Diseases of the Urinogenital System.*

Inflammation of the Bladder

Any inflammation of the bladder is known medically as *cystitis.* Factors such as urinary tract stones, injury, and obstructions to the normal flow of urine can aggravate or cause cystitis in either sex. Cystitis resulting from infectious organisms, however, is much more common in women than in men. This is understandable in view of the relative shortness of the female urethra—the tube through which urine is discharged from the bladder and through which infectious organisms can reach the bladder from the outside. In addition, the anus and the vagina, both of which may frequently be sources of infection, are situated relatively close to the external opening of the female urethra.

In women generally, the symptoms of cystitis may include a burning sensation around the edges of the vulva. There is usually a frequent urge to urinate and difficulty or pain (*dysuria*) associated with urination. Urinary retention and dehydration, which are generally under the control of the individual, can contribute to the spread of infection once it begins. The lining of the urinary bladder is relatively resistant to infection by most microorganisms as long as the normal flow of liquids through the urinary tract is maintained. In cases that do not yield quickly to copious fluid intake, there are medications that may be prescribed to cure the infection. Where urinary frequency or difficulty is accompanied by the appearance of blood in the urine, a physician should be consulted immediately.

Honeymoon Cystitis

One type of cystitis tends to occur mostly in young women during the first few weeks of frequent sexual activity, to which it is attributed. Sexual activity may result in swelling of the urethra and the neck of the bladder, making urination difficult. The inflammation of these tissues can in turn make them more susceptible to infection. A treatment recommended specifically for honeymoon cystitis is to drink large quantities of water or other fluids and to empty the bladder before and after engaging in sexual intercourse. Adequate lubrication, such as petroleum jelly, is also important. Medical care should be sought if the condition persists.

Urethral Disorders

The urethra is perforce involved in the inflammation of cystitis because it is the route by which infectious organisms reach the bladder. In addition, there are disorders that are essentially confined to the urethra.

Urethral Caruncle

Urethral caruncle is a rather uncommon urinary tract disorder that tends to be confined to women after the menopause. A *caruncle* (not to be confused with *carbuncle*) is a small, red, fleshy outgrowth. It may be visible near the opening of the urethra. A caruncle growing from the cells of the urethra may be a sign of a bacterial infection, a tumor, or any of several other possible conditions. Symptoms may include vaginal bleeding, pain, tenderness, painful sexual intercourse (dyspareunia), a whitish, viscid discharge, and difficulty in urinating. A physician should be consulted when such symptoms are present. A tissue biopsy and Pap smear may be taken to diagnose the condition. Caruncles are easily treated and of no long-term consequence.

Urethral Diverticulum

Another disorder of the urethra is a *urethral diverticulum,* or outpocket-

The Female Urinary System

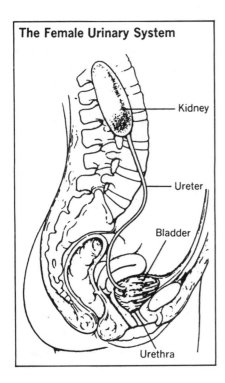

Kidney

Ureter

Bladder

Urethra

ing of the urethra. The problem can be caused by a developmental malformation, an injury, inflammation, a cyst, a urinary stone, or a venereal disease. Stones are a common cause, and in some patients there may be more than one diverticulum. The symptoms may include discomfort and urinary difficulty, as well as dyspareunia. The disorder can be diagnosed with the help of X-ray photographs of the region of the urethra and bladder after they have been filled with a radiopaque substance that flows into any diverticula that may be present.

Treatment of a urethral diverticulum includes antibiotics to stop infection, medications to relieve pain and discomfort, and douches. In some cases, surgery is needed to eliminate the diverticula.

Structural Anomalies

Various kinds of injury may be sustained by the female reproductive system and other abdominal organs, chiefly as a result of childbearing. The structural damage can generally be repaired by surgical measures.

Fistula

An abnormal opening between two organs or from an organ to the outside of the body is known as a *fistula*. Fistulas may involve the urinary and reproductive systems of a woman. Damage to the organs during pregnancy or surgery, for example, can result in a fistula between the urethra and the vagina, causing urinary incontinence. A similar kind of fistula can develop between the rectum and the vagina as a result of injury, complications of pregnancy, or surgery. Disorders of this sort must be repaired surgically.

Prolapsed Uterus

The uterus normally rests on the floor of the pelvis, held in position by numerous ligaments. Damage to the ligaments and other supporting tissues causes the uterus to descend, or *prolapse*, into the vagina. There are various degrees of prolapse, ranging from a slight intrusion of the uterus into the vagina to a severe condition in which the cervix of the uterus protrudes out of the vaginal orifice. Prolapse of the uterus resembles a hernia but is not a true hernia, because the opening through which the uterus protrudes is a normal one.

Backache and a feeling of heaviness in the pelvic region may accompany the condition. Many women complain of a "dragging" sensation. An assortment of complications may involve neighboring organ systems; bleeding and ulceration of the uterus are not uncommon. Coughing and straining can aggravate the symptoms.

Like the various types of hernia, a prolapsed uterus does not improve without treatment but tends instead to worsen gradually. The only permanent treatment is surgical repair. In mild cases, a woman may get relief from symptoms through exercises intended to strengthen the muscles of the pelvic region. Supporting devices, such as an inflatable, doughnut-shaped pessary, are available as temporary methods of correcting a prolapse. Preventive exercises may be recommended for childbearing women who want to avoid weakened muscles and ligaments leading to prolapse.

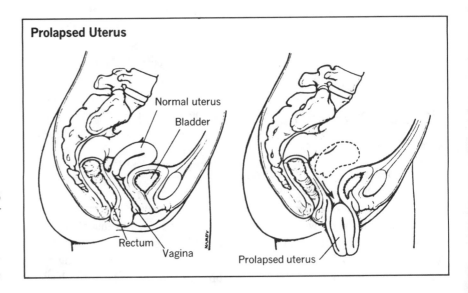

Prolapsed Uterus

Normal uterus

Bladder

Rectum

Vagina

Prolapsed uterus

Tipped Uterus

The uterus may be out of its normal position without being prolapsed. A malpositioned uterus may be "tipped" forward, backward, or otherwise be out of alignment with neighboring organs. A malpositioned uterus may cause no symptoms, or it may be associated with dysmenorrhea or infertility. If a malpositioned uterus causes pain, bleeding, or other problems, the condition can be corrected surgically, or a pessary support may relieve the symptoms. Displacement of the uterus occasionally is the result of a separate pelvic disease that requires treatment.

Hernias of the Vaginal Wall

The wall of the vagina may be ruptured in childbirth, especially in a multiple delivery or birth of a larger-than-average baby. The kind of hernia depends on the exact site of the rupture and what organ happens to lie against the vaginal wall at that point. The condition may be further complicated by a prolapsed uterus. Careful examination of the patient and X-ray pictures may be necessary to determine whether just one or several of the urinary, reproductive, and gastrointestinal organs in the pelvic cavity are involved.

Cystocele

Cystocele is a hernia involving the bladder and the vagina. Structurally, part of the bladder protrudes through the wall of the vagina. The symptoms, in addition to a feeling of pressure deep in the vagina, may be urinary difficulties, such as incontinence, a frequent urge to urinate, and inability to completely empty the bladder. Residual urine in the bladder may contribute to infection and inflammation of the bladder. Treatment includes

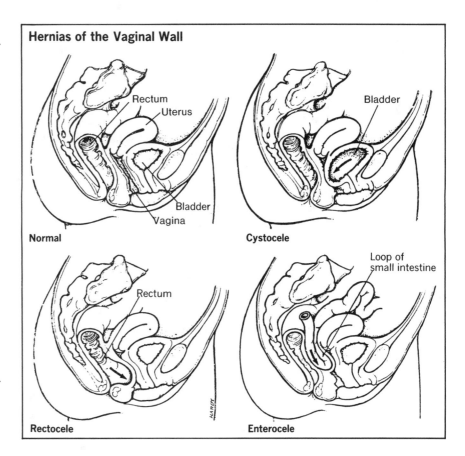

Hernias of the Vaginal Wall

Normal — Rectum, Uterus, Bladder, Vagina

Cystocele — Bladder

Rectocele — Rectum

Enterocele — Loop of small intestine

surgery to correct the condition, pessaries if needed to support the structures, and medications to control infection.

Rectocele

A hernia involving the tissues separating the vagina and the rectum, behind the vagina, is called a *rectocele*. The symptoms are a feeling of fullness in the vagina and difficulty in defecating. Enemas or laxatives may be needed to relieve constipation because straining, or even coughing, can aggravate the condition. Surgery is the only permanently effective treatment. Special diets, laxatives, and rectal suppositories may be prescribed pending surgery.

Enterocele

A herniation of the small intestine into the vagina is called an *enterocele*.

Some of the symptoms are similar to those of other hernias involving the vaginal wall, and in addition, a patient with an enterocele may experience abdominal cramps shortly after eating. An enterocele can be dangerous, as well as uncomfortable, because a segment of the small bowel can become trapped and obstructed, requiring emergency surgery.

Varicose Veins

Varicose veins of the vulva, vagina, and neighboring areas are another possible effect of pregnancy, although the legs are more often affected. Obesity, reduced physical activity during pregnancy, and circulatory changes associated with pregnancy can contribute to the development of varicose veins. The symptoms generally are limited to discomfort, although there can be bleeding, particularly at the time of childbirth.

Varicose veins that occur in the vulva and vagina during pregnancy and cause discomfort can be treated surgically during the early months of pregnancy. Some drugs and supportive therapy can be used to help relieve symptoms. But many physicians recommend that surgical stripping of veins be delayed until after the pregnancy has been terminated. A complication of untreated varicose veins can be development of blood clots in the abnormal blood vessels. For a discussion of varicose veins of the legs during pregnancy, see "Leg Cramps and Varicose Veins" in Ch. 4, *The Beginning of a Family.*

Benign Neoplasms

The word *neoplasm* refers to any abnormal proliferation of tissue that serves no useful function. There are numerous kinds of neoplasms but just two main groups—cancerous, or *malignant;* or noncancerous, or *benign.* In ordinary speech the word *benign* suggests some positive benefit, but a benign neoplasm, though noncancerous, may in fact be harmful to health or at least worrisome. Benign neoplasms that are of particular concern to women are discussed below.

Cysts

A *cyst* is a sac containing a gaseous, fluid, or semisolid material. (Certain normal anatomical structures, like the urinary bladder, are technically known as cysts—hence the term *cystitis* for inflammation of the bladder.) Abnormal, or neoplastic, cysts can develop at several sites within the urinary and reproductive systems.

Vaginal Cysts

A cyst may develop in a gland at the opening of the vagina as a result of infection with a venereal or other disease. Such a cyst can block the flow of secretions from the gland and produce swelling and pain. Dyspareunia, or painful intercourse, is sometimes a symptom. A vaginal-gland cyst usually is treated with antibiotics and hot packs. In some cases, it may be necessary for a physician to make an incision to drain the cyst.

Ovarian Cysts

Cysts in the ovaries may be caused by a malfunction of physiological process or by a pathological condition. Some pathological cysts are malignant. The cysts in the ovaries generally are filled with fluid that may range in color from pale and clear to reddish brown, depending upon the source of the fluid. Some cysts are too small to be seen with the naked eye, whereas others may be four or five inches in diameter when symptoms begin to cause discomfort. There are several different kinds of ovarian cysts.

Follicular Cyst

A *follicular,* or *retention,* cyst is a physiological cyst and is one of the most common types. It develops in an old follicle in which an ovum for some reason has failed to break out of its capsule during the ovulation process. Ordinarily, the contents of such a follicle are resorbed, but sometimes a cyst develops. It rarely grows larger than about two inches in diameter. It may rupture but usually disappears after a few months. The symptoms may include pain with some uterine bleeding and dyspareunia. Treatment consists of warm douches, analgesics, and hormone therapy designed to restore normal ovarian activity. If the

symptoms persist or the cyst continues to increase in size, or if serious complications occur, the physician may recommend exploratory surgery.

Occasionally such cysts, whether or not they rupture, produce symptoms that mimic those of appendicitis, with severe abdominal pain. The abdomen may become so tender that a physician cannot palpate the organs in order to distinguish between an ovarian cyst and appendicitis, particularly if the right ovary is involved. The symptoms occur at the time that ovulation would be expected. If the physician cannot be certain that the cause of the abdominal pain is indeed a cyst, for which surgery is not needed, he may recommend surgery anyway— just to be on the safe side.

Multiple follicular cysts, involving the ovaries on both sides (*bilateral polycystic ovaries*) can result in a syndrome (or group of symptoms) that includes infertility, obesity, and abnormal growth of body hair. All of these effects are related to a disruption of normal sex-hormone activity; they generally occur in young women, from teenagers to those in their 20s. The therapy includes both medical and surgical efforts to restore normal menstrual function, a diet to control obesity, and the use of various depilatory techniques to remove unwanted body hair.

Corpus Luteum Cyst

This kind of cyst may develop in the ovary following ovulation or during the early part of a pregnancy. The corpus luteum is a small, temporary gland that forms in the empty follicle after the ovum has been released from the ovary. Its function is to produce the hormone progesterone, which is important in preparing the endometrium, the lining of the uterus, to receive a fertilized ovum. The corpus luteum, however, also can be overproductive of a brownish fluid that fills the former follicular space, causing it to swell to a diameter of two or three inches. The cyst causes symptoms of pain and tenderness and may also result in a disruption of normal menstrual cycles in a woman who is not pregnant.

Most corpus luteum cysts gradually decrease in size without special treatment, except to relieve the symptoms. There may, however, be complications, such as torsion, or painful twisting of the ovary, or a rupture of the cyst. A ruptured corpus luteum cyst can result in hemorrhage and peritonitis, requiring immediate surgery.

Chocolate Cyst

So called because of their brownish-red color, chocolate cysts consist of misplaced endometrial tissue growing on the ovary instead of in its normal position lining the uterus. Chocolate cysts are among the largest of the ovarian cysts, ranging up to five or six inches in diameter. They cause symptoms associated with a variety of disorders of the reproductive system, including infertility, dyspareunia, and dysmenorrhea. Surgery usually is a favored method of therapy, the precise procedure depending upon the amount of ovarian tissue involved. A small chocolate cyst can be cauterized, but a large cyst may require removal of a portion of the ovary. See also "Cancer of the Ovary" later in this chapter.

Cysts of the Breast

Cysts may form in the milk glands or the ducts leading from the glands. They are caused by imbalances in ovarian hormones and they tend to develop in mature women approaching the menopause. The cysts tend to fluctuate in size, often enlarging just before or during menstruation, and there may be a discharge from the nipple. Pain and tenderness are usually present, although painless cysts are sometimes discovered only when a woman examines her breasts for possible lumps. Cysts may be almost microscopic in size or as large as an inch or more in diameter. It is not uncommon for more than one cyst to occur at the same time in one breast or both.

A medical examination is recommended when any kind of lump can be felt in the breast tissue. This is particularly important for women who have passed menopause. The physician frequently can determine whether a lump is a result of a cyst or cancer by the patient's history and by physical examination, especially when repeated at intervals of several weeks. Mammography and biopsy study of a small bit of tissue are used to confirm the diagnosis.

Women who are troubled by breast cysts may be helped by wearing a good brassiere at all times, even during sleep, to protect tender areas. The only medications available are those that relieve pain and discomfort—symptoms that usually subside when the menopause is reached.

Other Noncancerous Masses

A benign lump in the breast can be caused by either a fat deposit or an abscess. A fatty mass frequently forms if an injury to the breast damages adipose tissue. Because of a similarity of the symptoms to those of breast cancer, a biopsy is usually required to distinguish the lesion from a cancer. The involved tissue may in any case be removed surgically.

An abscess of the breast as a result of an infection, although a rare problem, may produce a lump that requires treatment with antibiotic medications or by an incision to drain the pus. Breast infections leading to abscesses are most likely to occur in nursing mothers but can also develop in women who are not lactating. When an infection develops in a breast being used to nurse a baby, nursing has to be discontinued temporarily while the infection is treated. See also "Cancer of the Breast" later in this chapter.

Polyps

A *polyp* is a strange-looking growth, even for an abnormal growth of tissue. It has been described as having the appearance of a tennis racket or a small mushroom. Polyps are found in many parts of the body, from the nose to the rectum. Usually they are harmless. But a polyp can result in discomfort or bleeding and require surgical excision. A polyp on the breast, for example, can become irritated by rubbing against the fabric of a brassiere. Although polyps generally are not cancerous, it is standard procedure to have the polyp tissue, like any excised tissue, tested in the laboratory. If malignant cells accompany a polyp, they are usually found at the base of the growth, which means that some of the tissue around the polyp must be excised along with the growth itself. Once a polyp is removed it does not grow again, although other polyps can occur in the same region.

Cervical Polyp

Polyps in the cervix are not uncommon, occurring most frequently in the years between menarche and menopause. A cervical polyp may be associated with vaginal bleeding or leukorrhea; the bleeding may occur after douching or sexual intercourse. In some cases, the bleeding is severe. Cervical polyps can usually be located visually by an examining physician and removed by minor surgery.

Endometrial Polyp

Endometrial polyps, which develop in the lining of the uterus, usually occur in women who are over 40, although they can develop at any age after menarche. They are frequently the cause of nonmenstrual bleeding. They tend to be much larger than polyps that grow in other organs of the body: an endometrial polyp may be rooted high in the uterus with a stem reaching all the way to the cervix. Such a polyp is usually located and removed during a D- and C- procedure. As in the case of a cervical polyp, the growth and a bit of surrounding tissue are studied for traces of cancer cells.

Benign Tumors

Tumors are rather firm growths that may be either benign or malignant. In practice, any tumor is regarded with suspicion unless malignancy is ruled out by actual laboratory tests. Even a benign tumor represents a tissue abnormality, and if untreated can produce symptoms that interfere with normal health and activity.

Fibromas

Among the more common of the benign tumors is the *fibroma,* commonly known as a *fibroid tumor,* composed of fibrous connective tissue. About one of every 20 ovarian tumors is a fibroma, and a similar growth in the uterus is the most common type of tumor found in that organ. Fibromas also occur in the vulva.

Ovarian Fibroma

Ovarian fibromas are usually small, but there are instances in which they have grown to weigh as much as five pounds. A large fibroma can be very painful and produce symptoms such as a feeling of heaviness in the pelvic area, nausea, and vomiting. The growth may crowd other organs of the body, causing enlargement of the abdomen and cardiac and respiratory symptoms. The only treatment is surgical removal of the tumor, after which there is usually a quick and full recovery.

Uterine Fibroma

Fibroid tumors of the uterus can also grow to a very large size, some weighing many pounds. Like ovarian fibromas, they can press against neighboring organs such as the intestine or the urinary bladder, producing constipation or urinary difficulty. More commonly, there is pain and vaginal bleeding, along with pelvic pressure and enlargement of the abdomen. It is possible in some cases for a fibroid tumor to grow slowly in the uterus for several years without causing serious discomfort to the patient. If the tumor obstructs or distorts the reproductive tract, it may be a cause of infertility.

Treatment of fibroid tumors varies according to their size, the age of the patient and her expectations about having children, and other factors. If the tumor is small and does not appear to be growing at a rapid rate, the physician may recommend that surgery be postponed as long as the tumor poses no threat to health. For an older woman, or for a woman who does not want to bear children, a hysterectomy may be advised, especially if symptoms are troublesome. If the patient is a young woman who wants to have children, the physician is likely to advise a *myomectomy,* a surgical excision of the tumor, since a fibroid tumor of the uterus can cause serious complications during pregnancy and labor. It can result in abortion or premature labor, malpresentation of the fetus, difficult labor, and severe loss of blood during childbirth. While fibroid tumors of the uterus are not malignant, special tests are made of the endometrial tissue as part of any myomectomy or hysterectomy to rule out the possibility that cancer cells may be involved in the disorder.

Endometriosis

Endometriosis is the medical term for a condition in which endometrial tissue, the special kind of tissue that lines the uterus, grows in various areas of the pelvic cavity outside the uterus. Endometrial cells may invade such unlikely places as the ovaries (the most common site), the bladder, appendix, Fallopian tubes, intestinal tract, or the supporting structure of the uterus. The external endometrial tissue may appear as small blisters of endometrial cells, as solid nodules, or as cysts, usually of the ovary, which may be four inches or more in diameter, like the chocolate cysts of the ovaries. Such a mass of sometimes tumorlike endometrial cells is called an *endometrioma.*

The misplaced endometrial tissue causes problems because it goes through menstrual cycles just as the endometrium does within the cavity of the uterus. The endometrial tissue proliferates after ovulation and may cause almost constant pain, wherever it is located, for a few days before the start of menstruation. The symptoms subside after the menstrual flow begins. The effects may include dyspareunia, rectal bleeding, backache, and generalized pain in the pelvic region as sensitive tissues throughout the pelvic cavity are irritated by monthly cycles of swelling and bleeding.

Because infertility is associated with endometriosis, which can become progressively worse, young women who want to bear children are sometimes encouraged to begin efforts to become pregnant as early as possible if they show signs or symptoms of the disorder. Treatment includes hormone medication and surgery to remove the lesions of endometriosis or the organ involved. For patients with extensive spread of endometrial tissue outside the uterus, the physician may recommend removal of one or both ovaries. Destruction of the ovaries surgically or by radiation therapy may be employed to eliminate the menstrual cycle activity that aggravates the symptoms of endometriosis. These procedures cause sterility and premature menopause, but some women prefer this to the discomfort of endometriosis. The hormone therapy inhibits the ovulation phase of the menstrual cycle. Without ovulation, the endometrial tissue does not proliferate. For this reason, pregnancy often eliminates or eases the symptoms of endometriosis during parturition and for a period of time thereafter.

Dyspareunia

Dyspareunia, or painful intercourse, is often associated with endometriosis and is attributed to irritation of nerve fibers in the area of the cervix from the pressure of sexual activity. There are many other possible causes of painful intercourse, some functional and some organic in nature. In addition to endometriosis, the problem may be owing to a vaginal contracture, a disorder involving the muscles of the pelvic region, inflammation of the vagina or urethra, prolapsed or malpositioned uterus, *cervicitis* (inflammation of the cervix), or a disorder of the bladder or rectum. A cause of dyspareunia in older women may be a degeneration of the tissues lining the vagina, which become thin and dry. Temporary therapy for dyspareunia may include water-soluble lubricants, anesthetic ointments, steroid hormones, analgesics, and sedatives.

In appropriate cases, surgery is effective in correcting an organic cause of painful sexual intercourse. Functional or psychogenic (of psychological origin) causes of dyspareunia usually require psychological counseling for the patient and her sexual partner.

Backache

Still another effect of endometriosis that can suggest other disorders is backache. When endometrial tissue invades the pelvic region, there may be a fairly constant pain in the back near the tailbone or the rectum. Usually the backache subsides only after the cause has been eliminated. Temporary measures include those advised for other kinds of backache: sleeping on a firm mattress, preferably reinforced with a sheet of plywood between springs and mattress; application of dry heat or warm baths; sedatives to relieve tension, and analgesics to relieve the pain.

A backache that radiates down the back and into a leg, following the path of a sciatic nerve, can be the result of a disorder of the ovaries or uterus. An ovarian cyst or infection of the Fallopian tubes can produce a backache that seems to be centered in the lumbosacral area of the spinal column. Such backaches, sometimes called gynecologic backaches, tend to occur most frequently during a woman's childbearing years and more often affect women who have had several children than women who have not been pregnant. Tumors also can produce backache symptoms. X-ray pictures, myelograms, and laboratory studies may be required in order to rule out the possibilities that the back pain may be caused by a tumor, a herniated or "slipped" disk, or a deformity of the spinal column that might have been aggravated by one or more pregnancies. Most backaches, however, relate to poor posture or mus-

cle tension. Anxiety or other kinds of emotional stress can aggravate the symptoms. See also "Backaches" in Ch. 23, *Aches, Pains, Nuisances, Worries,* and "Back Pain and Its Causes" in Ch. 25, *Women's Health.*

Cancers of the Reproductive System

Cancer of the Cervix

The cervix of the uterus is the ninth most common site of cancers affecting women. As compared with all cancers of the reproductive organs of women, it rates third, after uterine cancer and ovarian cancer. It has been estimated that about 13,000 cases of cervical cancer are found among American women each year, and approximately 4,500 deaths every year are a result of this disease.

The number of cases of preinvasive cervical cancer is down because of the increased number of women who undergo regular gynecological examination. When cancer is diagnosed early, the survival rate increases tremendously for the patient.

The actual causes of cervical cancer are still unknown. Current medical thinking suggests that there is no causal relationship between cervical cancer and the use of oral contraceptives.

Preinvasive Stage

The earliest signs of cervical cancer tend to appear between the ages of 25 and 45. At this early, *preinvasive* stage, the cancer is described as *in situ*—confined to its original site. If the cancer is not treated at this stage, the disease spreads and becomes a typical invasive cancer within five to ten years. Signs of bleeding and ulceration usually do not appear until this has occurred. However, because of the relatively slow growth of cervical cancer in the early stage, the disease usually can be detected by a Pap smear test before it becomes invasive.

Invasive Cancer

Cancer that has spread beyond the cervix is far more difficult to treat. Surgery, radiation or chemotherapy, and regular examinations to catch any recurrence of cancer will probably be necessary. It is unusual for anyone to develop invasive cancer without knowing it, if she has undergone regular, routine pelvic exams.

Diagnostic Methods

Pap Smear Test

The *Pap smear* test (named for Dr. George Papanicolaou, who developed the technique in 1928) is a quick and simple method of detecting cancerous cells in secretions and scrapings from mucous membrane. It requires the collection of small samples of cells from the surface of the cervix and from the cervical canal. Such samples are obtained by inserting a plastic spatula or a brush-tipped tube into the vagina, into which a speculum has been placed previously. The device is scraped gently over the area of the cervix. The physician may collect also a sample of vaginal secretions, which may contain possibly cancerous cells not only from the cervix but from the ovaries and uterus as well. (This is

the only way a Pap smear test can be done if a woman has had a complete hysterectomy and has no cervix.) All cell samples are placed (smeared) on microscope slides and treated with a chemical preservative. The slides are sent to a laboratory for study and a report is made to the examining physician, usually within a few days, on the findings.

Results from the Pap smear are reported as: normal, inadequate sampling, showing infection, or showing cell abnormalities. Except for the normal results, Paps will be done again to ensure accuracy. No one should wait more than six months for a follow-up reading on an infectious diagnosis and treatment. For all others, follow-up should be immediate. Cell abnormalities are divided into at least three categories: low-grade lesions (noncancerous), high-grade lesions (noncancerous), and cancer.

Other Diagnostic Tests

When a report of positive findings is returned by the laboratory, the physician immediately arranges for further studies. These involve examination of the cervix visually by a special microscopic technique known as *colposcopy,* and the removal of small tissue samples. These studies are usually done in a physician's office. In some cases a biopsy is necessary. The biopsy sample is taken when possible from the same location on the cervix as the Pap smear that resulted in positive findings. The Loop Electrosurgical Excision Procedure (LEEP) is a method of combining the biopsy and the excision of the diseased tissue. An electrified loop removes the abnormal tissue from the cervix. The small circle that is removed can then be examined for signs

of cancer. The electrical charge of the loop cauterizes the cut to prevent infection and bleeding. Treatment ordinarily is not started until all of the studies have verified that there is cancer in the tissues of the cervix; other disorders, such as cervicitis, venereal infection, and polyps, can mimic symptoms of cervical cancer.

Therapy

The kind of treatment recommended for a case of cervical cancer generally depends upon several factors, such as the stage of cancer development and the age and general health of the patient. For a young woman who wishes to have children despite cancer *in situ,* which is limited to the cervix, surgeons may excise a portion of the cervix and continue watching for further developments with frequent Pap smears and other tests. The treatment of choice for cervical cancer in the early stage, however, is surgical removal of the body of the uterus, as well as of the cervix—a procedure called a *total hysterectomy.* This is the usual treatment for women over the age of 40 or for those who do not wish to have children. Sometimes more extensive surgery is necessary.

Radiation treatment may be advised for women who are not considered to be good surgical risks because of other health problems. Radiation may be recommended along with surgery for women with advanced cervical cancer in order to help destroy cancer cells that may have spread by metastasis to other tissues.

The five-year cure rate for cervical cancer is about 99 percent when treatment is started in the early, preinvasive stage. The chances of a cure drop sharply in later stages, but the five-year cure rate is still as high as 65 percent if treatment is started when the cancer has just begun to spread to the vagina or other nearby tissues.

Cancer of the Body of the Uterus

Cancer of the body of the uterus, or *endometrial cancer,* is more common than cancer of the cervix. Uterine cancer is the most common type of cancer of the reproductive organs. Cervical cancer primarily affects women before middle age; uterine cancer occurs more frequently among women beyond the menopause, with its highest rate occurring among women between the ages of 50 and 70. Survival rate for cancer of the uterus is high, with 82 percent living 5 years after diagnosis. Risk factors for uterine cancer include obesity, diabetes, and ovarian cysts. Other potential risks are for women who have taken estrogen-only pills for menopausal symptoms and women who have taken tamoxifen for breast cancer.

Diagnostic Methods

Early symptoms usually include bleeding between menstrual periods or after menopause, and occasionally a watery or blood-stained vaginal discharge. Most patients experience no pain in the early stages, although pain is a symptom in advanced uterine cancer or when the disease is complicated by an infection. Unfortunately, there is no simple test, like the Pap smear for cervical cancer, that provides a good diagnostic clue to the presence of endometrial cancer. The Pap smear does occasionally pick up cells sloughed off by the endometrium, and laboratory tests can tell if they might be malignant. The best chance for early diagnosis is for a woman to report to her gynecologist or physician any signs of abnormal bleeding between periods, or postmenopausal bleeding. Unusual bleeding should be followed up by the doctor with examination of the uterine lining.

A physician who is suspicious of symptoms of endometrial cancer must depend upon direct methods to confirm or rule out the disease. The usual method is a dilatation and curettage (D and C), during which a small sample of uterine lining will be removed for biopsy, or a sample may be withdrawn by suction (aspirated) from the uterine cavity. The cervix is dilated (opened) and the uterine lining scraped with a curette. Aspiration can be done in the physician's office with local anesthesia of the cervix or with no anesthesia. There is little or no discomfort following aspiration.

Therapy

If the diagnostic D and C is done when the abnormal bleeding associated with uterine cancer first begins, the chances of a cure are very good. The first step, if the general health of the patient permits surgery, is complete removal of the uterus, ovaries, and fallopian tubes—a procedure called a *radical hysterectomy.* Radiation may also be administered to control the spread of cancer cells.

A hysterectomy should not affect a woman's normal sexual activity. Sexual relations usually can be resumed about six to eight weeks after the operation, or when the incision has healed. If the incision is made through the pubic region or vagina, there should be little or no visible scar. See "Family Planning," in Chapter 4.

Estrogen and Cancer

There is a higher incidence of cancer of the uterus among women who have tumors of the ovary that produce estrogen, as well as among women whose menopause begins later than the usual age (and hence who have produced estrogen naturally for a longer-than-usual period). Because of the statistical associations between uterine cancer and estrogen-producing tumors, as well as other factors, the American Cancer Society has cautioned that physicians should exert "close supervision of women on estrogen, with an awareness that sustained use [of estrogens] may stimulate dormant factors in the body and lead to development of endometrial cancer." For women who are prescribed estrogen for menopause, it is recommended that the estrogen be given in combination with a synthetic progestin. Unopposed estrogen increases the growth of cancerous tumors already present, and is suspected of increasing the risk of new cancer growths.

Among the conditions for which estrogen has been prescribed for women of middle age and beyond are uncomfortable effects of menopause, such as itching and irritation caused by dryness of the vagina, and what is commonly referred to as "hot flashes." See *The Middle Years,* Ch. 5, "Menopause" for more information.

Diethylstilbestrol

An estrogenlike synthetic compound has definitely been implicated in the development of a type of cancer, *adenocarcinoma,* which primarily affects epithelial tissue. The synthetic hormone known chemically as *diethylstilbestrol* (DES) or stilbestrol was taken for the most part in the late 1940s and through the 1960s by pregnant women for the treatment of such complications as bleeding and threatened miscarriage. Around 1971, physicians became aware that some of the daughters whose mothers had taken DES during their pregnancy had developed an unusual cell formation in vaginal tissue, vaginal and cervical cancers, and some anatomical abnormalities. Cancers have been discovered in daughters as young as seven years of age. An unknown but substantial number of women in the

United States alone received DES while pregnant, but approximately 1 in 1000 have been found to be afflicted with cervical or vaginal cancers. The National Cancer Institute has urged that all mothers and daughters who may have been exposed to DES during the mother's pregnancy arrange to be examined by a physician for possible effects of the drug.

The use of DES for pregnant women has been discontinued, although the compound is still available for treating certain cases of breast cancer and menopausal symptoms in nonpregnant women.

Cancer of the Ovary

Ovarian cancer is the fifth most common type of cancer in women, with an average of 21,000 new cases each year. It is second to uterine cancer in the number of cases of cancer of the reproductive system. It has, however, a much lower survival rate. Because of the difficulty in diagnosing ovarian cancer, the cancer is more likely than other forms to go unchecked until it has spread to other areas of the body. Less than 2 in 5 women will survive five years after diagnosis. There are several different kinds of malignant tumors of the ovary; some originate in the ovaries and others are caused by cells that have metastasized from a cancer at some other site, such as the uterus.

There are no age limits for cancer of the ovary, although most cases are detected in women between 50 and 70. A physician at a routine pelvic examination may notice a lump or other abnormal growth in the abdominal region. The symptoms reported by patients usually include abdominal discomfort or digestive problems, possibly because ovarian cancers often grow large enough to press on neighboring organs and cause urinary

difficulties, constipation, or other digestive disorders. A clue is given in some cases by endometrial bleeding as a result of abnormal hormone production by the affected ovary. However, the more common kinds of ovarian cancers do not produce hormones. Occasionally, cancer cells from an ovarian tumor will be found in a Pap smear sample. But there are no direct, simple tests for cancer of the ovary.

Treatment for ovarian cancer varies with the individual case. As with cancer at other sites, surgery is generally necessary. The extent of the surgery depends upon the type of lesion and other factors. In an advanced case of an older woman, total hysterectomy along with removal of the ovaries and fallopian tubes would be the treatment of choice. But if the patient is a young woman and the cancer is not extensive, the surgeon may excise the affected ovary and leave the remainder of the reproductive system intact. Radiation and chemotherapy are commonly applied in addition to surgery. The most important risk factor is having relatives who have had ovarian cancer. If a mother, grandmother, or sibling have been diagnosed with ovarian cancer, then the woman is recommended to undergo regular blood tests to check for malignancy. Let your doctor know if you have a family history of ovarian cancer.

Cancer of the Breast

Cancer of the breast is one of the oldest and best-known types of cancer. It is described in an ancient Egyptian papyrus of 5,000 years ago. The hormonal factors involved in the physiology of breast cancer have been

studied by physicians for more than 100 years. But it remains the most common of cancers affecting woman. It kills more women than any other kind of cancer, except lung cancer. About 150,000 women in the United States develop breast cancer each year, and 35 percent die of the disease. Nearly everyone knows a friend or relative who has been stricken by breast cancer. Yet the cause of breast cancer is still unknown.

Women whose female relatives have had breast cancer are more likely to be victims than women from families in which breast cancer is not present. The disease appears to be linked statistically also to women who do not have children before their 30s or who do not have any children; to mothers who do not nurse their babies; to women who reach the menopause later than normal; and to women who began menstruation earlier in life than normal. There is increasing evidence also that ovarian activity may play an important role in the development of breast cancer. Women with ovarian tumors and women who use supplementary estrogen have been shown by some studies to be at increased risk, while the process of having many children and nursing them, which suppresses estrogen hormone activity, is associated with a decreased risk of developing breast cancer. However, 55 percent of the diagnosed cases are for women who have no known risk factors.

Cancer of the breast may occur as early as the teens, but this is rare. It is generally not found before the age of 30, and the incidence peaks around the time of menopause. Then there is a second period after the age of about 65 when the incidence of breast cancer rises again.

Breast cancer usually begins in the ducts of the milk glands; the first noticeable sign is a lump in the breast.

The lump may appear anywhere in the breast, but the most common site is the upper, outer quadrant. Most lumps are not usually cancerous, but a biopsy (described below) must be performed to check the tissue involved.

In a typical case of breast cancer, a small tumor half an inch in diameter, large enough to be detected during careful self-examination, can grow to a cancer two inches in diameter in six months to a year. The lump generally causes no pain; pain is rarely associated with early breast cancer. If the tumor is allowed to grow unchecked, it may cause pulling of the skin from within. This effect may appear as a flattening of the breast or a dimpling of the skin, or a sinking, tilting, or flattening of the nipple. Less frequently, the tumor begins in a duct near the nipple, causing irritation of the skin of the nipple and a moist discharge. In such cases a scab eventually forms at that site. In time, cancer cells spread to the nearby lymph nodes and the danger becomes very serious of metastasis to any part of the body.

Detection of Breast Cancer

Fortunately, breast cancer can be treated effectively if it is detected early enough. Some 95 percent of breast cancers are discovered by the patient herself when she notices a lump. In all too many cases the discovery is made by chance and the lump may be quite large. The cure rate for breast cancer could be greatly improved if all women made a routine of monthly self-examination and then consulted a physician immediately if they found the least indication of a thickening or lump. Most such lumps are benign, but it is most important that the ones that are malignant be identified without delay.

The American Cancer Society and the National Cancer Institute recommend that every woman follow a prescribed method of self-examination just after the menstrual period, continuing every month after the menopause. The procedure consists of carefully looking at and feeling the breasts, and takes only a few minutes. A detailed description of the proper procedure is available in pamphlet form from the Superintendent of Documents, U.S. Government Printing Office, Washington, D.C. 20402. Ask for Public Health Service Publication No. 1730. A film entitled *Breast Self-Examination,* produced by the American Cancer Society and the National Cancer Institute, is also available.

If a tumor can be detected as even a small lump, it must have been developing for some time. There is a truism about breast cancer to the effect that a cancer that is undetectable is curable—leaving unspoken the implication that a cancer that is detectable may not be curable. In recent years, methods of early detection have been refined to the point that tumors once undetectable can now be detected before any lump becomes palpable.

Self-examination of the Breasts

Step 1

Step 2

Step 3

Self-examination of the breasts as recommended by the American Cancer Society. *(Step 1)* Examine breasts during a shower or bath; hands glide easier over wet skin. With fingers flat, move the left hand gently over every part of the right breast, then the right hand over the left breast. Check for any lump, hard knot, or thickening. *(Step 2)* Before a mirror, inspect the breasts with arms at the sides, then with arms raised. Look for any changes in the contour of each breast, a swelling, dimple of skin, or changes in the nipple. Then rest palms on hips and press down firmly to flex the chest muscles. Left and right breasts will not match exactly — few women's breasts do. But regular inspection will show what is normal for you. *(Step 3)* While lying down with a pillow or folded towel under the right shoulder and with the right hand behind the head, examine the right breast with the left hand. With fingers flat, press gently in small circular motions around an imaginary clock face. Begin at 12 o'clock, then move to 1 o'clock, and so on around back to 12. A ridge of firm tissue in the lower curve of each breast is normal. Next, move in an inch toward the nipple and keep circling to examine every part of the breast, including the nipple. This requires at least three more circles. Then repeat the procedure slowly on the left breast with the pillow under the left shoulder and left hand behind the head. Notice how the breast structure feels. Finally, squeeze the nipple of each breast gently between thumb and index finger. Any discharge, clear or bloody, should be reported to a physician immediately.

Thermography

One early warning detection technique involves the use of *thermography,* which is based on the fact that tumor cells produce slightly more heat than normal tissue. Hence a device that is sufficiently heat sensitive can detect and pinpoint the location of an incipient tumor. A harmless tumor, too, would have a higher-than-normal temperature. Further tests would be needed to determine the true cause of the "hot" tissue-reading.

Mammography

Mammography is an X-ray technique developed specifically for examination of breast tissue. A tumor shows up on a mammogram as an opaque spot because of mineral concentrations associated with the growth. However, like thermography, mammography cannot determine whether a tumor is benign or malignant or if the opaque spot on the film is because of some other mineral-rich tissue rather than a tumor. The examining physician uses mammography only as one among other diagnostic tools.

Guidelines from medical groups such as the American Medical Association and the American Cancer Society are as follows:

- Physical breast exams by doctors once a year, and monthly self-exams for all age groups from puberty to 40 onward.
- No known risk factors, ages 40-49, physical breast exam by doctor every year, mammogram every one to two years
- Risk factors ranked medium to high, ages 40-49, physical breast exams and mammograms once a year or more frequently with the advice of a physician
- Age 50, with or without risk factors, mammogram and physical breast exam every year

Some gynecologists recommend a mammogram at the age of 35 so that there is an opportunity for comparison when mammograms are done after the age of 40. Consult with your physician about his or her personal recommendations. Some insurance companies will pay for yearly mammograms; others pay for biannual mammogram exams. Some states require insurance companies by law to pay for at least one exam. Check with your insurance company about their policy. Medicare covers mammograms for women over the age of 65.

Xeroradiography

Xeroradiography is a method that, like mammography, uses X rays, but it entails only about half the exposure to radiation. The pictures are developed by xerography, the process made familiar by Xerox copying machines. The picture consists of dots in varying shades of blue. The process produces a sharp picture, making interpretation simpler and more accurate than is possible with X-ray photographs. When performed by experienced medical technicians, xeroradiography can detect from 85 to 95 percent of all breast cancer, including those too small to be located by palpation. The xeroradiography examination and the physician's examination of the breast usually take only about 20 minutes.

Other Methods

Other diagnostic tools have come into use. *Ultrasound* and *diaphanography,* for example, have reportedly proved their value, especially when combined with other techniques, including mammography. Ultrasound depends on sound waves that vibrate at frequencies beyond the range of human hearing; transmitted into the breast, ultrasound can distinguish between lumps that are cystic and fluid-filled—and therefore benign—and those that

are solid. Other tests, however, may be needed to differentiate between benign solid and malignant solid lumps. In diaphanography, or transillumination, a technician or physician shines an ordinary white light through the breast in the dark. An overhead camera takes pictures with infrared film. Diaphanography can determine whether breast lumps are fibrous, benign, or malignant.

Fine needle aspiration has also proved useful in diagnosing breast cancer. The surgeon uses a needle to draw out a sample approximately 0.5 cm in size. Microscopic examination of the sample follows.

Biopsy

When a physician believes there is good evidence of a cancer in a breast as a result of thermography, xeroradiography, mammography, palpation of lumps, and other factors, the next step is a biopsy study. The suspected lesion is located for the biopsy procedure and the exact position and extent of the planned incision is marked on the skin. The patient is then wheeled into the operating room and the tissue sample is excised while the patient is anesthetized. An entire nodule of breast tissue is removed for microscopic examination of the tissue cells. It is sent to the pathology department, which usually reports within 90 minutes whether the tissue is noncancerous or malignant. Provisional preparations are made for a mastectomy. If the lesion is not cancerous—and between 60 and 80 percent of biopsies of breast lumps are not—the patient is taken back to the recovery room and, as soon as possible, reassured that the tumor was benign. The incision made for the biopsy leaves an almost indiscernible scar. In some cases, a hollow needle may be used to withdraw tissue, leaving no scar. This is called a *needle biopsy.*

The Two-Step Procedure

Because of the psychological and physical problems associated with breast cancer, approaches to surgery have changed drastically in recent years. The patient today has a choice: if she desires, she can request that the test and operation take place in two separate stages. To make that choice, the woman simply does not sign a form granting permission to perform both the biopsy and the *mastectomy*, or breast removal, on the same day.

In many cases, it may be necessary to perform both operations on the same day. In such cases, experts say, the woman should insist that her surgeon refer her for presurgical *staging*.

Staging involves administration of various tests that are carried out before a mastectomy. The tests show whether the cancer has already spread, or metastasized, to parts of the body other than the breast and local lymph node regions. Staging is widely regarded as a necessary procedure in all cases of breast cancer. A mastectomy has the single purpose of preventing the spread of cancer; the patient has to know, for her own peace of mind, whether it has already spread.

A two-step procedure involves other choices. Where the biopsy is to be carried out separately, the patient may ask to have it done under local anesthesia, as an outpatient. That possibility can be explored with the surgeon. If a general anesthetic appears preferable, the patient may have to spend a night in the hospital. But the *diagnostic biopsy*—involving surgical removal of the entire tumor—and mastectomy can still be performed separately. After a biopsy specimen is removed, the specimen may be subjected to an estrogen-receptor assay. The assay tells the surgeon whether or not the cancer

depends on the female hormone estrogen for its growth. That information provides a clue to possible future treatment.

The two-step procedure offers some advantages insofar as diagnosis is concerned. In particular, it makes possible a "permanent section" in which excised tissue is chemically treated to produce a high-quality slide for microscopic examination. Such an examination is far more complete and accurate than the "frozen section" that is necessary in the one-step procedure. The freezing process may distort the cells, leading sometimes to inaccurate results. For many women, the one- to two-day wait for the results of a permanent-section biopsy is worth the time involved, especially because it may be possible to perform the biopsy under local anesthesia on an outpatient basis.

Following the biopsy, the patient receives the pathologist's report on whether the finding is positive or negative. If positive, precise information will usually be given on the type of cancer and where it is located in the breast. Then the patient may want to obtain a second opinion on the permanent-section pathology report and slides. The second opinion is also given by a pathologist. It helps in making decisions on surgery.

Mastectomy

If the lesion is malignant, the surgeon proceeds with the mastectomy. Depending upon the seriousness of the case and the procedure recommended by the surgeon and the pathologist, the operation may be a *simple mastectomy*, a *radical mastectomy*, a *modified radical mastectomy*, or any of a number of other forms of breast operation. In the United States until recently, radical mastectomy was the usual procedure for breast cancer treatment. Today, at least seven dif-

The striped areas show the tissue removed in a radical *(above)* and a simple *(below)* mastectomy, including the axillary lymph nodes in the former case.

ferent types of mastectomy, some more widely accepted than others, may be performed. All may be recommended in different cases depending upon the type of cancer, its invasive potential, or ability to spread, and other factors. The seven:

- *Wedge excision, lumpectomy,* or *segmental resection:* the tumor is removed along with some surrounding tissue

- *Simple (or total) mastectomy:* the breast alone is removed

- *Simple mastectomy* accompanied by *low axillary dissection:* the breast is removed along with some of the underarm nodes or glands

- *Modified-radical mastectomy* accompanied by *full axillary dissection:* the breast is removed along with all the lymph glands under the arm

- *Halsted-type radical mastectomy:* the breast is removed along with the underarm lymph glands and the chest muscles

- *Radical mastectomy* with *internal mammary node biopsy:* the same procedure as the Halsted-type radical mastectomy, except that the lymph nodes that lie under the ribs, next to the breastbone, are also sampled for biopsy

- *Super-radical mastectomy:* the same as the above, but all of the internal mammary nodes are removed

Most patients have deep concern about many aspects of breast surgery, including the cosmetic effects. For that reason, it is important to select the appropriate type of surgery. Survival rates depend as much on timely use of pre- and postoperative radiotherapy and postoperative chemotherapy as on the type of operation. But the kind of operation may determine whether the patient will be able to function normally in a relatively short period of time.

Some surgeries allow reconstruction of the breast either during or after a mastectomy, using artificial material to create a breast to match the natural one.

Postoperative Therapies

The type of surgery recommended in any given case of breast cancer has significance for postoperative therapy. Breast surgery may be less extensive or radical where the cancer has spread to the lymph nodes or to other parts of the body; the use of chemotherapy and radiation therapy may then be more aggressive.

More commonly, the cancer is localized. Options include:

- surgery only;

- surgery with radiation;

- surgery with chemotherapy;

- surgery with a combination of these treatments; or

- radiation or chemotherapy without surgery.

The choices of alternative therapies should be made with an eye to still other factors.

Radiation

A lumpectomy, or segmental mastectomy, is usually followed by radiation therapy. Treatments are typically given five days a week for five weeks. A "booster" treatment may follow completion of the initial series of treatments. Side effects from radiation therapy include fatigue; reddened, moist, or dry skin at the site of the radiation; decreased or heightened sensitivity; enlarged pores; and sometimes changes in breast size.

Chemotherapy

Adjuvant chemotherapy, which follows surgery, is the usual treatment where breast cancer has spread to the lymph nodes and the patient has not entered menopause. Postmenopausal women may be given tamoxifen, an antiestrogen drug, or may undergo chemotherapy. Except for some high-risk patients, adjuvant chemotherapy is not recommended for women with noncancerous nodes.

Hormone Therapy

Less toxic than chemotherapy, hormone treatments are normally given to women whose cancer has not spread to the underarm nodes and whose tumors were hormone-dependent. This is especially the case if a patient is postmenopausal. For these women tamoxifen would also be a standard treatment if the cancers had spread to the lymph nodes.

Other Alternatives

There are alternatives to the above therapies. Radiation alone may be recommended where the disease is so far advanced that surgery is not feasible, or where the patient's health is too poor to risk surgery. Radiation treatment may also be effective in reducing the pain in bones or areas of the central nervous system where cancer cells may have metastasized. Radiation also may be used in addition to chemotherapy in certain cases because X rays, or similar radiation, can reach areas where chemical medications cannot penetrate.

The Rape Victim

The woman who has been raped faces special problems. Authorities agree that long-term health threats can be minimized if the victim takes certain precautions. Complications arising from sexual assault include contracting sexually transmitted disease (STD) or other diseases; becoming pregnant; and experiencing the aftereffects of contusions and abrasions. Experts suggest that women try to protect themselves against rape and follow certain procedures in the event that a rape occurs.

Precautions

Because rapists generally attack without warning, the woman who feels that she is at risk can sometimes do little more than exercise vigilance in protecting herself. There are precautions, however, that women may take. Self-defense or martial-arts courses may be the answer for some. Although weapons may impart a sense of security, authorities are divided on the issue of their value. Additionally, the weapons themselves may be illegal in some cities or states. Noisemakers, including whistles and siren devices, may or may not be either available or effective, depending upon the circumstances.

Among the possible nonviolent methods of self-protection are the following:

- If you are being followed by a man who is more than 20 or so feet away, you can scream or use a noisemaker.
- Where possible, if followed, you should go into a store and tell the proprietor or clerk that you want to use a telephone.
- Again where possible, bring third parties into the situation—a chance pedestrian, perhaps another woman, or a passing group.
- Remain out of doors if your choice lies between entering a hallway or lobby or staying outside.
- Never go home if you know there is no one home. Instead ring all the door bells on apartment doors or go to a neighbor you know will be home.
- If you find it necessary to walk alone at night, walk in the street—again if possible and safe.
- Take a taxicab home if you have to travel late at night, and ask the driver to wait until you get indoors.
- Even when entering your own building, check the entrance and both sides before going inside.
- If you live alone, pretend you don't.

If a Rape Occurs

The rape victim may face a long period in which recovery and normal living seem impossible. The ability to enjoy life, sex, love, and work may appear to be elusive, even nonexistent. Six months or a year may pass without bringing relief from bad dreams, feelings of guilt, insomnia, and many other physical and psychological aftereffects. But authorities say that what a victim does after experiencing rape may make the transition to normal living easier while also protecting her against recurring health problems.

The Sympathetic Ear

Preferably before, but certainly after reporting to the police, the victim should confide in another person—whether husband, lover, close woman friend, counselor, pastor, hotline volunteer, or someone else trustworthy. The person confided in should go to the police station with the victim—if not the first time, then on any later occasions. The person confided in should be able to provide support, to make sure the victim's rights are protected, and to listen sympathetically to the victim's story.

Going to the Hospital

The rape victim should go as soon as possible to a hospital and undergo the pelvic and other examinations that physicians administer in such cases. If the woman goes to the hospital immediately, she should not wash herself or change clothes. A shower can remove valuable medical evidence. The pelvic examination is designed to find evidence of abrasions or internal damage, and for collection of any semen left by the rapist. Physicians will also examine for any of the rapist's hair, blood, skin, or semen. Any such evidence may be important in court later.

The hospital visit has other pur-

poses. A physician can also administer preventive injections for sexually transmitted diseases and, if desired, an antipregnancy medication. The latter medication must be taken within three days if it is to be effective.

Importantly, the hospital visit may or may not bring the rape case automatically to the attention of the police. That would be true in some areas but not in all. Ultimately, the victim has to report the crime.

Reporting to the Police

Failure to report a rape immediately or after a few days probably means the rapist will not be apprehended. Even so, as many as nine out of ten rapes go unreported simply because most victims cannot face the added trauma of being questioned in detail and, possibly, rude treatment. The woman who does report to the police should, however, do so as soon as possible; each passing day increases the possibility that the police will want to know the reasons for the delay. But reporting late, experts stress, is better than not reporting at all. Reporting a rape does not mean that the victim has to press charges later.

Rape Crisis Centers

Rape crisis centers operate in most communities of any size. The staffs of these centers include many rape victims who have decided to devote time to helping other victims. To find help or advice, or an experienced person to accompany you to the police station with, you can:

- Check the front of your telephone directory for the number of a rape hotline.
- Call Women Against Rape (WAR) if the group has an office in your area. WAR should be listed in the telephone book under "Women."
- Failing the other alternatives, the local YWCA or women's center should have a rape crisis number.

26

Physicians and Diagnostic Procedures

*M*edicine is the umbrella term for the entire profession dealing with the maintenance of health and treatment of disease. In a narrower sense, however, it is often used in distinction to *surgery,* which deals with the correction of disorders or other physical change by operation or by manual manipulation. Thus the term *medical* is often used in distinction to *surgical,* and a *physician,* who treats his patients by medical means, may likewise be distinguished from a *surgeon.* The term *physician,* however, is also used broadly to apply to any authorized practitioner of medicine, including surgeons.

The two kinds of physicians most likely to be encountered when we have an undefined symptom or ailment that requires professional diagnosis and treatment are general or family practitioners and internists. These are the generalists of the medical profession, physicians who treat a wide variety of disorders and illnesses. Unlike other specialists, they usually do not require a referral from another physician and are the first to interview a person about his condition and any complaints he may have.

Diagnosing diseases and disorders requires highly developed skill on the part of the physician or other medical professional. Usually, the diagnosis calls for systematic use of instruments and diagnostic aids, various tests, and, often, extremely sophisticated machines. Questions that the physician asks are designed to provide additional information on which to base the diagnosis.

Using new diagnostic tests, physicians can determine during pregnancy whether a woman will bear a child with a genetic disorder. Tests make it possible to detect prenatally more than 200 diseases, among them sickle-cell anemia, normally fatal blood disorders called *thalassemias,* and hemophilia.

New and growing understanding of the genetic code, the pattern of genes that determines each person's makeup, has made these revolutionary diagnostic tests possible. Scientists cataloging the more than 100,000 human genes can both identify individual genes and work out their structures. Such information is stored in "gene libraries" for the use of physicians and others seeking to identify diseases and health problems long in advance of their actual occurrence.

The General Practitioner

The *general practitioner,* or GP, is about the closest thing we have to the old country doctor who hung out his shingle in front of his small-town house and made midnight carriage rides to deliver babies. The GP not only delivers babies but also listens to our problems, treats skin rashes, sets broken bones, sees children through difficult diseases, dispenses antibiotics and painkillers, and does all the other things we expect a physician to do. He may also perform appendectomies.

Internal Medicine

The *internist* is really a specialist in the branch of medicine called *internal medicine.* He usually refers surgery, and may also refer special problems affecting specific body systems, to physicians specializing in such areas. The internist's training is longer and

Medical Specialties and Subspecialties

Allergy and Immunology
Anesthesiology
Colon and Rectal Surgery
Dermatology
Emergency Medicine
Family Practice
Internal Medicine
  Cardiology
  Endocrinology and Metabolism
  Gastroenterology
  Hematology
  Infectious Diseases
  Medical Oncology
  Nephrology
  Pulmonary Disease
  Rheumatology
Neurological Surgery
Nuclear Medicine
Obstetrics and Gynecology
Ophthalmology
Orthopedic Surgery
Otolaryngology

Pathology
  Blood Banking
Pediatrics
  Pediatric Cardiology
  Pediatric Endocrinology
  Pediatric Hematology-Oncology
  Neonatal-Perinatal Medicine
  Nephrology
Physical Medicine and Rehabilitation
Plastic Surgery
Preventive Medicine
Psychiatry and Neurology
  Psychiatry
  Neurology/Special Competence in
    Child Neurology
  Psychiatry and Neurology
  Child Psychiatry
Radiology
Surgery
Thoracic Surgery
Urology

---

more intensified than that of the GP. In addition, most internists spend one or two years of study in a subspecialty, such as cardiology (heart), hematology (blood), etc. An internist is usually associated with at least one major hospital, its specialists, and its operating and laboratory facilities.

The field of an internist has been defined as "medical diagnosis and treatment"—obviously a very broad definition, to which must be added the observation that one of the responsibilities of the internist is to know when his knowledge is insufficient and when he should refer a patient to another specialist.

An internist should not be confused with an *intern* (or *interne*), who is a medical school graduate serving a year in residence at a hospital. The intern is, in a sense, an apprentice physician, putting the finishing practical touches on the knowledge he has accumulated in medical school by first-hand diagnosis and treatment of patients under the supervision of an experienced physician.

The American Medical Association officially recognizes and licenses physicians and surgeons as specialists in 23 fields (listed below). Before becoming a certified specialist in any of these fields, a physician must qualify in training and pass examinations supervised by a board made up of physicians already practicing that specialty. This training is known as residency training.

Subspecialties of Internal Medicine

An internist may develop a special interest in any of a number of subspecialties, including *cardiology* (the study of the diseases of the heart) or *gastroenterology* (the study of disorders of the digestive tract). Both cardiology and gastroenterology are unusual subspecialties in that the internist must pass an examination for certification as a *cardiologist* or *gastroenterologist*.

A number of other subspecialties

of internal medicine probably sound familiar. *Hematology,* the scientific study of blood and blood-forming tissues, is the interest of the *hematologist. Endocrinology* is the study of the endocrine system, the network of ductless glands and other structures that secrete hormones directly into the bloodstream; the specialist is an *endocrinologist,* and may also specialize in metabolism, the chemical processes that take place to bring about growth, generation of energy, elimination of wastes, and other functions. The study of the connecting and supporting tissues of the body is called *rheumatology,* and the specialist is a *rheumatologist.*

Other specialties of internal medicine include infectious diseases; *medical oncology,* the study of tumors; *nephrology,* the study of the anatomy, physiology, and pathology of the kidneys; and pulmonary disease, disorders of the lungs or respiratory system.

Internists may also, of course, have satisfied the requirements of boards for both internal medicine and one of the other special branches of medicine.

Medical Specialties

The following major specialties are recognized by the American Medical Association:

Allergy and Immunology: The *allergist/immunologist* both diagnoses and treats allergies and specializes in the reactions of tissues of the immune system of the body to stimulation by antibodies (immunology).

Anesthesiology: The *anesthesiologist,* especially during major surgery, administers a patient's state of anesthesia (loss of the sensation of pain) either in parts of or all of the body.

Colon and Rectal Surgery: *Proctology* is the field dealing with diseases of the rectum and colon.

Dermatology: The *dermatologist* is a specialist in the diagnosis and treatment of skin diseases.

Emergency Medicine: The physician specializing in *emergency medicine* studies particularly those conditions that result from trauma or sudden illness.

Family Practice: The *family practice physician* specializes in family medicine, which is concerned with the diagnosis and treatment of health problems of people of either sex and any age. This specialist was once called a *general practitioner.*

Internal Medicine: The role of the *internist,* a kind of general specialist, is discussed above.

Neurological Surgery: The *neurological surgeon* deals with the diagnosis, treatment, and surgical management of disorders and diseases of the brain, spinal cord, and nervous systems.

Nuclear Medicine: The physician specializing in *nuclear medicine* is concerned with the use of radioactive material in the diagnosis and treatment of disease.

Obstetrics and Gynecology: A physician can be an *obstetrician,* a *gynecologist,* or both. The obstetrician's specialty is pregnancy and childbirth; the gynecologist specializes in the care and treatment of women and their diseases, especially of the reproductive system. In practice, he usually treats women who are not pregnant.

Ophthalmology: The *ophthalmologist* is a specialist in medical and surgical treatment of the eye.

Orthopedic Surgery: The *orthopedist,* or *orthopod,* specializes in diagnosing, treating, and surgically correcting, where possible, disorders and injuries associated with the bones, joints, muscles, cartilage, and ligaments.

Otolaryngology: The *otolaryn-gologist* is a specialist, with surgical competence, in practically all the cavities of the head except those holding the eyes and brain. He is the physician of the ear, nose, and throat, often abbreviated to ENT.

Pathology: The *pathologist* investigates the course and causes of diseases, using both laboratory devises and various established techniques.

Pediatrics: The *pediatrician* specializes in all medical aspects of child care. Subspecialties of pediatrics include *pediatric cardiology, pediatric endocrinology, pediatric hematology/ oncology, neonatal/perinatal medicine,* and *nephrology.*

Physical Medicine and Rehabilitation: This specialist deals with the full or partial restoration of use and function to body parts that have been affected by disease or injury, or have been defective at birth.

Plastic Surgery: The *plastic surgeon* specializes in operations designed to give a more normal appearance to parts of the body that are disfigured or that the owner feels are unsightly.

Psychiatry and Neurology: Broadly speaking, the *psychiatrist* deals with the subjective feelings of his patients; the *neurologist* deals with the facts of the nervous system.

Radiology: The *radiologist* is an expert in using electromagnetic radiations (e.g., X rays) for the diagnosis and treatment of diseases.

Surgery: The *general surgeon* has been trained to perform surgery anywhere on the body, but he usually specializes in a particular area.

Thoracic Surgery: A *thoracic surgeon* specializes in operations involving the organs of the chest, or thoracic cavity.

Urology: The *urologist* specializes in the diagnosis, treatment, and surgical management of diseases affecting the male urinogenital tract and female urinary tract.

The Physical Examination

The use of physical examinations to determine the health of people is not new. Medical literature reveals that periodic health examinations were required of the Spartans of ancient Greece. American physicians have encouraged periodic examinations of children and adults as a preventive health measure since the beginning of the Civil War. But only in the last few decades has the general public accepted the idea that many physical disorders can be detected in the earliest stages by an examining physician, and corrective measures prescribed to ensure the maximum number of productive years for the patient. Heart disease, cancer, diabetes, hypertension, and glaucoma are just a few examples of diseases that a physician can detect during a routine physical examination long before disabling symptoms begin to be noticeable to the patient. The Pap test for women is a specific example of an examination technique that can predict the development of cervical cancer several years before the woman might notice signs and symptoms of the insidious disease.

On the other hand, physical examinations may determine that bothersome symptoms do not herald a dangerous disease. A man who suffers from abdominal pains and fears he has stomach cancer would be relieved to learn after an examination that the problem is only nervous tension, which can be corrected by other means. Heart palpitations and breathlessness similarly might be found through a physician's examination to be symptoms of anxiety rather than of heart disease.

The Importance of Periodic Physicals

Health examinations for most Americans unfortunately tend to be sporadic. During infancy and upon entering school, there may be detailed physical examinations, possibly followed by additional checkups during later childhood when required by the local educational system, and finally, a thorough examination for persons entering the military service or applying for a job or an insurance policy. But there may follow a period of 30 to 40 "lost years" for many persons before they feel the need for a checkup because of the symptoms of one of the degenerative diseases that may appear when they have reached their 50s or 60s. Unfortunately, statistics show that nearly 30 percent of chronic and disabling diseases begin before the age of 35 and about 40 percent between the ages of 35 and 55, with evidence that many chronic disabilities actually developed more or less unnoticed by the patients during the "lost years" when periodic physical examinations were considered by them unnecessary.

Periodic physical examinations are now encouraged for persons of all age groups, with four objectives:

- To detect abnormalities so that early diagnosis and treatment can prevent disability and premature death, especially from chronic diseases

- To improve the individual's understanding of health and disease

- To establish good relations between patient and physician as a basis for continuing health maintenance

- To provide specific preventive health measures, such as immunizations and advice about such lifestyle matters as cigarette smoking and weight control

General Diagnostic Procedures

A typical physical examination will include a careful health appraisal by an examining physician, including a detailed health history of the patient and study of the patient's body appearance and functions, an X ray of the chest area, and electrocardiogram of the heart in some cases, and laboratory analysis of blood and urine samples. Other appropriate procedures, such as a Pap smear test, may be added to the routine. Because no two persons are exactly alike and the differences among patients are likely to increase with advancing years, the examining physician's interest in a set of signs and symptoms may vary with different patients as he pieces evidence together to come up with a complete evaluation of a particular patient.

Medical History

The examination almost invariably begins with the *medical history* and includes details that may seem trivial or unimportant to the patient. But the information sometimes can provide important clues to a physician compiling data about a patient. This information usually includes the age, sex, race, marital status, occupation, and birthplace of the patient. The examiner also may want to know about any previous contacts with the physician's medical group, clinic, hospital, or other medical facility, in the event that previous medical records of the individual are on file.

Symptoms

The physician may ask a simple, obvious question, like "What is bothering you?" or "Why did you want to see a doctor?" The answer given may become for examining purposes the chief complaint and usually will in-

volve any current or recent illness. If there is a current or recent illness to discuss, the physician will want to know more about it: when did it begin, how did it begin, and how has it affected you? If the physician asks about *symptoms,* he usually is probing for information about what the patient feels, and where. A symptom may be a pain, ache, bloated feeling, and so on. A *sign* is, in medical terminology, what somebody else, such as the physician, observes; signs and symptoms usually go together in solving a medical problem.

The physician's view of the importance of some symptoms may not be the same as the patient's. The physician may try to pursue complaints that may not seem important to the patient but actually can be more significant than the chief complaint. The physician's training and experience give him some advantages in concluding, for example, that a 45-year-old woman who has had a chronic cough for several years probably does not have lung cancer, even though that may be her chief concern.

Past Illnesses

Other details included in the medical history would be a list of childhood diseases, adult diseases such as pneumonia or tuberculosis, broken bones suffered, burns or gunshot wounds, unconsciousness as a result of an injury, a description of past operations, information about immunizations, medicines taken and side effects experienced from medications, and, for women, information about pregnancies, if any. Family history questions would cover information about the parents and blood relatives, including a variety of diseases they may have suffered.

Life-Style and Attitude

Next, the physician may review the

body systems, asking questions about any difficulties experienced with the head, eyes, ears, mouth, nose, lungs, heart, etc. Changes in body weight, hair texture, appetite, and other factors will be recorded, along with information about occupation, military service, and travel in foreign countries. Life-style questions could cover sleeping habits, sex life, use of coffee, tea, alcoholic beverages, vitamin tablets, sleeping pills, tobacco, exercise, and social activities. In addition to the answers given, the physician may record how the answers to questions are presented by a patient, since the patient's attitude can offer additional insight into the person's mental and physical health. For example, a patient who tries to dominate the examination interview or who answers the physician's questions with a response like "What do you mean by that?" may reveal more by the quality than the content of the answers.

Observation

After the medical history has been recorded or updated, the physician may begin a general inspection of the patient's body, beginning with the head and neck and working down to the feet. The physician looks for possible deformities, scars or wounds, including insect bites, or pulsations or throbbing areas. Bruises, areas of skin peeling or flaking, areas of heavy skin pigmentation or loss of pigmentation, hair distribution, perspiration or goose bumps, firmness or slackness of the skin, warts, calluses, and other features are noted.

Palpation

The physician usually checks the exterior of the body by a method known as *palpation*, which means feeling with the fingers and hands. Because some parts of the hand are more sen-

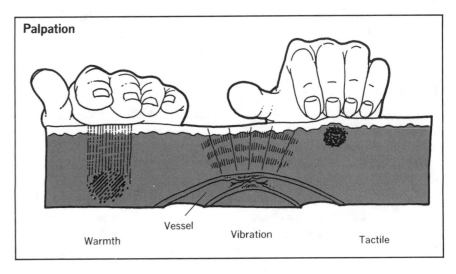

Palpation

Warmth　　Vessel　　Vibration　　Tactile

sitive to warmth and others are more sensitive to vibrations, the physician may shift from finger tips to palms at various times in his search for health clues. Rough vibrations from a disorder in the respiratory system, the trembling sensation of blood encountering an obstruction, or the grating feeling of a bone deformity can be detected during palpation. The physician also can tell from palpation where areas are tender or abnormally warm to the touch. If he finds a raised area of the skin, he can tell by palpation whether there is a growth within or beneath the skin.

Percussion and Auscultation

In addition to palpation, the examining physician may apply *percussion*, or tapping, of certain body areas. Tapping the chest, for example, gives the physician some information, from the sounds produced, about the condition of the lungs. He also uses a related technique of *auscultation*, or listening to sounds within the body, either with his ear against the body or through a stethoscope, the familiar Y-shaped instrument used to amplify internal sounds.

In percussion, the physician usually places one hand on the surface of the patient's body with the fingers slightly spread apart and taps on one

of the fingers with the middle finger of the other hand. By moving the lower hand around on various areas of the chest surface while tapping one finger on the other, the physician can get a fairly accurate "sound picture" of the condition of organs within the chest. He can outline the heart, and the distance moved by the diaphragm in filling and emptying the lungs, by listening for changes in percussion sounds that range from resonance

Percussion and Ausculation

over hollow spaces to dullness over solid or muscular areas. Lack of resonance over a normally resonant area of the lung might indicate fluid, pneumonia, or perhaps an abnormal mass. Percussion may also give the first sign of enlargement of organs, such as the liver, heart, or spleen.

During auscultation, the physician listens for normal or abnormal breathing sounds. He can usually detect specific aberrations in lung function by noises made as the air rushes in and out of the lungs through the bronchi. A sound of frictional rubbing can suggest a rough surface on the lining of the pleura, a membrane surrounding the lung tissue; a splashing or slapping sound would indicate the presence of fluid in the lungs. In auscultation of the heart, the physician listens for extra heartbeats, rubbing sounds, the rumbling noises of a heart murmur, or the sounds of normally functioning heart valves opening and closing.

An experienced physician may use his stethoscope for listening to sounds beyond the chest area. He may listen to the sounds of blood flowing through vessels of the neck, bowel sounds through the wall of the abdomen, and the subtle noises made by joints, muscles, and tendons as various limbs are moved.

During examination of the chest, the physician usually asks the patient to perform certain breathing functions: take a deep breath, hold your breath, inhale, exhale, etc. On one or more of the exhalation commands, the physician may make a quick check of the air exhaled from the lungs to determine if there is any odor suggesting a disease that might be unnoticed by the patient. Just as the physician learns to recognize the meaning of percussion and auscultation sounds, he learns the meaning of certain odors of bacterial activity or other disorders.

Body Structure and Gait

Weight and height are checked as part of any routine examination. These factors are important in a health examination for children to determine the rate of growth, even though youngsters of the same age can vary considerably in height and weight and still be within the so-called normal range. Sudden changes in the rate of growth or abnormal growth may be signs that special attention should be given to possible problems. Adults also can vary greatly in weight and height, but special concern may be indicated by the physician if the individual is exceptionally tall, short, fat, or skinny. In addition to a possible disease associated with unusual stature, the facts and figures obtained about body build can be important because certain disorders tend to develop in individuals of a particular body structure. Posture also provides clues to the true condition of a patient; a person who has a slouch or who holds one shoulder higher than the other may have an abnormal spinal curvature. The physician may watch the patient's manner of walking, because a person's gait can suggest muscle, bone, or nervous-system disorders; a person who seems to lean forward and take short steps, for example, may have muscles that do not relax normally during movement of the legs.

Blood Pressure

Blood pressure is measured with the help of a device called a *sphygmomanometer* and the stethoscope. The sphygmomanometer has either a dial with a face that shows the blood pressure reading in millimeters of mercury, or a column of mercury in a glass tube with numbers alongside it. Either kind of device also has attached to it an inflatable cuff, which is wrapped around the upper arm; a rub-

ber bulb is used to inflate the cuff and increase pressure in it so that it can control the blood flow in the arm. The physician or nurse places the bell-shaped end of the stethoscope on a point on the inside of the elbow where the pulse can be felt. The bulb is squeezed to increase the cuff pressure until the heartbeat, in the form of the pulse, can no longer be heard through the stethoscope. The reading on the sphygmomanometer at that stage may be well over 200. Then the physician slowly deflates the cuff and lets the reading on the gauge fall gradually until he hears the first beat of the heart. The reading on the gauge at that point is recorded as the *systolic pressure*. The physician continues to relax the pressure in the cuff and watches for the reading at the point where the thumping of the heart disappears. That number is recorded as the *diastolic pressure*.

If the systolic pressure is, for example, 130 and the diastolic pressure is 72, the physician may make a notation of "BP 130/72," which is the patient's blood pressure at the time of the examination. The records also may indicate whether the patient was sitting or lying down at the time and whether the pressure was taken on the right arm or the left arm. Sometimes the pressure is checked on both arms. If the patient appears tense or anxious, which could produce a higher than normal blood pressure reading, the physician may encourage the patient to relax for a few minutes and try again for a more meaningful reading.

Pulse Rate

The pulse itself usually is studied for rate and quality, or character, which means the force of the pulse beat and the tension between beats. The pulse beat for small children may be well over 100 per minute and still be con-

Pulse

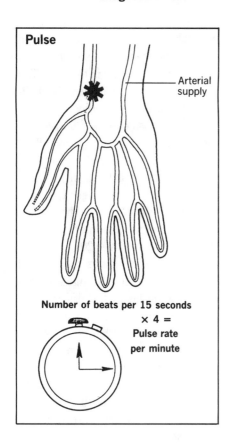

Arterial supply

Number of beats per 15 seconds
× 4 =
Pulse rate per minute

sidered normal. But in an adult who is relaxed and resting, any pulse rate over 100 suggests that something is wrong. An adult pulse rate of less than 60 also might indicate an abnormal condition.

Eyes

Inspection of the eyes is usually done with the aid of an *ophthalmoscope,* by means of which the physician can visualize the retina on the back inner surface of each eye, and its associated arteries, veins, and nerve fibers. Distended retinal veins may be a sign of a variety of disorders, including diabetes or heart disease; signs of hardening of the arteries also may be observed in the eyes before other indications are found elsewhere in the body. The condition of retinal blood vessels may, in addition, signal the development of hypertension.

Mouth, Nose, and Ears

The mouth, nose, and ears are in-

spected for signs of abnormalities. A device called an *otoscope* is inserted in the outer ear to examine the external auditory canal and eardrum. If the patient wears dentures, the physician may ask that they be removed during examination of the mouth so that the health of the gums can be checked. The condition of the tongue, teeth, and gums can reveal much about the health habits of the individual. An inadequate set of teeth, for example, can indicate that certain important food items that require chewing are being avoided. Tobacco stains obviously are a sign of tobacco use.

X Rays

A chest X ray is usually a routine part of the examination; the X ray usually covers the chest area, showing the condition of the heart and lungs. The finished X-ray picture looks something like a large photographic negative, but the film is designed so that areas filled with gas, such as the lungs or fatty tissues, appear almost trans-

parent, and bone or solid metal objects appear sharply opaque. Muscle, blood, and other objects, including gallbladder stones, can be identified through a hazy kind of contrast between opaque and translucent. A number of special kinds of X rays may be ordered if the physician wants to make a more detailed check of some possible disorder involving a specific body cavity, such as a peptic ulcer in the stomach wall.

Electrocardiogram

An increasing number of health examinations today include an electrocardiographic study of the heart. An *electrocardiogram,* or *EKG,* is made as a kind of "picture" traced by a pen on a moving sheet of paper, with the movements of the pen controlled by electrical impulses produced by the heart. All muscle activity produces tiny electrical discharges, and the rhythmic contractions of heart muscle result in a distinctive pattern of electrical pulsations that forms the elec-

Electrocardiogram

Electrocardiographic lead

trocardiogram picture. The tracing appears to the patient as simply a long, wavy line, but the physician can identify each of the wave crests and dips in terms of different parts of the heart muscle contracting or relaxing in proper sequence, or—if the heart is not functioning normally—not in proper sequence.

The electrocardiogram is recorded by attaching electrodes, or leads, to the chest, arms, and legs, in a series of differing arrangements depending upon the kind of heart picture the physician wants to record. The wires from the electrodes are connected to the machine that translates the heartbeat rhythms into the electrocardiogram. There is no danger of electrical shock, because the only electricity flowing through the wires is the current produced continuously by the human body as part of its natural functions.

It is always an advantage for the patient to have an electrocardiogram taken early in adult life and when in a good state of health, because that record can serve as a benchmark for comparing electrocardiograms made later in life when the condition of the heart may have changed. This rule applies to all other health examination records as well.

Urinalysis

No patient health evaluation is complete without the findings of laboratory tests of blood and urine. The physician or his assistant may give special instructions about food and water intake well in advance of the time for delivering a urine specimen, because those factors can influence the chemical makeup of the sample. The time of day of the collection also can affect the composition of the urine sample; urine voided early in the morning is likely to be more acid in content, while urine collected after a meal may be more alkaline. Thus, for a routine physical, the physician may advise that a urine sample be taken at his office at 9:00 A.M. but that nothing be eaten since the previous evening meal. The physician also may want not the first but the second specimen of the day. In some cases, depending upon the patient's complaint, the physician may request a collection of all the urine voided during a period of 12 or 24 hours.

Chemical Content of the Urine

A typical urine sample is, of course, mostly water. But it also may contain about two dozen identifiable minerals and other chemicals, including sodium potassium, calcium, sulfur, ammonia, urea, and several different acids. A urine sample can range in color from pale straw to dark amber, depending upon the concentration. It also can be other colors, including orange or blue, or even colorless, depending upon foods eaten, medications taken, diseases, or exposure to toxic substances.

Appearance and Acidity

The urine sample's general appearance, including color, is noted by the laboratory technician. The sample also is tested for acidity or alkalinity, normal urine being just slightly on the acid side of neutral. Urine that is definitely acidic can be a sign of a variety of disorders, including certain metabolic problems. Urine that is markedly on the alkaline side of neutral also can suggest a number of possible disorders, including an infection of the urinary tract. Alkalinity could also be caused by certain medications, or even by the patient's use of large doses of bicarbonate of soda. Foods rich in protein can make the urine more acidic, while citrus fruits and some vegetables may tend to make a patient's urine more alkaline.

What the Urine Shows

A thorough analysis of a person's urine can turn up some clues to the condition of almost every part of the body and verify or rule out the presence of any of a number of physical disorders. The specific gravity of the urine, for example, can indicate the general health of the urinary tract; protein (albumin) tests may tell something about the condition of the kidneys and prostate and, in a pregnant women, indicate toxemia; glucose (sugar) in the urine could suggest diabetes; the presence of ketone bodies could be a sign of metabolic disorders; bilirubin (bile) in the urine could be a sign of liver disease, and so on. Various urine tests check for the presence of red blood cells or white blood cells, tissue cells from the lining of organs, various hormones, traces of drugs taken, fat bodies, parasites, indications of renal calculi (kidney stones), and a variety of bits of tissue, often microscopic, called *casts*. One kind of cast might be a sign of heart failure or shock, another might be a warning of heavy-metal poisoning, a third might indicate a kidney infection.

Blood Tests

Laboratory blood studies also can reveal bits of information about organ systems throughout the body. For a simple blood test, a few drops may be drawn from a capillary through a finger prick; more detailed blood tests can require the equivalent of a couple of teaspoonfuls of blood drawn from a vein in the arm. The amount of blood taken for a laboratory test is not harmful; a normal body manufactures a couple of ounces of new blood every day, several times the amount used for a laboratory test.

Red Cells

For a count of red blood cells (RBC),

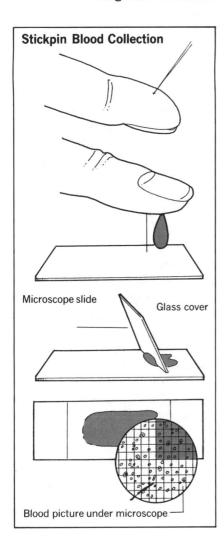

Stickpin Blood Collection

Microscope slide

Glass cover

Blood picture under microscope

or *erythrocytes*, a small part of the original blood sample may be diluted and a bit of the solution placed on a special microscope slide that enables the technician to estimate the average number of red blood cells per cubic millimeter of blood. The normal RBC range for a man is in the neighborhood of 4.8 to 5.8 million red blood cells per cubic millimeter of blood; for a woman, the RBC count is about 4.4 to 5.4 million. For a child, the normal figure is slightly less than that of a woman.

The blood sample also may be checked for the level of hemoglobin, an iron-protein substance that gives the blood its red color and makes it possible for blood to carry oxygen to all parts of the body. A below-normal level of hemoglobin could be a sign of anemia resulting from a number of possible causes, including actual loss of blood from hemorrhage, vitamin deficiencies, lack of iron in the diet, or a disease.

White Cells

White blood cell (WBC), or *leukocyte,* counts are made the same way as RBC counts. The total normal WBC count for both men and women ranges from 5,000 to 10,000 per cubic millimeter. A higher count would indicate the presence of an infection or other disease problem.

Other Factors

Other blood studies may be performed for information about the coagulation characteristics of a patient's blood sample, levels of calcium, sodium, potassium, and other chemicals present, presence of certain enzymes, acidity of the blood, levels of sugar, bilirubin, urea nitrogen, cholesterol and other fatty substances, alcohol and other drugs, and proteins, including albumin.

Not all of these tests are performed during a routine physical examination, but they could be used if needed to track down the cause of an otherwise elusive set of symptoms. By comparing the results of two blood enzyme tests, for example, it would be possible to sort out symptoms of six different kinds of liver disease, as well as a heart attack and infectious mononucleosis. The results might not be the final answer to a medical problem, but the laboratory test data could be important pieces of the jigsaw puzzle that the physician needs to complete the health picture that begins to take form when the patient enters the physician's office for a physical examination.

Specialties and Their Diagnostic Procedures

If a definite diagnosis cannot be made on the basis of the medical history and preliminary physical examination, more specialized tests are employed. These are usually made under the direction of a specialist. These specialists and some of the most important of their diagnostic procedures—there are literally hundreds of them—are described below, arranged according to the major body systems.

The Skeleton and the Muscles

The *orthopedic surgeon,* or *orthopedist,* is the major specialist in the diagnosis, treatment, and surgical correction of diseases and injuries of the bones, joints, and musculature. Because the healthy functioning of muscles is closely involved with the nervous system, the *neurologist* is frequently consulted. The branch of internal medicine called *rheumatology* is specially concerned with the joints.

The teeth and their supporting structures are, of course, the concern of *dentistry* and the *dentist.* The *orthodontist* is a dentist specializing in the alignment of teeth and their proper positioning in the mouth. A *pediatric dentist* specializes in teeth problems of young people up to the time that the second set of teeth erupt. An *oral surgeon* (dental surgeon) performs surgery within the oral cavity, including tooth extraction. He and the orthodontist have had additional training after receiving the dental degree, and the oral surgeon may have a medical degree (MD) as well. The *periodontist* treats gum disorders.

Diagnostic Procedures

X rays are probably relied upon more than any other technique for special investigations of the bones, joints,

The Human Skeleton

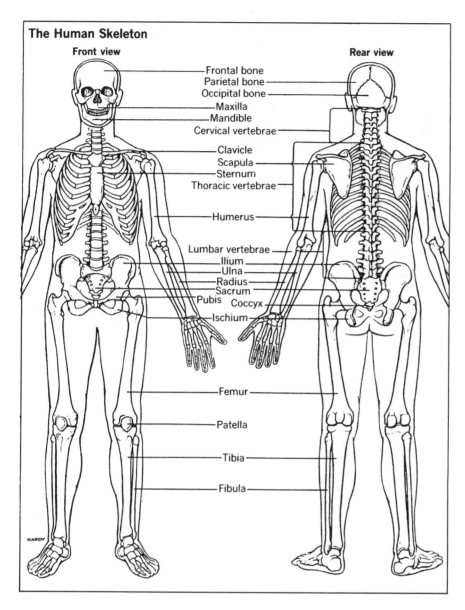

The Nervous System and the Brain

The *neurosurgeon*, sometimes popularly referred to as a brain surgeon, is qualified for diagnosis, treatment, and surgery of the brain and nervous system. The term *neurologist* is generally restricted to a physician who does not perform surgery. The neurologist may be an internist having neurology as a subspecialty.

Diagnostic Procedures

A *spinal fluid exam,* or spinal tap, involves the withdrawal by special needle under sterile conditions, and subsequent laboratory examination, of a small amount of cerebrospinal fluid for the diagnosis of polio, meningitis, brain tumors, and other conditions. The *electroencephalogram* (EEG) gives a picture of, and shows irregularities in, a person's "brain waves." The *echoencephalogram* uses ultrasonic waves, rather than the electric currents of the EEG, to investigate the functioning of the brain. A *brain scan* calls for the injection of a radioactive element into the brain tissue or fluid and records its movements on a photographic plate.

Recently, an X-ray technique utilizing a computer and known as *CT scanning* (for *computed tomography*) has proved to be most effective for visualizing "slices" of the brain that would otherwise be inaccessible, and no injection is necessary. Sometimes called a *brain scanner,* the device takes a series of pictures as it is rotated around the patient. From data fed into a computer, the computer generates composite pictures of the brain.

An even later development, *nuclear magnetic resonance* (NMR), or *magnetic resonance imaging,* utilizes two simple elements, a magnet and radio waves, to make sophisticated analyses. Like CT, NMR provides

and teeth. They can reveal a tiny tooth cavity, a hairline fracture of a major bone, a bony deposit, or an eroded surface around a joint. *Serum analysis*—laboratory investigation of the clear portion separated from a person's blood sample—can also reveal underlying chemical irregularities that accompany or precede bone and joint diseases.

Synovial aspiration (also called *synovial fluid exam*) involves the withdrawal of a tiny amount of fluid (synovial fluid) with a needle inserted into a joint. The laboratory analysis of the fluid can diagnose gout and some

forms of arthritis.

Electromyography can give an electrical tracing of muscle nerve function and reveal the presence of disorders.

Muscle biopsy is the surgical excision of a small piece of muscle tissue for laboratory examination and tests.

Skin, Hair, and Nails

The *dermatologist* is the principal specialist. *Skin biopsy,* the removal of a piece of skin tissue for laboratory testing and microscopic study, is used for difficult diagnoses.

Nervous System
Cranial Nerves

Optic nerve (vision)
Olfactory nerve (smell)
Oculomotor nerve (eye muscles)
Trigeminal nerve (face)
Trochlear nerve (eye muscles)
Facial nerve (facemuscles)
Acoustic nerve (hearing and balance)
Glossopharyngeal nerve (taste)
Vagus nerve (heart, lungs, abdomen)

Central Nervous System

Cerebrum

Cerebellum

Brachial plexus
Spinal cord

**Autonomic Nervous
System**

**Peripheral Nervous
System**

Thoracic nerves
Radial nerve
Ulnar nerve

Femoral nerve

Sciatic nerve

high-resolution pictures of the structures of various body parts and organs. But NMR does not utilize X rays and it can be used to examine the biochemistry of living cells.

The *cerebral arteriogram* is a method of visualizing and assaying brain damage by injecting a dye into the blood vessels serving the brain and then X-raying them. It is especially useful in judging the severity and location of hemorrhages and strokes. A *pneumoencephalogram* is an X-ray picture of the brain taken after air or gas has been injected into the ventricles of the brain.

The Circulatory System, the Heart, and Blood

The *cardiologist* is an internist who has special knowledge in the diagnosis and medical treatment of heart disease. The *hematologist* is an internist who has special training in the techniques of diagnosing and treating diseases of the blood (including lymph) and bone marrow.

The *thoracic surgeon* is a surgeon who has satisfied the requirements of licensing boards for both general surgery and thoracic (chest cavity) surgery. He has special training in the

surgical treatment of defects and diseases of the heart and large blood vessels. The *vascular surgeon* is a general surgeon specializing in the surgical treatment of diseases of blood vessels.

Diagnostic Procedures

The *electrocardiogram* graphically records the electrical activity of the heart associated with contraction of the cardiac muscle. It can provide valuable information regarding disorders of or damage to the heart muscle (i.e., heart attack), disturbances in rhythm, or enlargement of any of the four chambers of the heart. A *vectorcardiogram* is similar to the electrocardiogram but more specifically attuned to the magnitude and direction of the electrical currents of the heart. Abnormalities not apparent on the electrocardiogram may often be revealed by a vectorcardiogram.

The *phonocardiogram* is a recording on paper of the heart sounds, which enables the physician to evaluate murmurs and abnormal heart sounds with more accuracy than by listening with the stethoscope. The timing of the murmur with relation to the specific events of heart muscle contraction may also be precisely evaluated. The *echocardiogram* provides a paper tracing of sound waves that are directed toward, and subsequently bounced back from, various internal heart structures. The technique is useful in diagnosing abnormalities of the heart valves, as well as abnormal collections of fluid in the sac (pericardium) enveloping the heart.

The *fluoroscope* visualizes the heart in action by use of X rays. It is useful in the evaluation of heart and vessel pulsation, as well as of valve or vessel calcification. Plain *chest X rays* may reveal enlargement of the heart, abnormal calcification of vessels or heart valves, and signs of a congestive heart valve. These are only three examples of the great number of abnormalities that can be revealed by a routine chest X ray.

The *cardiac X-ray series* are a number of X rays of the chest taken in several positions as the patient swallows a liquid, for example, barium sulfate, which makes the esophagus stand out on the X ray. This is usually called a barium swallow. Indentation of the esophagus by abnormally enlarged heart chambers may be revealed by this technique. "Barium meals" are also important in the radiologic diagnosis of disorders of the esophagus, stomach, and small intestine.

Cardiac catheterization is the insertion of a small tubular surgical instrument via a vein in the arm or artery of the leg, through the blood vessels, directly into the right or left side of the heart. This procedure is employed to confirm suspected intracardiac (within the heart) anomalies, determine intracardiac pressures, and take blood samples. Catheterization enables the physician to confirm suspected defects in the walls dividing the heart chambers or to estimate the severity of a lesion and the need for corrective surgery.

Angiocardiography (or simply *angiography*), if warranted, is performed at the same time as cardiac catheterization. Its principle involves the injection of a contrast material (e.g., a substance visible on a fluoroscopy screen or X-ray film) by means of the catheter, with consequent visualization of the heart and major blood vessels. Angiography is not limited to investigation of the heart chambers but can reveal abnormalities of large vessels such as the aorta, coronary arteries, and renal arteries.

CT scanning, mentioned above, is becoming an increasingly important

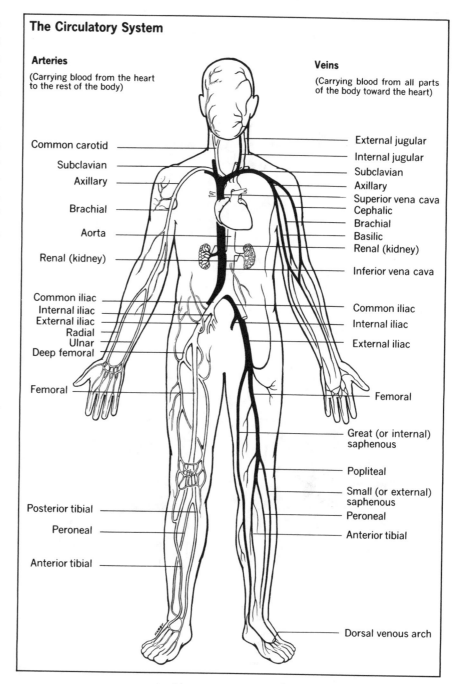

The Circulatory System

Arteries
(Carrying blood from the heart to the rest of the body)

Common carotid
Subclavian
Axillary
Brachial
Aorta
Renal (kidney)
Common iliac
Internal iliac
External iliac
Radial
Ulnar
Deep femoral
Femoral
Posterior tibial
Peroneal
Anterior tibial

Veins
(Carrying blood from all parts of the body toward the heart)

External jugular
Internal jugular
Subclavian
Axillary
Superior vena cava
Cephalic
Brachial
Basilic
Renal (kidney)
Inferior vena cava
Common iliac
Internal iliac
External iliac
Femoral
Great (or internal) saphenous
Popliteal
Small (or external) saphenous
Peroneal
Anterior tibial
Dorsal venous arch

diagnostic tool and may in many cases make angiocardiography unnecessary. Sometimes called a *body scanner*, the CT scanner takes a series of computer-assisted X-ray pictures as it slowly rotates around the patient, thus providing cross-sectional pictures of the target organ. It is a painless and safe procedure, and is capable of providing pictures of areas of the body that would be very difficult to visualize by any other means.

Hematological (Blood Sampling) Diagnostic Techniques

Routine laboratory tests performed in all hospital admissions are the *peripheral smear* and *complete blood count*. Approximately 5 milliliters (ml) of blood are *aspirated* (withdrawn by suction) from a vein, typically in the crease of the elbow. From this sample, a determination of the patient's hemoglobin and percentage of red

The Heart

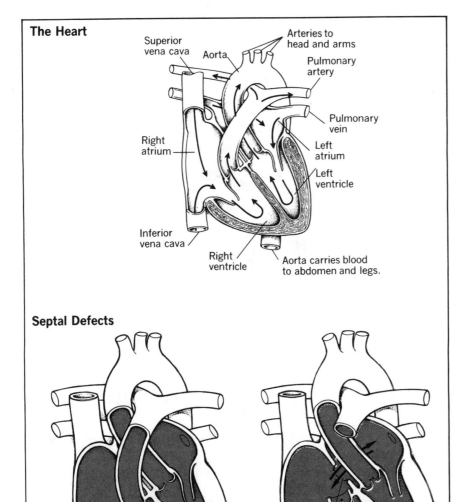

Superior vena cava

Aorta

Arteries to head and arms

Pulmonary artery

Pulmonary vein

Right atrium

Left atrium

Left ventricle

Inferior vena cava

Right ventricle

Aorta carries blood to abdomen and legs.

Septal Defects

Interventricular defect

Interatrial defect

A normal heart in cross section (*top*), shows the circulation of the blood. An interventricular defect (*bottom left*) allows blood to pass directly between the left and right ventricles. An interatrial defect (*bottom right*), with the aorta seen in cross section over the left atrium, allows blood to pass freely between the two atria. Any septal defect interferes with the effectiveness of the pumping action of the heart.

In suspected cases of *neoplastic diseases*—diseases involving abnormal growths that may be or may become malignant—a *lymph node biopsy* (surgical excision and microscopic examination of lymph node tissue) is performed. A *lymphangiogram* is used when tumors of the lymphatic system are suspected. A dye or contrast material visible on an X ray is injected into a lymphatic vessel, usually one on the top of the foot. X rays of the abdomen taken over the next several days are studied for abnormalities in the size and structure of internal lymph nodes.

There are numerous other hematological tests, including radioactive (radioisotope) tests, which are used in special situations when diagnosis by other means is inadequate.

The Digestive System and the Liver

The internist is generally able to treat most gastrointestinal disorders. The *gastroenterologist* is an internist who has special knowledge of disorders of the digestive tract. *Colon* and *rectal surgeons* operate on the large intestine, rectum, and anus; *proctology* deals with the diagnosis and treatment of disorders in this area. Surgeons and internists specializing in this region are called *proctologists*.

Diagnostic Procedures

Examination can be made of the esophagus, stomach, and duodenum, and sometimes of the entire length of the small intestine, by using a sequence of many fluoroscope, motion-picture, and X-ray pictures. This is called the *gastrointestinal series,* or simply the *GI series*. So that the internal walls of the digestive organs will stand out clearly in the pictures, the patient eats nothing for eight hours before, and when the exami-

corpuscles per milliliter of plasma may be calculated. Microscopic analysis of the number and character of the red cells, white cells, and platelets provides additional essential information.

If an abnormality such as decreased hemoglobin or overpopulation of white cells is noted on complete blood count and peripheral smear, the physician might request that a sample of the patient's bone marrow be ob-

tained for evaluation—a procedure called *bone marrow biopsy*. Following local anesthesia of the operative site, typically the hipbone, a biopsy needle is inserted into the marrow of the bone and a small sample of marrow is withdrawn. If performed by an experienced physician, the patient feels only some pressure and very slight pain as the marrow sample is aspirated.

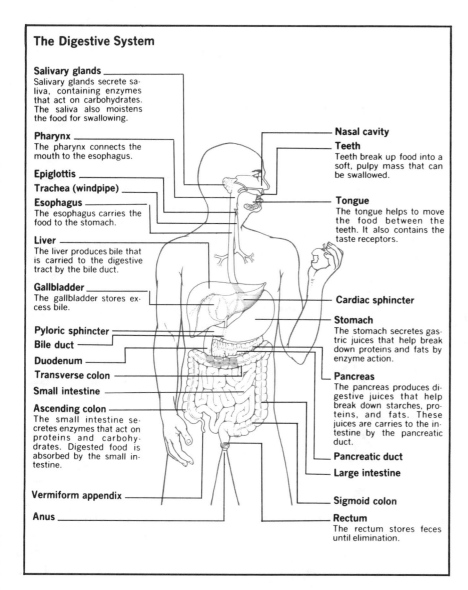

The Digestive System

Salivary glands
Salivary glands secrete saliva, containing enzymes that act on carbohydrates. The saliva also moistens the food for swallowing.

Pharynx
The pharynx connects the mouth to the esophagus.

Epiglottis

Trachea (windpipe)

Esophagus
The esophagus carries the food to the stomach.

Liver
The liver produces bile that is carried to the digestive tract by the bile duct.

Gallbladder
The gallbladder stores excess bile.

Pyloric sphincter

Bile duct

Duodenum

Transverse colon

Small intestine

Ascending colon
The small intestine secretes enzymes that act on proteins and carbohydrates. Digested food is absorbed by the small intestine.

Vermiform appendix

Anus

Nasal cavity

Teeth
Teeth break up food into a soft, pulpy mass that can be swallowed.

Tongue
The tongue helps to move the food between the teeth. It also contains the taste receptors.

Cardiac sphincter

Stomach
The stomach secretes gastric juices that help break down proteins and fats by enzyme action.

Pancreas
The pancreas produces digestive juices that help break down starches, proteins, and fats. These juices are carries to the intestine by the pancreatic duct.

Pancreatic duct

Large intestine

Sigmoid colon

Rectum
The rectum stores feces until elimination.

spaces of the body that would otherwise be inaccessible.

Special tests for the liver's health and function include the removal of a tiny piece of liver tissue, by means of a long needle inserted through the skin, and the tissue's subsequent laboratory examination; this procedure is called *needle biopsy of liver* and often is used to confirm diagnosis of cirrhosis. An injection of a chemical called *BSP,* followed later by analysis of a blood specimen, is used to investigate liver function. A *liver scan,* like a brain scan, employs a radioactive substance to visualize the function of the organ.

X-ray examination of the gallbladder, resulting in a *cholecystogram—cholecyst* is a medical name for "gallbladder"—is used to diagnose gallbladder disease and to locate gallstones. A dye is swallowed before the test.

The Respiratory System and the Lungs

The internist handles most nonsurgical disorders, and the thoracic surgeon specializes in surgical procedures involving the respiratory organs.

Diagnostic Procedures

In the *sputum exam* a number of bacteriological, chemical, and microscopic tests are peformed on the sputum (saliva, often mixed with mucus or other substances); these tests can detect a hidden abscess in the respiratory tract, pneumonia, tuberculosis, and other lung diseases.

Practically everybody is aware of the value of *chest X rays* in the diagnosis of diseases and disorders of the lungs, heart, and ribs. Many diseases of the lungs and respiratory system are also revealed by tests administered on the skin. For example, the skin's reaction to a substance called

nation begins, he is asked to swallow a glassful of chalky, sticky barium sulfate. The GI series is one of the first tests administered when an ulcer or cancer is suspected in the stomach or duodenum.

Gastric analysis is the extraction and study of stomach juices for clues to intestinal disorders.

A *barium enema* is the injection via the anus of a barium solution; it usually precedes X-ray examination of the large intestine for signs of cancer or other diseases. *Stool exams,* laboratory studies of the feces, may also reveal cancer, as well as the presence of parasitic worms and amebas.

There are a wide variety of slender, hollow, tubular instruments equipped with a light and a lens to enable the physician to see into the GI tract: the *esophagoscope* for insertion by way of the mouth into the esophagus; the *gastroscope* for inspection of the stomach; the *gastroduodenal fiberscope* for inspection of the stomach and duodenum. "Scopes" inserted via the anus include the *proctosigmoidoscope* for visual examination of the rectum and lower colon, and the *colonoscope* for investigating farther up the large intestine. These are called *fiberoptic* instruments because they transmit light by means of a bundle of fibers of glass or plastic that permit observation of curved interior

The Respiratory System

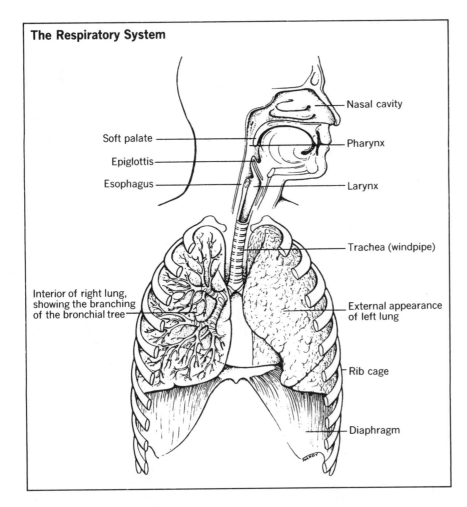

Nasal cavity

Soft palate

Pharynx

Epiglottis

Esophagus

Larynx

Trachea (windpipe)

Interior of right lung, showing the branching of the bronchial tree

External appearance of left lung

Rib cage

Diaphragm

PPD (*p*urified *p*rotein *d*erivative) is used in diagnosing tuberculosis. *Bronchoscopy* is inspection of the bronchial tubes with the tube and scope instrument called the *bronchoscope.*

Special tests that measure lung volume, capacity, and function have become more common as physicians have become conscious of the adverse effects of air pollution and the growing incidence of irreversible diseases, such as emphysema.

The Endocrine Glands

There is no AMA/licensed specialty, but the internist/endocrinologist is the expert.

Diagnostic Procedures

There are a great many tests, using both blood and urine samples, that suggest or confirm the excess or insufficiency of a specific hormone in the body. In turn, these tests point to the overactivity or underactivity of one of the hormone-secreting endocrine glands.

The Sense Organs—Eye, Ear, Nose

The two specialists in this area are both licensed to peform surgery in their special areas of competence. The *ophthalmologist* is the eye doctor. The *otolaryngologist* is the ear, nose, and throat specialist.

Diagnostic Procedures

We are all familiar with the lettered test charts that determine whether we are nearsighted or farsighted or have some other defect in our eyes'

focusing apparatus, such as an astigmatism. Color charts to test for color blindness are also commonly used.

With the *ophthalmoscope* and the *slit-lamp microscope,* which magnifies a beam of concentrated light, the ophthalmologist can examine the structures within the eye in great detail. The *retinoscope* reveals the actual structural abnormalities that account for nearsightedness or farsightedness. The *gonioscope* enables the ophthalmologist to inspect the angle between the cornea and the iris, which is of importance in diagnosing glaucoma. The fluid pressure itself within the anterior chamber can be measured by an extremely delicate spring-balance gauge called a *tonometer.* Finally, *perimeter* can be used to map boundaries of the visual field; the narrowing of these boundaries ("tunnel vision" is the extreme example) is a symptom of glaucoma and other eye disorders.

Hearing and hearing loss are measured by a device called the *audiometer,* with which a physician can measure accurately the whole range of vibrations heard as sound by the human ear. The *otoscope* is an instrument for examining the external auditory canal and eardrum.

The Urinogenital System and the Kidneys

The *urologist* is the acknowledged specialist. He does not deal, however, with the female reproductive organs, which are the specialty of the obstetrician and gynecologist.

Diagnostic Procedures

The collective name for a number of tests that analyze the contents of urine is *urinalysis.* These include tests of the urine's physical properties, as well as chemical and microscopic analysis. Telltale signs of diseases of the kidneys and bladder often show up in urine, and sugar in the urine may be an indication of diabetes. *Urine culture* is a test for microbial infections of the urinary tract.

Pyelograms are X-ray examinations of the interior of the kidney (kidney pelvis) and of the tube (ureter) carrying urine away from the kidney to the bladder. Pyelograms may involve the injection of a substance into the patient's bloodstream to facilitate viewing of the kidney area.

The special hollow tube, lens, and light instrument called a *cystoscope* is used to view the inside of the bladder after being inserted up the urethra. *Voiding cystometrics* test the condition and capacity of the bladder by pumping water into it, measuring the resulting pressures, and timing the onset of the desire to void.

The technique of *needle biopsy*, discussed in respect to the liver under "The Digestive System and the Liver" in this chapter, is also used to examine kidneys and prostate tissue.

For a discussion of diagnostic procedures for the female reproductive system, see "The Gynecological Examination" in Ch. 25, *Women's Health.*

Patients' Rights

Diagnostic procedures have raised many questions centering on patients' rights. The questions concern both physicians and hospitals and relate to the general right of a patient to know what is happening to him or her and why.

Efforts to develop lists of specific rights that the patient enjoys have gone far beyond the specific area of diagnosis and treatment. The lists touch on such matters as the patient's need to maintain privacy, his or her right to be informed of any surgical or other procedures to be peformed, and the right to refuse treatment to the extent permitted by law. One such "Bill of Rights" was issued by the American Hospital Association in 1973. It noted in part:

> Equitable and humane treatment at all times and under all circumstances is a right. This principle entails an obligation on the part of all those involved in the care of the patient to recognize and to respect his individuality and his dignity. This means creating and fostering relationships founded on mutual acceptance and trust.

Like other statements on patients' rights, the AHA list stressed *informed consent.* That meant the need on the part of the patient to be able to agree to medical and surgical treatment on the basis of complete, accurate information. Informed consent as a principle provided the foundation for many other specific or general rights. These include:

- The right to considerate and respectful care

- The right to take part in planning for one's own care

- The right to have records kept confidential

- The right to full explanation of the hospital bill

Questions to Ask the Physician

The various rights suggest some of the questions the patient may want to ask his physician—either at the time of the first visit or later. For example, most patients want to know the results of diagnostic tests and procedures. Patients may also ask about planned treatments, the risks and chances of success or failure with particular types of treatment, and the period of time for which the patient may be hospitalized.

Many other factors become impor-

tant. Where one patient may want to know about alternative forms of care or treatment, another may ask about the surgeons who may perform an operation, the specialists who may be called in, and so on. Typically, most questions relate to the patient's situation: how far it has progressed, whether danger to life or health is involved, the physician's estimate of the chances of recovery, and other points. Physicians themselves suggest that patients ask questions to find out:

- Whether hospitalization, if it has been recommended, is really necessary

- Whether consultation with another physician or other physicians may be called for

- Whether—if necessary—medical terms or wordings can be clarified

- Whether, in case the patient is in doubt, the physician understood what the patient reported about symptoms, history, prescriptions already taken, and similar data

Common sense usually indicates what other questions the patient should ask the physician. The patient may have to make allowances for medical procedures. For instance, a thorough physical examination always requires that the patient undress— but no invasion of privacy is intended. Most important, the patient's right to free communication should be respected, and the patient should understand that it is.

Diagnostic Tests and Patients' Rights

Many diagnostic tests and procedures have been discussed. Many others could be listed.

One reason is that as medical costs have risen in recent years, some persons have questioned the necessity of various diagnostic tests. Consumer advocates have insisted that patients in some hospitals have been charged for tests that only increased their hospital bills. In some cases the tests were given in *batteries,* or sets. The question that has come up: Did the patients actually understand all those tests and what they involved?

Another reason why questions about patients' rights have been raised centers on the nature of test batteries and the time available to physicians. The batteries can be complex, and the physician may often be short of time. He may find it difficult or impossible to explain every test he has ordered—and to do so in enough detail so that the patient knows what each test requires and what it means in terms of discomfort, risk, and cost.

Hospital admission tests may be simple or complex. They may involve only "vital signs" tests of temperature, pulse rate, respiratory rate, and blood pressure. But they can include the *admission labs*—screening tests done by automated machines. These tests may include a urinalysis (UA), a complete blood count (CBC), and serum chemistries—Simultaneous Multiple Analyzer tests of 12 (SMA-12) or 24 (SMA-24) factors. The SMA-12 would typically call for chemical analyses for calcium, inorganic phosphorous, glucose, and nine other body elements.

Admission labs usually also include a test for syphilis, a chest X ray, and an EKG. The latter is often considered essential for patients over 40. Together, the admission labs tell the physician a number of important facts about the state of the patient's health.

Literally dozens of other tests could be noted. All involve some degree of risk and discomfort for the patient. But for most admission tests, both risk and discomfort are minimal. When the patient agrees to undergo them in batteries, is his or her right of informed consent being violated?

The Physician's Challenge

That question cannot be answered in a single word. The physician faces a dilemma in nearly all cases. He or she has to ask how much information can and should be transmitted—and how much the patient can absorb without becoming confused. He or she has also to ask what degree of risk is involved in any test or series of tests. Then the physician has to weigh the advantages of having test readings against the disadvantage involved in not having those test results. For a woman under 35, a test for cancer such as a mammogram may entail some risk if administered regularly (annually). For an older woman the risk is considered minimal.

With some tests, the risk for the patient is slight to virtually non-existent. But all tests given in batteries involve some risk, however minor. Does that mean that administration of tests in batteries increases the risk element significantly? It may, say those who argue against administration of tests by sets or groups.

The protocols or understandings on patients' rights establish fairly loose standards. That applies particularly in the area of information to be given to the patient. Thus the physician has to make a judgment decision in many cases. He or she tries to find out what the patient wants to know and whether all the needed information is readily available. The physician may even have to do some "homework" to answer the patient's questions.

Authorities agree that physicians

A Guide to Some Home Medical Tests

Kind	Function	How It Works	Time Required
Blood glucose monitoring	Measures the level of glucose (a kind of sugar) in blood	Wash your hands thoroughly. Prick a finger or earlobe to obtain a drop of blood, then follow instructions.	1 to 2 minutes
Ovulation monitoring	Measures the quantity of luteinizing hormone (LH) in urine	A chemically treated strip is dipped in urine specimen and compared with a color guide.	20 minutes to 1 hour
Pregnancy	Detects human chorionic gonadotropin, produced by a developing placenta, in urine	Chemicals are mixed with a urine specimen in a small test tube. A ring formation or color change indicates pregnancy.	20 minutes to 2 hours
Urinary tract infections	Detects nitrite in urine	Chemically treated test strip is dipped in urine specimen on three consecutive mornings.	30 to 40 seconds
Occult fecal blood	Detects hidden blood in stools	A color change, appearing when stool specimen is brought into contact with peroxide and guaiac, indicates hidden blood.	30 seconds to 16 minutes
Gonorrhea	Detects the bacteria causing gonorrhea in the specimen of pus from the penis	Specimen, collected on a slide, is allowed to air-dry. Then follow directions.	Several days
Blood pressure	Measures the pressure of blood on the walls of the arteries	The center of a cuff is placed on the pulse point of the upper arm. With or without a microphone, the user listens for artery sounds.	2 to 5 minutes
Impotence	Detects, measures the rigidity of erections during sleep	Soft fabric band or stamps are placed around the penis before the subject goes to bed at night. The strips break at different degrees of pressure.	Overnight
Vision	Screens for visual acuity problems	Using three different tests, you read special eye charts.	2 to 3 minutes

should spend time with patients and their families to the extent necessary to clarify procedures, risks, and prognoses. Physicians are also advised to talk to patients in a direct and honest manner, and in layman's terms. By such means the patient's rights are protected. The physician also finds out what he or she needs to know to make an accurate diagnosis.

Home Testing

Various kinds of medical tests may be self-administered. In increasingly common use are tests designed to provide clues to vision problems, gastrointestinal diseases, ovulation, pregnancy, infections, diabetes, and other conditions. Generally the self-testing products fall into three categories. The first helps to diagnose a specific condition, such as pregnancy (for use after a missed menstrual period). A second type, for persons with obvious symptoms, is designed to identify such indications of disease as hidden blood in stools. A third class includes monitoring devices, used most often on the advice of a physician. Blood glucose test kits for diabetics are examples of the last.

Self-tests, while relatively cheap and effective, should be used cautiously. The tests may have the pos-itive benefit of motivating a person to see a physician; but users should remember that test results are not uniformly reliable. For that reason, no single positive test should be taken as a "diagnosis." Nor should a subsequent negative test result be accepted as evidence of a "cure."

Exceptions to such general rules may be made where specific products help a person maintain testing regimens either at home or while traveling—as in the case of glucose monitoring. Fecal occult (hidden) blood tests have also proved so useful that the American Cancer Society has distributed free test kits.

27

Nutrition and Weight Control

Just as it was for our earliest ancestors, food is an integral part of our daily lives. Not only is food essential for survival, but oftentimes the way in which we structure our lives—our work habits, our recreational activities—revolves around how, when, and where we get food and eat it.

Ironically, however, because most of us live a much faster-paced lifestyle than we did even twenty years ago, we spend less time choosing, preparing, and eating food. We grab breakfast on the run (if we eat it at all), hurry through lunch, and rarely take time to plan and prepare a leisurely, well-balanced dinner. Often everyone in the family is on a different schedule, with the result that all too often we rely on prepackaged microwave dinners or take out fast food. Consequently, many of us are not eating properly, spending money on expensive vitamins to make up for poor nutrition, starving ourselves to lose weight, or gaining extra pounds by filling up on empty calories.

Practicing good eating habits may take a little more time and planning than we think we can afford, but its benefits will pay off in the long run in a healthier, happier way of life.

Basic Nutritional Requirements

The process by which food is converted into useful energy is called *metabolism*. It begins with chemical processes in the gastrointestinal tract which change plant and animal food into less complex components so that they can be absorbed to fulfill their various functions in the body—growth, repair, and fuel. Different foods have different energy values, measured in calories. An ideal diet for the average healthy individual provides the highest nutritional benefits from the fewest number of calories. Information on the protein, fat, and carbohydrate content in specific foods, as well as the number of calories, may be obtained by consulting the table "Nutrients in Common Foods." The Metric Equivalents table converts spoon and cup measures into metric measures.

Protein

Of the several essential components of food, *protein* is in many ways the most important. This is so not only because it is one of the three principal sources of energy, but also because

much of the body's structure is made up of proteins. For example, the typical 160-pound man is composed of about 100 pounds of water, 29 pounds of protein, 25 pounds of fat, 5 pounds of minerals, 1 pound of carbohydrate, and less than an ounce of vitamins. Because the muscles, heart, brain, lungs, and gastrointestinal organs are made up largely of protein, and since the protein in these organs is in constant need of replacement, its importance is obvious.

The recommended dietary allowance for protein is 0.8 g/Kg of body weight per day for persons aged 15 and up and 1 g/Kg of body weight for children under 15. (To convert your weight from pounds to kilograms, divide by 2.2. Thus a woman weighing 130 pounds weighs about 59 kilograms and needs about 47 grams of protein a day. A man weighing 175 pounds needs about 64 grams of protein a day.) Most Americans, however, eat about twice the amount they need, and while more may sound better, too much is too much. Your body uses only what it needs. Some excess protein is excreted as urine; the rest is converted to fat.

Chemically, proteins are varying mixtures of amino acids that contain various elements, including nitrogen. There are 22 different amino acids that are essential for the body's protein needs. Nine of these must be provided in the diet and are thus called *essential* amino acids; the rest can be synthesized by the body itself.

Meat, fish, poultry, eggs, and milk or milk products are the primary protein foods and contain all of the necessary amino acids; they are therefore called *complete* proteins. Grains and vegetables are partly made up of protein, but more often than not, they do not provide the whole range of amino acids required for proper nourishment. When properly combined, however, vegetable proteins, too, can be complete. For example, mixing rice and dried beans provides the same quality of protein as a steak (with a lot less fat).

One gram of protein provides four calories of energy.

Carbohydrates

Carbohydrates are another essential energy source. Called *starches* or *sugars,* they are present in large quantities in grains, fruits, and nuts. As *complex carbohydrates,* or *polysaccharides,* they are found in the foods named and particularly in breads, breakfast cereals, flours, pastas, barley, legumes, rice, and starchy vegetables. *Simple carbohydrates,* or mono- or disaccharides, are found in such foods as table sugars, candy, pastries, and soft drinks.

Complex carbohydrates are primary sources of calories, nutrients, and fiber—for such purposes as muscle contraction, weight reduction, and control of sodium and cholesterol. Simple carbohydrates, on the other hand, are pure sources of calories and contain little nutritional value. It is for this reason that they are often termed "empty" calories. Lack of adequate

carbohydrates means the body will begin to convert body fat or protein into sugar.

Although there is no absolute dietary requirement for carbohydrates, it is generally recommended that more than half the energy requirement beyond infancy be provided by complex carbohydrates. One gram of carbohydrate provides four calories of energy. Thus the average man consuming about 2,900 calories per day should consume about 360 grams of carbohydrate. The average woman consuming about 2,200 calories per day should consume about 275 grams of carbohydrate.

Fats

Fats are a chemically complex food component composed of *glycerol* (a sweet, oily alcohol) and fatty acids. Fats exist in several forms and come from a variety of sources. One way to think of them is to group them as visible fats, such as butter, salad oil, or the fat seen in meat, and as invisible fats, which are mingled, blended, or absorbed into food, either naturally, as in nuts, meat, or fish, or during cooking. Another way is to think of them as solid at room temperature (fats), or as liquid at room temperature (oils).

Saturated and Unsaturated

Fats are also classified as *saturated* or *unsaturated.* This is a chemical distinction based on the differences in molecular structure of different kinds of fat. If the carbon atoms in a fat molecule are surrounded or boxed in by hydrogen atoms, they are said to be saturated. This type of fat tends to be solid at room temperature, and high consumption of it increases the cholesterol content of the blood, which can lead to heart disease. *Unsaturated* fats, such as those found in

fish and vegetable oils, contain the least number of hydrogen atoms and do not add to the blood cholesterol content. They are either *monounsaturated* or *polyunsaturated.* In general, fats in foods of plant origin are more unsaturated than in those of animal origin (except for coconut and palm oils, which are highly saturated). It is recommended that you consume no more than 30 percent of your daily calories from fats; 10 percent of each of the three types, or, for our average man, about 32 grams total; for our average woman, about 24 grams total.

Fats play several essential roles in the metabolic process. First of all, they provide more than twice the number of calories on a comparative weight basis than do proteins and carbohydrates (one gram of fat contains nine calories). They also can be stored in the body in large quantities (in adipose tissue) and used as a later energy source. They serve as carriers of the fat-soluble vitamins A, D, E, and K, and—of no little importance—they add to the tastiness of food.

Vitamins

Vitamins, which are present in minute quantities in foods in their natural state, are essential for normal metabolism and for the development and maintenance of tissue structure and function. In addition to the fat-soluble vitamins noted above, there are a number of B vitamins, as well as vitamin C, also called *ascorbic acid.* If any particular vitamin is missing from the diet over a sufficiently long time, a specific disease will result.

Vitamin A

Vitamin A is essential for vision, growth, cell growth and development, reproduction, a strong immune

Average Daily Calorie Consumption

Men	Calories
Sedentary	2,500
Moderately active	3,000
Active	3,500
Very active	4,250

Women	Calories
Sedentary	2,100
Moderately active	2,500
Active	3,000
Very active	3,750

Guidelines for average daily calorie consumption by men and women. With increasing use of labor-saving devices, most Americans fall into the sedentary category.

Calorie Consumption for Some Activities

Type of Activity	Calories Per Hour
Sedentary: reading, sewing, typing, etc.	30–100
Light: cooking, slow walking, dressing, etc.	100–170
Moderate: sweeping, light gardening, making beds, etc.	170–250
Vigorous: fast walking, hanging out clothes, golfing, etc.	250–350
Strenuous: swimming, bicycling, dancing, etc.	350 and more

Low Calarie Diet

Sample Menus

	800 calories		1,200 calories		1,600 calories	
	Weight grams	Household measure	Weight grams	Household measure	Weight grams	Household measure
Breakfast						
Orange, sliced	125	1 medium	125	1 medium	125	1 medium
Soft cooked egg	50	One	50	One	50	One
Toast	25	1 slice	25	1 slice	25	1 slice
Butter	5	1 teaspoon	5	1 teaspoon	5	1 teaspoon
Coffee or tea	—	As desired	—	As desired	—	As desired
Milk	240	1 cup skim	240	1 cup skim	240	1 cup whole
Luncheon						
Clear broth	—	As desired	—	As desired	—	As desired
Salad (cottage cheese, tomato, plain lettuce leaf)	90	½ cup	90	½ cup	90	½ cup
Egg			50	One	50	One
Green peas					100	½ cup
Baked apple, unsweetened	80	1 small	80	1 small	80	1 small
Bread			25	1 slice	25	1 slice
Butter			5	1 teaspoon	5	1 teaspoon
Milk	240	1 cup skim	240	1 cup skim	240	1 cup whole
Coffee or tea	—	As desired	—	As desired	—	As desired
Dinner						
Roast beef, lean	60	2 ounces	90	3 ounces	120	4 ounces
Carrots, plain	100	½ cup	100	½ cup	100	½ cup
Tossed vegetable salad with vinegar	50	¾ cup	50	¾ cup	50	¾ cup
Pineapple, unsweetened	80	½ cup	80	½ cup	80	½ cup
Bread			25	1 slice	25	1 slice
Butter			5	1 teaspoon	10	2 teaspoons
Coffee or tea	—	As desired	—	As desired	—	As desired
Nourishment						
Peach					100	1 medium

These diets contain approximately 800, 1,200, and 1,600 calories. The 800 calorie diet, even with variations in selections of food, will not meet the recommended daily allowances in iron and thiamine. The approximate composition is as follows:

	800 calories	1,200 calories	1,600 calories
Protein	60 gm.	75 gm.	85 gm.
Fat	30 gm.	50 gm.	80 gm.
Carbohydrate	75 gm.	110 gm.	130 gm.

From the *Clinical Center Diet Manual*, revised edition, prepared by the Nutrition Department. The Clinical Center, National Institutes of Health, Public Health Service, U.S. Department of Health, Education, and Welfare (Public Health Service Publication No. 989), pp. 67–68.

system, and healthy hair, skin, and mucous membranes.

Vitamin A is fat soluble and is therefore stored by the body (in the liver). It comes in two forms: retinol, found only in animal foods (chiefly liver), and beta-carotene, found in fruits and vegetables (chiefly deep green or orange ones like spinach and sweet potatoes). Retinol is instantly available for bodily use, while beta-carotene must be converted by the body into retinol before it can be used. (Because the body will not convert excess beta-carotene into retinol, there is no danger of overdosing on this form of vitamin A. Retinol, however, can be extremely toxic at high levels.)

Symptoms of vitamin A deficiency include dry rough skin, slow growth, night blindness, thickening of bone, and increased susceptibility to infection. Vitamin A deficiency is rare in the United States.

Formerly measured in International Units (IU), vitamin A content is now expressed retinol equivalents (RE). One RE equals 10 IU of beta-carotene and 3.33 IU of retinol. The Recommended Daily Allowance (RDA) for vitamin A for adult males is 1000 RE and for adult women, 800 RE.

Vitamin D

Vitamin D is essential for proper metabolism of calcium, which is primarily responsible for the healthy growth of bones and teeth.

Vitamin D is fat soluble and therefore excessive intake can be toxic. It is consumed chiefly as an addition to milk and is also manufactured by the body by a reaction of sunlight on sterols present in the skin.

The major deficiency disease of vitamin D in children is rickets (deformation of the skeleton) and in adults excessive bone loss and fractures.

The RDA for adults over 24 is 5 micrograms.

Vitamin E (tocopherol)

Vitamin E is essential for healthy nerve function and reproduction.

Vitamin E is found principally in plant oils, particularly wheat germ oil and nuts. It is fat soluble, but there is little danger of toxicity because absorption by the body is relatively inefficient.

Vitamin E is measured in tocopherol equivalents (TE). The RDA for adult males is 10 TE and for adult women 8 TE. Deficiencies in a normal diet are rare.

Vitamin K

Vitamin K is essential for proper clotting of the blood.

Vitamin K is fat soluble and is found primarily in green leafy vegetables. Another form of the compound is synthesized by intestinal bacteria. Like vitamin E, there is little danger from ingesting too much vitamin K, and most diets provide an adequate supply.

The RDA for adult males over age 24 is 80 micrograms and for adult women 65 micrograms.

Vitamin C (ascorbic acid)

Vitamin C is essential for healthy skin, bones, teeth, and muscles, for producing and maintaining collagen, and for fighting infection.

Vitamin C is water soluble and therefore must be ingested every day. It is widely available in a variety of colorful fruits and vegetables, such as peppers, broccoli, cabbage, oranges, strawberries, and tomatoes. Unfortunately, vitamin C is also the most unstable of all vitamins and minerals: it is easily destroyed by heat

Table 1

Desirable Weights for Men and Women Aged 25 and Over[1]
(in pounds by height and frame, in indoor clothing)

	MEN (in shoes, 1-inch heels)				WOMEN (in shoes, 2-inch heels)		
Height	Small Frame	Medium Frame	Large Frame	Height	Small Frame	Medium Frame	Large Frame
5' 2"	112–120	118–129	126–141	4' 10"	92– 98	96–107	104–119
5' 3"	115–123	121–133	129–144	4' 11"	94–101	98–110	106–122
5' 4"	118–126	124–136	132–148	5' 0"	96–104	101–113	109–125
5' 5"	121–129	127–139	135–152	5' 1"	99–107	104–116	112–128
5' 6"	124–133	130–143	138–156	5' 2"	102–110	107–119	115–131
5' 7"	128–137	134–147	142–161	5' 3"	105–113	110–122	118–134
5' 8"	132–141	138–152	147–166	5' 4"	108–116	113–126	121–138
5' 9"	136–145	142–156	151–170	5' 5"	111–119	116–130	125–142
5' 10"	140–150	146–160	155–174	5' 6"	114–123	120–135	129–146
5' 11"	144–154	150–165	159–179	5' 7"	118–127	124–139	133–150
6' 0"	148–158	154–170	164–184	5' 8"	122–131	128–143	137–154
6' 1"	152–162	158–175	168–189	5' 9"	126–135	132–147	141–158
6' 2"	156–167	162–180	173–194	5' 10"	130–140	136–151	145–163
6' 3"	160–171	167–185	178–199	5' 11"	134–144	140–155	149–168
6' 4"	164–175	172–190	182–204	6' 0"	138–148	144–159	153–173

[1]Adapted from Metropolitan Life Insurance Co., New York. New weight standards for men and women. *Statistical Bulletin* 40:3.

Table 2

Average Weights for Men and Women[1]
(in pounds by age and height, in paper gown and slippers)

				MEN			
Height	18–24 Years	25–34 Years	35–44 Years	45–54 Years	55–64 Years	65–74 Years	75–79 Years
5' 2"	137	141	149	148	148	144	133
5' 3"	140	145	152	152	151	148	138
5' 4"	144	150	156	156	155	151	143
5' 5"	147	154	160	160	158	154	148
5' 6"	151	159	164	164	162	158	154
5' 7"	154	163	168	168	166	161	159
5' 8"	158	168	171	173	169	165	164
5' 9"	161	172	175	177	173	168	169
5' 10"	165	177	179	181	176	171	174
5' 11"	168	181	182	185	180	175	179
6' 0"	172	186	186	189	184	178	184
6' 1"	175	190	190	193	187	182	189
6' 2"	179	194	194	197	191	185	194
				WOMEN			
4' 9"	116	112	131	129	138	132	125
4' 10"	118	116	134	132	141	135	129
4' 11"	120	120	136	136	144	138	132
5' 0"	122	124	138	140	149	142	136
5' 1"	125	128	140	143	150	145	139
5' 2"	127	132	143	147	152	149	143
5' 3"	129	136	145	150	155	152	146
5' 4"	131	140	147	154	158	156	150
5' 5"	134	144	149	158	161	159	153
5' 6"	136	148	152	161	164	163	157
5' 7"	138	152	154	165	167	166	160
5' 8"	140	156	156	168	170	170	164

[1]Adapted from National Center for Health Statistics: Weight by Height and Age of Adults, United States. *Vital Health Statistics*. PHS Publication No. 1000—Series 11, No. 14.

and oxygen, and thus care should be taken in cooking and storing of fruits and vegetables.

The classic vitamin C deficiency disease is scurvy, typified by the wasting away of muscles, wounds and bruises that don't heal, and bleeding, deteriorating gums. Milder forms of vitamin C deficiency produce milder versions of these symptoms. Vitamin C deficiency has also been linked to such health problems as the common cold, anemia, atherosclerosis, asthma, cancer of the stomach and esophagus, infertility in males, rheumatoid arthritis, and cataracts.

Vitamin C is measured in milligrams (mg). The RDA for adults is 60 mg. Megadoses of vitamin C are often recommended to fight colds or as a general preventive measure against disease, although the body only uses as much as it needs; the rest is excreted in the urine. Toxicity is rarely a problem.

Thiamin (vitamin B₁)

Thiamin is essential for the proper metabolism of carbohydrates and for a healthy nervous system.

Thiamin is water soluble and is found primarily in cereals, wheat germ, pork, and nuts. It is strongly susceptible to destruction during cooking. Deficiency is not common among the general population, but studies have shown heavy drinkers, pregnant women, and the elderly to be more deficient. Severe thiamin deficiency results in beriberi, a disease that weakens the body, disables the mind, and permanently damages the heart. Symptoms of deficiency include loss of appetite, nausea, vomiting, constipation, depression, fatigue, poor eye-hand coordination, irritability, headaches, and anxiety.

Thiamin is measured in milligrams. The RDA for adult males is 1.5 mg

and for adult women 1.1 mg. Danger of toxicity is rare as excess thiamin is excreted in urine.

Riboflavin (vitamin B₂)

Riboflavin is essential for growth and repair of tissues and aids in DNA synthesis. It helps metabolize proteins, fats, and carbohydrates.

Most Americans get plenty of this water-soluble vitamin, which is readily found in liver, eggs, and milk products. Studies have found that children in low-income families, however, are less likely to get enough riboflavin. Signs of deficiency include a purplish-colored tongue; cracks at the corners of the mouth; sores and burning of the lips, mouth, and tongue; itchy inflamed eyelids; flaky skin around the nose, ears, eyebrows, or hairline; and light sensitivity of eyes. Deficiency in riboflavin often means deficiency in other B vitamins as well. Cataracts, birth defects, and anemia have been linked to riboflavin deficiency.

Unlike vitamin C and thiamin, riboflavin is not easily destroyed by cooking, although adding baking soda to vegetables when cooking creates an alkaline solution that destroys it. Risk of toxicity is very low, and excess riboflavin is excreted in the urine.

Riboflavin is measured in milligrams. The RDA for adult males is 1.7 mg and for adult women 1.3 mg.

Niacin (vitamin B₃)

Niacin is essential for the release of energy from carbohydrates, fats, and proteins and for the formation of DNA.

Most Americans get plenty of niacin from their diets; only heavy drinkers are at risk of deficiency. Severe deficiencies of niacin result in pellagra, a disease virtually wiped out in

the United States since the 1930s with the advent of fortified flour and cereals with the vitamin.

Niacin is widely available in a variety of plant and animal foods, including fish, liver, turkey, cereals, and peanuts. The body is also able to convert the amino acid tryptophan into niacin, and thus proteins high in tryptophan also provide plenty of niacin.

Niacin is measured in milligrams (60 mg of tryptophan equal 1 mg of niacin). The RDA for adult males is 19 mg and for women 15 mg.

Vitamin B₆

Vitamin B₆ is essential for fat and carbohydrate metabolism and for the formation and breakdown of amino acids. It also helps regulate blood glucose levels and is needed to synthesize hemoglobin.

Vitamin B₆ occurs in three forms: pyridoxine, pyridoxal, and pyridoxamine, which are converted by the body into pyridoxal phosphate and pyridoxamine phosphate. It is most readily found in nuts, kidney, liver, eggs, pork, poultry, dried fruits, and fish.

Although few Americans get the full RDA of vitamin B₆, there is no evidence of corresponding overt deficiency symptoms. The following health problems, however, have been linked to B₆ deficiency: asthma, carpal tunnel syndrome, cancer (melanoma, breast, and bladder), diabetes, coronary heart disease, premenstrual syndrome, sickle-cell anemia, and aging and dementia.

In moderate doses B₆ is not toxic. Although excessive amounts of this water-soluble vitamin are to a great extent flushed out of the body in the urine, high doses have produced neurological disturbances such as numbness in the hands, feet, and mouth.

Vitamin B₆ is measured in milligrams. The RDA for adult men is 2 mg and for women 1.6 mg.

Vitamin B$_{12}$

Vitamin B$_{12}$ is important for normal growth, healthy nerve tissue, and normal blood formation.

Most Americans get plenty of B$_{12}$. It is found chiefly in animal foods: meat, fish, eggs, and milk products. Only strict vegetarians (vegans), who eat none of these foods are in danger of deficiency. Problems for everyone arise with age, however; the stomach may become less able to absorb B$_{12}$ and deficiency may result. Pernicious anemia is the classic B$_{12}$ deficiency disease and may take years to appear. Other health problems that may be linked to B$_{12}$ deficiency include infertility, nervous system disorders, and walking difficulties.

Cooking results in few losses of B$_{12}$, and toxicity is not a danger. The RDA for B$_{12}$ for adults is 2 micrograms.

Folacin (folic acid, or folate)

Folacin is essential for many metabolic processes, especially cell growth and division.

Women, especially pregnant women, and alcoholics are most likely to be folacin deficient. Signs of deficiency include anemia, weakness, pallor, headaches, forgetfulness, sleeplessness, and irritability. Vitamin B$_{12}$ deficiency can aggravate folacin deficiency because B$_{12}$ is essential to release folacin from bodily storage. Other health problems that may be associated with folacin deficiency include depression, dementia, neuropsychological disorders, toxemia of pregnancy, infections, and fetal damage.

Folacin is widely distributed in fruits and vegetables, but it is easily destroyed during cooking and storage. The RDA for folacin for adult men is 200 micrograms and for women, 180 micrograms.

Recommended Dietary Allowances for Fat-Soluble Vitamins

	Age	Vit. A (mcg RE)	Vit. D (mcg)	Vit. E (mgTE)	Vit.K (mcg)
Infants	0 to .5	375	7.5	3	5
	.5 to 1	"	10	4	10
Children	1 to 3	400	"	6	15
	4 to 6	500	"	7	20
	7 to 10	700	"	"	30
Males	11 to 14	1,000	"	10	45
	15 to 18	"	"	"	65
	19 to 24	"	"	"	70
	25 to 50	"	5	"	80
	51 +	"	"	"	"
Females	11 to 14	800	10	8	45
	15 to 18	"	"	"	55
	19 to 24	"	"	"	60
	25 to 50	"	5	"	65
	51 +	"	"	"	"
Pregnant		"	10	10	"
Nursing	1st 6 months	1,300	"	12	"
	2nd 6 months	1,200	"	11	"

Biotin

Biotin is essential for overall growth and well-being. It is important in the metabolism of fats and in the utilization of carbon dioxide.

The best sources of biotin are liver, egg yolks, soy flour, cereals, and yeast. It is also produced by intestinal bacteria, although it is not known whether this form is readily absorbed by the body. Deficiencies are most often produced by the ingestion of large amounts of raw egg white, which contains a biotin-binding protein called avidin that prevents the absorption of biotin. Symptoms of deficiency include nausea, vomiting, swelling of the tongue, pallor, depression, hair loss, and dry scaly dermatitis.

The RDA for adults is a wide range: from 30 to 100 micrograms. Toxicity from a normal diet is not a concern.

Pantothenic acid

Pantothenic acid is essential for general growth and well-being. It is an important component in a number of metabolic reactions such as the release of energy from carbohydrates, fats, and proteins and the synthesis of sterols and steroid hormones.

Pantothenic acid is widely distributed among foods, chiefly animal tissues, cereals, and legumes. Evidence of dietary deficiency of pantothenic acid has not been clinically recognized in humans, and there is no specific disease associated with pantothenic acid deficiency.

Pantothenic acid is measured in milligrams. There is no RDA, but daily consumption by adults of between 4 and 7 mg is considered safe. Toxicity from a normal diet is not a concern.

Minerals

Minerals are another component of basic nutritional needs. All living things extract them from the soil, which is their ultimate source. Like vitamins, they are needed for normal metabolism and must be present in the diet in sufficient amounts for the maintenance of good health. The essential minerals include calcium, phosphorus, magnesium, iodine, iron, zinc, selenium, molybdenum, copper, manganese, fluoride, and chromium.

Recommended Dietary Allowances for Water-Soluble Vitamins

	Age	Vit. C (mg)	Thiamin (mg)	Riboflav. (mg)	Niacin (mg)	Vit. B6 (mg)	Folate (mcg)	Vit. B12 (mcg)
Infants	0 to .5	30	0.3	0.4	5	0.3	25	0.3
	.5 to 1	35	0.4	0.5	6	0.6	35	0.5
Children	1 to 3	40	0.7	0.8	9	1	50	0.7
	4 to 6	45	0.9	1.1	12	1.1	75	1
	7 to 10	"	1	1.2	13	1.4	100	1.4
Males	11 to 14	50	1.3	1.5	17	1.7	150	2
	15 to 18	60	1.5	1.8	20	2	200	"
	19 to 24	"	"	1.7	19	"	"	"
	25 to 50	"	"	"	"	"	"	"
	51 +	"	1.2	1.4	15	"	150	"
Females	11 to 14	50	1.1	1.3	"	1.4	180	"
	15 to 18	60	"	"	"	1.5	"	"
	19 to 24	"	"	"	"	1.6	"	"
	25 to 50	"	1.1	"	"	"	"	"
51 +		"	1	1.2	13	"	"	"
Pregnant		70	1.5	1.6	17	2.2	400	2.2
Nursing	1st 6 months	95	1.6	1.8	20	2.1	280	2.6
	2nd 6 months	90	"	1.7	20	"	260	"

Calcium

Calcium is essential for bone growth, development, and retention as well as for proper nerve conduction, muscle contraction, blood clotting, and membrane permeability.

Dairy products are the primary sources of calcium, but the mineral is also found in green leafy vegetables and soft bones, such as those of sardines and salmon. Maximum calcium ingestion is extremely important during the years from birth to age 25, when the body reaches its peak bone mass. Deficiencies are most common in women and have been linked to the development of osteoporosis in the later years.

The RDA for calcium for children between the ages of 11 and 24 is 1,200 mg. For adults over 24 the RDA is 800 mg. Ingestion of very large amounts of calcium may inhibit the absorption of iron, zinc, and other essential minerals.

Phosphorus

Phosphorus is a structural component of all cells. It is a part of DNA, and is therefore essential in the growth, maintenance, and repair of all body tissues. It is also critical for energy transfer and production.

Phosphorus is present in nearly all foods, principally cereals and proteins. Deficiency is a serious concern only for premature infants fed exclusively human milk.

The RDA for phosphorus is the same as that for calcium, 800 mg for adults over 24. Toxicity from a normal diet is not a concern.

Magnesium

Like phosphorus, magnesium is a structural component in soft tissue cells and is therefore important in the growth, maintenance, and repair of these tissues. It is also important in energy production, lipid and protein synthesis, the formation of urea, muscle relaxation, and in the prevention of tooth decay.

The best sources of magnesium are nuts, legumes, unmilled grains, and green vegetables. Deficiencies from a normal diet are rare and are related instead to various diseases such as those of the gastrointestinal tract, kidney dysfunction, and malnutrition and alcoholism. Symptoms of deficiency include weakness, confusion, personality changes, muscle tremor, nausea, lack of coordination, and gastrointestinal disorders.

The RDA for adult men is 350 mg and for adult women 280 mg.

Iodine

Iodine is an essential component of thyroid hormone, which is important in cellular reactions, metabolism, and growth and development.

Iodized salt and water are the most common sources, and most animal foods contain adequate supplies depending on the soil quality and the amount of iodine added to animal feeds. Iodine is also added in the processing of bread dough. Deficiencies in the United States are not common. The classic deficiency disease in adults is goiter. Iodine deficient fetuses are at a risk of developing cretinism.

The RDA for iodine for adults is 150 micrograms.

Iron

As an essential component of hemoglobin and myoglobin, iron is necessary for the proper transfer of oxygen to cells and muscles. It is also important for energy production and collagen synthesis.

Many Americans don't get enough iron. Women and very young children get the least, followed by the elderly. Iron deficiency leads to anemia: muscles become weak, and fatigue, listlessness, and a tendency to tire easily set in. Even mild iron deficiency, however, can affect a person's intellectual capabilities, especially children's. Symptoms of deficiency in children include irritability, hyperactivity, learning problems, shortened attention span, poor motivation, and poor intellectual performance.

There are two types of iron, heme and nonheme. Heme comes from animal foods and is much more readily absorbed than nonheme iron, which comes from vegetables. When eaten together, however, the rate of absorption for nonheme iron increases significantly. Also, iron eaten with just a little vitamin C dramatically increases its absorption. Tannins (in tea and red wine) block iron absorption. Iron-rich foods include liver and other organ meats, beef, dried fruits, pumpkin and sunflower seeds, legumes, dark green leafy vegetables, prune juice, and whole grain cereals.

The RDA for adult males is 10 mg and for adult women 15 mg. There is little danger of toxicity from a normal diet, although some people have an inherited defect in regulating iron absorption and can easily get too much.

Zinc

Zinc is essential for cell multiplication, tissue regeneration, sexual maturity, and proper growth. It is also important as a cofactor in more than 20 enzymatic reactions and serves as a binder in many others.

Severe zinc deficiency is not a problem in the United States, but the effects of mild deficiency—common especially in children, women, and the elderly—on overall health are feared to be widespread. Signs of deficiency include loss of appetite, stunted growth in children, skin changes, small sex glands in boys, delayed sexual maturation, impotence, loss of taste sensitivity, white spots on fingernails, delayed wound-healing, and dull hair color.

Animal foods are good sources of zinc as are oysters, milk, egg yolks, wheat germ, pumpkin and sunflower seeds, nuts, cheese, dry beans, lentils, and whole grains. Toxicity is rare. The RDA for adults is 12 mg.

Selenium

Selenium functions in a similar way to vitamin E, as an antioxidant helping to protect cells from destruction by toxic agents. Its consumption has also been associated with lower incidences of cancer and heart disease.

Good sources of selenium include whole grains, seafood, liver, kidney, meat, seeds, and nuts. Deficiency may be a problem in areas with selenium-poor soils. Selenium is toxic at higher than trace amounts. The RDA for adult males is 70 micrograms and for adult women 55 micrograms.

Molybdenum

Molybdenum is essential in the function of certain enzyme systems and is also necessary in iron metabolism.

Sources of molybdenum include meats, whole grains, legumes, leafy vegetables, and organ meats. The molybdenum content of vegetables varies widely depending on the content of the soil in which they were grown. Deficiency is not known in humans. Ingesting more than trace amounts is not recommended. The RDA for adults is between 75 and 250 micrograms.

Copper

Copper is important as a cofactor in several enzyme systems and as a catalyst in the synthesis of hemoglobin. It also aids in collagen formation and is involved in the synthesis of phospholipids, which maintain healthy nerve fibers.

Copper deficiency is believed to be more common than once thought, and it has been linked to heart disease, central nervous system disorders, anemia, and bone disorders. Good sources of copper include shellfish, liver, nuts and seeds, meats, and green leafy vegetables. Copper sup-

plements are not recommended because they can interfere with other minerals, and copper is toxic at more than trace amounts. The RDA for copper is 1.5 to 3 mg.

Manganese

Manganese has a variety of functions, some that other minerals can perform in its place. It is known to play a role in such things as collagen formation, urea formation, synthesis of fatty acids and cholesterol, digestion of proteins, normal bone formation and development, and protein synthesis.

Manganese deficiency has not been observed in humans. Sources of manganese include liver, kidney, spinach, whole grain cereals and breads, dried peas and beans, and nuts. Excessive intake of manganese can interfere with iron absorption. More than trace amounts of manganese are not recommended. The RDA is 2 to 5 mg.

Fluoride

Fluoride is essential for the development of healthy teeth and bones and the prevention of tooth decay.

Fluoride deficiency shows up in increased incidences of tooth decay. Fluoridated water is the most common source of fluoride for many people. For those without access to such water fluoride tablets or toothpaste are helpful. Fish, tea, milk, and eggs are also sources of fluoride. The RDA for adults is between 1.5 and 4 mg.

Chromium

Chromium is important for maintaining normal glucose metabolism. It also acts as a cofactor for insulin.

Chromium deficiency can show up in the form of glucose intolerance in malnourished children and in some diabetics. Sources of chromium include whole grains, brewer's yeast, meats,

Recommended Dietary Allowances for Minerals

	Age	Calcium (mg)	Phospho. (mg)	Magnesium (mg)	Iron (mg)	Zinc (mg)	Iodine (mcg)	Selenium (mcg)
Infants	0 to .5	400	300	40	6	5	40	10
	.5 to 1	600	500	60	10	"	50	15
Children	1 to 3	800	800	80	"	10	70	20
	4 to 6	"	"	120	"	"	90	"
	7 to 10	"	"	170	"	"	120	30
Males	11 to 14	1,200	1,200	270	12	15	150	40
	15 to 18	"	"	400	"	"	"	50
	19 to 24	"	"	350	10	"	"	70
	25 to 50	800	800	"	"	"	"	"
	51 +	"	"	"	"	"	"	"
Females	11 to 14	1,200	1,200	280	15	12	"	45
	15 to 18	"	"	300	"	"	"	50
	19 to 24	"	"	280	"	"	"	55
	25 to 50	800	800	"	"	"	"	"
	51 +	"	"	"	10	"	"	"
Pregnant		1,200	1,200	320	30	15	175	65
Nursing	1st 6 months	"	"	355	15	19	200	75
	2nd 6 months	"	"	340	"	16	200	"

and cheeses. Hard water also contains chromium. Chromium intake should not exceed trace amounts. The RDA for adults is between 50 and 200 micrograms.

Fiber

Fiber in the diet is important for proper elimination. It provides bulk, and its use has been linked to the prevention of many health problems: constipation, appendicitis, colon cancer, diverticular disease, spastic colon, hiatal hernia, varicose veins, hemorrhoids, coronary heart disease, high blood pressure, gallstones, diabetes, obesity, ulcerative colitis, and Crohn's disease.

Fiber is found almost exclusively in plant foods and comes in basically two types: water soluble or water insoluble. Soluble fiber is found primarily in fruits and vegetables and in oat bran in the form of gums and pectin and affects the way the body metabolizes sugars and fats. Insoluble fiber is primarily associated with whole grains, the traditional "bran," such as wheat bran and rice bran, and is the fiber we think of when we think of laxatives. Generally, the less processed the food, the higher it is in either kind of fiber.

Fiber in high doses can affect the absorption of other vitamins and minerals as well as cause flatulence, bloating, nausea, diarrhea, and impaction or rupture of the bowl. Daily consumption of 35 to 40 grams of fiber is recommended for optimum health and safety.

Water

Water is not really a food in the fuel sense, but it is in many ways a crucial component of nutrition: the body's need for water is second only to its need for oxygen. It makes up from 55 to 65 percent of the body's weight, and is constantly being eliminated in the form of urine, perspiration, and expired breath. It must therefore be replaced regularly, for while a person can live for weeks without food, he can live for only a few days without water.

Normally, the best guide to how much water a person needs is his sense of thirst. The regulating mechanism of excretion sees to it that an excessive intake of water will be eliminated as urine. The usual water requirement is on the order of two quarts a day in addition to whatever amount is contained in the solids which make up the daily diet.

Basic Daily Diets

Everyone should have at least the minimal amount of basic nutrients for resting or basal metabolism. The specific needs of each individual are determined by whether he is still growing, and by how much energy is required for his normal activities. All those who are still growing—and growth continues up to about 25 years of age—have relatively high food needs.

For Infants

That food needs of an infant are especially acute should surprise no one. The newborn baby normally triples his birth weight during his first year and is very active in terms of calorie expenditure.

For his first six months, breast milk or formula, or a combination of both, fills his nutritional needs. The amount of milk he should get each day is about two and a half ounces per pound of his body weight. This provides 50 calories per pound, and in the early months is usually given in six feedings a day at four-hour intervals.

If his weight gain is adequate and he appears healthy, and if his stomach is not distended by swallowed air, his appetite is normally a satisfactory guide to how much he needs. The formula-fed baby should get a supplement of 35 milligrams of ascorbic acid each day and 400 international units of vitamin D if the latter has not been added to the milk during its processing.

Solid Foods

Between two and six months of age, the baby should begin to eat solid foods such as cooked cereals, strained fruits and vegetables, egg yolk, and homogenized meat. With the introduction of these foods, it is not really necessary to calculate the baby's caloric intake. Satisfaction of appetite, proper weight gain, and a healthy appearance serve as the guides to a proper diet.

By one year of age, a baby should be getting three regular meals a day, and as his teeth appear, his food no longer needs to be strained. By 18 to 24 months, he should no longer need baby foods. For further information on the care and feeding of infants, see under "Birth, Infancy, and Maturation" in Ch. 2, *The First Dozen Years.*

Basic Food Groups

The recommended daily amounts of food for people over the age of two have been established with reasonable accuracy, but they always contain a fairly generous safety factor.

The Four Group Division

In general, foods are divided into four major groups:

- Meat, fish, eggs
- Dairy products
- Fruits and vegetables
- Breads and cereals

The Seven Group Division

For purposes of planning daily requirements, a more detailed way of considering food groupings is the following:

- Leafy green and yellow vegetables
- Citrus fruits, tomatoes, and raw cabbage
- Potatoes and other vegetables and fruits
- Milk, cheese, and ice cream
- Meat, poultry, fish, eggs, dried peas, and beans
- Bread, flour, and cereals
- Butter and oils

The "Daily Food Guide" table can be used as a general guide to planning nutritionally balanced meals for preteens, teens, and adults of any age.

The Years of Growth

Even though a child will never again triple his weight in a single year as he did during his first, a proper diet is crucial during the years from 2 to 18, since this is a period of tremendous growth.

Other food goals that should be realized during the childhood and adolescent years are an awareness of what a balanced diet is, a reasonable tolerance for a variety of foods, decent manners at the table, and a sense of timing about when to eat and when not to eat.

These are also the years that a young person should begin to learn something about how to buy and prepare food, how to serve it attractively, and how to clean up after a meal.

Creating a Pleasant Atmosphere at Mealtime

Although a child's attitudes about food and eating can often be exasperating, it is up to the parent to make mealtime as pleasant as possible, and above all, to avoid any battles of will.

If a young child is too tired, too excited, or too hungry to cope with a meal without ending up in tears or a tantrum, he should not be forced to eat. There are several ways to help children develop a wholesome attitude toward food and eating; here are a few suggestions:

- Children should never be bribed with candy, money, or the promise of special surprises as a way of getting them to eat properly.
- They should not be given the idea that dessert is a reward for finishing the earlier part of the meal.
- Relatively small portions should be served and completely finished before anything else is offered.

Estimated Safe and Adequate Daily Dietary Intakes of Selected Vitamins and Minerals

		Biotin	Pant. acid	Copper	Manganese	Fluoride	Chromium	Molyb.
		(mcg)	(mg)	(mg)	(mg)	(mg)	(mcg)	(mcg)
Infants	0 to 0.5	10	2	0.4-.06	0.3-0.6	0.1-0.5	10-40	15-30
	0.5 to 1	15	3	0.6-0.7	0.6-1.0	0.2-1.0	20-60	20-40
Children/ Adolescents	1 to 3	20	"	0.7-1.0	1.0-1.5	0.5-1.5	20-80	25-50
	4 to 6	25	3-4	1.0-1.5	1.5-2.0	1.0-2.5	30-120	30-75
	7 to 10	30	4-5	1.0-2.0	2.0-3.0	1.5-2.5	50-200	50-150
	11 +	30-100	4-7	1.5-2.5	2.0-5.0	"	"	75-250
Adults		"	"	1.5-3.0	"	1.5-4.0	"	"

Metric Equivalents of Traditional Food Measures		
1 teaspoon	=	5 milliliters
1 tablespoon	=	15 milliliters
¼ cup	=	60 milliliters
⅓ cup	=	80 milliliters
½ cup	=	120 milliliters
⅔ cup	=	160 milliliters
¾ cup	=	180 milliliters
1 cup	=	240 milliliters
		or 0.24 liter

- Between-meal snacks should be discouraged if they cut down on the appetite at mealtime.

- From time to time, the child should be allowed to choose the foods that he will eat at a meal.

Parents should keep in mind that the atmosphere in which a child eats and the attitudes instilled in him toward food can be altogether as basic as the nourishment for his body.

Teenage Diet

From the start of a child's growth spurt, which begins at age 10 or 11 for girls and between 13 and 15 for boys, and for several years thereafter, adolescent appetites are likely to be unbelievably large and somewhat outlandish. Special care, however, should be taken with the youngster who is putting on too much weight as well as with the one who is attracted by a bizarre starvation diet: both instances could indicate emotional problems.

Adult Nutrition

Adult nutrition is concerned with more than 50 years of an individual's life span. In typical cases, there is a slow but steady weight gain that may go unnoticed at first; for some, there is an obesity problem that begins at about age 40.

Because it is never easy to lose weight, it is especially important for adults to eat sensibly and avoid excess calories. See under "Weight," for a discussion of weight control and obesity.

For Older People

People over 60 tend to have changes in their digestive system that are related to less efficient and slower absorption. Incomplete chewing of food because of carelessness or impaired teeth can intensify this problem. Avoiding haste at mealtimes ought to be the rule.

In cases where a dental disorder makes proper chewing impossible, food should be chopped or pureed. Older people occasionally have difficulty swallowing; for example, they may choke on a large piece of unchewed meat.

Food for older people should be cooked simply, preferably baked, boiled, or broiled rather than fried, and menus excessively rich in fats should be avoided. A daily multivitamin capsule is strongly recommended for those over 60. A poor appetite can be stimulated by an ounce or two of sherry before a meal unless there are medical reasons for avoiding alcoholic beverages of any kind. See under "Aging and What To Do About It" in Ch. 6, *The Later Years,* for a discussion of diet and eating habits in the later years.

During Pregnancy

A pregnant woman needs special foods to maintain her own health as well as to safeguard the health of her baby. She should have additional vitamin D, folic acid, and iron, usually recommended as dietary supplements. More important for most women is the provision of adequate protein in the diet to prevent toxemia of pregnancy or underweight babies. Between 70 and 85 grams of protein a day should be eaten during pregnancy, even if this results in a weight gain of as much as 25 pounds. Adequate nutrition is more important than restricting weight gain to 20 pounds or less.

Nursing Mothers

A nursing mother has special dietary needs in addition to those satisfied by the normal adult diet. She should drink an extra quart of milk and eat two more servings of citrus fruit or tomatoes, one more serving of lean meat, fish, poultry, eggs, beans, or cheese, and one more serving of leafy green or yellow vegetables.

Malnutrition

The classic diseases of nutritional deficiency, or malnutrition, such as scurvy and pellagra, are now rare, at least in the United States. The chief reason for their disappearance is the application of scientific knowledge gained in this century of the importance of vitamins and minerals in the diet. Thus most bread is fortified with vitamins and minerals, and in addition, commercial food processing has made it possible for balanced diets of an appealing variety to be eaten all year round.

Many people do not get an adequate diet, either through ignorance or because they simply cannot afford it. A number of food programs have been created to assist them, but unfortunately, the programs don't reach everyone who needs help.

Causes of Malnutrition

Some people, either because of ignorance or food faddism, do not eat a balanced diet even though they can afford to. There are also large numbers of people with nutritional deficiency diseases who can be described as abnormal, at least in regard to eating. Some are alcoholics; others live alone and are so depressed that they lack sufficient drive to feed themselves properly. Combination of any of these factors increase the likelihood of poor nutrition and often lead to health-damaging consequences.

Disease

People can also develop nutritional deficiencies because they have some disease that interferes with food absorption, storage, and utilization, or that causes an increased excretion, usually in the urine, of substances needed for nutrition. These are generally chronic diseases of the gastrointestinal tract including the liver, or of the kidneys or the endocrine glands.

Medications

Nutritional deficiencies can also result from loss of appetite caused by medications, especially when a number of different medications are taken simultaneously. This adverse affect on the appetite is a strong reason for not taking medicines unless told to do so by a physician for a specific purpose.

Most people are not aware of inadequacies in their diet until there are some dramatic consequences. Nor is it easy to recognize the presence of a disorder that might be causing malnutrition. A physician should be consulted promptly when there is a persistent weight loss, especially when the diet is normal. He should also be informed of any changes in the skin, mucous membranes of the mouth or tongue, or nervous system function, because such symptoms can be a warning of dietary deficiency.

The family or friends of a person with a nutritional deficiency can often

Nutrients in Common Foods

Food	Food energy Calories	Protein Grams	Fat Grams	Carbohydrate Grams
Milk and Milk Products				
Milk; 1 cup:				
Fluid, whole	165	9	10	12
Fluid, nonfat (skim)	90	9	trace	13
Buttermilk, cultured (from skim				
milk)	90	9	trace	13
Evaporated (undiluted)	345	18	20	24
Dry, nonfat (regular)	435	43	1	63
Yogurt (from partially skimmed				
milk); 1 cup	120	8	4	13
Cheese; 1 ounce:				
Cheddar or American	115	7	9	1
Cottage:				
From skim milk	25	5	trace	1
Creamed	30	4	1	1
Cream cheese	105	2	11	1
Swiss	105	7	8	1
Desserts (largely milk):				
Custard, baked; 1 cup, 8 fluid				
ounces	305	14	15	29
Ice cream, plain, factory packed:				
1 slice or individual brick, 1/8				
quart	130	3	7	14
1 container, 8 fluid ounces	255	6	14	28
Ice milk; 1 cup, 8 fluid ounces	200	6	7	29
Eggs				
Egg, raw, large:				
1 whole	80	6	6	trace
1 white	15	4	trace	trace
1 yolk	60	3	5	trace
Egg, cooked; 1 large:				
Boiled	80	6	6	trace
Scrambled (with milk and fat) ...	110	7	8	1
Meat, Poultry, Fish, Shellfish				
Bacon, broiled or fried, drained,				
2 medium thick slices	85	4	8	trace
Beef, cooked without bone:				
Braised, simmered, or pot-				
roasted; 3 ounce portion:				
Entire portion, lean and fat	365	19	31	0
Lean only, approx. 2 ounces	140	17	4	0
Hamburger patties, made with				
Regular ground beef; 3-ounce				
patty	235	21	17	0
Lean ground round; 3-ounce				
patty	185	23	10	0
Roast; 3-ounce slice from cut				
having relatively small amount				
of fat:				
Entire portion, lean and fat	255	22	18	0
Lean only, approx. 2.3 ounces	115	19	4	0
Steak, broiled; 3-ounce portion:				
Entire portion, lean and fat	375	19	32	0
Lean only, approx. 1.8 ounces	105	17	4	0
Beef, canned: corned beef hash: 3				
ounces	155	8	10	9
Beef and vegetable stew: 1 cup ...	220	16	11	15
Chicken, without bone: broiled; 3				
ounces	115	20	3	0
Lamb, cooked:				
Chops; 1 thick chop, with bone,				
4.8 ounces:				
Lean and fat, approx. 3.4				
ounces	340	21	28	0
Lean only, 2.3 ounces	120	18	5	0

Nutrients in Common Foods (continued)

Food	Food energy	Protein	Fat	Carbohydrate
	Calories	Grams	Grams	Grams
Roast, without bone:				
Leg; 3-ounce slice:				
Entire slice, lean and fat	265	20	20	0
Lean only, approx. 2.3 ounces	120	19	5	0
Shoulder; 3-ounce portion, without bone:				
Entire portion, lean and fat	300	18	25	0
Lean only, approx. 2.2 ounces	125	16	6	0
Liver, beef, fried; 2 ounces	120	13	4	6
Pork, cured, cooked:				
Ham, smoked; 3-ounce portion, without bone	245	18	19	0
Luncheon meat:				
Boiled ham; 2 ounces	130	11	10	0
Canned, spiced; 2 ounces	165	8	14	1
Pork, fresh, cooked:				
Chops; 1 chop, with bone, 3.5 ounces:				
Lean and fat, approx. 2.4 ounces	295	15	25	0
Lean only, approx. 1.6 ounces	120	14	7	0
Roast; 3-ounce slice, without bone:				
Entire slice, lean and fat	340	19	29	0
Lean only, approx. 2.2 ounces	160	19	9	0
Sausage:				
Bologna; 8 slices (4.1 by 0.1 inches each), 8 ounces	690	27	62	2
Frankfurter; 1 cooked, 1.8 ounces	155	6	14	1
Tongue, beef, boiled; 3 ounces	205	18	14	trace
Veal, cutlet, broiled; 3-ounce portion, without bone	185	23	9	0
Fish and shellfish:				
Bluefish, baked or broiled; 3 ounces	135	22	4	0
Clams: raw, meat only; 3 ounces	70	11	1	3
Crabmeat, canned or cooked; 3 ounces	90	14	2	1
Fishsticks, breaded, cooked, frozen; 10 sticks (3.8 by 1.0 by 0.5 inches each), 8 ounces	400	38	20	15
Haddock, fried; 3 ounces	135	16	5	6
Mackerel: broiled; 3 ounces	200	19	13	0
Oysters, raw, meat only; 1 cup (13–19 medium-size oysters, selects)	160	20	4	8
Oyster stew: 1 cup (6–8 oysters)	200	11	12	11
Salmon, canned (pink); 3 ounces	120	17	5	0
Sardines, canned in oil, drained solids; 3 ounces	180	22	9	1
Shrimp, canned, meat only; 3 ounces	110	23	1	–
Tuna, canned in oil, drained solids; 3 ounces	170	25	7	0
Mature Beans and Peas, Nuts				
Beans, dry seed:				
Common varieties, as Great Northern, navy, and others, canned; 1 cup:				
Red	230	15	1	42
White, with tomato or molasses:				
With pork	330	16	7	54
Without pork	315	16	1	60

detect his condition because they become aware of changes in his eating patterns. They can also note early signs of a deficiency of some of the B vitamins, such as cracks in the mucous membranes at the corners of the mouth, or some slowing of intellectual function.

Correction of Nutritional Deficiencies

Nutritional deficiencies are among the most easily preventable causes of disease. It is important to realize that even mild deficiencies can cause irreparable damage, particularly protein deprivation in young children, which can result in some degree of mental retardation. Periodic medical checkups for everyone in the family are the best way to make sure that such deficiencies are corrected before they snowball into a chronic disease. In most cases, all that is required is a change of eating habits.

Weight

Probably the most important dietary problem in the United States today is obesity. It is certainly the problem most talked about and written about, not only in terms of good looks, but more important, in terms of good health.

All studies indicate that people who are obese have a higher rate of disease and a shorter life expectancy than those of average weight. From a medical point of view, people who are too fat may actually suffer from a form of malnutrition, even though they look overnourished.

Being too fat and being overweight are not necessarily the same. Heavy bones and muscles can make a person overweight in terms of the charts, but only an excess amount of fat tissue can make someone obese. However, height and weight tables are generally used to determine obesity.

Table 1 lists standard desirable weights for people of various heights, calculated with indoor clothing and shoes on. Frame sizes are estimated in a general way. This table applies to anyone over the age of 25, indicating that weight gain for the rest of the life span is unnecessary for biological normalcy.

Table 2 gives average weights of American men and women, according to height and age. These measurements are made without clothing or shoes. Note that the weights are considerably higher than the corresponding ones of Table 1. There is a modest weight gain until the middle years and then a gradual loss.

To determine whether a person is obese according to the tables, the percent that he is overweight has to be calculated. An individual is usually considered obese in the clinical sense if he weighs 20 percent more than the standard tables indicate for his size and age.

The Pinch Test

Another method of determining obesity is to use the "pinch" test. In most adults under 50 years of age, about half of the body fat is located directly under the skin. There are various parts of the body, such as the side of the lower torso, the back of the upper arm, or directly under the shoulder blade, where the thumb and forefinger can pinch a fold of skin and fat away from the underlying bone structure.

If the fold between the fingers—which is, of course, double thickness when it is pinched—is thicker than one inch in any of these areas, the likelihood is that the person is obese.

Nutrients in Common Foods (continued)

Food	Food energy Calories	Protein Grams	Fat Grams	Carbohydrate Grams
Beans, dry seed:				
Lima, cooked; 1 cup	260	16	1	48
Cowpeas or black-eyed peas, dry,				
cooked; 1 cup	190	13	1	34
Peanuts, roasted, shelled; 1 cup	840	39	71	28
Peanut butter; 1 tablespoon	90	4	8	3
Peas, split, dry, cooked; 1 cup	290	20	1	52
Vegetables				
Asparagus:				
Cooked; 1 cup	35	4	trace	6
Canned; 6 medium-size spears	20	2	trace	3
Beans:				
Lima, immature, cooked; 1 cup	150	8	1	29
Snap, green:				
Cooked; 1 cup	25	2	trace	6
Canned; solids and liquid; 1				
cup	45	2	trace	10
Beets, cooked, diced; 1 cup	70	2	trace	16
Broccoli, cooked, flower stalks; 1				
cup	45	5	trace	8
Brussels sprouts, cooked; 1 cup ...	60	6	1	12
Cabbage; 1 cup:				
Raw, coleslaw	100	2	7	9
Cooked	40	2	trace	9
Carrots:				
Raw: 1 carrot (5½ by 1 inch) or				
25 thin strips	20	1	trace	5
Cooked, diced; 1 cup	45	1	1	9
Canned, strained or chopped; 1				
ounce	5	trace	0	2
Cauliflower, cooked, flower buds; 1				
cup	30	3	trace	6
Celery, raw: large stalk, 8 inches				
long	5	1	trace	1
Collards, cooked; 1 cup	75	7	1	14
Corn, sweet:				
Cooked; 1 ear 5 inches long	65	2	1	16
Canned, solids and liquid; 1 cup	170	5	1	41
Cucumbers, raw, pared; 6 slices (⅛-inch thick, center section)	5	trace	trace	1
Lettuce, head, raw:				
2 large or 4 small leaves	5	1	trace	1
1 compact head (4¾-inch diameter)	70	5	1	13
Mushrooms, canned, solids and liquid; 1 cup	30	3	trace	9
Okra, cooked; 8 pods (3 inches long, ⅝-inch diameter)	30	2	trace	6
Onions: mature raw; 1 onion (2½-inch diameter)	50	2	trace	11
Peas, green; 1 cup:				
Cooked	110	8	1	19
Canned, solids and liquid	170	8	1	32
Peppers, sweet:				
Green, raw; 1 medium	15	1	trace	3
Red, raw; 1 medium	20	1	trace	4
Potatoes:				
Baked or boiled; 1 medium, 2½-inch diameter (weight raw, about 5 ounces):				
Baked in jacket	90	3	trace	21
Boiled; peeled before boiling	90	3	trace	21
Chips; 10 medium (2-inch diameter)	110	1	7	10
French fried:				
Frozen, ready to be heated for serving; 10 pieces (2 by ½ by ½ inch)	95	2	4	15

Nutrients in Common Foods (continued)

Food	Food energy Calories	Protein Grams	Fat Grams	Carbohydrate Grams
Ready-to-eat, deep fat for entire process; 10 pieces (2 by ½ by ½ inch)	155	2	7	20
Mashed; 1 cup:				
Milk added	145	4	1	30
Milk and butter added	230	4	12	28
Radishes, raw; 4 small	10	trace	trace	2
Spinach:				
Cooked; 1 cup	45	6	1	6
Canned, creamed, strained; 1 ounce	10	1	trace	2
Squash:				
Cooked, 1 cup:				
Summer, diced	35	1	trace	8
Winter, baked, mashed	95	4	1	23
Canned, strained or chopped; 1 ounce	10	trace	trace	2
Sweet potatoes:				
Baked or boiled; 1 medium, 5 by 2 inches (weight raw, about 6 ounces):				
Baked in jacket	155	2	1	36
Boiled in jacket	170	2	1	39
Candied; 1 small, 3½ by 2 inches	295	2	6	60
Canned, vacuum or solid pack; 1 cup	235	4	trace	54
Tomatoes:				
Raw; 1 medium (2 by 2½ inches), about ⅓ pound	30	2	trace	6
Canned or cooked; 1 cup	45	2	trace	9
Tomato juice, canned; 1 cup	50	2	trace	10
Tomato catsup; 1 tablespoon	15	trace	trace	4
Turnips, cooked, diced; 1 cup	40	1	trace	9
Turnip greens, cooked; 1 cup	45	4	1	8
Fruits				
Apples, raw; 1 medium (2½ inch diameter), about ⅓ pound	70	trace	trace	18
Apple juice, fresh or canned; 1 cup	125	trace	0	34
Apple sauce, canned:				
Sweetened; 1 cup	185	trace	trace	50
Unsweetened; 1 cup	100	trace	trace	26
Apricots, raw; 3 apricots (about ¼ pound)	55	1	trace	14
Apricots, canned in heavy syrup; 1 cup	200	1	trace	54
Apricots, dried: uncooked; 1 cup (40 halves, small)	390	8	1	100
Avocados, raw, California varieties: ½ of a 10-ounce avocado (3½ by 3¼ inches)	185	2	18	6
Avocados, raw, Florida varieties: ½ of a 13-ounce avocado (4 by 3 inches)	160	2	14	11
Bananas, raw; 1 medium (6 by 1½ inches), about ⅓ pound	85	1	trace	23
Blueberries, raw; 1 cup	85	1	1	21
Cantaloupes, raw, ½ melon (5-inch diameter)	40	1	trace	9
Cherries, sour, sweet, and hybrid, raw; 1cup	65	1	1	15
Cranberry sauce, sweetened; 1 cup	550	trace	1	142
Dates, "fresh" and dried, pitted and cut; 1 cup	505	4	1	134
Figs:				
Raw; 3 small (1½-inch diameter), about ¼ pound	90	2	trace	22
Dried; 1 large (2 by 1 inch)	60	1	trace	15

The Problem of Overweight

The percentage of overweight people in this country has been increasing steadily, chiefly because people eat more and use less physical energy than they used to. Americans do very little walking because of the availability of cars; they do very little manual labor because of the increasing use of machines. They may eat good wholesome meals, but they have the time for nibbling at all hours, especially when sitting in front of the television screen.

These patterns usually begin in childhood. Youngsters rarely walk to school any more; they get there by bus or car. They often have extra money for snacks and soft drinks, and frequently parents encourage them to overeat without realizing that such habits do them more harm than good.

Most overweight children remain overweight as adults. They also have greater difficulty losing fat, and if they do lose it, tend to regain it more easily than overweight adults who were thin as children. Many adults become overweight between the ages of 20 and 30. Thus, by age 30, about 12 percent of American men and women are 20 percent or more overweight, and by age 60, about 30 percent of the male population and 50 percent of the female are at least 20 percent overweight. As indicated above, the phenomenon of weight gain while aging does not represent biological normalcy.

Why People Put On Weight

Why does weight gain happen? Excess weight is the result of the imbalance between caloric intake as food and caloric expenditure as energy, either in maintaining the basic metabolic processes necessary to sustain life or in performing physical activity. Calories not spent in either of these ways become converted to fat and accumulate in the body as fat, or *adipose* tissue.

A *calorie* is the unit of measurement that describes the amount of energy potentially available in a given food. It is also used to describe the amount of energy the body must use up to perform a given function.

Counting Calories

If an adult gets the average 3,000 calories a day in his food from the age of 20 to 70, he will have consumed about 55 million calories. About 60 percent of these calories will have been used for his basic metabolic processes. The rest—22 million calories—might have resulted in a gain of about 6,000 pounds of fat, since each group of 3,500 extra calories could have produced one pound of fat.

In some ways, it's a miracle that people don't become more obese than they do. The reason, of course, is that most or all of these extra calories are normally used to provide energy for physical activity. Elsewhere in this chapter are some examples of calorie expenditure during various activities.

A reasonably good way for an adult to figure his daily caloric needs for moderate activities is to multiply his desirable weight (as noted in Table 1) by 18 for men and 16 for women. If the typical day includes vigorous or strenuous activities, extra calories will, of course, be required.

Parental Influences and Hereditary Factors

Although there are exceptions, almost all obese people consume more calories than they expend. The reasons for this imbalance are complex. One has to do with parental weight. If the weight of both parents is normal, there is only a 10 percent likelihood that the children will be obese. If one

Nutrients in Common Foods (continued)

Food	Food energy Calories	Protein Grams	Fat Grams	Carbohydrate Grams
Fruit cocktail, canned in heavy syrup, solids and liquid; 1 cup	175	1	trace	47
Grapefruit:				
Raw; ½ medium (4¼-inch diameter, No. 64's)	50	1	trace	14
Canned in syrup; 1 cup	165	1	trace	44
Grapefruit juice:				
Raw; 1 cup	85	1	trace	23
Canned:				
Unsweetened; 1 cup	95	1	trace	24
Sweetened; 1 cup	120	1	trace	32
Frozen concentrate, unsweetened:				
Undiluted; 1 can (6 fluid ounces)	280	4	1	72
Diluted, ready-to-serve; 1 cup	95	1	trace	24
Frozen concentrate, sweetened:				
Undiluted; 1 can (6 fluid ounces)	320	3	1	85
Diluted, ready-to-serve; 1 cup	105	1	trace	28
Grapes, raw; 1 cup:				
American type (slip skin)	70	1	1	16
European type (adherent skin) ...	100	1	trace	26
Grape juice, bottled; 1 cup	165	1	1	42
Lemonade concentrate, frozen, sweetened:				
Undiluted; 1 can (6 fluid ounces)	305	1	trace	113
Diluted, ready-to-serve; 1 cup ...	75	trace	trace	28
Oranges, raw; 1 large orange (3-inch diameter)	70	1	trace	18
Orange juice:				
Raw; 1 cup:				
California (Valencias)	105	2	trace	26
Florida varieties:				
Early and midseason	90	1	trace	23
Late season (Valencias)	105	1	trace	26
Canned, unsweetened; 1 cup	110	2	trace	28
Frozen concentrate:				
Undiluted; 1 can (6 fluid ounces)	305	5	trace	80
Diluted, ready-to-serve; 1 cup	105	2	trace	27
Peaches:				
Raw:				
1 medium (2½-inch diameter), about ¼ pound	35	1	trace	10
1 cup, sliced	65	1	trace	16
Canned (yellow-fleshed) in heavy syrup; 1 cup	185	1	trace	49
Dried: uncooked; 1 cup	420	5	1	109
Pears:				
Raw; 1 pear (3 by 2½-inch diameter)	100	1	1	25
Canned in heavy syrup; 1 cup ...	175	1	trace	47
Pineapple juice; canned; 1 cup	120	1	trace	32
Plums:				
Raw; 1 plum (2-inch diameter), about 2 ounces	30	trace	trace	7
Canned (Italian prunes), in syrup; 1 cup	185	1	trace	50
Prunes, dried:				
Uncooked; 4 medium prunes	70	1	trace	19
Cooked, unsweetened; 1 cup (17–18 prunes and ⅓ cup liquid)	295	3	1	78
Prune juice, canned; 1 cup	170	1	trace	45
Raisins, dried; 1 cup	460	4	trace	124
Raspberries, red:				
Raw; 1 cup	70	1	trace	17

Nutrients in Common Foods *(continued)*

Food	Food energy	Protein	Fat	Carbohydrate
	Calories	Grams	Grams	Grams
Frozen; 10-ounce carton	280	2	1	70
Strawberries:				
Raw; 1 cup	55	1	1	12
Frozen; 10-ounce carton	300	2	1	75
Tangerines; 1 medium (2½-inch diameter), about ¼ pound	40	1	trace	10
Watermelon: 1 wedge (4 by 8 inches), about 2 pounds (weighed with rind)	120	2	1	29
Grain Products				
Biscuits, baking powder, enriched flour; 1 biscuit (2½-inch diameter)	130	3	4	20
Bran flakes (40 percent bran) with added thiamine; 1 ounce	85	3	1	22
Breads:				
Cracked wheat:				
1 pound (20 slices)	1,190	39	10	236
1 slice (½ inch thick)	60	2	1	12
Italian; 1 pound	1,250	41	4	256
Rye:				
American (light):				
1 pound (20 slices)	1,100	41	5	236
1 slice (½ inch thick)	55	2	trace	12
Pumpernickel; 1 pound	1,115	41	5	241
White:				
1–2 percent nonfat dry milk:				
1 pound (20 slices)	1,225	39	15	229
1 slice (½ inch thick)	60	2	1	12
3–4 percent nonfat dry milk:				
1 pound (20 slices)	1,225	39	15	229
1 slice (½ inch thick)	60	2	1	12
5–6 percent nonfat dry milk:				
1 pound (20 slices)	1,245	41	17	228
1 slice (½ inch thick)	65	2	1	12
Whole wheat, graham, or entire wheat:				
1 pound (20 slices)	1,105	48	14	216
1 slice (½ inch thick)	55	2	1	11
Cakes:				
Angel food: 2-inch sector (1/12 of cake, 8-inch diameter)	160	4	trace	36
Butter cakes:				
Plain cake and cupcakes without icing:				
1 square (3 by 3 by 2 inches)	315	4	12	48
1 cupcake (2¾-inch diameter)	120	2	5	18
Plain cake with icing:				
2-inch sector of iced layer cake (1/16 of cake, 10-inch diameter)	320	5	6	62
Rich cake:				
2-inch sector layer cake, iced (1/16 of cake, 10-inch diameter)	490	6	19	76
Fruit cake, dark; 1 piece (2 by 1½ by ¼ inches)	60	1	2	9
Sponge; 2-inch sector (1/12 of cake, 8-inch diameter)	115	3	2	22
Cookies, plain and assorted; 1 cookie (3-inch diameter)	110	2	3	19
Cornbread or muffins made with enriched, degermed cornmeal; 1 muffin 2¾-inch diameter)	105	3	2	18
Cornflakes: 1 ounce	110	2	trace	24
Corn grits, degermed, cooked: 1 cup	120	3	trace	27

parent is obese, there is a 50 percent probability that the children will be too, and if both are, the probability of obese offspring is 80 percent.

No one knows for certain why this is so. It is probably a combination of diet habits acquired in youth, conditioning during early years to react to emotional stress by eating, the absence of appropriate exercise patterns, and genetic inheritance.

Some obese people seem to have an impairment in the regulatory mechanism of the area of the central nervous system that governs food intake. Simply put, they do not know when to stop eating. Others, particularly girls, may eat less than their nonobese counterparts, but they are considerably less active. Some researchers think that obese people have an inherent muscle rhythm deficiency. A few people appear to have an abnormality in the metabolic process which results in the accumulation of fat even when the balance between calories taken in and expended is negative and should lead to weight loss.

Obesity and Health

There are many reasons why obesity is a health hazard. The annual death rate for obese people between the ages of 20 and 64 is half again as high as that for people whose weight is close to normal. This statistical difference is due primarily to the increased likelihood that the obese person will suffer from diabetes mellitus and from diseases of the digestive and circulatory systems, especially of the heart.

One possible reason for the increased possibility of heart disease is that there are about two-thirds of a mile of blood vessels in each pound of adipose tissue. Thus 20 or more pounds of excess weight are likely to impose a great additional work load on the heart.

Obese people are also poorer surgical risks than the nonobese, and it is often more difficult to diagnose and therefore to treat their illnesses correctly.

Permanent loss of excess weight makes the formerly obese person come closer to matching the life expectancy of the nonobese. However, losing and regaining weight as a repeated pattern is even more hazardous in terms of health than consistent obesity.

Psychological Consequences of Obesity

In ways that are both obvious and subtle, obesity often has damaging psychological consequences. This is particularly true for obese children, who tend to feel isolated and rejected by their peers. They may consider themselves victims of prejudice and blame their obesity for everything that goes wrong in their lives. In many cases, the destructive relationship between obesity and self-pity keeps perpetuating itself.

Obese adults are likely to experience the same feelings, but to a somewhat lesser degree. For some, obesity is an escape which consciously or unconsciously helps them to avoid situations in which they feel uncomfortable—those that involve active competition or relationships with the opposite sex.

Avoiding Excess Weight

Clearly, obesity is a condition that most people would like to avoid. Not putting on extra pounds does seem to be easier, in theory at least, than taking them off. One possible explanation for this is that additional adipose tissue consists of a proliferation of fat cells. Shrinking these cells is one thing, eliminating them is another. Our present lack of fundamental knowledge about the regulatory and

Nutrients in Common Foods (continued)

Food	Food energy Calories	Protein Grams	Fat Grams	Carbohydrate Grams
Crackers:				
Graham; 4 small or 2 medium ...	55	1	1	10
Saltines; 2 crackers (2-inch square)	35	1	1	6
Soda, plain: 2 crackers (2½-inch square)	45	1	1	8
Doughnuts, cake type; 1 doughnut	135	2	7	17
Farina, cooked; 1 cup	105	3	trace	22
Macaroni, cooked; 1 cup:				
Cooked 8–10 minutets (undergoes additional cooking as ingredient of a food mixture)	190	6	1	39
Cooked until tender	155	5	1	32
Noodles (egg noodles), cooked; 1 cup	200	7	2	37
Oat cereal (mixture, mainly oat flour), ready-to-eat; 1 ounce	115	4	2	21
Oatmeal or rolled oats, regular or quick cooking, cooked; 1 cup	150	5	3	26
Pancakes, baked; 1 cake (4-inch diameter):				
Wheat (home recipe)	60	2	2	7
Buckwheat (with buckwheat pancake mix)	45	2	2	6
Pies; 3½-inch sector (⅛ of 9-inch diameter pie):				
Apple	300	3	13	45
Cherry	310	3	13	45
Custard	250	7	13	27
Lemon meringue	270	4	11	40
Mince	320	3	14	49
Pumpkin	240	5	13	28
Pretzels; 5 small sticks	20	trace	trace	4
Rice, cooked; 1 cup:				
Converted	205	4	trace	45
White	200	4	trace	44
Rice, puffed or flakes; 1 ounce	110	2	trace	25
Rolls:				
Plain, pan (16 ounces per dozen); 1 roll	115	3	2	20
Hard, round (22 ounces per dozen); 1 roll	160	5	2	31
Sweet, pan (18 ounces per dozen); 1 roll	135	4	4	21
Spaghetti, cooked until tender; 1 cup	155	5	1	32
Waffles, baked, with enriched flour: 1 waffle (4½ by 5½ by ½ inches)	215	7	8	28
Wheat, puffed: 1 ounce	100	4	trace	22
Wheat, rolled, cooked; 1 cup	175	5	1	40
Wheat flakes; 1 ounce	100	3	trace	23
Wheat flours:				
Whole wheat; 1 cup, sifted	400	16	2	85
All purpose or family flour: 1 cup, sifted	400	12	1	84
Wheat germ; 1 cup, stirred	245	17	7	34
Fats, Oils, Related Products				
Butter; 1 tablespoon	100	trace	11	trace
Fats, cooking:				
Vegetable fats:				
1 cup	1,770	0	200	0
1 tablespoon	110	0	12	0
Lard:				
1 cup	1,985	0	220	0
1 tablespoon	125	0	14	0
Margarine; 1 tablespoon	100	trace	11	trace
Oils, salad or cooking; 1 tablespoon	125	0	14	0

Nutrients in Common Foods (continued)

Food	Food energy	Protein	Fat	Carbohydrate
	Calories	Grams	Grams	Grams
Salad dressings; 1 tablespoon:				
Blue cheese	90	1	10	1
Commercial, plain (mayonnaise type)	60	trace	6	2
French	60	trace	6	2
Mayonnaise	110	trace	12	trace
Thousand Island	75	trace	8	1
Sugars, Sweets				
Candy; 1 ounce:				
Caramels	120	1	3	22
Chocolate, sweetened, milk	145	2	9	16
Fudge, plain	115	trace	3	23
Hard	110	0	0	28
Marshmallow	90	1	0	23
Jams, marmalades, preserves; 1 tablespoon	55	trace	trace	14
Jellies; 1 tablespoon	50	0	0	13
Sugar; 1 tablespoon	50	0	0	12
Syrup, table blends; 1 tablespoon	55	0	0	15
Miscellaneous				
Beverages, carbonated, cola types; 1 cup	105	–	–	28
Bouillon cubes; 1 cube	2	trace	trace	0
Chocolate, unsweetened; 1 ounce	145	2	15	8
Gelatin dessert, plain, ready-to-serve; 1 cup	155	4	0	36
Sherbet, factory packed; 1 cup (8-fluid-ounce container)	235	3	trace	58
Soups, canned, prepared with equal amount of water; 1 cup:				
Bean with pork	168	8	6	22
Beef noodle	140	8	5	14
Bouillon, broth, and consomme	30	5	0	3
Chicken consomme	44	7	trace	4
Clam chowder, Manhattan style	80	2	3	12
Tomato	90	2	3	16
Vegetable beef	80	5	2	10
Vinegar; 1 tablespoon	2	0	–	1

Adapted from *Nutritive Value of American Foods* by Catherine F. Adams, Agriculture Handbook No. 456, U.S. Department of Agriculture, issued November 1975. The cup measure used in the following table refers to the standard 8-ounce measuring cup of 8 fluid ounces or one-half liquid pint. When a measure is indicated by ounce, it is understood to be by weight—1/16 of a pound avoirdupois—unless a fluid ounce is indicated. All weights and measures in the table are in U.S. System units.

metabolic mechanisms relating to obesity limits the technique of preventing overweight to recommending a balance between caloric intake and expenditure.

The real responsibility for preventing the onset of obesity in childhood rests with parents. It is important for the parents to set a good example and to instill early on all of the fundamentals of good nutrition and healthy eating habits; these are of the utmost importance in this connection. Caloric expenditure in the form of regular exercise is equally important.

Exercising by Habit

This does not necessarily mean that exercise should be encouraged for its own sake. What it does mean is making a habit of choosing an active way of approaching a situation rather than a lazy way: walking upstairs rather than taking the elevator; walking to school rather than riding; walking while playing golf rather than riding in a cart; running to get the ball that has rolled away rather than ambling toward it. These choices should be made consistently and not just occa-

sionally if obesity is to be avoided. Those people who naturally enjoy the more active way of doing things are lucky. Those who don't should make an effort to develop new patterns, especially if obesity is a family problem.

Anyone with the type of physical handicap that makes a normal amount of exercise impossible should be especially careful about caloric intake.

Weight Reduction

The treatment of obesity is a complicated problem. In the first place, there is the question of who wants or needs to be treated and how much weight should be lost. Except in unusual situations, anyone who wants to lose weight should be encouraged to do so. Possible exceptions are teenagers who are not overweight but who want to be as thin as they can possibly be—the boy who is involved in an athletic event such as wrestling, or the girl who has decided she wants to look like a fashion model.

Crash dieting is usually unwise if the goal is to lose too much weight too rapidly and should be undertaken only after consulting a doctor about its advisability. As for adolescents who have become slightly overweight during puberty, they may be ill-advised to try to take off the extra pounds that probably relate to a temporary growth pattern.

Losing Weight Must Be Self-Motivated

Unless there are compelling medical reasons for not doing so, anyone weighing 20 percent or more over the normal limit for his age and body build should be helped to slim down. It is extremely important, however, for the motivation to come from the person himself rather than from outside pressure.

Unless an overweight person really wants to reduce, he will not succeed in doing so, certainly not permanently, even though he appears to be trying. He must have convinced himself—intellectually and emotionally—that the goal of weight loss is truly worth the effort.

It is very difficult not only for his friends and family but for the person himself to be absolutely sure about the depth of his motivation. A physician treating an overweight patient has to assume that the desire to reduce is genuine and will try to reinforce it whenever he can. However, if a patient has made a number of attempts to lose weight over a period of years and has either been unable to reduce to any significant degree, or has become overweight again after reducing, it is probably safe to assume that the emotional desire is absent, or that there are emotional conflicts that stand in the way.

It is very possible that such a person could be harmed psychologically by losing weight, since he might need to be overweight for some deep-seated reason. This can be true for both children and adults. Occasionally it is possible for a psychiatrist or psychologist to help the patient remove a psychological block against losing weight, after which weight reduction can occur if the caloric balance is straightened out.

Effective Planning for Weight Loss

The ultimate key to successful weight reduction is proper eating combined with proper physical activity. This balance is extremely difficult for many people to achieve because it involves a marked change in attitudes and behavior patterns that are generally solidly established and of long duration. Furthermore, once the changes are made, they will have to endure for a

Effect of Fat Accumulation in Abdomen

Fat accumulating in the abdomen puts severe stress on the lower vertebral column and can lead to many back problems.

lifetime if the weight that has been lost is not to be regained.

It is therefore important that the reducing diet should be somewhat similar to the person's usual eating pattern in terms of style and quality. Intake of fat and calories should be reduced and that of fiber increased, and probably the word "dieting" should not be used to describe the process, since most people don't find the idea of permanent dieting congenial.

Similarly, the increased physical activity that must accompany the new eating style should be of a type that the person enjoys. It is virtually impossible for an overeating person to reduce merely by restricting his caloric intake, or merely by increasing his caloric expenditure. The two must go together.

Cutting Down Step by Step

The first thing to determine when planning to lose weight is the number of pounds that have to go. A realistic goal to set is the loss of about one pound a week. This may seem too slow, but remember that at this rate, fifty pounds can be lost in a year.

Getting Started

Start by weighing yourself on arising, and then for two weeks try to eat in your customary manner, but keep a careful record of everything that you eat, the time it is eaten, and the number of calories it contains. During this period, continue to do your usual amount of physical activity.

When the two weeks are over, weigh yourself again at the same time of day as before. If you haven't gained

Daily Food Guide				
	Child	Preteen and Teen	Adult	Aging Adult
Milk or milk products (*cups*)	2–3	3–4 or more	2 or more	2 or more
Meat, fish, poultry, and eggs (*servings*)	1–2	3 or more	2 or more	2 or more
Green and yellow vegetables (*servings*)	1–2	2	2	at least 1
Citrus fruits and tomatoes (*servings*)	1	1–2	1	1–2
Potatoes, other fruits, vegetables (*servings*)	1	1	1	0–1
Bread, flour, and cereal (*servings*)	3–4	4 or more	3–4	2–3
Butter or margarine (*tablespoons*)	2	2–4	2–3	1–2

1. The need for the nutrients in 1 or 2 cups of milk daily can be satisfied by cheeses or ice cream. (1 cup of milk is approximately equivalent to 1½ cups of cottage cheese or 2–3 large scoops of ice cream.)
2. It is important to drink enough fluid. The equivalent of 3–5 cups daily is recommended.
3. The recommended daily serving of meat, fish, and poultry (3 oz.) may be alternated with eggs or cheese, dried peas, beans, or lentils.
4. Iron-rich foods should be selected as frequently as possible by teenage and adult females to help meet their high requirement for this mineral (liver, heart, lean meats, shellfish, egg yolks, legumes, green leafy vegetables, and whole grain and enriched cereal products).

From *Your Age and Your Diet* (1971), reprinted with permission from the American Medical Association.

any weight, you are in a basal caloric state. Then check over your food list to see what might be eliminated each day without causing discomfort.

Try to think in terms of eliminating fats and simple carbohydrates first, because it is essential that you continue to get sufficient vitamins and minerals which are largely found in proteins and complex carbohydrates. The foods described in the "Daily Food Guide" chart should all continue to be included in your daily food consumption. If you are in the habit of having an occasional drink, remember that there are calories in alcohol but no nutrients, and that most alcoholic beverages stimulate the appetite.

Planning Meals

When you replan your meals, keep in mind that the items you cut down on must add up to between 300 and 400 calories a day if you are going to lose one pound a week.

Your total daily food intake should be divided among at least three meals a day, more if you wish. If you need to eat more food or to eat more often, try snacking on low calorie foods such as cabbage, carrots, celery, cucumber, and cauliflower. All of these can be eaten raw between meals.

There is definitely something to be said in favor of having breakfast every morning, or at least most mornings. This may be psychologically difficult, but try to do it, because it will be easier to control your urge to eat too much later in the day.

Increasing Exercise

At the same time that you begin to cut down on your food intake, start to increase your daily exercise in whatever way you find congenial so that the number of calories expended in increased exercise plus the number of calories eliminated from your diet comes to 500 or more. This is your daily caloric loss compared with your so-called basal caloric state.

Achieving Your Goal

You may wish to double your daily caloric loss so that you lose two pounds a week. Do not try to lose any more

than that unless you are under close medical supervision.

If you gained weight during your two-week experimental period, you will have to increase your daily caloric loss by 500 for every pound gained per week. Thus, if you gained one pound during the two weeks, you will have to step up your daily caloric loss to 750 to lose a pound a week.

You'll have to keep plugging away to achieve your goal. It will be trying and difficult in many ways. You may get moody and discouraged and be tempted to quit. Don't. You'll probably go on periodic food binges. All this is natural and understandable, so try not to brood about it. Just do the best you can each day. Don't worry about yesterday, and let tomorrow take care of itself.

In many ways it can help, and in some cases it's essential, to have the support and encouragement of family and friends, particularly of those with whom you share meals. You may find it helpful to join a group that has been formed to help its members lose weight and maintain their weight loss. This is a good psychological support.

Maintaining Your Weight Loss

Once you have achieved your desired weight, you can test yourself to see what happens if you increase your caloric intake. Clearly, anyone who can lose weight in the manner described can't stay in a state of negative caloric imbalance indefinitely. But you will have to be careful, or you'll become overweight again. It's a challenge, but people who stick to a disciplined program can be rewarded by success.

Special Problems

If you do not succeed in losing weight in spite of carrying out the program described above, you may need professional help because of some special problem. A qualified physician may try some special diets, or he may even suggest putting you into a hospital so that he can see to it that you have no caloric food at all for as long as three weeks.

Perhaps the situation is complicated by a metabolic abnormality that can be corrected or helped by medication. Although such conditions are rare, they are not unheard of.

Obesity is almost never caused by a "glandular" problem—which usually means an underactive thyroid. Do not take thyroid pills to reduce unless your thyroid has been found to be underactive on the basis of a specific laboratory test.

The indiscriminate use of pills to reduce, even when prescribed, is never helpful in the long run, although it may appear to be at first. The unsupervised use of amphetamines, for example, can be extremely dangerous. See Ch. 29, *Substance Abuse,* for further information about the dangers of amphetamine abuse.

Because so many people are eager to reduce, and because losing weight isn't easy, there are many unethical professionals who specialize in the problem. Avoid them. All they are likely to do for you is take your money and make your situation no better— and often worse—than it was to begin with.

Underweight

Weighing too little is a problem that is considerably less common than weighing too much. In fact, in many cases, it isn't accurate to call it a problem at all, at least not a medical one.

There are some times, however, when underweight may indicate the presence of a disease, especially when a person rather suddenly begins and continues to lose weight, even though there has been no change in his eating habits. This is a situation

---

Sodium Restricted Diets
Diets Moderately Restricted in Sodium

If only a moderate sodium restriction is necessary, a normal diet *without added salt* may be ordered. Such an order is interpreted to mean that the patient will be offered the regular salted food on the general selective menu with the following exceptions:

1. No salt will be served on the tray.
2. Soups that are salted will be omitted.
3. Cured meats (ham, bacon, sausage, corned beef) and all salted cheeses will be omitted.
4. Catsup, chili sauce, mustard, and other salted sauces will be omitted.
5. Salt-free gravies, sauces, and salad dressings will be substituted for the regular salted items.
6. Salted crackers, potato chips, nuts, pickles, olives, popcorn, and pretzels will be omitted.

This diet contains approximately 3 grams of sodium or 7.5 grams of sodium chloride, depending on the type and quantity of the food chosen.

---

that calls for prompt medical evaluation. Fortunately, such a person may already be under a physician's care at the time the weight loss is first noticed.

More often, however, underweight is a chronic condition that is of concern to the person who feels his looks would improve if he could only add some extra pounds. This is especially true in the case of adolescent girls and young women.

What To Do About Weighing Too Little

Chronic underweight is rarely a reflection of underlying disease. It is rather an expression of individual heredity or eating patterns, or a combination of both. Treatment for the condition is the opposite of the treatment for overweight. The achievement of a positive caloric balance comes first; more calories have to be consumed each day than are expended. An underweight person should record his food history over a two-week period in the manner described for an overweight one. Once this has been done, various adjustments can be made.

First of all, he should see that he eats at least three meals a day and that they are eaten in a leisurely way and in a relaxed frame of mind. All of

the basic foods should be represented in the daily food intake, with special emphasis on protein and complex carbohydrates. The daily caloric intake should then be gradually increased at each meal and snacks added, so long as the snacks don't reduce the appetite at mealtimes.

Carbohydrate foods are the best ones to emphasize in adding calories. Since the extra food intake may cause a certain amount of discomfort, encouragement and support from family and friends can be extremely helpful. Just as there may be psychological blocks against losing weight, there may well be a complicated underlying resistance to adding it.

Anyone trying to gain weight should remain or become reasonably active physically. Adding a pound or two a month for an adult—and a little more than that for a growing youngster—is an achievable goal until the desired weight is reached. When this happens, there will probably have to be some adjustments in eating and exercise patterns so that a state of caloric balance is achieved.

How Food Relates to Disease

Just as proper food is essential in the prevention of some diseases, it is helpful in the treatment of others. It also plays an important role in protecting and fortifying the general health of a patient while a specific illness is being treated.

The components of therapeutic diets are usually prescribed by the physician in charge, but some general principles will be presented here. Remember that diets designed to treat a given disease must supply the patient's basic nutritional requirements.

Ulcers

Special diet is a major treatment consideration in the case of peptic ulcer, whether located in the stomach (gastric) or in the small intestine (duodenal). A major aim of such a diet is the neutralizing of the acidity of gastric juices by the frequent intake of high protein foods such as milk and eggs. Foods which irritate an ulcer chemically, such as excessive sweets, spices, or salt, or mechanically, such as foods with sharp seeds or tough skins, and foods that are too hot or too cold, should be avoided. It is also advisable to eliminate gravies, coffee, strong tea, carbonated beverages, and alcohol, since all of these stimulate gastric secretion. Such a diet is called a *bland* diet. A soft diet is recommended for some forms of gastrointestinal distress and for those people who have difficulty chewing. It is often combined with the bland diet recommended for peptic ulcer patients to reduce the likelihood of irritation. See Ch. 11, *Diseases of the Digestive System,* for further information about ulcers.

Diabetes

As the section on diabetes mellitus indicates (see Ch. 15), the major objectives of the special diet are weight control, control of the abnormal carbohydrate metabolism, and as far as

possible, psychological adjustment by the patient to his individual circumstances. To some extent, he must calculate his diet mathematically. First, his daily caloric needs have to be determined in terms of his activities:

If he is overweight or underweight, the total calories per pound of body weight will have to be adjusted downward or upward by about five calories per pound.

After his total daily caloric needs have been figured out, he can calculate the number of grams of carbohydrate, protein, and fat he should have each day: 58 percent of the calories should come from carbohydrates, 12 percent from protein, and 30 percent from fat. One-fifth of the total should be obtained at breakfast and the rest split between lunch and dinner. Snacks that are taken during the day should be subtracted equally from lunch and dinner.

It is important that meals and planned snacks be eaten regularly and that no food servings be added or omitted. Growing children from 1 to 20 years of age who have diabetes will require considerably more daily calories. A rough estimate is 1,000 calories for a one-year-old child and 100 additional calories for each year of age.

Salt-Free Diets

There are a number of chronic diseases which are treated in part by restricting the amount of sodium in the diet. These diseases, which are associated with fluid retention in the body, include congestive heart failure, certain types of kidney and liver diseases, and hypertension or high blood pressure.

The restriction of sodium intake helps to reduce or avoid the problem of fluid retention. The normal daily diet contains about seven or more grams of sodium, most of it in the

form of sodium chloride or table salt. This amount is either inherent in the food or added during processing, cooking, or at mealtime. Half the weight of salt is sodium.

For people whose physical condition requires only a small restriction of the normal sodium intake, simply not salting food at the table is a sufficient reduction. They may decide to use a salt substitute, but before doing so should discuss the question with their physician.

A greater sodium restriction, for example, to no more than 5 grams a day, requires the avoidance of such high salt content foods as ham, bacon, crackers, catsup, and potato chips, as well as almost entirely eliminating salt in the preparation and serving of meals. Severe restriction—1 gram or less a day—involves special food selection and cooking procedures, as well as the use of distilled water if the local water has more than 20 milligrams of sodium per quart. In restricting sodium to this extent, it is important to make sure that protein and vitamins are not reduced below the minimum daily requirements. See "Sodium Restricted Diets."

Other Diseases Requiring Special Diets

There are several other disorders in which diet is an important consideration: all chronic gastrointestinal disorders, such as gallbladder stones, ulcerative colitis, enteritis, and diverticulitis; a variety of hereditary disorders such as phenylketonuria and galactosemia; atherosclerosis, especially when it is associated with elevated blood levels of cholesterol or triglycerides or both; liver disease such as cirrhosis; many of the endocrine diseases; kidney stones; and sometimes certain neurological diseases such as epilepsy. Diet also plays a special role in convalescence from most illnesses and in post-surgical care. A modified fat diet and low fat diet are recommended for some diseases of the liver and gallbladder. A minimal residue diet is recommended for some digestive troubles and before and after gastrointestinal surgery.

Diet and Individual Differences

Most discussions about food and eating tend to suggest that all normal people have identical gastrointestinal and metabolic systems. This is simply not true. There are many individual differences that explain why one man's meat is another man's poison. A person's intolerance for a given food may be caused by a disorder, such as an allergy or an ulcer, and it is possible that many of these intolerances will ultimately be related to enzyme deficiencies or some other biochemical factor.

More subtle are the negative physical reactions to particular foods as a result of psychological conditioning. In most such cases, the choice is between avoiding the food that causes the discomfort or eating it and suffering the consequences. Of course, compulsive overeating can also cause or contribute to discomfort. Practically no one can eat unlimited quantities of anything without having gastrointestinal discomfort or *dyspepsia.*

The establishment of so-called daily minimum food requirements suggests that every day's intake should be carefully balanced. Although this is beneficial, it is by no means necessary. Freedom from such regimentation can certainly be enjoyed during a holiday, or a trip to another country, or on a prolonged visit to relatives with casual food habits.

Sometimes a change in diet is dictated by a cold or an upset stomach or diarrhea. Liquids containing carbohydrates, such as tea with sugar and light soups, should be emphasized in treating a cold, while at the same time solid food intake should be somewhat reduced. In the case of an upset stomach or diarrhea, the discomfort may be eased by not eating or drinking anything at all for a whole day. This form of treatment may be helpful for an adult, but since children with diarrhea can become dehydrated in a day or so, professional advice is indicated when cutting down liquid intake.

Diet and Disease Prevention

More and more, medical specialists agree that diet can be helpful in preventing various diseases. Consensus has become general that a diet low in cholesterol and saturated fats can help prevent cardiovascular disease caused by atherosclerosis. Among the foods that reduce total cholesterol levels are rice bran and oat bran. Other sources of the soluble fiber that decreases blood cholesterol include peas, lentils, barley, and pectin fruits like apples, oranges, pears, and prunes. Also recommended are skinless poultry and fish, lean meat, and low-fat dairy products.

Food-Borne Diseases

There are several ways in which food can be the *cause* of disease, most commonly when it becomes contaminated with a sufficient amount of harmful bacteria, bacterial toxin, viruses, or other poisonous substances. The gastrointestinal diseases typically accompanied by nausea, vomiting, diarrhea, or stomach cramps that are produced in this way are not, strictly speaking, caused by the foods themselves, and are therefore called food-borne diseases.

Most food-borne illnesses are caused by a toxin in food contaminated by staphylococcal or salmonella bacteria. In general, milk, milk products, raw shellfish, and meats are the foods most apt to be contaminated. This is most likely to happen when such foods are left standing at room temperature for too long between the time they are prepared and the time they are eaten. However, food can also become contaminated at many different points in time and at various stages of processing. Standards enforced by federal and local government agencies provide protection for the consumer for foods bought for the home as well as for use in restaurants, although whether the protection is adequate is a matter of dispute.

Food Storage

Food is best protected from contamination when it is stored below 40 degrees Fahrenheit or heated to 145 degrees or more. Cold slows bacterial growth; cooking kills it. Bacteria present in food can double in number every 15 minutes at room temperature.

All food stored in the refrigerator should be covered except ripe fruits and vegetables. Leftover foods cannot be kept indefinitely, nor can frozen foods be stored beyond a certain length of time. Specific information about these time periods for individual items is available from the Agricultural Extension Service in each state.

Commercially processed foods sold in the United States are under government control and generally are safe. However, any food can spoil or become contaminated at any point in time, and the consumer should not buy or serve food whose container (package or can) has been broken, cracked, or appears unusual.

Food Additives

From time to time, concern is expressed about one or another food additive as a hazard to health. Most of these additives are put into foods during processing in order to increase their nutritional value, or to improve their chemical or physical characteristics, such as taste and color. Perhaps as many as 2,000 different substances are used in this way in the United States. Some are natural products such as vanilla, others are chemicals derived from other foods, and a few, like artificial sweeteners, are synthetic. Other additives are referred to as indirect, since they are residues in the food from some stage of growing, processing, or packaging. Although additives are controlled and approved by agencies such as the federal Food and Drug Administration, they continue to be a cause of concern to many people.

Pesticides

The pesticides and fertilizers used in growing fruits and vegetables and the additives given to livestock may pose additional health hazards to humans. The National Academy of Sciences, for example, in 1988 estimated the national risk of cancer from pesticide use alone at as many as 20,000 cases a year.

Although it is not known how much is too much, it only makes sense to try and eliminate as much of the risk as possible. This is fairly easy to do. First of all, eat a wide variety of foods to help minimize your exposure to any one pesticide. Eat what's in season and what's grown locally or domestically. (The right season and less transportation mean less chemicals to ripen and preserve food; food and animals from abroad are subject to different health standards that are hard to regulate and check.) Wash all meat and produce carefully; many toxins are easily removed with soap and water. Peel any fruit or vegetable with a wax coating. (Although it is generally

advisable to retain as much of the skin of produce as possible for higher vitamin content, wax coatings hold in toxic residues.) Trim produce.

You may also want to go further in reducing your chances of consumption of added toxins by buying organically grown and raised produce and meat. These foods are not widely available in all areas of the country, and they often cost quite a bit more than foods raised with chemicals, but many people not only feel safer eating these foods, but find them tastier as well. Home gardening without the use of chemical fertilizers and pesticides is another healthful option. Be sure to wash and trim carefully all organic or home-grown vegetables, however, to guard against ingestion of naturally occurring toxins such as fungus.

Psychological Aspects of Food and Meals

Food and meals play an important role in emotional well-being and interpersonal relationships as well as in physical health and appearance.

During Infancy

The infant whose needs are attended to by a loving family develops a general sense of trust and security. The major contribution to his emotional contentment is probably made at mealtimes, and perhaps in a special way if he is breast-fed.

For most infants, food comes to be identified with love, pleasure, protection, and the satisfaction of basic needs. If there is an atmosphere of tension accompanying his feeding times, his digestion can be impaired in such a way as to cause vomiting, fretting, or signs of colic. If the tension and the baby's reaction to it—and inevitably the mother's increasing tension as a consequence—become a

chronic condition, the result may be a failure to gain weight normally, and in extreme cases, some degree of mental retardation. Throughout life, good nutrition depends not only on eating properly balanced meals that satisfy the body's physiological requirements, but also on a reasonable degree of contentment and relaxation while eating.

Everybody develops individual emotional reactions and attitudes about food and its role as a result of conditioning during the years of infancy and childhood. These attitudes relate not only to food itself and to mealtimes in general, but also to other aspects of eating, including the muscle activities of sucking, chewing, and swallowing.

If food symbolized contentment during the early years, it probably will have the same role later on. If it was associated with conflict, then it may be associated throughout life with strife and neurotic eating patterns.

During Childhood

For the preschool child, mealtimes should provide the occasion for the development of interpersonal relationships, because they are a daily opportunity for both verbal and nonverbal self-expression. The child who eats with enthusiasm and obvious enjoyment is conveying one message; the one who dawdles, picks at food, and challenges his mother with every mouthful is conveying quite a different one.

Meals can become either positive or negative experiences depending in large part on how the adults in the family set the stage. Communication can be encouraged by relaxed conversation and a reasonably leisurely schedule. It can be discouraged by watching television or reading while eating, by not eating together, or by eating and running.

Reasonably firm attitudes about eating a variety of foods in proper quantities at proper times and avoiding excessive catering to individual whims can also help in the development of wholesome eating patterns.

Those who select and prepare the food can transmit special messages of love and affection by serving favorite dishes, by setting the table attractively, and by creating an atmosphere of grace and good humor. Or they can show displeasure and generate hostility by complaining about all the work involved in feeding everyone, or by constant criticism of table manners, or by bringing up touchy subjects likely to cause arguments at the table.

Diet Fads

There are many fads and fallacies about losing weight. Everyone wants an easy solution; cosmetic and food product manufacturers know this and develop products that play to this desire. Thus we have pills that are supposed to burn fat while we sleep; machines that are supposed to give us a "workout" while we're lying down by electrically stimulating our muscles; plastic suits that we wear while exercising that are supposed to produce dramatic weight loss; and special creams and body scrubbers that are supposed to take away unsightly cellulite.

The truth is that a pill will not burn calories for you, a machine will not do your exercise for you, a plastic suit will only make you lose water, not fat, and the idea that there is a special kind of fat called cellulite is a myth.

Cellulite, in fact, is fat, plain and simple; there are no special varieties. Much of the body's fat is stored directly beneath the skin where there is also a sheath of connective tissue, which tends to compartmentalize the fat cells. The more fat the more this

FOODS TO AVOID	FOODS TO EAT
High saturated fat percentages	Low or no saturated fat
Avocado 15-20%	Apples 0%
Biscuits 23%	Apricots 0%
Bread stuffing 25%	Cherries 0%
Sweet rolls 27 + %	Cranberry sauce 0%
Fried chicken 27%	Fruit 0%
Bran muffins 30%	Fruit juices 0%
Veal 30-50%	Herbs 0%
Chicken livers 33%	Peaches 0%
Ham 33%	Plums 0%
Lunch meats 35 + %	Rice, plain 0%
Duck 35%	Split peas 0%
Pancakes 35%	Vegetables, raw or steamed 0%
Pork 35%	Squid 1%
Beef brisket 40%	Cornmeal 10%
Ground beef 40%	Popcorn, plain 12%
Hotdogs 40%	Sweet and sour sauce 12%
Lamb 40-50%	Teriyaki sauce 14%
Rib roast 42%	Spaghetti, no egg 15%
Gravy 50 + %	Halibut 17%
Custard 50%	Chestnuts 19%
Cheese 50-80%	Salmon 19%
Cream 60%	Carp 20%
Ice cream 60 + %	Perch 20%
Beef heart 80%	Abalone 21%
Coconut 88%	Clams 21%
Cream substitute 90 + %	Trout 22%
Sour cream 91%	Octopus 27%

NOTE: The same percentage number may appear in both columns; the determining factor is then the grams of fat in each item. The left column has more grams of fat, even if the percentage is the same for an item in the right column.

tissue is stretched and the more the fat bulges around and through it, producing cellulite's characteristic dimpled effect. Women tend to have thinner skin and less flexible connective tissue, making them more "prone" to cellulite than men. There is no point in spending money on special creams or brushes; you cannot scrub away excess fat. You have to reduce your intake and burn it through exercise.

Similarly, most diet programs that consist of pills, powders, or foolish eating habits are ineffective and usually harmful. Many of them are addictive and those who benefit from the diet programs often gain back the weight lost once they return to their "normal" eating habits.

One controversial drug that appears frequently in pills is phenylpropanolamine hydrochloride (PPA). Producers of PPA claim that it acts as an appetite suppressant, though its effectiveness is questionable.

Taken in large doses, its effects resemble those of amphetamines. It can produce such side effects as anxiety, sleeplessness, headaches, irregular heart rhythm, and even lead to strokes or seizures.

Another diet drug, benzocaine, is present in chewing gum and candy. It deadens taste receptors, which supposedly suppresses one's appetite. It does not, however, stop the habit of munching, which is a great cause of weight gain.

Guar gum is another diet substance that gives the dieter a sense of fullness. It is a vegetable gum that swells when it absorbs moisture. When taken improperly, it can swell in the throat and cause an obstruction, resulting in suffocation. At least 1 death and 50 injuries have been reported as a result of ingesting guar gum diet products.

Anybody interested in losing a substantial amount of weight should consult with his or her physician. The physician will know of a nutritionist who can provide a healthy program for weight reduction. If a person chooses to try one of the over-the-counter diet programs, read the directions carefully.

Weight loss involves a complete change in one's lifestyle. The solution includes eating balanced meals, reducing the intake of fat, increasing proportionately the consumption of carbohydrates, and exercising three or four times a week. It is a slow process that does not offer the quick yet temporary loss offered by over-the-counter diet programs. Rather, it is a permanent commitment to a healthy way of life. Only then, can a person maintain an optimal weight.

28

Mental and Emotional Disorders

The ability to adapt is central to being emotionally fit, healthy, and mature. An emotionally fit person is one who can adapt to changing circumstances with constructive reactions and who can enjoy living, loving others, and working productively. In everyone's life there are bound to be experiences that are anxious or deeply disturbing, such as the sadness of losing a loved one or the disappointment of failure. The emotionally fit person is stable enough not to be overwhelmed by the anxiety, grief, or guilt that such experiences frequently produce. His sense of his own worth is not lost easily by a setback in life; rather, he can learn from his own mistakes.

Communication and Tolerance

Even the most unpleasant experiences can add to one's understanding of life. Emerging from a crisis with new wisdom can give a sense of pride and mastery. The emotionally fit person can listen attentively to the opinions of others, yet if his decision differs from that being urged by friends and relatives, he will abide by it and can stand alone if necessary, without guilt and anger at those who disagree.

Communicating well with others is an important part of emotional fitness. Sharing experiences, both good and bad, is one of the joys of living. Although the capacity to enjoy is often increased by such sharing, independence is also essential, for one person's pleasure may leave others indifferent. It is just as important to appreciate and respect the individuality of others as it is to value our own individual preferences, as long as these are reasonable and do not give pain to others.

Ways of Expressing Disagreement

Communication should be kept open at all times. Anger toward those who disagree may be an immediate response, but it should not lead to cutting off communication, as it so frequently does, particularly between husbands and wives, parents and children.

Emotional maturity enables us to disagree with what another says, feels, or does, yet make the distinction between that person and how we feel about his thoughts and actions. To tell someone, "I don't like what you are doing," is more likely to keep the lines of communication open than telling him "I don't like you." This is particularly important between parents and children.

It is unfortunately common for parents to launch personal attacks when children do something that displeases them. The child, or any person to whom this is done, then feels unworthy or rejected, which often makes him angry and defiant. Revenge becomes uppermost, and communication is lost; each party feels misunderstood and lonely, perhaps even wounded, and is not likely to want to reopen communication. The joy in a human relationship is gone, and one's pleasure in living is by that much diminished.

Function of Guilt

The same principles used in dealing with others can be applied to ourselves. Everyone makes mistakes, has angry or even murderous thoughts that can produce excessive guilt. Sometimes there is a realistic reason for feeling guilty, which should be a spur to take corrective action. Differentiate clearly between thoughts, feelings, and actions. Only actions need cause guilt. In the privacy of one's own mind, anything may be thought as long as it is not acted out; an emotionally fit person can accept this difference.

Role of the Subconscious

Emotional disorders are similar to other medical diseases and can be treated by physicians or other professionals just as any other disease can be treated. Fortunately, this truth is widely accepted today, but as recently as 200 years ago it was believed that the emotionally ill were evil, possessed by the devil. Their illness was punished rather than treated. The strange and sometimes bizarre actions of the mentally ill were feared and misunderstood.

Freud and Psychoanalysis

Although we have penetrated many of the mysteries of the mind, much remains to be discovered. Significant steps toward understanding mental functioning came about through the work of Sigmund Freud. Building upon the work of others before him and making his own detailed observations, Freud demonstrated that there is a subconscious part of the mind which functions without our awareness.

He taught that mental illness resulting from subconscious memories could be cured by *psychoanalysis,* which brings the memories out into consciousness. He believed that dreams are a major key to the subconscious mind and that thoughts, dreams, fantasies, and abnormal fears follow the rules of cause and effect and are not random. This is called *psychic determinism,* meaning that emotional disorders can be understood by exploring the subconscious. *Psychiatrists* help the patient understand how his mind works and why it

works that way—often the first step toward a cure.

Does psychic determinism rule out will power as a function of the mind? No, because the subconscious is only one part of the mind. Although it has an important influence, there are other forces influencing behavior and thought: the *id,* or instinctive force, the *superego,* or conscience, and the *ego,* or decision-maker. The more we know about how our minds work, what underlies our wishes and thoughts, the more control we can exercise in choosing how to behave in order to achieve our goals.

Role of Sexuality

Freud discovered that young children and even babies are aware of the sensations, pleasurable and painful, that can be experienced from all parts of the body. The sexual organs have a rich supply of nerves; the baby receives pleasure when these organs are touched, for example, during a bath or a diaper change. The child learns that when he touches these organs he obtains a pleasant feeling; therefore he repeatedly touches and rubs them (*infantile masturbation*).

This concept, that the child derives pleasure from his body and sex organs, is called *infantile sexuality.* It does not mean that the baby has adult sexual ideas or wishes. These do not develop until puberty. It does mean that parents have the responsibility to see to it that children learn early that sex is associated with tenderness and love between man and woman. Even young children are aware of what their parents do and how they treat each other.

Types of Mental Illness

Although there is considerable disagreement about the classification of mental disorders, a convenient sys-

tem used by many doctors divides mental illnesses into two general categories, organic and functional.

Some types of mental illness show little or no evidence of changes in brain tissue: these are called *functional* disorders. Another group of mental illnesses does involve some definable impairment of brain tissue resulting from disease, injury, the introduction of poisonous substances, malfunction of the body's metabolic processes, nutritional problems, or inherited defects. These are *organic* disorders. Organic brain damage may be *congenital*—that is, existing at or prior to birth—or *acquired.* Examples of congenital defects are *hydrocephalus,* an accumulation of fluid within the skull of a newborn infant that destroys brain tissue; *phenylketonuria* (PKU), a type of mental retardation associated with an inability of the child's body to metabolize a protein substance; and *Down's syndrome* (also called *Mongolism*), a form of retardation that occurs more frequently in children of older mothers and which is marked by certain physical features such as eyes that resemble those of Oriental people. Some examples of acquired defects are cerebrovascular accidents such as stroke; injuries to the brain, as from a fall or from the introduction of poisonous substances such as lead, arsenic, or mercury; and arteriosclerosis, resulting in senile psychosis in aged people.

This chapter will deal only with functional illness. Organic disorders are treated in the chapters on diseases of particular systems of the body and often in other sections as well. If you are in doubt about where to find information about a particular disorder, consult the index.

Who Is Mentally Ill?

Most people occasionally experience spells of anxiety, blue moods, or temper tantrums, but unless the psychological suffering they endure or inflict upon others begins to interfere with their job or marriage, they seldom seek professional guidance. There is no exacting scientific standard for determining when an eccentric pattern of behavior becomes a mental illness. Norms vary from culture to culture and within each culture, and, as every student of history and every parent know, norms also change from generation to generation.

Just how can a determination be made as to who is mentally ill? No temperature reading, no acute pain, no abnormal growth can be looked for as evidence of a serious problem. Yet there are warning signs, and among the common ones are these:

- Anxiety that is severe, prolonged, and unrelated to any identifiable reason or cause

- Depression, especially when it is followed by withdrawal from loved ones, from friends, or from the usual occupations or hobbies that ordinarily afford one pleasure

- Loss of confidence in oneself

- Undue pessimism

- A feeling of constant helplessness

- Uncalled for or unexplainable mood changes—for example, an abrupt switch from happiness to unhappiness when nothing has happened to warrant it

- Rudeness or aggression that is without apparent cause or which is occasioned by some trivial incident

- An unreasonable demand for perfectionism, not only in oneself but in one's loved ones, friends, business associates, and even from things or situations

- Habitual underachievement, especially if one is adequately equipped to do the work one is called upon to perform

- The inability to accept responsibility, often manifested by a recurrent loss of employment

- Phobias

- Unreasonable feelings of persecution

- Self-destructive acts

- Sexual deviation

- A sudden and dramatic change in sleeping habits

- Physical ailments and complaints for which there are no organic causes

If one or more of these warning signs occur frequently or in severe form, a mental illness may be present, and professional help should be sought to evaluate the underlying problem.

Types of Functional Mental Illness

Functional mental disorders may be broken down into four general categories: neuroses; psychophysiological (or psychosomatic) disorders; personality or character disorders; and psychoses.

Neurosis

A *neurosis* (or *psychoneurosis*) is characterized primarily by emotional rather than physical symptoms—although physical symptoms may be present. The neuroses are usually categorized according to the type of reaction that the patient exhibits in his attempt to resolve the underlying emotional conflict. All of them involve anxiety as a prominent symptom.

Anxiety Reaction

The *anxiety reaction* is probably the most widespread of all the neurotic response patterns. Although, as noted above, all the neuroses share anxiety as a symptom, the most common and outstanding characteristic of the anxiety reaction is a feeling of dread or apprehension that is not related to any apparent cause. The anxiety is caused by conflicts of which the patient himself is unaware but which may be stimulated by thoughts or events in his present life. For example, the junior executive who is constantly apprehensive that his employer will ridicule his work and dismiss his ideas may be expressing an anxiety reaction to a childhood fear that equated ridicule with abandonment or mutilation.

While anxiety reaction symptoms are primarily mental or emotional— the patient feels inadequate or ineffectual, or behaves irrationally—anxiety is always accompanied by physiological changes such as sweating and heart palpitations. Fatigue and feelings of panic are also common symptoms.

Conversion Reaction

The *conversion reaction* (or *conversion hysteria*) describes a type of neurotic behavior in which the patient, instead of coming to grips with his underlying psychic conflict, manages to convert it into physical symptoms involving functions over which he ordinarily exerts complete control. Sometimes the physical symptoms are unimportant, but often they are markedly dramatic. For example, the soldier who becomes deaf to the sound of explosions even though there is no organic defect that would account for a loss of hearing has effectively obliterated a sensation that evokes associations too painful to acknowledge.

Obsessive-Compulsive Reaction

A person beset by persistent, unwanted ideas or feelings (*obsessions*), who is impelled to carry out certain acts (*compulsions*) ritualistically, no matter how irrational they are, is reacting to a psychic conflict in an *obsessive-compulsive* manner. The obsession may involve a feeling of violence or sexuality directed toward a member of his own family. Usually the feeling will never lead to any overt action of the type imagined, but the idea is nevertheless persistent and painful.

Obsessive-compulsive patients are typically exceptionally meticulous and conscientious, often intelligent and gifted in their work. But they expend an enormous amount of energy and time in observing compulsive acts. For example, they may take a dozen or more showers every day because they are obsessed with the idea that they are dirty or carrying a contagious disease. By performing an apparently harmless compulsive act, the patient is temporarily relieved of the obsession.

Depressive Reaction

Most people have blue moods from time to time in their lives. Indeed, when faced with a personal tragedy like the death of a loved one, a normal healthy individual may well undergo a period of depression. A person suffering from the *depressive reaction*, however, has persistent feelings of worthlessness and pessimism unrelated to events that might depress a normal person. An inability to cope with problem situations is gradually magnified into an inability to cope with anything at all. Attempts to mask the crisis by putting on a "front"—feigning cheerfulness and optimism—give way to episodes of total hopelessness. Suicide is often considered and sometimes attempted. Threats of suicide

from a depressed person should always be regarded seriously.

Common physical symptoms accompanying depression are fatigue, loss of appetite, and insomnia.

Phobic Reaction

A *phobic reaction* is the result of an individual's attempt to deal with an anxiety-producing conflict, not by facing up to the actual source of that conflict but by avoiding something else. The substitute—whether it be an animal, closed places, or whatever—is responded to with the intense anxiety that is really felt for the true source of anxiety. This process is known as *displacement,* and the irrational fears or dreads are known as *phobias.*

Thus, a person who had been regularly punished as a child by having been forcibly confined in a closet might be unable to deal with the anxiety of the experience consciously. The anxiety might be displaced and emerge later in life in the form of terror of crowded or confined places—*claustrophobia.*

Phobias can involve almost anything one encounters in life—including things that go on in one's body and one's mind. Some of the most common phobias have to do with disease—*bacteriophobia,* for example, the fear of germs.

Scores of phobias exist, ranging alphabetically from *acrophobia,* the fear of heights, to *xenophobia,* the fear of strangers. Other well-known examples are *ailurophobia,* the fear of cats; *cynophobia,* the fear of dogs; *algophobia,* the fear of pain; *agoraphobia,* the fear of open spaces; *erythrophobia,* the fear of blushing; *mysophobia,* the fear of dirt and contamination; *nyctophobia,* the fear of the dark; and *lyssophobia,* the fear of rabies.

Dissociative Reaction

The *dissociative reaction* involves a

basic disruption of the patient's personality. The dissociative reaction permits a person to escape from a part of his personality associated with intolerable anxiety. The escape is made in various ways: by forgetfulness or absent-mindedness, dream states (including sleepwalking), amnesia, and—most seriously—the adoption of multiple personalities, in which the patient behaves like one person at certain times and like an altogether different person at other times.

Psychophysiological Disorders

It has been estimated that one-half or more of the patients of a general practitioner either do not have any organic illness or do not have any organic disease that could account for the severity or extent of the symptoms described. These patients are obviously not inventing their symptoms. The symptoms—whether they be itching, constipation, asthma, or heart palpitations—are real enough. But in many cases they are either wholly or partly of psychological origin—*psychogenic* is the medical term.

The psychological and physiological aspects of humans are so closely interwoven that the problem of *psychophysiological* (or *psychosomatic*) disorders must be considered with attention to both aspects. Consider how many physiological changes in normal people can be induced by psychological states: sweating, blushing, gooseflesh, sexual arousal, weeping, the feeling of "a lump in the throat," etc. It should hardly be surprising, then, that when someone has a physical illness there are profound concomitant psychological factors that can materially affect the physiological disease.

In many cases, however, as noted above, there is no detectable organic disease. Anxiety and other disturbing emotions such as rage are sometimes dealt with by the individual by constructing a pattern of defense that involves physiological reactions. Confronted with an emotional conflict that cannot be handled consciously, the individual may channel his feelings inward and deal with it by the formation of troublesome physical symptoms. It must be stressed that this strategy is not consciously engineered by the patient and that the symptoms are genuinely experienced.

Psychophysiological disorders affect many parts of the body, but certain organs and tissues seem more vulnerable than others. The digestive tract, for example, is frequently beset by disorders that are psychophysiological, including diarrhea, constipation, regional enteritis (inflammation of the intestine), ulcerative colitis (ulcers and inflammation of the colon), and peptic ulcers. Hypertension is frequently associated with psychogenic causes. Muscle cramps, recurrent stiff necks, arthritis, backaches, and tension headaches are other common complaints. Many skin conditions such as hives and eczema can be triggered by or are aggravated by psychological factors.

The symptoms of a psychophysiological illness appear to have no logical relation to the conflict that is responsible for them, nor do they relieve the underlying anxiety.

Personality or Character Disorders

Another group of mental illnesses is the *personality* or *character disorders,* so called because they appear to stem from a kind of defect in or arrested development of the personality. Unlike neurotic patients, individuals with personality disorders do not especially suffer from anxiety, nor is their behavior markedly eccentric. But when observed over a period of time,

the personality problem becomes evident.

Personality disorders fall into various categories including:

- The *passive-dependent* individual, needs excessive emotional support and reassurance from an authority figure.

- The *schizoid* individual is withdrawn from and indifferent to other people.

- The *paranoid* individual is exquisitely sensitive to praise or criticism and often suspicious of expressed or implied attitudes toward him, and who often is subject to feelings of persecution.

- The *cyclothymic* (or *cycloid*) individual is subject to sharply defined moods of elation or depression, seemingly without relation to external circumstances.

- The *sociopathic* individual is characteristically lacking in a sense of personal responsibility or of morality. Formerly called the *psychopathic* personality, the sociopath may be disposed to aggressive, hostile, sometimes violent behavior and frequently engages in self-destructive behavior such as alcoholism or addiction to drugs. Sociopathic behavior also includes sexual deviation.

Psychosis

The chief distinction between *psychosis* and neurosis is that a psychosis represents a more complete disintegration of personality and a loss of contact with the outside world. The psychotic is therefore unable to form relationships with people. Most people who suffer from nonpsychotic mental disorders are seldom, if ever, hospitalized, and then usually for very

brief periods. But many psychotics are so crippled by their illness that they are hospitalized repeatedly or for protracted periods of time.

Schizophrenic Reaction

Schizophrenia, the most common and destructive of the psychotic reactions, is characterized by withdrawal from external reality, inability to think clearly, disturbances in affective reaction (capacity to feel and express emotion), and a retreat into a fantasy life—all of these resulting in a progressive deterioration of the patient's ordinary behavioral patterns.

Simple Schizophrenia

The patient with *simple schizophrenia* experiences a gradual loss of concern and contact with other people, and a lessening of the motivation needed to perform the routine activities of everyday life. There may be some personality deterioration, but the presence of hallucinations and delusions is rare.

Hebephrenic Schizophrenia

This form of schizophrenia is marked by delusions, hallucinations, and regressed behavior. Hebephrenics babble and giggle, and often react in inappropriately childish ways. Their silly manner can make them seem happier than other schizophrenics, but this disorder often results in severe personality disintegration—more severe, in fact, than in other types of schizophrenia.

Catatonic Schizophrenia

In *catatonic schizophrenia* there are dramatic disturbances of the motor functions. Patients may remain in a fixed position for hours, days, or even weeks. During this time their muscles may be rigid, their limbs held in awkward positions. They may have to be fed, and their urinary and bowel functions may be abnormal. This stuporous state may be varied by an occasional period of frenzied but purposeless excitement.

Paranoid Schizophrenia

The *paranoid schizophrenic* is preoccupied with variable delusions of persecution or grandeur. Men working with pneumatic drills on the street, for example, are really sending out supersonic beams designed to destroy his brain cells; the water supply is being poisoned by visitors from other planets; any mechanical malfunction, as of a telephone or an elevator, is part of a deliberate plot of harassment or intimidation.

Paranoid schizophrenia is often marked by the presence of hallucinations, by disturbances in mental processes, and by behavioral deterioration. The disorder is regarded as particularly serious—hard to deal with and likely to become permanent.

Paranoid Reaction

The patient with this disorder suffers from delusions, usually of persecution, sometimes of grandeur. In this respect, *paranoia* is very similar to paranoid schizophrenia. However, in paranoid schizophrenia the delusions are often variable, and usually there is a breakdown of the patient's behavioral patterns.

A case of true paranoia, by contrast, is characterized by an invariable delusion around which the patient constructs and adheres to a highly systematized pattern of behavior. When the delusion is of such a nature that its persistence does not engender a conflict between the patient and

his surrounding social structure, the patient may never be suspected of mental illness, perhaps merely of eccentricity. If, however, the delusion does provoke conflict, the patient may react with destructive hostility, and hospitalization or some other kind of professional treatment will be necessary.

Manic-Depressive Reaction

This disorder, also called an *affective reaction,* is characterized by two phases—*mania* and *depression.* Patients are governed by one phase or another or by the alternation of both.

The manic phase may be mild and bring elation and a general stepping up of all kinds of activity. The patient tends to talk endlessly and in an associative rather than a logical way. If the disorder is more severe, he may act or dress bizarrely; he may be a whirlwind of activity and become so excited and agitated that he foregoes food and sleep and ends in a state of total collapse.

In a mild depressive phase, the individual feels dull and melancholy, his confidence begins to drain away, and he becomes easily fatigued by daily routines. When the depressive phase is more severe, the patient starts to retreat from reality, gradually entering into a state of withdrawal that is very much like a stupor. At this point he hardly moves or speaks. He may be unable to sleep. Eventually he begins to question his value as a human being and is crushed by feelings of guilt. He may refuse to eat. Symptoms may progress to the point where an attempt at suicide is a real possibility.

Although the manic-depressive psychosis may alternate from one of its phases to the other, one or the other phase is usually dominant for a prolonged period of time. Depression is more often dominant than mania.

Manic-depressive patients often recover spontaneously for periods of time, but relapses are fairly common.

Depressive Reaction

The *depressive reaction* is a disorder connected with aging and its attendant changes in sexual functioning; it usually occurs at the time of the menopause in women, in the middle or late 40s, and somewhat later in men. Formerly called *involutional melancholia,* it is characterized, as that name suggests, by a sense of hopeless melancholy and despair.

Patients begin to feel that life has passed them by. They experience real physical symptoms such as loss of vigor, and develop various hypochondriacal complaints. Their interests become narrower, and they begin to retreat from the world.

As the melancholy deepens, there are periods of senseless weeping, bouts of intense anxiety, feelings of worthlessness, and growing concern—coupled with delusions—about dying and death. The depth of the depression is overwhelming, and the danger of suicide greater than in any other psychosis.

Treatment of Emotional Problems and Mental Disorders

When should help be sought for an emotional problem? Sometimes individuals themselves realize that they need help and seek it without urging. They may have symptoms such as anxiety, depression, or troublesome thoughts that they cannot put out of their mind. But many others who need help do not know it or do not want to know that they need it. They usually have symptoms that disturb others rather than themselves, such as irritability, impulsive behavior, or excessive use of drugs or alcohol that interferes with their family relationships and work responsibilities.

Other people in need of psychological guidance are those who have a physical disease that is based on psychological factors. They react to stress internally rather than externally. Instead of displaying anger, they feel it inside. We are all familiar with headaches or heartburn caused by tension; more serious diseases clearly associated with emotional factors are asthma, certain skin disorders, ulcerative colitis, essential hypertension, hyperthyroidism, and peptic ulcer. Other physical symptoms that may be related to psychological factors are some types of paralysis, blindness, and loss of memory.

In all these situations the patient's enjoyment of life is curtailed. He has no feeling of control over what he does and little or no tolerance for himself and others. Such an existence is completely unnecessary today, with the many agencies and specialists, capable of effectively treating these problems.

Mental Health Professionals

Who can help those with emotional problems? Confusion about the different professions in the mental health field is understandable. To add to the muddle, self-appointed counselors without professional training and experience have set themselves up in this field, so it is necessary to know whom to consult to obtain the best help possible.

Psychiatrists

Psychiatrists are medical doctors; that is, they have graduated from a medical school, served internships and afterwards residencies specializing in emotional disorders. They are specialists in the same way that a surgeon or an eye doctor is a specialist. Most are members of the American Psychiatric Association. They are experienced in treating medical illnesses, having done so for many years before being certified as specialists in emotional disorders. Generally they can be relied upon to adhere to the ethical and professional standards of the medical field.

The American Psychiatric Association, 1400 K St., N.W., Washington, D.C. 20005, can supply the names of members. The American Board of Psychiatry and Neurology, One American Plaza, Suite 800, Evanston, Illinois 60201, examines and certifies psychiatrists who pass its tests, so that the term "board certified" means that the psychiatrist has passed its tests. If a family physician is consulted about an emotional problem, he will often refer the patient to a psychiatrist, just as he would to any other specialist.

Psychologists

Psychologists have gone to college, majored in psychology, and most often have advanced degrees, for example, a doctorate in psychology. They are not medical doctors and may get a degree in psychology without ever working with a human being, e.g., by working in animal behavior, experimental psychology, or other fields. They may or may not have clinical training, but many acquire this training and experience with human beings. There is no guarantee that a psychologist has this background, however, without looking into the qualifications of each individual.

Psychotherapists

Psychotherapy is the general term for any treatment that tries to effect a cure by psychological rather than physical means. A psychotherapist may be a psychiatrist, or he may be a psychologist, or may have no training at all. Anyone can set up an office and call himself a psychotherapist, psychoanalyst, marriage counselor, family therapist, or anything else he desires. It is up to the patient to check on the training and background of a therapist. Any reputable therapist should be pleased to tell patients his credentials and qualifications for helping them. A psychoanalyst, for example, may be a psychiatrist with several years of additional training in psychoanalysis, or may be someone whose qualifications consist of a college psychology courses.

Social Workers

Social workers are another group of trained persons who may also counsel those with emotional problems. They may work either with individuals, families, or groups after meeting the educational requirements for the profession, which include a bachelor's degree and two years of professional training leading to a master's degree in social work.

Professionals should be associated with recognized groups of their peers, or perhaps with a medical center or hospital. Generally a person with emotional problems should consult a psychiatrist first, who will then either treat the problem or be in a good position to advise what is necessary and who can best be available for treatment.

Types of Therapy

Functional mental illnesses are treated by a variety of tools, among them psychotherapy and chemotherapy (treatment with drugs).

Psychotherapy

As noted above, psychotherapy applies to various forms of treatment that employ psychological methods designed to help patients understand themselves. With this knowledge, or insight, the patient learns how to handle his life—with all its relationships and conflicts—in a happier and more socially responsible manner.

The best known form of psychotherapy is psychoanalysis, developed by Freud but modified by many others, which seeks to lift to the level of awareness the patient's repressed subconscious feelings. The information about subconscious conflicts is explored and interpreted to explain the causes of the patient's emotional upsets.

The technique employs a series of steps beginning with *free association,* in which the patient is encouraged to discuss anything that comes to mind, including things that the patient might be reluctant to discuss with anyone else but the analyst. Other steps include dream analysis and *transference,* which is the redirection to the analyst of repressed childhood emotions.

Group therapy is a form of therapeutic treatment in which a group of approximately six to ten patients, usually under the guidance of a therapist, participate in discussions of their mental and emotional problems. The therapist may establish the direction of the discussion or may remain mostly silent, allowing the patients' interaction to bring about the special cathartic benefits of this technique.

Family therapy is much like group therapy, with an individual family functioning as a group. It is felt that the family members may be better able to discuss the problems of relating to each other within the context of a group than they would be on an individual basis with a therapist.

Psychodrama is a therapeutic technique in which a patient or a group of patients act out situations centered about their personal conflicts. The psychodrama is "performed" in the presence of a therapist and, sometimes, other people.

Children are sometimes enrolled in programs of *play therapy* in which dolls, doll houses, and other appropriate toys are made available so that they can express their frustrations, hostilities, and other feelings through play. This activity, carried on under the observation of a therapist, is considered a form of catharsis in that it often prevents the repression of hostile emotions. In the case of a maladjusted child, it can also act as a helpful diagnostic tool—revealing the source of the child's emotional problem.

Chemotherapy

The relationship between body chemistry and mental illness has been studied for over half a century. The result of this study is the therapeutic technique known as *chemotherapy,* the treatment of disease with drugs or chemicals.

Early Uses of Chemical Agents

Sedatives to provide treatment of mental diseases were used during World War I for soldiers suffering from shell shock. *Sodium amytal,* one of the early chemicals used, offered a prolonged restful sleep, after which the army patients could tolerate some form of psychotherapeutic treatment.

In the 1930s, physicians introduced *insulin shock therapy* as a method for treating psychotic patients. The patients received injections of insulin in doses large enough to produce a deep coma, after which they were revived by doses of sugar. As with the use of sodium amytal, the insulin treatment was accompanied by psychotherapy for most effective results.

Present-Day Uses of Chemical Agents

More recently, the control of mental illness has taken a giant step forward with the development of *tranquilizers* and *antidepressants.* Tranquilizers counteract anxiety, tension, and overexcitement; they are used to calm patients whose behavior is dangerously confused or disturbed. Antidepressants help to stimulate the physiological activity of depressed patients, thereby tending to relieve the sluggishness that attends depression.

The treatment of the manic-depressive psychosis has been facilitated with the use of salts derived from lithium, a metal. Lithium salts seem to control the disease without producing the undesirable emotional and intellectual effects that resulted from the previous treatment with tranquilizers and antidepressants. The medication has been found to be particularly effective in treating patients with frequent manic episodes; it is also said to be effective as a preventive measure against future manifestations of mania or depression. Lithium may have adverse side effects and must be administered carefully.

Chemotherapy does not usually cure mental illness. It does, however, improve the patient's mental state, thereby enabling him to cope more effectively with the problems of everyday life.

Electroshock Treatment

Electroshock is a form of therapy in which a carefully regulated electric current is passed through a patient's head, thereby producing convulsions and unconsciousness.

Electroshock is primarily a treatment for the manic-depressive psychosis; to a lesser extent the therapy is used on schizophrenic patients. It often shortens depressed periods, and sometimes the patient seems totally free of the symptoms of his disorder. Unfortunately, the remission may be temporary; electroshock does not prevent further attacks. Also, transitory memory impairment often occurs.

Because of the recent advances in the techniques of chemotherapy, electroshock is used much less frequently than it was in the past.

Facilities Available for the Mentally Ill

The last decade has seen a number of hopeful changes in the facilities for treatment of mental disorders in the United States. The great majority of severely ill mental patients used to be cared for in county or state mental hospitals, many of which were crowded and able to offer custodial care but very little in the way of therapeutic programs. The picture has changed, however, and the extent and quality of care in these hospitals is expanding and improving.

Patients with mental illnesses are also being treated in greater numbers at general hospitals. As a matter of fact, more patients who need hospitalization for such illnesses are being admitted to general hospitals than to public mental hospitals.

Treatment for the mentally or emotionally disturbed is also provided in other facilities, including private mental hospitals, mental health clinics, and various social agencies.

Among the new facilities for treating mental illness is one which permits many patients who would formerly have been hospitalized, perhaps for the rest of their lives, to be served by community mental health centers. These centers offer both inpatient and outpatient care. The services they provide go beyond diagnosis and treatment to include rehabilitation, thus making it possible for more and more of today's mental patients to live at home, function in a job situation, and be a part of their own community.

Results of Treatment

What can be expected from treatment? Does a person who has been through treatment emerge bland, uncaring about others, with absolutely no problems, and without guilt for his misdeeds? Absolutely not. What treatment can do, said Freud, is to change neurotic misery into common unhappiness. There will always be things in life that are disappointing or otherwise upsetting. No treatment can eliminate such problems. After successful treatment, however, one should be better able to handle these stresses with flexible and constructive responses and to see his own difficulties in relation to the problems of others.

To feel emotionally fit is to have a capacity for enjoying life, working well, and loving others. Fear, shame, and guilt about undergoing needed treatment should not prevent anyone from reaching that potential.

29

Substance Abuse

"Drug-Related Deaths up 59%." "Driving-and-Drinking Accident Claims 5 Lives." "Teen Drug Abuse—The News Is Bad."

The headlines tell a story with a moral, or lesson. The lesson is that the United States has a major health and social problem. Once called by a number of names, including *alcoholism, drug addiction,* and *drug abuse,* the problem today goes by the designation *substance abuse.* In this usage, the phrase applies to all forms of addiction or abuse, whether the substance is alcohol or such vegetation-derived drugs as marijuana, cocaine, and heroin.

In a broad sense, substances include any material aside from food that can be imbibed, injected, or taken into the body in any way and that changes or affects the body or mind. This definition covers aspirin, many medications, tobacco, and a broad range of other substances. But *substance abuse* refers to unhealthy or excessive use of any material, alcohol, or addictive drugs at an individual's discretion and not according to a physician's prescription.

The dimensions of the substance-abuse problem are almost incalculable. Americans in 1986 spent an estimated $110 billion on addictive drugs alone. At least 40 percent of all Americans between the ages of 18 and 25 had experimented with one or more illegal substances. As one authority wrote,

Not only the poor, the uneducated, the deprived, or the shadow types are being destroyed. We're dealing with the privileged, the successful, the professional.

Alcohol Abuse

Alcohol abuse is not unique to the United States or to the twentieth century. Alcoholic beverages, and their use or abuse, have an ancient history. Long before humans began to keep records of any kind, these beverages were valued as food, medicine, and ceremonial drinks. When people today have a beer with dinner, or toast newlyweds with champagne, or share wine at a religious ritual or festival, they are continuing traditions that have deep roots in the past.

The consumption of alcoholic beverages has always been a fact of life.

So has, in a sense, alcohol abuse. The immigrants who came to the United States brought their ethnic ceremonies and drinking habits with them. The frontiersmen who moved continually west found liquor to be a source of release and comfort. Inevitably, alcohol use and abuse occurred.

Most drinkers have been, and are, able to control what they are doing and are none the worse for the habit. However, of the estimated 100 million drinkers in the United States, about 10 million have some kind of problem with alcohol: they are *alcohol abusers.* The 10 million alcoholics cost the economy some $60 billion annually. Drunken drivers are implicated in about half of the nearly 50,000 traffic deaths occurring yearly.

Scientists have come to believe that habitual alcohol abuse is a disease and should be treated as such. In 1956, the American Medical Association officially termed alcoholism an illness and a medical responsibility.

Kinds of Alcohol

The alcohol in beverages is chemically known as *ethyl alcohol.* It is often called *grain alcohol.* It is produced by the natural process of *fermentation:* When certain foods such as honey, fruits, grains, or their juices remain in a warm place, airborne yeast organisms begin to change the sugars and starches in these foods into alcohol. Ethyl alcohol is in itself a food in the sense that its caloric content produces energy in the body, but it contains practically no essential nutriments.

Methyl alcohol, also called *wood alcohol,* because it is obtained by the dry distillation of maple, birch, and beech, is useful as a fuel and solvent. It is poisonous if taken internally and can cause blindness and death. Other members of the same family of chemicals, such as *isopropyl alcohol,* are also used as rubbing alcohols—as cooling agents and skin disinfectants—and are also poisonous if taken internally.

Present-Day Drinking Trends

On a per capita basis, Americans drink twice as much wine and beer as they did a century ago, and half as much distilled spirits. Where the drinking takes place has also changed. There is less hard drinking in saloons and more social drinking at home and in clubs. The acceptance of drinking in mixed company has made it more a part of social situations than it used to be.

Here are some facts about the current consumption of alcoholic beverages in the United States:

- Drinking is more common among men than among women, but the gap is closing.

- It is more common among people who are under 40.

- It is more common among the well-to-do than among the poor.

- Beyond the age of 45, the number of drinkers steadily declines.

Teenagers and Alcohol

One fact emerges clearly and consistently from all the surveys of teenage drinking in all parts of the country: the drinking behavior of parents is more related to what children do about drinking than any other factor. It is more influential than children's friends, their neighborhoods, their religion, their social or economic status, or their local laws.

Statistics on teenage (and adult) drinking vary from one ethnic group or one part of the country to another. But overall, the statistics show that about two-thirds of all Americans 18 and older consume alcoholic beverages. Some three-quarters of all students in the tenth to twelfth grade range also drink.

In general, drinking is an activity that is associated with growing up. For boys, it represents manhood; for girls, sophistication.

Kinds of Alcoholic Beverages

The way any alcoholic drink affects the body depends chiefly on how much alcohol it contains. The portion of alcohol can range from less than 1/20th of the total volume, in the case of beer, to more than one-half in the case of rum. As a general rule, distilled drinks have a higher alcohol content than fermented ones.

The five basic types of beverages are beers, table wines, dessert or cocktail wines, cordials and liqueurs, and distilled spirits such as brandy and whisky. The labels of beers and wines usually indicate the percentage of alcohol by volume. The labels of distilled spirits indicate *proof.*

Proof

The proof number is twice the percentage of alcohol by volume. Thus a rye whisky that is 90-proof contains 45 percent alcohol, 80-proof bourbon is 40 percent alcohol, and so on. The word *proof* used in this way comes from an old English test to determine the strength of distilled spirits. If gunpowder soaked with whisky would still ignite when lighted, that fact was "proof" that the whisky contained the right amount of alcohol. The amount, approximately 57 percent, is still the standard in Canada and Great Britain.

How Alcohol Affects the Body

The overall effects of alcohol on the body and on behavior vary a great deal depending on many factors. One factor should be noted at once: if the blood reaching the brain contains a certain percentage of alcohol, there are marked changes in reaction. As the percentage increases, the functioning of the brain and central nervous system is increasingly affected. As the alcohol is gradually metabolized and eliminated, the process reverses itself.

If at any given time the blood contains a concentration of about 3/100 of one percent (0.03 percent), no effects are observable. This amount will make its way into the bloodstream after you have had a highball or cocktail made with one and one-half ounces of whisky, or two small glasses of table wine, or two bottles of beer. It takes about two hours for this amount of alcohol to leave the body completely.

Twice that number of drinks produces twice the concentration of alcohol in the bloodstream (0.06 percent) with an accompanying feeling of warmth and relaxation.

If the concentration of alcohol in the bloodstream reaches 0.1 percent—when one part of every thousand parts of blood is pure alcohol—the person is legally drunk in most states.

The motor areas of the brain are affected; there is a noticeable lack of coordination in standing or walking. If the percentage goes up to 0.15 percent, the physical signs of intoxication are obvious, and they are accompanied by an impairment of mental faculties as well.

A concentration of as much as 0.4 percent can cause a coma. At the level of 0.5 to 0.7 percent there may be paralysis of the brain centers that control the activities of the lungs and heart, a condition that can be fatal.

Alcohol affects the brain and nervous system in this way because it is a depressant and an anesthetic.

How Alcohol Moves through the Body

Although it is negligible as nourishment, alcohol is an energy-producing food like sugar. Unlike most foods, however, it is quickly absorbed into the bloodstream through the stomach and small intestine without first having to undergo complicated digestive processes. It is then carried to the liver, where most of it is converted into heat and energy. From the liver, the remainder is carried by the bloodstream to the heart and pumped to the lungs. Some is expelled in the breath and some is eventually eliminated in sweat and urine. From the lungs, the alcohol is circulated to the brain.

People who use good judgment when drinking rarely, if ever, get drunk. The safe and pleasurable use of alcoholic beverages depends on the drinker's weight and his or her physical condition and emotional state. Other factors include the following:

1. *The Concentration of Alcohol in the Beverage* The higher the alcohol content in terms of total volume, the faster it is absorbed. Three ounces of straight whisky—two shot glasses— contain the same amount of alcohol as 48 ounces (or four cans) of beer.

2. *Sipping or Gulping* Two shots of straight whisky can be downed in seconds or, more normally, in a few minutes. The same amount diluted in two highballs can be sipped through an entire evening. In the latter case, the body has a chance to get rid of much of the alcohol.

3. *Additional Components of the Drink* The carbohydrates in beer and wine slow down the absorption of alcohol in the blood. Vodka mixed with orange juice travels much more slowly than a vodka martini.

4. *Food in the Stomach* The alcohol concentration in two cocktails consumed at the peak of the hunger before dinner can have a nasty effect. Several glasses of wine with a meal or a brandy sipped after dinner get to the bloodstream much more slowly and at a lower concentration. The sensible drinker doesn't drink on an empty stomach.

The Hangover

The feeling of discomfort that sometimes sets in the morning after excessive drinking is known as a hangover. It is caused by the disruptive effect of too much alcohol on the central nervous system. The symptoms of nausea, headache, dry mouth, diarrhea, fatigue, dizziness, heartburn, and a feeling of apprehension are usually most acute several hours after drinking and not while there is still any appreciable amount of alcohol in the system.

Although many people believe that "mixing" drinks, such as switching from whisky drinks to wine, is the main cause of hangovers, a hangover can just as easily be induced by too much of one type of drink or by pure alcohol. Nor is it always the result of drinking too much because emotional stress or allergy may well be contributing factors.

Some aspects of a hangover may be caused by substances called *congeners*. These are the natural products of fermentation found in small amounts in all alcoholic beverages, among them tannic acid and fusel oil. Some congeners have toxic properties that produce nausea by irritating certain nerve centers.

In spite of accumulated lore about hangover remedies, there is no certain cure for the symptoms. Neither raw eggs, oysters, alkalizers, sugar, black coffee, nor another drink has any therapeutic value. A throbbing head and aching joints can sometimes be relieved by aspirin and bed rest. Stomach irritation can be eased by bland foods such as skim milk, cooked cereal, or a poached egg. Persons seeking relief may also try analgesics such as aspirin or acetaminophen for the headache, antacids if the problem is upset stomach, or over-the-counter medications for the diarrhea.

Alcohol and General Health

As a result of new studies of the effect of alcohol on the body, many myths have been laid to rest. In general, it is known that in moderate quantities, alcohol causes the following reactions: the heartbeat quickens slightly, appetite increases, and gastric juices are stimulated. In other words, a drink makes people "feel good." But drinking does have harmful effects when consumed in large quantities.

Tissue Impairment

Habitual drinking of straight whisky can irritate the membranes that line the mouth and throat. The hoarse voice of some heavy drinkers is the result of a thickening of vocal cord tissue. As for the effect on the stomach, alcohol doesn't cause ulcers, but it does aggravate them.

There is no evidence to support the belief that port wine or any other alcoholic beverage taken in moderation will cause gout. Studies have shown that as many as 60 percent of all patients with this disease had never drunk any wine at all.

Brain Damage

Alcohol abuse continued over many years has been found to contribute to cognitive defects. These may, in turn, indicate brain impairment. Researchers do not know what the defects represent—whether greater susceptibility to the problems of aging or an actual, alcohol-caused "premature aging" effect. Whatever the case, long-term chronic alcohol abuse leads to more rapid aging of the brain. Neuropsychologically, the alcoholic's brain resembles that of an older nonalcoholic.

Long-term abuse can have many other effects. These include withdrawal symptoms beginning 12 to 48 hours after a person stops drinking, sometimes followed by *delirium tremens* (DTs), which brings hallucinations and can be fatal; the Werner-Korsakoff syndrome, a type of beriberi characterized by a lack of the B vitamins; alcoholic peripheral neuropathy, involving damage to the nerve tissue outside the brain and spinal cord; and liver damage, including alcoholic hepatitis and cirrhosis. In the latter the liver becomes hard and yellowed.

Alcohol and Immunity to Infection

Moderate drinkers who maintain proper health habits are no more likely to catch viral or bacterial diseases than nondrinkers. But heavy drinkers, who often suffer from malnutrition, have conspicuously lower resistance to infection. Even well-nourished heavy drinkers have a generally lower immunity to infection than normal. When the blood-alcohol level is 0.15 percent or higher, the alcohol appears to weaken the disease-fighting white blood cells.

Alcohol and Stroke

Studies have shown that heavy drinkers face nearly three times the teetotaler's risk of hemorrhagic stroke. Light drinkers face twice the risk. About one stroke in four occurring in the United States is hemorrhagic, but these strokes are more likely to be fatal than those caused by blood clots.

Alcohol and Life Expectancy

It is difficult to isolate drinking in itself as a factor in longevity. One study reported the shortest life span for heavy drinkers, a somewhat longer one for those who don't drink at all, and the longest for moderate drinkers. But other factors, such as general health and heredity, play important roles.

Alcohol and Sex Activity

Alcohol in sufficient quantity depresses the part of the brain that controls inhibitions. This liberating effect has led some people to believe that alcohol is an aphrodisiac, in men. This is a conclusion that is far from the truth. At the same time that alcohol increases the sexual appetite, it reduces the ability to perform.

Alcohol as an Irritant

Many otherwise healthy people cannot tolerate alcoholic beverages of any kind, or of a particular kind, without getting sick. In some cases, the negative reaction may be psychological in origin—connected with a disastrous experience with drunkenness in the early years or with an early hatred for a drinker in the family. Some people can drink one type of beverage but not another because of a particular congener, or because of an allergy to a specific grain or fruit. People suffering from such diseases as peptic ulcers, kidney and liver infections, and epilepsy should never drink any alcoholic beverages unless allowed to do so by a physician.

Uses and Hazards

At practically all times and in many parts of the world today, alcoholic beverages of various kinds have been and are still used for medicinal purposes. This should not be taken to mean that Aunt Sally is right about the curative powers of her elderberry wine, or that grandpa knows best when he says brandy is the best cure for hiccups. Today an American physician may recommend a particular alcoholic beverage as a tranquilizer, a sleep-inducer, or an appetite stimulant.

Use of Alcohol with Other Drugs

Alcoholic beverages should be avoided by anyone taking barbiturates or other sedatives. See "Drug Use and Abuse" later in this chapter for a discussion of barbiturates.

Alcohol and Driving

For many people, coordination, alertness, and general driving skills are impaired at blood-alcohol levels below the legal limit (0.1 percent). There are some people who become dangerous drivers after only one drink. Attempts are constantly being made, but so far with less than perfect success, to educate the public about the very real dangers of drunken driving.

Possible Causes of Alcohol Abuse

A popular myth holds that alcohol causes alcohol abuse. It doesn't—any more than sugar causes diabetes. Various theories have been evolved to explain what does cause alcohol abuse.

Physiological Causes

Although several physiological factors seem to be involved in the progression of alcohol abuse, no single one can be pinpointed as the cause of the disease. Among the theories that have come under investigation are the following: abnormal sugar metabolism, disorders of the endocrine glands, and dietary deficiencies.

Psychological Causes

Recent studies have pointed to a possible relationship between personality and alcohol abuse. Researchers indicate that one definable segment of the alcoholic population has the character disorder known as *antisocial personality*. Once called a *sociopath,* the person with an antisocial personality is usually charming in a social sense, manipulative, impulsive and rebellious, and egocentric. An estimated 25 percent of the alcoholic population falls in this category; in the general population the prevalence of antisocial personalities is about 3 percent.

Sociological Factors

Practically all studies of alcohol abuse in the United States indicate that ethnic groups vary dramatically in their rates of problem drinkers. A great deal of attention has therefore been focused on *learned attitudes* toward alcoholic beverages and how they are used or abused. Generally, in the low-incidence groups attitudes toward drinking are clearly defined and understood by all the members of the group. Drunkenness is consistently frowned upon. In the high-incidence groups, researchers have found extensive conflict over alcohol. The basic rules aren't clearly defined, and there are no clear-cut standards for acceptable and unacceptable drinking behavior.

Genetic Factors

Research into the genetics of alcohol abuse has led to a theory of "familial abuse." The theory holds that the person with a close relative who is alcoholic is at far greater risk of succumbing to the disease than are others without such connections. Familial abuse or "familial alcoholism" characterizes as many as three in four of all abusers. Therapy has thus begun to focus on the families of alcohol abusers—particularly young sons—as the ones most susceptible to the disease.

Recognizing the Danger Signals of Problem Drinking

The chronic alcohol abuser shows physical symptoms that a physician can recognize. Among them are hand tremors, deterioration of eye functions, reduced bladder control, liver disorders, anemia, memory lapses, and others. But there are many other symptoms that family members and friends can observe, among them these:

- Alcohol use as a way of handling problems or escaping from them

- Increased use of alcohol with repeated occasions of unintended intoxication

- Sneaking drinks or gulping them rapidly in quick succession

- Irritation, hostility, and lying when the subject of alcohol abuse is mentioned

- A noticeable deterioration in appearance, health, and social behavior

- Persistent drinking in spite of such symptoms as headaches, loss of appetite, sleeplessness, and stomach trouble

Treatment

Methods of treating alcohol abuse fall generally into three categories. Choice of any one form of treatment depends on the particular needs of a client, including the degree of dependency. The three categories include the hospital, the intermediate, and the outpatient settings. Other approaches to treatment may be geared to individual or group needs.

The family physician can in most cases provide guidance on what kind of treatment would most benefit a particular patient. The alcohol abuser may be referred first to a toxicologist for an interview and recommendations on treatment. A review of the patient's history is a typical first step in treatment. Family involvement during therapy may be critically important. More than 4,200 centers offer treatment programs; of these, many are nonprofit clinics while others are units owned by for-profit health care chains. Many centers and clinics specialize in team approaches to therapy.

The Hospital Setting

Whether undertaken voluntarily or involuntarily (for example, by court order) the treatment formats offered in a hospital can be individualized.

Where some patients adjust best to inpatient care, others prefer partial hospitalization. In the latter case the patient is allowed to go home or to work at appropriate times, otherwise living in the hospital. In a hospital detoxification program, one designed to end physical addiction, the patient has a variable period, usually two weeks to a month, during which he or she undergoes a programmed regimen of activities. These may range from exercise classes to medications to bed rest and regulated diets.

The Intermediate Setting

The intermediate settings usually include at least halfway houses, quarterway houses, and residential care sites. The first of these offer not only living quarters but also job counseling, psychotherapy, and other services. In quarterway houses, the patient receives more attention in the form of counseling and psychotherapy. Residential care centers usually offer little beyond living quarters.

The Outpatient Setting

Again in the outpatient setting the patient has a range of treatment choices. Among them typically are individual counseling sessions held by a paraprofessional; individual therapy sessions with a professional who may have an advanced degree in social work, psychology, medicine, or a related specialty; and group therapy sessions supervised by either a paraprofessional or a professional.

Chemical Treatments

Some treatment programs utilize medications to help patients to "shake the habit." Tranquilizers may be used to reduce tensions and prepare the patient for a follow-up stage. In a program of *aversion therapy* a substance called emetine may be prescribed. Taken before an alcoholic drink, emetine causes nausea. The treatment should be undertaken only under medical supervision.

Where to Find Help

Volunteer organizations of various kinds offer the alcohol abuser and his or her family a wide range of services and programs. The best known is Alcoholics Anonymous (AA), which is supported by contributions from members. AA utilizes a group-support approach to treatment. Most larger communities have AA chapters as well as Al-Anon and Alateen units for family members, relatives, and friends of abusers. Alateen works with young people between 12 and 20 years of age. Counseling and referrals may be obtained from a local Alcoholic Treatment Center.

Information may also be obtained from the following national headquarters of organizations established to help alcohol abusers:

Alcoholics Anonymous World
  Services
P.O. Box 459
Grand Central Station
New York, NY 10163

National Association for Children of
  Alcoholics
31582 Coast Highway, Suite 201
South Laguna, CA 92677
(714/499-3889)

Al-Anon Family Group Headquarters
P.O. Box 862
Midtown Station
New York, NY 10018
(212/302-7240)

National Council on Alcoholism and
  Drug Dependence
12 W. 21 Street
New York, NY 10010
(212/206-6770)

Drug Abuse

Like alcohol abuse, drug abuse can wreck lives and break up families. But to many experts the problem of drug abuse is far more serious than alcohol abuse. The trade in addictive, harmful drugs is not only unlawful; it has grown year by year, to the point where many believe it is out of control. The U.S. government spent some $1.6 billion on efforts to combat illegal drug importation in 1986, calling on units of the military forces to join the campaign. Even so, heroin imports increased by about 10 percent and cocaine imports by about 4 percent.

The forms that drug abuse takes, and the numbers of drugs, are numerous and increasing. Many authorities believe we should examine our whole American society for the "pill-happy" context in which drug abuse occurs. Dr. Joel Fort, former consultant on drug abuse to the World Health Organization, called America

> "a drug-prone nation. . . . The average 'straight' adult consumes three to five mind-altering drugs a day, beginning with the stimulant caffeine in coffee, tea, and Coca Cola, going on to include alcohol and nicotine, often a tranquilizer, not uncommonly a sleeping pill at night and sometimes an amphetamine the next morning."

The social effects of drug abuse rank among the most alarming of all the symptoms of what has been called the drug crisis. By estimate, drugs are involved in one-third to one-half of all crimes committed in the United States in a typical year. In a single recent year, medical treatments for drug abusers cost the nation more than $2 billion. The costs of abuse to families, communities, and to abusers themselves cannot be calculated.

Making the problem of control of drug abuse unbelievably complex is the fact that literally thousands of drugs and drug combinations have basic roles in medical treatments. Legal and illicit uses may, because of the close connections, become confused. Physicians' instructions regarding use of such legal drugs as sleeping pills may be ignored or neglected. Legitimately prescribed drugs may, in some cases, unintentionally lead to abuse or dependency.

Other facts make it difficult to control drug abuse. More and more, for example, abusers are turning to multiple substance abuse. Cocaine "sniffers" may take alcohol in one form or another to soften the uncomfortable and even painful effects of cocaine withdrawal. Physicians report that "polydrug" abuse leads to progressive worsening of such medical symptoms as stomach ailments and liver problems.

Designer drugs add another complicating factor. Made in clandestine chemical laboratories, these drugs are imitations or analogs of such other drugs as cocaine, heroin, amphetamines, and many other basic substances. The new drugs are legal until declared illegal by the federal government's Drug Enforcement Administration because a chemist has altered their chemical compositions enough to take them out of the banned or controlled drug categories. Far more powerful than the basic drugs they imitate, the designer forms have been implicated in more than 200 deaths. Researchers indicate that there is no limit to the numbers of designer drugs that can be produced.

A designer drug called *new heroin* (*Ecstasy*) was, on analysis, found to contain the industrial chemical MPTP, a suspected causative element in cases of Parkinson's disease. A number of new-heroin abusers also had classic Parkinson's symptoms: rigidity, tremors in the arms, legs, and even the head, and slow or difficult movement. Thus new research has focused on MPTP as a possible clue to the degenerative brain processes that lead to Parkinson's.

Over-the-Counter Drugs

Americans consume over-the-counter (OTC) drugs in enormous quantities. Purchasable without a physician's prescription, these drugs have limited but real potential for abuse. They range from headache remedies to cold nostrums and from acne ointments to vitamins. In general, good practice is to use OTC drugs as seldom as possible, for short-term, minor illnesses. Medicines of proven effectiveness should be used exclusively: taking an aspirin for a headache is a good example. The U.S. Public Health Service offers these guidelines:

- Self-prescribed drugs should never be used continuously for long periods of time. . . . A physician is required for abdominal pain that is severe or recurs periodically; pains anywhere, if severe, disabling, persistent, or recurring; headache, if unusually severe or prolonged more than one day; a prolonged cold with fever or cough; earache; unexplained loss of weight; unexplained and unusual symptoms; *malaise* lasting more than a week or two. . . .

The Food and Drug Administration (FDA), a branch of the U.S. Public Health Service, is responsible for establishing the safety and usefulness of all drugs marketed in the United States, both OTC and prescription. You can be assured that OTC drugs are safe provided you take them in strict accordance with the label instructions. These indicate the appropriate dosages, among other things, and carry warnings against prolonged or improper use, such as "discontinue if pain persists," or "do not take if abdominal pain is present." This labeling information is regulated by the FDA.

Drug Classifications

In addition to alcohol, the drugs of potential abuse fall into six categories: stimulants, depressants, and narcotic preparations, all of which can have legitimate medical uses; hallucinogens; cannabinoids such as marijuana; and inhalants (or volatile inhalants) such as aerosol sprays, glues, and fuels. See the accompanying table:

Major Drug Classifications	
Type	**Examples**
Stimulants	Amphetamines Cocaine derivatives
Depressants	Valium Seconal
Narcotics (opioids)	Morphine Codeine
Hallucinogens	LSD Mescaline Psilocybin
Marijuana (cannabinoids)	Marijuana Hashish
Inhalants	Gasoline Amyl nitrate

Drug abuse can lead to at least three kinds of addiction or dependency. *Physical addiction* results in unpleasant withdrawal symptoms, including, nausea, headache, or cold sweats when the abuser does not take the drug. Sudden withdrawal from some physically addictive drugs can cause heart failure. *Psychological addiction,* more subtle, is a stage at which the abuser believes he or she cannot cope without the drug. In *functional addiction,* the abuser grows dependent on such drugs as decongestant nasal sprays to remain free of an annoying physical condition.

Definitions of Dependence and Addiction

Dependence and addiction is used to describe the compulsive and uncontrollable use of a substance. The use continues despite negative effects on health, lifestyle, work, or other aspects of one's life. Lack of the substance leads to craving, physical or psychological discomfort, and, at times, an overwhelming desire to obtain more of the substance to alleviate the negative sensations experienced from withdrawal.

Psychological dependence or addiction occurs when the user feels he or she cannot manage without the drug. This can occur for several reasons, with several types of drugs. The condition can be mild or can be extraordinarily severe.

Psychological addiction to painkillers—and this can include ibuprofen (Motrin), aspirin, and acetaminophen (Tylenol)—occurs when the user feels that pain may be too great without regular medication. As pain occurs without use, it fulfills the user's expectations. The pain may be real or may be psychosomatic (triggered by psychological expectations of pain), but it reassures the user that the drug is needed and does good. The problem is that with many types of drug, the effectiveness decreases as use increases.

Psychological addiction can accompany physical addiction, and it is usually difficult to distinguish where psychological needs leave off and physical needs begin. Many addictions are a combination of psychological and physical.

Physical dependence or addiction occurs when the body has developed a physical need for the drug. Physical dependence is usually recognized when the user stops taking the drug. Withdrawal symptoms occur when the body is denied the chemicals to which it has become habituated. Withdrawal symptoms can include dizziness, anxiety, restless sleep, dull ache, acute pain, heart tremors, seizures and convulsions, and heart attack. Sudden withdrawal from some physically addictive drugs can kill the user. Many of the street drugs, such as cocaine and heroin, and many of the prescription drugs, such as Xanax and codeine, can produce severe symptoms if withdrawal is sudden from quantities that were abusive.

Tolerance is the term used for the effect that occurs when the quantity of drug is progressively increased to achieve the desired result. For some chemicals, the body becomes habituated to one quantity and the dosage must be increased to maintain the same level of relief or pleasure experienced from the drug. Increased tolerance for some drugs is what frequently leads to levels that are physically addictive.

Three Classes of Prescription Drugs

Among the drugs that may be prescribed for you are some that have a tremendous potential for abuse. They include *stimulants,* such as amphetamines; *depressants,* such as sleeping pills; and *narcotic* painkillers, including morphine and codeine. When abused (that is, when taken in any way other than according to a physician's strict instructions) these drugs constitute a substantial part of America's burgeoning national drug problem.

Stimulant Drugs

The legitimate use of stimulant drugs and their great capacity for abuse stem from the same property: their ability to speed up the processes of the central nervous system. Physicians may prescribe amphetamines primarily to curb the appetites of patients who are dieting or to counteract mild depression. More rarely, they use stimulant drugs to treat *narcolepsy,* a disease in which the patient is subject to irresistible bouts of sleep, and to counteract the drowsiness caused by sedatives. Amphetamines and an amphetamine-like drug (Ritalin) may be used to treat some hyperactive children who are extremely excitable and easily distracted. For reasons that are imperfectly understood, the drug calms these children instead of stimulating them.

Amphetamines

The major forms of the amphetamines are: amphetamine (Benzedrine), the more powerful dextroamphetamine (Dexedrine), and methamphetamine (Methedrine, Desoxyn). The street name for these drugs is "speed."

The consumption of amphetamines is reportedly far greater than the prescription books indicate. Some 10 billion tablets are produced in the United States annually, enough for 50 doses for every man, woman, and child. Of this amount, probably half is diverted into illicit channels. Underground laboratories manufacture even more.

Abusers of amphetamines include students cramming for exams, housewives trying to get through the day without collapsing from exhaustion, and the businessman who has tossed and turned all night in a strange hotel bedroom and needs to be alert for a conference the next morning.

Used judiciously, amphetamines can improve performance, both mental and physical, over moderate periods of time. In effect, they delay the deterioration in performance that fatigue normally produces. Required to carry out routine duties under difficult circumstances and for extended periods, some astronauts have used amphetamines under long-range medical supervision.

Amphetamines give some persons feelings of self-confidence, well-being, alertness, and an increased ability to concentrate and perform. Others may experience an increase in tension ranging from the uncomfortable to an agonizing pitch of anxiety. High doses may produce dry mouth, sweating, palpitations, and raised blood pressure. Because amphetamines only defer the effects of fatigue, the letdown can be dangerous, especially for such users as long-distance truck drivers. In addition, the feelings of self-confidence about improved performance may be highly deceptive. Some college students who have crammed for exams while on speed have turned in blank examination books, or written a whole essay on one dense line.

Amphetamine abusers quickly develop a tolerance to the drug. They may have continually to increase dosages, and may undergo different kinds of drug experiences. Psychological dependence can build rapidly.

Amphetaminelike Stimulants

Several drugs that are chemically unrelated to the amphetamines produce very similar effects on the body. They are, also, equally amenable to abuse. Among them are methylphenidate (Ritalin) and phenmetrazine (Preludin). The latter has been commonly used as a diet pill.

Cocaine

Ranked as powerful stimulants to the central nervous system, cocaine and its derivatives have become the trendy drugs of the late 20th century. An alkaloid found in the leaves of the coca bush, *Erythroxylon coca,* cocaine in its crystalline form is a white powder that looks like moth flakes. Cocaine can be sniffed, smoked, or taken intravenously. Abusers of cocaine may or may not develop a tolerance for the drug. But some evidence indicates that the same dose repeated frequently will not produce similar effects over a period of time.

Very little street-purchased cocaine is pure. Usually, the drug is mixed, or cut, with other drugs or with substances that resemble it, such as talcum powder or sugar.

Physical dependence on cocaine is rare. Psychological dependence is much more common. When physical dependence occurs, the withdrawal symptoms may include hunger, irritability, extreme fatigue, depression, and restless sleep. With psychological dependence, abusers come to need the feeling of euphoria induced by cocaine. When a dose wears off, the abuser may go into a period of deep depression.

The use of cocaine as a legal anesthetic need not lead to addiction. It has been used particularly in surgical operations on the mouth, eyes, and throat because it can constrict blood vessels and because it is rapidly absorbed by the mucous membranes.

Cocaine's effects as a stimulant last only a short time. Generally, the effects depend on the size of the dose. A small dose may produce sensations of euphoria and illusions of increased strength and sensory awareness. A large dose may magnify these effects. The abuser may engage in irrational behavior, and may experience such physical side effects as sweating, di-

lation of the pupils, and rapid heartbeat.

In extreme cases abusers may have hallucinations and feelings of paranoia and depression. They may imagine that insects are crawling over their skins (formication) and may have chest pains. Injections by needle may produce skin abscesses. Both heavy and light users may develop runny noses, eczema around the nostrils, and deterioration of the nasal cartilage. The latter occurs because cocaine is usually "snorted" into the nostrils through a straw or a roll of paper, or from a spoon.

Death results, occasionally, from overdoses of cocaine, with respiratory arrest as a prime cause. The abuser may also have high fever, heart rhythm disturbances, or convulsions.

Crack Cocaine

By a simple process dealers in cocaine can convert cocaine in white powder form, cocaine hydrochloride, into cocaine alkaloid, called *freebase.* The process involves mixing powdered cocaine with baking soda and water to form a paste. Once the concoction hardens, it looks like lumpy, off-white granulated sugar. Unlike powdered cocaine, the drug in this form, called *crack* or *rock,* can be smoked, eliminating the need for needles.

However made, crack is a purified cocaine base that is usually smoked in a special pipe with wire screens, or sprinkled on a tobacco or marijuana cigarette. The drug produces a high that may start in eight seconds and last two minutes. By contrast, snorted cocaine takes effect after about five minutes.

Crack produces a very intense euphoria along with other physical symptoms. Because the drug in this form is far more potent than powdered cocaine, the heartbeat speeds up and the abuser's blood pressure may rise. Heart-lung problems may follow, and seizures can occur. Death may ensue. Because of the variations in the strength and purity of crack, and because of the variability of a body's response, death can occur on the first use or the thousandth. Abuse of crack may lead to physical addiction in weeks, with the victim needing continually larger doses to achieve a high.

Depressant Drugs

Making up a second class of medically useful drugs that are also widely abused, the depressants act as sedatives on the central nervous system (CNS). They may also act as hypnotic, or sleep-inducing, agents.

The depressants include mainly the barbiturates, which are both sedative and hypnotic, and the tranquilizers, which can calm without producing sleep. Though they are available as main or secondary constituents of more than 80 brand name preparations, the barbiturates are readily abused.

Tranquilizers act selectively on the brain and the central nervous system. Divided into major and minor tranquilizers, these drugs are similar to barbiturates in many ways, including their sedative or calming effect. The major tranquilizers, called *neuroleptics* because they are useful in the treatment of mental disorders, are *haloperidol* and *chlorpromazine*. These drugs lead to virtually no addiction or dependence even in long-term therapy.

The minor tranquilizers, among them *meprobamate* (Miltown), *chlordiazepoxide* (Librium), and *diazepam* (Valium), are, by contrast, highly addictive. Abusers take such drugs to achieve euphoric states as well as to offset the effects of alcohol, amphetamines, and other drugs.

Barbiturates

Barbiturates have many legitimate uses. For example, they may be prescribed to overcome insomnia, reduce high blood pressure, alleviate anxiety, treat mental disorders, and sedate patients both before and after surgery. Barbiturates may help to bring epileptic and other convulsions under control.

Barbiturates are metabolized, or broken down chemically, by the liver. They are then eliminated by the kidneys at different speeds depending on their types: slow- or long-acting, intermediate and short-acting, or ultra-short-acting. The first of these, primarily phenobarbital and barbital, take effect on the brain in one to two hours and last for six to 24 hours. The intermediate and short-acting barbiturates, including secobarbital and pentobarbital, take effect in 20 to 45 minutes and last five to six hours. The best known of the ultra-short-acting drugs, sodium pentothal or thiopental, can produce unconsciousness in a few minutes. Used mostly in hospitals as an anesthetic, pentothal is also injected by dentists to produce instant unconsciousness.

Abuse

Barbiturate abusers usually select the ultra-short-acting form of the drug because of the rapid action. Abusers as a group generally fall into four categories, with some overlap.

The "silent abuser" takes sleeping pills at first to get some sleep, probably with a physician's prescription. Progressively, the drug helps the abuser to deal with tension and anxiety. Indulging at home, he or she finds the barbiturates producing an alcohol-like high, with slurred speech, confusion, poor judgment and coordination, and sometimes wild emotional swings. Eventually the abuser is obtaining the drug through illicit channels. Some may end up spending most of their time in bed.

A second group, taking barbiturates for stimulation, has already developed a high tolerance that makes drug stimulation possible. Some other abusers find that the drug releases inhibitions.

Made up mostly of young people who are experimenting with various drugs, a third group uses barbiturates to "come down" from an amphetamine high. Members of this group may find themselves in a vicious cycle of stimulation and sedation. To obtain both effects at once, some abusers take the barbiturate-amphetamine combination in the same swallow—a so-called "set-up."

A fourth group, abusers of heroin and other narcotics, uses barbiturates as a substitute when drugs of choice are not available. They may also combine barbiturates with heroin to prolong its effect. In one hospital surveyed, 23 percent of the narcotics users said they were also dependent on barbiturates.

Effects and Dangers

Barbiturate abuse is generally considered to be far more dangerous than narcotic abuse. Every year brings some 3,000 deaths from barbiturate overdose, accidental or intentional. For such reasons many physicians believe barbiturates are the most dangerous of all drugs. Chronic abuse can lead to psychological dependence and increased tolerance, followed often by physical dependence of a particularly anguishing kind.

Abrupt withdrawal from barbiturates can be much more dangerous than withdrawal from heroin. Within a day the abuser withdrawing from barbiturates may experience headaches, muscle twitches, anxiety, weakness, nausea, and blood pressure drops. If the abuser stands up suddenly he or she may faint. Delirium and convulsions may come later. The latter can be fatal. Thus the withdrawal must always be undertaken under medical supervision. Even with supervision, a withdrawal from barbiturates may take two months.

Abuse of barbiturates presents other dangers. Unintentional overdosing frequently occurs when a person takes a regular dose to get to sleep and then remains awake or awakens soon afterward; tired and confused, the person may take another or repeated doses. Death may result. Mixing barbiturates and alcohol can produce the same outcome.

Other Barbiturate-Type Drugs

Some depressants are chemically unrelated to the barbiturates but have similar effects. These include *glutethimide*, *ethchlorvynol* (Placidyl), and *methyprylon* (Noludar). These too lead to tolerance when abused and sometimes to psychological and physical dependence.

Tranquilizers

The minor tranquilizers are manufactured as capsules and tablets in many sizes, shapes, and colors. They may also be purchased in liquid form for injection. Used legitimately to treat emotional tension and as muscle re-

Varieties of abused drugs		
Name	**Form**	**Drug**
amphetamine methamphetamine	capsule, pill, liquid, powder, tablet, lozenge; swallowed	stimulant
barbiturate	sleeping pills, capsules, tablets; swallowed; injected	depressant, sedative
cocaine	white powder; sniffed, smoked, injected	stimulant, local anesthetic
hashish	resin; smoked	relaxant, euphoriant, hallucinogen (in large or strong doses)
heroin	powder; injected, or sniffed	narcotic
inhalants (for example, gasoline, paint, glue, aerosols, amyl nitrite)	aerosols, volatile substances, solvents; sniffed	
LSD (d-lysergic acid diethylamide)	tablet, capsule, liquid; swallowed	hallucinogen (psychedelic)
marijuana, marihuana	dried leaves; smoked	relaxant, euphoriant, hallucinogen (in large or strong doses)
mescaline	tablet, capsule; swallowed	hallucinogen
PCP	powder; smoked, swallowed	anesthetic (used only with animals)

laxants, these tranquilizers have high abuse potential because they produce both psychological and physical dependence. Tolerance develops with prolonged abuse.

Miltown, Librium, and Valium produce effects similar to those of barbiturates. But the minor tranquilizers act more slowly and have longer duration. Once considered completely harmless, these drugs came into such vogue that in the 1970s the federal government intervened. Both Valium and Librium as well as some other drugs were placed under federal control. From 1975 on anyone requiring a prescription for these drugs was limited to five prescription refills within a six-month period following the initial prescription. If more of the medication was required after that, a new prescription had to be written.

Withdrawal from the minor tranquilizers can be as dangerous and painful as withdrawal from barbiturates. Combining the tranquilizing drugs with others, including alcohol, is a highly dangerous form of abuse. Each drug reinforces the effects of the other. The result may be greater than the combined effects of the different drugs.

Narcotics (Opiates)

Narcotics are drugs that relieve pain and induce sleep by depressing the central nervous system. Under U.S. law, narcotics are addictive drugs that produce rapid and severe physical and psychological dependence; that category includes opium and such opium derivatives as heroin, morphine, and codeine. The narcotics, or *opioids*, also include the so-called synthetic opiates, among them *meperidine* and *methadone*.

Opium

The seedpods of the opium poppy, *Papaver somniferum*, produce a gummy resin that has narcotic effects when eaten or smoked. Opium has been used in many lands and many cultures since prehistoric times. It was used medicinally in ancient Egypt. But not until recently did its addictive properties become known.

Of the more than two dozen active compounds, or *alkaloids,* that can be isolated from opium, the two most important are morphine and codeine.

Morphine

Morphine, named after Morpheus, the Roman god of dreams, is the chemical substance in opium that gives it sedative and analgesic properties. Isolated initially in the early 1800s, morphine was later synthesized in pure form. On the illicit drug market it appears usually as a white powder.

Morphine can relieve almost any kind of pain, particularly dull, continuous pain. It may also relieve the fear and anxiety that go with such suffering. In addition to drowsiness, euphoria, and impairment of mental and physical performance, morphine may have adverse effects including nausea, vomiting, and sweating. Intravenous injections of the drug may produce an orgasmic high sensation beginning in the upper abdomen and spreading throughout the body. Taken in overdose, morphine can lead to respiratory depression that is sometimes severe enough to cause coma and death. Morphine is highly addictive and is used only short-term in hospitals because longer exposure easily leads to problems. Naloxone (Narcan) may be administered intravenously as an antidote for morphine overdose.

Codeine

Taking its name from the Greek word *kodeia,* meaning poppyhead, codeine is a mild pain-reliever that can be produced from gum opium or through conversion from morphine. The effects of codeine peak in 30 to 60 min-utes; they disappear in three to four hours. Codeine is milder than either morphine or heroin in analgesic effect, and is an ingredient in some popular nonprescription cough syrups. All forms can induce addiction problems with regular use.

Heroin

Originally thought to be nonaddictive, heroin was for a time used as a cure for opium and morphine addiction. It was then found to be more addictive than either of those drugs. It was prohibited in the United States in 1924 and became a staple on the drug black market. Heroin is several times as powerful as morphine.

All of the opiates, including heroin, produce feelings of well-being or euphoria. They also lead to dulled senses and to reduction or elimination of normal fears, tensions, and anxiety. The drug also produces sleepiness and lethargy; *nodding* is one of the characteristic symptoms of abuse. Possible side effects include nausea, flushing, constipation, slowed respiration rates, retention of urine, and, eventually, malnutrition resulting from loss of appetite. When first injecting heroin, nausea and vomiting can occur almost immediately.

The heroin abuser rapidly develops tolerance to the drug. Continually larger doses are then required to produce the same degree of euphoria. Used chronically, heroin leads to both psychological and physical dependence. The former is far more important, and is more difficult to break.

Caught in a cycle involving desperate efforts to obtain enough money, often by criminal means, and getting high, the heroin abuser is not necessarily driven by the search for escape. He or she may want, equally, to avoid withdrawal symptoms. For the chronic abuser these symptoms can be difficult and painful, and may include anxiety, sweating, muscle aches, vomiting, and diarrhea.

Heroin sold on the streets is cut with quinine, milk sugar, or baking soda. It may be cut several times before reaching the abuser. A bag may contain only 1 to 5 percent heroin. If the addict unknowingly buys a dose containing 30 percent or more pure heroin, the higher concentration can spell grave illness or death.

Because heroin can be taken in different ways, the drug's narcotic effects are variable. Sniffing is the mildest form of abuse, followed by skin-popping or subcutaneous injection anywhere on the body, and mainlining, injection directly into a vein, usually the large vein inside the elbow. Abscesses at the preferred site of injection are common, and the vein may become inflamed.

Heroin use does not necessarily lead to dependence. Many persons have experimented with the drug without becoming addicted. Others "joy-pop"—use the drug on weekends, usually for recreational purposes or "kicks."

Little agreement exists regarding treatments for heroin abuse. A promising yet controversial method is the substitution of controlled doses of *methadone* for heroin. Methadone is a synthetic opiate that does not produce the euphoria of heroin. The substitution can help the abuser to lead a normal life, but he or she may still be addicted—to methadone.

Other forms of treatment utilize group psychotherapy, often in live-in communities modeled after the West Coast's *Synanon.* Some experts believe that only multiple-approach treatment formats, combining chemical treatment, psychiatry, user communities, and rehabilitation, can be effective. But the five-year cure rate for heroin abusers is low—only about one-third of that for alcoholics.

Synthetic Opiates

Prescription pain-relievers such as Demerol, Dilaudid, Pantopon, and other synthetic opiates can become addicting if used indiscriminately. They occasionally appear on the illicit drug market. With the increased availability of methadone in treatment clinics, methadone itself is used illicitly, often in combination with alcohol or other drugs, and especially when heroin is in short supply.

The Hallucinogens: LSD and Others

LSD (lysergic acid diethylamide) is one of a class of drugs legally classed as *hallucinogens*—agents that cause the user to experience hallucinations, illusions, and distorted perceptions. Others include *mescaline, psilocybin* and *psilocin, PCP, DMT* (dimethyltryptamine), and *DOM* or *STP.*

A colorless, tasteless, odorless compound, LSD is a semisynthetic acid of immense potency. A single effective dose requires, on the average, only 100 millionths of a gram. A quantity of LSD equivalent to two aspirin tablets would furnish 6,500 such doses. When sold on the street, LSD is generally mixed with colored substances. It may be manufactured in capsule, tablet, or liquid form.

History of LSD

With names such as *California sunshine, acid, purple haze,* and others, LSD reached a peak of popularity in the 1960s. Today it cannot be made legally except for use in certain supervised experiments. Physicians may use it to treat alcoholism and some mental disease, but without uniformly convincing results. It may be sold illegally in sugar cubes, candy, cookies, on the surfaces of beads, even in the mucilage of stamps and envelopes. One dose may produce a 4- to 18-hour *trip,* a hallucinogenic experience.

In the 1960s this trip made LSD the drug of choice for many substance abusers. Among those who claimed that LSD and other psychedelic drugs were consciousness-expanding were well-known public figures. The drugs, in brief, were supposed to enhance the user's appreciation of everything in the environment, to increase creativity, open the gates of awareness to mind-bending mystical or religious experiences, and perhaps to bring about profound changes, hopefully for the better, in the user's personality.

While some users reported such results, various studies suggested that the improvements were illusory. Members of some groups nonetheless felt that it was "in" to be an *acidhead,* an LSD user. One authority estimates that less than 1 percent of the total population have experimented with LSD. Partly because knowledge of dangers in LSD use has become common, the drug has passed the peak of its popularity even though it can still be obtained illegally.

Addictive Aspects

Abuse of LSD is difficult; the drug produces such a spectacular high that daily ingestion is virtually out of the question. Thus LSD use does not lead to physical dependence. But the heavy user can develop a tolerance for the drug very quickly. The tolerance disappears after a few days of abstinence.

Effects

Taking LSD, the individual is usually prepared for minor physical discomforts: a rise in temperature, pulse, and blood pressure; the sensation of hair standing on end; and some nausea, dizziness, and headache. The trip begins about an hour after the drug is first taken. Vision is affected the most profoundly. Colors become more intense and more beautiful; those in a painting may seem to merge and stream. Flat objects become three-dimensional.

The LSD user's reactions are closely related to his or her expectations. Thus one trip may be mind-expanding, filled with brilliant sights and sensations as well as euphoric feelings of oneness with the universe. Another trip may bring anxiety, panic, fear, and depression verging on despair. The latter experience can be terrifying; some bad trips have ended in psychiatric wards, with the tripper suffering from a severe mental disorder, a *psychosis.* An individual's body image may be distorted; in the LSD-induced vision he or she may have no head, for example. Such psychotic episodes, or breaks, may clear up within a day or two. Others can last for months or years.

Some trips have ended in tragedy. Convinced that they could fly or float through the air, some trippers have walked through high windows to their deaths. Others have walked in front of trains or cars.

In effect, no one can predict what psychological changes LSD use will produce. One reason is that no one really knows how LSD works inside the body to affect the mind. What is known is that the drug moves quickly to the brain and throughout the body, acting on both the central and autonomic nervous systems. But all traces of the drug disappear from the brain in some 20 minutes. The effects, as noted, last many more hours.

As with all drugs, LSD should not be ingested by persons who have psychotic tendencies or who are unstable. A disquieting side effect, usually occurring after chronic or heavy use, appears in the flashback, a reexperiencing of the effects of the drug weeks or months after a trip. One theory holds that flashbacks are induced by stress or fatigue, or by resort to other drugs, but the theory remains a theory.

Studies have reported some statistical findings. One research project found that the children of LSD users are 18 times more likely to have birth defects than the children of non-users. Some research also suggests that the drug may have toxic effects on some cells of the human body. An unproved, and possibly unprovable, theory indicates that there may be a link between LSD use and breaks in chromosomes that could conceivably lead to leukemia or to birth defects in users' children.

Other Hallucinogens

Many other substances, both natural and synthetic, are used as hallucinogens. Most of them produce effects similar to those of LSD, but are far less potent.

Mescaline

Mescaline is the active ingredient of *peyote,* a Mexican cactus that has been used by American Indians for centuries to achieve mystical states in religious ceremonies. Users consume cactus "buttons" either ground up or whole. Mescaline itself may be obtained as a powder or a liquid. It can also be synthesized in a laboratory.

Psilocybin and Psilocin

Psilocybin and psilocin are the active hallucinogenic ingredients in the Aztec mushroom *Psilocybe mexicana.* The mushroom grows in southern Mexico and has been eaten raw by

the natives since about 1500 B.C. Both derivatives can be made in the laboratory.

PCP (Phencyclidine Hydrochloride)

First developed in 1959 as an anesthetic, PCP in its pure form is a white crystalline powder that is readily soluble in water or alcohol. It appears on the drug black market as tablets, capsules, and colored powders. Abusers snort, smoke, or eat PCP. They can also inject the drug, but do not usually do so. PCP appears as an adulterant in many drug mixtures—in mescaline, psilocybin, or LSD, for example. PCP reportedly has as many or more undesirable effects as positive ones, among them forgetfulness, loss of behavior control, feelings of depersonalization, paranoid episodes, hallucinations, and suicidal impulses.

DMT (Dimethyltryptamine)

Called the "businessman's high" because its effects may last only 40 to 50 minutes, DMT is similar in structure to psilocin. DMT can be smoked or injected; in either case the effect is a powerful wave of exhilaration. An ingredient of various plants native to South America, DMT has long been used by Indian tribes in the form of intoxicating drinks or snuff, often very dangerous. In the United States, DMT is synthesized from tryptamine in the laboratory.

DOM or STP

DOM or STP is a synthetic compound originally developed by the Dow Chemical Company for possible use in the treatment of mental disorders. The drug was never released. Manufactured illicitly, it was allegedly given the name STP for Serenity, Tranquillity, Peace. The drug is powerful, it

produces vivid hallucinations, and it seems to last as long as LSD. It is also extremely poisonous, and can bring on fever, blurred vision, difficulty in swallowing, and occasionally death from convulsions. In some cases abusers suffer from manic psychoses lasting for days.

Marijuana (Cannabinoids)

Marijuana, or *marihuana,* is a Mexican-Spanish word originally used to refer to a poor grade of tobacco. Later it came to mean a smoking preparation made from the Indian hemp plant (*Cannabis sativa*). A tall, weedy plant related to the fig tree and the hop, cannabis grows freely in many parts of the world and in a variety of grades depending on climate and method of cultivation. The different grades produce drugs of varying strengths. Some 300 million people around the world obtain drug preparations of one kind or another from cannabis.

Drugs are obtained almost exclusively from the female hemp plants. The male plants produce the fiber for hemp. When the female plants are ripe, late in the summer, their top leaves and especially the clusters of flowers at their tops develop a minty, sticky, golden-yellow resin, which eventually blackens. This resin contains the highest concentrations of THC (tetrahydrocannabinol), the group of substances containing the active principles of the drug. The pure resin of carefully cultivated plants is the most potent form of cannabis. It is available in cakes, called *charas* in India, and as a brown powder called hashish in the Middle East.

An estimated 15,000 tons of marijuana are illegally smuggled into the United States annually. But cannabis cultivation has become a major underground business inside the United

States. Most illegal shipments of the drug come from Colombia, Jamaica, and Mexico.

Abuse Potential

Marijuana has puzzling aspects. Scientists have not succeeded in establishing exactly what substances in the cannabis plant produce drug effects, or how. THC is, of course, believed to be the most important active element, but chemists believe it is not the only one.

Beyond that, marijuana seems to be in a special class as a drug. It is classed as a hallucinogen, but is less potent than the true hallucinogens. It is not a narcotic, and it resembles both stimulants and depressants in some of its effects. Its use does not lead to physical dependence, nor does the user or abuser develop tolerance. Some users, in fact, find that with regular use they need less marijuana to achieve the desired high.

Users do acquire a slight to moderate psychological dependence—less, in some experts' opinions, than do regular users of alcohol or tobacco. Thus much of the theorizing about marijuana is conjecture despite the fact that millions of persons use it regularly or occasionally.

Effects

Experimenters and newcomers to marijuana smoking may experience little at the beginning. A sense of panic may accompany early exposure to the drug. More serious reactions have been reported, however, including *toxic-psychosis* (psychosis caused by a toxic agent) with accompanying confusion and disorientation. But such reports are rare. Experimenters using large doses of marijuana, hashish,

or THC have induced what they termed hallucinations and psychotic reactions.

The experienced smoker may feel halfway between elation and sleepiness. He or she may have some altered perceptions of sound or color, for example, and a greatly slowed-down sense of time. It is usually possible to control the extent of the high by stopping when a given point is reached. The smoker often experiences mild headache or nausea.

Medical Evidence

Research and medical use of marijuana have led to some relatively tentative findings. Some evidence indicates, for example, that the drug may produce genetic damage. More definitely, marijuana has been found to be effective for reducing the pressure of fluids in the eyes of patients suffering from glaucoma. In a 1976 case, the Food and Drug Administration (FDA) approved the use of marijuana for such treatment.

In 1985 the FDA licensed a small drug firm to manufacture THC for use in combating the nausea associated with cancer chemotherapy. Other studies indicated that the drug may also be useful in the treatment of such other diseases as multiple sclerosis.

The debate over full legalization of marijuana promises to continue. Few argue that all penalties for major suppliers should be dropped, at least as long as marijuana remains illegal. But many persons see a contradiction in sending a young person to prison for smoking a marijuana cigarette while his or her parents can drink three martinis every evening.

Inhalants

The inhalants as a class include solvents used in cleaning compounds,

aerosol sprays, fuels, and glues. Abusers of these substances sniff or inhale the fumes for recreational and mind-altering purposes. But the substances, primarily chemical compounds, were never meant for human consumption. With some exceptions, they are available commercially and thus have appeal for persons who cannot afford or cannot obtain the more conventional drugs.

Strictly speaking, tobacco, cocaine, and marijuana could be considered inhalants. But the term more commonly refers to three categories of products: solvents, aerosols, and anesthetics. Among the solvents are commercial items such as gasoline, transmission fluid, paint thinner, and airplane cement. The aerosol products include shoeshine compounds, insecticides, spray paints, and hair spray. The type of inhalant used appears to vary according to geographic location, the ethnic backgrounds of abusers, and availability.

Anesthetics comprise a special group of inhalants. Some of them, including nitrous oxide, ether, and chloroform, were used recreationally before medical applications were found for them. Because they are not widely available, they are not abused as much as solvents and aerosols.

Abuse Patterns

Young teenagers are primary inhalant abusers. But some groups or classes of adults, such as prisoners in institutions, also use inhalants. Reasons for abuse vary; among teenagers they range from hostility and lack of affection to peer pressure. Adults, say authorities, are attracted by the ready availability of many inhalants. Alcoholics may resort to inhalants while trying to forestall the symptoms of withdrawal from alcohol.

Effects

Among the active chemicals in many inhalants are toluene, naphtha, carbon tetrachloride, acetone, and others. The fumes from these chemicals enter the bloodstream quickly. They are then distributed to the brain and liver. Entering the central nervous system, the fumes depress such body functions as respiration and heartbeat.

Classed as depressants, inhalants are sometimes referred to as "deliriants." The reason is that they can produce illusions, hallucinations, and mental disturbances. These effects usually result in cases of overdose; in moderate doses, the abuser feels sedated, has changed perceptions and impaired judgment, and may experience fright or even panic. Depending on the dosage, the abuser may also feel intoxicated, and may have lowered inhibitions along with feelings of restlessness, uncoordination, confusion, and disorientation.

Prolonged abuse can lead to nausea, muscular weakness, fatigue, and weight loss. Other effects of such abuse can be extensive damage to the kidneys, bone marrow, liver, and brain. Inhalants have been implicated in some forms of cancer. A high can last from a few minutes to an hour or more. Repeated dosing can produce physical and psychological dependence; but inhalants are not considered as dangerously addictive as other depressants.

In the 1960s the many deaths resulting from glue-sniffing made inhalant abuse a matter of nationwide concern. Studies reported later that about two-thirds of these deaths came about because the abusers, usually children, put plastic bags over their heads to intensify the effect and suffocated.

More recently, deaths have occurred from children experimenting with all types of aerosol sprays and fumes and dying either from toxic poisoning or suffocating in their own vomit after they pass out.

Where to Find Help

Substance abuse has many disturbing aspects aside from the physical, psychological, and social damage that it can cause. With addictive medicines, the progression from a *therapeutic* dose—the amount prescribed by a physician—to a *toxic* dose may seem, to some persons, natural and even inevitable. Ingestion or injection of a *lethal* dose may follow as an unintended consequence.

Other factors are causes for concern. The proliferation of illicit street drugs, the rapidity with which dependence or addiction can develop, and the costs and complexity of treatment or detoxification programs all add to the dangers inherent in abuse as a spreading phenomenon. Researchers are discovering weapons that may help in some cases to make treatment more effective: *naloxone* (Narcan), for example, can be given intravenously to reduce the toxic effects of narcotics. But too often a drug has done irreversible harm in a human system before help arrives.

American society has begun to mobilize resources to aid those who need information, assistance, or counsel, for themselves or others, in cases of substance abuse. A National Partnership to Prevent Drug and Alcohol Abuse has established a network of community groups to inform teenagers about narcotics and their potentially disastrous effects. Among helplines and hotlines is one operated by Fair Oaks Hospital in Summit, New Jersey, with the toll-free number 800-COCAINE. Counselors serving with 800-COCAINE are linked to a network of treatment centers and hospitals throughout the country. The addresses and telephone numbers of four national groups, including Fair Oaks Hospital and its program, are:

National Federation of Parents for
  Drug-Free Youth
1423 N. Jefferson
Springfield, MO 65802
417/836-3709

American Counsel for Drug Education
204 Monroe, Suite 110
Rockville, MD 20850
301/294-0600

National Parent Resource Institute for
  Drug Education (PRIDE)
50 Hurt Plaza, Suite 210
Atlanta, GA 30303
404/577-4500

Fair Oaks Hospital
19 Prospect Street
Summit, NJ 07901
800/COCAINE

30

The Environment and Health

How pure is the soil in which the food grows? How clean is the air? How unpolluted the water? How healthy the animals that provide substantial portions of our diets?

Americans were asking such questions with increasing frequency in the 1980s. Their concern had a basis in historic fact. Newspaper reports had for years told of the spread of toxic wastes, of the threat of radiation from nuclear power plants, of seepages of poisonous chemicals, and of polluted drinking water. The Environmental Protection Agency (EPA), established in 1970, had the task of monitoring the environment, but the agency could not prevent such accidents as Three-Mile Island, leaks of toxic gases and liquids in at least four states in 1983, and a toxic gas leak at a chemical plant in West Virginia in 1985. The latter accident raised new fears concerning health that had been generated by a 1984 accident that took 2,000 lives in Bhopal, India.

It became obvious that individual and public health depended on factors that were, in part, beyond governmental control. No one suggested that the American economy should shut down until every possible source of contamination had been removed or neutralized. But because the health fears were so real and so widespread, the environment—all of it, natural and manmade—became the focus of intense interest.

Today's Challenges

Can the health hazards in the environment be reduced or eliminated without hurting the American system and without changing Americans' lifestyles? Most experts believe it is possible.

Harmful ingredients in the environment may be the result of pollution, accidental or intentional. But some toxic substances enter the environment as a result of deliberate planning. Asbestos, for example, a mineral fiber that will not burn, has been widely used to insulate and fireproof buildings. The EPA called a halt to the use of asbestos in construction in the 1970s, when researchers proved that the fiber caused diseases such as *asbestosis,* a lung ailment, and several forms of cancer. Excluding such problems, the major health hazards fall in four main categories: Air, water, and noise pollution and food contamination. Some other hazards, including toxic wastes, nuclear radiation, and workplace dangers, received special attention.

Air Pollution

Air pollutants can damage health in a number of ways. Even where little scientific proof links these pollutants to specific maladies, much statistical or circumstantial evidence suggests that air pollution can lead to various forms of respiratory disease. Some cases of air pollution outside the workplace and exclusive of nuclear radiation hazards have been documented.

Inversions

An inversion is a freak weather condition in which a mass of warm air rests like a lid on top of cooler air. The warm air traps the lower air and prevents the pollutants in it from being ventilated. The results can be deadly.

Donora, Pennsylvania, experienced an inversion in 1948. Situated in a valley, at the center of an industrial complex, the town found its air becoming more and more polluted over a six-day period. Residents eventually had difficulty breathing; more than half of the valley's 14,000 inhabitants were coughing and gasping for breath. Thousands were hospitalized. Twenty-two persons died. Physicians used adrenalin to keep older people alive. Daytime visibility dwindled to a few yards. Some residents collapsed on the streets and in their homes.

What had happened? The temperature inversion, trapping the smoke and fumes from smoldering slag heaps, trash fires, coal-fueled home heating plants, and smokestacks, had filled the valley's air with soot, sulfur dioxide, and other pollutants.

Sulfur Dioxide

Sulfur dioxide enters the air from many sources. In the main, however, it is spewed into the atmosphere when heavy fuel oil and coal are burned to provide heat, generate electricity, and provide industrial power. Large cities are especially vulnerable because of their concentrations of heavy industry.

Sulfur dioxide apparently irritates the lungs and leads to a reduction of the lungs' oxygen-handling capacity. Persons who are particularly susceptible to carbon and sulfur dioxide-filled smogs are those suffering from bronchial asthma, chronic bronchitis, and emphysema. The respiratory systems of such persons are already defective. In emphysema, for example, the elasticity of the air sacs in the lungs has progressively broken down, usually after prolonged infection or repeated bronchial irritation. Cigarette smoking can produce such irritation; the sulfur dioxide only worsens the situation.

Lead

Substantial evidence indicates that lead in the air can cause neurological harm and impair body chemistry and bone growth. Most of the airborne lead comes from auto and smelter emissions. These are inhaled directly or they may "soak" food crops. Children are most immediately affected because they have fewer natural defenses against toxic absorption than adults. But adults too may feel the effects of such absorption. They may, for example, feel tired, cramped, or confused.

Because their bodies absorb and metabolize substances rapidly, children may have rates of lead absorption four times as high as those of adults. Workers in some industries, including the ceramic, glass, and lead industries, are also at risk. One study showed that 44 percent of the lead workers in two U.S. smelters suffered from clinical poisoning.

Specific effects of lead poisoning range across a broad spectrum. The formation of red blood cells may be inhibited even by low-level exposure to lead in the air. At higher levels, lead may cause anemia. In children, bone cell growth may be stunted; in pregnant women, lead may prevent the normal development of the fetal skeleton. But lead affects the brain primarily, in some cases interfering with motor skills, auditory development, memory, and the nervous system. Children with higher levels of lead absorption have been found to have serious learning disabilities. Fortunately, lead levels may fluctuate, and the lead in blood and soft tissue may pass out of the human system four to six weeks after exposure ends. But lead remains in bone for periods lasting as long as three decades.

Other Fuel Contaminants

Auto exhausts are major sources of other air pollutants besides lead. Exhaust emissions, for example, may include nitrogen oxides, carbon monoxide, hydrocarbons, and soot. The latter is made up of visible particles of carbon suspended in the air.

How can these substances affect your health? Nitrogen oxides irritate the eyes and the respiratory tract. When nitrogen oxide and hydrocarbons mix in sunlight, they form other noxious substances in the typical photochemical smog that has a yellowish cast. The new ingredients include *ozone,* a poisonous form of oxygen, and peroxyacetyl nitrate (PAN), which is intensely irritating to the eyes. Los Angeles was the first city to experience these smogs; they now occur in many other cities as well.

Worst of all, auto exhaust hydrocarbons include varieties that are possible *carcinogens,* causes of cancer in susceptible individuals. Carbon monoxide, another major hazard, is a colorless, odorless gas that is lethal even in small concentrations because it combines with hemoglobin and thus readily replaces oxygen in the blood. In concentrations that have been measured in heavy city traffic, carbon monoxide can make you tired, headachy, drowsy, and careless.

Acid Rain

While so-called *acid rain* has not been found to harm humans directly, scientists say it has begun to damage the natural food chain in certain regions. As industrial smokestacks emit pollutants, including sulfur and nitrogen oxides, these rise into the upper atmosphere. Mixed with water vapor and other substances, the airborne chemicals are changed by sunlight, becoming tiny acid droplets. The droplets fall to earth as rain or snow, raising the acid content of freshwater lakes and damaging trees and other plants. Under conditions of extreme acidity, fish populations have disappeared; where the food web is disrupted, aquatic animals, algae, and bacteria may dwindle in number. The effects of acid rain on crops and trees are less apparent but are thought to be harmful.

To some extent, acid rain is a geographic phenomenon in North America. Factories in the midwestern industrial belt throw off most of the pollutants, which are then carried east and north. Southeastern Canada and the northeastern and eastern regions of the United States are the areas primarily affected.

Indoor Air Pollution

Reports of illness associated with office and other nonresidential buildings have given rise to what has been termed the "sick building syndrome." The causes of this syndrome, or complex of symptoms, have not been completely and precisely explained. Among the possible explanations are the following:

- Building ventilation has been reduced to conserve energy, with the result that ventilation is simply inadequate

- Indoor air has become contaminated by emissions from the building fabric and associated systems, furnishings, office equipment, or maintenance materials

- Entrainment or cross contamination has taken place, with contaminants generated in a different part of the building or in a separate building drawn in by an air-handling system

- Bioeffluents, or volatile human substances, spread throughout a building, polluting the air with pyruvic acid, lactic acid, acetaldehyde, butyric acid, carbon dioxide, and other body effluents

- Combustion byproducts from smoking tobacco have produced substances, smoke included, that contaminate indoor air

- Microorganisms or airborne particles from molds, dust mites, and other sources cause such illnesses as Legionnaires Disease

A common tendency has been to identify a public building's heating, ventilating, and air conditioning (HVAC) system as the cause of indoor air pollution. But that conclusion may be premature and overly nonspecific. The symptoms described by persons affected by the sick building syndrome should be studied closely. At least four separate illnesses have been isolated according to their symptoms and causes. Hypersensitivity Pneumonitis and Humidifier Fever usually produce such symptoms as coughing, wheezing, chest tightness, muscular aches, chills, headache, fever, and fatigue. While these conditions are rarely fatal, Legionnaires Disease, produced by the bacterium *Legionella pneumonophilae,* is notable because of its 15 to 20 percent mortality rate. Both Legionnaires Disease and the relatively less serious Pontiac Fever are identified by their pneumonialike symptoms.

Household Chemicals

Depending on its location, structural characteristics, and other factors, the typical home may have as many as 350 or more organic chemical pollutants in its interior air. Household chemical products like spray paints, insecticides, and furniture polish disperse tiny (and toxic) droplets into the air, adding the propellant to the chemicals in the basic product. Among the hazard-producing chemicals, some solvents in particular are known or suspected carcinogens. One of the worst is methylene chloride, found in paint sprays and paint strippers and in some hair sprays and insecticides. Product labels may identify methylene chloride as a "chlorinated solution" or as "aromatic hydrocarbons."

Radon

After cigarette smoking, say scientists, the second leading cause of lung cancer may be radon gas. Considered by many to be the most dangerous of all indoor air pollutants, radon, a naturally occurring radioactive gas, diffuses out of the ground into houses that happen to be built above subsurface sources.

Invading homes, according to the U.S. Environmental Protection Agency, radon causes between 5,000 and 20,000 lung cancer deaths annually. The gas breaks down into unstable elements called "radon daughters"; these become attached to particles of dust or other matter floating in the air. If breathed in, the radon daughters lodge in the linings of the lungs. Radioactive decay takes place almost at once, with the daughters emitting alpha particles that damage the adjacent lung cells, sometimes causing cancer.

Private homes can be tested for radon and, if hazardous levels are found, can be equipped with ventilation or other equipment to remove the health threat. A charcoal-based detector is available. Finally, many firms can conduct home radon checks for a fee.

Water Pollution

To an increasing extent, water pollution has prevented or limited use of many once-valuable sources of water. This progressive deterioration of the nation's water supply has resulted from years of abuse in which natural lakes and waterways were inundated with quantities of raw sewage, waste products of industrial plants and slaughterhouses, petroleum residues, poisonous herbicides and insecticides, and so on. But the pollutants generally fall into two categories: materials that change with time and contact with water, and materials that remain unchanged in form. Organic materials in sewage and such industrial wastes as pulp and paper effluents belong in the first group; inorganic salts like sodium sulfate and such inert inorganic materials as pesticides represent the second.

Where do the pollutants come from? Communities generate thousands of tons of municipal sewage daily. Industries, the greatest users of water, utilize more than half of all the water consumed in the United States for raw material, heating and cooling processes, and transporting, sorting, and washing operations. Agriculture, the second largest user, requires millions of gallons of water for irrigation and drainage; for spraying orchards and crops, often with insecticides, fungicides, or herbicides; for removal of animal and other organic wastes; and for manufacturing operations such as meat packing and canning.

Chemical Contamination

The continuing proliferation of chemicals, many of them toxic, suggests the dimensions of the problems relating to water pollution. One estimate by the EPA's Office of Toxic Substances indicated that more than 70,000 chemicals are manufactured or processed commercially in the United States. About 1,000 new chemical compounds are added annually. Literally hundreds of these compounds find their ways into the nation's water supply, some in potentially dangerous concentrations.

How directly and to what degree

chemical contaminants contribute to America's health bill cannot be gauged with accuracy. But the roles of these contaminants as carcinogens is widely accepted. Federal health officials have estimated that environmental carcinogens, including those in water, account for 55 to 60 percent of all U.S. cancer cases annually. Some estimates run much higher.

Heavy Metals

Attention has focused on the heavy metals. A study by the U.S. Geological Survey reported that small amounts of seven toxic metals were present in many of the nation's lakes and streams, with dangerous concentrations occurring occasionally. The metals are mercury, arsenic, cadmium, chromium, cobalt, lead, and zinc. Aside from being generally poisonous, some of these metals are implicated in specific health problems. Cadmium, as one example, has been linked to hypertension caused by kidney malfunction. Some other substances represent special situations.

Mercury

Because mercury is heavier than water, experts thought for years that it could be dumped into lakes, the oceans, and waterways. In theory, the mercury would lie harmlessly on the bottom. In reality, bacteria can convert some of the metallic part of the element into water-soluble form. The new compound enters the food chain and ends up in fish. When dangerous levels of this form of mercury were found in some waters and in food fish, warnings were issued regarding canned tuna and swordfish. The government later announced that 97 percent of the tuna on the market was safe to eat. But lakes and rivers across the country were closed to commercial and sport fishing.

An extremely toxic substance, mercury can, even in small concentrations, produce blindness, paralysis, and brain damage. The U.S. Food and Drug Administration has established the safe limit of mercury in food at half a part per million—about the equivalent of a thimbleful in an Olympic-sized swimming pool.

PCBs

Among the chief water pollutants today are the *polycholorinated biphenyls* (PCBs), highly toxic chemicals used industrially in carbonless copying paper and as an additive in lubricants, paints, printing inks, coatings, waxes, and many other products. PCBs, which are *biodegradable* (capable of decomposing) only over a period of years, have been found in unusually large quantities in waterways downstream from manufacturing plants. The EPA banned the direct discharge of PCBs into any U.S. waterway in 1977 after tests showed that fish in some rivers, like the Hudson, had levels of PCBs far higher than the permissible levels.

No one knows what the long-term effects of ingesting small quantities of PCBs will be. But the chemical is a suspected carcinogen. PCB's have also caused severe skin and eye irritations and have been implicated in reproductive disorders, kidney damage, and liver ailments. Researchers believe that the millions of pounds of PCBs in the nation's water or in landfills will take many years to dissipate.

Sludge

Sewage treatment plants around the country also face the major health challenge of disposing of the sludge, or solid matter, that is removed from sewage in the treatment process. Sludge contains not only human wastes but the residues of petroleum products, detergents, toxic heavy metals such as cadmium, lead, and zinc, and many other contaminants. Disposal methods range from dumping on land to burning and to composting for use as fertilizer. But environmental experts maintain that the use of sludge as fertilizer constitutes a health hazard; and major food processors will not accept food grown with sludge as fertilizer. In refusing such food, the companies are following guidelines set by the National Food Processors Association, which has expressed concern for farm workers' health and for the health of the consumer.

The sludge comes from an estimated 6.8 billion gallons of sewage flushed daily into America's sewers. The sewage itself contains microorganisms that can endanger health. You may be risking gastrointestinal upsets if you swim at a beach that is posted with a sign proclaiming "polluted water." Scientists warn that the fish caught in sewage-polluted coastal waters and harbors may not only be cancerous; they may also be carcinogenic. A number of states including Michigan and New York have restricted or banned sales of tainted fish such as naturally grown carp, catfish, and striped bass.

Oil Spills

With the increasing reliance on supertankers to carry industrial and heating oil from abroad, the danger of major water-polluting oil spills in coastal areas has grown substantially. Several of these huge ships have gone aground and broken apart under heavy pounding by sea waves. Their cargoes have spilled into the oceans, where currents usually carry them many miles before they float ashore or sink to the ocean floor. The oil reaching land fouls beaches and kills water birds. Similar accidents on inland waterways have polluted rivers and lakes, killing fish and spoiling recreational areas.

Noise Pollution

"Pollution" refers generally to the various forms of physical pollution by liquids, gases, or solids. Few persons realize that we are all threatened by a pollutant so common that it tends to be overlooked: noise.

Noise assails us nearly everywhere. It fills homes with loud music or the dog's barking or the grinding of the washing machine and the workplace with the chatter of drill presses and the roar of huge engines. Neither city dwellers nor country people can live noise-free today; none of us can escape car and truck horns, motorcycles that belch sound, and the noisy throb of machinery.

Effects of Sound on the Eardrum

Noise is not just annoying; it is potentially dangerous, both physically and mentally. It has been described as "a slow agent of death." A form of energy, sound or noise is caused by anything that vibrates, that moves back and forth. Our ears receive the effects of this vibrating motion from a distance, great or small, via sound waves. These waves are successive series of regions of compressed air and partial vacuums, or areas of high and low air pressure. Sound can also travel through liquids and solids. We *hear* sound because our eardrums are moved back and forth by the changes in air pressure. The eardrum, or *tympanic membrane*, may perceive a sound that moves it only one billionth of a centimeter—the threshold of hearing. If the intensity of sound pressure becomes too great, we experience pain, and the eardrum or the delicate structures inside the ear may be damaged.

The intensity of sounds is often measured in units called *decibels,* or *db.* These units are logarithmic, that is, 10 db is ten times as powerful as 1 db, 20 db is 100 times as powerful, 30 db is 1,000 times as powerful, and so on. On this scale, 0 db is at the threshold of hearing; rustling leaves, 20 db; a quiet office, about 50 db; conversation, 60 db; heavy traffic, 90 db; a pneumatic jackhammer six feet away, 100 db; a jet aircraft 500 feet overhead, 115 db; a Saturn rocket's takeoff, 180 db.

For most people, the pain threshold is about 120 db; deafening ear damage can result at 150 db. But damage of various kinds can come from much lower exposures. Temporary hearing impairment can result from sounds over the 85 db now found in modern kitchens with all appliances going. If the ears do not get a chance to recover, the impairment will become permanent.

Damage to the Inner Ear

Although very loud noise can damage the eardrum, most physiological damage from noise occurs in the snail-shaped, liquid-filled *cochlea,* or inner ear. Sound transmitted to the cochlea produces waves in the liquid, which in turn move delicate and minute structures called hair cells or *cilia* in that part of the cochlea known as the organ of Corti. The motion of the cilia is transformed into electrical impulses that conduct the sensation of sound to the brain.

The cilia can easily be fatigued by noise, causing a temporary loss of hearing, or a shift in the threshold of hearing. If they are not given a chance to recuperate, they will be permanently damaged, and irreversible hearing loss will result. There are some 23,000 cilia in the average cochlea; different sets of cilia respond to different frequency bands. The cilia responding to sound frequencies of

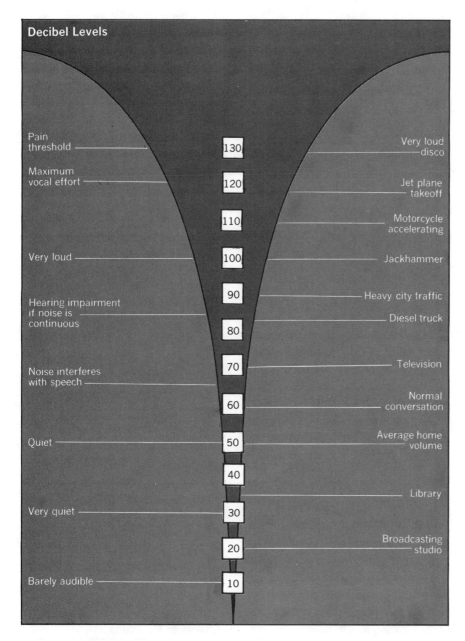

Decibel Levels

Pain threshold	130	Very loud —disco
Maximum vocal effort	120	Jet plane takeoff
	110	Motorcycle accelerating
Very loud	100	Jackhammer
	90	Heavy city traffic
Hearing impairment if noise is continuous	80	Diesel truck
	70	Television
Noise interferes with speech	60	Normal conversation
Quiet	50	Average home volume
	40	
Very quiet	30	Library
	20	Broadcasting studio
Barely audible	10	

4,000 to 6,000 cps (cycles per second) are especially vulnerable to damage. The region of 85 to 95 db is generally regarded as the beginning of dangerous sound intensities. In general, the louder the noise, the longer it lasts, the higher it is, and the purer in frequency, the more dangerous it is. Thus, jet engines and powerful sirens are particularly hazardous.

Noise and Stress

The EPA has estimated that some 20 million Americans live or work at noise levels that could cause hearing losses; about 18 million have experienced at least some hearing loss because of noise exposure. But sound, or noise, can lead to physical and psychological problems ranging from irritability to migraine headaches. Linked with many such problems is stress, which has been found to cause high blood pressure, insomnia, ulcers, digestive disorders, alcoholism, anxiety, and many other ills.

Excessive noise has been implicated in such problems as adrenaline flow, elevated heart rates, and blood pressure. All are associated with heart disease. Noise can also affect children in special ways. For example, researchers believe it can retard language development and impair reading ability. Pregnant women exposed to excessive noise may show symptoms of stress and may pass on the harmful effects to their unborn babies. Studies in several countries have shown that the newborns of women living near airport runways experience a higher than normal incidence of birth defects.

Noise-related stress has a definite effect on mental well-being. No one knows exactly how, but noise can produce irritability, tension, and nervous strain. More seriously, British medical authorities have reported a significantly higher incidence of mental illness among people exposed constantly to aircraft noise.

Workplace Noise

Workplace noise presents special problems. Persons working in such industries as construction, mining, steel, lumber, and textiles are almost universally exposed to loud noises. Certain operations in other industries expose workers to high decibel levels. Overexposure takes place when employees work eight hours a day at sites with noise levels exceeding 90 decibels. Such standards, established by the government's Occupational Safety and Health Administration (OSHA), provide also that overexposure occurs where workers are subjected to higher decibel levels for shorter periods.

Workplace noise can lead to problems similar to those produced by overexposure elsewhere. But many workers have little choice as regards the places where they work. For their parts, companies may have limited options insofar as noise control or abatement is concerned. Changing the gears of a machine or building an enclosure around it may not always be feasible.

Some professional musicians find it difficult or impossible to avoid excessive noise on the job. Rock music artists, for example, spend hours at a stretch in enclosed places that magnify sound that is already greatly amplified. Such persons may be at serious risk of incurring hearing losses.

Food Hazards

Contaminants found in water often make their way into food products in the cooking and packaging processes, so that many of the comments on water pollution apply here. Some dilute water pollutants become highly concentrated as they pass up the food chain and end in fish or other foods for man. Mercury was cited earlier as one example. Contamination of food with harmful microorganisms is an everpresent concern wherever standards of cleanliness and sanitation are low.

Additives

Food entails a whole new set of problems because of the thousands of new ingredients that have been added to it, directly and indirectly, in recent years. These substances include many that have been deemed necessary because of the revolution in food technology: the rise of packaged convenience foods of all kinds. Labels on today's convenience foods list preservatives, nutrients, flavors, colors, and processing agents. The trouble with food additives is that we have had little time to learn about their long-term effects on the body. The Food and Drug Administration does set standards in this area; but in the opinion of many experts, these safeguards are inadequate.

What do the additives do and what are they? What kinds of health hazards do they present? The principal kinds are explained below.

Nutrients

Some additives are simply vitamins and minerals that increase the nutritional value of food. Iodine is added to salt as a goiter preventative; vitamins A and D go into fortified milk. The vitamin and mineral additives are generally beneficial.

Preservatives

Preservatives do what the name implies: they protect against spoilage from molds, yeasts, or bacteria, or prevent oxidation. In the first category are such substances as salt, sugar, vinegar, and—among the controversial additives—sodium nitrate, sodium nitrite, and the sulfiting agents. Where some of these substances guard against illnesses like salmonella and *Clostridium botulinum*, or botulism, a deadly form of food poisoning, the controversial types may cause serious illnesses and even cancers. For example, nitrates and nitrites can combine with the amines in protein to become nitrosamines, powerful carcinogens.

The antioxidants include lecithin from soybeans, ascorbic acid (vitamin C), and *butylated hydroxytoluene* (BHT) and *butylated hydroxyanisole* (BHA). The latter two have been studied because they appear to protect against stomach cancer and liver damage.

Flavors

Of the more than 1,500 different flavors used in food, some are natural and some synthetic. Among the natural flavors are cinnamon, vanilla, and citrus oils. The synthetics, some of

which, like vanillin, have exactly the same chemical compositions as their originals, include monosodium glutamate (MSG), hydrolyzed vegetable protein, and maltol. MSG in particular has become controversial because it can cause "Chinese restaurant syndrome," with temporary headaches, dizziness, and other unpleasant symptoms.

Colors

As a group, the color additives are the most controversial. But they range from beta carotene, a yellow coloring that is used in carrots and sweet potatoes and is beneficial, to a number of coal tar dyes. The FDA has banned as unsafe more than a dozen of the latter in recent years. Others are readily available and are widely used in cereals, baked goods, ice cream, and beverages.

Processing Agents

Many useful processing agents, including yeast and baking soda, are standard kitchen items. They help to control stability, moisture, texture, and other food qualities and characteristics.

Chemical Residues

Some toxic substances found in food appear in the natural environment. An example: the trace amounts of arsenic in cow's milk. Other poisons are introduced into the environment by humans. These, including fungicides, herbicides, and pesticides, have aroused deep concern among environmentalists and a growing number of private physicians.

American farmers use more than 350 approved agricultural chemicals, including about one billion pounds of insecticides annually. Because of such heavy use, about 52 percent of the average American's diet contains one or more kinds of chemical residues. Measured often in parts-per-billion, these can collect in human bodies. Permanent damage can result, according to researchers. Among the compounds are not only weed- and bug-killers like parathion but also growth-enhancers like daminozide.

Researchers warn of other problems with contaminated food. The use of antibiotics in livestock feed, for example, promotes the development of bacteria that resist antibiotics. As one result, humans who eat beef or pork that is improperly cooked may acquire infections that resist penicillin or tetracycline.

Irradiated Foods

Consumer groups have urged further study and cautious use of irradiation as a means of preserving many foods. At least 30 countries have approved radiation exposure to retard spoilage and aging; but concerns remain. They focus particularly on the nutritional losses thay may occur if foods are exposed to more than one kind of preservative, on the effects of radiation exposure on workers handling irradiated foods, and on environmental hazards that could emerge in the transport, storage, and handling of radioactive food-processing wastes.

The possible long-term effects of irradiation have led to other concerns. Radiation kills the salmonella microorganism, but may not affect more virulent and dangerous bacteria such as those responsible for botulism and may, over time, strengthen those other organisms. Irradiation might even produce dangerous mutations of some bacteria. Researchers point out further that meat can become contaminated after irradiation, indicating that other preservatives might have to be used.

Other Hazards

Toxic Wastes

Various estimates place the number of toxic-waste disposal sites in the United States at 14,000 to 20,000. Poisonous substances left over from industrial processes are buried or simply dumped at these sites, many of which present serious health hazards. Primarily, according to scientists, the open dumps, landfills, bulk storage containers, and surface impoundments at the thousands of sites spill toxic chemicals into the surrounding soil and through it into groundwater systems. Noxious fumes and even flames burst from some sites at unpredictable moments. The wastes include a huge variety of substances, among them chlorinated solvents, aromatic hydrocarbons, pesticides, trace metals, and PCBs.

The locations of many waste disposal sites remain unknown, often, until a health or environmental problem is detected. Thus the health threats posed by waste dumps may lie dormant for years and may surface only after a container has rusted through or seepage has brought poisonous slush into contact with drinking-water sources.

Waste chemicals can enter the body through skin contact and inhalation as well as ingestion. But the latter is the most common method. Where dosage is substantial, ingestion usually leads to toxic effects on the liver and kidneys. Other parts of the body may be affected as well. Skin contact may produce lesions while inhalation can have direct respiratory effects.

Improved methods of disposing of toxic wastes have combined with public awareness and governmental action to build hopes of reduced waste problems in the future. In the mean-time, as environmentalists contend, the thousands of existing toxic-waste sites pose continuing health hazards.

Nuclear Radiation

Among the most dangerous of all pollutants is nuclear or "ionizing" radiation. Made up of particles of energy, this radiation can attack the atoms that form the body's cells, causing both short- and long-term damage. Human tissues like skin, bone-marrow, and intestinal cells, all of which reproduce rapidly, feel the impact of radiation most intensely. But different isotopes in ionizing radiation concentrate in different body tissues, sometimes causing cancer or genetic mutations many years after exposure. Of the most common radioactive elements in radiation from a nuclear power plant, barium resembles calcium and therefore concentrates in the bones while iodine 131 concentrates in the thyroid.

Completely invisible, radiation reaches the earth from various natural and manmade sources. Some comes from the sun and outer space; larger amounts are given off by radioactive materials, including waste from nuclear power plants, the fallout from nuclear weapons explosions, and various electronic devices. The numbers of such devices are increasing steadily; among them are lasers, X-ray machines, TV sets, and microwave ovens.

The damage done to the human body as a result of exposure to radiation varies with the intensity of the "dose" and the isotopes involved. A dose of radiation above 1,000 rem, a unit of measurement, is always fatal. Smaller doses, with exposure over an extended period of time, may also be fatal. Victims can protect themselves to a limited degree if given time. For example, they can guard against thyroid cancer by taking potassium iodide. Ingested in pill form, the medication loads the thyroid gland with iodine, thus "blocking" the iodine 131 isotope and preventing its concentration in the thyroid.

In a simple operation physicians can transplant marrow into persons exposed to the barium isotope, and thus reduce the possibility of bone-marrow syndrome. This illness cripples the body's immune system. But donor marrow must match that of the victim, and the relatives of a victim are those most likely to supply marrow that is a genetic match. If the relatives have also been exposed to radiation, no donors may qualify.

Workplace Dangers

Air and noise pollution are, as noted, common in certain industries. The materials and machines used in manufacturing processes are the usual causes of such pollution. Many controls have been mandated by the federal Occupational Safety and Health Administration, but researchers have reported that some industries are experiencing increased health hazards, largely because of the materials they use.

High-tech microelectronics plants are especially threatened. According to scientists, many such plants use toxic chemicals that have been linked to reproductive disorders in both men and women. Among the high-tech hazards usually cited are glycol ethers, widely used as a solvent by manufacturers of printed circuit boards; arsenic, an element in the manufacture of some semiconductor chips; and lead, used in soldering and other operations. Some semiconductor plants are also employing radio-frequency radiation in potentially dangerous amounts to etch and clean silicon wafers.

31

Health Insurance

Health insurance has two basic purposes. It provides for reimbursement to families or individuals for health care costs. It may also guarantee replacement income when a person is unable to work because of sickness or injury. Reimbursement insurance can cover virtually all types of expenses connected with hospital care, medical treatment, and related services. Disability insurance usually calls for periodic payments to make up for lost income.

From another perspective, health insurance offers protection to both groups and individuals. The groups may be company work forces that have *group insurance* as a benefit. Individuals can buy insurance from as many as 1,000 commercial insurance companies offering a huge variety of plans.

Some insurers are general insurance companies. Others are hospital and medical service plans such as Blue Cross and Blue Shield, group medical prepayment plans such as health maintenance organizations (HMOs), and others.

What Health Insurance Is and Does

"Health insurance" means a number of things. It may be called "accident and health insurance" or "disability insurance." Various types of policies have other names. The different descriptions indicate that the policies vary as regards the types of expenses covered. While some policies cover hospital expenses only, others may cover virtually all kinds of medical expenses.

Two Types of Coverage

In general, private health insurance coverage is one of two kinds: *group* and *individual*. Employers, unions, and other kinds of organizations typically provide group insurance as an employee or membership benefit. An individual can buy individual insurance whether or not he or she is covered under a group policy. But a good group policy usually covers all the major health problems or contingencies that a person could face under normal circumstances.

Group insurance has a number of specific advantages over individual coverage, among them the following:

- Because a number of people can be included under a single contract, with consequent savings to the insurer in sales, administrative, and claims costs, the insurer can charge less per individual covered.

- In most cases the company, union, or organization holding the group contract pays part or all of the individual premiums.

- With group insurance the health of the individual insured person is usually not a major factor in determining eligibility. The insurance company is more interested in the average age and overall health status of the group. The health of individuals may become a selection factor, however, where small groups, 10 or fewer persons, are involved.

- Unless an individual leaves a job or gives up a membership, his or her group coverage cannot be canceled. Termination of the group plan itself would, of course, terminate coverage.

Despite such advantages, individual and family policies fulfill at least two fundamental needs. First, they provide coverage for persons who are not members of an insured group. Such policies may also cover those who cannot, for whatever reason, obtain group coverage. Second, the individual or family policy can provide supplementary coverage where a group plan does not meet all basic health insurance needs.

Group and individual plans differ in basic ways. Where a group policy establishes the level of benefits for all group members, the individual policy can more easily be tailored to specific requirements.' With the individual policy, too, each person or family is enrolled separately. The cost of individual insurance is usually substantially higher because the insurer considers the age, health status of the insured, and other factors when setting premium rates.

Principles of Health Insurance

Private or commercial health insurance programs function according to some key principles. Primarily, these programs are based on the theory that a relatively small, regular payment, the premium, can protect the insured against what might be a sizable loss.

A companion principle holds that the insured must pay the expenses of operating an insurance system. These expenses include the costs of maintaining offices, investigating claims, and otherwise administering the system as well as paying benefits.

Two other principles underlie the operation of most health insurance programs:

- The *large-loss principle,* which holds that the insured should try to obtain protection only against those costs or losses that he or she could not bear financially. Under this principle the contract may exclude from reimbursement some specific kinds of costs. Most such policies contain a "deductible" clause specifying that the insured must pay a certain amount of initial costs.

  Major medical insurance plans probably exemplify best the large-loss, or large-risk, principle. These policies nearly always provide for a deductible. The higher the deductible, as a rule, the lower the premium.

- The *first-dollar principle,* under which the policy pays the full cost of all covered hospital and medical expenses. Policies of this kind have no deductible clauses.

  Advocates of first-dollar policies stress the need for preventive health care. The policy in theory encourages the insured to see a physician and obtain treatment before a health problem becomes worse or even unmanageable.

Kinds of Insurance Plans

Voluntary or private health insurance plans offer protection against a broad range of hospital and medical expenses. Some policies offer protection against a single illness such as cancer while others insure individuals, families, or groups against nearly all medical contingencies. Some of the many kinds of coverage are as follows:

Hospital

Blue Cross plans and most other commercial plans provide room benefits at a specified rate per day. Usually, they also cover miscellaneous hospital services, including drugs, operating room, and laboratory services up to a given cost level. Some commercial plans and most Blue Cross plans cover all costs in a semiprivate, or shared, room.

Surgical

Typically, health insurance policies cover the costs of surgery according to a schedule that establishes specified amounts for listed procedures. The insurance contract sets a payment of so many dollars for an appendectomy or a tonsillectomy, for example, with that payment going toward coverage of the surgeon's bill. In the case of Blue Shield, certain surgeons perform surgical operations for low-income subscribers for no additional charge.

Regular Medical

This is a form of insurance that provides coverage of physicians' fees in cases that do not involve surgery. The medical care may be provided in the home, in a hospital, or in a physician's office. A regular medical policy may also cover diagnostic X-ray and other laboratory expenses.

Major Medical

As noted, major medical policies usually provide for deductibles. After an insured has reached a specified hospital-medical expense level, the insurer will also pay, for example, 80 percent of all remaining expenses to a set maximum. The maximum may be $1 million or more. Some policies offer unlimited coverage. In some cases the policy sets a maximum, perhaps $5,000, $10,000, or $25,000, for a given illness in a one- or three-year period. Where an insurance company and the insured pay percentages of all costs beyond a deductible, the policy is said to be a form of "coinsurance."

Comprehensive or Comprehensive Major Medical

This kind of health policy combines hospital, major medical, and surgical coverage in one contract. Generally, little or no deductible applies to hospital and surgical charges. But the major medical coverage ordinarily comes with a deductible.

Dental

Basic or comprehensive protection, covering the costs of hospital care, surgery, and physicians' services, may also include dental insurance. A basic plan may establish a set of allowances for each procedure to an annual maximum of, for example, $500 or $1,000. A comprehensive policy would cover, typically, 80 percent of all dental expenses above a specified minimum.

Special Perils

While frowned upon by many insurance experts, "special perils" plans continue to appear. They cover such specific health hazards as cancer, polio, and vision problems.

Auto and Travel

Many insurance companies offer auto and travel policies that cover insured persons in the event of injury or death in an accident. Such policies may provide protection against almost any travel accident in various kinds of vehicles.

Income

Insurance against loss of income gives the insured person a flow of cash if, because of illness or disability, he or she cannot work. A commercial policy that limits coverage to accidental disability usually costs much less than broader coverage, or it provides for greater benefits. Accidental disability payments, usually monthly, may continue for life. Payments for disability resulting from illness are commonly limited to 6, 12, or more months depending on the terms of the contract.

Many policies provide only for *hospital income insurance*. Such insurance pays a stipulated cash payment for every day of hospitalization. Insurance companies offer these policies to individuals only, not to groups.

Basic Protection

Of the various kinds of comprehensive health insurance, the so-called "basic protection" plan ranks among the most common. Basic protection offers coverage for the costs of hospital care and services and physicians' services.

Most basic protection policies specify that hospital room and board benefits will be paid in one of two ways. One kind of policy provides for reimbursement for actual room and board charges up to a set daily maximum. Another kind offers a service type of benefit equaling the hospital's established semiprivate room and board rates. If the insured occupies a private room, he or she pays the additional room charge.

Surgical-Expense Insurance

Basic policies that provide hospital expense coverage generally offer surgical-expense benefits as well. That means coverage may extend to operations and postoperative, inpatient physicians' visits. The policy then becomes a "hospital-and-surgical-expense" or "hospital-surgical" plan.

Surgical-expense insurance normally pays benefits whether illness or accident makes the surgery necessary. Coverage may include benefits for anesthetics. A schedule of surgical procedures and specified maximum benefits for each may be part of such a policy. Physicians' fees may be covered to a "reasonable and customary" level for the particular city or region. In this case the policy would not contain a surgical schedule.

Physician's-Expense Insurance

The counterpart of the surgical-expense policy is the physician's-expense plan. This policy offers benefits to help cover the costs of nonsurgical physicians' services in a hospital, home, or office. The terms of the policy usually provide for maximum payments for specified services. The latter may include diagnostic X-ray and other laboratory expenses.

Policy Provisions

Purchasing health insurance calls for close attention to the provisions of any given policy. Little standardization exists among the hundreds of types of policies, a factor that makes the buyer's task a difficult one. In four areas in particular the buyer should scrutinize closely the "fine print" in an individual, but not a group, policy.

Provisions Relating to Other Policies

Many policies include clauses that limit or prohibit payments where the policyholder has other insurance covering the same loss or expense. In this way insurers protect themselves against overpayments for specific losses. A typical clause of this kind reduces benefits payments to the policy's prorated share of the insured person's actual expenses.

Preexisting Conditions

Most individual health insurance policies exclude preexisting conditions. That means they do not cover at all, or do not cover for a stated period, physical or health problems that existed before the policy became effective. The waiting period that must elapse before coverage for a preexisting condition begins may be 30, 60, or more days.

Cancellation and Renewal

All health policies contain cancellation and renewal provisions. One type, the most favorable to the policyholder, specifies that the insurer cannot cancel or refuse to renew the policy before the insured turns 65. The same clause may state that the premium cannot be increased. Because it provides guaranteed coverage, this kind of policy is usually the most expensive.

Many policies contain a widely used modification of the no-cancel, guaranteed renewal clause. This alternative provides that the company must continue the coverage until the insured reaches 65, but that the premium can be increased for entire groups of insured persons. In a third variation, some policies permit the insurer to cancel or refuse to renew the coverage at any time by giving written notice to the policyholder. This kind of policy is the least advantageous to the insured.

"Good-Health" Discounts

Increasingly, the disability, hospital, or medical policy provides for discounts for persons in good health. For example, the policy may specify that the applicant be a nonsmoker who exercises three to five times a week and does not have a high-risk job or hobby. Race-car driving would fall in the latter category.

Discounts of 5 to 15 percent have been available to nonsmokers since the 1960s. New discount arrangements broaden the range of qualifying factors and increase the discount levels. The new trend takes as a model the life insurance plan that may offer discounts of up to 50 percent if the applicant observes basic rules of health and safety. These include, in addition to those named, adhering to a nutritious diet, using seat belts while riding in a car, and avoiding excess salt in diet.

Meeting Special Needs

Some health insurance policies are designed to meet special needs. One common kind of coverage protects persons who are above-average risks: persons with poor health histories, existing problems or illnesses, or chronic disorders of one kind or another. Other types of policies serve other purposes.

Existing Health Problems

Because persons with existing health problems are not average risks, insurance for them may be costly. But an approach to insurance may be made in at least three ways.

1. A policy may exclude entirely the usual benefits for the specified existing condition. The insurance may then provide protection for all or many other conditions. Standard rates or premiums may be charged.

2. Charging a standard rate, the insurer may amend the policy to provide for a longer waiting period before coverage begins. In such a case standard benefits may be available.

3. The policy may call for a higher than normal premium to compensate for the greater degree of risk. Regular benefits might be available.

Some special health coverages have become relatively common. For example, dental-expense insurance helps pay for normal dental care as well as accidental damage. Insurance companies, prepayment plans, and some state dental associations make such coverage available, usually providing for a deductible and for coinsurance.

Special coverage may, finally, be provided for eye care. Many group policies have such coverage.

Insuring the Unemployed and Divorced

Most Americans have health insurance as a job-related benefit. Coverage terminates, however, if an individual quits his or her job, is laid off, or loses the job for whatever reason.

An employee who is leaving a job should find out how long, if at all, coverage will continue after employment terminates. A normal period would be 30 days. In that period the employee is usually allowed to convert the coverage from group to individual. The conversion option means the employee can remain insured by the same company while retaining, usually, reduced benefits. The premium payments generally increase, sometimes dramatically. Where a group policy permits conversion, the insured has the right to convert regardless of existing health problems. No medical examination is required.

Many group policies provide for conversion from group to individual coverage where a divorced person was dependent for protection on the former spouse's group plan. The person needing health coverage has to apply within the specified period, but cannot be rejected for health reasons.

By the middle 1980s, some 25 states had laws requiring "group continuance." By the terms of these laws a divorced spouse or unemployed person could remain in the group and receive the same benefits as before. The insured had only to assume the group cost formerly contributed by the employer for each insured individual. The effect of the group continuance laws was to make it possible for divorced or unemployed persons to retain group coverage for about half of what an individual policy would cost. With some exceptions, state laws limited group continuance periods to a year or less.

"Medigap" Insurance

An estimated 95 percent of all Americans over 65 are protected by Medicare. But the government program covers only a portion of all possible physician and hospital expenses—less than 50 percent. To help bridge the gap between Medicare and the 100 percent coverage that most persons need and want, private insurance companies have developed "medigap" policies.

What do the medigap policies cover? Their terms vary. Most help insured persons to expand existing Medicare coverages. But few offer even partial protection against hospital and medical costs that Medicare does not cover, or does not cover fully. These areas include: routine physical checkups; most prescription drugs; hearing tests and hearing aids; eye examinations and eyeglasses; most dental care, including dentures; private nursing care; and custodial home nursing care.

Because neither Medicare nor medigap insurance covers these areas thoroughly, many elderly persons remain vulnerable. But some medigap policies, including those offered by Blue Cross/Blue Shield and some associations for the elderly, provide for good hospital and physician coverage.

Congress set minimum standards for medigap insurance in 1980. But the Better Business Bureau has warned that the older person in need of additional insurance should shop carefully. Some groups, the BBB states, offer insurance as a means of building membership rolls. The BBB also advises as follows:

- Older buyers should make sure they have the Medicare medical insurance (Part B) as well as the hospital coverage (Part A).

- Insurance buyers should check the reputation of any potential private insurer with the state insurance department and the local Better Business Bureau. Insurance companies are also rated according to their financial health in *Best's Insurance Reports: Life and Health Insurance,* available in most libraries.

- The practice of switching from one insurance company to another because of premium levels can be hazardous: rates charged by any company can increase.

- As a rule, premiums should not be paid for years in advance. Your needs may change.

Five Innovative Plans

Pressures to cut the costs of medical care have given rise to basic changes in the methods of delivering such care in the United States. No longer do most persons simply call their family physicians and, if the physician so advises, go to a specific hospital. More and more, insurance plans and programs offer both choices and restrictions. Five innovative programs in particular have gained in popularity.

Health Maintenance Organizations (HMOs)

Operating clinic-style facilities, HMOs require that their subscribers pay a set monthly premium. In return the HMO provides full medical care. But members have to select their physicians from a list provided by the HMO. If hospitalization is necessary, the subscriber goes to a hospital selected by the organization.

Charging premiums that may be 10 to 20 percent lower than those for equivalent insurance coverage, HMOs provide incentives to avoid unnecessary expenses or treatments. HMOs, for example, encourage subscribers to make use of preventive care to stay healthy. Thus most HMOs offer eye and hearing checkups, as well as podiatry and dental services, at little or no cost beyond a monthly fee.

Many subscribers point to the convenience of HMOs as their major attraction. Subscribers not only have the convenience of full medical and hospital services at one facility; they pay no deductibles and have no claim forms to fill out.

HMOs have won federal support. New rules published in 1985 encouraged Medicare recipients to drop out of the government's medical insurance program and to join HMOs. The usual HMO restrictions on choices of physicians and hospitals would apply; applicants would join a central hospital facility, with its own physicians and specialties, and would be directed to specific physicians approved for HMO patients. Those who make the change have to retain the Medicare Part B coverage.

Former Medicare beneficiaries have various ways to report grievances. They can, for example, write to the U.S. Department of Health and Human Services Office of Health Maintenance Organizations, Compliance Division, Room 9-11, Parklawn Building, 5600 Fishers Lane, Rockville, MD 20857.

Preferred Provider Organizations (PPOs)

In the PPO, subscribers receive care at a discount if they go to physicians and hospitals recommended by the insurer. Generally, the insurance company underwriting the PPO allows employees in insured groups to go to a nonparticipating physician. But in such a case the costs of care rise considerably, sometimes to twice those charged by the listed physicians.

Under the PPO arrangement, physicians, hospitals, and insurers work together to keep down overall costs. A PPO hospital provides care for insured persons at reduced rates. In exchange, the hospital enjoys increased utilization of its facilities.

Managed Care

Unlike the HMO and the PPO, a managed care program gives members the freedom to pick the physicians and hospitals they prefer. But severe cost-containment rules apply. The restrictions may include the following:

- Preadmission reviews of hospital stays by panels of physicians and nurses. A panel would have to agree in all cases, except for maternity care and emergencies, that hospitalization and the proposed care are necessary.

- Reviews during hospitalization to ensure that continued inpatient care is necessary.

- Mandatory second opinions before some operations to make certain a particular procedure is necessary.

- As in some newer group plans,

surgery is performed on an outpatient basis where possible.

Companies adopting managed care plans may offer HMO and PPO plans as well. An eligible employee in such a firm then has a choice of program.

Hospital Chains

Competition among health care providers has led to still another approach to both cost control and hospital utilization. Some for-profit hospital chains have bought insurance companies to obtain insurance licenses, then provided health insurance programs that required the insured to use the chain's facilities.

A variation on the HMO and PPO systems, the hospital chain approach makes possible insurance costs that are 10 to 15 percent lower than those of traditional plans. Chain officials contend that the lower charges are justified by more efficient hospital operation.

Insurance experts note characteristics of the hospital chains' programs that appear to justify caution on the part of the potential buyer. For example, the policies sold by the chains usually impose limits on lifetime benefits. Unlike the plans of such nonprofit groups as Blue Cross/Blue Shield, the chains' policies provide for the termination of certain benefits at specified ages.

Nursing Home Care

Increasingly, major insurance companies have begun to devise policies that would cover the costs of nursing home care for the elderly. Such spe-

cialized plans face a double difficulty. First, the insurance company needs to make a profit off the program of coverage. Second, nursing home costs ranging generally from $15,000 to $50,000 and more per year raise the possibility of enormous claims that could continue for years.

Long-term care insurance marks a start toward a solution. Major insurers have begun to market policies that differ on such points as home health care benefits and the right to renew. But because no actuarial figures are available to show, for example, how many younger policyholders would be needed to offset older beneficiaries, the companies have worked through organizations such as the American Association of Retired Persons (AARP). The memberships of such groups are usually numerous enough to reduce the risks of major claims.

If given a choice, the person shopping for a long-term care policy should ask at least these questions:

- Does the policy put a ceiling on benefits, and at what point?

- Exactly what does the policy cover? No such policies provide coverage for *all* the ills of aging.

- To be eligible for benefits, must the patient be hospitalized before he or she enters a long-term care facility?

- Must a patient's diagnosis cite an organic disease before eligibility can begin?

- Are "mental health" problems, possibly including Alzheimer's disease and senility, excluded from coverage?

32

Home Care of the Sick

Patients suffering from serious illnesses or from certain communicable diseases should be hospitalized. Home care facilities do not normally include the expensive and delicate medical equipment required for the complete care of these diseases.

If, however, the physician in charge of a case decides that his patient does not need hospitalization and that adequate home nursing care can be provided, the well-being of the patient can be greatly enhanced by his being cared for in the comfortable and familiar surroundings of his own home.

When the decision to treat a patient at home is made, it must be understood that the physician's orders regarding rest, exercise, diet, and medications have to be rigorously adhered to. Nursing responsibilities assigned to the patient and whoever else is tending to the patient's recovery should be carried out as conscientiously as they would be if the patient's care were entrusted to a team of medical professionals in a hospital environment.

The physician in charge of a case should, of course, be notified of any significant changes in the condition of the patient. The physician should be contacted if, for example, the patient complains of severe pain, pain of long duration, or pain that apparently is not directly related to an injury or surgical procedure. The location and characteristics of the pain should be noted, and the physician will want to know whether the pain is affected by changing the position of the patient or if it seems to be related to the intake of food or fluids.

In addition to being informed of such potentially dangerous developments, the physician should get daily or frequent reports on the patient's progress. The easiest and best way to see that this is done is to keep a written record of the following functions, symptoms, and conditions of the patient:

- Morning and evening body temperature, pulse rate, and respiration rate

- Bowel movements—frequency, consistency of stools, presence of blood

- Urination—amount, frequency, presence of burning sensation, color

- Vomiting or nausea

- The amount and kind of solid foods and liquids taken by the patient

- Hours of sleep

- Medications given (should be administered only on the instructions of the physician)

- Patient's general appearance (includes any unusual swelling, skin rash, or skin discoloration)

- General mental and psychological condition of the patient, such as signs of irritability or despondency

Checking the Pulse and Respiration

The pulse and respiration are usually checked in the morning and again in the evening; the physician may recommend other times as well.

Pulse

The home nurse should learn how to measure the pulse rate in beats per minute. A watch with a second hand or a nearby electric clock will help count the passage of time while the pulse beat is counted. The pulse can be felt on the inner side of the wrist, above the thumb; the pulse also can be checked at the temple, the throat, or at the ankle if for some reason the wrist is not conveniently accessible.

The patient should be resting quietly when the pulse is counted; if the patient has been physically active the pulse count probably will be higher than normal, suggesting a possible disorder when none actually exists. Temperature extremes, emotional upsets, and the digesting of a meal also can produce misleading pulse rates.

What is a normal pulse rate? The answer is hard to define in standard or average terms. For an adult male, a pulse rate of about 72 per minute is considered normal. The pulse of an adult woman might range around 80 per minute and still be normal. For children, a normal pulse might be one that is regularly well above 100 per minute. Also, a normal pulse may vary by a few beats per minute in either direction from the average for the individual. The home nurse with a bit of practice can determine whether a patient's pulse is significantly fast or slow, strong or weak, and report any important changes to the physician.

Respiration

The patient's respiration can be checked while his pulse is taken. By observing the rising and falling of the patient's chest, a close estimate of the rate of respiration can be made. An average for adults would be close to 16 per minute, with a variation of a few inhalations and exhalations in either direction. The rate of respiration, like the pulse rate, is higher in children.

Sometimes the respiration rate can be noted without making it obvious to the patient that there is concern about the information; many persons alter their natural breathing rate uncon-

sciously if they know that function is being watched.

Body Temperature

A fever thermometer, available at any drugstore, is specially shaped to help the home nurse read any tiny change in the patient's temperature, such changes being measured in tenths of a degree. Instead of being round in cross-section like an ordinary thermometer, a fever thermometer is flat on one side and ridge-shaped on the other. The inner surface of the flat side is coated with a reflective material and the ridge-shaped side actually is a magnifying lens. Thus, to read a fever thermometer quickly and properly, one looks at the lens (ridged) side.

How To Take the Temperature

The usual ways of taking temperature are by mouth (oral) or by the rectum (rectal), and fever thermometers are specialized for these uses. The rectal thermometer has a more rounded bulb to protect the sensitive tissues in the anus. Normal body temperature taken orally is 98.6° F. or 37° C. for most people, but slight variations do occur in the normal range. When the temperature is taken rectally, a normal reading is about 1° F. higher— 99.6° F. or about 37.5° C.—because rectal veins in the area elevate the temperature slightly.

Before a patient's temperature is taken, the thermometer should be carefully cleaned with soap and water, then wiped dry, or sterilized in alcohol or similar disinfectant. The thermometer should then be grasped firmly at the shaft and shaken briskly, bulb end downward to force the mercury down to a level of 95° F. or lower—or 35° C. or lower if the thermometer is calibrated according to the Celsius temperature scale. See the chart *Body*

Body Temperature in Degrees		
Fahrenheit		**Celsius**
105.5		40.8
105		40.6
104.5		40.3
104		40
103.5		39.7
103		39.4
102.5		39.2
102		38.9
101.5		38.6
101		38.3
100.5		38.1
100		37.8
99.5		37.5
99	Normal	37.2
98.6	Range	37.0
97.8		36.6

Temperature in Degrees for comparative values of the Fahrenheit and Celsius scales.

If the temperature is taken orally, the thermometer should be moistened in clean fresh water and placed well under the tongue on one side. If the temperature is taken rectally, the thermometer should be dipped first in petroleum jelly and then inserted about one inch into the opening of the rectum. If an oral thermometer is used in the rectum, special care should be taken to make sure that the lubrication is adequate and that it is inserted gently to avoid irritating rectal tissues. Whichever method is used, the thermometer should be left in place for at least three minutes in order to get an accurate reading.

If circumstances preclude an oral or rectal temperature check, the patient's temperature may be taken under the arm; a normal reading in that area is about 97.6° F. or 36.5° C.

Above-Normal Temperature

If the patient's temperature hovers around one degree above his normal reading, the home nurse should note the fact and watch for other signs of a fever that would indicate the presence of an infection or some other bodily disorder. A mild fever immediately after surgery or during the course of an infectious disease may not be cause for alarm. Also, the normal body temperature of a mature woman may vary with hormonal changes during her menstrual cycle. But when oral temperatures rise above 100° F. the change should be regarded as a warning signal. A rise of as much as three degrees above normal, Fahrenheit, for a period of several hours or more, could be critical, and a physician should be notified immediately.

Sleep

Another item to be checked each day for the at-home medical records is the patient's sleeping habits. While there is no standard number of hours of sleep per day preferred for healthy individuals, a regular pattern of sleep is very important during recovery from disease or injury, and an obvious change from such a pattern can suggest tension, discomfort, or other problems. Typical daily sleep periods for most adults range from 7 to 9 hours, while children and infants may sleep as much as 12 to 20 hours per day and be considered normal; sleep in the form of naps should be included in total amounts per day.

Making the Patient Comfortable

A good deal of the patient's time at home will be devoted to sleep or rest, most or all of it in bed. The bed should give firm support to the body; if the mattress does not offer such support, place a thick sheet of plywood between the springs and mattress. Pillows can be placed under the head and shoulders of the patient to raise those parts of the body from time to time. When the patient is lying on his back,

a small pillow can be slipped under the knees to provide support and comfort. A small pillow can also be placed under the small of the back if necessary. Additional pillows may be placed as needed between the ankles or under one foot or both feet.

If the pressure of bed clothing on the feet causes discomfort, a bridge made from a grocery carton or similar box can be placed over the feet but beneath the blankets. To help maintain muscle tone and circulation in the feet and legs, a firm barrier can be placed as needed at the foot of the bed so the patient can stretch his legs and push against the barrier while lying on his back.

Changing Position

Helping the patient change position in bed is an important home-nursing technique. Unless a definite effort is made to help the patient change positions at regular intervals, the sick person may tend to curl up into a sort of fetal position, with the hips and knees flexed and the spine curved. While this position may be preferred by the patient in order to increase body warmth or to relieve pain, the practice of staying in one position for longer periods of time can lead to loss of muscle tone and even deformities.

Moving or positioning the patient in bed should, of course, be done according to directions outlined by the doctor for the specific medical problem involved. Body movements should not aggravate any injury or other disorder by placing undue strain or stress on a body part or organ system that is in the healing stage. At the same time, the patient should be stimulated and encouraged to change positions frequently and to use as much of his own strength as possible.

If the patient is likely to need a very long period of bed rest, and the family can afford the modest expense,

it may be wise to purchase or rent a hospital-type bed. The basic hospital bed is higher from the floor than ordinary beds, making the tasks of changing bed linens, taking temperatures, etc., easier for the home nurse. More sophisticated hospital beds have manual or electrical controls to raise the head and foot of the bed.

Helping the Patient Sit Up

The patient can be helped to a sitting position in bed by placing one arm, palm upward, under the patient's shoulder while the patient extends an arm around the nurse's back or shoulders. The nurse also may slip both hands, palms facing upward, under the patient's pillow, raising it along with the patient's head and shoulders. The same procedures can be used to help move a patient from one side of the bed to the other if the patient is unable to move himself.

When the patient has been raised to a sitting position, he should try to brace his arms behind him on the bed surface with elbows straightened. If the patient feels dizzy or faint as a result of the effort, he can be lowered to the back rest position again by simply reversing the procedure.

When the patient is able to support himself in a sitting position, he should be encouraged to dangle his legs over the side of the bed, and—when his strength permits—to move to a chair beside the bed and rest for a while in a seated position.

Bathing the Patient

A patient who is unable to leave the bed will require special help in bathing. When bath time comes, the nurse will need a large basin of warm water, soap, a washcloth, and several towels, large and small. A cotton blanket also should be used to replace the regular blanket during bathing, and pillows should be removed from the bed unless they are necessary at the time.

One large towel should be placed under the patient's head and another should be placed on top of the bath blanket, with part of the towel folded under the bath blanket. This preliminary procedure should help protect the bed area from moisture that may be spilled during the bathing procedure.

The bath should begin at the area of the eyes, using only clear water and brushing outward from the eyes. Soapy water can be applied to the rest of the face, as needed, with rinsing afterward. After the face, bathing and rinsing are continued over the chest and abdomen, the arms and hands, the legs and feet, and the back of the body from the neck downward to the buttocks. The external genitalia are washed last.

During the washing procedure, the nurse uses firm strokes to aid circulation and checks for signs of pressure areas or bed sores. Skin lotions or body powders may be applied, and a back rub given, after washing. The teeth may be brushed and the patient may want to use a mouthwash. After the personal hygiene routine is completed, a fresh pair of pajamas can be put on. If bed linen needs to be changed, the bathing period provides a good opportunity for that chore.

Changing the Bed Linen

Changing the bed linen while the patient is in bed can be a challenge for any home nurse. However, there are a few shortcuts that make the task much easier. First, remove all pillows, or all but one, as well as the top spread if one is used. Loosen the rest of the bedding materials on all sides and begin removing the sheets from

Changing Patients Bed

New sheet   Old sheet   New sheet   Old sheet

the head of the bed, top sheet first. By letting the patient hold the top edge of the blanket, or by tucking the top edges under his shoulder, the blanket can remain in place while the top sheet is pulled down, under the blanket, to the foot of the bed. If the top sheet is to be used as the next bottom sheet, it can be folded and placed on the side with the top spread.

Next, the patient must be moved to one side of the bed and the bottom sheet gathered in a flat roll close to the patient. Then the clean bottom sheet is unfolded on the mattress cover and the edges, top, and bottom, tucked under the mattress. The rest of the clean sheet is spread over the empty side of the bed and pushed in a flat roll under the soiled sheet next to the patient's back.

The next step is to roll the patient from one side of the bed onto the clean sheet that has been spread on the other side. The soiled bottom sheets can be pulled out easily and the new bottom sheet spread and tucked in on the other side.

The new top sheet can be pulled up under the blanket, which has been used to cover the patient throughout the change of bed linens. Finally, the top spread and pillows can be replaced, after the pillow cases have been changed. A special effort should be made, meanwhile, to keep the mattress cover and bottom sheet of the patient's bed as flat and smooth as possible and to allow room for the feet to move while the sheets are firmly tucked in at the foot of the bed.

The home nurse should handle the soiled linens carefully if the patient is being treated for an infectious disease; they should never be held close to the face.

Bowel Movements and Urination

If the patient is expected to remain bedridden for a long period of time, the home nurse should acquire a bedpan and perhaps a urinal from a drugstore. A sheet of oilcloth, rubber, or plastic material should also be provided to protect the bed during bowel movements and urination.

If the patient is unable to sit up on a bedpan because of weakness, his body can be propped up with pillows. If he is capable of getting out of bed but is unable to walk to the bathroom, a commode can be placed near the bed and the patient can be helped from the bed to the commode and back. Another alternative is to use a wheelchair or any chair with casters to move the patient between the bedroom and bathroom.

Administering an Enema

Occasionally, a physician may recommend an enema to help the patient empty his bowels or to stimulate the peristaltic action associated with normal functioning of the intestinal tract.

Since enemas are seldom an emergency aspect of home nursing, there usually is time to purchase disposable enema units from a drugstore. The disposable enema contains about four or five ounces of prepared solution packaged in a plastic bag with a lubricated nozzle for injecting the fluid into the patient's rectum. The entire package can be thrown away after it has been used, thus eliminating the need to clean and store equipment. The alternative is to use a traditional enema bag filled with plain warm water or a prescribed formulation.

An enema is best administered while the patient is lying on his side with his knees drawn up toward his chest. When using the disposable enema unit, the home nurse simply squeezes the solution through the lubricated nozzle that has been inserted into the rectum. When using an enema bag, the home nurse should lubricate the nozzle before insertion. After insertion of the nozzle, the enema bag should be held or suspended above the patient so that, upon the opening of the valve that controls the flow of the enema, the liquid will flow easily into the patient's rectum.

Feeding the Patient

It may be necessary at times for the home nurse to feed a patient unable to feed himself. An effort should be made to serve meals to the patient in an attractive and, when possible, colorful manner. The bedding should be protected with towels or plastic sheeting and the patient made as comfortable as possible with his head raised.

Liquids should be offered in a spoon filled about two-thirds full with any drops on the bottom of the spoon carefully wiped off. The spoon should be held so that the area between the tip and the side touch the patient's lower lip. Then the spoon is tilted toward the tip so the liquid will run into the patient's mouth. The process takes time, and much patience is required of the nurse. The patient may be slow to swallow and in no hurry to finish the meal.

If the patient can take liquids through a glass tube or plastic straw, the home nurse should see to it that the end of the tube inserted in the container of liquid is always below the surface of the fluid so that the patient will swallow as little air as possible.

A patient who can drink liquids from a spoon or tube may be able to drink from a cup. In making the step from tube or spoon to cup, the home nurse can help the patient by holding the cup by its handle and letting the patient guide the cup to his lips with his own hands.

The nurse should always make sure the patient is fully alert before trying to put food or liquid into his mouth; a semiconscious person may not be able to swallow. The nurse also should test the temperature of the food; cold foods should be served cold and warm foods should be served warm. But foods should never be too hot or too cold for the patient. Finally, the dishes, tubes, or other devices used to feed the patient should be carefully cleaned before storing them.

Ice Bags and Hot-Water Bottles

Ice bags and hot-water bottles frequently are used in home nursing to relieve pain and discomfort. The temperature of the water in a hot-water bottle or bag should be tested before it is placed near a patient's body. The maximum temperature of the water should be about 130° F., and preferably a few degrees cooler. The hot-water container should never be placed directly against the skin of a patient; it must be covered with soft material, such as a towel, to protect the patient against burns. A patient who is receiving pain-killing medications could suffer serious tissue damage from a hot-water bottle without feeling severe pain.

When ice is the preferred method of relieving pain, it can be applied in a rubber or plastic bag sealed to prevent leakage and covered with a soft cloth. Cold applications to very young and old persons should be handled cautiously and with medical consultation, particularly if ice packs are to be applied to large body areas for long periods of time; individuals at both age extremes can lack the normal physiological mechanisms for coping with the effects of cold temperatures.

Steam Inhalators

If the at-home patient suffers from a respiratory ailment that is relieved by steam inhalation, there are several devices to provide the relief he needs. One is the commercial electric inhalator that boils water to which a few drops of a volatile medication are added to provide a pleasantly moist and warm breathing environment. If a commercial inhalator is not available, a similar apparatus can be made by fashioning a cone from a sheet of newspaper and placing the wide end of the cone over the top and spout of a teapot containing freshly boiled water. The narrow end of the cone will direct the hot water vapor toward the face of the patient. If a medication is to be added, it can be applied to a ball of cotton placed in the cone; the steam or water vapor will pick up the medication as it passes through the cone.

If medicated vapor is intended for a small child or infant, the end of the cone can be directed into a canopy or tent made of blankets placed over a crib or the head of a bed. This arrangement should produce an effective respiratory environment for the child while keeping his body safely separated from the hot teakettle.

Still another method of providing steam inhalation for a patient requires only an old-fashioned washstand pitcher and bowl plus a grocery bag. An opening is cut in one corner of the bottom of the bag which is placed upside down over the pitcher filled with hot steaming water and, if needed, a medication. The patient simply breathes the hot moist air seeping through an opening in the bag. The pitcher of steaming water is placed in a bowl or basin as a safety precaution.

Sickroom Devices

With a bit of imagination, many sickroom devices can be contrived from items already around the house. A criblike bed railing can be arranged, for example, by lining up a series of ordinary kitchen chairs beside a bed; if necessary, they can be tied together to prevent a patient from falling out of bed. The bed itself can be raised to the level of a hospital bed by placing the bed legs on blocks built from scrap lumber. Cardboard boxes can be shaped with scissors and tape into bed rests, foot supports, bed tables, or other helpful bedside aids.

Plastic bags from the kitchen can be used to collect tissues and other materials that must be removed regularly from the sickroom. Smaller plastic bags may be attached to the side of the bed to hold comb, hairbrush, and other personal items.

Keeping Health Records

The family that keeps good records of past injuries and illnesses, as well as immunization information and notes on reactions to medications, has a head start in organizing the home care of a member who suddenly requires nursing. The file of family health records should include information about temperatures and pulse rates taken during periods of good health; such data can serve as benchmark readings for evaluating periods of illness. Also, if each member of the family can practice taking temperatures and counting pulse and respiration rates during periods of good health, the family will be better able to handle home nursing routines when the need arises.

Home Care Equipment Checklist

Following is a convenient checklist of basic supplies needed for home care of the sick:

1. Disinfectants for soaking clothing and utensils used by the sick. Not all disinfectants are equally effective for every purpose. For clothing and food utensils, corrosive or poisonous disinfectants are to be avoided. Antiseptics do not kill bacteria; they only retard their growth. Among the common disinfectants that can be used in the home are:

- Alcohol, 75 percent by weight, used for disinfecting instruments and cleaning the skin

- Lysol, for decontaminating clothing and utensils

- Soap with an antibacterial agent for scrubbing the hands

- Carbolic acid (phenol) for disinfecting instruments and utensils (it is corrosive, poisonous, and very effective if used in 5 percent solution)

- Cresol in 2.5 percent solution for disinfecting sputum and feces (less poisonous than phenol and can be obtained as an alkali solution in soap)

- Boric acid, a weak antiseptic eyewash

- Detergent creams, used to reduce skin bacteria

2. Disposable rubber gloves, to be used when handling patients with open wounds or contagious diseases, as well as for cleaning feces.

3. Paper napkins and tissues for cleaning nasal and oral discharges.

4. Rectal and oral thermometers. The former is used primarily for infants, while the latter is used for adults and older children. Thermometers should always be thoroughly disinfected after use by soaking in isopropyl alcohol, and they should be washed prior to reuse.

5. Eating and drinking utensils to be used only by the patient. Disposable utensils are preferable.

6. Urinal, bedpan, and sputum cup for patients who cannot go to the toilet. After use, they should be thoroughly disinfected with cresol and washed with liquid soap containing an antibacterial agent.

7. Personal toilet requisites: face cloths and towels, toilet soap, washbasin, toothbrush and toothpaste, comb, hairbrush, razor, and a water pitcher (if running water is not accessible to the patient).

8. Measuring glass graduated in teaspoon and tablespoon levels for liquid medication.

9. Plastic waste-disposal bags that can be closed and tied.

33

Health Care Delivery

A Changing Service

Unending change has characterized American health care in recent decades. The general practitioner in private practice, once the institutionalized symbol of medical care in the United States, has largely given way to specialists of many kinds. Where the general practitioner once sent a handwritten bill for services to the family home, he or she may now send a computerized invoice to an insurance company or a government agency. The "house call" has virtually disappeared.

Technology has taken over. Hospitals and other health care institutions may pay sums in seven figures for equipment that can save lives but that also demands to be used. A "technological imperative" requires that the new approach or instrument or drug at least be tried—experimented with, proven useful or useless, and made available to those who need it. In diagnosis and therapy in particular, physicians and other professionals are continually seeking the new and better.

Some seven million people work in the American health care system. Half a million of those are physicians. The facilities in which the system's personnel work range from rural clinics to high-technology urban medical centers. On balance, the consumer dealing with this system has many choices. Understanding those choices may make the difference between a beneficial experience and a frustrating search for help.

Health care reaches the American public at three broadly defined levels. The three are primary, secondary, and tertiary care.

Primary Care

Essentially, *primary care* refers to "first contact" care as provided in physicians' offices or hospitals. Such care may also be provided in emergency rooms and outpatient clinics. The individual can obtain primary care without referral by a physician, but referrals from this level of care are generally necessary to ensure that the patient will receive treatment at the next higher level. Among the types of services provided at the primary care level are health maintenance for infants and children, screening for infectious and communicable diseases, and treatment for minor injuries.

Secondary Care

At the *secondary care* level the patient usually comes under the care of a specialist, often in a community hospital or other, similar setting. Secondary level specialties include such well-known areas of medicine as obstetrics and gynecology, dermatology, otolaryngology, and cardiology. While physicians often refer their patients for secondary level care, many persons "refer themselves."

Tertiary Care

At the tertiary care level, the patient receives highly specialized, high-technology care and treatment. Complex programs and unusual procedures, among them open heart surgery, heart or kidney transplantation, and neurological surgery, are provided by physicians with extensive training and the advantages of sophisticated equipment for diagnosis and treatment. Often, care at this level is obtainable only if the patient enters a hospital with specialized facilities. Of the various tertiary care institutions, three key ones are hospitals specializing in a certain disease or a group of diseases, hospitals associated with medical schools, and large regional referral centers. Many such institutions would be expected to have diagnostic equipment for such procedures as cardiac catheterization, nuclear magnetic resonance testing, and CT scanning.

Importantly, the three levels of care overlap. The distinctions among them are not always clearly drawn or defined. For the patient, the most important factor may be the need for referrals at some levels and not at others.

Health Care Delivery Formats

The average American visits a physician five times a year. That statistic appears in a U.S. Public Health Service survey that also defines a visit as an encounter with a physician or other health professional under a physician's direction or supervision. The "encounter" can take place in the physician's office, in the patient's home, by telephone, or in some other ambulatory care setting. The physician initiates about half of the encounters, usually as part of follow-up care.

Office and Clinic Care

In the main, the patient sees his or her physician in an office or at a site reserved for group practice; in a hospital outpatient department; in an ambulatory surgical center; or in a freestanding surgical center.

Office-Based Practice

Most physicians practice on their own; even so, the solo practice is declining as a way of medical life. The solo practitioner survives in isolated or rural areas, but hardly at all elsewhere. For the physician, solo practice is both simpler because of the independence and freedom it

guarantees and more complex because the service responsibility may continue 24 hours a day, seven days a week. For the patient, the main advantage of solo practice is both the closer relationship that can develop and less fragmented care.

Partnerships

Very common today is the partnership, an agreement between two or more physicians under which the participants share office space, staff, and equipment. The physicians retain their independence in the sense that they have their own practices, but they usually share patient responsibilities under given circumstances. A physician who has to be out of contact with the office may, for example, give a patient another partner's number so as to have continuous backup. Spreading the care responsibilities and reducing the workload, each physician may also have more time for each patient.

The patient may find major advantages in the partnership. He or she can become acquainted with the physician's partner and in this way obtain personalized care at all times. Backup support may be especially important in obstetrics, where deliveries may occur without warning, and in cardiology, where emergencies are equally unscheduled.

Groups

Where three or more physicians associate in an arrangement that is normally less formal than a partnership, it is termed a *group*. The physicians belonging to the group may practice in a single specialty or in diverse fields of medicine. An example of the latter would be a group of three doctors offering internist, obstetrics-gynecological, and pediatric services. In other

ways the group shares the advantages and disadvantages of the typical partnership. Like the partnership, the group has one particular advantage, however: other physicians are available for consultation and education. The group format may also make possible relatively sophisticated laboratory and other facilities.

Health Maintenance Organizations

The health maintenance organization (HMO) ranks as a special kind of group practice, one that involves a fixed monthly or annual fee system rather than a fee-for-service arrangement. The fixed fee ensures that the HMO member will receive, at no additional charge, all necessary health services, including hospitalization and the care of specialists. Preventive medicine at no extra cost to the member is a feature of the HMO that has ensured reduced usage of hospital facilities.

Preferred Provider Organizations

Like the HMO, the preferred provider organization (PPO) is at least partly a response to rising health-care costs. Forming a PPO, a group of physicians contracts individually with an insurance company or employer to provide health services for fees that are usually lower than those prevailing in the community or area. The PPO does charge on a fee-for-service basis, but employees making use of the organization's medical services save money because they avoid the copayments of conventional insurance plans and the standard deductibles. Physicians belonging to the PPO have a stable pool of employed members whose health problems may be extremely diverse. For the employer or insurance company, a particular advantage is the ability to bargain for lower fees.

Three Alternative Systems

Obviously, office and clinic care takes many forms. Three alternatives that provide relatively minor, low-level services are the hospital outpatient department, the ambulatory surgical center, and the freestanding emergency center. Each plays a particular role in the health care delivery network.

Hospital Outpatient Departments

Outpatient departments once offered free services as a means of training medical students and residents or because physicians volunteered their services for such departments. Today, outpatient departments charge for their services while delivering health care that varies broadly as regards quality. One hospital in three has an outpatient department or a clinic for ambulatory care while nine of ten community hospitals offer outpatient care in their emergency departments.

Ambulatory Surgical Centers

Sometimes called surgicenters, the ambulatory surgical center may be attached to a hospital or be completely independent. In either case, the surgicenter may be an effective alternative in the traditional situation where a patient needs an abortion, a dilatation and curettage (D & C), hernia repair, or tissue biopsy. Because they perform lower-risk procedures, ambulatory surgical centers can keep costs down. Local anesthesia is the norm, and usually the patient goes home on the day of the operation.

Freestanding Emergency Centers

Sometimes called *urgicenters,* freestanding emergency centers resemble hospital emergency departments. But private, for-profit groups usually run them. Open from 12 to 24 hours daily, they operate on a drop-in basis, meeting a definite need where a hospital emergency room is far away or when all physicians' offices have shut down for the day. Typically, emergency centers treat sprains and bruises, cuts that require stiches, and upper respiratory infections. Charges for such services usually range from visits to physicians' offices on the low side to hospital emergency rooms on the high side.

Community Health Care Facilities

Providing more evidence of the complexity of the United States' health care delivery complex, community health facilities fill a void in health services at a very basic level. At least five different modes of providing health care need to be considered as community facilities.

School and College Health Programs

Once concerned primarily with the control of communicable diseases and screenings for dental, vision, and hearing problems, school and college health programs have taken on new functions. At the elementary and high-school levels, they may help with health and sex education programs, keep vaccination records, and consult with parents. Colleges and universities generally provide infirmary services, meaning inpatient care for acute illness. At larger schools, programs may deal with contraception and pregnancy problems, substance abuse, and neuroses.

Industrial Health Programs

Treatment of work-related injuries and minor illnesses remains a key function of industrial health programs. The programs also continue to give minor physical exams and to provide general medical and dental care. But they have expanded their services in recognition of the value of preventive medicine. Newer or more modern programs offer comprehensive worksite education and screening programs, alcohol abuse counseling, stop-smoking clinics, and aerobic fitness classes.

Health Screening

Provided by local health departments and voluntary health agencies (see Chapter 36), health screening varies from community to community as regards both availability and reliability. Depending on community funding, a local health department may or may not provide tests that screen for infectious or parasitic diseases, including sexually transmitted diseases (see Chapter 17), and chronic disorders such as high blood pressure, sickle cell anemia, or diabetes. Many health departments make referrals to follow-up medical care.

Neighborhood and Primary Health-Care Centers

Neighborhood and primary health-care centers were established first in the 1960s to provide ambulatory care in underserved communities, both rural and urban. Staffed often by U.S. Public Health Service medical personnel or by nurse practitioners, the centers either limited their services according to income requirements or served specific communities. Because of cuts in federal spending, experts note, many such centers have been or are being phased out.

Women, Infant, and Child Care

Also federally funded, the women, infant, and child care program emphasizes provision of well-baby care, nutritious food, and nutrition education for pregnant women, infants, and children under three. Estimates indicate that the program saves three dollars for every dollar spent. But federal budget cuts have begun seriously to scale back the program.

Disease Prevention and Control

County or city health departments usually establish disease prevention and control programs to help control the spread of communicable diseases. Methods used include immunization, screening, and follow-up. Typical concerns include immunization for childhood diseases like diphtheria, measles, and polio; tuberculosis and sexually transmitted diseases; and influenza immunization for older persons.

Hospitals

Viewed a century ago as a death-house, the hospital has a new image in the 1980s. With an entirely revised role built on its ability to provide comforts and even amenities, the hospital has added a "hotel" function to its fundamental "healing" function. But the hotel role does not affect the hospital's main medical purpose: to provide, within budgetary and other limits, sophisticated, technologically up-to-date care. The hospital has become the place to go for diagnostic and therapeutic care that a physician's office cannot provide.

A basic method of classifying hospitals is by length of the patient's stay. Viewed this way, hospitals fall into two groups, long-term or extended-care institutions and short-term hospitals. The former will be discussed later; the second group includes community, teaching, and public hospitals.

Community Hospitals

Most Americans receive medical care in community hospitals. Usually quite small, with 50 to 500 beds, this kind of hospital generally provides good to excellent secondary-level care. Traditionally, community hospitals were nonprofit corporations that depended heavily on community support. Today, the community hospital is increasingly likely to be proprietary. That means it is run for profit by investor-owned groups or corporations.

The costs of medical care at a proprietary community hospital may not be significantly different from those charged by a voluntary or nonprofit hospital.

Teaching Hospitals

Ranging in size from a few hundred to a few thousand beds, teaching hospitals universally offer training for undergraduate medical students, postgraduate students, or fellows. Also, nearly all have ties to major medical schools. A state government may own a teaching hospital that is used by state medical schools; others are owned by the associated university or by a nonprofit corporation. Teaching hospitals provide care at all three levels.

Public Hospitals

Public hospitals include not only county hospitals but others supported by public funds, among them public health service hospitals, Veterans Administration (VA) hospitals, and municipal short-term-stay hospitals. Many such institutions that are owned by federal, state, or city governments are teaching hospitals, and many also have associated rehabilitation units and nursing homes.

The Elderly: Home Care

Surprisingly, most elderly persons live at home and receive care from relatives and others who may visit the home to help out. Younger family members may need home care because of illness or injury, but typically the disabled or ill older person is the one receiving such care. A number of community resources are available to make home care—or self-care for those living alone—easier. These resources include home health workers, such services as Meals-on-Wheels, and various day-care programs.

Invaluable aids for those responsible for home care for an aging relative are unskilled companions and temporary help. With this kind of assistance, the elderly person may be able to enjoy continuity of care and independence while maintaining ties with family, home, and community.

Home Health Services

Some 2,500 home health agencies operate under the general direction of physicians to provide two kinds of services: skilled and supportive. Of the many types of home health service providers, the best known are private, either profit-making or nonprofit; public health agencies such as neighborhood health centers; hospital-based services; and local or county health department or community and church programs. The nationwide Visiting Nurses Association is perhaps the most familiar.

Different communities and areas enjoy different levels and types of home health services. But most such agencies provide care to anyone who requests it. Fees vary, and may be paid by the individual or the family accepting the care. In other cases the government or individual insurance plans may reimburse the family, partially or totally, for the fees charged.

Hospital social workers or discharge-planners, the Area Agency on Aging, the local office of the Social Security Administration, day-care centers, and churches and synagogues normally provide information on home health services.

Voluntary Health Agencies

Many voluntary health agencies provide aid and support to the disabled or sick elderly person (see Chapter 36). Such groups and organizations as the American Cancer Society and the Easter Seal Society may even offer "friendly visitor" services in specific communities. Most of the groups see education of the public as functional to their roles. Thus they may provide films, lecturers, books and pamphlets, and other materials of interest to groups and organizations of many kinds. Many such agencies have specialized equipment for those who need it as well as listings of community resources.

Drugstores and Medical Supply Houses

Two other basic sources of specialized equipment and sickroom supplies, the medically oriented drugstore and the medical supply house, play important roles. In many cases the family discharging home care responsibilities can obtain wheelchairs, walkers, portable oxygen equipment, and hospital beds from one source or the other. Often, the supplier will rent or sell the specialized equipment; the choice may be the family's to make.

Community Facilities for the Aged

An entire new category of health care facilities has come into being in recent years in response to the needs of the elderly. These community facilities are designed specifically for those elderly persons living at home who are not housebound.

Adult Day Care

A broad variety of community-based centers schedule adult day-care programs for the elderly. To some extent the programs provide an alternative to institutionalization. In each case the programs are tailored to meet specific needs. Each type has a basic therapeutic objective.

Day Hospitals

Generally located at an extended-care facility or hospital, the day hospital provides medical care and supervision for persons recovering from acute illnesses. A physician's referral is normally required; fees closely parallel those charged for other hospital services. The day hospital that treats primarily patients discharged from an institution is sometimes called an after-care clinic.

Medical Day Care

Where chronically ill or disabled persons do not require frequent or intensive medical intervention, the medical day care service may be the solution. Located usually in a long-term care institution or freestanding center, such a care service may include nursing and other supports. A physician's referral is required, and rehabilitation and maintenance are primary therapeutic goals. Reimbursement is by third-party (insurance company) payments on a sliding scale. Medicaid pays for medical day care in some states.

Mental Health Day Care

Offering a supervised environment along with mental health services to adults with organic or functional mental illness, the mental health day care service is usually located in a psychiatric institution or freestanding center. Referral by a psychiatrist is required. Three basic therapeutic goals are supervision, assistance with coping skills, and safety for the patient. Reimbursement is by third-party payment.

Social Adult Day Care

Title XX of the Social Security Act provides for funding of many social adult day care facilities, all of which are geared to the needs of adults who have difficulty functioning independently. Both families and health facilities can make referrals, but examination by a physician is normally required before admission. Third-party reimbursement is the norm. Program objectives and services vary widely, and are usually formulated by the funding source and the sponsoring organization. Program participants may attend part-days or full days five days a week; the facility may provide a midday meal and transportation within a specified area.

Nutrition Services

Nutrition ranks as a critical need for both homebound and more independent elderly persons. Meals-on-Wheels, a community service offered under voluntary auspices but funded partly by public funds, caters to the homebound. For a reasonable charge the service provides at least one hot meal daily for persons 60 and older. For the elderly attending senior centers, the Area Agency on Aging provides both adequate nutrition and a chance to socialize. Agency personnel can keep in touch with clients' physical and social situations, giving the program an important outreach and prevention dimension.

Extended-Care, Long-Term Care, Nursing Homes

Closely related, the extended-care facility, long-term care facility, and nursing home nonetheless meet different needs. A relatively recent innovation, the extended-care facility provides a service that falls between that given in an acute-care hospital and that provided in a skilled nursing facility or nursing home.

Extended-Care Facility

Despite its name, the extended-care facility provides short-term inpatient care. This type of facility is designed mainly to aid patients who have been hospitalized but no longer need the full complement of hospital services. Such patients still require professional nursing and medical supervision. Typically attached to a hospital, the extended-care facility may also serve those who are not acutely ill but who require skilled care.

Because most extended-care facilities are physically attached to hospitals, patients often simply move from one hospital wing to another. Some nursing homes also meet the standards set for qualification as extended-care facilities by the Joint Commission on the Accreditation of Hospitals (JCAH). For the most part, extended-care facilities charge much less than the typical hospital.

Long-Term Care Facilities

Patients with chronic conditions that cannot be treated effectively in a general hospital generally qualify for care in a long-term care facility. Such conditions range from tuberculosis to mental retardation. The facilities also include chronic disease hospitals, rehabilitation hospitals, and psychiatric hospitals for both children and adults.

Nursing Homes

Also falling in the category of long-term care facilities, nursing homes comprise a special group of facilities of different kinds. They offer services ranging from sheltered living arrangements to around-the-clock nursing care. All nursing homes rank as residential facilities.

The approximately 18,000 nursing homes in the United States have between 1.3 and 1.5 million beds. Three-quarters of these nursing homes are proprietary, or for-profit, institutions that house about two-thirds of all the beds. Nonprofit organizations operate 15 percent of all the nation's nursing homes and make available about 20 percent of the beds. The government operates the remaining homes.

Nursing homes accommodate persons of all ages. A few younger residents have serious congenital illnesses or disorders, or have been recently discharged from a hospital. Others are recovering from recent surgery. But most patients are the chronically ill elderly. Typically, a nursing home resident is a woman in her 80s, single or widowed. Afflicted with three or more serious chronic illnesses, she has very likely exhausted all her assets except her monthly Social Security payments.

Residential-Care Facilities

Standing at the lowest level of nursing home care, the residential-care facility is usually appropriate for the person who can no longer live alone and manage household chores. This "typical" resident does not need extensive medical attention but does require sheltered living, prepared meals, and some medical monitoring. The latter may include supervision of medications and tracking of signs and symptoms.

Intermediate-Care Facilities

The intermediate-care facility supplements typical RCF services with regular, but not round-the-clock, nursing care for residents who are unable to survive on their own. The intermediate-care facility may also make provision for social and recreational activities. Programs of physical therapy and rehabilitation, occupational therapy, speech therapy, and social work services may also be offered.

Skilled Nursing Facilities

With staffs of registered nurses, licensed practical nurses, and nurses' aides, skilled nursing facilities can provide 24-hour care. They are, thus, appropriate for persons in need of intensive nursing care and rehabilitation. Like intermediate-care facilities, skilled nursing facilities are state-certified for the most part, a factor that makes them eligible for public funds as payment for services. Lack of certification may mean that an ICF or SNF has serious deficiencies.

Hospices

Described sometimes as more a philosophy than a type of physical facility, the hospice is a form of care for the terminally ill. The family and the patient merit equal consideration in the typical hospice; the purpose is to minimize the twin fears associated with dying, fear of isolation and fear of pain. Typical palliative care involves the careful control of pain and the management of other symptoms of terminal disease or illness.

A growing number of communities have hospice facilities. But no pattern appears in the types of institutions— or sections of institutions—devoted to the care of the terminally ill. A hospice may be a wing in a hospital or simply a group of hospital beds that can be made available as needed. A hospice may also be a separate building or institution. While families provide much of the care as long as patients are at home, a team including a physician, nurses, counselors, home health aides and others may be continually on call. The team provides continuity between home and hospice when patients must be institutionalized. At all times, the individual patient's comfort is a prime consideration.

Patients enter hospice programs at their own requests. A physician's referral, indicating that the prognosis is no more than six months, may also be required.

34

Voluntary Health Agencies

Major Agencies

The establishment of more than 100 voluntary health agencies since the beginning of this century has been a major factor in the growth of health services to the American public. These agencies, whose activities are made possible by donations of time and money from the public, occasionally augmented by government grants for special projects, have the following objectives: spreading information about various diseases to the professional and lay public; sponsoring research; promoting legislation; and operating referral services on the community level to patients in need of diagnosis, treatment, and financial aid.

Some of these agencies, such as the American Diabetes Association or the Arthritis Foundation, focus on a particular disease; others deal with problems arising from related disorders, such as the National Association for Mental Health and the American Heart Association. Still others, such as Planned Parenthood and the American Social Health Association, have programs vital not only to individuals, but to society as a whole.

To coordinate the activities of these many groups, to promote better health facilities, and to establish standards for the organization and conduct of these agencies, the National Health Council was founded in 1920. Its membership includes government, professional, and community associations, as well as the 21 voluntary health agencies described below, which command a total budget of almost $1.5 billion and involve the services of almost 12 million volunteers.

All of these organizations function on the national, state, and community level. Information and literature may be obtained through local chapters or by writing to the national office of the organization. Volunteers may offer their services in a variety of ways: as office workers, fund raisers, speakers, and community coordinators.

On the following pages, voluntary health agencies are discussed under the subjects with which they are concerned; the subjects are arranged alphabetically. Following these agencies is a brief discussion of other voluntary health agencies. Because of limitations of space, however, many worthwhile organizations have had to be omitted.

Accident Prevention

The National Safety Council, 444 North Michigan Avenue, Chicago, Illinois 60611, was founded in 1913 to improve factory safety but soon broadened its activities to preventing every type of accident. The Council is now composed of groups and individuals from every part of the population: business, industry, government, education, religion, labor, and law. Its main efforts are devoted to building strong support for official safety programs at the national, state, and community levels in specific areas, such as traffic, labor, and home.

The Council believes that practically all accidents can be prevented with the application of the right safeguards. These safeguards include public education and awareness of danger, enforcement of safety laws and regulations, and improved design standards for machines, farm equipment, and motor vehicles.

It maintains the world's largest library of accident prevention materials, distributes a wide variety of safety literature, and issues awards for outstanding safety achievements. It also serves as a national and international clearing house of information about the causes of accidents and how they can be prevented.

In addition to campaigning for increased safety legislation on the national and state level, the Council's current programs include a defensive driving course, which provides effective adult driver training on a mass scale; a safety training institute; environmental and occupational health and "Right-to-Know" educational materials; and several approaches to the alcohol and driving problem.

Its publication, *Family Safety and Health,* has record circulation of more than two million readers, and its manual called *Fundamentals of Industrial Hygiene* provides more than 1,000 pages of material essential to the safety of factory workers.

The Council in recent years has expanded its safety promotion work to include both on- and off-the-job safety for workers and their families, as well as 24-hour-a-day safety for all persons in all activities.

Alcoholism

The National Council on Alcoholism and Drug Dependence, 12 W. 21st Street, New York, New York 10010, is the only national voluntary health agency founded to combat alcoholism as a disease by an extensive program on the professional and community level. The Council is completely independent of Alcoholics Anonymous, although the two organizations cooperate fully.

In nearly 200 cities where the Council has affiliates, alcoholism information centers have been established that provide referral services for alcoholics and drug addicts and their families as well as educational materials for all segments of the community, including physicians and nurses, the clergy, the courts, social workers, and welfare agencies. Local affiliates also help to develop labor-management programs that provide help for employees who suffer from the disease.

The Council also sponsors research, professional training, and legislative action. Its publications department distributes a variety of fact sheets, pamphlets, posters, and videos. For a listing of publications or information on the Council's programs, write the national headquarters or contact the nearest local affiliate.

Arthritis

The Arthritis Foundation, 1314 Spring Street N.W., Atlanta, Georgia 30309, was established to help arthritis sufferers and their physicians through programs of research, patient services, public health information, and education on the professional and popular level. Its long-term goal is to find the cause, prevention, and cure for the nation's number one crippling disease.

The Foundation operates local chapters throughout the United States whose chief concern is the patient who has or might have arthritis. These chapters are centers for information about the disease itself and also serve as referral centers for treatment facilities. In addition, they distribute literature and sponsor forums on the latest developments in research and patient care.

Some chapters support arthritis clinics and home care programs; most conduct patient self-help programs such as discussion groups and exercise classes. Parent groups are often maintained for parents of children with arthritis.

Two special groups work within the Foundation: the Arthritis Health Professions Association which devotes itself to continuing education for health professionals caring for arthritis patients and the American Juvenile Arthritis Organization for those with a special interest in arthritis in children.

A major part of the Foundation's work at the national level is providing funds for fellowships to young physicians and scientists so that they may continue their work in arthritis research and in funding through annual grants research at major institutions throughout the United States.

Cancer

The American Cancer Society, 1599 Clifton Rd. N.E., Atlanta, Georgia 30329, was established in 1913 by a small group of physicians and volunteer workers to inform the public about the possibility of saving lives through the early diagnosis and treatment of cancer. The Society now has 57 regional groups, one in each state plus one in the District of Columbia and six other metropolitan areas, devoted to the control and eradication of cancer. In addition to the physicians, research scientists, and other professional workers engaged in the Society's activities, more than two million volunteers are connected with its many programs.

The American Cancer Society conducts widespread campaigns to educate the public in the importance of annual medical checkups so that cancerous symptoms can be detected while they are still curable. Such checkups should include an examination of the rectum and colon and, for women, examination of the breasts and a Pap test for the detection of uterine cancer.

In another of its campaigns, the Society emphasizes the link between cigarette smoking and lung cancer. It also sponsors an extensive program to persuade teenagers not to start smoking. During its annual April Crusade against Cancer, the Society distributes approximately 40 million copies of a leaflet containing lifesaving information on early detection of cancer.

On the professional level, the major objective of the Society is to make every physician's office a cancer-detection center. To achieve this goal, it publishes a variety of literature, offers refresher courses, sponsors seminars, and cooperates closely with local and state medical societies and health departments on the diagnosis and treatment of cancer. It also arranges national and international conferences for the exchange of information on the newest cancer-fighting techniques, and finances a million-dollar-a-year clinical fellowship program for young physicians.

Among its special services to patients are sponsorship of the International Association of Laryngectomies, for people who have lost their voices to cancer; and Reach to Recovery, a program for women who have had treatment for breast cancer and who need support and guidance to return to normal living. On the community level, the American Cancer Society operates a counseling service for cancer patients and their families, referring them to the proper medical facilities and social agencies for treatment and care. Through its "loan closets," it provides sickroom necessities, hospital beds, medical dressings, and so on.

Some local divisions offer home care programs through the services of the Visiting Nurse Association or a similar agency. Although the Society does not operate medical facilities, treat patients, or pay physicians' fees, some of the chapters support cancer detection programs and professionally supervised rehabilitation services.

Cerebral Palsy

The United Cerebral Palsy Associations, 7 Penn Plaza, Suite 804, New York, New York 10001, founded in 1948 by a small group of concerned parents, now has 203 affiliates across the country where those who have the condition may obtain treatment referral, therapy, and education. The Associations also play an important role in vocational training, job placement programs, housing, and recreational services.

The Research and Educational Foundation of this organization supports studies investigating possible causes of cerebral palsy. The Foundation also gives grants to universities and medical schools for research into the causes and prevention of cerebral palsy and new methods of therapy, for training medical and other professional personnel in the management of this condition.

Cystic Fibrosis

The Cystic Fibrosis Foundation, 6931 Arlington Road, No. 200, Bethesda, Maryland 20814, was organized in 1955 by a group of concerned parents whose children were born with this lung disease. The Foundation now concerns itself with all serious lung ailments of children regardless of their medical names, and it engages in a broad program of research, medical education, public information, and the sponsorship of diagnostic and treatment centers.

The Foundation's 58 local chapters offer advice and information to parents of children with severe lung disease, and have direct connections with the more than 120 Cystic Fibrosis Centers throughout the country. They refer patients to sources of financial aid, make arrangements for the purchase of drugs at a discount, and lend home treatment equipment to families who cannot afford to buy it.

The national organization makes grants for research activities, conducts professional conferences, and publishes literature for physicians and the general public on various aspects of childhood lung diseases.

Diabetes

The American Diabetes Association, National Service Center, P.O. Box 25757, 1660 Duke Street, Alexandria, Virginia 22314, was established as a professional society in 1940. In recent years it has enlarged its scope so that it currently has 800 affiliated local chapters throughout the country that promote the creation of better understanding of diabetes among patients and their families; the exchange of knowledge among physicians and other scientists; the spreading of accurate information to the general public about early recognition and supervision of the disease; and the sponsorship of basic research.

Since 1948, the American Diabetes Association has conducted an annual Diabetes Detection Drive supported by widespread publicity in all news media. During this drive, approximately three million testing kits are provided to state and county medical societies to facilitate the early detection and prompt treatment of the disorder. This annual activity hopes to find the estimated 1,600,000 people who are unaware that they have diabetes.

Among the Association's publications of special interest to diabetics and their families are the *Diabetes Forecast,* a national magazine that presents news items on research and treatment; *Meal Planning with Exchange Lists,* prepared with the cooperation of the American Dietetic Association and the U.S. Public Health Services; and *A Cookbook for Diabetics,* which contains attractive recipes for meals that can be served to diabetics.

Other activities of the Association include encouraging the employment of diabetics and providing special groups such as teachers, police, and social agencies with information on the condition. It also established a classification of the disease according to its severity. Guidelines on emergency medical care and the scientific journal *Diabetes* are available to physicians.

Drug Abuse

The American Social Health Association, which was organized originally to combat the spread of venereal disease, expanded its program in 1960 to include drug abuse education. For information about its activities in this field, see below under "Sexually Transmitted Diseases."

Eye Diseases

The National Society to Prevent Blindness, 79 Madison Avenue, New York, New York 10016, was founded in 1908 to reduce the number of cases of infants born with impaired sight. In subsequent years, it merged with the American Association for the Conservation of Vision and the Ophthalmological Foundation. The Society is now concerned with investigating all causes of blindness and supports measures and community services that will eliminate them. It also distributes information on the proper care and use of the eyes.

The organization's first and most significant victory was the adoption of laws by almost all states requiring that silver nitrate solution be routinely dropped into the eyes of all newborn babies to counteract the possibility of congenital blindness. This resulted in a dramatic drop in the number of children suffering from eye impairment dating from birth.

For almost half a century, the Society has actively campaigned to reduce the number of people suffering from glaucoma, one of the leading causes of blindness in the United States. It has also conducted a national program to educate the elderly in the ease, safety, and advantages of surgery for cataracts, the leading cause of blindness among the aged.

Since 1926, the Society has been conducting preschool vision screening programs administered by teams that travel from big cities to isolated rural communities. Current activities also include research into the cause, treatment, and prevention of eye diseases leading to blindness; assembling data and publishing reports; cooperating with community agencies to improve eye health; promoting conditions in schools and industry to safeguard vision; and advocating eye examinations in early childhood so that disorders can be properly and promptly corrected.

Family Planning

Planned Parenthood Federation of America, 810 Seventh Avenue, New York, New York 10019, is the nation's oldest and largest voluntary family planning organization. Tracing its origins to 1916, when Margaret Sanger founded the first U.S. birth control clinic in Brooklyn, New York, Planned Parenthood maintains that every individual has the fundamental right to choose when or whether to have a child.

Planned Parenthood has five key goals:

- To increase the availability and accessibility of high-quality and affordable reproductive health care services and information, especially for underserved groups

- To reduce adolescent pregnancy and unwanted births to teens

- To meet the challenge of changes in health care delivery systems and maintain high-quality, efficiently run, and creative Planned Parenthood programs

- To further Planned Parenthood's role in the provision of education of human sexuality, reproduction, and population, and on the bioethical and legal implications of reproductive technology

- To increase access to safe and effective methods of voluntary fertility regulation for individuals in developing countries

Each year, more than three million individuals in 49 states and the District of Columbia obtain medical, educational, and counseling services through more than 900 clinics operated by Planned Parenthood's 171 affiliates. The organization is active in more than 100 developing countries throughout the world. In addition, Planned Parenthood conducts clinical research, provides professional training of health and education personnel, and serves as a resource to health agencies, government agencies at the state and federal levels, legislators and other policy makers, and the media.

Heart Disease

The American Heart Association, 7320 Greenville Avenue, Dallas, Texas 75231, was founded in 1924 as a professional organization of cardiologists. It was reorganized in 1948 as a national voluntary health agency to promote a program of education, research, and community service in the interests of reducing premature death and disability caused by diseases of the heart and blood vessels. The complex of heart disorders, including atherosclerosis, stroke, high blood pressure, kidney diseases, rheumatic fever, and congenital heart disturbances, is by far the leading cause of death in the United States.

Since its first Annual Heart Fund Campaign in 1949, the Association has contributed more than $150 million to research and has been a major factor in the reduction of cardiovascular mortality statistics. It has spent more than $2 million since 1959 studying human heart transplantation procedures, and has contributed to the development of an artificial heart, plastic heart valves, and synthetic arteries.

Public and professional education programs designed to reduce the risk of heart attack through avoidance of cigarette smoking, obesity, and foods high in cholesterol are conducted on a nationwide and community level by the Association's affiliates throughout the country. The local chapters are also engaged in service programs for rheumatic fever prevention, stroke rehabilitation, school health, cardiopulmonary resuscitation, and industrial health. In addition, they conduct information and referral services for patients and their families.

The American Heart Association publishes many technical and professional journals as well as material designed for the general public.

Hemophilia

The National Hemophilia Foundation, 110 Green Street, Room 406, New York, New York 10012, was established in 1948 to serve the needs of hemophiliacs and their families by ensuring the availability of treatment and rehabilitation facilities. It is estimated that there are as many as 100,000 males suffering from what is popularly known as "bleeder's disease," an inherited condition passed from mothers to sons.

The long-term goal of the Foundation is to develop a national program of research and clinical study that will provide new information about early diagnosis and effective treatment of the disorder as well as trained professional personnel to administer patient care.

The development in recent years of blood-clotting concentrates is the most important advance to date in the treatment of the disease. This development, supported in part by the Foundation's 48 chapters, makes it possible for patients to have elective surgery and dental work, and to eliminate much of the pain, crippling, and hospitalization of those suffering from hemophilia.

The need for blood supplies from which to extract the clotting factor caused the Foundation to embark on an extensive campaign for blood donations. For this purpose, it has been working closely since 1968 with the American Red Cross and the American Association of Blood Banks. It also maintains close ties with various laboratories and research groups in the development of more powerful concentrates that can be manufactured and sold at the lowest possible cost.

The organization's activities include a national network of facilities with blood banks, clinics, and treatment centers as well as referral services. It has also established a Behavioral Science Department to explore the nonmedical aspects of hemophiliacs' problems, such as education, vocational guidance, and psychological needs.

Kidney Disease

The National Kidney Foundation, 30 E. 33rd Street, Suite 1100, New York, New York 10016, formerly the National Kidney Disease Foundation, was founded in 1950 by a group of parents whose children had a disease with no cure—nephrosis. The ultimate goal was the total eradication of all diseases of the kidney and urinary tract. Today, although there remains no cure for nephrosis, the disease is almost totally treatable. In the past two decades the National Kidney Foundation and its 49 affiliates nationwide have supported more than $20 million in research to find the answers to kidney and urinary tract related diseases.

The National Kidney Foundation and its affiliates sponsor a wide variety of programs in treatment, service, education, and prevention that are designed to aid the patient in the community. Examples of some affiliate programs include: information and referral programs for patients and their families, drug banks, support groups, summer camp programs for children on dialysis and transplantations, transportation services, counseling and screening, and direct financial assistance to needy patients.

The National Kidney Foundation seeks continually to increase the number of organs available for transplantation through its nationwide Organ Donor Program. To date, more than 50 million donor cards have been distributed by the Foundation and its affiliates. Distribution of public and professional educational materials continues to heighten public awareness of organ donation and the "Gift of Life" it can provide to thousands of people waiting for a kidney transplant.

Mental Health

The National Mental Health Association, 1021 Prince Street, Alexandria, Virginia 22314-2971, was founded in 1909 to work toward the improved care and treatment of people with mental illnesses, the promotion of mental health, and the prevention of mental disorders. The original National Committee for Mental Hygiene merged with the National Mental Health Foundation and the Psychiatric Foundation in 1950 to create the organization as it now stands.

The association implements its service programs through its 650 affiliates (local chapters and larger state divisions) across the country. These mental health associations tailor their efforts to the needs of their communities.

The National Mental Health Association is composed of one million volunteers and supporters who have a keen interest in mental health. They include family members whose loved ones have been affected by mental illnesses, current or former consumers, mental health professionals, and lay citizens.

Recent and ongoing activities include:

- Coordinated a national coalition to address the needs of people with mental illnesses who are homeless.

- Serves as a prime source of referral and educational information on mental illnesses and mental health issues through the NMHA Mental Health Information Center.

- Assists local and state MHA affiliates in serving communities through patient and family support groups, housing programs, suicide-prevention hotlines, and school mental health education programs.

- Helped extend the civil rights protection of the 8th and 14th Amendments to the U.S. Constitution to the mentally disabled by representing persons with severe mental illnesses before the Supreme Court.

- Specified a "state-of-the-art" program to prevent severe mental and emotional disabilities in a landmark 1986 report by its National Commission on the Prevention of Mental-Emotional Disabilities.

- Serves as the public-interest policy voice for mental health issues in the Congress and state legislatures.

Multiple Sclerosis

The National Multiple Sclerosis Society, 205 East 42nd Street, New York, New York 10017, was founded in 1946 with the primary goal of supporting research on this chronic neurological disease whose cause and cure are unknown. Some 250,000 Americans are estimated to have multiple sclerosis (MS).

Research aimed at finding the cause and methods of arresting MS is being conducted worldwide. From the beginning the Society has made every effort to increase professional and public awareness of the symptoms of MS and the best ways of treating them. This is done through a network of 143 chapters and branches and some 470,000 active members. The chapters, which are either affiliated with or support MS clinics around the country, provide home and hospital visits, recreational programs, referrals for medical care, job counseling, and other services. The chapters also arrange educational programs for physicians and social workers as well as for patients and their families. The society sponsors public education awards in magazine, radio, and television writing and conducts Project Rembrandt, a biennial competition for artists with MS.

The national office distributes publications for physicians and the interested public, including guides for the development of patient services and a quarterly magazine, *Inside MS.*

Films, slide presentations, videocassettes and audiocassettes are available for purchase or loan.

Physical Disabilities

The National Easter Seal Society, 70 East Lake Street, Chicago, Illinois 60601, has grown from its pioneering origins in 1919 to a national organization that serves more than one million disabled people of all ages. Among its network of facilities are comprehensive rehabilitation centers, treatment and diagnostic centers, and vocational training workshops, residential camps, special education programs, and transportation services in many different parts of the country.

Because many disabled children and adults in rural areas and small communities are unaware of the services available to them, the Society gives top priority to publicizing its information, referral, and follow-up activities. In recent years, it has also established mobile treatment units in hospitals and nursing homes in rural areas.

Other innovative activities include screening and testing programs to detect hearing loss in newborns and learning disabilities in preschool children, and providing treatment and referral for those who are disabled by respiratory diseases.

The Society collaborates with federal and professional agencies in all programs designed to eliminate architectural barriers to the disabled, and was instrumental in the enactment of legislation making it mandatory that all buildings constructed with government funds be fully and easily accessible to the disabled. It also initiates and supports significant studies in rehabilitation procedures as well as scientific research in bone transplant techniques.

Extensive literature is distributed to professionals, the public, parents, and employers. It also assembles special educational packets for parents of the disabled.

Sexually Transmitted Diseases

The American Social Health Association, P.O. Box 13827, Research Triangle Park, North Carolina 27709, was organized in 1912 to promote the control of venereal disease and to combat prostitution. In the mid-1980s the Association faced new challenges in the field of sexually transmitted diseases (STDs) while also developing new strategies to augment and complement existing AIDS information programs, promote attention to chlamydia, the most widespread STD in the United States, exert influence in Congress for additional federal funding for STD prevention and control programs, and place STD information in the hands of high-school students.

The Association is in close touch with government agencies such as the Public Health Service, the National Institutes of Health, and the various branches of the armed forces. Through these channels, it promotes its program for STD education in the schools and for research toward the discovery of an immunizing vaccine against syphilis and gonorrhea.

It is the major national voluntary repository for information and consultation on STDs, and maintains the world's most comprehensive collection of source workshops, residential camps, special education programs, and materials on STDs. It constantly helps communities in diagnosing their problems and produces a number of publications for teachers, guidance counselors, and youth workers.

The Association stresses the importance of introducing family life education into the curriculum of elementary and secondary schools and of establishing training programs on this subject in teachers' colleges. These efforts have resulted in the inclusion of family life education in an increasing number of school systems throughout the United States.

Tuberculosis and Respiratory Diseases

The American Lung Association, 1740 Broadway, New York, New York 10019, is the direct descendant of the first voluntary health organization to be formed in the United States. In 1904, when the National Association for the Study and Prevention of Tuberculosis was organized, this disease was the country's leading cause of death. Since 1973, with the sharp increase in the problems relating to smoking and air pollution, the association has been known by its present name, which was adopted to reflect the broader scope of its activities.

It now concerns itself not only with the elimination of tuberculosis but with chronic and disabling conditions, such as emphysema, and with acute diseases of the respiratory system, such as influenza. Through its affiliates and nationwide state organizations, it is actively engaged in campaigns against smoking and air pollution.

The early endeavor of the association to have tuberculosis included among the reportable diseases was accomplished state by state, and since the 1920s all states have required that every case in the country be brought to the attention of local health officials.

Public awareness of better care and the development of effective drugs have dramatically reduced the number of TB patients, but the association continues to concern itself with the fact that provisional data indicate that there are still about 22,000 new cases each year.

Through its local affiliates, the American Lung Association initiates special campaigns to combat smoking and air pollution, using radio and television announcements, car stickers, posters, and pamphlets, as well as films and exhibits. Educational materials on respiratory diseases are regularly distributed by the national office to local associations for physicians, patients, and the general public. Funds raised by the annual Christmas Seal drive also support research and medical education fellowships.

Other Voluntary Health Agencies

In addition to those voluntary health agencies that are members of the National Health Council, many other organizations function on a national scale and offer specialized services as well as literature and guidance to professionals, patients, parents, and concerned families. The following is a partial list.

Alcoholics Anonymous World Services, P.O. Box 459, Grand Central Station, New York, New York 10163, is a fellowship of men and women who share their experiences and give each other support in overcoming the problem of alcoholism. Chapters exist throughout the country and offer referral services, literature, and information about special hospital programs.

Al-Anon Family Group Headquarters, Inc., P.O. Box 862 Midtown Station, New York, New York 10016, is not affiliated with Alcoholics Anonymous, but cooperates closely with it. Al-Anon, which includes Alateen for younger members, is a primary community resource and self-help fellowship for the families and friends of alcoholics. Members share their experiences, strength, and hope at regularly held meetings, and learn to cope with the effects of being close to an alcoholic. Headquarters registers, services, and provides literature to 33,000 groups worldwide, of which 19,000 are in the United States.

Asthma and Allergy Foundation of America, 1835 K Street, N.W., Suite P-900, Washington, D.C. 20006, was established to help solve all health problems related to allergic diseases by sponsoring research and treatment facilities. It also grants scholarships to medical students specializing in the study of allergy.

Alzheimer's Association, 70 E. Lake Street, Suite 600, Chicago, Illinois 60601, was founded in 1980 to heighten public awareness of this degenerative brain disorder, provide support for patients and their families, aid research efforts, advocate for legislation that responds to the needs of Alzheimer's disease patients and their family members, and commemorate National Alzheimer's Disease Awareness Month each November. The network includes more than 200 chapters and affiliates across the country representing over 1,000 Family Support Groups. To obtain the most up-to-date information on Alzheimer's disease legislation and research, and for referral to local chapters, call the Association's toll-free information and referral number, 800-621-0379 (in Illinois only, 800-572-6037) or write to the Association.

The *American Foundation for AIDS Research* (AmFAR), 5900 Wilshire Blvd., 2nd Floor, East Satellite, Los Angeles, California 90036, was created in the fall of 1985 as a result of the unification of two not-for-profit public foundations: the AIDS Medical Foundation (AMF), incorpo-

rated in the State of New York in April 1983; and the National AIDS Research Foundation (NARF), incorporated in the State of California in August 1985. AmFar is an independent, national organization whose directors, committee members, and staff are professionals in the field of AIDS.

The Foundation has two main missions. First, it supports and facilitates laboratory and clinical research projects selected on the basis of scientific merit and relevance to achieve an understanding of the pathogenesis of AIDS, its prevention through the use of a vaccine, and its treatment. Second, the Foundation works to develop data and to serve as a source of accurate and up-to-date information about an epidemic that has profound psychosocial repercussions in our society.

American Foundation for the Blind, 15 West 16th Street, New York, New York 10011, is a national nonprofit organization working with local and national services to improve the quality of life for all blind and visually impaired persons. It stocks many different consumer products and publications and has recorded and produced millions of talking book records for the Library of Congress.

Through its staff of national consultants and its regional offices, the Foundation maintains a direct liaison with state, regional, and local agencies.

The *Association for Voluntary Surgical Contraception,* 122 East 42nd Street, New York, New York 10168, was founded in 1943 to promote the right of each individual to choose sterilization as a method of birth control. A nonprofit membership organization, the AVSC has increasingly collaborated with governmental and private sector providers to ensure effective access to sterilization facilities. The Association also sponsors training,

education, and program support for sterilization and family planning counselors and others; prepares annual estimates of male and female voluntary sterilizations in the United States; issues a quarterly newsletter, the *AVSC News,* and other publications, and initiates and monitors research into medical, legal, psychological, ethical, and public health aspects of voluntary sterilization.

The Epilepsy Foundation of America, 4351 Garden City Drive, Landover, Maryland 20785, is the result of a merger in 1967 of two similar organizations. At present, the Foundation has 85 local affiliates that provide information, referral services, and counseling. It conducts a research grant program for medical and psychosocial investigation and distributes a wide variety of literature on request to physicians, teachers, employers, and the interested public on such subjects as anticonvulsant drugs, insurance, driving laws, and emergency treatment. The national office also maintains an extensive research library.

The Leukemia Society of America, 733 Third Avenue, New York, New York 10017, was organized in 1949 and now has 57 chapters. It supports research in the causes, control, and eventual eradication of the disease that, though commonly thought of as a disorder of the blood, is in fact a disorder of the bone marrow, lymph nodes, and spleen, which manufacture blood. The society has a continuing program of education through special publications directed to physicians, nurses, and the public. Through its local affiliates, it conducts patient-aid services that provide counseling, transportation, and—to those who need financial assistance— drugs, blood transfusions, and laboratory facilities.

The Muscular Dystrophy Association, Inc., 810 Seventh Avenue, New

York, New York 10019, has as a primary goal the scientific conquest of muscular dystrophy and related neuromuscular diseases. The Association supports scientific investigators worldwide. In addition, through its 170 chapter affiliates nationwide, MDA provides a comprehensive patient and community services program to individuals diagnosed with any one of 40 neuromuscular disorders. The Association maintains a network of some 240 MDA clinics coast to coast to provide diagnostic services and therapeutic and rehabilitative follow-up care as well as genetic, vocational, and social service counseling to patients and their families. MDA also sponsors a summer camping program for youngsters aged 6 to 21 as well as adult outings, with activities geared to the special needs of those with neuromuscular diseases.

The Association for Retarded Citizens of the United States, P.O. Box 6109, Arlington, Texas 76006, established in 1950, is the nation's largest voluntary organization specifically devoted to promoting the welfare of children and adults with mental retardation. It is estimated that there are six million such persons in the United States. Through its 1,500 affiliates the association conducts and supports research, sponsors employment programs, advocates for progressive public policy, and works for better community services. Counseling and referral services, as well as extensive literature for professionals and concerned families, are available on request.

The March of Dimes Birth Defects Foundation, 1275 Mamaroneck Avenue, White Plains, New York 10605, was founded in 1938 to combat infantile paralysis (polio). In the 30 years since the conquest of polio, through the development of the Salk and Sabin polio vaccines, the March of Dimes has dedicated itself to the prevention of birth defects, the nation's number one child health problem. It does this through programs of birth defects research and medical service and education that provide new knowledge and understanding of birth defects and their prevention. More than a quarter-million babies are born with one or more of the 3,000 known birth defects each year. The Foundation also has established the Salk Institute in La Jolla, California, directed by Dr. Jonas Salk, for the purpose of carrying on basic research in life processes to discover what causes birth defects and other diseases. Special Health Services and Agencies

Many factors have contributed to the growth of the American system of health services. Specialists in various medical specialties have tried to meet needs for new types of health care. Medical care has become so effective that individual life expectancy has increased enormously; as one result, the number of Americans aged 65 and older tripled in the three-quarters of a century between 1900 and 1975. As the population of the United States has grown older, in percentage terms, the problems of the aged have received more attention. New methods and devices have been developed for the care and assistance of the ill or disabled of any age.

Special health services and agencies help to fill such needs. Many older persons have utilized the services of trained individuals who make survival possible—sometimes at home—or slow down the rate of deterioration. Other institutions and agencies perform simple maintenance tasks for the aged or the seriously ill or handicapped, or help with rehabilitation. Social service agencies and groups with health roles, for example, provide adult day care, homemaker assistance, and home health services that may include the following:

- Part-time or occasional nursing care, often under the supervision of a registered nurse

- Physical, occupational, or speech therapy

- Medical social services that help the patient and his or her family to adjust to the social and emotional conditions accompanying illness or disability of any kind

- Assistance from a home health aide, including help with such tasks as bathing and going to the bathroom, taking medications, exercising, and getting into and out of bed

- Under some circumstances, medical attention from interns or residents in training

35

Medical Emergencies

Anyone attempting to deal with a medical emergency will do so with considerably more confidence if he has a clear notion of the order of importance of various problems. Over and above all technical knowledge about such things as tourniquets or cardiac massage is the ability of the rescuer to keep a cool head so that he can make the right decisions and delegate tasks to others who wish to be helpful.

Cessation of Breathing

The medical emergency that requires prompt attention before any others is cessation of breathing. No matter what other injuries are involved, artificial respiration must be administered immediately to anyone suffering from respiratory arrest.

To determine whether a person is breathing naturally, place your cheek as near as possible to the victim's mouth and nose. While you are feeling and listening for evidence of respiration, watch the victim's chest and upper abdomen to see if they rise and fall. If respiratory arrest is indicated, begin artificial respiration immediately.

Time is critical; a human body has only about a four-minute reserve supply of oxygen in its tissues, although some persons have been revived after being submerged in water for ten minutes or more. Do not waste time moving the victim to a more comfortable location unless his position is life threatening.

If more than one person is available, the second person should summon a physician. A second rescuer can also assist in preparing the victim for artificial respiration by helping to loosen clothing around the neck, chest, and waist, and by inspecting the mouth for false teeth, chewing gum, or other objects that could block the flow of air. The victim's tongue must be pulled forward before artificial respiration begins.

Normal breathing should start after not more than 15 minutes of artificial respiration. If it doesn't, you should continue the procedure for at least two hours, alternating, if possible, with other persons to maintain maximum efficiency. Medical experts have defined normal breathing as eight or more breaths per minute; if breathing resumes but slackens to a rate of fewer than eight breaths per minute, or if breathing stops suddenly for more than 30 seconds, continue artificial respiration.

Mouth-to-Mouth and Mouth-to-Nose Artificial Respiration

Following is a description of the techniques used to provide mouth-to-mouth or mouth-to-nose artificial respiration. These are the preferred methods of artificial respiration because they move a greater volume of air into a victim's lungs than any alternative method.

After quickly clearing the victim's mouth and throat of obstacles, tilt the victim's head back as far as possible, with the chin up and neck stretched to ensure an open passage of air to the lungs. If mouth-to-mouth breathing is employed, pull the lower jaw of the victim open with one hand, inserting your thumb between the victim's teeth, and pinch the nostrils with the other to prevent air leakage through the nose. If using the mouth-to-nose technique, hold one hand over the mouth to seal it against air leakage.

Next, open your own mouth and

Cardiopulminary Resuscitation (CPR)

(1) Open airway: **tilt the head back** by the forehead and **lift the chin**. (2) If not breathing, begin rescue breathing. **Pinch nose, give 2 full breaths**, each of about five seconds in duration. If passage is blocked, reposition head and try again. If still no air enters the lungs, perform the Heimlich maneuver abdominal thrusts. (3) **Check pulse** at the carotid artery. (4) If heart is beating, continue mouth-to-mouth until breathing is started. **If no pulse, begin chest compressions**. Perform 15 compressions to every 2 full breaths. Check pulse after four cycles of compressions/breaths. **Warning:** Performing CPR is not recommended unless you have training. CPR incorrectly performed can cause physical injury and death. The American Red Cross and other organizations offer CPR certification. Mouth-to-mouth resuscitation can be performed, but classes are also available for training. CPR and resuscitation should be performed continuously until medical help arrives.

take a deep breath. Then blow forcefully into the victim's mouth (or nose) until you can see the chest rise. Quickly remove your mouth and listen for normal exhalation sounds from the victim. If you hear gurgling sounds, try to move the jaw higher because the throat may not be stretched open properly. Continue blowing forcefully into the victim's mouth (or nose) at a rate of once every three or four seconds. (For infants, do not blow forcefully; blow only small puffs of air from your cheeks.)

If the victim's stomach becomes distended, it may be a sign that air is being blown into the stomach; press firmly with one hand on the upper abdomen to push the air out of the stomach.

If you are hesitant about direct physical contact of the lips, make a ring with the index finger and thumb of the hand being used to hold the victim's chin in position. Place the

ring of fingers firmly about the victim's mouth; the outside of the thumb may at the same time be positioned to seal the nose against air leakage. Then blow the air into the victim's mouth through the finger-thumb ring. Direct lip-to-lip contact can also be avoided by placing a piece of gauze or other clean porous cloth over the victim's mouth.

Severe Bleeding

If the victim is not suffering from respiration failure or if breathing has been restored, severe bleeding is the second most serious emergency to attend to. Such bleeding occurs when either an artery or a vein has been severed. Arterial blood is bright red and spurts rather than flows from the body, sometimes in very large amounts. It is also more difficult to control than blood from a vein, which

can be recognized by its dark red color and steady flow.

Emergency Treatment

The quickest and most effective way to stop bleeding is by direct pressure on the wound. If heavy layers of sterile gauze are not available, use a clean handkerchief, or a clean piece of material torn from a shirt, slip, or sheet to cover the wound. Then place the fingers or the palm of the hand directly over the bleeding area. The pressure must be *firm and constant* and should be interrupted only when the blood has soaked through the dressing. *Do not remove the soaked dressing.* Cover it as quickly as possible with additional new layers. When the blood stops seeping through to the surface of the dressing, secure it with strips of cloth until the victim can receive medical attention. This procedure is almost always successful in stopping blood flow from a vein.

If direct pressure doesn't stop ar-

Pressure Points

(Adapted with permission from an American Red Cross illustration.)

Two major pressure points: in the arm, the brachial artery; in the leg, the femoral artery. Continue to apply direct pressure and elevate the wounded part while utilizing pressure points to stop blood flow.

Pressure Points

(Top) Use the femoral artery for control of severe bleeding from an open leg wound. Place the victim flat on his back, and put the heel of your hand directly over the pressure point. Apply pressure by forcing the artery against the pelvic bone. *(Bottom)* Use the brachial artery for control of severe bleeding from an open arm wound. Apply pressure by forcing the artery against the arm bone. Continue to apply direct pressure over the wound, and keep the wounded part elevated.

(Adapted with permission from American Red Cross illustrations.)

terial bleeding, two alternatives are possible: pressure by finger or hand on the pressure point nearest the wound, or the application of a tourniquet. No matter what the source of the bleeding, if the wound is on an arm or leg, elevation of the limb as high as is comfortable will reduce the blood flow.

Tourniquets

A tourniquet improperly applied can be an extremely dangerous device, and should only be considered for a hemorrhage that can't be controlled in any other way.

It must be remembered that arterial blood flows away from the heart and that venous blood flows toward the heart. Therefore, while a tourniquet placed on a limb between the site of a wound and the heart may slow or stop arterial bleeding, it may actually increase venous bleeding. By ob-

structing blood flow in the veins beyond the wound site, the venous blood flowing toward the heart will have to exit from the wound. Thus, the proper application of a tourniquet depends upon an understanding and differentiation of arterial from venous bleeding. Arterial bleeding can be recognized by the pumping action of the blood and by the bright red color of the blood.

Once a tourniquet is applied, it should not be left in place for an excessive period of time, since the tissues in the limb beyond the site of the wound need to be supplied with blood.

Shock

In any acute medical emergency, the possibility of the onset of shock must always be taken into account, especially following the fracture of a large bone, extensive burns, or serious wounds. If untreated, or if treated too late, shock can be fatal.

Shock is an emergency condition in which the circulation of the blood is so disrupted that all bodily functions are affected. It occurs when blood pressure is so low that insufficient blood supply reaches the vital tissues.

Types of Circulatory Shock and Their Causes

- *Low-volume shock* is a condition brought about by so great a loss of blood or blood plasma that the remaining blood is insufficient to fill the whole circulatory system. The blood loss may occur outside the body, as in a hemorrhage caused by injury to an artery or vein, or the loss may be internal because of the blood loss at the site of a major fracture, burn, or bleeding ulcer. Professional treatment involves replacement of blood loss by transfusion.

Arterial Bleeding

Severe arterial bleeding can be controlled by the correct application of a tourniquet. (1) A long strip of gauze or other material is wrapped twice around the arm or leg above the wound and tied in a half-knot. (2) A stick, called a windlass, is placed over the knot, and the knot is completed. (3) The windlass is turned to tighten the knot and finally, (4) the windlass is secured with the tails of the tourniquet. Improper use of a tourniquet can be very dangerous.

- *Neurogenic shock,* manifested by *fainting,* occurs when the regulating capacity of the nervous system is impaired by severe pain, profound fright, or overwhelming stimulus. This type of shock is usually relieved by having the victim lie down with his head lower than the rest of his body.
- *Allergic shock,* also called *anaphylactic shock,* occurs when the func-

tioning of the blood vessels is disturbed by a person's sensitivity to the injection of a particular foreign substance, as in the case of an insect sting or certain medicines.

- *Septic shock* is brought on by infection from certain bacteria that release a poison which affects the proper functioning of the blood vessels.
- *Cardiac shock* can be caused by any circumstance that affects the pumping action of the heart.

Symptoms

Shock caused by blood loss makes the victim feel restless, thirsty, and cold. He may perspire a great deal, and although his pulse is fast, it is also very weak. His breathing becomes labored and his lips turn blue.

Emergency Treatment

A physician should be called immediately if the onset of shock is suspected. Until medical help is obtained, the following procedures can alleviate some of the symptoms:

1. With a minimum amount of disturbance, arrange the victim so that he is lying on his back with his head somewhat lower than his feet. (**Exception:** If the victim's breathing is difficult, or if he has suffered a head injury or a stroke, keep his body flat but place a pillow or similar cushioning material under his head.) Loosen any clothing that may cause constriction, such as a belt, tie, waistband, shoes. Cover him warmly against possible chill, but see that he isn't too hot.

2. If his breathing is weak and shallow, begin mouth-to-mouth respiration.

3. If he is hemorrhaging, try to control bleeding.

4. When appropriate help and transportation facilities are available, quickly move the victim to the nearest hospital or health facility in order to begin resuscitative measures.

5. *Do not* try to force any food or stimulant into the victim's mouth.

Cardiac Arrest

Cardiac arrest is a condition in which the heart has stopped beating altogether or is beating so weakly or so irregularly that it cannot maintain proper blood circulation.

Common causes of cardiac arrest are heart attack, electric shock, hemorrhage, suffocation, and other forms of respiratory arrest. Symptoms of cardiac arrest are unconsciousness, the absence of respiration and pulse, and the lack of a heartbeat or a heartbeat that is very weak or irregular.

Cardiac Massage

If the victim of a medical emergency manifests signs of cardiac arrest, he should be given cardiac massage at the same time that another rescuer is administering mouth-to-mouth resuscitation. Both procedures can be carried on in the moving vehicle taking him to the hospital.

It is assumed that he is lying down with his mouth clear and his air passage unobstructed. The massage is given in the following way:

1. The heel of one hand with the heel of the other crossed over it should be placed on the bottom third of the breastbone and pressed firmly down with a force of about 80 pounds so that the breastbone moves about two inches toward the spine. Pressure should not be applied directly on the ribs by the fingers.

2. The hands are then relaxed to allow the chest to expand.

3. If one person is doing both the cardiac massage and the mouth-to-mouth respiration, he should stop the massage after every 15 chest compressions and administer two very quick lung inflations to the victim.

4. The rescuer should try to make the rate of cardiac massage simulate restoration of the pulse rate. This is not always easily accomplished, but compression should reach 60 times per minute.

The techniques for administering cardiac massage to children are the same as those used for adults, except that much less pressure should be applied to a child's chest, and, in the case of babies or young children, the pressure should be exerted with the tips of the fingers rather than with the heel of the hand.

Caution

Cardiac massage can be damaging if applied improperly. Courses in emergency medical care offered by the American Red Cross and other groups are well worth taking. In an emergency in which cardiac massage is called for, an untrained person should seek the immediate aid of someone trained in the technique before attempting it himself.

Obstruction in the Windpipe

Many people die each year from choking on food; children incur an additional hazard in swallowing foreign objects. Most of these victims could be saved through quick action by nearly any other person, and without special equipment.

Food choking usually occurs because a bite of food becomes lodged at the back of the throat or at the

opening of the trachea, or windpipe. The victim cannot breathe or speak. He may become pale or turn blue before collapsing. Death can occur within four or five minutes. But the lungs of an average person may contain at least one quart of air, inhaled before the start of choking, and that air can be used to unblock the windpipe and save the victim's life.

Finger Probe

If the object can be seen, a quick attempt can be made to remove it by probing with a finger. Use a hooking motion to dislodge the object. Under no circumstances should this method be pursued if it appears that the object is being pushed farther downward rather than being released and brought up.

Back Blows

Give the victim four quick, hard blows with the fist on his back between the shoulder blades. The blows should be given in rapid succession. If the victim is a child, he can be held over the knee while being struck; an adult should lie face down on a bed or table, with the upper half of his body suspended in the direction of the floor so that he can receive the same type of blows. A very small child or infant should be held upside down by the torso or legs and struck much more lightly than an adult.

The Heimlich Maneuver

If the back blows fail to dislodge the obstruction, the Heimlich maneuver should be given without delay. (Back blows may loosen the object even if they fail to dislodge it completely; that is why they are given first.) The lifesaving technique known as the *Heimlich maneuver* (named for Dr. Henry J. Heimlich) works simply by

Back Blows for Treatment of Strangulation

Children may be placed over the knee and struck sharply between the shoulders.

Adults may be placed over the edge of a table, supported by grasping the waist, and struck sharply between the shoulders with the fist.

squeezing the volume of air trapped in the victim's lungs. The piece of food literally pops out of the throat as if it were ejected from a squeezed balloon.

To perform the Heimlich maneuver, the rescuer stands behind the victim and grasps his hands firmly over the victim's abdomen, just below the victim's rib cage. The rescuer makes a fist with one hand and places his other hand over the clenched fist. Then, the rescuer forces his fist sharply inward and upward against the victim's diaphragm. This action compresses the lungs within the rib cage. If the food does not pop out on the first try, the maneuver should be repeated until the air passage is unblocked.

The Heimlich Maneuver

(Left) The rescuer stands behind the victim and grasps his hands firmly over the victim's abdomen just below the rib cage *(top right)*. The position of the rescuer's hands and the direction of thrust are shown at the bottom right.

When the victim is unable to stand, he should be rolled over on his back on the floor. The rescuer then kneels astride the victim and performs a variation of the Heimlich maneuver by placing the heel of one open hand, rather than a clenched fist, just below the victim's rib cage. The second hand is placed over the first. Then the rescuer presses upward (toward the victim's head) quickly to compress the lungs, repeating several times if necessary.

The Heimlich maneuver has been used successfully by persons who were alone when they choked on food; some pressed their own fist into their abdomen, others forced the edge of a chair or sink against their abdomen.

Poisoning

In all cases of poisoning, it is imper-

ative to get professional assistance as soon as possible.

Listed below are telephone numbers for Poison Control Centers throughout the United States. These health service organizations are accessible 24 hours a day to provide information on how best to counteract the effects of toxic substances.

In the event of known or suspected poisoning, call the center nearest you immediately. Give the staff member to whom you speak as much information as possible: the name or nature of the poison ingested, if you know; if not, the symptoms manifested by the victim.

If for any reason it is impossible to telephone or get to a Poison Control Center (or a doctor or hospital), follow these two general rules:

1. If a strong acid or alkali or a petroleum product has been ingested,

dilute the poison by administering large quantities of milk or water. Do not induce vomiting.

2. For methanol or related products such as window cleaners, antifreeze, paint removers, and shoe polish, induce vomiting—preferably with syrup of ipecac.

Calling for Help

Every household should have a card close by the telephone—if possible attached to an adjacent wall—that contains the numbers of various emergency services. In most communities, it is possible to simply dial the operator and ask for the police or fire department. In many large cities, there is a special three-digit number that can be dialed for reaching the police directly.

An ambulance can be summoned either by asking for a police ambulance, by calling the nearest hospital, or by having on hand the telephone numbers of whatever private ambulance services are locally available. Such services are listed in the classified pages of the telephone directory.

Practically all hospitals have emergency rooms for the prompt treatment of accident cases. If the victim is in good enough physical condition, he can be placed in a prone position in a family station wagon for removal to a hospital. However, under no circumstances should a person who has sustained major injuries or who has collapsed be made to sit upright in a car. First aid must be administered to him on the spot until a suitable conveyance arrives.

Every family should find out the telephone number of the nearest Poison Control Center (see section in this chapter) and note it on the emergency number card.

The Emergency-Free Home

Every year, hundreds of thousands of Americans go to hospital emergency rooms to obtain treatment for injuries or illnesses incurred in their homes. But many of these emergency health problems could have been prevented. In too many cases, no one took action to eliminate home hazards simply because they were easy to overlook or were not readily detectable.

Millions more Americans suffer less serious home injuries and do not go to hospitals.

With a little forethought, many of these home accidents can be prevented. This chapter provides basic guidelines for home safety.

Medical Supplies and Equipment

Can you "immunize" your home against accidents, illnesses, and injuries resulting from misuse of medicines and medical equipment? Yes, and the effort is worth taking.

First Aid Needs

The first step toward home safety is preparedness. This means ensuring that basic first aid equipment and medications are in the home, readily available.

Both materials and medicines should be chosen with care. Key considerations are the ages of those who live in the home, special requirements of particular family members, the seasons of the year, and other factors that may suggest a need for certain products or preparations.

First aid supplies should be kept in a medicine cabinet or in a larger storage place such as a bathroom closet or a cabinet beneath a sink. Basic first aid items include:

- Assorted bandages
- Sterile gauze pads (for compresses)
- Waterproof adhesive tape
- 3% hydrogen peroxide (for cleaning cuts, wounds)
- 5% hydrocortisone ointment (for local pain, itching)
- Ice pack
- Tweezers (for removing splinters, debris)
- Oral fever thermometer
- Rectal thermometer (for children)
- Heating pad

Medicines and Medications

With the nondrug necessities stocked, you can turn your attention to pills, medications, ointments, powders, drugs, and others.

A first rule is: Don't overstock. Many medicine cabinets contain things that only help to delay proper medical attention.

"One such hazardous medicine is syrup of ipecac," according to a medical authority. "A preparation that induces vomiting, it's a basic need in a household with children. But it should never be used unless a physician approves. Use of ipecac after ingestion of some liquids can be very damaging and even fatal."

Leftover antibiotics may present another problem. Because these medications can be costly, many householders keep in their medicine cabinets (or on their dressers or nightstands) any supplies that are left after an initial bout with illness. *Antibiotics should never be used a second time without consulting a physician.*

Taking leftover antibiotics can cause severe allergic reactions. Self-medication may also make it difficult or impossible for a physician to diagnose an illness.

Antibiotics prescribed in series should be taken until the series is completed. As a final rule, no such medications should be passed on to friends or relatives for their use. Borrowed medications could harm, rather than help, the recipient.

What drugs or medications should be in your medicine cabinet? Some basic items are:

- Cold and allergy medications, including an antihistamine, a decongestant, a cough suppressant, an expectorant
- An antacid for indigestion
- An anti-odor foot cream or powder
- An anti-diarrheal medicine
- A laxative
- Eyedrops
- Aspirin or an aspirin-free pain reliever
- Other items as required for chronic conditions.

Here are some additional safety rules regarding medicine cabinets:

- If possible, locate the medicine cabinet in a cool, dry, dark place, out of the reach of children.
- Check the contents periodically and throw away out-of-date or spoiled items (including aspirin that smells like vinegar).
- Remove the cotton from any medicine cabinet containers that may

use cotton stoppers (because the cotton can absorb a medication's active ingredients).

- If even one pill in a bottle has deteriorated or spoiled, throw out the entire batch.

- Keep liquids in their amber containers to protect the contents from light.

- To discard medications, flush them down the toilet, then remove the labels on the containers to prevent others from refilling the prescriptions.

- Keep emergency phone numbers (physician, pharmacist, fire, police, and so on; see the list of emergency phone numbers on the inside front cover of this volume) on the medicine cabinet or near it. When in doubt about which medication to use, call a doctor or pharmacist.

Reducing the Risk of Medicine Poisoning

Following certain safety rules can help ensure against the possibility of medicine poisoning. The rules are most important in homes where there are very young children or very old family members.

Medicines or preparations that are potentially harmful should be kept in a locked cabinet. If there are a number of such preparations in the home, they should probably be kept in a separate, locking storage place. If this is not possible, they should at least be stored out of the reach of young children.

Other safety rules are simply common sense. For example, one should never transfer a medicine into an unlabeled container. Old medicine containers should be thrown away. Special care should be taken with the dosages of both liquid and solid drugs. Sleeping tablets, tranquilizers, and

even aspirin can, if taken in overdose, seriously harm the body.

If children resist taking their medicine, parents should never encourage them by pretending that the medicine is candy. Nor should parents rely too heavily on anti-tamper packaging. The shrink-wraps, push-and-turn bottle caps, foil inner seals, and other anti-tamper devices are valuable but not foolproof.

In any case of medicine poisoning, do not wait to seek help. Stay calm, call your physician or the nearest hospital or poison control center, and get instructions on correct procedures. If you take a poisoned family member to a hospital or elsewhere for help, you should bring with you the container(s) from which pills or liquid were taken. Do not administer salt and water to induce vomiting; the mixture is potentially fatal.

Dangers of Alternative Medicines and Quack Remedies

Americans spend billions of dollars each year on "alternative" medicinal supplies and equipment. In too many cases the quack remedies not only do not help, they may do serious harm.

Examples of items that flood the marketplace but should not be found in your home are numerous. Among the many unproved procedures and preparations are hair analysis and cytotoxic tests for food allergies; oral chelation therapy, with vitamin and mineral capsules or tables for cardiovascular disease; and various "metabolic" programs, "non-toxic holistic medicines," radical dietary changes and regimens, and programs calling for massive doses of vitamins.

Still others include detoxification and drastic "cleansing" enemas, herbal mixtures to be applied to a sore or inflamed area, immune boosters that once were sold as cancer cures and now are promoted as treatments

for AIDS, and laetrile, an unproven cancer treatment.

The following guidelines can help protect your family from such noneffective medications:

- Beware of testimonials in ads or on labels that purportedly come from satisfied users.

- Do not believe any promises of "money-back guarantees." They are rarely dependable.

- Be wary of advertising that claims a product is effective against numerous ailments.

- Be wary of promises of a "cure" or of "complete relief" from pain.

- Discount any "FDA-tested" or "FDA-recommended" testimonials. Federal law states that the Food and Drug Administration cannot be mentioned as giving marketing approvals.

- Beware of mentions of "natural" ingredients. The definition of natural is elusive, and the word is often abused.

- Think twice before buying *anything* that is advertised with such terms as these: "amazing," "vanish," "discovery," "breakthrough," "painless," "exclusive," or "instant."

- Finally, warns the FDA, "If the product sounds too good to be true, it probably is."

Emergency-Proofing Your Home

The modern home is a marvel of devices and appliances, such as space heaters, washers, dryers, refrigerators, gas and electric furnaces, and many others. To a great extent, the hazards of large or small appliances are associated with fire. But householders should also take precautions against the dangers of electrocution, falls caused by poorly placed electrical cords, and other accident-producers.

Household items that are most likely to be hazardous are heating-cooling equipment, cooking equipment, heat tapes and humidifiers, and small electrical appliances.

Heating-Cooling Equipment

In the first category are furnaces, air conditioners, space heaters, and similar equipment. The primary safety rule with heating equipment is to make sure it is operating properly and efficiently. For furnaces of any kind, an annual checkup—usually in the summer or fall—is advisable. Many homeowners have maintenance policies that include such checkups.

All *space heaters* come with instructions for installation and operation. These instructions should be followed closely. Space heaters should be located so that they have plenty of room around them. They should be placed at a safe distance from all papers, clothing, draperies, furniture, and children. Manufacturers' labels usually indicate what the proper clearance is for a particular model.

As with furnaces, space heaters should be kept in good working condition. Missing controls should be replaced; so should missing or defective guards or screens.

Electric space heaters should have tip-over shutoff switches that turn off the current if the unit is knocked over. These heaters should also have guards around their coils. The guard can be a wire grille or other protective "fence" that keep fingers or fabrics away from the heating element.

If an extension cord is used with the space heater, the cord should have a power rating at least as high as the heater's rating. The cord should be in a safe place and out of the reach of children.

An important rule: Do not use a portable electric heater in a bathroom, near a sink, or close to water. This presents the risk of electrocution.

Gas space heaters may be vented or unvented. Both kinds need special care and attention.

If a gas space heater is vented, it should be vented correctly. That is, the vent pipe should be properly sized and free of cracks, leaks, and blockages, with tight joints and crack-free heat exchanger (to prevent leakage of carbon monoxide). If in doubt about the venting, call a servicer or your gas supplier.

When using an unvented gas space heater, you should always have a door or window slightly open in the room where the heater is located.

With either kind of gas heater, light the match *first* before you turn on the gas for the pilot light. This prevents flareups due to accumulated gas.

Woodburning, kerosene, or oil space heaters not only need to be installed properly; it would also be wise to have them inspected by a local fire safety official. Then you should use only the fuel, and in some cases the *grade* of fuel, for which the heater was designed.

The chimney of the heater or stove should be cleaned regularly, once every couple of months at least. In the case of a woodburning heater, it is best to use only paper or wood for kindling. *Never* use gasoline or another flammable or combustible fluid to start a woodburning stoves.

Cooking Equipment

The U.S. Consumer Product Safety Commission (CPSC) reports that more than 100,000 fires each year are associated with cooking equipment, especially stoves. These fires cause an estimated $300 million in property losses.

Some basic safety precautions can prevent most of these fires. For example, householders can avoid storing flammable or combustible items above the stove, including potholders, plastic utensils, or towels. Children's favorite foods, including cookies or candy, should never be kept above the range or in its immediate vicinity.

Clothing can be a trap for the unwary. Loose-fitting sleeves should not be worn while cooking. Also, you should never leave a stove unattended, especially when a burner is turned to a high setting.

Heat Tapes and Humidifiers

Heat tapes and ultrasonic humidifiers can pose home safety and health hazards. Heat tapes, used to keep exposed water pipes from freezing, present fire hazards. Ultrasonic humidifiers filled with tap water may discharge dangerous mineral particles into the air.

Electric heat tapes, or pipe heating cables, plug into wall or floor outlets. Once plugged in, they emit heat through their molded plastic insulation. Used in crawl spaces and in the substructures of homes and mobile homes, many tapes remain plugged in year-round. A thermostat in the power supply cord turns the tape on when the temperature falls below a certain level.

Improper installation of heat tapes has become a major cause of home fires in recent years. In many cases, lack of attention to the instructions that come with the product has resulted in faulty installation. Some homeowners lap the tape over itself when winding the tape around the pipe. Others ignore manufacturers' warnings that specific lengths of tape be used to protect pipes of given diameters and lengths.

If your home has heat tapes already installed you should (1) inspect all tapes, or have a licensed electrician inspect them, for proper installation or deteriorated installation; (2) check older tapes for cracks in the plastic insulation or bare wires, and replace worn tapes at once; (3) make certain, if you have plastic pipes, that the tapes you are using are recommended specifically for your kind of plastic piping; and (4) inspect all tapes to make sure none is wrapped over the thermal insulation on a pipe or near flammable objects.

Ultrasonic humidifiers using tap water have been found to spread such impurities as lead, aluminum, asbestos, or dissolved organic gases into the air. All these substances can be health hazards. To avoid such problems, use bottled, demineralized water or install demineralizing filters on your tap-water supply.

Other humidifiers pose no such mineral particle threat.

Home Electrical Safety

Have you conducted an audit of the connections, cords, gadgets (aside from major appliances), and other electrical equipment in your home? If not, such an audit is virtually a must.

You can start checking all lighting, including bulbs and sockets, all cords and extension cords, and all TV or audio equipment. Bulbs with wattages too high for the size of a fixture may overheat and cause a fire, so you should replace oversized bulbs with others of appropriate wattages. If the correct wattage is not indicated, use a bulb no larger than 60 watts.

Make sure all electrical cords are placed out of traffic areas so that people will not trip or fall over them. Stepping on cords can damage them, too, and produce fire hazards. Also check to make sure that cords do not have furniture resting on them. Cords should not be frayed, should not be wrapped around themselves or any

object, and should *never* be attached to walls with nails or staples.

Extension cords should be equipped with safety covers and should never carry more than their proper loads. Cords and electrical devices will normally have electrical ratings.

Wall outlets and switches should be checked to make sure they are working properly and fixed if they are not. You can test them by touching: an unusually warm outlet or switch may indicate an unsafe wiring condition. Plugs should fit into outlets snugly, and all outlets should have face plates so that no wiring is exposed.

Kitchen countertop appliances should be placed so that they remain dry. If they give off heat, as does a toaster, they should have some space to "breathe." Countertop appliances should be unplugged when not in use.

Cords for countertop appliances are critically important. These should never be placed so that they can come into contact with hot surfaces; especially cords around toasters, ovens, and ranges. The same rule holds with water or wet surfaces.

Because ground fault circuit interrupters (GFCIs) can prevent many electrocutions, the Consumer Product Safety Commission recommends that all countertop outlets be equipped with them. They should also be used in bathrooms and other areas where there is a risk of electrical shock. Test your GFCIs regularly in accordance with the manufacturers' instructions.

Most current building codes require that bathrooms be equipped with GFCIs. Older homes may not have them.

Other electrical appliances and equipment require safety care. These items can include hair dryers, curling irons, and electric blankets. A universal rule is that such devices be unplugged when not in use. Plugged in

and allowed to fall into water, they can cause an electrocution. They should also be in good operating condition, with no damaged wiring or other parts.

Do not use portable electric heaters in the bathroom or other rooms where they may come into contact with water. Keep *any* use of electrical devices or appliances in such rooms to a minimum.

Electric blankets also have to be used with care. They should be in good condition and have no charred spots on either the upper or the lower blanket surface. Before using them, look for cracks or breaks in wiring, connectors, and plugs.

To prevent overheating, do not cover electric blankets with other blankets, comforters, or other bedding. They should also be used flat, not folded back, and should not be tucked in except in accordance with the manufacturers' instructions.

Basement, garage, and workshop power tools and outlets constitute another extremely important area of safety concern. Power tools should have three-pronged plugs to indicate that they are double insulated. These plugs reduce the risk of electric shock.

Check your fuse box or circuit breaker. A fuse of the wrong size can present a fire hazard. If you do not know what sizes are correct, an electrician can tell you. Your circuit breakers should be "exercised" periodically if they are to remain in good working order. This procedure is simple:

1. Turn off your freezer, refrigerator, and air conditioner.

2. Flip each circuit breaker off and on three times.

3. Turn the appliances back on.

Repeat this routine at least once a year. Also check the GFCIs on your basement, garage, or workshop equipment to make sure they are working properly.

Receptacles located outdoors represent a final stage in your electrical audit. These receptacles or outlets should have waterproof covers that keep water out and prevent malfunctions. The covers should be *closed* when not in use. If your home has no GFCIs on outside receptacles, have them installed.

As regards electric lawn movers and other electric garden tools and appliances, the basic rules of safety apply. But remember: extension cords used outside should be specifically designed for such use, or you may be risking a fire or a serious shock.

Home Fire Prevention and Protection

Many home fires have nothing to do with gadgets or appliances. Both the simplest and the most complex of our daily amenities can be fire hazards. Extremely flammable liquids provide power for our cars. Fabrics and upholstered furniture can ignite and burn. Some of us carry fire sources, matches or cigarette lighters, in our pockets.

In the sections that follow, effort will be made to call attention to the most important of these hazards.

Matches, Lighters, and Cigarettes

Some prohibitions that help to immunize your home against accidental fires are matters of common sense. Others have more technical origins.

Some 140 young children die each year in fires that they or their friends or siblings started. Children start thousands more home fires while playing with matches or lighters. Thus a basic rule is that children should not have access to either matches or cigarette lighters. Both

should be kept out of sight and reach.

Adults should never use either matches or lighters as toys or sources of amusement. Cigarette butts should not be left burning in ashtrays that children can reach.

Ashtray and cigarette discipline is always appropriate. Lighted butts should not be thrown into the trash. A lighted butt can start a major fire. Ashtrays should not be placed on the arms of chairs, where they can be knocked off. As a precaution, check the furniture where smokers have been sitting to make sure that no lighted cigarettes have fallen unnoticed behind or between cushions or under furniture.

In a recent year, 46,700 mattress and bedding fires took some 700 lives. Thus, "No smoking in bed" represents a cardinal rule of home safety.

Furniture Precautions

Because many home fires start on pieces of furniture, you should take special care when selecting the items you need. In particular, you should look for furniture designed to reduce the likelihood of furniture fires that may be started by cigarettes.

This task has become simpler in recent years. Manufacturers are making upholstered furniture far more fire resistant than they have in the past. All furniture that meets the standards of the Upholstered Furniture Action Council (UFAC) carries a gold-colored tag with red letters that states, "Important Consumer Safety Information from UFAC."

Other precautions help reduce the risks of injury or death from furniture fires. For example, look for upholstery fabrics made primarily from such thermoplastic fibers as nylon, polyester, acrylic, and olefin. These resist ignition by burning cigarettes better than do rayon or cotton, both cellulose fabrics.

Flammable Liquids

The federal Hazardous Substances Act establishes three labeling categories for liquid products:

1. *Extremely flammable liquids* include gasoline, the white gas commonly used in camping stoves, contact adhesives, and wood stains that produce ignitable vapors at room temperature. Once ignited, the vapors act as wicks to carry the fire to the container of the liquid.

2. *Flammable liquids* produce ignitable vapors at higher temperatures. This group includes paint thinners, some paints, and automotive products such as brake fluids.

3. *Combustible liquids* can be ignited but are less likely to catch fire than the other kinds. This category includes furniture polishes, oil-based paints, fuel oil, diesel oil, and kerosene.

Remember: some products do not carry *flammable* labels because they will not catch fire in liquid form as they come from the container (such as paint strippers). Once they are applied, however, they become quite flammable because their flame-suppressant chemicals evaporate.

Use solvent-based products with adequate moving air ventilation, and ventilate the work area. These precautions will keep fumes from building up and igniting. They will also protect you from the toxic effects of invisible and sometimes explosive vapors.

Wise Use of Flammable Liquids

At one time or another, nearly everyone has to use flammable liquids. Here are some fundamental rules for wise use:

● Never use such liquids near flames or a source of sparks, including pilot lights.

- Use gasoline only as a fuel, not as a cleaning fluid.

- Always shut off power mowers, chain saws, or other gas-powered equipment before refueling them. Refuel outdoors and wait for hot parts to cool before adding fuel.

- Use only liquids identified as *charcoal starters* to get charcoal fires going. Never pour on additional fluid after starting the fire.

Proper Storage

Gasoline and other extremely flammable liquids should be stored outside your house or apartment, but they should *not* be stored in the trunk of your car. Children should not be able to reach your safe-storage place. For added insurance, lock up all flammable liquids.

Never keep gasoline in glass bottles, plastic jugs, or other makeshift containers. If possible, invest in a gasoline container with such safety features as a pressure release valve or a flame arrester.

Flammable Fabrics

There are four basic safety principles regarding the flammability of fabrics:

1. All fibers used in ordinary clothing can burn. But some catch fire and burn less readily than others. The more-fire-resistant fabrics are fire-resistant cotton, wool, rayon, polyester, and modacrylic. Fabrics that burn most readily are acetate, untreated cotton and rayon, and linen.

2. The way in which a fabric is made determines the way it burns. As a rule, heavy, tightly constructed fabrics ignite with difficulty and burn more slowly than fabrics that are light, open, or fuzzy. Once ignited, however, the heavier fabrics burn longer than the lightweights and can cause very serious injuries.

3. "Flame resistant" does not mean "noncombustible." The phrase only indicates that a fabric is designed to resist ignition and burning. Fabrics are incapable of providing you with protection if you reach into a fireplace, a wood-burning stove, or an oven. To maintain a fabric's flame-resistant qualities, follow the manufacturer's instructions regarding care and cleaning.

4. A garment's style has much to do with safety. The safest clothes are those that fit closely, have large neck openings and quick release closures, and are wrap-style.

Remember the three rules for extinguishing a clothing fire:

1. Don't run.

2. Do try to remove the burning article of clothing.

3. If that fails, drop to the floor or ground and roll back and forth.

Smoke Detectors

There are two basic rules regarding smoke detectors. First, every home should have at least one smoke detector, approved by a recognized national testing laboratory. Second, at least one smoke detector should be placed on each floor of your home.

Both types of detectors, ionization and photoelectric detectors, if well designed and engineered, are effective. The particular layout of your home may determine whether you need plug-in or battery-powered devices. Both have advantages and disadvantages.

The battery-powered smoke detector can run out of power, usually after about a year. It then gives a warning sound, at which time you need to install new batteries.

The plug-in detector operates like a permanently burning lamp. However, it cannot operate if fire or some other interference breaks the electrical circuit that powers the detector. Other tips:

- Place detectors high up, on a ceiling or wall, close to where people sleep. Otherwise the alarm may not be heard.

- Never place a smoke detector in the kitchen or very near it. Airborne kitchen grease and cooking fumes can easily activate the device, touching off a false alarm.

- Even if a battery-powered detector does not give a signal that its batteries are running down, change the batteries at least once a year.

- With a photoelectric detector, the light source should be replaced as soon as it burns out.

- Test photoelectric detectors regularly with real smoke—from a just-extinguished candle, for example. Test ionization detectors using a *lighted* candle. Test detectors every two to four weeks.

Fire Extinguishers

Fire extinguishers complement your smoke alarms and should be part of your home "immunization" program. The extinguishers should be kept in areas where fires are most likely to occur: the kitchen, home workshop, or rooms where flammable materials are kept, where people may be smoking, or where there are hazard-producing activities or materials.

Fire extinguishers are rated according to size. A five-pound extinguisher rated ABC (meaning it can be used to fight fires of any kind) is considered minimal for home protection. Many homeowners, however, buy two-and-one-half-pound extinguishers specifically to fight small kitchen fires.

The best protection against home fires may be a common garden hose.

Using extensions, it can be made long enough to reach every room in the house. You can also attach nozzles that make it possible to sprinkle, spray, or direct a solid stream. Keep the hose in one place so that it is always ready to use.

An Escape Plan

Fire causes most home emergencies, but other conditions can be just as disastrous. An accident outside the home may force immediate evacuation; so may natural disasters such as storms or floods.

An escape plan should be part of your program for immunizing your home against emergencies. The plan can save lives by preventing panic.

For Fires

In cases of fire, you need to have two exits from each part of the house. You may want to consider installing rope or chain safety ladders outside windows that are too high above the ground for safe jumping. If you live in an apartment, you should obtain escape instructions from your building management or landlord or your local fire department.

Through informal fire drills, you can help to ensure that each member of your household understands the escape plan. You should include small children in all rehearsals, and repeat them periodically. Everyone should know where they are to meet to be sure everyone got out safely.

Young children should understand clearly that they have to evacuate when everyone else does. They *must* escape; they cannot hide under a bed or in a closet.

Three rules are critically important:

1. *Stay low.* Since most smoke rises, you need to keep low, crawling on hands and knees when necessary, to pass safely through a smoke-filled hallway or room.

2. *Feel doors before you open them.* If you find that the door panels, the knob, or the molding surrounding the door are hot to the touch, it may mean that the fire is just outside. Move toward another exit.

3. *Use wet cloths.* To avoid excessive smoke inhalation, a major cause of fire-related deaths, you can wet pillow cases, towels, or other fabrics and hold them over your face while you make your way to an exit.

For Natural Disasters

In case of natural disasters, you need to obtain accurate, current information as well as warnings, advice, or instructions from agencies. Disregarding such instructions or advice can endanger you and your family.

Your home should be equipped with a battery-powered portable radio. The radio could mean the difference between disaster and survival if your power is interrupted. You should have spare, sealed-in-the-package batteries for the radio. To prolong their lives, you can keep them in a refrigerator freezer.

Other avenues of communication in an emergency are available in most communities in the United States. These include amateur radio, citizens' band (CB) radio, community disaster warnings, special signals and communications methods, and (of course) the telephone.

Amateur radio or "ham" operators have proven to be unusually helpful in emergencies. To locate such an operator in your community, you can inquire among your neighbors or write, enclosing a self-addressed, stamped envelope, to the Amateur Radio Relay League, 225 Main St., Newington, CT 06111.

Poisonous or Harmful Substances

Each year, more than 100,000 children under the age of five become victims of accidental ingestion of poisonous or harmful substances. These include medicines and such flammable liquids as gasoline, but they also include a vast range of liquids, solids, and gases that find their ways into the home.

Substances that require special precautions range from carbon monoxide to spoiled food, cleaning fluids, detergents, and pesticides. Some general guidelines are as follows:

- Bring such substances into your home only if necessary, and then in the smallest possible quantity.

- Keep all products in their original containers, never in containers customarily used for food or drinks.

- If a product comes in a child-resistant container, never transfer it to a container that has no such protection.

- Carefully separate foods from potentially harmful products.

- After using a product that comes in a child-resistant container, resecure the cap or other closure.

- Make sure that all products that entail any risk or hazard are properly labeled, and turn on lights before using such products.

- Store potentially hazardous products in a separate area from other household products, preferably in a locked cabinet.

Because not all the harmful substances that enter your home have warnings on their containers, you should make it your business to learn whether hazards exist.

Contamination from Pets

The case of a one-year-old boy in Columbus, Ohio alerted the U.S. government to some of the hazards that can enter your home with pets.

Four days after his mother gave him a baby turtle, the child became ill with fever, abdominal pain, and bloody diarrhea. The following day, his brother showed similar symptoms. Analysis of stool cultures showed that the children had been infected with salmonella, a disease-causing organism carried by the turtle.

The children recovered. Subsequently, however, the U.S. Food and Drug Administration (FDA) banned the sale and public distribution of small turtles with shells less than four inches long. Included in the ban are turtle eggs. Aside from salmonella, turtles can introduce into your home other bacteria that can cause fever, diarrhea, and various gastrointestinal problems. Infection can lead to additional complications and even death.

Almost any kind of pet can introduce disease-causing organisms into the home. "Some pet store owners may . . . be ignorant of the potential diseases and illnesses that can be caused not only by turtles, but by other reptiles, birds, and mammals sold as pets," according to an FDA official.

Among household pets, dogs are susceptible to infection by a variety of worms and other parasites. Worms present a particularly insidious problem because the host pets can become seriously sick unless owners take curative steps. Also, many varieties of worms can infect dogs, and the symptoms can be extremely diverse and complex.

Generally, humans cannot be infected by dog-borne illnesses. But hookworm is an exception. As the FDA notes, "Although canine hookworms can't mature in people, the larvae can migrate through the skin and subcutaneous tissue, causing serious skin lesions."

Lead Poisoning

Many ceramic-ware products sold in the United States are coated with glazes that are applied and fused onto a shaped piece of clay. Cadmium may be used to enhance the vividness of the colors.

Both cadmium and lead are toxic metals. Both can, under given conditions, leach into foods stored in some glazed ceramic containers.

Since 1971, the FDA has limited the amounts of lead that can leach or soak out of ceramic ware into foods. But cases of lead poisoning and various studies have renewed concerns about lead from all sources and from many different consumer products. These products include the 60 percent of all ceramic foodware imported into the United States from foreign countries.

Lead can, however, invade the home environment in other ways or from other sources. Some paints manufactured before 1978 contained lead (see Lead Poisoning, pp. 163–4). That paint still covers the walls, floors, and furniture of many older apartments and homes. In some communities, water reaches homes by way of old lead service pipes and water system mains.

You can reduce the risks to a safe minimum and avoid the stomach disorders and other problems, including brain damage in severe cases, that lead can produce.

Ceramic-ware Lead Poisoning

The following precautions can help prevent lead poisoning from ceramic ware:

1. *Avoid storing foods in ceramic ware.* Much preferred and far safer are glass or plastic containers. The high acid content of many foods increases the amounts of lead that the food can absorb.

2. *Be especially wary of products imported from or bought in foreign countries.* Manufacturers in those countries do not necessarily adhere to high safety standards. You may be wise either to avoid purchasing dinnerware made in other countries or to use such products for other purposes, such as decoration.

3. *Avoid using antiques or collectibles to hold food and vegetables.* They may be family heirlooms, or they may have been bought at garage or rummage sales, antique shops, or flea markets, but ceramic ware of uncertain origin may be dangerous.

4. *Beware of ceramic items made by amateurs or hobbyists.* Hobbyists can obtain safe glazes today, but you may not be able to tell whether the maker actually used such a glaze.

You have another choice if you want to use ceramic items to store foods or liquids: you can have your ceramic ware tested by a qualified commercial laboratory. Check your local health department or the telephone book for laboratories in your area.

Paint Lead Poisoning

Parents of young children should learn to recognize the symptoms of such poisoning and to consult as quickly as possible with a doctor, local hospital or clinic, or public health department. Delay can, in serious cases, lead to mental retardation, paralysis, and even death.

A difficulty in recognizing paint lead poisoning is that the symptoms are similar to those of many other childhood ailments. A child with lead poisoning may complain of stomachaches or may vomit. Headaches, a loss of appetite, crankiness, and excessive tiredness may be other symptoms. The child may lose interest in normal play.

A second problem is that a child can be poisoned by chewing on or eating dirt, dust, newspapers, some pottery, some furniture, or many other nonfood substances containing lead. But hospital or clinic blood tests for lead poisoning take only minutes. If a high concentration of lead is found in the blood, treatment may be necessary. Follow the directions and guidance of your doctor or local health department.

Depending on your child's age, you may be able to explain that he or she should eat nothing but food. Babysitters should be instructed about lead poisoning hazards and should keep children in their care from eating paint, newspapers, or other nonfood substances.

To remove the threat of paint lead poisoning, keep your home in good shape, free of water leaks from faulty plumbing, defective roofs, or exterior holes that could admit rain or dampness. Repaint the interior surfaces of your home every four to five years. Here are some further precautions:

1. Replaster any plaster walls that may be cracking or peeling.

2. Using a broom or stiff brush, remove all the pieces of loose paint from the walls.

3. Sweep up and put into a paper bag all the pieces of paint and plaster and place them in a trash can. *Do not burn them.*

4. While removing lead-based paint by scraping or sanding, keep children and pregnant women away (preferably outside the home) and take precautions to protect yourself. The dust you raise may be harmful.

The Allergen-Free Environment

Some 35 million Americans suffer from allergies. They may have hay fever, asthma, food intolerances or sensitivities, or adverse skin reactions to the stings of hornets, bees, or wasps. While medical scientists do not completely understand the causes and workings of allergies, great progress is being made in this area.

One result of allergy research is that most people with allergies are able to lead normal lives in spite of diverse symptoms and reactions. For hay fever sufferers, doctors can prescribe drugs to relieve irritating nasal inflammation, or allergic rhinitis. Cromolyn sodium may be prescribed to relieve the symptoms of asthma; the sodium can be inhaled through a spinhaler, nebulizer machine, or metered dose inhaler.

For most allergy victims, the best defense is to avoid the substances or circumstances that bring on attacks or symptoms. If there are allergy sufferers in your family, you may want to establish a home environment that is as allergen-free as possible. Furry pets are a major cause of allergic reactions. Carpeting, unless laid on a cement floor, serves as the perfect incubator for dust mites. Books can also harbor mites. Both feather and foam rubber pillows can be hazards. The best protection is cleanliness.

Radon, A Special Case

Radon is a colorless, odorless, radioactive gas that is almost impossible to detect without instruments. It seeps through the crevices or spaces in the soil or rock on which a home is built. It can enter your home through cracks, drains, and the tiny holes or pores in walls.

Persons exposed to radon face serious health risks, specifically lung cancer. Also, continued exposure to radon increases the risk of illness.

Many persons never realize that the gas is invading their homes.

Detection of radon requires special equipment but moderate cost. Two commercially available radon detectors are the charcoal canister and the alpha track detector. The former calls for a test period of three to seven days, and the latter requires two to four weeks. Trained personnel can provide other methods of detection. Reports on measurements of radon gas are made in terms of picocuries per liter (pCi/l).

Readings of above 1.0 WL (working level) or above 200 pCi/l, require immediate follow-up measurements.

Doing it yourself to close off the radon entry points in your basement begins with caulking. Using urethane or silicone caulk, seal up the gap (if any) between the basement floor and all walls; fill cracks in the mortar joints between concrete blocks; and lay a thick bead of caulk around the perimeter of sump openings. Treated plywood or a metal sheet can then be used to cover the sump, with more caulk used as a sealant.

Use ready-mix concrete to seal any large openings around pipes, pipe-chase openings, and spaces along the top rows of concrete-block walls. Inject insulation into the top rows of concrete-block walls before sealing them. Foam backing can be applied before the concrete sealing is applied to pipe-chase openings.

Ventilation supplements your efforts to close all gaps and holes in your basement's floors and walls. Without creating uncomfortable drafts, you can ventilate under your basement slab *if:* (1) you have a continuous slab with no large, unsealed openings to the earth beneath, and (2) there is a sufficiently porous bed under the slab to permit ventilating air to circulate through it. Given both conditions, you can create your own subslab vent system with pipes and a fan; the air intake and exhaust pipes should be located in opposite corners of the basement.

Other methods of ventilating your basement include forced-air systems using fans to maintain a balanced air exchange rate; heat-recovery ventilators that replace radon-tainted air with outside air; and use of a product called Enka-drain, which traps radon in a nylon mesh airspace that is then vented through an exhaust pipe.

Because it is a gas, radon always moves from a higher pressure area (the ground) to a lower-pressure one (your house). That means you have a final alternative to ventilation: pressurize your basement and home by providing outside air supplies for wood stoves, fireplaces, gas dryers, and furnaces.

Safety for the Old and the Young

Some precautions can help prevent home accidents. Older persons need special consideration because they may not be as mobile or as observant as they once were. Young children tend to actively and continuously explore what they see as their world.

Safety for Children

Some steps that will make home life safer for children are obvious. Toy boxes or chests should not have lids that can crush small fingers, for example. Windows should have safety locks so that children cannot open them more than two or three inches.

The bars of a child's bed should not be more than two-and- one-half inches apart. Baby carriages should not tip over easily, and should have safety harnesses.

Other precautions: High chairs should not have sharp edges or points, open tubes that might trap small limbs, or mechanisms that could pinch. Night clothes *must* be flame-resistant, and all clothes should be free of cords or other ties. Clothing for toddlers should allow free movement and growth.

Examine your child's room. Beds or cots should be solid and smooth, with no sharp projections and no horizontal bars that could make it easy for your child to climb out. If you are using a baby bed, it should have a dropside mechanism that is child-proof. Avoid plastic sheets in favor of absorbent cotton, and the sheets should be fitted or tightly tucked in.

Children's furniture should be soft, low, and free of sharp edges. The furniture should be positioned so that young children cannot climb onto shelves or window sills.

Toys should be selected carefully and maintained in a safe condition. The Consumer Product Safety Commission notes that all toys that come into your home should be adapted to your child's age, interests, and skill level. They should have quality design and construction. Instructions of use should be read carefully and followed. Labels can guide you to some extent. Plastic wrappings, if any, should be discarded immediately.

Check periodically for breakage or wear and tear that makes toys unsafe. Check, too, for surfaces with splinters. Repaint toys only with lead-free paint, and look for and remove rust or weak parts on outdoor toys in particular. Here are some important safety measures regarding toys:

- Teach your child to put his toys away when they are not in use. It's safer.

- Make sure all toys conform to laws that ban small, swallowable parts.

- Prohibit toy caps, some noise-making guns, and other toys that can produce loud noises that might damage hearing. (The law requires labels on boxes or caps that explode with a sound above a certain level: "WARNING: Do not fire closer than one foot to the ear. Do not use indoors.")

- Avoid leaving long strings or cords, on toys or off, in cribs or where young children can get at them.

- Keep out of your home dangerous projectiles such as guided missiles, dart guns, flying toys, and lawn darts. If you have very young children, exercise caution with balloons and other toys that may be best suited for older children.

- Monitor any electric toys so that they cannot shock or burn. Electric toys have to meet specific requirements for maximum surface temperatures, electrical construction, and appropriate warning labels. Electric toys with heating elements are not recommended for children under eight years old.

- Make sure infants' toys, such as rattles and teethers, are large enough that they cannot be swallowed.

A house check is in order if you have children. Is all furniture safe? Are stairs fitted with a handrail? Are there safety gates at the top and bottom? Are the stairs well lighted and free of ill-fitting carpets? In the bathroom, are all bath toys safe? Are they plastic? (They should be.) Have hand grips and rubber mats been properly placed, and are they also safe? Do you have non-slip flooring?

In the kitchen, in addition to the safety tips already noted, you will want to make sure that heavy items are out of the reach of little children; that only safe-to-play-with items are kept in children's-level cupboards; that doors have locks or bolts, where necessary; and that you use table mats instead of cloths if you eat at the kitchen table.

In the garage, do-it-yourself materials and tools should be kept in locked toolboxes, on safe, high shelves, or hanging out of reach. Discarded refrigerators or freezers should either be padlocked or have their doors removed.

Safety for the Elderly

Make your home safe for older family members or visitors before someone falls and incurs the most common of all injuries for older people: a broken hip. In addition to the safety measures that make your home safe for children, you can take further steps to protect older people in your home:

- Provide night lights in rooms that may need them, and make sure bathrooms and other rooms have light switches near entry doors.

- If possible, eliminate extension cords.

- Install light switches at the top and bottom of stairways.

- Provide toilet facilities on the same floor as an older person's bedroom.

- If necessary, install a higher toilet seat.

- Install handrails or grab bars for the toilet, bathtub, and stairway, and apply non-slip appliqués to tub bottoms and shower floors.

- Remove casters from furniture, or keep castered furniture against a wall.

- Where possible, give floors and carpets non-slip surfacing.

- Make the top and bottom stair step a different color than the others.

- Tape or tack down the edges of area rugs, runners, and mats that have a tendency to roll up or curl, or simply get rid of them.

- To prevent scalds, keep temperatures in your water heater below 120° F.

Examine your home through the eyes of an older person. Would you have access to a telephone if you were to fall? Can you install at least one telephone that could be reached if you were unable to stand? In the kitchen, are towels or dishcloths hanging close to the toaster or the stove? Do you have good, even lighting over the stove, sink, and countertop? Do you need additional lighting under a cabinet or over a countertop where you slice or cut foods?

Because hundreds of elderly persons are treated annually for injuries resulting from falls from boxes or chairs, a step-stool can be an extremely practical item of furniture. But the stool itself should be safe. It should have tight screws and braces, and it should have a handrail to hold while standing on the top step. If the stool has broken parts, it should be discarded.

Before stepping up, the stool should be fully opened and stable.

Clothing

Clothing can present a number of safety hazards for older people. The CPSC has estimated that 70 percent of all persons who die from clothing fires are over 65 years of age.

Some of those fires have started when older persons reached over hot or burning stove or range surfaces. It is safest not to wear clothes that have loose, flowing sleeves, or at least to tie or pin the sleeves snugly to your arm and wrist. Loose sleeves present another hazard: they can catch on pot or pan handles, overturning hot water or food and causing scalds. Awareness of how clothing can contribute to home safety also extends to the selection of nightwear.

Any program for making the home safe for older persons should include most of the other steps noted in this chapter, including those referring to electrical safety and flammable fabrics.

The Food Department

Threats to your health can enter your home in a grocery bag. They can develop in your home in the forms of mold or bacteria on food. Poor food handling practices, inside and outside the home, contribute to these health hazards. The greatest threats are a lack of sanitation, insufficient cooking, and improper storage (see also "Food Hazards," pp. 967–970).

Bacteria cause about 95 percent of all cases of food poisoning. People can ingest illness-producing bacteria in contaminated foods; the bacteria then multiply and spread infections in the digestive tract or the bloodstream. Such digestive problems occur most often in warm weather, when food may be taken to picnics or on cookout without proper refrigeration.

Contamination may also take place if parasitic animals such as the roundworm, found sometimes in pork, enter the body. The roundworm produces a disease called trichinosis.

There are four main kinds of bacteria that can contaminate foods and cause diseases: salmonella; "staph," or *staphylococcus aureus;* botulism; and *clostridium perfringens,* which causes diarrhea. However, you can avoid contamination if you take precautions. The four kinds of bacteria can produce symptoms as mild as an upset stomach or as severe as death, as in the case of botulism.

Food-Borne Poisons and Allergens

When shopping, you usually have to take on faith the food manufacturer's and the grocer's claims that their food is safe. But you can certainly be selective. You may want to avoid foods that touch off negative or allergic reactions. If certain foods have given you gastrointestinal or other problems in the past, it would be wise to avoid those foods when shopping.

You may have allergies—for example, to sulfites, the additives in many foods that can cause serious or even fatal reactions. Today, the labels on food packaging provide an abundance of dietary information to aid consumers in making choices.

Buying intelligently and carefully constitutes your first line of defense against food-borne illness and disease. Here are some guidelines for the conscientious shopper:

- Watch for possible spoilage in everything you buy, and *never* purchase food in a torn package or a dented or bulging can.

- Exercise your right to doubt: check display cases to make sure frozen foods are stored above the frost lines or load lines. Never buy frozen food that has softened.

- Always pick up meat, poultry, and dairy products last when making your grocery rounds.

- Never leave a sackful of groceries in the car on a hot day. Make the grocery store your last stop on the way home, and make sure perishable groceries are wrapped in an insulated bag for the trip home.

- Once home, put everything away quickly in the appropriate storage place, whether refrigerator, freezer, or storage cupboard.

Different foods require different storage methods. The labels on many packaged or canned foods provide instructions for storage procedures.

Food preparation under the wrong conditions creates many of the problems that Americans face when they sit down to eat. The wrong conditions range from unclean hands, hair, fingernails, and clothing to failure to wash one's hands thoroughly after us-

ing the toilet. You should wash your hands thoroughly after smoking or blowing your nose. You should also wash your hands after handling raw meat, poultry, or eggs and before working with other foods. Other precautions: Do not use your hands to mix foods; use clean utensils instead. Avoid using the same spoon more than once to taste food while preparing it. Never eat any food directly from the jar or can; this could contaminate the can's contents. Scrub potatoes and other raw foods before cooking them. Carefully clean all utensils, work surfaces, dishes, and kitchen equipment before using them. And drink only pasteurized milk.

It is best to serve foods soon after they are cooked; otherwise, refrigerate them. You can refrigerate hot or warm foods if you are sure they will not raise the refrigerator temperature above 45° F.

The temperatures at which you keep foods affect directly your home's level of food safety. Hot foods should be kept above 140 degrees for safety while cold foods should be stored at 40 degrees or lower. The danger zone in which foods can develop bacteria, sometimes in the space of two or three hours, lies between 60° and 125°. Keeping food warm for several hours in an oven can be hazardous if the oven's temperature is between 60° and 125°.

Some foods require special attention. Eggs, for example, should be used only if they are fresh, clean, uncracked, and odor-free. You may make exceptions if the eggs are unspoiled and if they are to be used in recipes that call for thorough cooking. When serving a dish that has eggs as a major ingredient, cool the dish quickly after it is cooked, preferably in cold water, if it is not to be served hot. Then refrigerate it.

Meat, poultry, and fish are also sensitive. If frozen, they should be

thawed in the refrigerator. If you need to thaw these products more quickly, you can place them, sealed in watertight wrappers, in cold water. To cook frozen items of these types, allow about one-and-one-half times the ordinary cooking times for thawed products of the same weight and shape.

Meats, poultry, or fish should be stuffed just before they are cooked, not a day or two ahead of time. The stuffing should reach a temperature of at least 165° F. during cooking. Use reliable timetables or follow package directions when cooking these products, and take extra care with ground meat. Because it is handled several times in packaging, ground meat should be cooked thoroughly and never eaten raw. Some *hams* need to be cooked, and should be if you have any doubt.

Fish, meat, and poultry should be cooked entirely in a single process, not cooked partially one day and then finished on another. Poultry should always be cooked thoroughly. If you store poultry products before the day on which you plan to cook them, you should store the giblets and the rest of the bird separately in the refrigerator. Use the hot dogs and cold meat within a few days after purchasing, and never more than a week later.

Freezer practices should be grounded in common sense. A fundamental rule is that freezing does not kill the bacteria in food; it only keeps existing bacteria from multiplying. Thawing enables those bacteria to begin to proliferate again.

Do not refreeze food that has been frozen and thawed. To protect frozen foods, wrap or package each item carefully to keep air away from the product. Different items can be kept safely in a freezing compartment for different periods of time, depending on the product. Label each item with the date it went into the freezer and the type of food.

Emergency Transport

In the majority of situations, the transfer of an injured person should be handled only by experienced rescue personnel. If you yourself must move a victim to a physician's office or hospital emergency room, here are a few important rules to remember:

1. Give all necessary first aid before attempting to move the victim. Do everything to reduce pain and to make the patient comfortable.

2. If you improvise a stretcher, be sure it is strong enough to carry the victim and that you have enough people to carry it. Shutters, doors, boards, and even ladders may be used as stretchers. Just be sure that the stretcher is padded underneath to protect the victim and that a blanket or coat is available to cover him and protect him from exposure.

3. Bring the stretcher to the victim, not the victim to the stretcher. Slide him onto the stretcher by grasping his clothing or lift him—if enough bearers are available—as shown in the illustration.

4. Secure the victim to the stretcher so he won't fall off. You may want to tie his feet together to minimize his movements.

5. Unless specific injuries prevent it, the victim should be lying on his back while he is being moved. However, a person who is having difficulty breathing because of a chest injury might be more comfortable if his head and shoulders are raised slightly. A person with a severe injury to the back of his head should be kept lying on his side. In any case, place the patient in a comfortable position that will protect him from further injury.

6. Try to transport the patient feet first.

(Adapted with permission from American Red Cross illustrations.)

How to lift an injured or unconscious person to place him on a stretcher. Three bearers on each side of the victim kneel on the knee closer to the victim's feet. The bearers work their hands and forearms gently under the victim to about the midline of the back. On signal, they lift together as shown; on a following signal, they stand as a unit, if that is necessary. In lowering the victim to a stretcher or other litter, the procedure is reversed.

The proper way to carry a victim on a stretcher. One bearer is at the head, one at the foot, and one at either side of the stretcher. The victim should be carried feet first.

7. Unless absolutely necessary, don't try to put a stretcher into a passenger car. It's almost impossible to get the stretcher or injured person into a passenger car without further injuring him. If there is no ambulance, a station wagon or truck makes a good substitute.

8. When you turn the patient over to a doctor or take him to an emergency room of a hospital, give a complete account of the situation to the person taking charge. Tell the doctor what you've done for the patient and what you suspect might cause further problems.

Alphabetic Guide to Medical Emergencies

Abdominal Wound

Abdominal wounds can result from gunshots during hunting or working with firearms, from falling on a knife or sharp object at home or work, or from a variety of other mishaps ranging from automobile accidents to a mugging attack. Such a wound can be a major emergency requiring surgery and other professional care. Call a physician or arrange for quick transportation to a hospital as quickly as possible.

Emergency Treatment

If there is severe bleeding, try to control it with pressure. Keep the victim lying on his back with the knees bent; place a pillow, coat, or a similar soft object under the knees to help hold them in the bent position. If abdominal organs are exposed, do not touch them for any reason. Cover the wound with a sterile dressing. Keep the dressing moistened with sterile water or the cleanest water available. Boiled water can be used to moisten the dressing, but be sure it has cooled before applying.

If the victim is to be moved to a hospital or physician's office, be sure the dressing over the wound is large enough and is held in place with a bandage. In addition to pain, you can expect the victim to experience nausea and vomiting, muscle spasms, and severe shock. Make the victim as comfortable as possible under the circumstances; if he complains of thirst, moisten his mouth with a few drops of water, but do not permit him to swallow the liquid.

Abrasions

Emergency Treatment

Wash the area in which the skin is scraped or rubbed off with soap and water, using clean gauze or cotton. Allow the abrasion to air-dry, and then cover it with a loose sterile dressing held in place with a bandage. If a sterile dressing is not available, use a clean handerchief.

Change the dressing after the first 24 hours, using household hydrogen peroxide to ease its removal if it sticks to the abrasion because of clotted blood. If the skinned area appears to be accompanied by swelling, or is painful or tender to the touch, consult a physician.

Acid Burns

Among acids likely to be encountered at work and around the home are sulphuric, nitric, and hydrochloric acids. Wet-cell batteries, such as automobile batteries, contain acid powerful enough to cause chemical destruction of body tissues, and some metal cleaners contain powerful acids.

Emergency Treatment

Wash off the acid immediately, using large amounts of clean, fresh, cool water. Strip off or cut off any clothing that may have absorbed any of the acid. If possible, put the victim in a shower bath; if a shower is not available, flood the affected skin areas with as much water as possible. However, do not apply water forcefully since this could aggravate damage already done to skin or other tissues.

After as much of the acid as possible has been eliminated by flooding with water, apply a mild solution of sodium bicarbonate or another mild alkali such as lime water. Caution should be exercised, however, in neutralizing an acid burn because the chemical reaction between an acid and an alkali can produce intense heat that would aggravate the injury; also, not all acids are effectively neutralized by alkalis—carbolic acid burns, for example, should be neutralized with alcohol.

Wash the affected areas once more with fresh water, then dry gently with sterile gauze; be careful not to break the skin or to open blisters. Extensive acid burns will cause extreme pain and shock; have the victim lie down with the head and chest a little lower than the rest of the body. As soon as possible, summon a physician or rush the victim to the emergency room of a hospital.

Aerosol Sprays

Although aerosol sprays generally are regarded as safe when handled according to directions, they can be directed accidentally toward the face with resulting contamination of the eyes or inhalation of the fumes. The pressurized containers may also contain products or propellants that are highly flammable, producing burns when used near an open flame. When stored near heat, in direct sunlight, or in a closed auto, the containers may explode violently.

Emergency Treatment

If eyes are contaminated by spray particles, flush the eye surfaces with water to remove any particles of the powder mist. Then carefully examine eye surfaces to determine if chemicals appear to be imbedded in the surface of the cornea. If aerosol spray is inhaled, move the patient to a well-ventilated area; keep him lying down, warm, and quiet. If breathing fails, administer artificial respiration. Victims of exploding containers or burning contents of aerosol containers should be given appropriate emergency treatment for bleeding, burns, and shock.

The redness and irritation of eye injuries should subside within a short time. If they do not, or if particles of spray seem to be imbedded in the surface of the eyes, take the victim to an ophthalmologist. A physician should also be summoned if a victim fails to recover quickly from the effects of inhaling an aerosol spray, particularly if the victim suffers from asthma or a similar lung disorder or from an abnormal heart condition.

Alkali Burns

Alkalis are used in the manufacture of soap and cleaners and in certain household cleaning products. They combine with fats to form soaps and may produce a painful injury when in contact with body surfaces.

Emergency Treatment

Flood the burned area with copious amounts of clean, cool, fresh water. Put the victim under a shower if possible, or otherwise pour running water over the area for as long as is necessary to dilute and weaken the corrosive chemical. Do not apply the water with such force that skin or other tissues are damaged. Remove clothing contaminated by the chemical.

Neutralize the remaining alkali with diluted vinegar, lemon juice, or a similar mild acid. Then wash the affected areas again with fresh water. Dry carefully with sterile gauze, being careful not to open blisters or otherwise cause skin breaks that could result in infection. Summon professional medical care as soon as possible. Meanwhile, treat the victim for shock.

Angina Pectoris

Angina pectoris is a condition that causes acute chest pain because of interference with the supply of oxygen to the heart. Although the pain is sometimes confused with ulcer or acute indigestion symptoms, it has a distinct characteristic of its own, producing a feeling of heaviness, strangling, tightness, or suffocation. Angina is a symptom rather than a disease, and may be a chronic condition with those over 50. It is usually treated by placing a nitroglycerine tablet under the tongue.

An attack of acute angina can be brought on by emotional stress, overeating, strenuous exercise, or by any activity that makes excessive demands on heart function.

Emergency Treatment

An attack usually subsides in about ten minutes, during which the patient appears to be gasping for breath. He should be kept in a semireclining position rather than made to lie flat, and should be moved carefully only in order to place pillows under his head and chest so that he can breathe more easily. A physician should be called promptly after the onset of an attack.

Animal Bites/Rabies

Wild animals, particularly bats, serve as a natural reservoir of rabies, a disease that is almost always fatal unless promptly and properly treated. But the virus may be present in the saliva of any warm-blooded animal. Domestic animals should be immunized against rabies by vaccines injected by a veterinarian.

Rabies is transmitted to humans by an animal bite or through a cut or scratch already in the skin. The infected saliva may enter through any opening, including the membranes lining the nose or mouth. After an incubation period of about ten days, a person infected by a rabid animal experiences pain at the site of infection, extreme sensitivity of the skin to temperature changes, and painful spasms of the larynx that make it almost impossible to drink. Saliva thickens and the patient becomes restless and easily excitable. By the time symptoms develop, death may be imminent. Obviously, professional medical attention should begin promptly after having been exposed to the possibility of infection.

Emergency Treatment

The area around the wound should be washed thoroughly and repeatedly with soap and water, using a sterile gauze dressing to wipe fluid away from—not toward—the wound. Another sterile dressing is used to dry the wound and a third to cover it while the patient is taken to a hospital or physician's office. A tetanus injection is also indicated, and police and health authorities should be promptly notified of the biting incident.

If at all possible the biting animal should be indentified—if a wild animal, captured alive—and held for observation for a period of 10 to 15 days. If it can be determined during that period that the animal is not rabid, further treatment may not be required. If the animal is rabid, however, or if it cannot be located and impounded, the patient may have to undergo a series of daily rabies vaccine injections lasting from 14 days for a case of mild exposure to 21 days for severe exposure (a bite near the head, for example), plus several booster shots. Because of the sensitivity of some individuals to the rabies vaccines used, the treatment itself can be quite dangerous.

Recent research, however, has established that a new vaccine called HDCV (human diploid cell vaccine), which requires only six or fewer injections, is immunologically effective and is not usually accompanied by any side effects. The new vaccine has been used successfully on people of all ages who had been bitten by animals known to be rabid.

Appendicitis

The common signal for approaching appendicitis is a period of several days of indigestion and constipation, culminating in pain and tenderness on the lower right side of the abdomen. Besides these symptoms, appendicitis may be accompanied by nausea and a slight fever. Call a physician immediately and describe the symptoms in detail; delay may result in a ruptured appendix.

Emergency Treatment

While awaiting medical care, the victim may find some relief from the pain and discomfort by having an ice bag placed over the abdomen. Do not apply heat and give nothing by mouth. A laxative should not be offered.

Asphyxiation

See GAS POISONING.

Asthma Attack

Emergency Treatment

Make the patient comfortable and offer reassurance. If he has been ex-amined by a physician and properly diagnosed, the patient probably has an inhalant device or other forms of medication on his person or nearby.

The coughing and wheezing spell may have been triggered by the presence of an allergenic substance such as animal hair, feathers, or kapok in pillows or cushions. Such items should be removed from the presence of the patient. In addition, placing the patient in a room with high humidity, such as a bathroom with the shower turned on, may be helpful.

Asthma attacks are rarely fatal in young people, but elderly persons should be watched carefully because of possible heart strain. In a severe attack, professional medical care including oxygen equipment may be required.

Back Injuries

In the event of any serious back injury, call a physician or arrange for immediate professional transfer of the victim to a hospital.

Emergency Treatment

Until determined otherwise by a physician, treat the injured person as a victim of a fractured spine. If he complains that he cannot move his head, feet, or toes, the chances are that the back is fractured. But even if he can move his feet or legs, it does not necessarily mean that he can be moved safely, since the back can be fractured without immediate injury to the spinal cord.

If the victim shows symptoms of shock, do not attempt to lower his head or move his body into the usual position for shock control. If it is absolutely essential to move the victim because of immediate danger to his life, make a rigid stretcher from a wide piece of solid lumber such as a door and cover the stretcher with a blanket for padding. Then carefully slide or pull the victim onto the stretcher, using his clothing to hold him. Tie the body onto the stretcher with strips of cloth.

Back Pain

See SCIATICA.

Black Eye

Although a black eye is frequently regarded as a minor medical problem, it can result in serious visual problems, including cataract or glaucoma.

Emergency Treatment

Inspect the area about the eye for possible damage to the eye itself, such as hemorrhage, rupture of the eyeball, or dislocated lens. Check also for cuts around the eye that may require professional medical care. Then treat the bruised area by putting the victim to bed, covering the eye with a bandage, and applying an ice bag to the area.

If vision appears to be distorted or lacerations need stitching and antibiotic treatment, take the victim to a physician's office. A physician should also be consulted about continued pain and swelling about the eye.

Black Widow Spider Bites

Emergency Treatment

Make the victim lie still. If the bite is on the arm or leg, position the victim so that the bite is lower than the level of the heart. Apply a rubber band or similar tourniquet between the bite and the heart to retard venom flow toward the heart. The bite usually is marked by two puncture points. Apply ice packs to the bite. Summon a physician or carry the patient to the nearest hospital.

Loosen the tourniquet or constriction band for a few seconds every 15 minutes while awaiting help; you should be able to feel a pulse beyond the tourniquet if it is not too tight. Do not let the victim move about. Do not permit him to drink alcoholic beverages. He probably will feel weakness, tremor, and severe pain, but reassure him that he will recover. Medications, usually available only to a physician, should be administered promptly.

Bleeding, Internal

Internal bleeding is always a very serious condition; it requires immediate professional medical attention.

In cases of internal bleeding, blood is sometimes brought to the outside of the body by coughing from the lungs, by vomiting from the stomach, by trickling from the ear or nose, or by passing in the urine or bowel movement.

Often, however, internal bleeding is concealed, and the only symptom may be the swelling that appears around the site of broken bones. A person can lose three or four pints of blood inside the body without a trace of blood appearing outside the body.

Some Symptoms of Internal Bleeding

The victim will appear ill and pale. His skin will be colder than normal, especially the hands and feet; often the skin looks clammy because of sweating. The pulse usually will be rapid (over 90 beats a minute) and feeble.

Emergency Treatment

Serious internal bleeding is beyond the scope of first aid. If necessary

treat the victim for respiratory and cardiac arrest and for shock while waiting for medical aid.

Bleeding, Minor

Bleeding from minor cuts, scrapes, and bruises usually stops by itself, but even small injuries of this kind should receive attention to prevent infection.

Emergency Treatment

The injured area should be washed thoroughly with soap and water, or if possible, held under running water. The surface should then be covered with a sterile bandage.

The type of wound known as a puncture wound may bleed very little, but is potentially extremely dangerous because of the possibility of tetanus infection. Anyone who steps on a rusty nail or thumbtack or has a similar accident involving a pointed object that penetrates deep under the skin surface should consult a physician about the need for antitetanus inoculation or a booster shot.

Blisters

Emergency Treatment

If the blister is on a hand or foot or other easily accessible part of the body, wash the area around the blister thoroughly with soap and water. After carefully drying the skin around the blister, apply an antiseptic to the same area. Then sterilize the point and a substantial part of a needle by heating it in an open flame. When the needle has been thoroughly sterilized, use the point to puncture the blister along the margin of the blister. Carefully squeeze the fluid from the blister by pressing it with a sterile gauze dressing; the dressing should soak up most of the fluid. Next, place a fresh

sterile dressing over the blister and fasten it in place with a bandage. If a blister forms in a tender area or in a place that is not easily accessible, such as under the arm, do not open it yourself; consult your physician.

The danger from any break in the skin is that germs or dirt can slip through the natural barrier to produce an infection or inflammation. Continue to apply an antiseptic each day to the puncture area until it has healed. If it appears that an infection has developed or healing is unusually slow, consult a doctor. Persons with diabetes or circulatory problems may have to be more cautious about healing of skin breaks than other individuals.

Blood Blisters

Blood blisters, sometimes called hematomas, usually are caused by a sharp blow to the body surface such as hitting a finger with a hammer while pounding nails.

Emergency Treatment

Wash the area of the blood blister thoroughly with soap and water. Do not open it. If it is a small blood blister, cover it with a protective bandage; in many cases, the tiny pool of blood under the skin will be absorbed by the surrounding tissues if there is no further pressure at that point.

If the blood blister fails to heal quickly or becomes infected, consult a physician. Because the pool of blood has resulted from damage to a blood vessel, a blood blister usually is more vulnerable to infection or inflammation than an ordinary blister.

Boils

Boils frequently are an early sign of diabetes or another illness and should be watched carefully if they occur often. In general, they result from germs or dirt being rubbed into the skin by tight-fitting clothing, scratching, or through tiny cuts made during shaving.

Emergency Treatment

If the boil is above the lip, do not squeeze it or apply any pressure. The infection in that area of the face may drain into the brain because of the pattern of blood circulation on the face. Let a physician treat any boil on the face. If the boil is on the surface of another part of the body, apply moist hot packs, but do not squeeze or press on the boil because that action can force the infection into the circulatory system. A wet compress can be made by soaking a wash cloth or towel in warm water.

If the boil erupts, carefully wipe away the pus with a sterile dressing, and then cover it with another sterile dressing. If the boil is large or slow to erupt, or if it is slow to heal, consult a physician.

Bone Bruises

Emergency Treatment

Make sure the bone is not broken. If the injury is limited to the thin layer of tissue surrounding the bone, and the function of the limb is normal though painful, apply a compression dressing and an ice pack. Limit use of the injured limb for the next day or two.

As the pain and swelling recede, cover the injured area with a foam-rubber pad held in place with an elastic bandage. Because the part of the limb that is likely to receive a bone bruise lacks a layer of muscle and fat, it will be particularly sensitive to any pressure until recovery is complete.

Botulism

The bacteria that produce the lethal toxin of botulism are commonly present on unwashed farm vegetables and thrive in containers that are improperly sealed against the damaging effects of air. Home-canned vegetables, particularly string beans, are a likely source of botulism, but the toxin can be found in fruits, meats, and other foods. It can also appear in food that has been properly prepared but allowed to cool before being served. Examples are cold soups and marinated vegetables.

Emergency Treatment

As soon as acute symptoms—nausea, diarrhea, and abdominal distress—appear, try to induce vomiting. Vomiting usually can be started by touching the back of the victim's throat with a finger or the handle of a spoon, which should be smooth and blunt, or by offering him a glass of water in which two tablespoons of salt have been dissolved. Call a physician; describe all of the symptoms, which also may include, after several hours, double vision, muscular weakness, and difficulty in swallowing and breathing. Save samples of the food suspected of contamination for analysis.

Prompt hospitalization and injection of antitoxin are needed to save most cases of botulism poisoning. Additional emergency measures may include artificial respiration if regular breathing fails because of paralysis of respiratory muscles. Continue artificial respiration until professional medical care is provided. If other individuals have eaten the contaminated food, they should receive treatment for botulism even if they show no symptoms of the toxin's effects, since symptoms may be delayed by several days.

Brown House (or Recluse) Spider Bites

Emergency Treatment

Apply an ice bag or cold pack to the wound area. Aspirin and antihistamines may be offered to help relieve any pain or feeling of irritation. Keep the victim lying down and quiet. Call a physician as quickly as possible and describe the situation; the physician will advise what further action should be taken at this point.

The effects of a brown spider bite frequently last much longer than the pain of the bite, which may be comparatively mild for an insect bite or sting. But the poison from the bite can gradually destroy the surrounding tissues, leaving at first an ulcer and eventually a disfiguring scar. A physician's treatment is needed to control the loss of tissue; he probably will prescribe drugs and recommend continued use of cold compresses. The victim, meanwhile, will feel numbness and muscular weakness, requiring a prolonged period of bed rest in addition to the medical treatments.

Bruises/Contusions

Emergency Treatment

Bruises or contusions result usually from a blow to the body that is powerful enough to damage muscles, tendons, blood vessels, or other tissues without causing a break in the skin.

Because the bruised area will be tender, protect it from further injury. If possible, immobilize the injured body part with a sling, bandage, or other device that makes the victim feel more comfortable; pillows, folded blankets, or similar soft materials can be used to elevate an arm or leg. Apply an ice bag or cold water dressing to the injured area.

A simple bruise usually will heal without extensive treatment. The swelling and discoloration result from blood oozing from damaged tissues. Severe bruising can, however, be quite serious and requires medical attention. Keep the victim quiet and watch for symptoms of shock. Give aspirin for pain.

Bullet Wounds

Bullet wounds, whether accidental or purposely inflicted, can range from those that are superficial and external to those that involve internal bleeding and extensive tissue damage.

Emergency Treatment

A surface bullet wound accompanied by bleeding should be covered promptly with sterile gauze to prevent further infection. The flow of blood should be controlled as described under "Severe Bleeding" in this chapter. *Don't* try to clean the wound with soap or water.

If the wound is internal, keep the patient lying down and wrap him with coats or blankets placed over and under his body. If respiration has ceased or is impaired, give mouth-to-mouth respiration and treat him for shock. Get medical aid promptly.

Burns, Thermal

Burns are generally described according to the depth or area of skin damage involved. First-degree burns are the most superficial. They are marked by reddening of the skin and swelling, increased warmth, tenderness, and pain. Second-degree burns, deeper than first-degree, are in effect open wounds, characterized by blisters and severe pain in addition to redness. Third-degree burns are deep enough to involve damage to muscles and bones. The skin is charred and there may be no pain because nerve endings have been destroyed. However, the area of the burn generally is more important than the degree of burn; a first- or second-degree burn covering a large area of the body is more likely to be fatal than a small third-degree burn.

Emergency Treatment

You will want to get professional medical help for treatment of a severe burn, but there are a number of things you can do until such help is obtained. If burns are minor, apply ice or ice water until pain subsides. Then wash the area with soap and water. Cover with a sterile dressing. Give the victim one or two aspirin tablets to help relieve discomfort. A sterile gauze pad soaked in a solution of two tablespoons of baking soda (sodium bicarbonate) per quart of lukewarm water may be applied.

For more extensive or severe burns, there are three first-aid objectives: (1) relieve pain, (2) prevent shock, (3) prevent infection. To relieve pain, exclude air by applying a thick dressing of four to six layers plus additional coverings of clean, tightly woven material; for extensive burns, use clean sheets or towels. Clothing should be cut away—never pulled—from burned areas; where fabric is stuck to the wound, leave it for a physician to remove later. Do not apply any ointment, grease, powder, salve, or other medication; the physician simply will have to remove such material before he can begin professional treatment of the burns.

To prevent shock, make sure the victim's head is lower than his feet. Be sure that the victim is covered sufficiently to keep him warm, but not enough to make him overheated; exposure to cold can make the effects of shock more severe. Provide the victim with plenty of nonalcoholic liquids such as sweetened water, tea, or fruit juices, so long as he is conscious and able to swallow.

To prevent infection, do not permit absorbent cotton or adhesive tape to touch the wound caused by a burn. Do not apply iodine or any other antiseptic to the burn. Do not open any blisters. Do not permit any unsterile matter to contact the burn area. If possible, prevent other persons from coughing, sneezing, or even breathing toward the wound resulting from a burn. Serious infections frequently develop in burn victims from contamination by microorganisms of the mouth and nose.

Long-Term Treatment

A highly effective method of treating serious burns involves, first, removal of samples of uninjured skin from victims' bodies. Laboratory workers then "grind up" the healthy skin samples and separate them into groups of cells. Placed in flasks and bathed in a growth-stimulating solution, the cells grow rapidly; while the colonies are small, they double in size every 17 hours. New skin appears. The procedure can be repeated until enough has been grown to cover the burned areas.

Because the "test-tube skin" is developed from samples of a victim's own skin, the body does not reject it. It can be grafted onto a burned area in patches until the entire burn is covered. The new skin has no hair follicles or sweat glands, and is thinner than normal skin. But it offers hope to some 10 to 15 percent of those persons who are hospitalized with burn injuries.

See also CHEMICAL BURNS OF THE EYE.

Carbuncles

Carbuncles are quite similar to boils

except that they usually develop around multiple hair follicles and commonly appear on the neck or face. Personal hygiene is one factor involved in the development of carbuncles; persons apparently susceptible to the pustular inflammations must exercise special care in cleansing areas in which carbuncles occur, particularly if they suffer from diabetes or circulatory ailments.

Emergency Treatment

Apply moist hot packs to the boil-like swelling. Change the moist hot packs frequently, or place a hot-water bottle on the moist dressing to maintain the moist heat application. Do not handle the carbuncle beyond whatever contact is necessary to apply or maintain the moist heat. The carbuncle should eventually rupture or reach a point where it can be opened with a sterile sharp instrument. After the carbuncle has ruptured and drained, and the fluid from the growth has been carefully cleaned away, apply a sterile dressing.

Frequently, carbuncles must be opened and drained by a physician.

Cat Scratch Fever

Although the scratch or bite of a house cat or alley cat may appear at first to be only a mild injury, the wound can become the site of entry for a disease virus transmitted by apparently healthy cats. The inflammation, accompanied by fever, generally affects the lymph nodes and produces some aches and pains as well as fatigue. Although the disease is seldom fatal, an untreated case can spread to brain tissues and lead to other complications.

Emergency Treatment

Wash the scratch thoroughly with water and either soap or a mild detergent. Apply a mild antiseptic such as hydrogen peroxide. Cover with a sterile dressing.

Watch the area of the scratch carefully for the next week or two. If redness or swelling develop, even after the scratch appears healed, consult your physician. The inflammation of the scratch area may be accompanied by mild fever and symptoms similar to those of influenza; in small children, the symptoms may be quite serious. Bed rest and antibiotics usually are prescribed.

Charley Horse

A charley horse occurs because a small number of muscle fibers have been torn or ruptured by overstraining the muscle, or by the force of a blow to the muscle.

Emergency Treatment

Rest the injured muscle and apply an ice pack if there is swelling. A compression dressing can be applied to support the muscle. Avoid movement that stretches the muscle, and restrict other movements that make the victim uncomfortable. If pain and swelling persist, call a physician.

During the recovery period, which may not begin for a day or two, apply local heat with a hot water bottle or an electric heating pad, being careful not to burn the victim. A return to active use of the muscle can begin gradually as pain permits.

Chemical Burns of the Eye

Emergency Treatment

Flush the victim's eye immediately with large quantities of fresh, clean water; a drinking fountain can be used to provide a steady stream of water. If a drinking fountain is not available, lay the victim on the floor or ground with his head turned slightly to one side and pour water into the eye from a cup or glass. Always direct the stream of water so that it enters the eye surface at the inside corner and flows across the eye to the outside corner. If the victim is unable, because of intense pain, to open his eyes, it may be necessary to hold the lids apart while water pours across the eye. Continue flushing the eye for at least 15 minutes. (An alternate method is to immerse the victim's face in a pan or basin or bucket of water while he opens and closes his eyes repeatedly; continue the process for at least 15 minutes.)

When the chemical has been flushed from the victim's eye, the eye should be covered with a small, thick compress held in place with a bandage that covers both eyes, if possible; the bandage can be tied around the victim's head. **Note:** Apply nothing but water to the eye; do not attempt to neutralize a chemical burn of the eye and do not apply oil, ointment, salve, or other medications. Rush the victim to a physician as soon as possible, preferably to an ophthalmologist.

Chemicals on Skin

Many household and industrial chemicals, such as ammonia, lye, iodine, creosote, and a wide range of insecticides can cause serious injury if accidentally spilled on the skin.

Emergency Treatment

Wash the body surface that has been affected by the chemical with large amounts of water. Do not try to neutralize the chemical with another substance; the reaction may aggravate the injury. If blisters appear, apply a sterile dressing. If the chemical is a refrigerant, such as Freon, or carbon dioxide under pressure, treat for frostbite.

If the chemical has splashed into the eyes or produces serious injury to the affected body surface, call a physician. The victim should be watched closely for possible poisoning effects if the chemical is a pesticide, since such substances may be absorbed through the skin to produce internal toxic reactions. If there is any question about the toxicity of a chemical, ask your doctor or call the nearest poison control center.

Chigger Bites

Emergency Treatment

Apply ice water or rub ice over the area afflicted by bites of the tiny red insects. Bathing the area with alcohol, ammonia water or a solution of baking soda also will provide some relief from the itching.

Wash thoroughly with soap, using a scrub brush to prevent further infestation by the chiggers in other areas of the body. Rub alcohol over the surrounding areas and apply sulfur ointment as protection against mites that may not have attached themselves to the skin. Continue applications of ice water or alcohol to skin areas invaded by the insects. Clothing that was worn should be laundered immediately.

Chilblains

Emergency Treatment

Move the victim to a moderately warm place and remove wet or tight clothing. Soak the affected body area in warm—but not hot—water for about ten minutes. Then carefully blot the skin dry, but do not rub the skin. Replace the clothing with garments that are warm, soft, and dry.

Give the victim a stimulant such as tea or coffee, or an alcoholic beverage, and put him to bed with only light blankets; avoid the pressure of heavy blankets or heavy, tight garments on the sensitive skin areas. The victim should move the affected body areas gently to help restore normal circulation. If complications develop, such as marked discoloration of the skin, pain, or blistering and splitting of the skin, call a physician.

Cold Sores/Fever Blisters

Emergency Treatment

Apply a soothing ointment or a medication such as camphor ice. Avoid squeezing or otherwise handling the blisters; moisture can aggravate the sores and hinder their healing. Repeated appearances of cold sores or fever blisters, which are caused by the herpes simplex virus, may require treatment by a physician.

Concussion

See HEAD INJURIES.

Contusions

See BRUISES.

Convulsions

Emergency Treatment

Protect the victim from injury by moving him to a safe place; loosen any constricting clothing such as a tie or belt; put a pillow or coat under his head; if his mouth is open, place a folded cloth between his teeth to keep him from biting his tongue. Do not force anything into his mouth. Keep the patient warm but do not disturb him; do not try to restrain his convulsive movements.

Send for a physician as quickly as possible. Watch the patient's breathing and begin artificial respiration if breathing stops for more than one minute. Be sure that breathing actually has stopped; the patient may be sleeping or unconscious after an attack but breathing normally.

Convulsions in a small child may signal the onset of an infectious disease and may be accompanied by a high fever. The same general precautions should be taken to prevent self-injury on the part of the child. If placed in a bed, the child should be protected against falling onto the floor. Place him on his side—not on his back or stomach—if he vomits. Cold compresses or ice packs on the back of the neck and the head may help relieve symptoms. Immediate professional medical care is vital because brain damage can result if treatment is delayed.

See also EPILEPTIC SEIZURES.

Cramps

See MUSCLE CRAMPS.

Croup

Croup is a breathing disorder usually caused by a virus infection and less often by bacteria or allergy. It is a common condition during childhood, and in some cases, may require brief hospitalization for proper treatment.

The onset of a croup attack is likely to occur during the night with a sudden hoarse or barking cough accompanied by difficulty in breathing. The coughing is usually followed by choking spasms that sound as though the child is strangling. There may also be a mild fever. A physician should be called immediately when these symptoms appear.

Emergency Treatment

The most effective treatment for croup is cool moist air. Cool water vaporizers are available as well as warm steam vaporizers. Another alternative is to take the child into the bathroom, close the door and windows, and let the hot water run from the shower and sink taps until the room is filled with steam.

It is also possible to improvise a croup tent by boiling water in a kettle on a portable hot plate and arranging a blanket over the back of a chair so that it encloses the child and an adult as well as the steaming kettle. A child should never be left alone even for an instant in such a makeshift arrangement.

If the symptoms do not subside in about 20 minutes with any of the above procedures, or if there is mounting fever, and if the physician is not on his way, the child should be rushed to the closest hospital. Cold moist night air, rather than being a danger, may actually make the symptoms subside temporarily.

Diabetic Coma and Insulin Shock

Diabetics should always carry an identification tag or card to alert others of their condition in the event of a diabetic coma—which is due to a lack of insulin. They also should advise friends or family members of their diabetic condition and the proper emergency measures that can be taken in the event of an onset of diabetic coma. A bottle of rapid-acting insulin should be kept on hand for such an emergency.

Emergency Treatment

If the victim is being treated for diabetes, he probably will have nearby a supply of insulin and a hypodermic apparatus for injecting it. Find the insulin, hypodermic syringe, and needle; clean a spot on the upper arm or thigh, and inject about 50 units of insulin. Call a physician without delay, and describe the patient's symptoms and your treatment. The patient usually will respond without ill effects, but may be quite thirsty. Give him plenty of fluids, as needed.

If the victim does not respond to the insulin, or if you cannot find the insulin and hypodermic syringe, rush the victim to the nearest physician's office.

Insulin shock—which is due to a reaction to too much insulin and not enough sugar in the blood—can be treated in an emergency by offering a sugar-rich fluid such as a cola beverage or orange juice. Diabetics frequently carry a lump of sugar or candy that can be placed in their mouth in case of an insulin shock reaction. It should be tucked between the teeth and cheek so the victim will not choke on it.

If you find a diabetic in a coma and do not know the cause, assume the cause is an insulin reaction and treat him with sugar. This will give immediate relief to an insulin reaction but will not affect diabetic coma.

Diarrhea

Emergency Treatment

Give the victim an antidiarrheal agent; all drugstores carry medications composed of kaolin and pectin that are useful for this purpose. Certain bismuth compounds also are recommended for diarrhea control.

Put the victim in bed for a period of at least 12 hours and withhold food and drink for that length of time. Do not let the victim become dehydrated; if he is thirsty, let him suck on pieces of ice. If the diarrhea appears to be subsiding, let him sip a mild beverage like tea or ginger ale; cola syrup is also recommended.

Later on the patient can try eating bland foods such as dry toast, crackers, gelatin desserts, or jellied consomme. Avoid feeding rich, fatty, or spicy foods. If the diarrhea fails to subside or is complicated by colic or vomiting, call a physician.

Dizziness/Vertigo

Emotional upsets, allergies, and improper eating and drinking habits—too much food, too little food, or foods that are too rich—can precipitate symptoms of dizziness. The cause also can be a physical disorder such as abnormal functioning of the inner ear or a circulatory problem. Smoking tobacco, certain drugs such as quinine, and fumes of some chemicals also can produce dizziness.

Emergency Treatment

Have the victim lie down with the eyes closed. In many cases, a period of simple bed rest will alleviate the symptoms. Keep the victim quiet and comfortable. If the feeling of dizziness continues, becomes worse, or is accompanied by nausea and vomiting, call a physician.

Severe or persistent dizziness or vertigo requires a longer period of bed rest and the use of medicines prescribed by a physician. While recovering, the victim should avoid sudden changes in body position or turning the head rapidly. In some types of vertigo, surgery is required to cure the disorder.

Drowning

Victims of drowning seldom die because of water in the lungs or stomach. They die because of lack of air.

Emergency Treatment

If the victim's breathing has been impaired, start artificial respiration immediately. If there is evidence of cardiac arrest, administer cardiac massage. When the victim is able to breathe for himself, treat him for shock and get medical help.

Drug Overdose (Barbiturates)

Barbiturates are used in a number of drugs prescribed as sedatives, although many are also available through illegal channels. Because the drugs can affect the judgment of the user, he may not remember having taken a dose and so may take additional pills, thus producing overdose effects.

Emergency Treatment

If the drug was taken orally, try to induce vomiting in the victim. Have him drink a glass of water containing two tablespoons of salt. Or touch the back of his throat gently with a finger or a smooth blunt object like the handle of a spoon. Then give the victim plenty of warm water to drink. It is important to rid the stomach of as much of the drug as possible and to dilute the substance remaining in the gastrointestinal tract.

As soon as possible, call a physician or get the victim to the nearest hospital or physician's office. If breathing fails, administer artificial respiration.

Drug Overdose (Stimulants)

Although most of the powerful stimulant drugs, or pep pills, are available only through a physician's prescription, the same medications are available through illicit sources. When taken without direction of a supervising physician, the stimulants can produce a variety of adverse side effects, and when used frequently over a period of time can result in physical and psychological problems that require hospital treatment.

Emergency Treatment

Give the victim a solution of one tablespoon of activated charcoal mixed with a small amount of water, or give him a glass of milk, to dilute the effects of the medication in the stomach. Then induce vomiting by pressing gently on the back of the throat with a finger or the smooth blunt edge of a spoon handle. Vomiting also may be induced with a solution made of one teaspoonful of mustard in a half glass of water. Do not give syrup of ipecac to a victim who has been taking stimulants.

As soon as possible call a physician or get the victim to the nearest hospital or physician's office. If breathing fails, administer artificial respiration.

Earaches

An earache may be associated with a wide variety of ailments ranging from the common cold or influenza to impacted molars or tonsillitis. An earache also may be involved in certain infectious diseases such as measles or scarlet fever. Because of the relationship of ear structures to other parts of the head and throat, an infection involving the symptoms of earache can easily spread to the brain tissues or the spongy mastoid bone behind the ear. Call a physician and describe all of the symptoms, including temperature, any discharge, pain, ringing in the ear, or deafness. Delay in reporting an earache to a doctor can result in complications that require hospital treatment.

Emergency Treatment

This may incude a few drops of warm olive oil or sweet oil held in the ear by a small wad of cotton. Aspirin can be given to help relieve any pain. Professional medical treatment may include the use of antibiotics.

Ear, Foreign Body in

Emergency Treatment

Do not insert a hairpin, stick, or other object in the ear in an effort to remove a foreign object; you are likely to force the object farther into the ear canal. Instead, have the victim tilt his head to one side, with the ear containing the foreign object facing upward. While pulling gently on the lobe of the ear to straighten the canal, pour a little warmed olive oil or mineral oil into the ear. Then have the victim tilt that ear downward so the oil will run out quickly; it should dislodge the foreign object.

Wipe the ear canal gently with a cotton-tipped matchstick, or a similar device that will not irritate the lining of the ear canal, after the foreign body has been removed. If the emergency treatment is not successful, call a physician.

Electric Shocks

An electric shock from the usual 110-volt current in most homes can be a serious emergency, especially if the person's skin or clothing is wet. Under these circumstances, the shock may paralyze the part of the brain that controls breathing and stop the heart completely or disorder its pumping action.

Emergency Treatment

It is of the utmost importance to break the electrical contact *immediately* by unplugging the wire of the appliance involved or by shutting off the house current switch. **Do not touch the victim of the shock while he is still acting as an electrical conductor.**

If the shock has come from a faulty wire out of doors and the source of the electrical current can't be reached easily, make a lasso of dry rope on a long sturdy dry stick. Catch the victim's hand or foot in the loop and drag him away from the wire. Another way to break the contact is to cut the wire with a dry axe.

If the victim of the shock is unconscious, or if his pulse is very weak, administer mouth-to-mouth respiration and cardiac massage until he can get to a hospital.

Epileptic Seizures

Epilepsy is a disorder of the nervous system that produces convulsive seizures. In a major seizure or *grand mal,* the epileptic usually falls to the ground. Indeed, falling is in most cases one of the principal dangers of the disease. Then the epileptic's body begins to twitch or jerk spasmodically. His breathing may be labored, and saliva may appear on his lips. His face may become pale or bluish. Although the scene can be frightening, it is not truly a medical emergency; the afflicted person is in no danger of losing his life.

Emergency Treatment

Make the person suffering the seizure as comfortable as possible. If he is on a hard surface, put something soft under his head, and move any hard or dangerous objects away from him. **Make no attempt to restrain his movements, and do not force anything into his mouth.** Just leave him alone until the attack is over, as it should be in a few minutes. If his mouth is already open, you might put something soft, such as a folded handerchief, between his side teeth. This will help to prevent him from biting his tongue or lips. If he seems to go into another seizure after coming out of the first, or if the seizure lasts more than ten minutes, call a physician. If his lower jaw sags and begins to obstruct his breathing, support of the lower jaw may be helpful in improving his breathing.

When the seizure is over, the patient should be allowed to rest quietly. Some people sleep heavily after a seizure. Others awake at once but are disoriented or confused for a while. Treat the episode in a matter-of-fact way. If it is the first seizure the person is aware of having had, advise him to see his physician promptly.

Eye, Foreign Body in

Emergency Treatment

Do not rub the eye or touch it with unwashed hands. The foreign body usually becomes lodged on the inner surface of the upper eyelid. Pull the upper eyelid down over the lower lid to help work the object loose. Tears or clean water can help wash out the dirt or other object. If the bit of irritating material can be seen on the surface of the eyeball, try very carefully to flick it out with the tip of a clean, moistened handkerchief or a piece of moistened cotton. Never touch the surface of the eye with dry materials. Sometimes a foreign body can be removed by carefully rolling the upper lid over a pencil or wooden matchstick to expose the object.

After the foreign object has been removed, the eye should be washed with clean water or with a solution made from one teaspoon of salt dissolved in a pint of water. This will help remove any remaining particles of the foreign body as well as any traces of irritating chemicals that might have been a part of it. Iron particles, for example, may leave traces of rust on the eye's surface unless washed away.

If the object cannot be located and removed without difficulty, a small patch of gauze or a folded handkerchief should be taped over the eye and the victim taken to a physician's office—preferably the office of an ophthalmologist. A physician also should be consulted if a feeling of irritation in the eye continues after the foreign body has been removed.

Fever

Emergency Treatment

If the fever is mild, around 100°F. by mouth, have the victim rest in bed and provide him with a light diet. Watch closely for other symptoms, such as a rash, and any further increase in body temperature. Aspirin usually can be given.

If the temperature rises to 101° F. or higher, is accompanied by pain, headache, delirium, confused behavior, coughing, vomiting, or other indications of a severe illness, call a physician. Describe all of the symptoms in detail, including the appearance of any rash and when it began.

Fever blisters

See COLD SORES.

Finger Dislocation

Emergency Treatment

Call a physician and arrange for inspection and treatment of the injury. If a physician is not immediately available, the finger dislocation may be reduced (put back in proper alignment) by grasping it firmly and carefully pulling it into normal position. Pull very slowly and avoid rough handling that might complicate the injury by damaging a tendon. If the dislocation cannot be reduced after the first try, go through the procedure once more. But do not try it more than twice.

Whether or not you are successful in reducing the finger dislocation, the finger should be immobilized after your efforts until a physician can examine it. A clean flat wooden stick can be strapped along the palm side of the finger with adhesive tape or strips of bandage to hold it in place.

Fingernail Injuries/Hangnails

Emergency Treatment

Wash the injured nail area thoroughly with warm water and soap. Trim off any torn bits of nail. Cover with a small adhesive dressing or bandage.

Apply petroleum jelly or cold cream to the injured nail area twice a day, morning and night, until it is healed. If redness or irritation develops in the adjoining skin area, indicating an infection, consult a physician.

Fish Poisoning

Emergency Treatment

Induce vomiting in the victim to remove the bits of poisonous fish from the stomach. Vomiting usually can be started by pressing on the back of the throat with a finger or a spoon handle that is blunt and smooth, or by having the victim drink a solution of two tablespoons of salt in a glass of water.

Call a physician as soon as possible. Describe the type of fish eaten and the symptoms, which may include nausea, diarrhea, abdominal pain, muscular weakness, and a numbness or tingling sensation that begins about the face and spreads to the extremities.

If breathing fails, administer mouth-to-mouth artificial respiration; a substance commonly found in poisonous fish causes respiratory failure. Also, be prepared to provide emergency treatment for convulsions.

Food Poisoning

Emergency Treatment

If the victim is not already vomiting, try to induce it to clear the stomach. Vomiting can be started in most cases by pressing gently on the back of the throat with a finger or a blunt smooth spoon handle, or by having the patient drink a glass of water containing two tablespoons of salt. If the victim has vomited, put him to bed.

Call a physician and describe the food ingested and the symptoms that developed. If symptoms are severe, professional medical treatment with antibiotics and medications for cramps may be required. Special medications also may be needed for diarrhea caused by bacterial food poisoning.

Fractures

Any break in a bone is called a fracture. The break is called an *open* or *compound fracture* if one or both ends of the broken bone pierce the skin. A *closed* or *simple fracture* is one in which the broken bone doesn't come through the skin.

It is sometimes difficult to distinguish a strained muscle or a sprained ligament from a broken bone, since sprains and strains can be extremely painful even though they are less serious than breaks. However, when there is any doubt, the injury should be treated as though it were a simple fracture.

Emergency Treatment

Don't try to help the injured person move around or get up unless he has slowly tested out the injured part of his body and is sure that nothing has been broken. If he is in extreme pain, or if the injured part has begun to swell, or if by running the finger lightly along the affected bone a break can be felt, *do not* move him. Under no circumstances should he be crowded into a car if his legs, hip, ribs, or back are involved in the accident. Call for an ambulance immediately, and until it arrives, treat the person for shock.

Splinting

In a situation where it is imperative to move someone who may have a fracture, the first step is to apply a splint so that the broken bone ends are immobilized.

Splints can be improvised from anything rigid enough and of the right length to support the fractured part of the body: a metal rod, board, long cardboard tube, tightly rolled newspaper or blanket. If the object being used has to be padded for softness, use a small blanket or any other soft material, such as a jacket.

The splint should be long enough so that it can be tied with a bandage, torn sheet, or neckties beyond the joint above and below the fracture as well as at the site of the break. If a leg is involved, it should be elevated with pillows or any other firm support after the splint has been applied. If the victim has to wait a considerable length of time before receiving professional attention, the splint bandaging should be checked from time to time to make sure it isn't too tight.

In the case of an open or compound fracture, additional steps must be taken. Remove that part of the victim's clothing that is covering the wound. Do not wash or probe into the wound, but control bleeding by applying pressure over the wound through a sterile or clean dressing.

Frostbite

Emergency Treatment

Begin rapid rewarming of the affected tissues as soon as possible. If possible, immerse the victim in a warm bath, but avoid scalding. (The temperature should be between 102°F. and 105°F.) Warm wet towels also will help if changed frequently and applied gently. Do not massage, rub, or even touch the frostbitten flesh. If warm water or a warming fire is not available, place the patient in a sleeping bag or cover him with coats and blankets. Hot liquids can be offered if available to help raise the body temperature.

For any true frostbite case, prompt medical attention is important. The depth and degree of the frozen tissue cannot be determined without a careful examination by a physician.

Gallbladder Attacks

Although gallstones can affect a wide variety of individuals, the most common victims are overweight persons who enjoy rich foods. The actual attack of spasms caused by gallstones passing through the duct leading from the gallbladder to the digestive tract usually is preceded by periods of stomach distress including belching.

X rays usually will reveal the presence of gallstones when the early warning signs are noted, and measures can be taken to reduce the threat of a gallbladder attack.

Emergency Treatment

Call a physician and describe in detail the symptoms, which may include colic high in the abdomen and pain extending to the right shoulder; the pain may be accompanied by nausea, vomiting, and sweating. Hot water bottles may be applied to the abdomen to help relieve distress while waiting for professional medical care. If the physician permits, the victim may be allowed to sip certain fluids such as fruit juices, but do not offer him solid food.

Gas Poisoning

Before attempting to revive someone overcome by toxic gas poisoning, the most important thing to do is to remove him to the fresh air. If this isn't feasible, all windows and doors should be opened to let in as much fresh air as possible.

Any interior with a dangerous concentration of carbon monoxide or other toxic gases is apt to be highly explosive. Therefore, gas and electricity should be shut off as quickly as possible. **Under no circumstances should any matches be lighted in an interior where there are noxious fumes.**

The rescuer needn't waste time covering his face with a handkerchief or other cloth. He should hold his breath instead, or take only a few quick, shallow breaths while bringing the victim to the out-of-doors or to an open window.

Emergency Treatment

Administer artificial respiration if the

victim is suffering respiratory arrest. Arrange for medical help as soon as possible, requesting that oxygen be brought to the scene.

Head Injuries

Accidents involving the head can result in concussion, skull fracture, or brain injury. Symptoms of head injury include loss of consciousness, discharge of a watery or blood-tinged fluid from the ears, nose, or mouth, and a difference in size of the pupils of the eyes. Head injuries must be thought of as serious; they demand immediate medical assistance.

Emergency Treatment

Place the victim in a supine position, and, if there is no evidence of injury to his neck, arrange for a slight elevation of his head *and* shoulders. Make certain that he has a clear airway and administer artificial respiration if necessary. If vomitus, blood, or other fluids appear to flow from the victim's mouth, turn his head gently to one side. Control bleeding and treat for shock. Do not administer stimulants or fluids of any kind.

Heart Attack

A heart attack is caused by interference with the blood supply to the heart muscle. When the attack is brought on because of a blood clot in the coronary artery, it is known as *coronary occlusion* or *coronary thrombosis.*

The most dramatic symptom of a serious heart attack is a crushing chest pain that usually travels down the left arm into the hand or into the neck and back. The pain may bring on dizziness, cold sweat, complete collapse, and loss of consciousness. The face has an ashen pallor, and there may be vomiting.

Emergency Treatment

The victim **must not be moved** unless he has fallen in a dangerous place. If no physician is immediately available, an ambulance should be called at once. No attempt should be made to get the victim of a heart attack into an automobile.

Until help arrives, give the victim every reassurance that he will get prompt treatment, and keep him as calm and quiet as possible. Don't give him any medicine or stimulants. If oxygen is available, start administering it to the victim immediately, either by mask or nasal catheter, depending on which is available.

If the victim is suffering from respiratory arrest, begin artificial respiration. If he is suffering from cardiac arrest, begin cardiac massage.

Heat Exhaustion

Heat exhaustion occurs when the body is exposed to high temperatures and large amounts of blood accumulate in the skin as a way of cooling it. As a result, there is a marked decrease in the amount of blood that circulates through the heart and to the brain. The victim becomes markedly pale and is covered with cold perspiration. Breathing is increasingly shallow and the pulse weakens. In acute cases, fainting occurs. Medical aid should be summoned for anyone suffering from heat exhaustion.

Emergency Treatment

Place the victim in a reclining position with his feet raised about ten inches above his body. Loosen or remove his clothing, and apply cold, wet cloths to his wrists and forehead. If he has fainted and doesn't recover promptly, smelling salts or spirits of ammonia should be placed under his nose. When the victim is conscious, give him sips of salt water (approximately one teaspoon of salt per glass of water), the total intake to be about two glasses in an hour's time. If the victim vomits, discontinue the salt solution.

Heatstroke/Sunstroke

Heatstroke is characterized by an acutely high body temperature caused by the cessation of perspiration. The victim's skin becomes hot, dry, and flushed, and he may suffer collapse. Should the skin turn ashen gray, a physician must be called immediately. Prompt hospital treatment is recommended for anyone showing signs of sunstroke who has previously had any kind of heart damage.

Emergency Treatment

The following measures are designed to reduce the victim's body temperature as quickly as possible and prevent damage to the internal organs:

Place him in a tub of very cold water, or, if this is not possible, spray or sponge his body repeatedly with cold water or rubbing alcohol. Take his temperature by mouth, and when it has dropped to about 100°F., remove him to a bed and wrap him in cold, wet sheets. If possible, expose him to an electric fan or an air conditioner.

Hiccups

Emergency Treatment

Have the victim slowly drink a large glass of water. If cold water is not effective, have him drink warm water containing a teaspoonful of baking soda. Milk also can be employed. For babies and small children, offer sips of warm water. Do not offer carbonated beverages.

Another helpful measure is breathing into a large paper bag a number of times to raise the carbon dioxide level in the lungs. Rest and relaxation are recommended; have the victim lie down to read or watch television.

If the hiccups fail to go away, and continued spastic contractions of the diaphragm interfere with eating and sleeping, call a physician.

Insect Stings

Honeybees, wasps, hornets, and yellow jackets are the most common stinging insects and most likely to attack on a hot summer day. Strongly scented perfumes or cosmetics and brightly colored, rough-finished clothing attract bees and should be avoided by persons working or playing in garden areas. It should also be noted that many commercial repellents do not protect against stinging insects.

Emergency Treatment

If one is stung, the insect's stinger should be scraped gently but quickly from the skin; don't squeeze it. Apply Epsom salt solution to the sting area. Antihistamines are often helpful in reducing the patient's discomfort. If a severe reaction develops, call a physician.

There are a few people who are critically allergic to the sting of wasps, bees, yellow jackets, or fire ants. This sensitivity causes the vocal cord tissue to swell to the point where breathing may become impossible. A single sting to a sensitive person may result in a dangerous drop in blood pressure, thus producing shock. Anyone with such a severe allergy who is stung should be rushed to a hospital immediately.

A person who becomes aware of having this type of allergy should consult with a physician about the kind of medicine to carry for use in a crisis.

Insulin Shock

See DIABETIC COMA AND INSULIN SHOCK.

Jaw Dislocation

The jaw can be dislocated during a physical attack or fight; from a blow on the jaw during sports activities; or from overextension of the joint during yawning, laughing, or attempting to eat a large mouthful of food. The jaw becomes literally locked open so the victim cannot explain his predicament.

Emergency Treatment

Reducing a dislocated jaw will require that you insert your thumbs between the teeth of the victim. The jaw can be expected to snap into place quickly, and there is a danger that the teeth will clamp down on the thumbs when this happens, so the thumbs should be adequately padded with handkerchiefs or bandages. Once the thumbs are protected, insert them in the mouth and over the lower molars, as far back on the lower jaw as possible. While pressing down with the thumbs, lift the chin with the fingers outside the mouth. As the jaw begins to slip into normal position when it is pushed downward and backward with the chin lifted upward, quickly remove the thumbs from between the jaws.

Once the jaw is back in normal position, the mouth should remain closed for several hours while the ligaments recover from their displaced condition. If necessary, put a cravat bandage over the head to hold the mouth closed. If difficulty is experienced in reducing a jaw dislocation, the victim should be taken to a hospital where an anesthetic can be applied. A dislocated jaw can be extremely painful.

Jellyfish Stings

Emergency Treatment

Wash the area of the sting thoroughly with alcohol or fresh water. Be sure that any pieces of jellyfish tentacles have been removed from the skin. Aspirin or antihistamines can be administered to relieve pain and itching, but curtail the use of antihistamines if the victim has consumed alcoholic beverages. The leg or arm that received the sting can be soaked in hot water if the pain continues. Otherwise, apply calamine lotion.

If the victim appears to suffer a severe reaction from the sting, summon a doctor. The victim may experience shock, muscle cramps, convulsions, or loss of consciousness. Artificial respiration may be required while awaiting arrival of a doctor. The physician can administer drugs to relieve muscle cramps and provide sedatives or analgesics.

Kidney Stones

Emergency Treatment

Call a physician if the victim experiences the agonizing cramps or colic associated with kidney stones. Discuss the symptoms in detail with the doctor to make sure the pain is caused by kidney stones rather than appendicitis.

Comforting heat may be applied to the back and the abdomen of the side affected by the spasms. Paregoric can be administered, if available, while waiting for medical care; about two teaspoonsful of paregoric in a half glass of water may help relieve symptoms.

Knee Injuries

Emergency Treatment

If the injury appears to be severe, including possible fracture of the kneecap, immobilize the knee. To immobilize the knee, place the injured leg on a board that is about four inches wide and three to four feet in length. Place padding between the board and the knee and between the board and the back of the ankle. Then use four strips of bandage to fasten the leg to the padded board—one at the ankle, one at the thigh, and one each above and below the knee.

Summon a physician or move the patient to a physician's office. Keep the knee protected against cold or exposure to the elements, but otherwise do not apply a bandage or any type of pressure to the knee itself; any rapid swelling would be aggravated by unnecessary pressure in that area. Be prepared to treat the patient for shock.

Laryngitis

Laryngitis is associated with colds and influenza and may be accompanied by a fever. The ailment can be aggravated by smoking, and it is possible that the vocal cords can be damaged if the victim tries to force the use of his voice while the larynx is swollen by the infection.

Emergency Treatment

Have the victim inhale the warm moist air of a steam kettle or vaporizer. A vaporizer can be improvised in an emergency by pouring boiling water into a bowl and forming a "tent" over the steaming bowl with a large towel or sheet, or by placing a large paper bag over the bowl and cutting an opening at the closed end of the bag so the face can be exposed to the steam. The hot water can contain a bit of camphor or menthol, if available, to make the warm moist air more soothing to the throat, but this is not necessary.

Continue the use of the vaporizer for several days, as needed. The victim should not use the vocal cords any more than absolutely necessary. If the infection does not subside within the first few days, a physician should be consulted.

Leeches

Emergency Treatment

Do not try to pull leeches off the skin. They will usually drop away from the skin if a heated object such as a lighted cigarette is held close to them. Leeches also are likely to let go if iodine is applied to their bodies. The wound caused by a leech should be washed carefully with soap and water and an antiseptic applied.

Lightning Shock

Emergency Treatment

If the victim is not breathing, apply artificial respiration. If a second person is available to help, have him summon a physician while artificial respiration is administered. Continue artificial respiration until breathing resumes or the physician arrives.

When the victim is breathing regularly, treat him for shock. Keep him lying down with his feet higher than his head, his clothing loosened around the neck, and his body covered with a blanket or coat for warmth. If the victim shows signs of vomiting, turn his head to one side so he will not swallow the vomitus.

If the victim is breathing regularly and does not show signs of shock, he may be given a few sips of a stimulating beverage such as coffee, tea, or brandy.

Motion Sickness

Emergency Treatment

Have the victim lie down in a position that is most comfortable to him. The head should be fixed so that any view of motion is avoided. Reading or other use of the eyes should be prohibited. Food or fluids should be restricted to very small amounts. If traveling by car, stop at a rest area; in an airplane or ship, place the victim in an area where motion is least noticeable.

Drugs, such as Dramamine, are helpful for control of the symptoms of motion sickness; they are most effective when started about 90 minutes before travel begins and repeated at regular intervals thereafter.

Muscle Cramps

Emergency Treatment

Gently massage the affected muscle, sometimes stretching it to help relieve the painful contraction. Then relax the muscle by using a hot water bottle or an electric heating pad, or by soaking the affected area in a warm bath.

A repetition of cramps may require medical attention.

Nosebleeds

Emergency Treatment

Have the victim sit erect but with the head tilted slightly forward to prevent blood from running down the throat.

Apply pressure by pinching the nostrils; if bleeding is from just one nostril, use pressure on that side. A small wedge of absorbent cotton or gauze can be inserted into the bleeding nostril. Make sure that the cotton or gauze extends out of the nostril to aid in its removal when the bleeding has stopped. Encourage the victim to breathe through the mouth while the nose is bleeding. After five minutes, release pressure on the nose to see if the bleeding has stopped. If the bleeding continues, repeat pressure on the nostril for an additional five minutes. Cold compresses applied to the nose can help stop the bleeding.

If bleeding continues after the second five-minute period of pressure treatment, get the victim to a physician's office or a hospital emergency room.

Poison Ivy/Poison Oak/Poison Sumac

Emergency Treatment

The poison of these three plants is the same and the treatment is identical. Bathe the skin area exposed to poison ivy, poison oak, or poison sumac with soap and water or with alcohol within 15 minutes after contact. If exposure is not discovered until a rash appears, apply cool wet dressings. Dressings can be made of old bed sheets or soft linens soaked in a solution of one teaspoon of salt per pint of water. Dressings should be applied four times a day for periods of 15 to 60 minutes each time; during these periods, dressings can be removed and reapplied every few minutes. The itching that often accompanies the rash can be relieved by taking antihistamine tablets.

Creams or lotions may be prescribed by a physician or supplied by a pharmacist. Do not use such folk remedies as ammonia or turpentine; do not use skin lotions not approved by a physician or druggist. Haphazard application of medications on poison ivy blisters and rashes can result in complications including skin irritation, infection, or pigmented lesions of the skin.

Rabies

See ANIMAL BITES.

Rape

Rape has been defined as any unlawful sexual intercourse or sexual contact by force or threat. Most commonly, men commit rape against women; but homosexual rape involving men only may occur, for example, in a prison.

Of the million or more Americans who are raped each year, one in five is under the age of 12. Boys are the victims of sexual assault as often as girls. In seven to ten percent of all reported adult cases, men are the victims.

Emergency Response

The victim of rape may not always be able to help him- or herself. Because violence may accompany the rape, the victim may find it impossible to seek help at once. But where possible, the recommended course of action is to go to a hospital for physical examination. Reporting to a hospital in itself may reduce the feelings of shock, depression, anxiety, and revulsion that generally follow a sexual assault. The physical examination that takes place at the hospital may produce evidence that could be important in a court trial if the rapist is later apprehended. Victims are also advised to report the rape to the police as soon as possible.

For additional information on ways to avoid rape and what to do if it occurs, see "The Rape Victim" in Ch. 25, *Women's Health.*

Sciatica/Lower Back Pain

Although lower back pain is frequently triggered by fatigue, anxiety, or by strained muscles or tendons, it may be a symptom of a slipped or ruptured disk between the vertebrae or of a similar disorder requiring extensive medical attention.

Emergency Treatment

Reduce the pressure on the lower back by having the victim lie down on a hard flat surface; if a bed is used there should be a board or sheet of plywood between the springs and mattress. Pillows should be placed under the knees instead of under the head, to help keep the back flat. Give aspirin to relieve the pain, and apply heat to the back. Call a physician if the symptoms do not subside overnight.

Scorpion Stings

Emergency Treatment

Apply ice to the region of the sting, except in the case of an arm or leg, in which event the limb may be immersed in ice water. Continue the ice or ice-water treatment for at least one hour. Try to keep the area of the sting at a position lower than the heart. No tourniquet is required. Should the breathing of a scorpion sting victim become depressed, administer artificial respiration. If symptoms fail to subside within a couple of hours, notify a physician, or transfer the victim to a doctor's office or hospital.

For children under six, call a physician in the event of any scorpion sting. Children stung by scorpions may become convulsive, and this condition can result in fatal exhaustion unless it receives prompt medical treatment.

Snakebites

Of the many varieties of snakes found in the United States, only four kinds are poisonous: copperheads, rattlesnakes, moccasins, and coral snakes. The first three belong to the category of pit vipers and are known as *hemotoxic* because their poison enters the bloodstream. The coral snake, which is comparatively rare, is related to the cobra and is the most dangerous of all because its venom is *neurotoxic*. This means that the poison transmitted by its bite goes directly to the nervous system and the brain.

How to Differentiate among Snakebites

Snakes of the pit viper family have a fang on each side of the head. These fangs leave characteristic puncture wounds on the skin in addition to two rows of tiny bites or scratches left by the teeth. A bite from a nonpoisonous snake leaves six rows—four upper and two lower—of very small bite marks or scratches and no puncture wounds.

The marks left by the bite of a coral snake do not leave any puncture wounds either, but this snake bites with a chewing motion, hanging on to the victim rather than attacking quickly. The coral snake is very easy to recognize because of its distinctive markings: wide horizontal bands of red and black separated by narrow bands of yellow.

Symptoms

A bite from any of the pit vipers produces immediate and severe pain and darkening of the skin, followed by weakness, blurred vision, quickened pulse, nausea, and vomiting. The bite of a coral snake produces somewhat the same symptoms, although there is less local pain and considerable drowsiness leading to unconsciousness.

If a physician or a hospital is a short distance away, the patient should receive professional help *immediately*. He should be transported lying down, either on an improvised stretcher or carried by his companions—with the wounded part lower than his heart. He should be advised to move as little as possible.

Emergency Treatment

If several hours must elapse before a physician or a hospital can be reached, the following procedures should be applied promptly:

1. Keep the victim lying down and as still as possible.

2. Tie a constricting band *above* the wound between it and the heart and tight enough to slow but not stop blood circulation. A handkerchief, necktie, sock, or piece of torn shirt will serve.

3. If a snakebite kit is available, use the knife it contains; otherwise, sterilize a knife or razor blade in a flame. Carefully make small cuts in the skin where the swelling has developed. Make the cuts along the length of the limb, not across or at right angles to it. The incisions should be shallow because of the danger of severing nerves, blood vessels, or muscles.

4. Use the suction cups in the snakebite kit, if available, to draw out as much of the venom as possible. If suction cups are not available, the venom can be removed by sucking it out with the mouth. Although snake venom is not a stomach poison, it should not be swallowed but should be rinsed from the mouth.

5. This procedure should be continued for from 30 to 60 minutes or until the swelling subsides and the other symptoms decrease.

6. You may apply cold compresses to the bite area while waiting for professional assistance.

7. Treat the victim for shock.

8. Give artificial respiration if necessary.

Splinters

Emergency Treatment

Clean the area about the splinter with soap and water or an antiseptic. Next, sterilize a needle by holding it over an open flame. After it cools, insert the needle above the splinter so it will tear a line in the skin, making the splinter lie loose in the wound. Then, gently lift the splinter out, using a pair of tweezers or the point of the needle. If tweezers are used, they should be sterilized first.

Wash the wound area again with soap and water, or apply an antiseptic. It is best to cover the wound with an adhesive bandage. If redness or irritation develops around the splinter wound, consult a physician.

Sprains

A sprain occurs when a joint is wrenched or twisted in such a way that the ligaments holding it in position are ruptured, possibly damaging the surrounding blood vessels, tendons, nerves, and muscles. This type of injury is more serious than a strain and is usually accompanied by pain, sometimes severe, soreness, swelling, and discoloration of the affected area. Most sprains occur as a result of falls, athletic accidents, or improper handling of heavy weights.

Emergency Treatment

This consists of prompt rest, the application of cold compresses to relieve swelling and any internal bleeding in the joint, and elevation of the affected area. Aspirin is recommended to reduce discomfort. If the swelling and soreness increase after such treatment, a physician should be consulted to make sure that the injury is not a fracture or a bone dislocation.

Sting Ray

Emergency Treatment

If an arm or leg is the target of a sting ray, wash the area thoroughly with salt water. Quickly remove any pieces of the stinger imbedded in the skin or flesh; poison can still be discharged into the victim from the sting-ray sheath. After initial cleansing of an arm or leg sting, soak the wound with hot water for up to an hour. Apply antiseptic or a sterile dressing after the soak.

Consult a physician after a sting-ray attack. The physician will make a thorough examination of the wound to determine whether stitches or antibiotics are required. Fever, vomiting, or muscular twitching also may result from an apparently simple leg or arm wound by a sting ray.

If the sting occurs in the chest or abdomen, the victim should be rushed to a hospital as soon as possible because such a wound can produce convulsions or loss of consciousness.

Strains

When a muscle is stretched because of misuse or overuse, the interior bundles of tissue may tear, or the tendon that connects it to the bone may be stretched. This condition is known as strain. It occurs most commonly to the muscles of the lower back when heavy weights are improperly lifted, or in the area of the calf or ankle as the result of a sudden, violent twist or undue pressure.

Emergency Treatment

Bed rest, the application of heat, and gentle massage are recommended for back strain. If the strain is in the leg, elevate the limb to help reduce pain and swelling, and apply cold compresses or an ice bag to the area. Aspirin may be taken to reduce discomfort.

In severe cases of strained back muscles, a physician may have to be consulted for strapping. For a strained ankle, a flexible elastic bandage can be helpful in providing the necessary support until the injured muscle heals.

Stroke

Stroke, or apoplexy, is caused by a disruption of normal blood flow to the brain, either by rupture of a blood vessel within the brain or by blockage of an artery supplying the brain. The condition is enhanced by hardening of the arteries and high blood pressure, and is most likely to occur in older persons. A stroke usually occurs with little or no warning and the onset may be marked by a variety of manifestations ranging from headache, slurred speech, or blurred vision, to sudden collapse and unconsciousness.

Emergency Treatment

Try to place the victim in a semireclining position, or, if he is lying down, be sure there is a pillow under his head. Avoid conditions that might increase the flow of blood toward the head. Summon a physician immediately. Loosen any clothing that may be tight. If the patient wears dentures, remove them.

Before professional medical assis-

tance is available, the victim may vomit or go into shock or convulsions. If he vomits, try to prevent a backflow of vomitus into the breathing passages. If shock occurs, do not place the victim in the shock position but do keep him warm and comfortable. If convulsions develop, place a handkerchief or similar soft object between the jaws to prevent tongue biting.

Sty on Eyelid

Sties usually develop around hair follicles because of a bacterial infection. Like cold sores, they are most likely to develop in association with poor health and lowered resistance to infection.

Emergency Treatment

Apply warm, moist packs or compresses to the sty for periods of 15 to 20 minutes at intervals of three or four hours. Moist heat generally is more penetrating than dry heat.

The sty should eventually rupture and the pus should then be washed carefully away from the eye area. If the sty does not rupture or is very painful, consult a physician. Do not squeeze or otherwise handle the sty except to apply the warm moist compresses.

Sunburn

Emergency Treatment

Apply cold wet compresses to help relieve the pain. Compresses can be soaked in whole milk, salt water, or a solution of cornstarch mixed with water. The victim also may get some relief by soaking in a bathtub filled with plain water. Soothing lotions, such as baby oil or a bland cold cream, can be applied after carefully drying

the skin. Don't rub the burn area while drying. Avoid the use of "shake" lotions, like calamine, which may aggravate the burn by a drying action. The victim should, of course, avoid further exposure to sunlight.

If pain is excessive, or extensive blistering is present, consult a physician. Avoid application of over-the-counter topical anesthetics that may cause allergic skin reactions.

A severe or extensive sunburn is comparable to a second-degree thermal burn and may be accompanied by symptoms of shock; if such symptoms are present the victim should be treated for shock. See also BURNS, THERMAL.

Sunstroke

See HEATSTROKE.

Tick Bites

Emergency Treatment

Do not try to scrape or rub the insect off the skin with your fingers; scraping, rubbing, or pulling may break off only part of the insect body, leaving the head firmly attached to the skin. Rubbing also can smear disease organisms from the tick into the bite. To make the tick drop away from the skin, cover it with a heavy oil, such as salad, mineral, or lubricating oil. Oil usually will block the insect's breathing pores, suffocating it. If oil is not readily available, carefully place a heated object against the tick's body; a lighted cigarette or a match that has been ignited and snuffed out can serve as a hot object.

Carefully inspect the bite area to be sure that all parts of the tick have been removed. Use a pair of tweezers to remove any tick parts found. Then carefully wash the bite and surrounding area with soap and water and apply an antiseptic. Also, wash your hands and any equipment that may have come in contact with the tick. Consult a physician if symptoms of tick fever or tularemia, such as unexplained muscular weakness, occur following a bite.

Toothaches

Emergency Treatment

Give an adult one or two aspirin tablets; a young child should be given no more than one-half of an adult tablet. The aspirin should be swallowed with plenty of water. Do not let it dissolve in the mouth or be held near the aching tooth. Aspirin becomes effective as a painkiller only after it has gone through the digestive tract and into the bloodstream; if aspirin is held in the mouth, it may irritate the gums.

Oil of cloves can be applied to the aching tooth. Dip a small wad of cotton into the oil of cloves, then gently pack the oil-soaked cotton into the tooth cavity with a pair of tweezers. Do not let the tweezers touch the tooth.

If the jaw is swollen, apply an ice bag for periods of 15 minutes at a time, at intermittent intervals. Never apply heat to a swollen jaw when treating a toothache. Arrange to see your dentist as soon as possible.

Tooth, Broken

Emergency Treatment

Apply a few drops of oil of cloves to the injured tooth to help relieve pain. If oil of cloves is not available, give an adult one to two regular aspirin tablets. One-half of a regular tablet can be given to a young child.

Make an emergency filling from a wad of cotton containing a few drops of oil of cloves. An emergency filling also can be made from powdered chalk; it is important to protect the cavity from infection while providing pain relief.

If the tooth has been knocked out of the socket, retrieve the tooth, because it can be restored in some cases. Do not wash the tooth; ordinary washing can damage dental tissues. A dentist will take care of cleaning it properly. Wrap the tooth in a damp clean handkerchief or tissue or place the tooth in a container of slightly salty warm water for the trip to the dentist.

Unconsciousness

Unconsciousness is the condition that has the appearance of sleep, but is usually the result of injury, shock, or serious physical disturbance. A brief loss of consciousness followed by spontaneous recovery is called *fainting*. A prolonged episode of unconsciousness is a *coma*.

Emergency Treatment

Call a physician at once. If none is available, get the victim to the nearest hospital. If the loss of consciousness is accompanied by loss of breathing, begin mouth-to-mouth respiration. If the victim is suffering cardiac arrest, administer cardiac massage. Don't try to revive the victim with any kind of stimulant unless told to do so by a physician.

Vertigo

See DIZZINESS.

36

Commonly Prescribed Generic Drugs

Name	Action	Prescribed for
Trade Names (CD) = combined drug)		
Acetaminophen	Believed to reduce concentration of chemicals involved in production of pain, fever, and inflammation (analgesic; antipyretic)	Relief of mild to moderate pain; reduction of fever

Anacin-3	Co-Tylenol (CD)	Excedrin (CD)	Penaphen (CD)	Tylenol Infant
Bancap (CD)	Darvocet-N (CD)	Hycomine (CD)	Protid (CD)	Drops
Capital (CD)	Datril	Hyco-Pap (CD)	Repan (CD)	Tylenol Junior
Codalan (CD)	Dolacet (CD)	Lorcet (CD)	Sinarest (CD)	Strength
Co-Gesic (CD)	Dorcol (CD) for	Midrin (CD)	Sine-Aid (CD)	Tylox (CD)
Comtrex (CD)	children	Pacaps (CD)	Sinutab (CD)	Unisom (CD)
Congesprin (CD)	Dristan (CD)	Percocet (CD)	Talacen (CD)	Vicodin (CD)
for children	Esgic (CD)	Percogesic (CD)	Tylenol	Wygesic (CD)

Name	Action	Prescribed for
Alprazolam	Believed to depress the central nervous system, slowing nervous response, and relieving nervousness and tension	Relief of anxiety attacks and insomnia; reduction of symptoms of chronic anxiety
Xanax		
Amitriptyline	Believed to restore to normal levels the constituents of brain tissue that transmit nerve impulses (antidepressant)	Relief of emotional depression; gradual improvement of mood
Elavil Endep Etrafon (CD)	Limbitral (CD) Triavil (CD)	
Ampicillin	Interferes with ability of susceptible bacteria to produce new protective cell walls as they grow and multiply (antibiotic)	Elimination of infections responsive to action of this drug
Omnipen Polycillin	Principen Unasyn	

Name	Action	Prescribed for
Trade Names (CD = combined drug)		
Antacids (Aluminum Hydroxide) (Calcium Carbonate) (Sodium Bicarbonate)	Neutralizes stomach acid; reduces action of digestive enzyme pepsin (relief from gastric hyperacidity)	Relief of heartburn, sour stomach, acid indigestion, and discomfort associated with peptic ulcer, gastritis, esophagitis, hiatal hernia
Absorbable: Sodium bicarbonate:	Alka-Seltzer Brioschi Bromo-Seltzer	Less absorbable: Aluminum hydroxide:	Amphojel Calcium carbonate:	Alka-2 Amitone
Aspirin (Acetylsalicylic Acid)	Dilates blood vessels in skin, thus hastening loss of body heat (antipyretic); reduces tissue concentration of inflammation and pain (analgesic; antirheumatic)	Reduction of fever; relief of mild to moderate pain and inflammation; prevention of blood clots, as in phlebitis, heart attack, stroke
Bayer Easprin Empirin St. Joseph's Children's Aspirin Alka-Seltzer (CD) Anacin (CD)	Ascriptin (CD) Axotal (CD) Buff-A Comp (CD) Bufferin (CD) Congespirin (CD) for children Darvon (CD)	Ecotrin Equagesic (CD) Excedrin (CD) 4-Way Cold Tablets (CD) Fiorinal (CD) Midol (CD)	Norgesic (CD) Percodan (CD) Robaxisal (CD) Soma Compound (CD) Supac (CD) Synalgos-DC (CD)	Talwin (CD) Zorprin
Atropine (Belladonna, Hyoscyamine)	Prevents stimulation of muscular contractions and glandular secretions in organ involved (antispasmodic [anticholinergic])	Relief of discomfort associated with excessive activity and spasm of digestive tract; irritation and spasm of lower urinary tract; painful menstruation
Antrocol (CD) Arco-Lase Plus (CD)	Donnagel-PG (CD) Donnatal (CD)	Donnatal Donnazyme (CD) Lomotil (CD)	Ru-Tuss (CD) SK-Diphenoxylate (CD)	Urised (CD)
Bendroflumethiazide	Increases elimination of salt and water (diuretic); relaxes walls of smaller arteries, allowing them to expand; combined effect lowers blood pressure (antihypertensive)	Elimination of excessive fluid retention (edema); reduction of high blood pressure
Naturetin	Corzide (CD)	Rauzide (CD)		
Beta-Adrenergic Blocking Agents	Decreases physical responses at beta-adrenergic receptors, slowing heart rate, dilating the vascular and bronchial systems (antihypertensive); believed to reduce cardiac output and nervous system responses in some forms of the medication	Treatment of high blood pressure; medication to reduce the incidence of another attack in heart attack patients; prevention of migraine headaches in chronic sufferers of migraines
Blocadren Corgard	Lopressor Normodyne	Sectral Tenormin	Visken	
Brompheniramine	Blocks action of histamine after release from sensitized tissue cells, thus reducing intensity of allergic response (antihistamine)	Relief of symptoms of hay fever (allergic rhinitis) and of allergic reactions of skin (itching, swelling, hives, rash)
Dimetane Bromfed (CD) Dimetapp (CD)	Poly-histine-DX (CD)			
Butabarbital	Believed to block transmission of nerve impulses (hypnotic; sedative)	Low dosage: relief of moderate anxiety or tension (sedative effect); higher dosage: at bedtime to induce sleep (hypnotic effect)
Butisol Pyridium Plus (CD)				

Name	Action	Prescribed for
Trade Names (CD = combined drug)		
Butalbital	Affects the actions of the central nervous system, relieving anxiety (anxiolytic), and relaxing muscles (barbiturate sedative)	Relief of headaches related to tension or stress, psychic tension; relaxation of muscle strain and contraction in the head, neck, and shoulders
Esgic (CD) Medigesic (CD) Sedapap (CD) Fioricet (CD) Phrenilin (CD) Fiorinal (CD) Repan (CD)		
Caffeine	Constricts blood vessel walls; increases energy level of chemical systems responsible for nerve tissue activity (cardiac, respiratory, psychic stimulant)	Prevention and early relief of vascular headaches such as migraine; relief of drowsiness and mental fatigue
No-Doz Esgic (CD) Fiorinal (CD) Pacaps (CD) Anacin (CD) Excedrin Extra Maximum Strength Wigraine (CD) Cafergot (CD) Strength (CD) Midol (CD) Vivarin		
Carisoprodol	Believed to block transmission of nerve impulses and/or to produce a sedative effect (muscle relaxant)	Relief of discomfort caused by spasms of voluntary muscles
Soma (CD) Soma Compound (CD)		
Chloral Hydrate	Believed to affect wake-sleep centers of brain (hypnotic)	Low dosage: relief of mild to moderate anxiety or tension (sedative effect); higher dosage: at bedtime to relieve insomnia (hypnotic effect)
SK-Chloral Hydrate		
Chloramphenicol	Prevents growth and multiplication of susceptible bacteria by interfering with formation of their essential proteins (antibiotic)	Elimination of infections responsive to action of this drug
Chloromycetin Ophthochlor Ophthocort		
Chlordiazepoxide	Believed to reduce activity of some parts of limbic system (tranquilizer)	Relief of mild to moderate anxiety and tension without significant sedation
Libritabs Limbitrol (CD) Librium Menrium (CD) Librax (CD)		
Chlorpheniramine	Blocks action of histamine after release from sensitized tissue cells, thus reducing intensity of allergic response (antihistamine)	Relief of symptoms of hay fever (allergic rhinitis) and of allergic reactions of skin (itching, swelling, hives, rash)
Chlor-Trimeton PediaCare (CD) Teldrin for children Comtrex (CD) Tylenol Cold Med- Contac ication (CD) Dristan (CD)		
Chlorpromazine	Believed to inhibit action of dopamine, thus correcting an imbalance of nerve impulse transmission thought to be responsible for certain mental disorders (antiemetic; tranquilizer)	Relief of severe anxiety, agitation, and psychotic behavior
Thorazine		
Chlorzoxazone	Inhibits nerve responses that trigger muscle contractions	Pain relief of muscle tension and injuries to the muscles and joints; relaxation of muscular tension for use in combination with physical therapy
Paraflex Parafon (CD) Remular		

Name	Action	Prescribed for
Trade Names (CD = combined drug)		
Codeine	Believed to affect tissue sites that react specifically with opium and its derivatives (antitussive; narcotic analgesic)	Relief of moderate pain; control of coughing
Acetaco (CD) Actifed with Codeine (CD) Ambenyl (CD) Calcidrine Syrup (CD) Codalan (CD) Codimal PH (CD)	Dimetane-DC (CD) Empirin with Codeine (CD) Fiorinal with Codeine (CD) IoTuss (CD) Naldecon-CX (CD) Novahistine DK (CD) Nucofed (CD) Pediacof (CD) Phenaphen with Codeine (CD) Phenergan with Codeine (CD)	Promethazine (CD) Robitussin A-C (CD) Soma Compound (CD) Triaminic with Codeine (CD) Tussar (CD) Tylenol with Codeine (CD)
Dexamethasone	Believed to inhibit several tissue mechanisms that induce inflammation (adrenocortical steriod [anti-inflammatory])	Symptomatic relief of inflammation (swelling, redness, heat, pain)
Decadron Dalalone Hexadrol Neodecadron		
Dextroamphetamine (d-Amphetamine)	Increases release of nerve impulse transmitter (central stimulant); this may also improve concentration and attention span of hyperactive child (primary calming action unknown); alters chemical control of nerve impulse transmission in appetite control center of brain (appetite suppressant [anorexiant])	Reduction or prevention of sleep epilepsy (narcolepsy); reduction of symptoms of abnormal hyperactivity (as in minimal brain dysfunction); suppression of appetite in management of weight reduction
Dexedrine	Biphetamine (CD)	
Diazepam	Believed to reduce activity of some parts of limbic system (tranquilizer)	Relief of mild to moderate anxiety and tension without significant sedation
Valium		
Dicyclomine	Believed to produce a local anesthetic action that blocks reflex activity responsible for spasm (antispasmodic)	Relief of discomfort from muscle spasm of the gastrointestinal tract
Bentyl		
Digitoxin	Increases availability of calcium within the heart muscle, thus improving conversion of chemical energy to mechanical energy; slows pacemaker and delays transmission of electrical impulses (digitalis preparations [cardiotonic])	Improvement of heart muscle contraction force (as in congestive heart failure); correction of certain heart rhythm disorders
Crystodigin		
Digoxin	Same as above	Same as above
Lanoxicaps Lanoxin		
Diphenhydramine	Blocks action of histamine after release from sensitized tissue cells, thus reducing intensity of allergic response (antihistamine)	Relief of symptoms of hay fever (allergic rhinitis) and of allergic reactions of skin (itching, swelling, hives, rash)
Ambenyl (CD) Benadryl Benadryl DM (CD) Bromanyl (CD) Dytuss (CD)	Tylenol Cold Night Time (CD) Unisom Dual Relief (CD)	
Doxylamine	Same as above	Same as above
Unisom	Cremacoat 4 (CD) Nyquil (CD)	

Name	Action	Prescribed for
Trade Names (CD = combined drug)		
Ephedrine	Blocks release of certain chemicals from sensitized tissue cells undergoing allergic reaction; relaxes bronchial muscles; shrinks tissue mass (decongestion) by contracting arteriole walls in lining of respiratory passages (adrenergic [bronchodilator])	Prevention and symptomatic relief of bronchial asthma; relief of congestion of respiratory passages
Primatene Mist / Bronkolixir (CD) / Bronkotabs (CD)	Medicone-Derma HC (CD) / Marax (CD) Mudrane (CD) / Nyquil (CD) / Primatene (CD)	Quadrinal (CD) Tedral (CD) / Quelidrine (CD) / Rynatuss (CD)
Ergotamine	Constricts blood vessel walls, thus relieving excessive dilation that causes pain of vascular headaches (migraine analgesic [vasoconstrictor])	Prevention and early relief of vascular headaches such as migraines or histamine headaches
Ergomar / Ergostat	Medihaler Ergotamine Bellergal (CD) / Cafergot (CD)	Wigraine (CD)
Erythromycin	Prevents growth and multiplication of susceptible bacteria by interfering with formation of their essential proteins (antibiotic)	Elimination of infections responsive to action of this drug
A/T/S / E.E.S. / E-Mycin / ERYC	EryDerm / Erymax / EryPed / Ery-Tab Erythrocin / Ilosone / Ilotycin / P.C.E.	Staticin/T-Stat / Wyamycin S / SK-Erythromycin / Pediazole (CD)
Estrogens (Estrogenic Substances) Conjugated Estrogens, Esterified Estrogens (Estrone and Equilin) Estradiol Mestranol	Prepares uterus for pregnancy or induces menstruation by cyclic increase and decrease in tissue stimulation; when taken regularly, blood and tissue levels increase to resemble those during pregnancy, thus preventing pituitary gland from producing hormones that induce ovulation; reduces frequency and intensity of menopausal symptoms (female sex hormone)	Regulation of menstrual cycle; oral birth control; prevention of pregnancy; relief of symptoms of menopause
Estratab / Premarin / Estratest (CD)	Mediatric (CD) / Menrium (CD) / PMB (CD) Brevicon (CD) / Demulen (CD) / Enovid (CD)	Modicon (CD) Ortho-Novum (CD) / Norethin (CD) / Norinyl (CD)
Fluoxetine	Believed to inhibit nerve uptake of serotonin to reduce depression (antidepressant, sedative)	Relief from acute depression or major depressive episodes
Prozac		
Griseofulvin	Believed to prevent growth and multiplication of susceptible fungus strains by interfering with their metabolic activities (antibiotic; antifungal)	Elimination of fungus infections responsive to actions of this drug
Fulvicin-U/F	Fulvicin P/G Grifulvin V	Grisactin Gris-PEG
Guaifenesin	Loosens phlegm and mucous from the bronchial passages by reducing viscosity and adhesiveness (expectorant)	Relief of painful coughs due to colds and influenzas; usually taken in conjunction with a decongestant
Codiclear (CD) / Codimal (CD)	Dilaudid (CD) / Donatussin (CD) Guaifed (CD) / Mudrane (CD)	Naldecon (CD) Quibron (CD) / Robitussin (CD) Triaminic (CD)
Hydralazine	Lowers pressure of blood in vessels by causing direct relaxation and expansion of vessel walls—mechanism unknown (antihypertensive)	Reduction of high blood pressure
Apresoline / Apresazide (CD) / Apresoline-Esidrex (CD)	Ser-Ap-Es (CD) / Serpasil- Apresoline (CD)	

Name	Action	Prescribed for
Trade Names (CD = combined drug)		
Hydrochlorothi-azide	Increases elimination of salt and water (diuretic); relaxes walls of smaller arteries, allowing them to expand; combined effect lowers blood pressure (antihypertensive)	Elimination of excessive fluid retention (edema); reduction of high blood pressure
Esidrix HydroDIURIL Oretic Aldactazide (CD) Aldoril (CD) Apresazide (CD)	Apresoline-Esidrix (CD) Dyazide (CD) Esimil (CD) Hydropres (CD) Inderide (CD) Maxzide (CD) Moduretic (CD) SK-Hydro- chlorothiazide Timolide (CD)	
Hydrocodone	Believed to affect opiate receptors in the nervous system, reducing pain and relaxing muscles (narcotic analgesic)	Relief of moderate to severe pain; severe cough and cold symptoms
Anexsia (CD) Azdone (CD) Bancap (CD) Codiclear (CD)	Codimal (CD) Co-Gesic (CD) Donatussin (CD) DuoCet (CD) Entuss (CD) Hyco-Pap (CD) Hydrocet (CD) Lorcet (CD)	Lortab (CD) Ru-Tuss with Hy- drocodone (CD) Triaminic (CD)
Hydrocortisone (Cortisol)	Believed to inhibit several tissue mechanisms that induce inflammation (adrenocortical steroid [anti-inflammatory])	Symptomatic relief of inflammation (swelling, redness, heat, pain)
Aeroseb-HC Carmol HC Cortef Eldecort F-E-P Hydrocortone Hytone	Penecort Synacort Vanoxide-HC Vioform- Hydrocortisone VōSoL HC Corticaine (CD) Cortisporin (CD) Derma-Sone (CD) Di-Hydrotic (CD) Hill Cortac (CD) Hysone (CD) Iodo-Cortifair (CD) Oticol (CD)	Otocort (CD) Proctocort Proctocream (CD) Proctofoam (CD)
Hydroxyzine	Believed to reduce excessive activity in areas of brain that influence emotional health (antihistamine; tranquilizer)	Relief of anxiety, tension, apprehension, and agitation
Atarax Vistaril Marax (CD) SK-Hydroxyzine		
Ibuprofen	Believed to inhibit prostaglandin sythetase production, acting as an anti-inflammatory agent; reduces fever (antipyretic), reduces inflammation and pain (antirheumatic, analgesic)	Relief of inflammation and pain from rheumatoid arthritis, osteoarthritis, and primary dysmenorrhea
Advil Children's Advil	IBU-TAB Medipren Motrin Nuprin	PediaProfen for Rufen children SK-Ibuprofen
Insulin (Human, beef, pork)	Facilitates passage of sugar through cell wall to interior of cell (hypoglycemic)	Control of diabetes
Humulin Iletin Insulatard NPH	Lente Insulin Mixtard Novolin NPH Insulin Regular Insulin Semilente Insulin	Ultrlente Insulin Velosulin
Isoniazid	Believed to interfere with several metabolic activities of susceptible tuberculosis organisms (antibacterial; tuberculostatic)	Prevention and treatment of tuberculosis
INH Laniazid Rifamate (CD)		
Isopropamide	Prevents stimulation of muscular contraction and glandular secretion in organ involved (antispasmodic [anticholinergic])	Relief of discomfort from excessive activity and spasm of digestive tract
Darbid		

Name	Action	Prescribed for
Trade Names (CD = combined drug)		
Isoproterenol/ Isoprenaline	Dilates bronchial tubes by stimulating sympathetic nerve terminals (Isoproterenol: adrenergic [bronchodilator]; Isoprenaline: sympathomimetic)	Management of acute bronchial asthma, bronchitis, and emphysema
Isuprel Medihaler-Iso Norisodrine Duo-Medihaler (CD)	Isuprel Hydrochloride (CD)	
Isosorbide Dinitrate	Acts directly on muscle cells to produce relaxation which permits expansion of blood vessels, thus increasing supply of blood and oxygen to heart (coronary vasodilator)	Management of pain associated with angina pectoris (coronary insufficiency)
Dilatrate Iso-Bid Isordil Sorbitrate		
Levodopa	Believed to be converted to dopamine in brain tissue, thus correcting a dopamine deficiency and restoring more normal balance of chemicals responsible for transmission of nerve impulses (anti-Parkinsonism)	Management of Parkinson's disease
Larodopa Sinemet		
Liothyronine (T-3)	Increases rate of cellular metabolism and makes more energy available for biochemical activity (thyroid hormone)	Correction of thyroid hormone deficiency (hypothyroidism)
Cytomel Euthroid (CD) Thyrolar (CD)		
Lithium	Believed to correct chemical imbalance in certain nerve impulse transmitters that influence emotional behavior (antidepressant)	Improvement of mood and behavior in chronic manic-depression
Eskalith Cibalith-S Lithane Lithobid		
Meclizine	Blocks transmission of excessive nerve impulses to vomiting center (antiemetic)	Management of nausea, vomiting, and dizziness associated with motion sickness
Antivert Bonine Meclizine HCl		
Meperidine/ Pethidine	Believed to increase chemicals that transmit nerve impulses (narcotic analgesic)	Relief of moderate to severe pain
Demerol Mepergan (CD)		
Meprobamate	Not known (tranquilizer)	Relief of mild to moderate anxiety and tension (sedative effect); relief of insomnia resulting from anxiety and tension (hypnotic effect)
Equanil Miltown	Deprol (CD) Meprospan Equagesic (CD) PMB (CD)	
Methadone	Believed to increase chemicals that transmit nerve impulses (narcotic analgesic)	Treatment of heroin addiction; sometimes for relief of moderate to severe pain
Dolophine Methadone Hydrochloride		

Name	Action	Prescribed for
Trade Names (CD = combined drug)		
Methyclothiazide	Increases elimination of salt and water (diuretic); relaxes walls of smaller arteries, allowing them to expand; combined effect lowers blood pressure (antihypertensive)	Elimination of excess fluid retention (edema); reduction of high blood pressure
Aquatensen	Enduron	Diutensen (CD)	Enduronyl (CD)
Methylphenidate	Believed to increase release of nerve impulse transmitter, which may also improve concentration and attention span of hyperactive child (primary action unknown) (central stimulant)	Management of fatigue and depression; reduction of symptoms of abnormal hyperactivity (as in minimal brain dysfunction)
Ritalin		
Nicotinic Acid/ Niacin	Corrects a deficiency of nicotinic acid in tissues; dilation of blood vessels is believed limited to skin—increased blood flow within head has not been demonstrated; reduces initial production of cholesterol and prevents conversion of fatty tissue to cholesterol and triglycerides (vitamin B-complex component; cholesterol reducer)	Management of pellagra; treatment of vertigo, ringing in ears, premenstrual headache; reduction of blood levels of cholesterol and triglycerides
Niacor Nicobid Nicolar Nicotinex Elixir Slo-Niacin		
Nitrofurantoin	Believed to prevent growth and multiplication of susceptible bacteria by interfering with function of their essential enzyme systems (antibacterial)	Elimination of infections responsive to action of this drug
Furacin	Macrodantin	
Nitroglycerin	Acts directly on muscle cells to produce relaxation which permits expansion of blood vessels, thus increasing supply of blood and oxygen to heart (coronary vasodilator)	Management of pain associated with angina pectoris (coronary insufficiency)
Nitro-Bid Nitrodisc Nitro-Dur Nitroglyn Nitrol	Nitrong Nitrostat Transderm-Nitro Tridil	
Nystatin	Prevents gorwth and multiplication of susceptible fungus strains by attacking their walls and causing leakage of internal components (antibiotic; antifungal)	Elimination of fungus infections responsive to action of this drug
Mycostatin Nilstat Nystex	Mycolog (CD) Myco-Triacet (CD) Mytrex (CD)	
Oral Contraceptives	Suppresses the two pituitary gland hormones that produce ovulation (oral contraceptives)	Prevention of pregnancy
Ovcon Brevicon Demulen Enovid-E	Loestrin LO/Ovral Micronor Medicon	Nordette Norinyl Norlestrin Ortho-Novum	Ovral Triphasil Ovrette Ovulen Tri-Norinyl
Oxycodone	Believed to affect tissue sites that react specifically with opium and its derivatives (narcotic analgesic)	Relief of moderate pain; control of coughing
Percocet (CD) Percodan (CD) SK-Oxycodone with Acetaminophen (CD)	SK-Oxycodone with Aspirin (CD) Tylox (CD) Roxicet (CD)	Roxicodone Roxiprin (CD)	

Name	Action	Prescribed for
Trade Names (CD = combined drug)		
Oxytetracycline	Prevents growth and multiplication of susceptible bacteria by interfering with their formation of essential proteins (antibiotic)	Elimination of infections responsive to action of this drug
Terra-Cortril (CD) Terramycin Urobiotic (CD)		
Papaverine	Causes direct relaxation and expansion of blood vessel walls, thus increasing volume of blood which increases oxygen and nutrients (smooth muscle relaxant; vasodilator)	Relief of symptoms associated with impaired circulation in extremities and within brain
SK-Papaverine Pavabid		
Paregoric (Camphorated Tincture of Opium)	Believed to affect tissue sites that react specifically with opium and its derivatives to relieve pain; its active ingredient, morphine, acts as a local anesthetic and blocks release of chemical that transmits nerve impulses to muscle walls of intestine (antiperistaltic)	Relief of mild to moderate pain; relief of intestinal cramping and diarrhea
Donnagel-PG (CD) Parepectolin (CD)		
Penicillin G	Interferes with ability of susceptible bacteria to produce new protective cell walls as they grow and multiply (antibiotic)	Elimination of infections responsive to action of this drug
Bicillin C-R SK-Pencillin G Pentids Wycillin Pfizerpen		
Penicillin V	Same as above	Same as above
Betapen-VK SK-Pencillin VK Pen-Vee K Veetids Ledercillin		
Pentobarbital	Believed to block transmission of nerve impulses (hypnotic; sedative)	Low dosage: relief of mild to moderate anxiety or tension (sedative effect); higher dosage: at bedtime to induce sleep (hypnotic effect)
Cafergot PB (CD) Nembutal		
Phenazopyridine	Acts as local anesthetic on lining of lower urinary tract (urinary-analgesic)	Relief of pain and discomfort associated with acute irritation of lower urinary tract as in cystitis, urethritis, and prostatitis
Azo Gantanol (CD) Pyridium Azo-Standard Thiosulfil-A (CD) Urobiotic (CD)		
Pheniramine	Blocks action of histamine after release from sensitized tissue cells, thus reducing intensity of allergic response (antihistamine)	Relief of symptoms of hay fever (allergic rhinitis) and of allergic reactions of skin (itching, swelling, hives, and rash)
Triaminic Poly-Histine-D Ru-Tuss with Hy- Tussagesic (CD) Citra Forte (CD) (CD) drocodone (CD) Tussirex (CD) Dristan (CD) Robitussin AC S-T Forte (CD) Fiogesic (CD) (CD) Triaminicin (CD)		
Phenobarbital/ Phenobarbitone	Believed to block transmission of nerve impulses (anticonvulsant; hypnotic; sedative)	Low dosage: relief of mild to moderate anxiety or tension (sedative effect); higher dosage: at bedtime to induce sleep (hypnotic effect); continuous dosage: prevention of epileptic seizures (anticonvulsant effect)
SK-Phenobarbital Bellergal-S (CD) Mudrane (CD) Primatene (CD) Solfoton Bronkolixir (CD) Mudrane GG (CD) Quadrinal (CD) Antrocol (CD) Bronkotabs (CD) Phazyme (CD) T-E-P (CD)		

Name	Action	Prescribed for
Trade Names (CD = combined drug)		
Phentermine	Believed to alter chemical control of nerve impulse transmitter in appetite center of brain (appetite suppressant [anorexiant])	Suppression of appetite in management of weight reduction
Adipex-P Fastin Ionamin		
Phenylbutazone	Believed to suppress formation of chemical involved in production of inflammation (analgesic; anti-inflammatory; antipyretic)	Symptomatic relief of inflammation, swelling, pain, and tenderness associated with arthritis, tendinitis, bursitis, superficial phlebitis
Butazolidin		
Phenylephrine	Shrinks tissue mass (decongestion) by contracting arteriole walls in lining of nasal passages, sinuses, and throat, thus decreasing volume of blood (decongestant [sympathomimetic])	Relief of congestion of nose, sinuses, and throat associated with allergy
Codimal (CD) Comhist (CD) Cogespirin (CD) for children Coryban-D Cough Syrup (CD) Dallergy (CD) Dimetapp (CD) Donatussin (CD) Dristan, Advanced Formula (CD)	Dura-Tap/PD (CD) Dura-Vent/PD (CD) Entex (CD) Extendryl (CD) 4-Way Nasal Spray (CD) Histor-D (CD) Hycomine (CD) Korigesic (CD) Naldecon (CD) Neo-Synephrine (CD) P-V-Tussin (CD) Pediacof (CD) Phenergan VC (CD) Protid (CD) Quelidrine (CD) Ru-Tuss (CD) Rynatan (CD) Rynatuss (CD)	Sinarest (CD) S-T Decongest (CD) S-T Forte (CD) Tamine S.R. (CD) Tussar DM (CD) Tussirex (CD)
Phenylpropano-lamine	Same as above	Same as above
Help Propagest Rhindecon Alka-Seltzer Plus (CD) Allerest (CD) Appedrine, Maxi- mum Strength (CD) Bayer Children's Cold Tablets (CD) Bayer Cough Sy- rup for Children (CD) Codimal Expecto- rant (CD) Comtrex (CD)	Conex (CD) Congesprin (CD) for children Contac (CD) Control (CD) Coryban-D (CD) CoTylenol Chil- dren's Liquid (CD) Cremacoat 3 (CD) Dehist (CD) Dexatrim (CD) Dieutrim (CD) Dimetane (CD) Dimetapp (CD) Dura-Tapp/PD (CD) Dura-Vent (CD) Dura-Vent/A (CD) Entex (CD) 4-Way (CD) Fiogesic (CD) Heat & Chest (CD) Histalet (CD) Hycomine (CD) Naldecon (CD) Nolamine (CD) Ornacol (CD) Ornade (CD) Poly-Histine (CD) Prolamine, Extra Strength (CD) Quadrahist (CD) Resaid (CD) Rescaps (CD)	Rhinolar (CD) Ru-Tuss (CD) S-T Decongest (CD) S-T Forte (CD) Sinubid (CD) Sinulin (CD) Sinutab (CD) Tamine S.R. (CD) Tavist-D (CD) Triaminic (CD) Triaminicin (CD) Triaminicol (CD) Tuss-Ade (CD) Tuss-Ornade (CD)
Phenytoin (formerly Diphenylhydan- toin)	Believed to promote loss of sodium from nerve fibers, thus lowering their excitability and inhibiting spread of electrical impulse along nerve pathways (anticonvulsant)	Prevention of epileptic seizures
Dilantin		
Pilocarpine	Lowers internal eye pressure (antiglaucoma [miotic])	Management of glaucoma
Almocarpine	Isopto Carpine Pilocar	
Potassium	Maintains and replenishes potassium content of cells (potassium preparations)	Management of potassium deficiency
Kaon Kay Ciel	K-Lor Kaochlor	Klorvess Pima Syrup

Name	Action	Prescribed for
Trade Names (CD = combined drug)		
Prednisolone	Believed to inhibit several mechanisms that induce inflammation (adrenocortical steroid [anti-inflammatory])	Symptomatic relief of inflammation (swelling, redness, heat, and pain)
Delta-Cortef Hydeltra-T.B.A. Metimyd Metreton Predate		
Prednisone	Same as above	Same as above
Deltasone Liquid Pred SK-Prednisone Sterapred		
Probenecid	Reduces level of uric acid in blood and tissues; prolongs presence of penicillin in blood (antigout [uricosuric])	Management of gout
Benemid SK-Probenecid ColBENEMID (CD) Col-Probenecid (CD) Polycillin-PRB (CD)		
Promethazine	Blocks action of histamine after release from sensitized tissue cells, thus reducing intensity of allergic response (antihistamine); blocks transmission of excessive nerve impulses to vomiting center (antiemetic); action producing sedation and sleep is unknown (sedative)	Relief of symptoms of hay fever (allergic rhinitis) and of allergic reactions of skin (itching, swelling, hives, rash); prevention and management of nausea, vomiting, and dizziness associated with motion sickness; production of mild sedation and light sleep
Phenergan	Mepergan (CD)	
Propantheline	Prevents stimulation of muscular contraction and glandular secretion within organ involved (antispasmodic [anticholinergic])	Relief of discomfort associated with excessive activity and spasm of digestive tract
Pro-Banthine	SK-Propantheline	
Propoxyphene	Increases chemicals that transmit nerve impulses, somehow contributing to the analgesic effect (analgesic)	Relief of mild to moderate pain
Darvon Darvocet-N (CD) Darvon Compound (CD) Dolene (CD)	SK-65 APAP (CD) SK-65 Compound (CD) Wygesic (CD)	
Pseudoephedrine (Isoephedrine)	Shrinks tissue mass (decongestion) by contracting arteriole walls in lining of nasal passages, sinuses, and throat, thus decreasing volume of blood (decongestant [sympathomimetic])	Relief of congestion of nose, throat, and sinuses associated with allergy
Sudafed Actifed (CD) Ambenyl-D (CD) Anafed (CD) Anamine (CD) Brexin (CD) Bromfed (CD) Chlor-Trimeton (CD) Chlorafed (CD)	Codimal-L.A. (CD) Gunifed (CD) Congess (CD) Histalet (CD) CoTylenol Cold Isoclor (CD) Medication (CD) Kronofed-A (CD) Deconamine (CD) Novafed (CD) Dimacol (CD) Novahistine (CD) Dorcol (CD) Nucofed (CD) Extra-Strength Phenergan (CD) Sine-Aid (CD) Poly-Histine-DX Fedahist (CD) (CD)	Respaire-SR (CD) Robitussin-DAC (CD) Sine-Aid (CD) Triafed (CD) Tussend Expectorant (CD) Zephrex (CD)

Name	Action	Prescribed for
Trade Names (CD = combined drug)		
Pyrilamine/ Mepyramine	Blocks action of histamine after release from sensitized tissue cells, thus reducing intensity of allergic response (antihistamine)	Relief of symptoms of hay fever (allergic rhinitis) and of allergic reactions of skin (itching, swelling, hives, and rash)
Albatussin (CD) Kronohist (CD) Ru-Tuss (CD) Citra Forte (CD) Mydol PMS (CD) Triaminic (CD) Codimal (CD) P-V-Tussin (CD) Triaminicin (CD) 4-Way Nasal Poly-Histine-D Triaminicol (CD) Spray (CD) (CD) Fiogesic (CD) Primatene-M (CD)		
Quinidine	Slows pacemaker and delays transmission of electrical impulses (cardiac depressant)	Correction of certain heart rhythm disorders
Cardioquin Duraquin Quinaglute Quinidex SK-Quinidine		
Reserpine	Relaxes blood vessel walls by reducing availability of norepinephrine (antihypertensive; tranquilizer)	Reduction of high blood pressure
Sandril Demi-Regroton Diutensen-R (CD) Serpasil (CD) Hydromox R (CD) SK-Resperine Diupres (CD) Hydropres (CD)		Regrotin (CD) Salutensin (CD) Ser-Ap-Es (CD)
Rifampin	Prevents growth and multiplication of susceptible tuberculosis organisms by interfering with enzyme systems involved in formation of essential proteins (antibiotic; tuberculostatic)	Treatment of tuberculosis
Rifadin Rifamate Rimactane		
Secobarbital	Believed to block transmission of nerve impulses (hypnotic; sedative)	Low dosage: relief of mild to moderate anxiety or tension (sedative effect); higher dosage: at bedtime to induce sleep (hypnotic effect)
Seconal		
Sulfamethox-azole	Prevents growth and multiplication of susceptible bacteria by interfering with their formation of folic acid (antibacterial)	Elimination of infections responsive to action of this drug
Gantanol Azo Gantanol (CD) Bactrim (CD) Septra (CD)		
Sulfisoxazole	Same as above	Same as above
Gantrisin SK-Soxazole Azo Gantrisin (CD) Pediazole (CD) for children		
Tetracycline	Prevents growth and multiplication of susceptible bacteria by interfering with their formation of essential proteins (antibiotic)	Elimination of infections responsive to action of this drug
Achromycin V Robitet SK-Tetracycline Topicycline Sumycin (CD)		

Name	Action	Prescribed for
Trade Names (CD = combined drug)		
Theophylline (Aminophylline, Oxtriphylline)	Reverses constriction by increasing activity of chemical system within muscle cell that causes relaxation of bronchial tube (bronchodilator)	Symptomatic relief of bronchial asthma
Accurbron Bronkodyl Constant-T Elixicon LABID Respbid Somophyllin	Sustaire Theo-Organidin Synophylate Theophyl Theobid Aerolate (CD) Theoclear Amesec (CD) Theo-Dur Aquaphyllin (CD) Theolair Brondecon (CD) Theon Bronkolixir (CD)	Bronkotabs (CD) Slo-bid (CD) Elixophyllin (CD) Slo-Phyllin (CD) Marax (CD) T.E.H (CD) Primatene (CD) T-E-P (CD) Quadrinal (CD) Tedral (CD) Quibron (CD) Theozine (CD)
Thyroid Liothyronine Thyroglobulin Levothyroxine	Makes more energy available for biochemical activity and increases rate of cellular metabolism by altering pocesses of cellular chemicals that store energy (thyroid hormones)	Correction of thyroid hormone deficiency (hypothyroidism)
Armour Thyroid Cytomel Euthroid Levothroid	Proloid Choloxin S-P-T L-Thyroxine Synthroid Thyrolar (CD) Thyrolar	
Tolbutamide	Stimulates secretion of insulin by pancreas (hypoglycemic)	Correction of insulin deficiency in adult diabetes
Orinase		
Trimethoprim	Prevents growth and multiplication of susceptible organisms by interfering with formation of proteins (antibacterial)	Elimination of infections responsive to action of this drug
Proloprim Trimpex Bactrim (CD)	Cotrim (CD) Septra (CD) Sulfatrim (CD)	
Triprolidine	Blocks action of histamine after release from sensitized tissue cells, thus reducing intensity of allergic response (antihistamine)	Relief of symptoms of hay fever (allergic rhinitis) and of allergic reacitons of skin (itching, swelling, hives, and rash)
Actidil Actifed (CD) Actifed-C (CD) Triafed (CD) Trifed (CD)		
Vitamin C (Ascorbic Acid)	Believed to be essential to enzyme activity involved in formation of collagen; increases absorption of iron from intestine and helps formation of hemoglobin and red blood cells in bone marrow; inhibits growth of certain bacteria in urinary tract; enhances effects of some antibiotics (vitamin)	Prevention and treatment of scurvy; treatment of some types of anemia; maintenance of acid urine
Cetane Cevalin Cevi-Bid Cevi-Fer (CD) Mediatric (CD)		

Index